D1289294

# Essentials of
# Diagnostic
# Microbiology

*Lisa Anne Shimeld • Anne T. Rodgers*

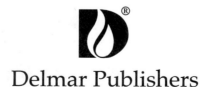

## Delmar Publishers

*an International Thomson Publishing company* I(T)P®

Albany • Bonn • Boston • Cincinnati • Detroit • London • Madrid
Melbourne • Mexico City • New York • Pacific Grove • Paris • San Francisco
Singapore • Tokyo • Toronto • Washington

# NOTICE TO THE READER

Cover Design: Charles Cummings Advertising/Art, Inc.

**Delmar Staff**

Publisher: Susan Simpfenderfer
Acquisitions Editor: Marlene McHugh Pratt
Developmental Editor: Jill Rembetski/Melissa Riveglia
Project Editor: William Trudell

Art and Design Coordinator: Rich Killar
Production Manager: Linda Helfrich
Marketing Manager: Darryl L. Caron
Editorial Assistant: Maria Perretta

COPYRIGHT © 1999
By Delmar Publishers
*an International Thomson Publishing company* I(T)P®

The ITP logo is a trademark under license.
Printed in the United States of America

For more information, contact:

Delmar Publishers
3 Columbia Circle, Box 15015
Albany, New York 12212-5015

International Thomson Publishing Europe
Berkshire House
168-173 High Holborn
London, WC1V7AA
United Kingdom

Nelson ITP, Australia
102 Dodds Street
South Melbourne,
Victoria, 3205 Australia

Nelson Canada
1120 Birchmount Road
Scarborough, Ontario
M1K 5G4, Canada

International Thomson Publishing France
Tour Maine-Montparnasse
33 Avenue du Maine
75755 Paris Cedex 15, France

International Thomson Editores
Seneca 53
Colonia Polanco
11560 Mexico D. F. Mexico

International Thomson Publishing GmbH
Königswinterer Straße 418
53227 Bonn
Germany

International Thomson Publishing Asia
60 Albert Street
#15-01 Albert Complex
Singapore 189969

International Thomson Publishing Japan
Hirakawa-cho Kyowa Building, 3F
2-2-1 Hirakawa-cho, Chiyoda-ku,
Tokyo 102, Japan

ITE Spain/Paraninfo
Calle Magallanes, 25
28015-Madrid, España

1 2 3 4 5 6 7 8 9 10 XXX 03 02 01 00 99 98

**Library of Congress Cataloging-in-Publication Data**

Essentials of diagnostic microbiology / [edited by] Lisa Anne Shimeld , Anne T. Rodgers.
    p. cm.
    Includes bibliographical references and index.
    ISBN 0-8273-7388-0
    1. Diagnostic microbiology. I. Shimeld, Lisa Anne.
    [DNLM: 1. Microbiological Techniques. 2. Laboratory Techniques and procedures. QW 25 E778 1998]
    QR67.E85 1998
    616.07′581—dc21
    DNLM/DLC
    for Library of Congress        98-17226
                          CIP

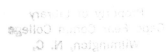

# ▶ CONTENTS

# Section II / Bacteriology

## Part 1 General Methods for Identification of Bacteria

# Section III / Mycology

# Section IV / Parasitology

**PREFACE**

Educators and practitioners working in the clinical microbiology field developed *Essentials of Diagnostic Microbiology* with a unique focus in mind. Other publishers try to cross-market microbiology texts as both a text and a reference, often including extraneous information today's busy students do not need in a textbook. *Essentials of Diagnostic Microbiology* instead presents the essential, entry-level skills and information medical laboratory technology students will need to enter the workforce. This text also teaches learners to use their critical thinking skills to explore topics further, seeking additional information when necessary. This approach saves both learners and educators valuable time otherwise spent extracting essential information from the volume of material found in other texts.

## TEXT ORGANIZATION

*Essentials of Diagnostic Microbiology* contains 51 chapters that focus on the fundamental principles and techniques involved in the study of microorganisms, as well as their application in the diagnosis of infectious disease. A unique feature of this text is its continuous emphasis on *essential* information presented in short, easy-to-understand segments. Five sections further subdivide the material into manageable parts. Each of the four subspecialty areas, Sections II–V, include short introductory chapters that lay the groundwork of basic technical, biological, and chemical principles related to that specialty. Subsequent chapters within each section then build upon this information by describing the characteristics of microorganisms recovered in the clinical laboratory and the practical approach to their identification. The chapters cover the collection and processing of clinical specimens and the interpretation of laboratory investigative results, tracing the application of basic principles of microbiology and characteristics of microorganisms to the recovery and identification of infectious agents in the clinical laboratory. This simple to complex organization allows learners to build knowledge and confidence gradually, applying what they learn to the identification of microorganisms and the diagnosis of infectious diseases.

**Section I, General Topics in Microbiology** provides students with a concise overview of diagnostic microbiology. *Chapter 1* introduces the learner to the study of microorganisms, while *Chapters 2–7* focus on key topics such as the infectious disease process, laboratory safety, immunologic and molecular techniques,

quality assurance, automation, and antimicrobial agents and antimicrobial susceptibility testing.

**Section II, Bacteriology** contains two parts: *General Methods for Identification of Bacteria* and *Isolation and Identification of Bacteria from Clinical Specimens.* Part 1 begins with an introductory chapter *(Chapter 8)* to ground learners in the basics of microscopic morphology, methods, techniques, and identification. *Chapters 9–23* introduce students to the identification of the most common bacteria they may encounter on the job. Part 2 begins with a similar introductory chapter *(Chapter 24)* to introduce students to techniques in processing and interpreting cultures from clinical specimens. *Chapters 25–33* take a body-systems approach to introduce the common resident flora of that system, specimen collection, specimen processing, related pathogenic microorganisms, and diseases.

**Section III, Mycology** begins with two introductory chapters *(Chapters 34 & 35)* that present the basic concepts and techniques related to mycology, including a review of fungi, approaches to identifying fungi, and media techniques, specimen collection and transport, and direct examination of specimens. *Chapters 36–41* cover superficial and subcutaneous mycoses, dimorphic, opportunistic, and saprobic fungi and yeasts.

**Section IV, Parasitology** also begins with an introductory chapter *(Chapter 42)* that reviews basic concepts and techniques related to parasitology, including symbiotic relationships, hosts, disease transmission, life cycles, and an overview of important parasites. *Chapters 43–47* next cover specimen collection and processing, protozoans, and helminths.

**Section V, Virology** begins with an introductory chapter *(Chapter 49)* on basic virology concepts, followed by chapters on specimen collection and processing *(Chapter 50)* and a unique chapter on emerging viral infections *(Chapter 51)*.

The text also includes a comprehensive glossary comprised of all of the chapters' key terms.

The unique learning aids included in *Essentials of Diagnostic Microbiology* are detailed in the **Key Features** section. These features, along with the text's focus on critical thinking and problem based learning, makes this the ideal textbook for medical laboratory technology students, or any undergraduate student enrolled in an allied health microbiology course. By introducing learners not only to microbiology, but also to the concepts important in clinical microbiology, this text could help prepare any student of medically oriented microbiology to better fulfill their role in the health care setting.

## ANCILLARIES

Supplements for *Essentials of Diagnostic Microbiology* include a student study guide/laboratory manual, an instructor's manual, and a computerized testbank.

- *Study Guide and Laboratory Manual to Accompany Essentials of Diagnostic Microbiology* reinforces concepts presented in the text through numerous multiple choice, matching, short answer, labeling, and critical thinking questions corresponding to each of the 51 text chapters. The second half of this workbook serves as a laboratory manual and contains step-by-step instructions on how to perform over 50 of the most common procedures done in a microbiology lab.

- *Instructor's Manual to Accompany Essentials of Diagnostic Microbiology* includes answers to the text's review questions and suggested responses to the case studies. Teaching tips and information on additional resources are also included.
- *Computerized Testbank to Accompany Essentials of Diagnostic Microbiology* includes over 1,500 test true/false, multiple choice, and short answer test questions based on the contents of the 51 text chapters.

## REVIEWERS

**Shirley Adams, MT**
Greenville Technical College
Greenville, SC

**Daniel Amsterdam, PhD**
Director of Laboratory Medicine
Erie County Medical Center
Buffalo, NY

**Sally McLaughlin Bauer**
Biology Department
Hudson Valley Community College
Troy, NY

**Judith Kaley Clark, MEd, MT (ASCP)**
IOP Coordinator
Pinnacle Health System
Harrisburg, PA
Dover, PA

**James E. Daly, M.Ed., MT (ASCP)**
Assistant Professor
Clinical Laboratory Science Technology
Lorain County Community College
Elyria, Ohio

**Ellen Digan, MA, MT (ASCP)**
Professor of Biology
Coordinator, MLT Program
Medical Laboratory Technical Program
Manchester Community-Technical College
Manchester, CT

**James Griffith, PhD, CLS (NCA)**
Professor and Chairperson
Department of Medical Laboratory Science
UMASS-Dartmouth
North Dartmouth, MA

**Lynette Hobbs**
Medical Technology
Tyler Junior College
Tyler, TX

**Karen Ingham**
Coordinator, MLT Program
Dutchess Community College
Poughkeepsie, NY

**Catherine A. Lencioni, MS, MT, (ASCP)**
Assistant Professor/Director
Medical Laboratory Technician Program
Phlebotomy Technician Program
Harrisburg Area Community College
Harrisburg, PA

**Mary Beth Murphy**
Houston Community College
MLT Program
Houston, TX

**John M. O'Leary, MS, MT (ASCP)**
MLT Program Director
Hudson Valley Community College
Biology Department
Troy, NY

**Phyllis Pacifico**
Sheridan Vocational Technical Center
Delray Beach, FL

**Suzanne Rohrbaugh, MS, MT (ASCP)**
Director of MLT, Phlebotomy and Medical Assisting
  Programs
Davidson Community College
Health Technology Division
Lexington, NC

## ABOUT THE AUTHOR

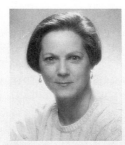 Lisa Shimeld earned her MS degree in Biology (Microbiology and Genetics emphasis) at California State University, San Bernardino. Her research interests include parasitic protozoans and the development of techniques for the karyotyping of insects. She is a Professor of Microbiology and the Chairperson of Biological Sciences and Chemistry at Crafton Hills College, a community college located in Southern California. Lisa teaches three levels of Microbiology at CHC and the two semester Biology for Majors series (Cell and Molecular Biology and Populations and Organisms). In addition to journal articles, Lisa has written a microbiology laboratory manual and numerous ancillaries for microbiology, biology, and biochemistry textbooks. Lisa is committed to the development of pedagogical materials that foster the ability to apply the skills and concepts learned in the classroom to real life situations.

## ACKNOWLEDGMENTS

So many extraordinary people helped make this book a reality that I'm afraid I might not remember to mention them all. I hope they will forgive me if I do, and know that I will always be grateful for all they have done. I have particularly enjoyed working with the many talented contributing authors who wrote chapters for this text. I appreciate the time they took out of their busy schedules for this project.

Everyone at Delmar Publishers has been wonderful to work with throughout the past three years. They are true professionals in every sense of the word. I would especially like to thank Jill Rembetski for helping me stay on top of the millions of issues, large and small, inherent to a project of this magnitude. I would also like to thank Melissa Riveglia who did so much since she joined the team that I don't know how we managed before then. Sarah Holle's organizational skills and keen sense of humor were also an invaluable asset. I hope we have an opportunity to work together in the future.

Thank you, Dave Molnar, for the excellent work you did in producing the high-quality photographs. I appreciate the time and care you took to always get the best shot, and the late nights you put in to make sure everything met deadline. Thank you, Ella and Paul Hayashi, for your generous contribution of film and photographic services.

I don't think I'll ever be able to adequately thank Bill Nauschuetz for all he did to help me find so many of the contributing authors for this book. I think you just might know everyone on the planet, Bill. And by the way, I did manage to take your advice and "keep smiling."

Thanks to Anne Rogers. It was your vision of an "essentials" text that led to making this book a reality. I especially appreciate your assistance in helping me to decide what to leave "in" and what to leave "out."

Most of all, I want to thank my husband, Brad Johnson, for making the largest contribution of all. It was your unshakable faith in me that kept me going throughout this enormous project. Oh, and by the way, are you ready to start the next book, Brad?

## SPECIAL MENTION

The contributors and I would also like to thank Becton Dickinson, bio Merieux Vitek, Inc., BION Enterprises, Ltd., Organon Teknika Corporation, remel, the Scripps Clinic and Wampole Laboratories for providing research assistance, photographs, and advice. Special thanks to all of the reviewers, Kim Barber, BS, Ann Doggert, MT (ASCP), Naomi Eberly, SFC, Dean Fagan, Wendy F. George, MS, W. Duayne Harrison, Michael Joyce, MM, Andrea Kubacki, Patricia A. Myers, Major William Nauschuetz, PhD, David A. Power, PhD, Bernie Trieber, A.F. Vega, Major A. Christian Whelen, and Christine Yinger.

# ► CONTRIBUTORS

**Jeffrey J. Adamovicz, PhD**
Research Investigator
United States Army Medical
    Research Institute of Infectious
    Disease
Fort Detrick
Frederick, MD
**Chapter 47: Blood and Tissue
    Helminths**

**Gloria T. Anderson, MT (ASCP)**
Medical Technologist (ASCP)
University of Texas at Pan
    American University
Edinburgh, TX
**Chapter 19: Gram-Negative
    Anaerobic Bacteria**

**Susan Barber, BS, MT (ASCP), SM**
Technical Coordinator
Scripps Clinic
La Jolla, CA
**Chapter 24: Processing and
    Interpretation of Cultures
    from Clinical Specimens**

**Rev. Dr. Geneva Burch, BS, MT
    (ASCP, CLS, NCA), MLT
    (ASCP)**
West Virginia Northern
    Community College
Wheeling Campus
Wheeling, WV
**Chapter 21: *Mycobacteria***
**Chapter 31: The
    Gastrointestinal Tract**

**Vivian Chantakrivat, MBA, MT
    (ASCP)**
California State University
Long Beach, CA
**Chapter 11: Aerobic Gram-
    Positive Bacilli, Coccobacilli,
    and Coryneform Bacilli**

**David W. Craft, PhD**
Lieutenant Colonel, Medical
    Service Corps
U.S. Army Medical Department
    Center & School
Ft. Sam Houston, TX
**Chapter 19: Gram-Negative
    Anaerobic Bacteria**
**Chapter 20: Gram-Positive
    Anaerobic Bacteria**

**James E. Daly, MEd, MT (ASCP)**
Assistant Professor, Clinical
    Laboratory Science Technology
Lorain County Community
    College
Elyria, Ohio
**Chapter 15: Miscellaneous
    Fastidious Aerobic and
    Facultative Gram-Negative
    Bacilli and Coccobacilli**

**Anne Delaney. MT (ASCP)**
Medical Technologist
Tripler Army Medical Center
Honolulu, HI
**Chapter 51: Emerging Viral
    Infections**

**Bardwell J. Eberly, MT (ASCP),
    SM**
Supervisor, Microbiology
Education Coordinator for UH at
    Manoa, Medical Technology
    Division
Tripler Regional Medical Center
Honolulu, HI
**Chapter 12: Aerobic
    Actinomycetes**
**Chapter 43: Specimen Collec-
    tion and Processing for
    Parasite Examinations**

**Susan L. Fraser, MD**
Infectious Diseases Fellow
Brooke Army Medical Center
Fort Sam Houston, TX
**Chapter 33: Deep Tissue and
    Internal Organ Sites**

**Daila S. Gridley, PhD**
Professor of Microbiology &
    Molecular Genetics and
    Radiation Medicine
Loma Linda University School of
    Medicine
Loma Linda, CA
**Chapter 14: *Haemophilus***
**Chapter 16: Gram-Negative
    Enteric Bacilli**
**Chapter 17: Nonfermenting
    Aerobic Gram-Negative
    Bacilli**
**Chapter 18: *Vibrio* and Other
    Curved Aerobic Gram-
    Negative Bacilli**
**Chapter 23: Chlamydia,
    Mycoplasma, and Rickettsia**

**James Griffith, PhD, CLS (NCA)**
Professor and Chairperson
Department of Medical Laboratory
    Science
UMASS-Dartmouth
North Dartmouth, MA 02747-2300
**Chapter 7: Antimicrobial
    Agents and Antimicrobial
    Susceptibility Testing**

**Linda S. Harrison, MS, MT
    (ASCP)**
Supervisory Microbiologist
Brooke Army Medical Center
Fort Sam Houston, TX
**Chapter 9: Staphylococcus and
    Related Aerobic Gram-
    Positive Cocci**

**Judith S. Heelan, PhD**
Director of Microbiology,
    Memorial Hospital of Rhode
    Island

Clinical Assistant Professor of
    Pathology and Laboratory
    Medicine, Brown University
    School of Medicine
Providence, RI
**Chapter 13: *Neisseria* and
    Other Aerobic Gram-
    Negative Cocci**
**Chapter 30: The Genital Tract**

**S. Vern Juchau, PhD, MPH, MA**
Chief, Bureau of Laboratory
    Services
Houston Department of Health &
    Human Services
Houston, TX
**Chapter 32: Skin Infections**

**James D. Kettering, PhD**
Professor of Microbiology
Loma Linda University School of
    Medicine
Loma Linda, CA
**Chapter 23: Chlamydia,
    Mycoplasma, and Rickettsia**
**Chapter 48: Basic Concepts
    and Techniques in Virology**
**Chapter 49: Specimen Collec-
    tion and Processing of Viral
    Specimens**
**Chapter 50: Clinically
    Significant Viruses and
    Their Identification**

**Judith A. Kjelstrom, MT (ASCP)
    PhD**
Professor of Microbiology/
    Anatomy and Physiology
American River College
Sacramento, CA
**Chapter 2: The Infectious
    Disease Process**

**Steven Mahlen, MS, M(ASCP),
    RM (AAM)**
Chief, Microbiology &
    Immunology
William Beaumont Army Medical
    Center
El Paso, TX
**Chapter 6: Automation in the
    Clinical Microbiology
    Laboratory**

**James A. Miller, MD**
**Chapter 34: Basic Concepts
    and Techniques in Mycology**
**Chapter 35: Collection and
    Processing of Fungal
    Specimens**
**Chapter 36: Dermatophytes
    and Other Agents of
    Superficial Mycoses**
**Chapter 37: Agents of
    Subcutaneous Mycoses**
**Chapter 38: Systemic
    Dimorphic Fungi**
**Chapter 39: Opportunistic
    Fungi**

**Chapter 40: Saprobic Fungi Encountered in Clinical Specimens**
**Chapter 41: Yeasts**

**James O. Murray, SM (AAM), CLS (NCA), MS**
Microbiologist
U.S. Army Medical Department Center and School
Fort Sam Houston, TX
**Chapter 26: Blood Cultures**

**Bill Nauschuetz, PhD**
Major, United States Army
Chief and Medical Director, Microbiology Section
Department of Pathology and Area Laboratory Services
Tripler Regional Medical Center
Honolulu, HI
and
Adjunct Assistant Professor
Department of Microbiology
University of Hawaii—Manoa
**Chapter 29: The Urinary Tract**
**Chapter 51: Emerging Viral Infections**

**Kathryn Nollar, MT (ASCP)**
Microbiology Supervisor
Redlands Community Hospital
Redlands, CA
**Chapter 5: Quality Assurance in the Clinical Microbiology Laboratory**

**Anne T. Rodgers, MT (ASCP), PhD**
Professor of Medical Technology
Armstrong Atlantic State University
Savannah, GA
**Chapter 3: Safety in the Clinical Microbiology Laboratory**
**Chapter 7: Antimicrobial Agents and Antimicrobial Susceptibility Testing**

**Chapter 31: The Gastrointestinal Tract**
**Chapter 34: Basic Concepts and Techniques in Mycology**
**Chapter 35: Collection and Processing of Fungal Specimens**
**Chapter 36: Dermatophytes and Other Agents of Superficial Mycoses**
**Chapter 37: Agents of Subcutaneous Mycoses**
**Chapter 38: Systemic Dimorphic Fungi**
**Chapter 39: Opportunistic Fungi**
**Chapter 40: Saprobic Fungi Encountered in Clinical Specimens**
**Chapter 41: Yeasts**

**Lynn L. Russell, MA, CLS (NCA)**
Springfield College
Springfield, MA
**Chapter 3: Safety in the Clinical Microbiology Laboratory**
**Chapter 28: Eye, Ear, and Sinus Tracts**

**Mark Shapiro, MS (ASCP), BS**
Clinical Microbiology Laboratory
Memorial Medical Center
Savannah, GA
**Chapter 27: The Respiratory Tract**

**Lisa Anne Shimeld, MS**
Professor of Microbiology
Biological Sciences Chairperson
Crafton Hills College
Yucaipa, CA
**Chapter 1: Introduction to the Study of Microorganisms**
**Chapter 22: *Spirochetes***
**Chapter 27: The Respiratory Tract**

**Chapter 42: Basic Concepts and Techniques in Parasitology**
**Chapter 44: Intestinal and Atrial Protozoans**
**Chapter 45: Plasmodia and Other Blood and Tissue Protozoans**
**Chapter 46: Intestinal Helminths**

**Diane K. Tamanaha, MS, MT (ASCP)**
Microbiologist
Tripler Army Medical Center
Honolulu, HI
**Chapter 25: Cerebral Spinal Fluid and Other Body Fluids**

**Helen B. Viscount, PhD**
United States Army Medical Research Institute for Infectious Diseases
Fort Detrick
Frederick, MD
**Chapter 4: Immunologic and Molecular Techniques**
**Chapter 10: *Streptococcus* and Related Aerobic Gram-Positive Cocci**

**A. Christian Whelen, PhD, D (ABMM)**
Director of Microbiology
Brooke Army Medical Center
San Antonio, TX
**Chapter 19: Gram-Negative Anaerobic Bacteria**

**Sheryl. A. Whitlock, MA, MT (ASCP), BB**
Laboratory Instructor
Swarthmore College
Swarthmore, PA
**Chapter 8: Microscopic and Cultural Techniques for Bacterial Identification**

# KEY FEATURES

Microbiology is an exciting and challenging subject. Delmar's *Essentials of Diagnostic Microbiology* presents the fundamental principles and techniques involved in the study of microorganisms, as well as their application in the diagnoses of infectious disease. The text provides the essential, entry-level skills and information medical laboratory students will need to enter the workforce. The text has many unique features that will make it easier for you to learn and integrate theory and practice, including:

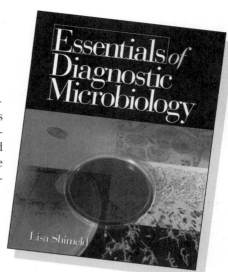

## CHAPTER 6

### Automation in the Clinical Microbiology Laboratory

Steven Mahlen, MS, M (ASCP), RM (AAM)

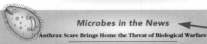

#### Microbes in the News

**Anthrax Scare Brings Home the Threat of Biological Warfare**

In February of 1998 two American men were arrested in Las Vegas, Nevada and charged with possession of the anthrax bacterium (*Bacillus anthracis*) for use as a deadly weapon. The incident made international headlines as the threat of biological terrorism seemed to materialize on American soil. Examination of vials containing the suspected weapons grade anthrax material by FBI and military experts revealed it to be a harmless anthrax vaccine. The men's attorneys said their clients were carrying anthrax vaccine for use in the testing of a device that would neutralize bacterial toxins in the human body. It is not illegal to possess bacteria, even serious pathogens, if criminal intent cannot be proven.

Although the charges against both men were dropped, one was kept in custody for violation of his parole. The man had been convicted in Ohio on wire fraud charges of illegally obtaining bubonic plague bacteria in 1997. He was sentenced to 18 months parole and was forbidden to conduct any experiments with, or obtain any infectious disease agents. He faces up to five years in prison if he is found to have violated his parole.

*Bacillus anthracis* is a gram-positive endospore-forming bacillus that causes anthrax in grazing animals including sheep, cattle, and

is highly lethal and is almost always fatal if treatment does not begin until symptoms are exhibited. With 100 million lethal doses per gram of anthrax material it is 100,000 times deadlier than the deadliest chemical warfare agent. The production of a stable, dry anthrax powder is low cost and does not require high technology. The material is easy to disseminate and is a silent, invisible killer.

Symptoms of anthrax begin after a 1 to 6 day incubation period and are nonspecific for inhalation anthrax. The infected individual develops a low grade fever, a dry hacking cough, and feels weak. After briefly improving, respiratory distress is followed by shock and usually death. If treatment is to be successful antibiotics such as penicillin or doxycycline, and a vaccine **must** be administered **prior** to the onset of symptoms. The antibiotics keep the patient alive while they build immunity in response to the vaccination. Anthrax can be prevented by vaccination with the FDA-licensed vaccine.

Sources:

*Time*: Catching a 48-Hour Bug. By Tamala M. Edwards. March 2, 1998 vol. 151 No. 8. Glossary

### Microbes in the News

**1** A snapshot of a real life news story showing a topic in microbiology "in action" appears at the beginning of chapters.

### Outline

A list of the main topics and subtopics at the beginning of each chapter allows you to preview its major points. Review these topic headings before you study the chapter. They'll be a roadmap to the material in the chapter. You may also use the outline as study guide for tests, in conjunction with the learning objectives. **2**

**INTRODUCTION**

**STREPTOCOCCUS PNEUMONIAE**
Organism Characteristics
Clinical Significance
Cultural Characteristics and Identification
Antibiotic Susceptibility Characteristics

**STREPTOCOCCUS PYOGENES**
Organism Characteristics
Clinical Significance
Cultural Characteristics and Identification
Antibiotic Susceptibility Characteristics

**STREPTOCOCCUS AGALACTIAE**
Organism Characteristics
Clinical Significance

Cultural Characteristics and Identification
Antibiotic Susceptibility Characteristics

**ENTEROCOCCI**
Organism Characteristics
Clinical Significance
Cultural Characteristics and Identification
Antibiotic Susceptibility Characteristics

**OTHER GROUP D STREPTOCOCCI**
Organism Characteristics
Clinical Significance
Cultural Characteristics and Identification
Antibiotic Susceptibility Characteristics

**VIRIDANS STREPTOCOCCI**
Organism Characteristics
Clinical Significance
Cultural Characteristics and Identification
Antibiotic Susceptibility Characteristics

**OBSCURE OR RARELY ISOLATED ORGANISMS**
Nutritionally Variant Streptococci
Other β-Hemolytic Streptococci

**SPECIAL CONSIDERATIONS FOR IMMUNOCOMPROMISED HOSTS**

### Key Terms

Unfamiliar or critical vocabulary words are listed alphabetically at the beginning of each chapter and appear in bold on their first use within that chapter. These terms are later defined in the **Glossary** at the end of the text. **3**

#### KEY TERMS

Bacteremia
Bacteriocins
CLED medium
Dysentery
Enteric fever
Enteroaggregative *E. coli* (EAEC)
Enterocolitis
Enterohemorrhagic *E. coli* (EHEC)

Enteroinvasive *E. coli* (EIEC)
Enteropathogenic *E. coli* (EPEC)
Enterotoxigenic *E. coli* (ETEC)
Heat-stable exotoxin (ST)
Heat-labile exotoxin (LT)
Lipopolysaccharide
Mesenteric adenitis
MUG test
Nephropathogenic *E. coli* (NPEC)

O, K, H, and Vi antigens
Plague
R plasmids
Shiga toxin
Swarming
Typhoid fever
Verotoxin
Widal test

### Learning Objectives

The objectives identify the key information to be gained from the chapter. Use these objectives, together with the review questions, to test your understanding of the chapter's content. **4**

#### LEARNING OBJECTIVES

Upon successful completion of this chapter, the student should be able to:

1. Discuss normal, anaerobic flora of humans by the four major anatomic locations.
2. Describe circumstances in which "normal" anaerobic flora cause disease.
3. Explain the three levels of identification in conventional clinical anaerobic bacteriology.
4. Describe common anaerobic media and primary culture strategies.
5. Describe the special potency disk patterns of major gram-negative anaerobes.
6. Based on Gram stain, colonial morphology, special potency disk pattern, determine which of the six additional level two tests are necessary for common identifications.
7. Solve case studies in anaerobic bacteriology.

## Procedures

Abbreviated instructions on how to perform specific laboratory procedures appear in text boxes throughout the text, where appropriate. Each procedure includes an overview of the procedure, principle, method, quality control, expected results, and references. See the end of this text for a complete listing of these procedures. All of the procedures contained in the text, plus many others, are included in more detail in *Study Guide and Laboratory Manual to Accompany Essentials of Diagnostic Microbiology*.

**5**

### PROCEDURE 9-1
#### Catalase

**Principle:**

Catalase is present in many bacterial cells to counteract the toxic buildup of the metabolic end-product, hydrogen peroxide. Catalase converts hydrogen peroxide into water and oxygen, creating a bubbling effect.

$$2\ H_2O_2 + catalase \rightarrow 2\ H_2O + O_2\ (bubbles)$$

**Method:**

To perform the test, place a drop of 3% hydrogen peroxide onto a slide. Using an applicator stick, gently pick a colony from the primary isolation plate and add to the drop of hydrogen peroxide. Hold the stick down and observe for vigorous bubbling.

**Expected Results:**

Staphylococci will be catalase positive and pr bubbles, whereas streptococci will be catalas ative.

**Limitations:**

Some organisms, along with red blood cells, p other enzymes that can also break down hyc peroxide, but the reaction will not be vigorc with catalase.

**Reference:**

Koneman, E. W., Allen, S. D., Janda, W. M., Sc enberger, P. C., & Washington, C. W., Jr. ( The gram-positive cocci part I: *Staphyloc* and related organisms. *Color atlas and textb* (6th ed.). Philade

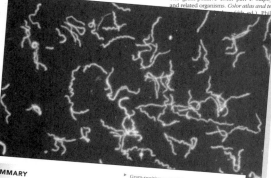

## Color Plates

An insert of color plates of many of the organisms discussed within the chapters, plus detailed captions, is included. The plates are numbered consecutively and referenced within the chapters as appropriate for ease of use.

**6**

### SUMMARY

- Anaerobic bacteria are often normal flora of the mucous membranes and frequently recovered in mixed cultures.
- Many gram-positive anaerobic infections are polymicrobial, flourishing in a localized environment with decreased or no oxygen.
- Gram-positive anaerobes are most likely to be recovered from abscess, body fluid, or wound specimens.
- Gram-positive anaerobic cocci (*Peptostreptococci*) are second only to the anaerobic gramnegative bacilli as the most commonly isolated anaerobic bacteria. They are most often recovered in blood cultures.
- *Propionibacterium acnes* is a diphtheroid and is the most commonly isolated from positive anaerobic bacilli...
- *Actinomycosis* species... sulfur granules that... jaw, and often exhi... phology.

- Gram-positive anaerobic spore-forming bacilli may be invasive and histotoxic or noninvasive and toxin-mediated such as botulism, tetanus, gastroenteritis, or antibiotic-associated pseudomembranous colitis.
- Egg yolk agar is a primary isolation media for the gram-positive, spore-forming anaerobic bacilli in which proteolytic enzyme activity, such as lipase and lecithinase, is exhibited.
- *Clostridium perfringens* is the most frequent clostridial isolate, exhibiting large boxcar-shaped rods on Gram stain, double zone ß-hemolysis, nonmotility, and positive Nagler and reverse CAMP tests.
- *C. perfringens* causes a histolytic myeonecrosis (gas gangrene) and is also the third most common cause of food poisoning (gastroenteritis) in the United States.
- There are four clinical forms of botulism, all...

## Summary

The summary for each chapter is presented in a bulleted format, emphasizing the key points from the chapter, to help you focus your study.

**7**

### CASE STUDY: PRIMARY ATYPICAL PNEUMONIA IN A CHILD

A 12-year-old girl was admitted with fever, a persistent nonproductive cough, and night sweats; she appeared mildly dyspneic. Four weeks previously, the patient had been well. During the course of illness, she experienced episodic pain in the subscapular region and shoulder. On admission her vital signs were: temperature, 38.5°C; pulse 98/min; respirations, 29/min; and blood pressure, 125/65 mm Hg. Other laboratory tests indicated a leukocyte count of 6.3 × 10⁹/L, white blood cell populations within normal limits, an increased blood sedimentation rate, and a high value for C-reactive protein. Chest radiographs showed bilateral lower lobe involvement. Blood cultures were negative and routine cultures of bronchial washings revealed no pathogens. An immunoblot for anti-I IgM was strongly positive and a complement fixation assay gave a serum antibody titer of >1:512 using M. pneumoniae antigen. Oral erythromycin and intravenous cefuroxime were administered. The patient turned afebrile within 2 days; improvement was slow, but uneventful. She was discharged from the hospital 5 days after admission.

**Questions:**

1. What does the strong positive for IgM antibodies suggest?

2. Is a slow recovery typical for pneumonia due

3. Is the patient immune to *M. pneumoniae* after this episode of illness?

## Case Study

The case studies in each chapter provide a critical thinking scenario for you to put your knowledge of the chapter content into practice.

**8**

### Review Questions

1. The presence of viable bacteria in the bloodstream is referred to as:
   a. bacteruria.
   b. bacteremia.
   c. septicemia.
   d. sepsis.

2. The type of bacteremia that occurs when bacteria periodically enter the bloodstream from an established abscess is:
   a. transient.
   b. continuous.
   c. intermittent.

3. A blood culture medium that would NOT be appropriate for the recovery of aerobic bacteria would be:
   a. soybean casein digest broth with 0.05% SPS.
   b. Brucella broth with 5% $CO_2$ gaseous atmosphere.
   c. brain-heart infusion broth with 0.025% SPS.
   d. thioglycollate broth with 5% carbon dioxide.

4. Which of the following is most significant in recovering clinically significant isolates from blood cultures?
   a. Scrub the venipuncture site with alcohol and iodine compounds.
   b. Include one anaerobic bottle in each set.
   c. Agitate the broth while incubating

## Review Questions

Multiple choice questions at the end of each chapter challenge you on the material you have just learned for quick reinforcement. The answers appear in the *Instructor's Manual*.

**9**

### REFERENCES & RECOMMENDED READING

Baron, E. J., Peterson, L. R., & Finegold, S. M. (1994). *Bailey and Scott's diagnostic microbiology* (9th ed.). St. Louis: Mosby–Year Book.

Fagan, M. D., Levy, R. M., & Murray, J. M. (1996). *Inflammation associated with acne* (Lesson Plan No. SMML-19F. Anaerobic Bacteriology). Fort Sam Houston, TX: US Army Medical Department Center and School.

Finegold, S. M., Baron, E. J., & Wexler, H. M. (1992). *A clinical guide to anaerobic infections*. Belmont, CA: Star Publishing.

Finegold, S. M., Rosenblatt, J. E., Sutter, V. L., & Attebery, H. R. (1974). *Scope monograph on anaerobic infections.* Kalamazoo, MI: Upjohn Company.

Gilligan, P. H., Shapiro, D. S., & Smiley, M. L. (1992). *Cases in medical microbiology and infectious diseases.* Washington, DC: American Society for Microbiology Press.

Gorbach, S. L. (1979). Other *Clostridium* species (including gas gangrene). In G. L. Mandell, R. G. Douglas, Jr., & J. E. Bennett (Eds.). *Principles and practice of infectious diseases* (pp. 1876–1885). New York: Wiley.

Hathaway, D. L. (1990). Toxigenic clostridia. *Clinical microbiology reviews, 3,* 66–98.

Knoop, F. C., Owens, M., & Crocker, I. C. (1993). *Clostridium difficile:* Clinical disease and diagnosis. *Clinical Microbiology Reviews, 6,* 251–265.

Koneman, E. W., Allen, S. D., Janda, W. M., Schreckenberger, P. C., & Winn, W. C. Jr. (1994). *Introduction to diagnostic microbiology.* Philadelphia: Lippincott.

Mangels, J. I. (Sec. Ed.). (1992). Anaerobic bacteriology. In H. D. Isenberg (Chief Ed.). *Clinical microbiology procedures handbook* (Vol. 1, Sec. 2). Washington, DC: American Society for Microbiology Press.

Midura, T. F. (1996). Update: Infant botulism. *Clinical Microbiology Reviews, 9,* 119–125.

Murray, P. R., Baron, E. J., Pfaller, M. A., Tenover, F. C., & Yolken, R. H. (Eds.). (1995). *Manual of clinical microbiology.* (6th ed.). Washington, DC: American Society for Microbiology.

Pezzlo, M. (Sec. Ed.) (1992). Aerobic bacteriology. In H. D. Isenberg (Chief Ed.). *Clinical microbiology procedures handbook* (Vol. 1, Sec. 1). Washington, DC: American Society for Microbiology Press.

Summanen, P., Baron, E. J., Citron, D. M., Strong, C. A., Wexler, H. M., & Finegold, S. M. (1993). *Wadsworth anaerobic bacteriology manual* (5th ed.). Belmont, CA: Star Publishing.

Talaro, K., & Talaro, A. (1996). *Foundations in microbiology* (2nd ed.). Dubuque, IA: William C. Brown Publishers.

## References & Recommended Reading

This listing includes both the references used in each chapter, plus additional sources for further study.

**10**

# General Topics in Microbiology

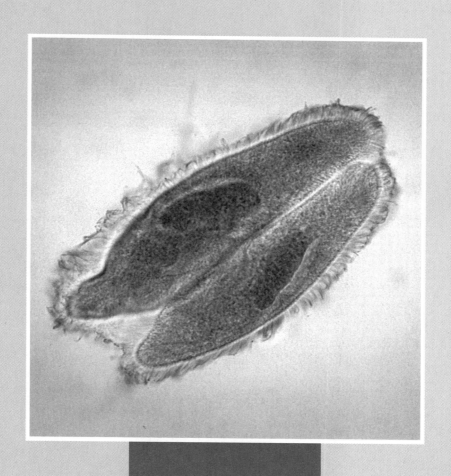

# CHAPTER 1

# Introduction to the Study of Microorganisms

Lisa Shimeld, MS

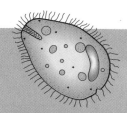

## Microbes in the News

### World Health Organization declares war on leprosy

Leprosy, a disease that has been surrounded by fear and superstition since biblical times, is targeted by the World Health Organization (WHO) for elimination by the year 2000. The goal is to reduce the prevalence rate to less than 1 case per 10,000 population worldwide.

The cause of leprosy, or Hansen's disease, is the gram-positive, acid-fast bacillus, *Mycobacterium leprae.* Much still remains unknown about the pathology and epidemiology of leprosy due to the lack of success in culturing the organism in vitro. It has, however, been grown in the footpads of mice and can occur in armadillos, suggesting that these animals could serve as models for development of the disease.

*Mycobacterium leprae* causes a chronic disease of the skin, mucous membranes, and peripheral nerves. There are two forms of the disease. Tuberculoid leprosy produces large, flattened plaques called macules on the face, trunk, and limbs. In this form, the disease is slow growing and infectivity is low; incubation is measured in years or decades. In lepromatous leprosy the organism is relatively fast growing. Extensive skin lesions develop, especially on the face, resulting in thickening of the loose skin of the lips, forehead, and ears. Infection with leprosy is associated with prolonged, close contact with an infected person and probably occurs through contamination of the nasal mucosa or minor skin lesions. The disease is diagnosed by Ziehl-Neelsen staining of skin scraping and detection of acid-fast bacilli.

As of July 1994, WHO estimated that there were still about 2.5 million people in the world with leprosy, representing about a 70% decline from the 1985 estimate of 10 to 12 million cases. This remarkable improvement is attributed primarily to a scheme introduced by WHO in 1981 that treats the disease with a combination of drugs. This strategy is called multidrug therapy (MDT) and is also used to treat diseases such as tuberculosis, caused by another resistant species of *Mycobacterium.* Some of the drugs used to treat leprosy include rifampin, dapsone, and clofazimine.

Despite these advances, elimination of leprosy represents a formidable problem. Eighty countries still have a prevalence rate greater than 1/10,000. Southeast Asia has two-thirds of the world's estimated cases and rates over 10/10,000 prevail; Africa's rate is 5.3/10,000. The biggest problem associated with the elimination of leprosy lies in the fact that of the estimated 2.5 million infected persons about 800,000 are not receiving any treatment. WHO estimates an additional 600,000 new cases every year, meaning that more than 5 million patients will have to undergo MDT to meet WHO's target for the year 2000. The elimination of leprosy is further complicated by the need for antibiotic therapy lasting from 6 months to 2 years, making the task both expensive and difficult to monitor.

Source: *Los Angeles Times,* an article issued in July 1994.

**PROCARYOTIC AND EUCARYOTIC MICROORGANISMS**

**PROCARYOTIC MICROORGANISM**
Bacteria
Morphology and Arrangement of
  Bacterial Cells

Bacterial Cell Walls
Criteria for Classification
Major Characteristics

**THE EUCARYOTIC MICROORGANISMS**
Fungi
Protozoans
Metazoans
Helminths
Viruses

## KEY TERMS

Apicomplexa
Aschelminthes
Ascomycota
Axial filament
Bacillus
Basidiomycota
Binomial
Cestoda
Chitin
Ciliophora
Class
Classification
Coccus (pl. cocci)
Coenocytic
Conjugation
Cyst
Definitive host
Deuteromycota
Dioecious
Division
Emerging diseases
Endospore
Eubacteria
Eucaryotic
Germ theory of disease

Hemaphroditic
Histone proteins
Hyphae
Intermediate host
International Code of
  Bacterial Nomenclature
International Journal of
  Systematic Bacteriology
Microspora
Monecious
Mycelia
Mycosis
Nematoda
Nomenclature
Nonhistone proteins
Normal flora
Nucleoid
Opportunistic pathogens
Pasteurization
Pellicle
Peptidoglycan
Phylogeny
Phylum (pl. phyla)
Plasmids

Platyhelminthes
Procaryotic
Pseudohyphae
Robert Whittaker
Rust
Sarcomastigophora
Septate
Smut
Species
Spirillum (pl. spirilla)
Spirochete
Staphylococci
Strain
Streptococci
Taxa
Taxonomy
Transduction
Transformation
Tremotoda
Trophozoite
Type strain
Vaccination
Yeast
Zygomycota

## LEARNING OBJECTIVES

**Upon successful completion of this chapter, the student should be able to:**

1. List individuals who made contributions to the field of microbiology and explain their contribution.
2. Compare and contrast procaryotic and eucaryotic cells.
3. List and describe the morphologies of procaryotic cells and describe the possible ways in which those cells may be arranged.
4. List and describe the different types of eucaryotic cells.

5. Compare and contrast the different types of eucaryotic cells.
6. Describe the major characteristics and give examples of different types of fungi, protozoans, and metazoans.
7. Describe the viruses and explain how they differ from cellular organisms.
8. List the five kingdoms, their major characteristics, and examples of representative members.
9. Explain the hierarchy of groups used in the classification of organisms.

## LEARNING OBJECTIVES (cont.)

10. Define scientific nomenclature and explain the importance of scientific names.

11. List and explain the criteria used for classification of bacteria, protozoans, fungi, and helminths. Describe their major characteristics.

## INTRODUCTION

Microorganisms are relevant to all of our lives in a multitude of ways. Sometimes the influence of microorganisms on human life is beneficial, whereas other times it is not. For example, a variety of bacteria and fungi are responsible for the spoilage of foods, yet others are required to produce such delights as cheese, bread, pickles, wine, and beer. Microbes are also an essential component of the ecosystem. Bacteria and fungi play a critical role in the decay of organic material and in the recycling of valuable resources, making them available to other organisms. Bacteria referred to as "nitrogen-fixers" live in the soil where they convert the vast quantities of nitrogen in air into a form that plants can use. Humans and other animals obtain much of their nitrogen by consuming these plants or by consuming other animals that have consumed plants. In many ways all other forms of life depend on microorganisms.

The relationship between microbes and humans is a close one. **Normal flora**, or normal microbiota, are microorganisms that begin to colonize the body at birth. These organisms live on or in the body, this being a normal and healthy state under most circumstances (see Figure 1-1). Many different environments exist on the body and over 100 species of microorganism may reside there. A variety of microbes are acquired from the environment and remain with their host throughout life. Others are transient and remain for days, weeks, or longer but eventually disappear.

Although some viruses can coexist with humans without causing harm most normal flora consists of bacteria and yeasts. The age and health of the host are just two of the factors that play a role in determining the exact composition of the population.

Just as microbes play a role in good health they can under certain circumstances become **opportunistic pathogens**. An opportunistic pathogen is an organism that does not usually cause disease. If, however, normal flora gain entry into a normally sterile site and the host's natural defenses are compromised, the result may be disease. After the introduction of antibiotics into general use, it appeared for a time that the threat of infectious disease would fade into the pages of history. Recently, bacterial infections resistant to all known antibiotics have shown that these predictions were but hopeful thinking and **emerging diseases** are often in the news. Rather than diminishing, the list of potentially pathogenic organisms continues to grow.

Some basic concepts in microbiology are introduced in this chapter. A brief history of microbiology and a discussion of taxonomy are followed by an introduction to procaryotic and eucaryotic microorganisms, and some metazoans that cause disease in humans. Finally, an overview of the diverse microorganisms relevant to the clinical microbiologist introduces the student to the four subspecialities of microbiology covered in the remaining chapters: bacteriology, mycology, parasitology, and virology.

## A BRIEF HISTORY OF MICROBIOLOGY

Some of the earliest observations of the microscopic world were recorded in 1665 by the English scientist, Robert Hooke. Hooke was a curious man who viewed many small objects and creatures using a simple lens that magnified approximately 30×. Among his specimens were the eye of a fly, a bee stinger, and the shell of a protozoan. Hooke also examined thin slices of cork, the bark of a particular type of oak tree. He found that cork was made of tiny boxes that Hooke referred to as "cells." Although Hooke found the "cells" interesting, he thought they were phenomenon unique to cork tissue. It was not until 1839 that two German biologists, Matthias Schleiden and Theodore Schwann, realized the significance of Hooke's observations. They examined a variety of organisms and found they were all made of the same cells Hooke had described. Schleiden and Schwann concluded that "all forms of life are comprised of cells," an observation that later became the foundation of the "cell theory." The cell theory has since been modified to "all life is comprised of cells that originate from other cells."

Unicellular life was first described just a few years after Hooke recorded his observations of the microscopic world. Anton van Leeuwenhoek was a Dutch merchant and a minor city official who built microscopes as a hobby. Van Leeuwenhoek polished grains

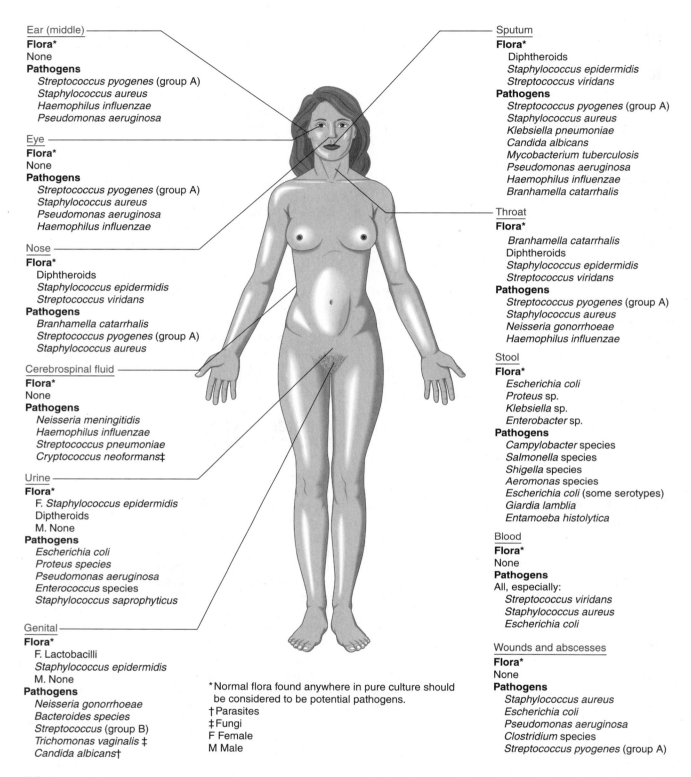

**Ear (middle)**
**Flora***
None
**Pathogens**
  *Streptococcus pyogenes* (group A)
  *Staphylococcus aureus*
  *Haemophilus influenzae*
  *Pseudomonas aeruginosa*

**Eye**
**Flora***
None
**Pathogens**
  *Streptococcus pyogenes* (group A)
  *Staphylococcus aureus*
  *Pseudomonas aeruginosa*
  *Haemophilus influenzae*

**Nose**
**Flora***
  Diphtheroids
  *Staphylococcus epidermidis*
  *Streptococcus viridans*
**Pathogens**
  *Branhamella catarrhalis*
  *Streptococcus pyogenes* (group A)
  *Staphylococcus aureus*

**Cerebrospinal fluid**
**Flora***
None
**Pathogens**
  *Neisseria meningitidis*
  *Haemophilus influenzae*
  *Streptococcus pneumoniae*
  *Cryptococcus neoformans*‡

**Urine**
**Flora***
  F. *Staphylococcus epidermidis*
  Diptheroids
  M. None
**Pathogens**
  *Escherichia coli*
  *Proteus species*
  *Pseudomonas aeruginosa*
  *Enterococcus* species
  *Staphylococcus saprophyticus*

**Genital**
**Flora***
  F. Lactobacilli
  *Staphylococcus epidermidis*
  M. None
**Pathogens**
  *Neisseria gonorrhoeae*
  *Bacteroides species*
  *Streptococcus* (group B)
  *Trichomonas vaginalis* ‡
  *Candida albicans*†

**Sputum**
**Flora***
  Diphtheroids
  *Staphylococcus epidermidis*
  *Streptococcus viridans*
**Pathogens**
  *Streptococcus pyogenes* (group A)
  *Staphylococcus aureus*
  *Klebsiella pneumoniae*
  *Candida albicans*
  *Mycobacterium tuberculosis*
  *Pseudomonas aeruginosa*
  *Haemophilus influenzae*
  *Branhamella catarrhalis*

**Throat**
**Flora***
  *Branhamella catarrhalis*
  Diphtheroids
  *Staphylococcus epidermidis*
  *Streptococcus viridans*
**Pathogens**
  *Streptococcus pyogenes* (group A)
  *Staphylococcus aureus*
  *Neisseria gonorrhoeae*
  *Haemophilus influenzae*

**Stool**
**Flora***
  *Escherichia coli*
  *Proteus* sp.
  *Klebsiella* sp.
  *Enterobacter* sp.
**Pathogens**
  *Campylobacter* species
  *Salmonella* species
  *Shigella* species
  *Aeromonas* species
  *Escherichia coli* (some serotypes)
  *Giardia lamblia*
  *Entamoeba histolytica*

**Blood**
**Flora***
None
**Pathogens**
All, especially:
  *Streptococcus viridans*
  *Staphylococcus aureus*
  *Escherichia coli*

**Wounds and abscesses**
**Flora***
None
**Pathogens**
  *Staphylococcus aureus*
  *Escherichia coli*
  *Pseudomonas aeruginosa*
  *Clostridium* species
  *Streptococcus pyogenes* (group A)

*Normal flora found anywhere in pure culture should
 be considered to be potential pathogens.
†Parasites
‡Fungi
F Female
M Male

**FIGURE 1-1** Microorganisms commonly found in the human body. (Adapted from *Clinical Procedures for Medical Assisting* by M. A. Frew and D. R. Frew, 1990, p. 69, Philadelphia: F. A. Davis Company. Adapted with permission.)

of sand into lenses able to magnify 300× and added a simple focus mechanism (see Figure 1-2). With his microscope van Leeuwenhoek viewed rain and pond water, infusions made from peppercorns, and scrap-ings from his teeth. Surprisingly, he was able to observe bacteria and protozoans at this low magnification. Figure 1-3 shows some of van Leeuwenhoek's drawings of what have since been identified as bacteria.

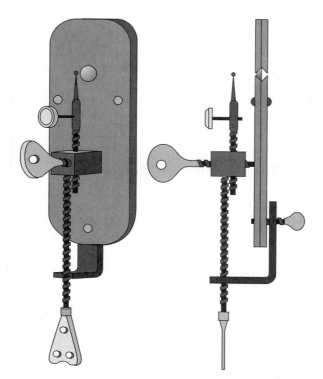

**FIGURE 1-2** Anton van Leeuwenhoek's microscope.

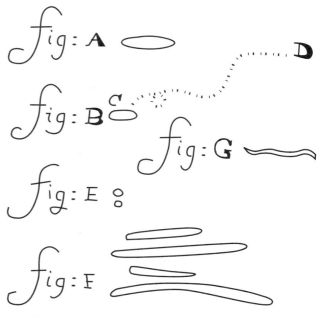

**FIGURE 1-3** Anton van Leeuwenhoek's drawings of cells that were later identified as bacteria.

## Spontaneous Generation

Discovery of the microscopic world in the 1600s raised some interesting questions and eventually led scientists to question of some long-held beliefs. At that time in history the scientific community used a theory known as "spontaneous generation" to explain the apparently magical origins of life. This theory was widely accepted by laypersons and by most members of the scientific community. Spontaneous generation proposed that simple life arose spontaneously from nonliving materials and had its basis in the teachings of Aristotle in the fourth century BC. Early ideas of spontaneous generation proposed that some mystical, "vital force" in air caused, for example, mice to arise from grain, worms from horse hairs, and maggots from decaying meat.

Although most people accepted spontaneous generation, the theory did have some strong opponents, such as the Italian physician Francisco Redi. In 1668, before van Leeuwenhoek's discovery of microscopic life, Redi developed an experiment designed to disprove that maggots arose spontaneously from decaying meat. Redi began by putting pieces of meat into six jars. Three of the jars he covered with lids, the other three he left open. Predictably, the meat in the closed jars decayed but no maggots appeared; however, maggots and eventually flies appeared in the open jars. Redi had a difficult audience to convince; his experiment did not convert the supporters of spontaneous generation. His critics argued that the experiment was not valid; the lids excluded air and, therefore, the magical, "vital" force necessary for spontaneous generation to occur.

Undaunted, Redi modified his experiment by putting netting rather than lids on some of the jars. Just as Redi predicted, no maggots appeared. These results provided a strong blow to the belief in the spontaneous generation of large forms of life, but many people still believed that microscopic forms of life were generated from nonliving substances.

The theory of spontaneous generation was finally laid to rest in 1861 by the French microbiologist, Louis Pasteur. Pasteur designed a series of experiments intended to prove that although microorganisms were present in air they were not spontaneously produced. He hypothesized that these "organized bodies" were carried by dust in the air. When the particles fell into seemingly sterile solutions their growth resulted in contamination. If they were prevented from coming in contact with the sterile solution then no contamination would occur.

Pasteur filled several round-bottomed flasks with broth and boiled the contents (see Figure 1-4). Some of the flasks were left open and within a few days became turbid, an indication that they were teeming with microbial life. Pasteur heated the necks of some of the other flasks and drew the glass into a long, S-shaped curve open at the end. This long neck allowed air to enter the flask freely but any microorganisms carried in the air were trapped in the neck. The broth in these flasks did not become contaminated and showed no signs of life after months or even years. These experiments showed that microorganisms present on

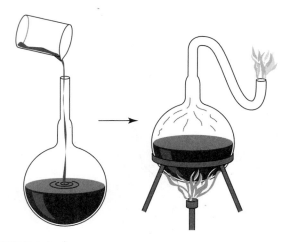

**FIGURE 1-4** Pasteur's experiment disproving the theory of spontaneous generation.

or in nonliving materials such as dust or water were responsible for the contamination of sterile solutions. Pasteur's experiments were simple and easy to reproduce making them especially convincing. Some of Pasteur's original flasks are still on display today at the Pasteur Institute in Paris.

## Fermentation

Superstition also surrounded the production of wine. Wine making was an important industry in many French villages during the 1600s and 1700s just as it is today. At that time in history the influence of microorganisms on fermentation was unknown.

It was not until the 1800s that scientists determined that living organisms, and not some mystical force, were responsible for fermentation.

Pasteur was a well known figure in France during the 1860s due to his earlier work on spontaneous generation and fermentation. Anxious to find a method to prevent the souring of beer and wine, a group of French merchants approached Louis Pasteur for help. Through a series of now classic experiments Pasteur determined that bacteria were responsible for the spoilage of wine after fermentation. He found that bacteria converted the alcohol into vinegar (acetic acid) in the presence of air. After further research Pasteur determined that mild heating of beer or wine after alcoholic fermentation would kill the bacteria and prevent souring. Mild heating rather than boiling was sufficient to kill the undesirable organisms without ruining the taste of the product; the process was named **pasteurization**. This was one of the first steps in establishing a connection between microorganisms and the spoilage of foods (Tortora, Berdell, & Case, 1995, p. 10).

Pasteur's discoveries rocked the scientific and med-

ical communities. Although physicians were aware of bacteria in diseased patients, they considered them a product of the disease rather than its cause. If, however, these microorganisms could cause food spoilage then perhaps they could also cause disease. This led to the development of the **germ theory of disease** or specifically the idea that bacteria are the cause of infectious disease.

## The Germ Theory of Disease

The understanding that the activity of microorganisms caused physical and chemical changes in organic substances gave credence to those who proposed that bacteria could cause disease. As early as 1546, Girolamo Francastoro discussed the concept of "contagion," an infection that passes from one individual to another. Francastoro speculated that infection is caused by very small, imperceptible particles passed by contact with an infected person, by fomites, or in the air. This was a difficult concept for people to accept. Most of them believed that disease was the punishment due to those who committed crimes or behaved immorally. They thought that infectious disease was spread by "miasma" or "vapors" that arose from decaying or diseased bodies and "altered the chemical quality of the atmosphere." The miasma theory persisted well into the 1800s.

Gradually though, through repeated studies, the evidence accumulated and physicians and scientists began to accept the germ theory. They realized that these infectious agents could be transmitted as suggested by Francastoro and Pasteur. Further evidence that this was indeed true was provided in the 1840s by the Hungarian physician, Ignaz Semmelweis.

Semmelweis supervised two separate maternity clinics; one was run by midwives, the other by obstetricians. He observed a significantly higher rate of childbed fever in the clinic run by obstetricians. Although unknown at that time, childbed fever, or puerperal fever, is caused by a hemolytic streptococcus. The organism reproduces rapidly causing sepsis that often results in death. After analyzing the two clinics for differences, Semmelweis concluded that the obstetricians themselves were transmitting the disease. The doctors made frequent examinations of many women and did not wash their hands between patients. In response to his findings Semmelweis implemented a policy requiring the physicians to wash their hands with a solution of lime chloride. The results were impressive—the incidence of childbed fever dropped to the same level as experienced in the clinic run by midwives. Although Semmelweis's experiment clearly showed that the physicians were transmitting childbed fever, many of his colleagues refused to accept his conclusions. Semmelweis was scorned and even lost his job because of his insistence that he was right. Not until several years later were his theories generally accepted and put into practice (Brock, 1961, p. 82).

## The Application of Aseptic Principles to Medical Issues

Joseph Lister was an English physician who applied the germ theory to medical issues. Influenced by the work of Semmelweis and Pasteur, he sought a way to reduce the incidence of infection after surgery. Lister was aware of disinfectants and that carbolic acid, or phenol, killed bacteria. In 1867, he wrote a paper describing the effects of soaking surgical dressings in carbolic acid before applying them to the surgical wound. Lister's results were so impressive that his techniques were quickly adopted by other physicians.

## Edward Jenner and Immunization

Edward Jenner was a young English physician who was anxious to find a way to protect people from smallpox. Smallpox is caused by a virus, a term that Jenner used for the infectious agent long before they were ever observed. The disease caused by the smallpox virus is highly infectious and often fatal. Survivors are often marked by devastating scars caused by the fluid-filled pustules, or "pox," that form as the disease progresses. Smallpox epidemics were common in the 1790s and were greatly feared. Thousands were killed in Europe as the disease swept across the land. European settlers traveling to the New World carried smallpox with them where it killed about 90% of the Native American population on the East coast.

In 1798, Jenner developed an immunization against smallpox despite the fact that he could not explain the cause of the disease. Jenner learned from a milkmaid that she was safe from infection by smallpox due to an earlier infection with cowpox. Cowpox is a milder disease caused by a closely related virus. In the process of investigating her claim Jenner determined that inoculation of a patient with scrapings from cowpox blisters provided protection against smallpox. Eventually the process was named **vaccination**, based on the Latin word "vacca" meaning "cow." Jenner's method was adopted throughout Europe replacing the risky technique of immunizing with actual smallpox material (see Figure 1-5).

## Robert Koch and Anthrax

Now that most members of the European scientific community accepted the connection between microorganisms and disease, the race was on to determine the causes of specific diseases. Robert Koch, a young German physician with no formal research training, was the first to do so. Koch was anxious to determine the etiology of the disease anthrax. Anthrax is primarily a

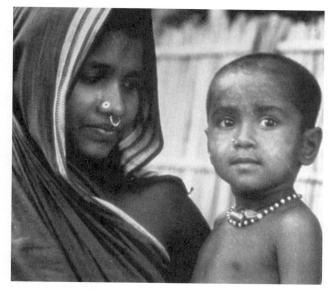

**FIGURE 1-5** The last known victim of smallpox in Asia was a three-year-old girl from Bangladesh. (Courtesy Dr. D. J. M. Tarantola, World Health Organization.)

disease of grazing animals such as sheep and cattle, but it can be transmitted to humans. It is caused by a bacterium now referred to as *Bacillus anthracis*. In his examination of animals that had died from anthrax, Koch discovered rod-shaped bacteria in their blood. Koch isolated the bacteria from the blood and cultured them on nutrients in the laboratory. A sample of the culture was then injected into a healthy animal, which became sick and died from anthrax. Finally, Koch isolated the same rod-shaped bacteria from the blood of the second animal establishing a link between the bacterium and anthrax.

## Magic Bullets and Modern Chemotherapy

After Koch established the relationship between microorganisms and disease intensive work by many physicians and scientists began to discover or develop substances that would kill pathogens without harming the patient. In 1910, Paul Ehrlich was the first to do so. He discovered an arsenic compound called salvarsan that was an effective treatment for syphilis. This marked the beginnings of the era of "modern chemotherapy," or the treatment of disease with chemicals.

An enormous advance in the search for "magic bullets" came in the form of a fortunate accident. While working with variants of *Staphylococcus* organisms, the Scottish physician and bacteriologist Alexander Fleming noticed that some of his plate cultures were contaminated with a variety of microorganisms. Fleming observed that surrounding the growth of a contaminating mold the *Staphylococcus* growth was inhibited (see Color Plate 1-6). He speculated that the mold was producing a substance that inhibited the bacterial growth as it diffused through the agar. Fleming isolated and subcultured the mold for further study.

Fleming wondered if other molds produced the antimicrobial substance and if it was active against other microorganisms. He tested a number of different molds and found that a strain of *Penicillium* produced the inhibitory substance and was culturally identical to the one he had isolated. He named the substance "penicillin." The mold was later identified as *Penicillium notatum*.

The significance of penicillin was not realized until after the 1939 discovery of two other antibiotics, gramicidin and tyrocidine, by the French microbiologist Rene Dubos. Both of these antibiotics are produced by species of the bacterium, *Bacillus brevis*. (Antibiotics are substances produced by some bacteria and fungi that inhibit the growth of or kill other species of bacteria.) In the 1940s, sufficient quantities of penicillin were produced for use in clinical studies. Synthetic drugs called the sulfonamides were discovered in 1935 by Dogmagk.

## TAXONOMY AND NOMENCLATURE OF MICROORGANISMS

An incredible diversity of life is present on our planet with new species of all types being constantly discovered. It has long been recognized that any attempts to study living things and their relationships to each other could only be achieved by the use of an orderly system of **taxonomy**. Aristotle (4th century BC) was probably the first to group all organisms, and categorized them as either plants or animals. In 1735, Carolus Linnaeus developed the basic rules for the system of taxonomy and **nomenclature** that we still use today. This system provides each organism with a unique name and arranges them into groups called **taxa** (categories) with other similar organisms to reflect their **phylogeny**, or evolutionary relatedness. The primary goals of taxonomy are **classification**, nomenclature, and identification, and over 2 million organisms have been categorized since Linnaeus's time. This chapter discusses the classification of bacteria, fungi, protozoans, and helminths that are human pathogens (disease causing) or potential human pathogens. The classification of viruses is covered in Chapter 51.

The classification of microorganisms began in 1674 with the invention of the light microscope (Howard, Keiser, & Smith, 1994, p. 3) and today is a discipline based on increasingly complex criteria. It was not, however, until 1866 that the German naturalist Ernest Haeckel proposed that the bacteria, fungi, and protists be removed from the plant and animal kingdoms. They were finally separated into three kingdoms early in the 1960s and into five kingdoms by Whittaker in 1969.

### The Five-Kingdom System of Classification

Although several systems of classification have been developed, the one that is most often used, and that is used in this book, was developed in 1969 by **Robert Whittaker** of Cornell University. Whittaker's system divided all life (except for the viruses) into five kingdoms based on cellular organization and nutritional patterns. The five kingdoms, their major characteristics, and some examples of each are shown in Table 1-1.

### The Taxonomic Hierarchy

Kingdoms are the largest taxa and contain several smaller groups called **phyla** or **divisions**. The term, division, is used in the classification of plants and fungi. Phylum is used for the remaining three kingdoms. Each phylum is in turn divided into several **classes**, and so on, down to **species**, the smallest taxon. There are seven levels in this hierarchy of classification that are arranged into descending ranks. In

### Table 1–1 ▶ The Five-Kingdom System

| Kingdom | Cellular Organization | Nutrition Type | Examples |
|---|---|---|---|
| Monera (or Procaryotae) | procaryotic, unicellular | varies | eubacteria, archaeobacteria |
| Fungi | eucaryotic unicellular or multicellular | heterotrophic, absorptive | molds, yeasts, mushrooms, smuts, rusts |
| Protista | eucaryotic unicellular or colonial | heterotrophic (a few autotrophic species) | protozoans, slime molds, some algae |
| Animalia | eucaryotic multicellular | heterotrophic, ingestive | invertebrates, vertebrates |
| Plantae | eucaryotic multicellular | autotrophic | some algae, mosses, ferns, all other plants |

order, they are kingdom, phylum (or division), class, order, family, genus, and species. Kingdom is the least specific taxon and species is the most specific. The naming of taxa in this hierarchy is subject to a set of rules, or a code. Bacteriologists, for example, use the **International Code of Bacterial Nomenclature**. Changes and additions are published in the **International Journal of Systematic Bacteriology**.

All members of the same kingdom share a few general characteristics; members of the same species are the same kind of organism. This is not a perfect system and not all organisms fit neatly into the seven taxa. Additional levels above (super) or below (sub) a taxa are used in these cases. Two examples of the hierarchy of classification applied to an organism are seen in Table 1-2 and Figure 1-6. Several taxonomic categories that fall below species are listed in Table 1-3.

## Nomenclature

Nomenclature refers to the naming of organisms. The **binomial** system of nomenclature that Linnaeus developed assigns a genus and species name to each organism. These standardized names are recognized around the world and provide scientists with a common language. They are less confusing than local names whose meaning can vary in different areas. When writing scientific names the genus name is always capitalized and the species name begins with a lower case letter. Both names are underlined or printed in italics.

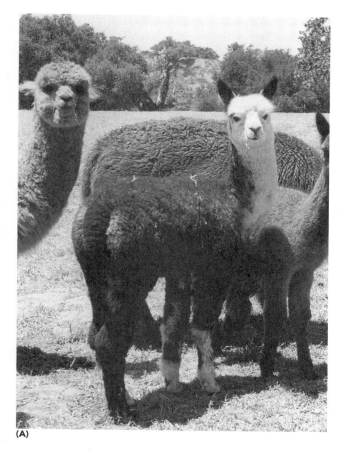

**(A)**

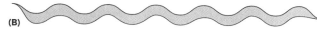

**(B)**

**FIGURE 1-6** (A) Alpaca and (B) *Treponema pallidum*, a spiral organism. (Photo courtesy Joan Speirs, El Ranchito, Santa Ynez, CA.)

Scientific names are derived from Latin, or latinized Greek (the language of scholars in Linnaeus's time), and are often descriptive of the organism. For example, the bacterium named *Staphylococcus epidermidis* is appropriately named. "Staphylo" refers to "grape-like" clusters of cells while a "coccus" is a spherical bacterial cell. Both of these are characteristics of the bacterium. The species name, epidermidis, reflects the fact that this organism is a common resident of the skin. The genus name of *Escherichia coli* is the latinized form of

| Table 1–2 ▶ The Hierarchy of Classification Using Examples from Kingdoms Animalia and Procaryotae | | |
|---|---|---|
| **Taxonomic Rank** | | |
| Kingdom | Animalia | Procaryotae |
| Phylum (Division) | Chordata | Gracilicutes |
| Class | Mammalia | Scotobacter |
| Order | Artiodactyla | Spirochaetales |
| Family | Camelidae | Spirochaetaceae |
| Genus | *Lama* | *Treponema* |
| species | *L. pacos* (alpaca) | *T. pallidum* |

| Table 1–3 ▶ Subspecific Ranks of Bacteria | | |
|---|---|---|
| **Taxonomic Rank** | **Alternate Name** | **Unique Features** |
| Biovar | Biotype | Special biochemical or physiological properties |
| Serovar | Serotype | Distinctive antigenic properties |
| Pathovar | Pathotype | Pathogenic properties for certain hosts |
| Phagovar | Phagotype | Can be lysed by certain bacteriophages |
| Morphovar | Morphotype | Special morphological features |

Escherich, the last name of the scientist who first described the bacterium. "Coli" refers to the colon and is appropriate because this organism is an enteric resident of humans and many other animals.

## PROCARYOTIC AND EUCARYOTIC MICROORGANISMS

Two basic types of cells differ greatly in their ultrastructure when viewed with an electron microscope. They are called **procaryotic** and **eucaryotic** cells. Besides their different sizes, procaryotic and eucaryotic cells differ most significantly in nuclear structure and organization. Procaryotic cells have a single, circular chromosome that is associated with **nonhistone proteins**. It is located in a part of the cytoplasm referred to as the **nucleoid** or nuclear area. The procaryotic chromosome undergoes division by binary fission and is not surrounded by a nuclear envelope. Eucaryotic cells have more than one chromosome that are surrounded by a nuclear envelope. These chromosomes are arranged in a linear fashion and are associated with a group of proteins referred to as the **histone proteins**. Eucaryotic cells undergo division by mitosis. Other differences between procaryotic and eucaryotic cells include the lack of membrane-bound organelles in procaryotes and the presence of **peptidoglycan** in most procaryotic cells.

Despite these differences procaryotic and eucaryotic cells also have many similarities. Both cell types have similar chemical compositions and use many similar metabolic pathways. Research has shown that the two cell types are related. It is generally accepted that eucaryotic cells evolved from procaryotes. Procaryotic and eucaryotic cells are compared in Table 1-4.

## PROCARYOTIC MICROORGANISM

### Bacteria

Procaryotes, the bacteria, are smaller and simpler than the protozoans and the fungi. They have one circular chromosome and reproduce primarily by asexual, binary fission. Many bacteria have in addition to the main chromosome, small, circular molecules of DNA called **plasmids**. These plasmids are self-replicating and code for traits that assist survival of adverse conditions. They can be transferred from cell to cell and between species by **conjugation**, **transduction**, or **transformation**. Most bacteria range in size from 0.2 to 2.0 µm in diameter and 2.0 to 8.0 µm in length, there are of course, larger and smaller species (Figure 1-7 and Table 1-5).

Six genera of gram-positive bacteria, including *Bacillus* and *Clostridium,* form a dormant stage called an **endospore**. Endospores are extremely resistant to adverse conditions including heat, lack of water, and exposure to some toxic substances. Endospores are clinically significant because they allow the microorganism to survive for an extended period of time separated from the host. Several species of endospore-forming bacteria are serious pathogens causing diseases such as botulism, gangrene, and anthrax.

### Table 1–4 ▶ Comparison of Procaryotic and Eucaryotic Cells

| Characteristic | Procaryotic | Eucaryotic |
|---|---|---|
| Average size of cells | 0.20–2.0 µm in diameter | 10–100 µm in diameter |
| Nucleus | No nuclear envelope or nucleoli | Membrane-bound, nucleoli present |
| Location/type of genetic material | Single, circular chromosome in cytoplasm; some have plasmids | Multiple, linear chromosomes in nucleus; other DNA in organelles |
| Membrane-bound organelles | Not present | Present (examples include mitochondria and endoplasmic reticulum) |
| Flagella | Hollow, made of protein, attached by basal body | Complex, 9+2 arrangement of microtubules |
| Glycocalyx | Exists as capsule or slime layer | Exists in animal cells |
| Cell wall | Usually present; many contain peptidoglycan | Present in plant cells, no peptidoglycan |
| Plasma membrane | No carbohydrates, most lack sterols | Sterols and carbohydrates present |
| Cytoskeleton | Not present | Present |
| Ribosomes | 70S | 80S (70S in organelles) |
| Cell division | Binary fission | Mitosis |
| Sexual reproduction | Transfer of DNA fragments by conjugation, transformation, or transduction | Involves meiosis |

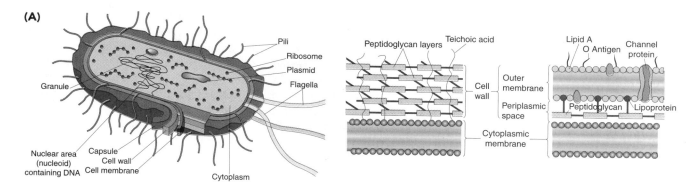

**FIGURE 1-7** (A) A Typical procaryotic cell. (B) Gram-positive and gram-negative cell walls.

## Morphology and Arrangement of Bacterial Cells

There are three basic morphologies of bacterial cells including **cocci** (singular, coccus), or round cells, **bacilli** (singular, bacillus), or rodlike cells, and helical or spiral-shaped cells (see Figure 1-8).

Cocci are round or oval, and they may be flattened on one side. Bacilli may be short or long, having either rounded or tapered ends. Some bacilli are short and oval and are easily mistaken for cocci. They are called coccobacilli. Curved rods are called vibrios. Helical or spiral-shaped cells having fairly rigid bodies are referred to as **spirilla**. Most are motile by means of flagella. Others are fairly flexible and have structures called **axial filaments** that are contained in an external sheath, they are called **spirochetes**.

| Table 1–5 ▶ Structures Found in a Typical Procaryotic Cell | | |
|---|---|---|
| **Structure** | **Characteristics** | **Function** |
| Glycocalyx (capsule or slime layer) | Gelatinous polysaccharide polypeptide layer | Surrounds the cell wall |
| | | May protect against phagocytosis and dessication |
| | | Aids in adherence to surfaces |
| Fimbriae and pili | Short, thin, hollow appendages attached to the cell wall | Fimbriae—attachment to surfaces |
| | | Pili—conjugation |
| Flagella | Long, thin, hollow structures consisting of a filament, hook, and basal body | Flagella rotate to push the cell |
| | | Attach to the cell wall |
| Axial filaments | Similar to flagella but wrapped around the cell, associated with spirochetes | Provides motility to spirochetes |
| Cell wall | Two types, gram-positive and gram-negative | Surrounds the plasma membrane and protects cell from environmental stress |
| | | Contains peptidoglycan |
| Cell membrane | Selectively permeable, phospholipid bilayer and protein | Surrounds cytoplasm and contains enzymes involved in metabolic reactions |
| Cytoplasm | Gelatinous matrix located inside the cell membrane | Made of water, organic and inorganic molecules |
| | | Contains ribosomes, DNA and inclusions |
| Ribosomes | 70S, contain rRNA and protein | Site of protein synthesis |
| Nucleoid | Contains the bacterial chromosome (DNA molecule) | Area in the cytoplasm where the main chromosome is located |
| Plasmids | Small, circular, extrachromosomal DNA molecules | Found in some cells in addition to the main chromosome |
| Inclusions | Reserve deposits of various materials found in the cytoplasm | Examples include sulfur granules and metachromatic granules |
| Endospores | The dormant, resistant stage of some bacteria (6 genera of gram-positive bacteria) | Assist survival of adverse conditions |

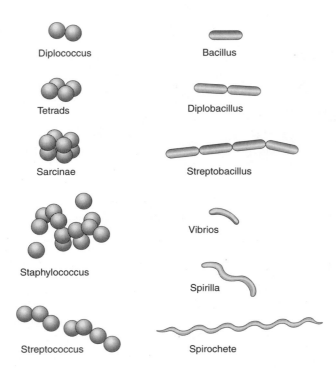

**FIGURE 1-8** Morphology and arrangment of bacterial cell.

In some species bacterial cells exist singly, but in many other cases the cells remain attached to each other after division resulting in arrangements of cells that can be characteristic. Some gram-positive cocci form long chains and are called **streptococci**. Grape-like clusters, or broad sheets of cocci, are known as **staphylococci**. Gram-positive bacilli sometimes form chains. Various arrangements of bacterial cells are shown in Figure 1-9. The medically significant bacteria are discussed in Section 2.

## Bacterial Cell Walls

Most species of the **eubacteria** (true bacteria) have cell walls. There are, however, exceptions such as the wall-less species of the genus *Mycoplasma*. The cell wall surrounds the plasma membrane and protects the cell from environmental stresses such as changes in osmotic pressure. Two types of cell walls exist and are distinguished on the basis of a differential staining technique. The technique is referred to as Gram staining and was developed in 1884 by the Danish bacteriologist, Hans Christian Gram.

Cell walls designated as gram-positive walls retain the primary dye, crystal violet, after decolorization and stain purple or blue. The crystal violet is washed away from gram-negative cell walls by decolorization, which are then colored red, or pink, by the safranin counterstain used in the last step of Gram staining. The Gram staining procedure is discussed in Chapter 8.

## Criteria for Classification

Classification of the bacteria is a difficult undertaking that is further complicated by the simple nature of these organisms. The basic taxonomic group in bacterial classification is the species, a taxon that is difficult to define at this level. Other, more complex forms of life, such as plants and animals, can be classified on the basis of reproductive compatibility as well as morphologic similarities. The bacteria have traditionally been categorized based on a variety of morphologic and physiologic features with more emphasis placed on physiology.

Bacterial species are actually a collection of **strains** that are the descendants of a single cell. One of these strains is selected as the **type strain** and serves as the example of the species. It also plays an important role in the classification of the species. A species, then, consists of the type strain and all other strains that are sufficiently similar to warrant inclusion of it in the species (*Bergey's Manual,* vol. 1, p. 1). One problem associated with this definition of species is that it involves subjective judgments and does not always accurately reflect phylogenetically relatedness of bacterial species. It is important that any truly usable classification scheme be reliable and stable and new work emphasizing genetic relatedness promises to be both. Studies that examine, for example, ribosomal RNA sequences that already resolved many confusing cases of bacterial taxonomy. Although there is no "official" classification of bacteria, the one that is presented in *Bergey's Manual of Systematic Bacteriology* is the most widely accepted scheme.

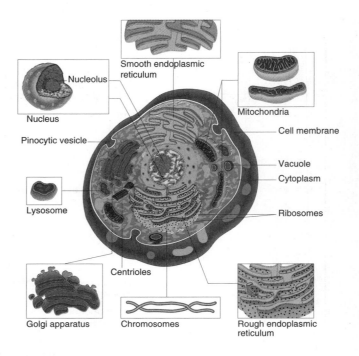

**FIGURE 1-9** A typical eucaryotic (animal) cell.

## Major Characteristics

*Bergey's Manual* divides the bacteria into four divisions (Table 1-6). The eubacteria make up three of these divisions while the archaeobacteria make up the fourth. Each division is separated into classes for a total of seven classes of bacteria. These are groups of convenience, really, and do not always reflect phylogenetic relationships between the organisms.

# THE EUCARYOTIC MICROORGANISMS

All other organisms are eucaryotic including the fungi, the protozoans, the plants, and the animals. The protozoans and some of the fungi are unicellular; the plants and animals are multicellular. Figure 1-9 shows the structure of typical eucaryotic cells, which are further delineated in Table 1-7.

## Fungi

The fungi are a diverse group of organisms that include the unicellular yeasts and the multicellular molds, mushrooms, **smuts**, and **rusts**; all are members of the kingdom, Fungi. The cell walls of fungi contain a complex carbohydrate called chitin. Fungi are nonphotosynthetic, and they obtain their nutrients by absorbing solutions of organic materials. **Yeasts** are oval cells, larger than the bacteria, having a distinct nucleus. Yeasts reproduce by budding and sometimes short chains of yeast cells called **pseudohyphae** form as cells divide.

Molds are multicellular and form long, filamentous chains of cells called **hyphae**. Hyphae can be **septate**,

| Table 1–6 ▶ The Four Divisions of Kingdom Procaryotae | | |
|---|---|---|
| **Division** | **Description** | **Examples of Classes** |
| Gracilicutes | Thin, gram-negative cell walls | Nonphotosynthetic bacteria, cyanobacteria |
| Firmucutes | Thick, gram-positive cell walls | Rods and cocci, Actinomycetes and related organisms |
| Tenericutes | Wall-less eubacteria | Mycoplasmas |
| Mendosicutes | Unusual cell walls | Archaeobacteria |

meaning that there are crosswalls (septa) separating the nuclei, or **coenocytic** (aseptate), which means that these crosswalls are absent. Hyphae twist and tangle together to form a fuzzy mass called a **mycelium**. Fungi reproduce sexually or asexually by the production of spores. They are classified into phyla according to the type of sexual spore they produce. Many of the fungi that cause disease in humans are dimorphic (having two growth forms—mold and yeast) and **mycoses** (fungal infections) are often difficult to cure.

**Criteria for Classification.** Although the fungi were once erroneously classified as plants, the 50,000 to 100,000 species that are recognized today are grouped into their own kingdom. Only a small fraction of these many species are pathogens, or opportunists, under certain circumstances. Pathogenic or potentially pathogenic species are almost always members of three phyla: **Zygomycota**, **Ascomycota**, and **Deuteromycota**. Rarely, a clinical isolate will be identified as a member

## Table 1–7 ▶ Structures in Eucaryotic (Animal) Cells

| Structure | Composition | Function |
|---|---|---|
| Cell membrane | Phospholipid bilayer with proteins | Selective barrier between the cell and its environment |
| Nucleus | Bilayer membrane surrounds chromosomes, nucleoplasm and nucleoli | Controls reproduction and synthesis of cellular materials |
| Nucleolus | Dark body in nucleus made of chromatin, RNA and protein | Production of ribosomes |
| Centriole | Microtubules | Give rise to spindle fibers, cilia and flagella |
| Golgi complex | A stack of flattened, membranous disks | Processing and packaging of cellular products |
| Endoplasmic reticulum | Membranous series of channels and canals | Synthesis and transport of various substances |
| smooth | | Lipid synthesis |
| rough | | Protein synthesis |
| Mitochondrion | Bilayer membranous structure with many enzymes; extensive folding of inner membrane | Aerobic respiration—production of adenosine triphosphate |
| Cytoskeleton | Microfilaments and microtubules in the cytoplasm | Shape, support, and movement of the cell |
| Vacuoles | Membranous sacs | Storage of cellular products |
| Lysosome | Membranous sac filled with digestive enzymes | Intracellular digestion |
| Cilia and flagella | Made of microtubules | Movement of the cell |

| Table 1–8 ▶ Classification of Zygomycota, Ascomycota, and Deuteromycota | |
|---|---|
| **Phylum I** | **Zygomycota** |
| Class | Zygomycetes |
| Genera | *Absidia* |
| | *Cunninghamella* |
| | *Mucor* |
| | *Rhizopus* |
| | *Rhizomucor* |
| Class | Trichomycetes |
| **Phylum II** | **Ascomycota** |
| Class | Hemiascomycetes |
| Genera | *Saccharomyces* |
| | *Schizosaccharomyces* |
| Class | Loculoascomycetes |
| Genus | *Piedraia* |
| Class | Plectomycetes |
| Genus | *Pseudallescheria* |
| **Phylum III** | **Deuteromycota (Fungi Imperfecti)** |
| Class | Blastomycetes |
| Genera | *Blastoschizomyces* |
| | *Candida* |
| | *Cryptococcus* |
| | *Malassezia* |
| | *Phaeoannellomyces* |
| | *Rhodotorula* |
| | *Torulopsis* |
| | *Trichosporon* |
| Class | Coelomycetes |
| Class | Hyphomycetes |
| Genera | *Acremonium* |
| | *Aspergillus* |
| | *Bipolaris* |
| | *Blastomyces* |
| | *Cladosporium* |
| | *Coccidioides* |
| | *Curvularia* |
| | *Epidermophyton* |
| | *Exophiala* |
| | *Fonsececaea* |
| | *Fusarium* |
| | *Geotrichum* |
| | *Histoplasma* |
| | *Madurella* |
| | *Microsporum* |
| | *Paracoccidioides* |
| | *Penicillium* |
| | *Phialophora* |
| | *Scedosporium* |
| | *Scopulariopsis* |
| | *Sporothrix* |
| | *Wangiella* |

of the phylum **Basidiomycota**. The fungi are classified into phyla according to the type of sexual spore that they produce, or by the lack of sexual reproduction as in phylum Deuteromycota. Members of this phylum are often called the "Fungi Imperfecti" due to the lack of an observed sexual stage in their life cycle. Separation into classes and genera is based on structural and physiologic characteristics. A commonly accepted classification of the fungi is shown in Table 1-8.

**Major Characteristics.** The fungi are eucaryotic organisms that have a nucleus, endoplasmic reticulum, mitochondria, and 80S ribosomes. They are very different from the plants, lacking chloroplasts and photosynthetic pigments. Also, the main component of the cell wall of fungi is the complex polysaccharide, **chitin**, rather than cellulose as in the plants. Several morphologic forms are found in kingdom Fungi (see Figure 1-10).

## Protozoans

Several species of protozoans parasitize humans and other species of animals. Life-threatening protozoal diseases are more common in third world nations than they are in developed parts of the world. Some, however, such as *Giardia lamblia,* are the cause of significant morbidity even in the United States.

The protozoans are eucaryotic and unicellular and are found living in many environments such as water and moist soil. They are members of the kingdom, Protista.

**Criteria for Classification.** The protozoans are classified into phyla according to their mode of locomotion (motility) and type of reproduction. The classification scheme used in this book recognizes four phyla. They are **Sarcomastigophora**, **Apicomplexa**, **Ciliophora**, and **Microspora**. The major features of the phyla are listed in Table 1-9. Other classification decisions, such

| Table 1–9 ▶ Protozoan Phyla and Their Major Features | | |
|---|---|---|
| **Phylum** | **Mode of Locomotion** | **Type of Reproduction** |
| Sarcomastigophora subphyla | Pseudopods, flagella or both | Asexual binary fission |
| Sarcodina | Pseudopods | |
| Mastigophora | Flagella | |
| Ciliophora | Rows of cilia | Mitotic fission |
| | | Sexual conjugation |
| Apicomplexa | Nonmotile when mature | Alternation of generations (asexual and sexual reproduction) |
| Microspora | Nonmotile when mature | Alternation of generations |

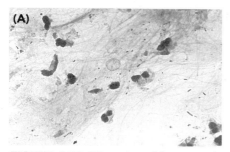
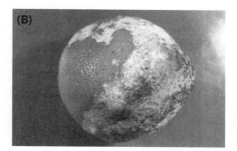
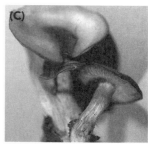

**FIGURE 1-10** Diversity of forms in the kingdom Fungi. (A) *Candida albicans* in Sputum. (B) A moldy orange. (C) The mushroom *Hygrophorus*.

as placement into classes or families, is based on such features as morphology, physiology, and habitat.

**Major Characteristics.** The protozoans are unicellular eucaryotes that are members of the kingdom Protista. Other members of this kingdom include the unicellular algae and the simple, colonial kelps. Although some of the algae and kelps are economically significant, none of them are pathogenic in humans. One characteristic that is shared by all of the protists is the lack of organized tissues.

Many protozoan species are free-living in soil or water. Others are facultative or obligate parasites of a variety of organisms. Most protozoans are able to reproduce asexually by fission, or schizogony (multiple fission), whereas others reproduce sexually by conjugation or the production of gametocytes. Some protozoans are able to produce a protective capsule referred to as a cyst to survive adverse environmental conditions and increase the likelihood of transfer to a suitable host. Although the protozoans lack cell walls most cells are covered by a flexible **pellicle**. We will limit our discussion to those species that spend all or part of their life cycle as human parasites.

Although thousands of species of protozoans have been classified only about two dozen species are parasites or occasional human parasites. A few species are harmless commensals of humans and other animals. Some of the protozoans have two or more stages in their life cycle including in many, a vegetative **trophozoite** and a dormant **cyst** (see Figure 1-11). Some species, such as those in phylum Apicomplexa, have complex life cycles with several morphologic stages and one or more intermediate hosts (see Figure 1-12). Examples of diseases caused by a variety of protozoan parasites include malaria, African sleeping sickness, and toxoplasmosis. Most protozoan species are heterotrophic although a few species such as *Euglena* have photosynthetic pigments and are autotrophic. The protozoans are discussed in more detail in Section 4, Parasitology.

## Metazoans

The metazoans are all eucaryotic and multicellular and are members of the kingdom Animalia. This "catch all" group of organisms includes the flatworms and roundworms, also referred to as the helminths, and the arthropods. Only those species that spend all or parts of their lives as human parasites are of medical signifi-

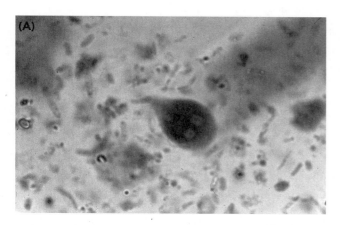
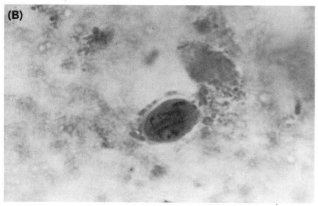

**FIGURE 1-11** *Giardia lamblia*. (A) Trophozoite. (B) Cyst.

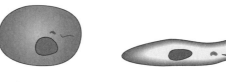

Amastigote    Epimastigote

**FIGURE 1-12** Life cycle stages of trypanosomes.

cance and are considered here. In this book, our discussion of arthropods is limited to those that act as intermediate hosts or vectors of other infectious agents.

## Helminths

Helminths are often referred to as the "worms." Their detection, for example in feces, has always been the source of great distress to the victim. Helminths have specialized organ systems, some of which are modified according to where the adult worm resides.

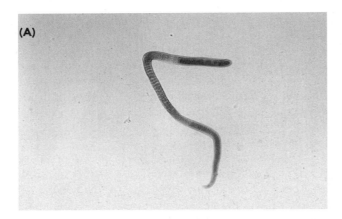

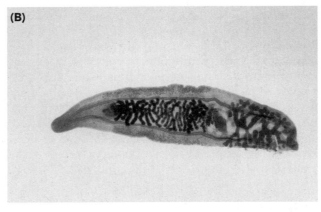

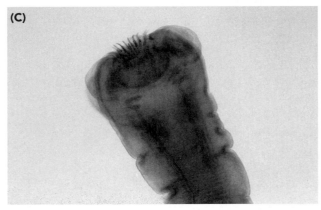

**FIGURE 1-13** Representative helminths. (A) Nematode. (B) Fluke. (C) Tapeworm.

These highly evolved organisms are well suited to their specialized lifestyle within their host species.

The parasitic helminths are highly evolved for a specialized style of life inside their hosts. Some of their body systems have become greatly simplified, or are completely lacking, unneeded in the protected environment provided by the host. For example, the tapeworms, or cestodes, lack a digestive system because they are able to absorb predigested nutrients from the host's intestinal contents. On the other hand, many helminths have more complex reproductive systems that produce large numbers of fertilized eggs. This strategy increases the chances of transfer to an appropriate host and survival of the species.

Adult helminths may be **dioecious**, having separate sexes, or **monecious**, or **hermaphroditic**, meaning that one individual has both male and female reproductive organs. Sexual reproduction occurs in both situations but dioecious species require that two adults of the opposite sex be present in the same host. Adult hermaphrodites may self-fertilize, or copulate with another individual and fertilize each other. Some helminths undergo asexual reproduction during one or more larval stages.

**Criteria for Classification.** The helminths are a diverse group of eucaryotic, multicellular organisms and are members of kingdom Animalia. They are classified into phyla according to their body shape. Schmidt and Roberts state in *Foundations of Parasitology* that the two phyla of helminths containing species that are human parasites are **Aschelminthes** (the round worms) and **Platyhelminthes** (the flat worms) (see Figure 1-13). The only class in Aschelminthes with members that parasitize humans is **Nematoda**. Phylum Platyhelminthes has two classes with parasitic members: **Trematoda** (the flukes) and **Cestoda** (the tape worms). Although some flukes are free-living for all or part of their life cycle, all of the cestodes are parasitic. All of the trematodes that are commonly human parasites are members of order Digenea. Members of Digenea have multiple hosts in their life cycle including at least one species of mollusk (snail) and one vertebrate (Howard).

**Major Characteristics.** One characteristic of the helminths that is not observed in any other group of infectious agents (except for the arthropods) is the presence of specialized organ systems. These systems and their adaptations for parasitic life are discussed in Chapters 46 and 47. Some of the major features of Aschelminthes and Platyhelminthes are listed in Table 1-10. The specific features of nematodes, trematodes, and cestodes are discussed in Chapters 46 and 47.

Many parasitic life cycles are extremely complex requiring two or more specific hosts. A **definitive host** harbors the adult parasite and one or more **intermediate hosts** may be required by the larval stages. The parasitic helminths are discussed in Chapters 46 and 47.

| Table 1–10 ▶ Some Major Features of Aschelminthes and Platyhelminthes | | | |
|---|---|---|---|
| **Phylum or Class** | **Body Shape** | **Digestive System** | **Diecious** |
| Phylum Aschelminthes (Class Nematoda) | Round | Complete | Yes |
| Phylum Platyhelminthes | Flattened | Simple, saclike or lacking | Some species |
|     Class Digenea | Leaf-shaped | Simple, saclike | Some species |
|     Class Cestoda | Long and segmented | Lacking | No |

## Viruses

Simpler than even the bacteria are the viruses. These filterable agents are nonculturable in the laboratory and can only be viewed by electron microscopy. This diverse group of infectious agents are obligate, intracellular parasites of bacteria (bacteriophages), plants, or animals and are usually species-specific in their ability to cause infection. The viral genome consists of a few genes of one type of genetic information, either DNA or RNA, and a few enzymes. A protein capsid and, perhaps, an envelope made of carbohydrates, lipids, and protein often surrounds the nucleic acid core (see Figure 1-14). The viruses are discussed in Chapters 48 through 51.

The viruses do not fit readily into any of the classification systems used for the procaryotic and eucaryotic organisms. The viruses are often referred to as subcellular or acellular due to their simple structures. Their apparent lack of many of the basic characteristics associated with life, such as respiration and metabolism, has led some to question whether or not the viruses are alive.

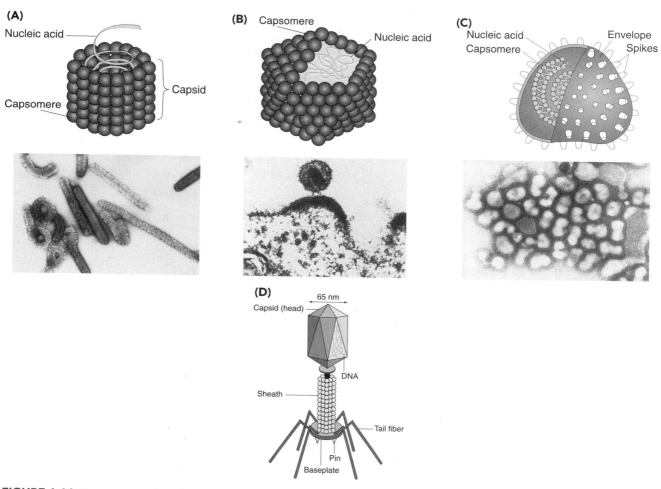

**FIGURE 1-14** Some examples of viral morphology. (A) A helical virus may look like long or coiled threads; Ebola virus showing helical rods; (B) A polyhedral virus (icosahedral); HIV budding out of a T cell. (C) An enveloped helical virus; Influenza. (D) T-even bacteriophage. (Photos for A & C courtesy Centers for Disease Control and Prevention, Atlanta, GA; Photo for B courtesy National Institute of Allergy and Infectious Diseases.)

## SUMMARY

▶ Microorganisms are relevant to all forms of life. Some microbes are beneficial to humans, such as those that play a role in the production of certain foods, whereas others cause disease.

▶ The expression, normal flora, refers to microbes that live on and in humans and other organisms, usually a normal and healthy state.

▶ Some early observations in microbiology were made by Robert Hooke (coined the term "cell"), Schleiden and Schwann (developed the "cell theory"), and Anton van Leeuwenhoek (built first simple microscopes).

▶ Spontaneous generation, an early theory to explain the origins of life, was finally disproved by Louis Pasteur in the mid-1800s, who then developed a process called pasteurization.

▶ The germ theory of disease stated that microbes are the cause of infectious disease. Semmelweis, Lister, Jenner, Koch, and Fleming were early pioneers in using the germ theory to explain and prevent disease.

▶ Taxonomy is the orderly classification of organisms into groups that reflect relationships between them and other organisms; the five-kingdom system is widely accepted and is used in this text.

▶ The taxonomic hierarchy consists of kingdoms, phyla, classes, orders, families, genera, and species. Each organism is assigned a genus and species name.

▶ The two basic cell types are procaryotic and eucaryotic cells.

▶ The procaryotic microorganisms are the bacteria, which are classified based on many criteria including morphology, physiology, and genetic characteristics.

▶ Bacteria are unicellular and have a simple structure. They reproduce mainly by asexual binary fission.

▶ The three basic morphologies of bacteria are cocci, bacilli, and spirilla, which may be arranged in various ways.

▶ Most eubacteria have cell walls, the two types of which can be differentiated by Gram staining into gram-positive and gram-negative cells.

▶ Eucaryotic microbes include fungi, protozoans, and metazoans.

▶ Fungi are diverse organisms and include yeast, molds, and others. They are classified into phyla according to the type of sexual spore they produce. Most pathogenic species are members of Zygomycota, Ascomycota, and Deuteromycota.

▶ Unicellular fungi are the yeasts. Multicellular fungi include molds, mushrooms, rusts, and smuts.

▶ Molds are made of long strands of cells called hyphae. A mycelium is a visible, tangled mass of hyphae.

▶ Protozoans are classified into phyla based on their mode of motility. This text recognizes four phyla—Sarcomastigophora, Apicomplexa, Ciliophora, and Microspora.

▶ Protozoans are eucaryotic and unicellular, free-living or parasitic.

▶ Metazoans are multicellular and include the flat worms, roundworms, and arthropods.

▶ Helminths are eucaryotic and multicellular, classified into phyla based on body shape. Aschelminthes are roundworms; parasitic roundworms are in the class Nematoda.

▶ Viruses do not fit into any of the classification systems used for procaryotic and eucaryotic organisms. They are simple, filterable agents that are nonculturable and can only be viewed with an electron microscope. All viruses are parasitic.

## Review Questions

1. Gram-positive cells are purple after decolorization because:
   a. the alcohol reacts with the safranin to stain the cells that color.
   b. they retain the safranin through decolorization.
   c. the iodine prevents the cells from losing the crystal violet through decolorization.
   d. they retain the crystal violet through decolorization.

2. The term "coenocytic" refers to:
   a. fungal hyphae that lack septa between nuclei.
   b. fungal hyphae that have septa between nuclei.
   c. mycelia that are fuzzy and white in appearance.
   d. mycelia that form when yeast cells are grown at 37°C in potato dextrose agar.

3. In the classification of life kingdoms represent _____ taxonomic group.
   a. the smallest and least specific
   b. the largest and least specific
   c. the smallest and most specific
   d. the largest and most specific

4. A pellicle is:
   a. common to viruses that contain RNA.
   b. a symptom that is common to most AIDS patients.

c.   a fungal structure that helps them produce carbohydrates from sunlight.

d.   a flexible covering found on some protozoans.

**5.** A microbiologist examines a preparation of cells. Even when magnified 1000X the cells are tiny, with no apparent nucleus or organelles. The majority of these cells are arranged in chains. What kind of cells are they?

a.   Human liver cells
b.   Diplobacilli
c.   Plant tracheid cells
d.   Streptococci

**6.** The dramatic decline in leprosy cases that occurred between 1985 and 1994 can be primarily attributed to:

a.   the loss of pathogenicity that has been observed in most species of *Mycobacterium* worldwide.

b.   the development of drugs against which *Mycobacterium* is unable to develop resistance.

c.   the implementation multidrug therapy introduced by WHO.

d.   the evolution of human resistance to leprosy.

**7.** Chitin is:

a.   a protein that is found only in certain species of procaryotic organisms.

b.   a lipid that causes *mycobacterium* to stain acid fast.

c.   a carbohydrate that is a component of mold cell walls.

d.   an antibiotic that inhibits the growth of some species of bacteria.

**8.** Plasmids are:

a.   organelles found in plant cells such as chloroplasts and tonoplasts.

b.   what eucaryotic chromosomes are called prior to their condensation in preparation for mitosis.

c.   viruses that infect plants.

d.   small, circular DNA molecules found in some bacteria.

**9.** Which of the following is found in most procaryotic cells but is never found in eucaryotic cells?

a.   A cell wall
b.   DNA
c.   RNA
d.   Peptidoglycan

**10.** Endospores are produced by:

a.   eucaryotic cells when they are faced with a lack of moisture.

b.   eight genera of gram-negative bacilli.

c.   six genera of gram-positive bacteria.

d.   plant cells and are the reproductive structure common to terrestrial dwellers.

**11.** "Bacterial species" is a difficult concept to define. Which of the following contributes to the problem?

a.   It is not possible (or relevant) to evaluate reproductive compatibility between bacteria because they usually reproduce asexually by binary fission.

b.   It is impossible to identify all of the strains making up one species and thereby fully describe that species.

c.   Bacterial species mutate quickly making classification impossible.

d.   No system for defining a bacterial species has been accepted by the microbiology community.

**12.** A protozoan is detected in a blood specimen. The organisms are elongated, leaf-shaped, and possess a flagellum. The organism is a member of which phylum and subphylum?

a.   Apicomplexa, sporozoa
b.   Sarcomastigophora, mastigophora
c.   Mastigophora, sarcomastigophora
d.   Microspora, apicomplexa

**13.** Multicellular organisms with flattened bodies divided into segments are likely to have which of the other following characteristics?

a.   A complete digestive system
b.   No digestive system
c.   Separate sexes
d.   A leaf-shaped form

**14.** Which of the following is a characteristic of fungi but not plants?

a.   Chitin cell walls
b.   No chlorophyll
c.   Filamentous growth
d.   All of the above

**15.** The identity of isolates of a clinical sample is determined by:

a.   comparison of the isolate to all of the known strains of a similar species.

b.   a consensus of all the technicians in the laboratory.

c.   comparing the characteristics of the isolate to those of known organisms until a match is achieved.

d.   All of the above are true.

**16.** Members of the same class are also members of the same _____.

a.   Species
b.   Genus
c.   Family
d.   Phylum

**17.** Which of the following are criteria used to classify fungi into phyla?
a.   Mode of motility
b.   Body shape
c.   Type of sexual spore produced
d.   Type of reproduction

**18.** Specialized organ systems will be present in:
a.   fungi (molds but not yeasts).
b.   protozoans that have more than one stage in their life cycle.
c.   helminths.
d.   the eubacteria.

**19.** Tapeworms possess:
a.   leaf-shaped bodies.
b.   segmented bodies.
c.   complex digestive systems.
d.   a resistant trophozoite form.

**20.** Which of the following is NOT one of the five kingdoms proposed by Whittaker?
a.   Animalia
b.   Viridae
c.   Plantae
d.   Monera

▶ **REFERENCES & RECOMMENDED READING**

Alcamo, E. L. (1994). *Fundamentals of microbiology* (4th ed.). Redwood City, CA: Benjamin/Cummings.

Brock, T. D. (Ed.). (1961). *Milestones in microbiology.* Englewood Cliffs, NJ: Prentice-Hall.

Garcia, L. S., & Bruckner, D. A. (1993). *Diagnostic medical parasitology* (2nd ed.). Washington, DC: American Society for Microbiology.

Howard, B. J., Keiser, J. F., Smith, T. F., Weissfeld, A. S., & Tilton, R. C. (1994). *Clinical and pathogenic microbiology* (2nd ed.). St. Louis: Mosby.

Krieg, N. R. (Ed.). (1986). *Bergey's manual of systematic bacteriology: Vol. 1.* (1986). Baltimore: Williams & Wilkins.

Mader, S. S. (1994). *Laboratory manual: Biology* (4th ed.). Dubuque: Wm. C. Brown.

Madigan, M. T., Martinko, J. M., & Parker, J. (1997). *Brock: Biology of microorganisms* (8th ed.). Englewood Cliffs, NJ: Prentice-Hall.

Markell, E. K., Voge, M., & John, D. T. (1992). *Medical parasitology* (7th ed.). Philadelphia: Saunders.

Sneath, P. H. A. (Ed.). (1986). *Bergey's manual of systematic bacteriology: Vol. 2.* Baltimore: Williams & Wilkins.

Tortora, G. J., Berdell R. F., & Case, C. L. (1995). *Microbiology: An introduction.* Redwood City, CA: Benjamin/Cummings.

# CHAPTER 2
# The Infectious Disease Process

Judith A. Kjelstrom, MT (ASCP), PhD

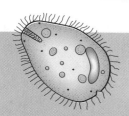

## Microbes in the News

In *ASM News* (May 1997), Alessio Fasano presented a fascinating, complex relationship between a bacterium, bacteriophage, and mammalian host. Pathogenic *Vibrio cholerae* and other *Vibrio* species produce diarrhea in mammals via the secretion of powerful exotoxins: cholera toxin (ctx), zona occludens toxin (zot), ace (accessory cholera toxin), and others.

According to Walder and Mekalanos at Harvard University Medical School, this set of virulence genes (ctx operon) came as a "gift package" from a filamentous bacteriophage designated CTX theta. An interesting finding is that a bacterial gene, toxR coregulates the transcription and translation of the ctx gene on the viral DNA, as well as the pili gene on its DNA. The pili are used to adhere to mammalian intestinal epithelium as well as acting as receptors for the virus. In addition, the protein product of the zot gene, not only assembles new virions, but also affects the permeability of tight junctions between mammalian intestinal epithelial cells!

This symbiotic relationship between the bacterium and its virus may enhance the survival of the bacterium, when ingested by a mammal. We usually think of diarrhea as a defense mechanism of the host, but there may be an alternative explanation. Ordinarily, *V. cholerae* lives in aquatic environments. When it is ingested by humans, it enters a new and hostile world. If this actively motile bacterium can induce diarrhea, it can speed its escape from the host and return to its preferred niche.

**INTRODUCTION**

**HOST RESISTANCE FACTORS**
Innate Resistance
Adaptive Resistance

**MICROBIAL MECHANISMS OF PATHOGENICITY**
Routes of Entry
Adherence and Invasion
Toxins
Avoidance of Host Defense
  Mechanisms
Dissemination

**PATHOLOGIC MECHANISMS IN THE HOST**
Minimal Cellular Damage
Direct Damage by the Microbe
Hypersensitivity Reactions by
  the Host
Host Susceptibility Factors

## KEY TERMS

Acquired immunity
Adhesin
Antibody
Antigen
Antigen-presenting cell
Antigenic variation
Antimicrobic
Asymptomatic carrier

Bacteriocin
Capsule
Colonization
Commensalism
Complement system
Cytokines
Disease
Endotoxin

Exotoxin
Host
Immunoglobulin
Infection
Inflammation
Innate resistance
Interferons
Interleukin

## KEY TERMS (cont.)

| | | |
|---|---|---|
| **Microbial pathogenicity** | **Parasitism** | **Superantigen** |
| **Molecular mimicry** | **Pathogen** | **Symbiosis** |
| **Mucociliary apparatus** | **Phagocytosis** | **Virulence** |
| **Mutualism** | **Phase variation** | **Zoonosis** |

## LEARNING OBJECTIVES

**Upon successful completion of this chapter, the student should be able to:**

1. Distinguish between colonization, infection, and disease.

2. Distinguish between innate and adaptive resistance mechanisms in the host.

3. Describe how endotoxin differs from exotoxins in both structure and effect on host.

4. List various survival tactics used by pathogens to avoid host defenses.

## INTRODUCTION

Infectious diseases (those caused by microbes) continue to be a leading cause of morbidity and mortality worldwide, accounting for 33% of the 52 million deaths per year. This chapter explores the complex relationships that exist between living organisms. It is a battle of wills, each struggling to survive. Microorganisms have a survival advantage because they can adapt to new environments quickly due to rapid expression of mutants. This is primarily due to their small genome size, rapid cell division, and acquisition of exogenous DNA (plasmid, phage, or free DNA).

This chapter examines various host–microbe relationships and levels of pathologic effects. Host defense mechanisms are explored as well as common themes of microbial entry, adherence, invasion, and possible dissemination.

In discussing the infectious disease process, one must define some terms. **Microbial pathogenicity** is defined as "the biochemical mechanism, whereby microorganisms cause disease" (Finlay & Falkow, 1989). The term **infection** is used to describe the successful persistence or multiplication of a **pathogen** (disease-causing microbe) on or within the **host** (in human medicine, the host is the human organism). **Disease** is an infection that causes overt damage (clinical symptoms) in the host. Infection and subsequent disease are dependent on the status of the host as well as the **virulence** (degree of pathogenicity) of the microbe (virus, bacteria, fungus, protozoan, or multicellular parasitic helminth). An infected host, showing no clinical symptoms, may be an unknowing source of a disease in a population. These persons are referred to as **asymptomatic carriers**.

By contrast, **colonization** is the persistence of microorganisms in a body site without causing disease, as seen with resident microflora or normal flora. This type of **symbiotic** (host–microbe) relationship is **mutualistic** (both organisms benefit) or **commensal** (no harm is done to the host), rather than **parasitic** (the microbe benefits at the expense of the host). It should be stressed that only a small proportion of the microorganisms associated with humans give rise to pathologic changes (Mims, 1987; Salyers & Whitt, 1994). Vast numbers of bacteria inhabit the mouth and intestines, or live on the skin, yet few cause any detectable illness (Figure 2-1). From an evolutionary viewpoint, this should be expected. A successful microbe must persist and leave descendants to avoid extinction (Mims, 1987).

The concept of balanced pathogenicity is important in understanding the process of infectious disease. Well established infectious agents cause the least amount of damage to the host, which is necessary to enter, multiply, and exit from the body. Many pathogens have not yet had time to reach this ideal state. As each microbe evolves, occasional virulent mutants emerge and cause extensive cellular damage and possible death in susceptible hosts. In addition, some microbes that originally appeared in one region of the world and selected for a more resistant host population, may "accidentally" be spread to a new geographical area and more susceptible hosts. Examples of such diseases are malaria, tuberculosis, measles, and influenza (Finlay & Falkow, 1994).

Finally, some microorganisms never evolve to a less virulent state because the human is not relevant to its survival. **Zoonoses** (animal-to-human transmission) such as rabies, plague, scrub typhus, and leptospirosis

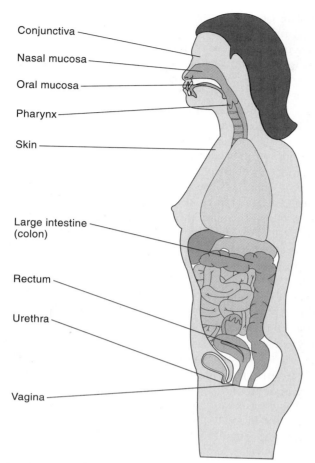

**FIGURE 2-1** Locations of resident microflora of the body.

are examples of such diseases. Occasionally a microbe may adapt to a new species of hosts, but with lower virulence (Finlay & Falkow, 1994).

## HOST RESISTANCE FACTORS

Resistance factors include both nonspecific or innate defenses and specific or adaptive immunity.

### Innate Resistance

**Innate resistance** includes physical and chemical barriers, phagocytic leukocytes, fever, acute inflammation, complement cascade, and natural killer (NK) cells. These defenses are genetically determined and do not improve with repeated exposure to the infectious agent, but may be more important to survival than acquired immunity.

**Physical Barriers.** Human skin seems fragile compared to the shell of a turtle or the hide of a rhinoceros, but it is an extremely effective barrier against most microorganisms. Normal intact skin has a number

of characteristics that make colonization difficult. One of the best defenses is epidermal sloughing of dead keratinized epithelial cells. Desquamation constantly removes microbes that may have begun to colonize. Keratin (a water-proofing protein produced by underlying keratinocytes) is a poor carbon source for most bacteria and fungi. An important exception are the fungi (Dermatophytes) that cause ringworm.

Another physical barrier is blockage of adhesion receptors by normal resident flora of the skin and mucous membranes of body openings (mouth, vagina, urethra, nose, anus). Pathogens must be able to attach to the host to cause disease.

Mucous membranes are comprised of layers of nonkeratinized living cells. These warm and wet membranes could be easy targets for invasion, if not for various defense mechanisms. One of the best is the **mucociliary apparatus**. Goblet cells, which produce mucus (a thick, sticky substance made of the protein mucin and polysaccharides), and ciliated epithelial cells provide a good defense for the respiratory tract. The mucus traps the microbes and the beating action of the cilia sweeps the mucus to the outside. In addition, the respiratory tract from the nose to lungs is curved and branched, which also helps to protect the sterile lungs from the external environment (Salyer & Whitt, 1994) (see Figure 2-2).

Other physical barriers are tearing by lacrimal glands, blinking of the eyes to wash away microbes, and peristalsis (rhythmic smooth muscle contractions) in the gastrointestinal tract and urinary tract. This flushing action expels microbes before most can adhere to mucosal receptors. In addition, mucosal epithelium has

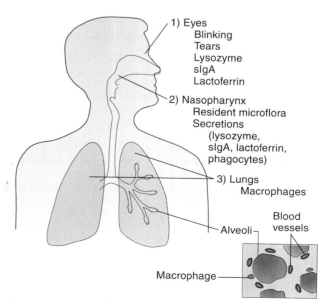

**FIGURE 2-2** Special defenses of respiratory tract and eyes.

tight junctions between cells, which prevent leakage of bacteria from the lumen into the inner part of the body.

**Chemical Barriers.** Skin has chemical barriers to microbial invasion as well. The water content is low (with the exceptions of skin folds, armpits, and groin), the temperature is below 37°C, and the pH is slightly acidic (approximately 3 to 5) due to the presence of lactic acid in sweat and fatty acids in sebum (product of oil glands). Both lactic acid and sebum have antimicrobial properties.

Saliva and tears contain various antimicrobial chemicals such as lysozyme (enzyme that cleaves the peptidoglycan backbone of the cell wall of some bacteria), lactoferrin (iron-binding protein, which prevents microbe access to free iron), lactoperoxidase (enzyme that produces superoxide radicals, a toxic substance to many bacteria), and secretory immunoglobulin A (sIgA). Gastric hydrochloric acid in the stomach is very toxic to most microorganisms and intestinal secretions contain bile salts (toxic to most gram-positive bacteria), lysozyme, and other chemicals. Urine is usually acidic (in nonvegetarians) and has a very wide range of osmolalities; both are inhibitory to microbial multiplication. Blood contains transferrin (iron-binding protein) as well as many other nonspecific and specific factors that are discussed later. Table 2-1 lists the major defenses of skin and mucous membranes.

Many normal flora bacteria produce **bacteriocins**, antimicrobial chemicals that usually kill closely related microbes. Polymorphonuclear neutrophils (PMNs, phagocytic granulocytic leukocytes) produce **antimi-crobic** cationic peptides called defensins, in addition to respiratory burst chemicals (to be discussed below). Paneth cells in the crypts of the small intestines produce lysozyme and toxic peptides called cryptdins. Macrophages (aggressively phagocytic white blood cells derived from monocytes) produce chemicals called **cytokines** after ingestion of bacteria. One cytokine, **interleukin** 6 (IL-6), induces the liver to produce mannose-binding proteins, which bind to the surface of the bacteria and cause activation of the complement system as discussed later (Salyer & Whitt, 1994). Figure 2-3 lists the major innate defenses of the gastrointestinal tract.

A class of similar antiviral proteins called **interferons** (IFN) are produced by certain animal cells after viral stimulation. They are host cell specific but not viral specific. Interferons are produced by the infected cell, then diffuse to neighboring cells. These proteins induce the uninfected cells to manufacture mRNA for the synthesis of antiviral proteins (AVPs), which disrupt viral multiplication.

**Phagocytes.** The host has white blood cells or leukocytes, which are adapted specifically to engulf and destroy bacteria, fungi, and other foreign substances (**phagocytosis**). These professional killers include PMNs and macrophages (transformed monocytes that leave the blood to move to the tissues). The phagocyte traps and engulfs its prey by forming a membrane-encased sac called a phagosome. Once inside the cytoplasm, the phagosome fuses with a lysosome (organelle with lysozyme, defensins, lactoferrin, hydrolases, acids,

## Table 2-1 ▶ Defenses of Skin and Mucosa

| Site | Defense | Function |
|---|---|---|
| Skin | Dry, acidic, keratin | Limit microbial growth |
| | Sloughing of cells | Remove microbes |
| | Resident microflora | Competition for adhesion receptors produce bacteriocins |
| Sebaceous and sweat glands | Lysozyme, toxic lipids, acidic | Kill many bacteria |
| Langerhan's cells of SALT | Phagocytosis | Kill microbes, present antigens to T cells |
| Mucous membrane | Sloughing cell | Removes microbes |
| | Tight junctions | Stop leakage of lumen contents between cells |
| | Resident microflora | Competition for adhesion receptors produce bacteriocins |
| Mucus, tears and saliva | Lysozyme | Cytolysis of bacteria |
| | sIgA | Prevent attachment |
| | | Enhance phagocytosis |
| | | Help trap microbes |
| | Lactoferrin | Bind iron, prevent microbial growth |
| | Lactoperoxidase | Superoxide radicals kill many microbes |
| MALT in submucosa | Phagocytosis | Kill microbes, present antigens to T cells |

MALT, mucosa-associated lymphoid tissue; SALT

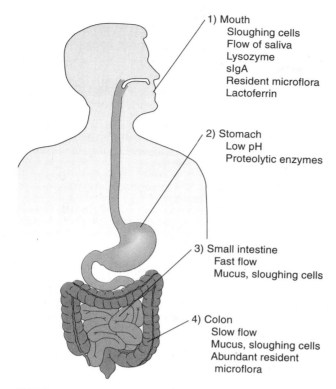

1) Mouth
   Sloughing cells
   Flow of saliva
   Lysozyme
   sIgA
   Resident microflora
   Lactoferrin

2) Stomach
   Low pH
   Proteolytic enzymes

3) Small intestine
   Fast flow
   Mucus, sloughing cells

4) Colon
   Slow flow
   Mucus, sloughing cells
   Abundant resident
   microflora

**FIGURE 2-3** Defenses of the gastrointestinal tract.

and enzymes that form reactive nitrogen). This is called phagolysosome fusion, which contributes to the killing of the prey. Another killing mechanism, which involves the uptake of oxygen, is the oxidative or respiratory burst. This results in the production of reactive oxygen intermediates: superoxides, hydroxyls, peroxides, and hypochlorous acid. An equally important killing system is the reactive nitrogen intermediates such as nitrous oxide, nitrates, and nitrites (see Figure 2-4).

**Fever Response.** Fever is defined clinically as any temperature above 37.8°C when taken orally and 38.4°C when measured rectally. Fever accelerates the mobilization and deployment of host inflammatory cells and inhibits the growth of some microbes. It commonly occurs in conjunction with microbial infection. **Endotoxin** (lipid A of lipopolysaccharide) in the cell walls of gram-negative bacteria, some proteinaceous **exotoxins**, and other pyrogens (fever inducers) induce macrophages to release cytokines: interleukin 1 (IL-1) and tumor necrosis factor-α (TNFα). IL-1 induces the hypothalamus to secret prostaglandins, which reset the body temperature to a higher level. The fever response is also induced by release of leukocyte-endogenous mediator (LEM) from cells. LEM also decreases the availability of free iron in the blood. Without iron, growth of microorganisms is slowed. One of the effects of TNFα is to lower blood pressure with subsequent symptoms of shock (Black, 1996; Youmans, Paterson, & Sommers, 1985).

**Inflammatory Response.** When the body is injured, a series of cellular and chemical events occur. There is a prompt and vigorous change in the microcirculation to increase blood to the injured area. The affected area shows four cardinal signs of acute inflammation: redness, heat, swelling, and pain. There may also be a loss of function. Vasodilation of the capillaries (due to histamines, leukotrienes, and the like released by mast cells and platelets) causes the first two signs. Subsequent increase in tissue fluid due to leaky capillaries leads to edema (swelling). Pain is due to pressure buildup and stimulation of pain receptors as well as release of bradykinins (pain mediators). Acute **inflammation** functions to rapidly kill the invading microbe, clear away tissue debris, and repair damaged tissue. Sometimes an acute inflammatory response becomes chronic (long-term), if the microbe cannot be cleared. The host attempts to confine the region of inflammation, by laying down fibroblasts, macrophages, lymphocytes, and collagen fibers. It may develop into a granuloma (a local accumulation of densely packed macrophages, T lymphocytes, and giant cells). Over time, calcium is deposited within granulomas (opaque on x-rays).

If inflammation becomes more severe or widespread, it is generally modulated by increased production of corticosteroid hormones as well as a general metabolic response by the body. IL-6 released by macrophages cause the liver to release various acute phase proteins: C-reactive protein (a ß-globulin detected by precipitating with the C carbohydrate of *Streptococcus pneumoniae*), mannose-binding protein, fibrinogen, haptoglobin, and protease inhibitors. Their presence in the blood is associated with an increased erythrocyte sedimentation rate (ESR). C-reactive protein and mannose-binding protein act as opsonins; they coat the microbe, thus enabling phagocytosis (Black, 1996; Mims, 1987).

**Complement Cascade.** The **complement system** is a set of 30 or more regulatory proteins that play a key

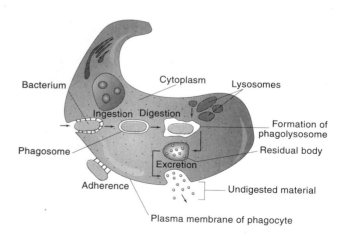

**FIGURE 2-4** The phagocytic process.

role in innate resistance. They are produced in the liver and then circulate in the plasma (in an inactive form). The system works as a cascade: a set of reactions that amplify some effect. There are two pathways in this system:

1. Classical pathway: triggered by antibody binding to the microbe
2. Alternative pathway: induced by chemicals in cell wall of microbe

The general functions of the complement cascade are:

▶ Cytolysis—membrane attack complex pokes holes in cell walls of bacteria (see Figure 2-5)
▶ Opsonization—binding of the complement component, C3b, enhances phagocytosis by PMNs and macrophages
▶ Generation of peptide fragments (C3a and C5a) enhances the inflammatory response

**Natural Killer (NK) Cells.**  The NK cells are a subpopulation of lymphocytes, which are neither T or B cells. They attack tumor cells and virally infected cells. Their activity is increased by exposure to interferon-γ and IL-2. NK cells secrete cytotoxic proteins, which trigger the death of the cell. They are part of innate resistance because, unlike T and B lymphocytes, their response does not improve after exposure to the foreign agent.

## Adaptive Resistance

Adaptive resistance is also called the specific immune response or **acquired immunity**. This powerful, complex system of immune effector cells, cytokines, im-

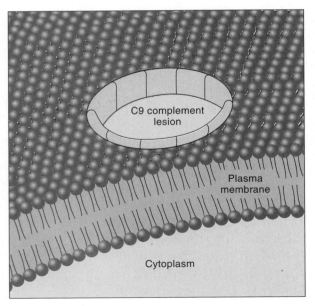

**FIGURE 2-5** Membrane attack complex of complement cascade.

munoglobulins (**antibodies**), and lymphoid tissues and organs provides the final line of defense against microbial invaders. To be successful, it must accomplish three tasks:

1. Immune recognition—respond to and identify the invading microbe (usually surface proteins or peptides called **antigens**)
2. Immune activation—bring in all the appropriate forces via chemical (cytokine) communication between cells
3. Immune response—to counterattack, destroy or contain the invader

Acquired immunity is developed during a person's lifetime (beginning at about 3 months of age). One of the key features of this system is immunologic memory. Its response is enhanced with repeated exposure to the foreign antigens. Another unique quality is its specificity. There are two main arms of this immune system: humoral (antibody mediated) and cellular (involves specialized white blood cells called T lymphocytes and macrophages).

**Humoral Immunity.**  Humoral immunity involves B lymphocytes (B cells), plasma cells, and secreted antibodies (immunoglobulins). B cells develop from lymphoid stem cells in bursal-equivalent tissue such as bone marrow and fetal liver. B cells develop in the bursa of Fabricius in birds (hence the name "B" cells), but there is no such organ in mammals. Mature B cells migrate to the lymphoid tissue (lymph nodes, gut-associated lymph tissue [GALT], spleen, tonsils, adenoids, etc.). When immunocompetent B lymphocytes (equipped with a unique antigenic receptor) encounter its specific antigen, they undergo rapid cell division (clones of identical cells) and transformation. This mechanism is called clonal selection. Some cells become nonmitotic effector cells (plasma cells), which produce and secrete specific antibodies into the blood, breast milk, mucus, and cerebrospinal fluid to fight the infection. A few B cells become memory cells, which are held in reserve in lymphoid tissue. These cells can quickly respond to future invasions by this species of microbe and are the basis of immunologic memory.

It is interesting that we are born with millions of B lymphocytes, each capable of producing antibodies of a unique specificity. **Antibodies** or **immunoglobulins** (Ig) are composed of Y-shaped glycoproteins with antigen-binding sites. The five classes of immunoglobulins are IgG, IgM, IgA, IgE, and IgD. Each class has a specific function, but most are involved in forming complexes with the antigen with subsequent inactivation and elimination of the foreign substance.

**Cellular Immunity.**  Cellular immunity or cell-mediated immunity (CMI) involves sensitized T lymphocytes (T cells bearing receptors for the antigen), cytokines, and activated macrophages. T cells also develop from lymphoid stem cells in the bone marrow. Before migrating to the lymphoid tissue, they infiltrate the thymus gland for education. Deletion of T cell clones with receptors for self-antigens normally occurs in the thymus.

Ninety percent of T cells have the type 2 receptor and can be divided into subpopulations of CD4+ and CD8+ T cells (CD refers to cluster of differentiation, cell markers bound by specific monoclonal antibodies). The main CD4+ T cells are the helper T ($T_H$) lymphocytes, which help or induce the immune response. They recognize antigenic peptides that are presented with major histocompatibility complex (MHC) class II molecules. The major CD8+ subset is the cytotoxic T ($T_C$) cells. These lymphocytes mainly kill tumor cells and cells displaying viral antigens or other foreign MHC antigens (host versus graft reaction).

The **antigen-presenting cells** (APCs) are found primarily in the skin (Langerhan cells), liver (Kupffer cells) lymph nodes, spleen, and thymus (interdigitating cells and follicular dendritic cells). APCs present processed antigenic peptides, in association with the class II MHC antigen, on its cell membrane to $T_H$ cells. These activated T cells secrete cytokines, express new surface receptors, and undergo clonal expansion. The various cytokines induce activation and proliferation of other lymphocytes with the same antigen specificity as well as activating macrophages and NK cells.

There are two functional subsets of T helper cells. $T_H1$ cells secrete IL-2 and γ-interferon. These cytokines induce cytoxicity and local inflammation (CMI). The $T_H2$ subset produces IL-4, IL-5, IL-6 and, IL-10, which activate B cells to clonally expand (humoral immunity) as well as increase productions of mast cell and eosinophils (Roitt, Brostoff, & Male, 1993).

Table 2-2 summarizes the major defense mechanisms of blood and tissue.

## MICROBIAL MECHANISMS OF PATHOGENICITY

For an organism to cause disease, it must accomplish three tasks: entry, adherence, and invasion or secretion of toxic substances.

### Routes of Entry

For a microbe to colonize and infect the host, it must first enter and adhere to host cells. The conjunctiva, breaks in the skin, and the alimentary, respiratory, and urogenital tracts offer pathways for infection by microbes. Some organisms cause disease via toxins; they do not have to invade the body to exert their pathogenic effect.

## Table 2–2 ▶ Defenses of Blood and Tissue

| Site | Defense | Function |
|------|---------|----------|
| Blood | Transferrin | Limits iron access to microbes |
| Blood, or injured tissue | Phagocytosis by PMNs | Ingest and kill microbes<br>Defensin production |
| Blood | Phagocytosis by monocytes | Ingest and kill microbes<br>Cytokine production |
| Injured tissue lymph system | Phagocytosis by macrophages | Ingest and kill microbes<br>Cytokine production |
| | Antigen presentation by APCs | Present antigens to T lymphocytes |
| Blood, or injured tissue | Complement cascade | Cytolysis of bacteria<br>Opsonization<br>Enhance inflammation |
| Liver | Acute phase proteins MBP, CRP, etc. | Binds to bacterial cell<br>Activate complement and acts as opsonin |
| Blood, lymph system, or injured tissue | T lymphocytes<br>Helper T cells<br>Cytotoxic T cells<br>DTH lymphocytes | Specific immunity: activate system<br>Kill virally infected cells and cancer cells<br>Chronic inflammation<br>Granulomas |
| | γ-interferon | Innate resistance: antiviral activity |
| | NK lymphocytes | Innate resistance: kill virally infected cells and cancer cells |
| | B lymphocytes | Specific immunity: opsonization, neutralization of toxin and viruses |
| | Plasma cells and antibodies | Complement activation |

APC, antigen-presenting cell; CRP, C-reactive protein; DTH, delayed-type hypersensitivity; MBP, mannose-binding protein; NK, natural killer; PMN, polymorphonuclear neutrophils.

## Adherence and Invasion

There are three groups of infections, based on mechanisms of adherence and invasion:

1. Those in which the microbe has a specific mechanism for adhering to and often penetrating normal healthy cells. The most common mechanism is via rod-shaped surface proteins called fimbria or pili. There are also afimbrial **adhesins** that mediate tight binding between bacteria and host cell.

2. Organisms that are carried in an arthropod and enter healthy cells via bite wounds

3. Opportunistic microorganisms that can only invade damaged cells or a host with impaired defenses

## Toxins

Some microbes do not actually invade tissues themselves. They produce toxic substances that induce disease symptoms. There are two general types of toxins: exotoxins and endotoxins.

**Exotoxins.** Exotoxins are toxic proteins secreted by the microbe or released during cell lysis. They can be classified into three groups: (1) A-B toxins, which get their name from the fact that two types of proteins make up the structure of the toxin. Receptor-binding B subunit(s) bind the toxic A portion. Binding of the B subunit(s) to a carbohydrate or protein moiety of a membrane receptor allows entry of the A subunit via endocytosis. Most of the well characterized bacterial toxins (cholera toxin, diphtheria toxin, pertussis toxin, Shiga toxin, botulism and tetanus toxins) fall into this category. The effects of the A subunit vary from disrupting cyclic AMP (cAMP) control, inhibiting protein synthesis, or interfering with neuron impulses. (2) Membrane-disrupting toxins (RTX family) are also called cytotoxins or hemolysins because they cause cell lysis. There are two types: pore (channel)-forming such as listeriolysin (*Listeria monocytogenes* toxin) and phospholipases as with alpha toxin in gas gangrene (*Clostridium perfringens* toxin). (3) **Superantigens** are unusual toxins that exert their effect by bridging an MHC class II molecule to a T-cell receptor, by non-specifically binding to external surfaces of the two molecules. No peptide antigen is involved in this interaction. Superantigens do not have to be processed by the APC to exert their effect on $T_H$ cells. As a consequence, 1 in 5 $T_H$ cells can be stimulated as compared to the normal 1 in 10,000. Massive amounts of IL-2 are released as a result of T-cell activation. Superantigens can be produced by viruses and bacteria, including *Mycoplasma* species. Among the best characterized superantigens are those of *Staphylococcus aureus* and *Streptococcus pyogenes* (group A ß-hemolytic streptococcus) (Kotb, 1995; Salyers & Whitt, 1994).

**ENTEROTOXINS.** Exotoxins that act on the intestinal tract are called enterotoxins. Enterotoxins that cause fluid loss without mucus and cells (diarrhea) are produced by *Vibrio cholerae*, enterotoxigenic *Escherichia coli*, *Campylobacter jejuni*, *C. perfringens*, and others. These bacteria secrete a heat-labile cholera toxin (CT) that disrupts cAMP activity. The pertussis toxin (PTX) of *Bordetella pertussis* (whooping cough agent) resembles the cholera toxin of *V. cholerae*, but it causes increased respiratory secretions rather than diarrhea.

Shiga toxin and Shiga-like toxins, enterotoxins produced by *Shigella dysenteriae*, strains of *E. coli* and *C. jejuni*, and others cause a more severe form of diarrhea called dysentery. It includes leukocytes, erythrocytes, epithelial cells, and mucus, along with increased fluid loss. These toxins inhibit ribosome function, thus prevent protein synthesis and result in cell death. The enterotoxins of *Clostridium difficile* (an anaerobic spore-forming gram-positive bacillus) are associated with diarrhea following the administration of broad-spectrum antibiotics. Without proper treatment, the toxins (toxin A and toxin B) cause cell death of epithelial cells and the infiltration of neutrophils, mucin, and fibrin, called pseudomembranous colitis.

Enterotoxins of *S. aureus* primarily induce nausea, abdominal cramping and vomiting, with some diarrhea. Within hours after ingestion of toxin-laden food, symptoms occur. The toxin does not target intestinal epithelial cells, but rather helper T lymphocytes. It acts as a superantigen, stimulating 1 in 5 T cells (normal antigens activate approximately 1 in 10,000). As a result, massive amounts of IL-2 are produced by these activated lymphocytes as well as increasing T cell multiplication. High levels of IL-2 do not act locally; IL-2 travels in the blood to activate centers in the brain stem and hypothalamus to give rise to fever, shock, nausea and gastric upset (Johnson, 1992).

**EXOTOXIN-INDUCED CELL DEATH.** Exotoxins may cause cell death in other body locations. They may disrupt the cell membrane, inhibit protein synthesis, or induce apoptosis (programmed cell death). Gas gangrene (tissue necrosis) due to *C. perfringens* is primarily due to alpha toxin, which damages cell membranes of the host. Inhibition of protein synthesis with subsequent cell death is seen with diphtheria toxin of *Corynebacterium diphtheriae* and exotoxin A of *Pseudomonas aeruginosa*. Severe invasive group A streptococci ("flesh-eating streptococci") secrete proteases that destroy muscle cells along with toxic shock-like toxins in necrotizing fasciitis.

**NEUROTOXINS.** Exotoxins that interfere with nerve transmission are called neurotoxins. Two examples of neurotoxin effects are seen in botulism and tetanus. *Clostridium botulinum* produces botulinum toxins (serotypes: A, B, $C_{1-3}$, D, E, F, and G), which are some of the most toxic substances known to humankind. Types A and B are the most common serotypes seen in the United States. These neurotoxins (usually acquired by ingestion of contaminated food) act primarily on peripheral nerves, preventing release of the neurotransmitter, acetylcholine, at neuromuscular junctions and causing flaccid paralysis of muscles (botulism). These toxins are zinc-requiring endopeptidases, which cleave a set of proteins (called synaptobrevins) found in synaptic vesicles. This results in blockage of exocytosis of acetylcholine into the synapse. Clinical signs of botulism include vertigo, cranial nerve palsies (difficulties with swallowing, speaking, keeping eyelids open), with subsequent respiratory failure and death in a few days.

*Clostridium tetani* produces tetanus toxin, which is also a zinc-requiring endopeptidase. This toxin is acquired through deep wound contamination by this soil-dwelling spore-forming bacteria. Germination of the spores releases this potent toxin, which passes up the axon of peripheral nerves (retrograde axonal transport) to the central nervous system. Tetanus toxin blocks transmission of inhibitory impulses in motor neurons, producing prolonged muscular spasms of both flexor and extensor (antagonists) muscle groups. This toxin prevents the release of inhibitory neurotransmitters such as γ-aminobutyric acid (GABA). Because flexor muscles are usually dominant, a person with advance tetanus will show generalized flexion contractures. The motor nerves in the brain stem are short and thus the cranial nerves are among the first to be affected. Early clinical signs are spasms of the eye muscles and jaw muscles (lockjaw). Generalized muscle spasms of the entire body show the classic symptoms of arched back and clenched fists and jaw. Spasms are so severe that bones often break. Without proper treatment with antitoxin, respiratory and heart failure leads to death (Mims, 1987; Salyers & Whitt, 1994).

**Endotoxin.** Endotoxin (lipid A of lipopolysaccharide) is an integral part of the outer membrane of cell walls of gram-negative bacteria. Because lipid A is embedded in the cell wall, it exerts its effects only after cell lysis. The release of endotoxin activates the complement cascade and the release of cytokines by monocytes, macrophages, and endothelial cells. The major chemicals secreted are IL-1 and TNFα, which lead to fever and shock symptoms. This condition is commonly referred to as septic shock, which often leads to collapse of the circulatory system, multiple organ failure and death. Gram-positive cell walls may also contain substances that induce septic shock.

These types of clinical symptoms are seen in toxic shock syndrome of severe invasive *S. pyogenes* and *S. aureus*. In addition, exfoliation of skin from the palms and soles of feet is seen. The inducing agents are exotoxins called toxic shock syndrome toxin-1 (TSST-1) in *S. aureus* and streptococcal pyogenic exotoxin A

(SpeA). Both toxins are also superantigens. Figure 2-6 demonstrates the activation of T cells by superantigens.

Gram-positive bacteria do not have lipopolysaccharide, but still can cause septic shock. It is believed that peptidoglycan fragments and teichoic acids of the cell wall can elicit the same response in the host (Salyers & Whitt, 1994).

## Avoidance of Host Defense Mechanisms

Evasion is another way that microbes can establish themselves within the host. Many novel survival mechanisms have evolved.

**Antigenic or Phase Variation.** This is a mechanism of changing major surface molecules (at a rate much higher than the rate of mutation) to thwart preexisting immune defenses of the host by creating new serotypes. This chameleon ability is seen among various pathogenic microbes such as the hemoflagellated protozoans *Trypanosoma,* the relapsing fever spirochaetal bacteria *Borrelia,* gram-negative bacilli *Salmonella typhimurium* and uropathogenic *E. coli,* gram-negative diplococci, *Neisseria gonorrhoeae* and *Neisseria meningitidis,* and the retrovirus, human immunodeficiency virus (HIV). These changes may involve "on or off" switching of genes (**phase variation**) for flagellar proteins, pilin types or outer membrane proteins. **Antigenic variation** usually involves changes in gene sequences due to homologous recombination, transformation, or plasmid exchange. Changes in the envelope proteins of HIV usually result from RNA transcriptional errors (Nassif & So, 1985; Roitt et al., 1993, Seifert & So, 1988).

**Molecular Mimicry.** **Molecular mimicry** refers to the situation in which surface proteins of a microbe are similar to host's proteins or the microbe covers itself with host proteins. Consequently, antibodies formed against the microbe may cross-react with host tissue (autoimmunity) or a poor immune response may be generated by the host, respectively. *Schistosoma* species (parasitic helminths) acquire a surface layer of blood group and MHC molecules of the host, thus becoming resistant to attack by antibodies and complement.

*Treponema pallidum,* the cause of syphilis, has very few outer membrane proteins and in addition, coat themselves with host proteins such as albumin, IgG, MHC class I antigens, and transferrin. These conditions slow the quick activation of the adaptive immune system. Some bacterial **capsules** are composed of polysaccharides that do not trigger an antibody response because they resemble host tissue polysaccharides, sialic acid and hyaluronic acid (Mims; Roitt et al., 1993; Salyers & Whitt, 1994).

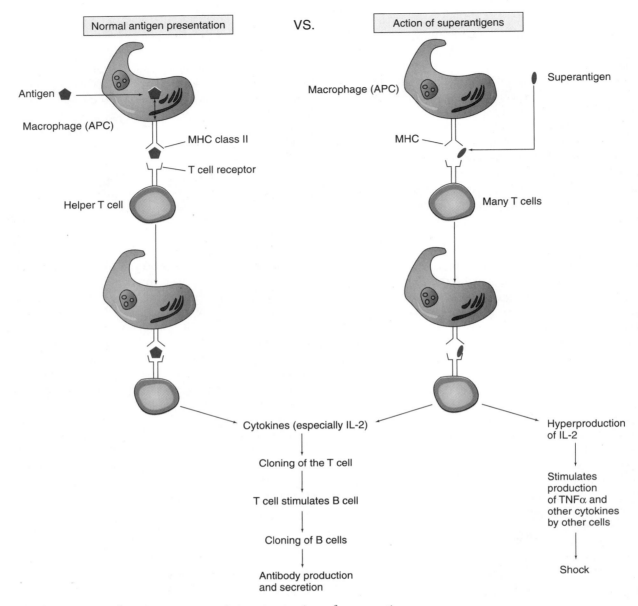

**FIGURE 2-6** Normal antigen presentation versus action of superantigens.

**Secretory IgA Protease.** Production of antibody-destroying enzymes by bacteria is an effective survival mechanism of certain bacteria such as *N. meningitidis*. Bacteria that enter via mucosal surfaces can avoid sIgA-mediated trapping and clearing. The extracellular enzyme cleaves human $sIgA_1$, which is the predominant immunoglobulin isotype found in these sites.

**Capsule Production.** Capsules can protect the bacteria from immune recognition. In addition, this loose covering usually has a net negative charge, which repels phagocytes (Figure 2-7). Anticapsular antibodies or complement proteins must coat the bacterium, before it can be phagocytosed. This process is called opsonization. The yeast-like fungus *Cryptococcus neoformans* is a prime example of a slick organism. It pro-

duces a thick capsule of polysaccharides and glycoprotein as well as secreting these substances into the bloodstream to bind anticapsular antibodies. In addition, this fungus produces melanin and mannitol, which may overwhelm the host's oxidative defense mechanisms (Hogan, Klein, & Levitz, 1996; Murphy, 1996).

**Resistance to Stomach Acid.** Stomach acid is usually an effective barrier to food-borne microbes. Tolerance to low pH is a feature of some food- and water-borne pathogens. This survival mechanism may involve cyst or spore formation as with *Giardia intestinalis (lamblia)* cysts, *C. botulinum* endospores, *Entamoeba histolytica* cysts, and others. *Helicobacter pylori* (the curved bacteria associated with gastric ulcers) produces urease, with resulting ammonia formation.

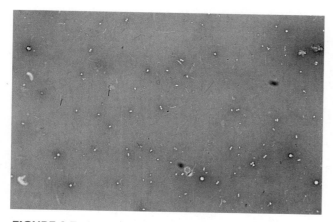

**FIGURE 2-7** Capsules of *Streptococcus pneumoniae*.

This alkaline chemical neutralizes the caustic HCl of the stomach and protects the bacteria in their niche.

The overuse of antacid medications or hyposecretion of HCl may increase host susceptibility to intestinal pathogens such as *V. cholerae, Salmonella* species, and so on.

**Resistance to Mannose-Binding Proteins.** Mannose-binding proteins (such as Tamm-Horsfall glycoprotein) of the urinary tract usually prevent adherence to epithelial cells by bacteria. Pathogenic *E. coli* can resist binding (mannose resistant), and thus are free to bind to mannose-containing cell receptors via their pili or adhesins.

**Iron-Scavenging Mechanisms.** The acquisition of iron is a must for any pathogenic organism. Iron is essential for growth, but iron concentrations in nature are generally quite low. One mechanism is the production of siderophores, small molecules that chelate iron with high affinity. Some bacteria can use transferrin, lactoferrin, and hemin as iron sources. Others produce toxins that kill cells, with subsequent release of their iron stores (ferritin or heme).

**Intracellular Parasitism.** Surviving after being phagocytosed is an excellent mechanism for avoiding the immune system. There are three basic mechanisms:

1. Inhibition of phagosome–lysosome fusion is seen with *Mycobacterium tuberculosis*, virulent *Nocardia asteroides, Toxoplasma gondii*, and others.
2. Escape from the phagolysosome is the method of choice of *Rickettsia rickettsiae, Trypanosoma cruzi*, and *Mycobacterium leprae*.
3. Survival in the acid environment of phagolysosomes is observed with *Listeria monocytogenes, Coxiella burnetii, Yersinia pestis, S. typhimurium*, and others (Mims, 1987).

## Dissemination

Relocation of the microbe after entry and adherence to host cells enables the microorganism to establish itself in the host. It may involve direct spread through tissue (via secretion of hyaluronidases, proteases, hemolysins, etc.) or hitchhiking in lymph and blood or cerebrospinal fluid (as in meningitis).

Table 2-3 summarizes the various virulence factors used by pathogenic microbes.

## PATHOLOGIC MECHANISMS IN THE HOST

The spectrum of clinical disease varies depending on the virulence factors produced by the microbe as well as the immune status of the host and the tissue infected (Mims, 1987).

### Minimal Cellular Damage

These types of infections are most commonly due to certain viruses. Infections with enterovirus, reovirus,

| Table 2–3 ▶ Virulence Factors of Pathogens | |
|---|---|
| **Factor** | **Function** |
| Pili, fimbriae and adhesins | Binding to receptors on host cells |
| Capsules, or surface proteins | Avoid phagocytosis |
| Antigenic or phase variation | Evade specific immune response |
| Exotoxins:<br>Enterotoxins<br>Neurotoxins<br>Superantigens | Disrupt normal cellular functions:<br>Effect is on gastrointestinal tract<br>Effect is on neurons<br>nonspecific T-cell activation and overproduction of IL-2 |
| Endotoxin (lipid A) | Induce IL-1 and tumor necrosis factor-α production<br>Fever and shock, possible disseminated intravascular coagulation |
| sIgA protease | Inactivates mucosal IgA, avoids microbial trapping in mucin |
| Siderophores, surface proteins that bind transferrin, lactoferrin, and ferritin | Iron acquisition by microbe |
| Inhibition of phagolysosome fusion or resistance to lysosomal enzymes and acids | Intracellular survival in macrophages or escape and dissemination |
| Formation of spores, cysts, or endospores | Resist killing by stomach acid or other toxic chemicals |
| Molecular mimicry of host | Avoid triggering immune response |
| Toxic proteins or substances | Kill phagocytes or inhibit oxidative burst by phagocytes or damage tissue |

and myxovirus are often asymptomatic. Detection of antibodies to these types of agents is often the only sign that an infection has occurred. Bacteria, such as *N. meningitidis, Streptococcus pneumoniae, Moraxella catarrhalis,* spend most of their time as resident flora of the human nasopharynx. Only when the host's immune status falters, do these microbes invade the body (lungs, meninges, blood, middle ear).

## Direct Damage by the Microbe

Cytopathic effects and cell death are seen with the invasion by many microorganisms. When poliovirus grows inside motor neurons, it causes shutdown of RNA, DNA, and protein synthesis with subsequent cell death. The skeletal muscles being served by these neurons cannot function, thus paralysis develops. Dental caries (destruction of tooth enamel) is due to plaque and lactic acid production by microcolonies of *Streptococcus mutans.* Most bacteria damage the cell in which they multiply. Intracellular bacteria such as *Mycobacteria, Listeria, Nocardia,* and *Brucella* species live in phagocytic cells such as monocytes and macrophages. As the bacteria slowly increase in number, the phagocyte eventually dies.

## Hypersensitivity Reactions by the Host

The immune response to the microbe by the host may actually induce local tissue damage or systemic disease. These responses are referred to as hypersensitivity reactions, of which four types exist.

Type I involves activation of IgE on mast cells, with subsequent release of histamine, heparin, and leukotriene. Dust mites, salivary proteins from insect bites, or common cold viruses can induce this type of host response. The effects range from local wheal and flare reaction, with itching and urticaria, or bronchospasms in airways to systemic anaphylaxis with hypotension, shock, and asphyxia.

Type II reactions involve antibody binding to cells bearing foreign antigens and results in cytolysis (cell lysis). Examples would include erythrocytes infected with *Plasmodium* species (the protozoan that causes malaria) and liver necrosis due to hepatitis B virus.

Type III hypersensitivity reactions are due to formation of immune complexes between antibody and soluble antigens, such as heat shock proteins. These complexes may deposit in small blood vessels of the kidney, joints, choroid plexus, or the ciliary body of the eye. Pain, swelling, and loss of function may result. An example of this phenomenon is acute glomerulonephritis following a skin or throat infection with group A streptococcus, or *S. pyogenes.*

Type IV reactions include Jones-Mote response, contact dermatitis, tuberculin, delayed-type, and granulomatous reactions. With the exception of the Jones-Mote reaction with basophil infiltration, type IV responses represent an inflammatory reaction by sensitized lymphocytes, macrophages, fibroblasts, and giant cells after 72 hours. The delayed-type response is induced by intracellular bacteria such as *M. tuberculosis* and *M. leprae,* most helminthic parasite larvae and ova, and systemic fungi such as *Coccidioides immitis* and *Histoplasma capsulatum.* Continued presence of antigen often induces the formation of granulomas (the most damaging effect to the host).

Some microbes actually induce autoimmune disease, when microbial antigens mimic host tissue. This results in the production of antibodies to tissues bearing these cross-reactive microbial antigens. Rheumatic heart disease after infection with group A streptococcus is believed to involve epitopes of certain serotypes of M protein in cell wall of group A streptococcus (see Figure 2-8). Anti-M protein antibodies cross-react with cardiac muscle (specifically: myosin and sarcolemmal membrane proteins).

## Host Susceptibility Factors

Susceptibility of the host plays a significant role in the extent of pathogenesis by a microbial agent. The genetic constitution of the host often determines whether a microbe causes disease. Usually, the host generates an effective immune response and clears the microbe. A powerful example of this phenomenon occurred in 1942, when more than 45,000 U.S. military personnel were vaccinated against yellow fever. The vaccine was contaminated with live hepatitis B virus. Only 914 clinical cases of hepatitis occurred: 580 were mild, 301 were moderate, and 33 resulted in severe disease. The incubation period varied from 10 to 20 weeks. Although

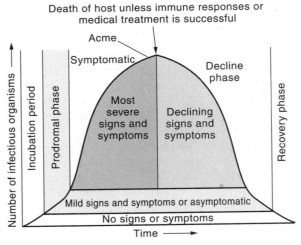

**FIGURE 2-8** Stages in the course of an infectious disease.

other physiologic factors may have been involved, genetic differences played a crucial role (Mims, 1987).

The age and sex of the host are also involved. Men over 40 years of age exhibit a gradual decline in both humoral and cell-mediated immunity. Therefore, there is an increased incidence of activation of healed pulmonary tuberculosis (trapped in granulomas) and

varicella-zoster virus in dorsal root ganglia, leading to the condition called shingles (Mims, 1987).

Other factors contributing to increased susceptibility include malnutrition, chronic stress, and administration of glucocorticoid hormones, which depress leukocyte function along with many other systemic effects (see Figure 2-8).

## SUMMARY

▶ Levels of host–microbe interactions are identified: colonization, infection, and disease.
▶ General types of host defenses are described—innate and adaptive resistance.
▶ Common themes for microbial entry and attachment and invasion of the host are described.

▶ Virulence mechanisms used by microbes to escape claring by the host's immune system are defined.
▶ Pathologic effects of microbial invasion or toxins are presented.

## CASE STUDY 1: VARIATION IN HOST SUSCEPTIBILITY TO *Listeria*

From January to August 1985, a county hospital in Los Angeles documented 142 cases of symptomatic listeriosis. The source of the bacteria was a certain brand of Mexican-style soft goat cheese. Ninety-three of the infected individuals were fetuses or newborns; the other 49 were adults (75% were pregnant women). Thirty infants and 18 adults died as a result of the infection. Forty-eight of the 49 infected adults were immunosuppressed (due to pregnancy, drugs, or illness) or elderly.

Many female goats and sheep harbor *Listeria monocytogenes* in their genital tracts and mammary glands. These hardy bacteria can grow at refrigerator temperatures and can survive within phagocytic leukocytes. The cheese plant followed safety regulations during the pasteurization process of the milk. The problem appeared to be that the flow of milk through the pasteurization equipment was too fast. Consequently, some raw milk got into the final product. (Adapted from Schuchat, A., et al. [1991]. Epidemiology of human listeriosis. *Clin Microbiol Rev.*, 4:169–183.)

**Questions:**

1. Propose possible changes in the processing procedures that could reduce or eliminate the risk of future contamination problems with *L. monocytogenes*.

2. Why did this disease affect only pregnant women, infants, and fetuses?

3. Explain why a microbiologist might place a portion of a food specimen at 4°C for 5 to 7 days, before subculturing onto selective media for *Listeria*.

## CASE STUDY 2: BACTERIAL ENDOPHTHALMITIS CAUSED BY A SOIL BACTERIUM, *AGROBACTERIUM RADIOBACTER.*

The pathogenicity of an organism is related to the site of infection as well as the immune status of the host. A 70-year-old man underwent uneventful outpatient cataract surgery with sutures. Four days later, he returned to the eye clinic with orbital swelling, a purulent discharge, and pain in the sutured eye. He did not have a fever. He did report that he had worked in his garden on the evening of his discharge.

Vitreous fluid was aspirated and submitted for Gram stain and culture (aerobic and anaerobic). The Gram stain showed a moderate number of short pleomorphic gram-negative rods with leukocytes. No growth was seen on the anaerobic cultures, but a heavy, pure growth of nonhemolytic colonies was seen on the sheep's blood agar as well as the MacConkey's plates (incubated aerobically). The Vitek GNI card identified the bacteria as *Agrobacterium tumefaciens* (A. radiobacter); 98% probability. The patient was given empirical therapy: steroids to reduce inflammation and a combination of vancomycin and gentamicin. He recovered completely.

Human infections with Agrobacterium are rare. They are soil organisms and those that contain the Ti plasmid produce crown gall disease or hairy root disease in plants. Although the two species are indistinguishable biochemically, human isolates are referred to as *A. radiobacter.* (Excerpts from case study by Miller, Novy, & Hiott [1996]. *J Clin Microbiol* [1996]. 34:3212–3213.)

**Questions:**

1. Discuss the factors involved in the development of this rare bacterial infection.

2. Why did the lab set up anaerobic as well as aerobic cultures on the vitreous fluid?

3. Discuss the pros and cons of outpatient surgeries.

## Review Questions

1. Which of the following mechanisms is NOT part of the host's innate resistance?
   a. Mucociliary apparatus of the trachea
   b. Phagocytosis by neutrophils
   c. Secretion of immunoglobulins by plasma cells
   d. Interferon production

2. Endotoxin is:
   a. a toxic protein secreted by a bacterial cell.
   b. a superantigen that activates 1 of 5 helper T lymphocytes.
   c. a toxic substance that forms during endospore formation.
   d. a toxic lipid that is a component of the outer membrane of gram-negative bacteria.

3. *Cryptococcus neoformans* avoids phagocytosis by:
   a. producing a large polysaccharide capsule.
   b. having toxic lipid A in its cell wall.
   c. killing NK cells as well as neutrophils.
   d. none of the above; this yeast is easily engulfed.

4. The ability of a microbe to cause disease depends on the host's:
   a. genetic makeup.
   b. nutritional status.
   c. level of stress.
   d. all of the above

5. When microbial antigens mimic host tissue they may:
   a. induce autoimmune disease.
   b. inhibit the production of antibody molecules.
   c. make the host more susceptible to secondary infection.
   d. all of the above

6. Superantigens are:
   a. A-B toxins that disrupt cAMP control in host cells.
   b. hemolysins or membrane-disrupting exotoxins.
   c. unusual exotoxins that bind nonspecifically to receptors on helper T lymphocytes and cause overproduction of IL-2.
   d. toxic lipids found in the outer membrane of gram-negative bacteria.

7. *Helicobacter pylori* can survive in the stomach because they:
   a. form resistant endospores.
   b. produce a thick polysaccharide capsule.
   c. produce catalase and form hydrogen peroxide.
   d. produce urease and form ammonia.

8. *Mycobacterium tuberculosis* avoid killing by the cells of the immune system by:
   a. producing powerful exotoxins.
   b. surviving within phagocytic white blood cells.
   c. forming dormant endospores.
   d. secreting lipid A, which kills lymphocytes.

9. Phase variation:
   a. is common among the pathogenic fungi.
   b. involves the switching "on or off" of genes for various characteristics.
   c. involves changes in nucleic acid sequence in RNA.
   d. is the result of degeneration of teichoic acid in gram-positive bacteria.

10. *Treponema pallidum* slow the activation of acquired immunity by:
    a. coating themselves with albumin.
    b. remaining dormant for long periods of time.
    c. deactivating antibodies.
    d. both a and c

## ▶ REFERENCES & RECOMMENDED READING

Black, J. (1996). *Microbiology, principles & applications.* Englewood Cliffs, NJ: Prentice-Hall.

Dale, B., & Dragon, E. A. (1994). Polymerase chain reaction in infectious disease diagnosis. *Lab Med, 25,* 637–641.

Finlay, B. B. (1995, May–June). Bacterial virulence factors. *Sci Am SCIENCE & MEDICINE,* 16–21.

Finlay, B. B., & Falkow, S. (1989). Common themes in microbial pathogenicity. *Microbiol Rev, 53,* 210–230.

Hogan, L. H., Klein, B. S., & Levitz, S. M. (1996). Virulence factors of medically important fungi. *Clin Microbiol Rev, 9,* 469–488.

Ingraham, J., & Ingraham, C. (1995). *Introduction to Microbiology.* San Francisco: Wadsworth.

Kauffmann, S. H. E. (1997). The roles of conventional and unconventional T cells in antibacterial immunity. *ASM News, 63,* 251–255.

Kotb, M. (1995). Bacterial pyogenic exotoxins as superantigens. *Clin Microbiol Rev, 8,* 411–426.

Mims, C. A. (1987). *The pathogenesis of infectious disease.* San Diego: Academic Press.

Murphy, J. W. (1996). Slick ways *Cryptococcus neoformans* foils host defenses. *ASM News, 62,* 77–80.

Nassif, X., & So, M. (1995). Interaction of pathogenic Neisseriae with nonphagocytic cells. *Clin Microbiol Rev, 8,* 376–388.

O'Brien, A. D., & Holmes, R. K. (1987). Shiga and shiga-like toxins. *Microbiol Rev 51,* 206–220.

Roitt, I., Brostoff, J., & Male, D. (1993). *Immunology.* St. Louis: Mosby.

Salyers, A. A., & Whitt, D. D. (1994). *Bacterial pathogenesis: A molecular approach.* Washington, DC: ASM Press.

Seifert, H. S., & So, M. (1988). Genetic mechanisms of bacterial antigen variation. *Microbiol Rev, 52,* 327–336.

Youmans, G. P., Paterson, P. Y., & Sommers, H. M. (1985). *The biologic and clinical basis of infectious diseases.* Philadelphia: Saunders.

# CHAPTER 3

# Safety in the Clinical Microbiology Laboratory

Lynn L. Russell, MA, CLS (NCA) with Anne T. Rodgers, MT (ASCP), PhD

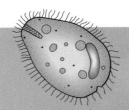

## Microbes in the News

### Laboratory Accident Causes Throat Infection

In the United Kingdom, an experienced medical laboratory scientific officer became infected with a toxigenic strain of *Corynebacterium diphtheriae*, the organism that causes diptheria, while handling a sample. Laboratories were informed that this sample came from a patient with a severe sore throat who had recently returned from Russia. The laboratory worker already had a sore throat and a cold when preparing a heavy suspension of organisms on the open bench for biochemical tests. The worker developed severe tonsillitis seven days after setting up these tests. A toxigenic strain of *C. diphtheriae* var gravis was isolated from a throat swab. Throat swabs were taken from close contacts of the laboratory worker and all other laboratory staff. They were all negative. A booster dose of diphtheria toxoid was given to all laboratory staff.

It is recommended that people who may be exposed to diphtheria in the course of their work be fully immunized and their levels of antibody tested at least three months after completion of immunization. Booster doses should be given at intervals of 10 years. Immunization protects people from the effects of the toxin, but it will not necessarily prevent acquisition and carriage of *C. diphtheriae*. Appropriate working practices are required to protect staff from acquiring infection in the laboratory and subsequently transmitting it to others.

Source: CDR (UK) Vol. 8 / No. 7, 13 February, 1998.

## KEY TERMS

Arthropod vector
Bacteriocidal
CDC
Containment
Decontamination
Disinfection

EPA
Epidemiology
HEPA
Immunocompromised
Mucous membrane

Nosocomial
Pathogen
Prophylaxis
Sharps
Standard Precautions

## LEARNING OBJECTIVES

**Upon successful completion of this chapter, the student should be able to:**

1. Use Standard Precautions and the Bloodborne Pathogens Standard in all their laboratory work.

2. Identify all warning signs and labels that indicate hazards for healthcare workers.

3. Discuss in detail the general requirements for personal safety and the management of laboratory accidents.

4. Describe the current precautions for tuberculosis control and hazardous waste disposal and to revise practices as new guidelines are issued.

5. Review and update personal knowledge of laboratory safety to successfully answer the study questions and work safely in a microbiology laboratory.

## INTRODUCTION

Laboratory workers are subject to unique occupational hazards. More than half a million cases of hospital-acquired illnesses (**nosocomial** infections) are reported annually. Of the cases that can be tracked there is a 4% fatality rate.

In examining the safety of microbiology laboratory workers one should look at the rules and regulations plus rational and common sense actions. The concept of universal standards is applied in all clinical laboratories now as good laboratory practice. Education is the best defense.

Regulations and guidelines for handling specimens have been created in response to public and worker concern with the **pathogens** in the news. These pathogenic microorganisms may be better known by their initials: hepatitis B virus (HBV), human immunodeficiency virus (HIV), and tuberculosis (TB). HBV, HIV, and TB are transmitted in the body fluids frequently handled by laboratory workers. Each of these pathogens can produce illnesses with potential morbidity and mortality. The regulations and guidelines related to these pathogens were written, approved, and put into practice to reduce the economic impact of loss of worker productivity and loss of workers.

The older and perhaps better known safety measures in the laboratory are sterilization and disinfection. Precautions should be taken when handling specimens from collection to disposal. When laboratory workers are busy processing specimens, identifying organisms, and making reports, it may seem like a waste of time to take extra steps, such as **decontamination**. However, these precautions protect them, their coworkers, family, and community contacts from direct or indirect contact with pathogens. When some unusual organisms are suspected additional precautions may be instituted. Again, though the steps or personal protective equipment (PPE) may be cumbersome, they could be essential for the safety and health of laboratory workers.

In addition to microscopic pathogens, macroscopic hazards also exist in the laboratory. One should be aware of fire hazards, dangerous chemicals, and other problems. There are specific rules for preventing these physical hazards.

Education is an essential element of laboratory safety. Essentially, every specimen should be treated with respect. To maintain a safe environment, laboratorians should apply the principles in good practice, perform the work necessary on the microbiology specimens, produce accurate results for the patient, and maintain a safe environment for themselves and those around them.

## METHODS OF STERILIZATION

Sterilization, or the removal or destruction of harmful organisms, is an important and necessary process. Sterilization methods may be physical, mechanical, or chemical. Physical methods include moist and dry heat and ultraviolet radiation. Mechanical methods include ultrasonic and sonic (sound) waves and filtration. Chemical methods include a variety of chemical agents such as acids and alkalis, phenols, halogens, and alkylating agents such as ethylene dioxide gas.

With so many options available, it is important to consider the factors involved in choosing a process. These include characteristics of the organism, agent to be used, object to be sterilized, and environmental aspects. We must also decide the purpose of the process. For example, if we want to preserve and reuse the object to be sterilized, incineration would NOT be a good choice! However, if we are only interested in disinfecting, a chemical method might be the best choice.

## Physical Methods

Heat is the most common of the physical methods and may be moist heat or dry heat. Dry heat in ovens is used to sterilize objects that would be damaged by exposure to moisture. This includes glassware and some metal objects. Cloth is not suitable for this method because it would become brittle. Dry heat sterilization is carried out at a temperature of 160°C for 1 to 2 hours.

The most common moist heat sterilization method is the autoclave. An autoclave is essentially a large pressure cooker that uses steam under pressure to achieve temperatures capable of sterilizing (see Figure 3-1). The standard temperature and time are 121°C for 15 to 20 minutes. This temperature can be achieved near sea level by pressures of 15 psi (pounds per square inch). At altitudes of 5,000 feet, the pressure must be increased by about 3 psi to achieve the required temperature. The proper temperature will only be achieved if the flowing steam is allowed to displace air in the chamber of the autoclave. In addition, to ensure complete penetration, the "load" in the autoclave must be arranged so that the steam can circulate. The time of exposure may be increased to ensure that items in the center of the load achieve a temperature of 121°C. The lower temperature for moist heat as compared with dry heat is possible because water/moisture increases the disruption of hydrogen bonds between peptide groups and thus promote protein denaturation. Denaturation will occur at the higher temperatures but the process takes more time. It is extremely important to follow each individual manufacturer's instructions for operation of the autoclave and to use a method of verifying sterility such as steritape or "Kilit" spore test ampules.

Ultraviolet or ionizing radiation is another example of a physical method of sterilization. Ultraviolet light and ionizing radiation are used both in the hospital setting and in the food industry. The radiation kills bacterial cells by causing alterations in the DNA of the

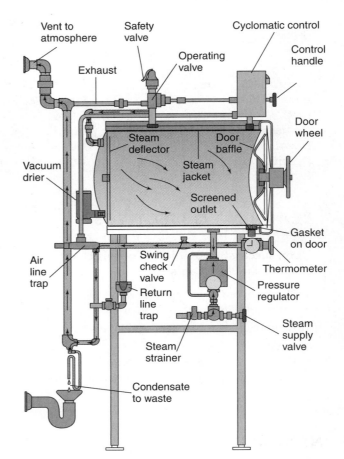

**FIGURE 3-1** Steam autoclave.

organism, resulting in blocking of the functions of DNA. When DNA cannot function, cell death occurs. Ultraviolet lamps are usually used in closed spaces such as rooms and bacteriologic hoods. Airborne contamination is significantly reduced with the use of this method but not all organisms may be killed. One disadvantage is that ultraviolet light causes irritation of the cornea and workers must be protected with safety glasses. Ionizing radiation is primarily used to sterilize food.

## Mechanical Methods

Ultrasonic and sonic (sound) waves may be used to sterilize objects. Sound waves denature proteins and cause fragmentation, resulting in cell death. As a practical, useful method, ultrasound as a sterilization method has few applications. Filtration, using cellulose membrane filter disks can be used to prepare bacteria-free solutions. Generally, filters are used to prepare bacteria-free solutions of components that would be destroyed by heat. This includes such solutions as urea media or media containing specific amounts of sugars.

## Chemical Methods and Disinfection

Chemical methods are the most commonly used means of sterilizing and disinfecting other than moist heat. Use of most chemical agents is considered **disinfection** rather than sterilization because they may not kill all forms of life present in or on a material. They reduce the infectivity of a material. Because many chemicals are used for disinfecting areas where people live and work and also are used on human skin, the ideal agent must be pleasant to use and have limited toxicity for living tissue but maximum toxicity for microorganisms. The agent must also be stable and remain active when exposed to changes in the environment. For example, a disinfectant that is used to disinfect tables should continue to be effective when it dries on the surface.

One of the first disinfectants used was phenol. Phenol certainly does not fit with the guidelines listed above because it is toxic to skin and has an unpleasant odor. However, it is extremely effective and its **bacteriocidal** (killing) ability is used as a standard to measure the effectiveness of chemical disinfectants. The phenol coefficient is the ratio of the minimum concentration of phenol to sterilize to the minimal sterilizing concentration of the substance being tested. The closer to 1 this value is, the better the more effective the disinfectant. Another way of expressing the phenol coefficient in the formula:

$$\text{Phenol coefficient} = \frac{\text{activity of test agent}}{\text{activity of phenol}}$$

The phenol coefficient is a measure of the activity of a given disinfectant compared to a standard concentration of phenol that can kill a standard concentration of test organisms in 10 minutes at about 20°C. The phenol coefficient is considered a good measure of effectiveness, but the value should be interpreted with care when evaluating disinfectants other than phenolic compounds. Some chemicals such as the halogens and surfactants vary in their activity and stability in the environment.

Chemical agents include halogens, alkylating agents, surface active agents (surfactants), phenols, and alcohols. Halogens include tincture of iodine and chlorine. Chlorine is used in the food industry and in water treatment. Chlorine is less effective when large amounts of organic matter are present. Tincture of iodine is no longer used routinely because it tends to burn exposed tissue and many patients have allergic reactions to it. The most common alkylating agent used in the hospital setting today is ethylene oxide. As a gas, it is very effective in sterilizing heat- or moisture-sensitive materials such as clothing, bedding, plastic, or surgical instruments. Sterilization with ethylene oxide gas takes more time than heat and is significantly more expensive. Workers involved in this type of sterilization must be carefully protected due to the potential for this substance to act as a carcinogen.

Surfactants, especially the quaternary ammonium compounds such as benzalkonium chloride, are effective bacteriocidal agents. They are pleasant to use and nontoxic but must be used carefully because they are neutralized by soaps. Alcohols are fair disinfectants. Ethanol and isopropyl alcohol are in widest use. Alcohols are most effective in concentrations from 50% to 70% because water is necessary for alcohol to denature proteins. Absolute (100%) alcohol is not effective as a disinfectant.

Table 3-1 summarizes the mode of action, advantages, and disadvantages of several of the more common disinfecting agents. Choosing a method of sterilization or disinfection is no easy task. To make an informed decision, you must consider all of the factors discussed in this section—nature of the organism, characteristics of the items to be sterilized or disinfected, and environmental factors. In addition, today we must add other factors such as cost, ease of use, and effectiveness.

## INFECTIOUS WASTE MANAGEMENT

Infectious waste management is an important part of general infection control in a hospital setting. Infectious waste may be defined as any waste that has the potential of transmitting infectious microorganisms. The protocols developed for handling infectious waste

### Table 3–1 ▶ Characteristics of Chemical Agents of Sterilization and Disinfection

| Agent | Mode of Action | Advantages | Disadvantages |
|---|---|---|---|
| Halogens | Combines with proteins Oxidizer | Wide spectrum of activity | Toxic to skin, allergic reactions |
| Ethylene oxide gas | Lethal disruption of cell metabolism | Can be used for items sensitive to heat | Requires safety precautions—carcinogenic and explosive |
| Quaternary ammonium compounds | Disruption of cell membranes | Stable, pleasant to use, broad spectrum of activity | Inactivated by soaps More expensive than others |
| Alcohols | Denature proteins | Easy to use, not toxic | Concentration is important, not effective against spores |
| Phenolic compounds | Coagulation of proteins, cell lysis | Powerful bactericide at proper concentrations | Toxic, strong odor |

are based on various local, state, and federal regulations. Most Federal regulations are monitored by the Environmental Protection Agency (**EPA**). Most states also regulate hazardous chemical waste. Radioactive waste disposal is regulated by the federal Nuclear Regulatory Commission (NRC). All of the regulations address definitions, storage, packaging, transportation, and control of the various types of waste—infectious, radioactive, chemical, and physical. Each type of waste has specific guidelines that must be followed. It should be remembered that even though infectious waste is defined as a separate waste category by regulatory agencies, any of the other types of waste (radioactive, chemical, physical) may be infectious. Hospitals and other health care facilities are required to have a waste disposal guide.

Precautions and guidelines for handling hazardous waste are grouped according to the type of hazard (see Table 3-2). These include: chemical, biologic, radiation, and mechanical hazards. **Sharps** would be considered mechanical hazards under the standard definitions, but in a lab setting would also pose a biologic risk because of possible contamination with blood. Laboratory waste may be categorized as chemical, infectious, radioactive, or physical. Guidelines for disposal are based on these categories and must adhere to the regulations that apply to the situation.

| Table 3–2 ▶ Types of Hazards and Hazardous Waste | |
| --- | --- |
| **Hazard** | **Hazardous Waste** |
| Mechanical | Sharp objects, needles, glass, lancets |
| Chemical | Flammable poisonous liquids or solids, corrosive unstable |
| Biologic | Materials that are contaminated with infectious agents |
| Radiation | All materials that are radioactive |

From an **epidemiologic** standpoint, disposal of infectious waste is an important issue because of the risk to the environment and to the community at large. Infections may be transmitted by many routes. Handling and disposal of waste can "open" many of these routes such as aerosols, contact, or the fecal-oral route if water or food is contaminated. Education of health care practitioners about the proper procedures for disposal of any potentially infectious waste is another important role for infection control personnel.

## LEGISLATIVE AND REGULATORY CONTROLS

Many government and nongovernment agencies have set regulations for microbiology laboratories. These are shown in Table 3-3.

| Table 3–3 ▶ Governmental and Nongovernmental Agencies That Set Regulations for Microbiology Laboratories |
| --- |
| **Federal** |
| Health Care Financing Administration (HCFA) |
| Centers for Disease Control and Prevention (CDC) |
| National Institutes of Occupational Safety and Health (NIOSH) |
| Environmental Protection Agency (EPA) |
| Food and Drug Administration (FDA) |
| Post Office |
| Health Resource Service Administration |
| Agency for Toxic Substances and Disease Registry |
| Nuclear Regulatory Commission (NRC) |
| Department of Transportation (DOT) |
| Department of Agriculture |
| |
| **State and Local** |
| Laboratory Licensure Division |
| Laboratory Licensure Division (Medicaid) |
| Health Department |
| |
| **Nongovernmental** |
| Joint Commission on Accreditation of Healthcare Organizations (JCAHO) |
| College of American Pathologists (CAP) |
| National Committee for Clinical Laboratory Standards (NCCLS) |
| American College of Physicians |
| Association for Practitioners of Infection Control |
| American Society for Microbiology (ASM) |
| Infectious Diseases Society of America |

## Centers for Disease Control and Prevention (CDC) Guidelines

With the increasing concern for the well-being of health care employees the **CDC** developed Universal Precautions guidelines in 1987. These were revised in the mid-1990s and are now known as **Standard Precautions**. These guidelines regard all blood and body fluids as potentially infectious.

### Potential Infectious Materials Other than Blood
▶ Semen
▶ Vaginal secretions
▶ Cerebrospinal fluid
▶ Synovial fluid
▶ Peritoneal fluid
▶ Pericardial fluid
▶ Amniotic fluid

### Less Commonly Encountered Infectious Materials
▶ Saliva in dental procedures
▶ Any body fluid contaminated with blood
▶ Any unfixed tissue or organ
▶ Cell or tissue culture with HIV or HBV

The concept of Standard Precautions as proposed by the CDC required all health care workers to follow certain practices when handling blood and body fluids. As the potential for infection cannot be known in advance, all specimens and contaminated materials are treated in such a manner as to minimize risk to the laboratory worker. Standard Precautions covers barrier protection, the use of gloves, vascular puncture procedures, precautions for laboratory workers with skin lesions, and pregnant workers. Other sections deal with body substance isolation (BSI) and warning labels on specimens.

## Occupational Safety and Health Administration

The Occupational Safety and Health Administration (OSHA) was created in 1970 and is a branch of the U.S. Department of Labor. The regulations of OSHA often come directly from standards and guidelines from the National Institute for Occupational Safety and Health (NIOSH), another group within the CDC. The biggest effect of OSHA on the microbiology laboratory is the Final Rule on Occupational Exposure to Bloodborne Pathogens.

Four years after universal precautions, the Bloodborne Pathogens Standards were published in the *Federal Register* to protect employees from exposure to infectious materials. Bloodborne pathogens are the most common microbiologic hazard facing clinical laboratorians. Several control measures are part of the bloodborne pathogens standard to minimize all occupational exposure to blood and other potentially infectious material. Included in the plan are an infection control focus and guidelines for a written exposure control plan.

The OSHA Standard is a federal regulation. Compliance is mandatory. Failure to comply can result in penalties and fines.

▶ It is not limited by type of facility or number of employees.
▶ It does not depend on quantities of infectious material.

The Bloodborne Pathogens Standard has several components. For example, under "methods of compliance, the engineering and work practice section," the use of sharps disposal containers are a required recommendation. Injuries from sharps are the number one way in which bloodborne pathogens enter the bodies of health care workers. Needles, scalpels, broken glass, and other sharp objects that can penetrate skin are the culprits and should be disposed of in designated sharps containers. The needles shall not be bent or recapped.

Handwashing is required after contact with blood or infectious material. Employers have the responsibility of providing accessible handwashing facilities and for ensuring that employees wash their hands after each exposure. Figure 3-2 provides a comprehensive review of the Standard Precautions.

Other exposure control measures in the OSHA Standard include:

▶ Prohibiting eating, drinking, smoking, applying cosmetics, or handling contact lenses in work areas
▶ Transporting specimens in clean break-resistant containers marked with a biohazard label
▶ Placing warning labels on regulated waste and on appliances and containers used to store blood and other infectious materials
▶ Storing food and drinks separately from laboratory items and specimens
▶ Prohibiting mouth pipetting of blood or other materials
▶ Using a biologic safety cabinet for procedures likely to produce aerosols
▶ Using centrifuge caps when processing specimens

Personal protective equipment (PPE) should be worn to cover the skin, clothing, and **mucous membranes** of laboratorians from blood-borne pathogens. Appropriate PPE includes gloves, laboratory coats, masks, and eye protection. The protective equipment that has been worn must be removed before leaving the work area. The used equipment is placed in a designated area or container.

When infectious material is discarded it becomes infectious waste. More than one federal agency has defined and regulated medical waste, which includes:

1. Microbiologic material
2. Pathologic material
3. Animal carcasses
4. Blood
5. Sharps
6. Waste from patients with communicable diseases

A discussion on a plan for waste management will be found later in the chapter.

The OSHA Standard has very specific wording on medical waste. Other components detailed are those of hepatitis B vaccination, postexposure evaluation, and follow-up. It is the responsibility of the employer to inform the employee/student and to make the vaccination available. If necessary, a postexposure evaluation and follow-up program must be made available to the employee.

Communication of hazards to employees is another requirement for employers. This is done with labels and signs. The universal biohazard symbol (see Figure 3-3) should be affixed to containers, appliances/equipment, storage containers and certain work areas such as HIV/HBV research laboratories.

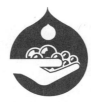

**Wash Hands** (Plain soap)
Wash after touching **blood, body fluids, secretions, excretions,** and **contaminated items.**
Wash immediately **after gloves are removed** and **between patient contacts.**
Avoid transfer of microorganisms to other patients or environments.

**Wear Gloves**
Wear when touching **blood, body fluids, secretions, excretions,** and **contaminated items.**
Put on **clean** gloves just **before touching mucous membranes** and **nonintact skin.**
Change gloves between tasks and procedures on the same patient after contact with material
that may contain high concentrations of microorganisms. Remove gloves promptly after use, before
touching noncontaminated items and environmental surfaces, and before going to another patient,
and wash hands immediately to avoid transfer of microorganisms to other patients or environments.

**Wear Mask and Eye Protection or Face Shield**
Protect mucous membranes of the eyes, nose and mouth during procedures and patient-care
activities that are likely to generate **splashes** or **sprays of blood, body fluids, secretions,** or
**excretions.**

**Wear Gown**
Protect skin and prevent soiling of clothing during procedures that are likely to generate **splashes**
or **sprays** of **blood, body fluids, secretions,** or **excretions.** Remove a soiled gown as promptly
as possible and wash hands to avoid transfer of microorganisms to other patients or environments.

**Patient-Care Equipment**
Handle used patient-care equipment soiled with **blood, body fluids, secretions,** or **excretions** in
a manner that prevents skin and mucous membrane exposures, contamination of clothing, and
transfer of microorganisms to other patients and environments. Ensure that reusable equipment is
not used for the care of another patient until it has been appropriately cleaned and reprocessed
and single use items are properly discarded.

**Environmental Control**
Follow hospital procedures for routine care, cleaning, and disinfection of environmental surfaces,
beds, bedrails, bedside equipment and other frequently touched surfaces.

**Linen**
Handle, transport, and process used linen soiled with **blood, body fluids, secretions,** or
**excretions** in a manner that prevents exposures and contamination of clothing, and avoids
transfer of microorganisms to other patients and environments.

**Occupational Health and Bloodborne Pathogens**
Prevent injuries when using needles, scalpels, and other sharp instruments or devices; when handling
sharp instruments after procedures; when cleaning used instruments; and when disposing of used needles.

**Never recap used needles using both hands** or any other technique that involves directing the point
of a needle toward any part of the body; rather, use either a one-handed "scoop" technique
or a mechanical device designed for holding the needle sheath.

Do not remove used needles from disposable syringes by hand, and do not bend, break, or otherwise manipulate used needles by hand. Place used disposable syringes and needles, scalpel
blades and other sharp items in puncture-resistant sharps containers located as close as practical
to the area in which the items were used, and place reusable syringes and needles in a puncture-
resistant container for transport to the reprocessing area.

Use **resuscitation devices** as an alternative to mouth-to-mouth resuscitation.

**Patient Placement**
Use a **private room** for a patient who contaminates the environment or who does not (or
cannot be expected to) assist in maintaining appropriate hygiene or environmental control. Consult
Infection Control if a private room is not available.

**FIGURE 3-2** Standard Precautions for infection control issued by the CDC in 1996. (Courtesy Brevis Corp.)

**FIGURE 3-3** Biohazard symbol.

# ENVIRONMENTAL CONTROLS

## Facilities

Environmental safety focuses on the design of the laboratory, the provision of appropriate equipment and the adoption of containment techniques.

The CDC biosafety level (BSL) of a laboratory depends on the type of work being done there. The biosafety level also determines the design of the laboratory. However, in general a laboratory should be:

1. Isolated from patient care areas
2. Able to limit access to visitors
3. Able to restrict airflow
4. Easy to clean
5. Equipped with handwashing and eye wash sinks
6. Using biologic safety cabinets
7. Using resistant materials for workbenches
8. Posted with an evacuation plan

These would be part of the secondary barriers. Equipment, especially that for containment, is of concern for laboratorians who are working with hazardous materials. Several items are considered here. The most important is the biological safety cabinet (BSC). The particular work of the laboratory determines the class of the BSC necessary. Centrifuges, particularly those used in the TB area, are also part of the barrier system. Blenders, grinders, refrigerators, and pipets are other pieces of equipment to evaluate for safety considerations.

**Containment.** To protect laboratory workers, other persons, and the outside environment from potentially hazardous agents, **containment** is used. The term describes safe methods for managing the agent in the area where hazardous materials are being handled.

There are two types of containment. Primary containment covers the personnel and the immediate laboratory and generally includes:

▶ Good microbiologic technique
▶ Use of appropriate safety equipment
▶ Vaccines for personnel

Specific primary barriers are protective garments, gloves, procedures to minimize aerosols, and good handwashing. Secondary containment refers to the environment external to the laboratory and is provided by a combination of safety equipment and facility design.

**Warning Signs and Labels.** Specific, recognizable signs and labels are a uniform way of informing people in the laboratory of potential hazards. Usually these are permanent signs. There may be certain areas that have a higher risk than others in the laboratory. The risk assessment may be based on fire, microbiologic, or chemical hazards.

There are very specific labels for containers of chemicals. There are rules for what should be on labels, what should be added to the manufacturer's label, and how unlabeled chemicals should be handled. Labels are required in several microbiologic situations:

1. The refrigerators and freezers containing blood and other infectious materials
2. Containers used to store, transport, and ship blood and other infectious materials and infectious waste
3. Sharps disposal containers
4. Contaminated equipment

The label for these situations is the universal biohazard symbol. The color is fluorescent orange with the symbol in black affixed to a container. An adaptation of this is the red bag or the red molded plastic containers used for disposal in the laboratories. (More specific conditions would be applied for the HIV and HBV research areas.)

Specific signs are used to communicate laboratory hazards. Signs are used for radionuclides. Signs are used on refrigerators and freezers to distinguish their use for flammable liquids. Signs are also used on refrigerators and freezers to designate whether or not they can tolerate explosions. Signs are on laboratory refrigerators to indicate which ones can be used for storage of food.

OSHA has specifications for general signs and the colors for various categories:

DANGER—red, black and white
CAUTION—yellow and black
SAFETY INSTRUCTION—green and white

# CLASSIFICATION OF BIOHAZARDOUS AGENTS

The CDC in association with the National Institutes of Health (NIH) has developed guidelines for safely handling biohazardous agents that are detailed in the document *Biosafety in Microbiological and Biomedical Laboratories (BMBL)*. In stating the principles of biosafety, the publication emphasizes that "the most important element of containment is strict adherence to standard microbiological practices and techniques."

In focusing on the laboratory practice and techniques, in addition to the basics listed earlier in this chapter, each laboratory should have a biosafety manual. The laboratory director is responsible for arranging training of personnel on safe practices and techniques. All personnel should be advised on hazards and required to follow established practices and procedures. Orientation and training of new employees in the microbiology laboratory is reinforced by the microbiology supervisor through continuing education and by monitoring employee compliance. The safe operation of the laboratory is a responsibility of the laboratory director, but requires the compliance of each worker in the laboratory.

Confucius said, "There are three ways of avoiding being eaten by a tiger: to wear a suit of armor, to go out and shoot the tiger, or to keep it in a well-barred cage." His wisdom can be applied to safety in the microbiology laboratory. Safety equipment, considered primary barriers, includes BSCs, safety centrifuge cups, gloves, gowns, face shields, and safety glasses or goggles. The PPE can be used in conjunction with the BSCs.

Facility design, the secondary barriers, protect persons working in the facility and persons and animals in the community. Secondary barriers include separation of the work area from public access, availability of an autoclave, handwashing facilities, and specialized ventilation systems. Good laboratory practice should dictate that the workplace be kept clean and uncluttered.

## Biologic Safety Levels

The BMBL referred to above describes four biosafety levels or BSLs. Each level consists of a combination of laboratory practices and techniques, safety equipment, and laboratory facilities. Each combination is especially appropriate for the operations performed, the documented or suspected routes of transmission of the infectious agents, and for the laboratory function or activity.

The higher the number of the class of the agents, the greater the hazard. The general scheme of combinations provides only for the minimal safety conditions. Therefore, when information indicates that factors have been altered then more stringent practices in a higher BSL could be used.

**BSL 1.** Work involves agents of no known or of minimal potential hazard. The work practices are appropriate for teaching laboratories and other laboratories that work with defined strains of microorganisms not known to cause disease in healthy adult humans. (Many agents may cause infection in the young, the old, or the other-

wise **immunocompromised**.) Work is conducted on open bench tops with access to an open bench top sink. Personnel and the supervisor should have appropriate training in the procedures to be performed.

**BSL 2.** Work involves agents of moderate risk. The work practices are appropriate for clinical, diagnostic, teaching, and other facilities. Work is done in an open bench with precautions for splashes and aerosols, which may include gloves, gowns, and BSCs. Laboratory personnel have specific training in handling pathogenic agents and are directed by scientists competent in this biosafety level. Access to the laboratory is limited when work is in progress. Secondary barriers, such as handwashing and waste decontaminating facilities, must be available.

**BSL 3.** Work involves a variety of indigenous and exotic agents with a potential for respiratory transmission and that may cause serious and potentially lethal infections. The work practices are appropriate for clinical, diagnostic, teaching, research, or production facilities. Laboratory personnel have specific training in handling pathogenic and potentially lethal agents and are supervised by competent, experienced scientists. More emphasis is placed on the primary and secondary barriers. All laboratory work should be performed in a BSC.

**BSL 4.** Work involves dangerous and exotic agents with life-threatening potential, which may be transmitted via the aerosol route, and for which there is no available vaccine or therapy. Laboratory personnel have specific and thorough training in handling extremely hazardous infectious agents, and they comprehend special containment practices. Access to the laboratory is strictly controlled. The work may be in a class III BSC or in a "moon" suit that completely surrounds the worker. The BSL 4 is usually in a separate building. The laboratory director is specifically responsible for the safe operation of the laboratory. This is the maximum level of containment and is limited to a few facilities across the country.

## Classification of Biologic Agents

The CDC has published a list of biologic agents classified according to risk. There is a general description for bacterial, fungal, parasitic, viral, rickettsial, and chlamydial agents not included in the higher classes. There are also specific viruses for BSL 1: influenza virus A/Pr8/34, Newcastle virus, and parainfluenza virus 3, SF4 strain. Many specific agents are listed for bacterial (40), fungal (4), parasitic (7) infections and 33 viral, rickettsial, and chlamydial agents are listed for BSL 2. Under BSL 3 are specific lists for bacterial (10), fungal (2), parasitic (1), and 11 viral, rickettsial, and chlamydial agents. *Mycobacterium tuberculosis* is listed in BSL 3, as are biphasic fungi. Work with HIV must be done using BSL 3 procedures also. The list for BSL 4 specifies 9 viral, rickettsial, and chlamydial agents, such as the hemorrhagic fever agents.

## CREATING A SAFE LABORATORY ENVIRONMENT

When a laboratory director develops a safe laboratory environment in a microbiology laboratory he or she may wish to consider the levels listed above as a basis for the plan. The BSL procedures would be applied to the amount of exposure.

### Biosafety in Microbiologic Laboratories

**Transmission.** In the microbiology laboratory the greatest safety risks are associated with the processing of the initial specimens and working with the isolated or concentrated organisms. Four basic elements are necessary to initiate an infection:

1. Susceptible host
2. Infectious agent
3. Concentration of the agent
4. Suitable route of transmission

The route of transmission is the element most receptive to control through biosafety guidelines. The most common routes of transmission include:

1. Aerosols
2. Ingestion
3. Inoculation (accidental)
4. Mucous membranes
5. Arthropod vectors

These play a major role in safety rules and regulations.

### Protection Techniques

Gloves are frequently used in the laboratory. They are worn to work with specimens or to protect in special procedures. Gloves should not be worn everywhere. After they have been used or "contaminated," they should NOT be worn to use objects in "clean" or uncontaminated areas: telephones, terminal keyboards, doorknobs, and water fountains, for example.

Long hair should be kept back and secured. This is to (1) prevent the hair from brushing across contaminated surfaces, (2) avoid shedding organisms from the hair onto the work surface, and (3) keep the hair out of equipment with moving parts. Beards come under this same precaution. Disposable covers are available to cover hair and beards. Beards are of additional concern when respirators must be worn.

Handwashing should be done frequently. This safety procedure would be done *immediately* after contact with blood or body fluids. It would be done also after removing gloves, before leaving the work area, and before eating or smoking on breaks. Handwashing is the single best precaution in most situations.

Another related step would be to keep work surfaces decontaminated. This is accomplished easily by cleaning the surfaces with a 1:10 dilution of sodium hypochlorite (or household bleach). Surfaces would be cleaned after any spills *and* at the end of each shift.

An extension of personal protection would be certain items available in the microbiology work area. These safety items include face shields, respirators, and pipetting aids that would be used directly by laboratorians. Respirators may require special instruction before they are first used. Also in this group would be splash guards, eye wash stations, emergency showers, and containers for sharps, all to be installed in the laboratories and kept functional by the employer.

### Management of Laboratory Accidents

Despite educational sessions, following Standard Precautions, and using protective techniques, accidents do occur. There can be accidents of two types: (1) spills of blood and body fluids, and (2) skin puncture or contamination with those fluids. The institution should have a written policy for each situation.

For spills, wear a gown and gloves to protect yourself while cleaning up the container and contents. Follow the policies and use the designated materials for absorbing the spill, cleaning and washing the area. All contaminated materials should be disposed of according to biohazard regulations.

As stated earlier, needle sticks would be the most common laboratory accident. Also exposure occurs when blood and body fluids splash in eyes, mouth, conjunctival or other mucous membranes, or nonintact skin (such as acne, dermatitis, or an open cut). When an incident occurs report it to the teacher or supervisor and follow the policies for the institution. The immediate action would be the appropriate first aid for that exposure.

A next step the employer makes available would be a postexposure examination by a physician. As part of the medical examination and follow-up the HIV and HBV antibody status should be determined for the injured health care worker and for the blood or body fluid source patient. **Prophylaxis** as prescribed by the U.S. Public Health Service should be given, and counseling offered. Gamma globulin may be used as immunoprophylaxis if there is a likelihood of exposure to hepatitis. Zidovudine (AZT) may be used as a chemoprophylaxis if there is a likelihood of exposure to HIV.

The documentation of the accident report, blood tests, vaccination, if done, and medical records of the health care worker are required. OSHA requires the recording of needle sticks that "require medical treatment . . . and are identified as causes of diagnosed occupationally related AIDS, AIDS related complex, or hepatitis."

Another situation to consider is the exposure of a patient to infected laboratory workers. Most of the possible situations involve invasive medical or dental procedures and therefore exclude laboratory staff in their routine duties. If laboratorians have strep throat, chickenpox or other communicable illness, or have been exposed to such an illness, they should avoid contact with patients until their infectious period is past. If a patient does have an exposure the same procedures for follow-up medical examinations, testing, and treatment would apply.

## Reporting of Incidents

OSHA requires the reporting of work-related injuries and illnesses. In reporting the exposure incidents or accidents, the routes of entry and the circumstances should be thoroughly documented. Each institution should have forms available for the incident reports. The basic information should identify the employee and along with the description of the accident, a statement as to whether the accident could have been prevented, and an evaluation of the steps to be taken for corrective action. Each employer, under OSHA, must display a poster that explains their obligation to employees. The employer must report to OSHA any fatalities or incidents that cause the hospitalization of five or more employees.

Along with the microbiology laboratory in a hospital, the infection control practitioner, the employee health service, and the safety committee work together to study hospital epidemiology, arrange for appropriate care of employees, review incidents, and reduce the number of missed work days due to illness and accidents. These departments should provide oversight education programs, physical examinations, tests, and vaccinations for continued safety and good health.

## Exposure Control Plan

The OSHA Standard states that there be a plan to control exposures to employees. This exposure control is accomplished through work practice controls, PPE, and proper disinfection and cleaning practices.

There are several "musts" for the full plan:

1. Adherence to Standard Precautions
2. Prevention of transmission from microbial culture and infectious waste
3. Training in Standard Precautions before starting employment

4. Annual retraining in Standard Precautions
5. Documentation of all training
6. Annual evaluation for compliance with Standard Precautions

## Infection Control Plan

The infection control plan (ICP) is the hospital's best means of guarding against the spread of disease within its walls. Such a plan would include isolation precautions, institution-wide infection control procedures, and employee health programs. Under the ICP come both the UP and PPE.

An ICP can be unique to the facility but must contain the elements stated in the OSHA Standard on Bloodborne Pathogens. There are protocols for observing UP, hazard communication or HAZCOM (labels), and for training personnel. These are being repeated to emphasize their necessity in protecting workers, reducing risk to patients and community, and saving financial losses for the institution.

The federal government has two reporting systems to track the effectiveness of ICPs. Both systems or lists are part of CDC. One list indicates diseases that are reported to local and state health departments, and then in turn to CDC's National Notifiable Disease Surveillance System (NNDSS). Examples of notifiable diseases are aseptic meningitis, gonorrhea, poliomyelitis, and tetanus. Another list is for diseases and conditions that do not have to be reported to NNDSS but on which CDC maintains surveillance. Examples of the conditions under surveillance are genital herpes simplex virus infection, giardiasis, mucopurulent cervicitis, and spinal cord injury.

## Personal Safety

To focus on personal safety, laboratorians should be well informed about the sources of infection in the workplace and the factors that affect disease susceptibility and pathogen transmission. There are basically four routes of transmission: contact transmission, vehicle transmission, **arthropod vector** transmission, and airborne transmission.

*Contact transmission* is the most frequent and can be by direct contact, indirect contact, or droplet contact. Droplet contact involves the airborne transfer of pathogens from one person to another as a result of coughing, sneezing, or talking. The droplets or aerosol can spread 10 to 20 feet from these actions. This airborne transfer can also be created when opening a stoppered tube. Particles are so small they evaporate as they settle, others dry and often are invisible; surgical masks do not provide protection here. Accidents involving aerosols in laboratory operations may be classified as:

### Most Severe

▶ Fluid ejected with force from a pipette
▶ Blending in a high-speed blender
▶ Leakage in a centrifuge carrier (due to poor work practice)

### Severe

▶ Opening lyophilized cultures
▶ Vortexing unstoppered tubes (due to poor work practice)

### Less Severe

▶ Grinding with mortar and pestle
▶ Decanting supernatant after centrifuging
▶ Releasing the vacuum on a freeze dryer
▶ Inserting an inoculation loop in a culture
▶ Withdrawing a sample through a stoppered vial

*Vehicle transmission,* a second route of transmission, can be by food, water, drugs, or blood. *Airborne transmission* is the means by which pathogens are carried on larger droplets or on dust particles. They can be redistributed in turn by other forces and can serve as markers for smaller particles. They must be able to survive in the environment to transmit disease and would be picked up by touch rather than inhaled.

*Vector transmission* would usually be by an insect or arachnid, and would be of concern to health care workers inside the facilities, especially if they are working with research animals.

For the first half of the twentieth century, the microorganisms of concern to laboratory scientists were bacteria (e.g., *Salmonella typhae*). With better isolation and identification techniques, viruses became the organisms of concern, primarily hepatitis and HIV. The dread of genetically engineered organisms and the rare exotic fevers, such as Ebola, has best been left to the movies at this time because they have not been demonstrated to be of widespread concern.

Protozoa and helminths have been named in some cases of laboratory-acquired infections. Several factors affect the severity of such infections, including the immune status of the laboratory worker. Women of childbearing age and persons of lowered immunocompetency should exercise special precautions or avoid working with live organisms. Thorough training of workers new to the parasitology area should be conducted. Because needle sticks and aerosolization were the reported cause of many accidental infections, BSL 2 and good laboratory practices should be strictly enforced when working with parasitology specimens.

The organisms of major concern to laboratorians in the 1990s are HIV, HBV, other viruses, *M. tuberculosis, Corynebacterium diphtheriae, Bordetella pertussis,* and group A and group B *Streptococcus.* To combat nosoco-mial infections and ensure personal safety, illness with the above organisms and others should be reported and treated. To repeat the precautions already cited, educating staff in the use of PPE, use of BSL, and adherence to UP is vital. You cannot go wrong with ample training and frequent handwashing.

## TRANSPORTATION OF INFECTIOUS AGENTS

Collecting, handling, transporting, and storing patient specimens is an important job of the clinical laboratorian. These four steps in the process are considered the preanalytical phase of laboratory testing. These steps can have profound effects on the results of specimen testing.

### Specimen Collection

Some specimens are collected at one site and shipped to a remote location for analysis. Specific regulations cover this type of situation and are issued by the U.S. Public Health Service (USPHS) and the U.S. Department of Transportation (DOT). These regulations are for packing, insulating, packaging, labeling, and shipping specimens by courier, mail, or air. The regulations are intended to protect the integrity of the specimen en route and to protect the handlers and health care workers if the specimen breaks in transit. (In addition to the international and national transporting regulations, there may be state and local regulations for the laboratory to be aware of also.)

There are points to keep in mind when considering the handling of specimens:

1. Treat all specimens with Standard Precautions.
2. Consider the changes in temperature and pressure along the route, which may have an impact on the specimen.
3. Fluid-resistant bags and proper labeling are necessary for diagnostic specimens in transit.
4. The status of the specimens should be checked on arrival.
   a. The laboratory should notify the sender immediately if there is a problem.
   b. If the package came from the outside and is broken, call CDC at 800-232-0124.

### Packaging

The American Type Culture Collection (ATCC) has published a guide (Brown & Simione, 1994) to packaging and shipping of specimens. ATCC is devoted to research and education on microorganisms and cell lines. Their publication has combined good laboratory practices and government regulations in one easy printed guide for the laboratorian who has to ship specimens to reference laboratories. There is a thorough discussion of the various permits and licenses, packaging and labeling requirements, guides to choosing a shipper, and rules for importation. Other sections cover the classification of cultures, and the new (1990) related regulations from the *Federal Register*.

## SPECIAL PRECAUTIONS IN THE CLINICAL MICROBIOLOGY LABORATORY

### Tuberculosis Control

For a few decades OSHA has been concerned with *M. tuberculosis* as an occupational hazard. They are enforcing old guidelines and writing new ones as they attempt to deal with a new strain of TB in the workplace. The new strain is multidrug-resistant tuberculosis or MDR-TB. This organism is resistant to more than one and up to nine drugs currently available for the treatment of TB.

The TB bacilli are easily transmitted in aerosols from coughs and their waxy coat enables them to survive in the environment for years. The route of airborne disease transmission can be traced from patient to health care worker or coworkers or family. One of the prime concerns with MDR-TB is the speed with which it can kill.

Emphasis is placed on the safety items discussed previously, such as the design of the laboratory, the proper use of BSCs, proper performance of laboratory procedures on initial specimens for TB, the safe manipulation of specimen to media and slides, and later when subculturing and disposing of the contaminated materials.

This organism is classified at BSL 3, one level higher than other mycobacteria. *M. tuberculosis* is thought to be capable of producing an infection following inhalation of a single viable organism. Gowning would always be required for this work. The safe work practices specified for the BSC should be strictly observed when working with this organism. In the larger picture there should be specific education and skin testing for employees working with TB.

A new inclusion in the rules for TB control is the use of respirators. Respirators were included in our list of PPE. Those for use in the TB laboratory would be the negative-pressure respirators with high-efficiency particulate airflow (**HEPA**) filters (and coded purple by leading manufacturers). The powered air-purifying positive-pressure respirators are available for special circumstances. The "who" and "when" of the use of respirators by laboratory personnel is still the subject of discussion, awaiting the publication of new OSHA guidelines to update those of 1993.

The laboratories handling TB cultures should review

the three basic areas of biosafety and containment: (1) laboratory practice and technique, (2) primary barriers or safety equipment, and (3) secondary barriers or facility design. For many laboratories, the engineering controls are adequate to contain aerosols without resorting to special PPE.

### Hazardous Waste Disposal

The clinical laboratory generates most of the hazardous waste in a health care facility and therefore must be aware of how to handle and how to dispose of the waste. The hazardous waste can injure the people who handle it and it can pollute the environment.

There are guidelines for the disposal of clinical laboratory waste as well as federal, state, and local regulations. Federal laws apply to clean air, clean water, solid waste disposal, and the transportation of hazardous waste among others. State regulations on hazardous waste in the EPA arena are equal to or greater than the federal regulations. This is true of dealing with radioactive materials and incinerators also. Local regulations cover sanitary sewage (liquid wastes from the laboratory put into the sewer), fire codes (storage of flammable materials), transportation of waste, incinerator emissions, and sanitary landfills.

Hospitals are required to have a waste disposal guide. NCCLS Document GP5-P is a good reference for information on this subject.

**Waste.** In the laboratory there are five general groups of waste: (1) chemical, (2) infectious, (3) radioactive, (4) sharps, and (5) nonhazardous. Materials from the laboratory that do not fit into groups 1 through 4 are put into the last group, nonhazardous. The name of the group may be misleading because it is not without risk.

Most of the hazardous waste by volume is chemical or radioactive. Medical or infectious waste is of concern to the people who come in contact with it along its route from generation to disposal. This could be considered the health problems or realistic problems. The environmental or perceived problems would relate to the public's idea of health risks. Although there have been cases reported in the news of exposure to medical waste, such as used syringes on the East Coast beaches, there has been no documentation of actual disease resulting from that contact.

There has not been an accepted definition of infectious waste yet, though it can be thought of in general terms as medical waste that can produce disease. The EPA would include specimens from laboratories; cultures of organisms and their containers; tissues and blood removed during autopsy, biopsy, or surgery; blood and blood products; contaminated needles; scalpel blades and broken glass; and fluids and excreta from patients with communicable diseases (NCCLS, GP5-A, 1986). The individual institution would have specific provisions for each of the categories that they would deal with, and must comply with state and local regulations also.

**Segregation.** Handling of infectious waste requires PPE, usually with utility gloves that are selected for that category of waste being handled. *The various categories of waste should be kept segregated and in appropriate containers. This makes it easier to decontaminate and much less expensive to dispose of if each is separate.* This also means NOT putting paper towels in medical waste containers. Because sharps figure prominently in laboratory accidents and exposure to hepatitis B and HIV, they have their own rigid containers to protect health care workers.

Labeling is vital when dealing with infectious material. The biohazard symbol should be on red bags and containers. Other labeling may be required by local, state, or federal regulations. Packaging must be sufficient to contain the infectious material be it liquid or solid, sharp or soft. The packaging would have to withstand compacting, tossing, and autoclaving.

**Treatment.** Treatment of infectious waste can be handled in one of several methods. The goal of the treatment, whatever the method, is to reduce the pathogenic organisms to a level below that which can transmit disease. New technologies are being introduced for treatment. They must meet the regulatory standards and the institution's needs and budget.

An institution must also plan for storage, transportation, and disposal of infectious waste. The facility may employ an outside contractor for these duties, particularly the last two. The options for disposal are subject to regulations and to owner requirements. The major options are landfill, incineration, and sanitary sewer. Each of these involves attention to protection of the workers performing any of these tasks and the concerns of the neighbors near any of these sites. Workers involved in any aspect of infectious waste treatment should be educated in the techniques of proper handwashing, barrier protection, sterilization, disinfection, decontamination, and Standard Precautions.

The incidence of accidents with sharps and spills is higher for the workers who collect infectious waste within the facilities and those who transport it to the treatment site. Accidents with infectious waste would be handled as accidents in the laboratory are handled.

## SUMMARY

▸ Standard Precautions from CDC and the Bloodborne Pathogens Standard from OSHA are the primary controls governing practice when health care workers are handling specimens.

▸ All facilities must meet specific biosafety levels depending on the microbiology work done there.

▸ There are published guidelines for working with potential pathogens.

▸ Handwashing and personal protective equipment should be used as well as other protection techniques to create a safe laboratory environment.

▸ Training on infection control plans is an important means of avoiding the spread of disease inside a health care facility.

▸ The collection, handling, transporting, and storing of patient specimens have implications for the integrity of the specimens and the safety of the laboratorians.

## Review Questions

1. When investigating infections, the route of transmission would be of prime importance. The most common routes of transmission in the laboratory are:
   a. breathing, bleeding, and food poisoning.
   b. chemicals, radiation, and laboratory animals.
   c. eating, drinking, smoking, and applying cosmetics.
   d. oral, respiratory, percutaneous, and cutaneous.

2. As indicated by the focus of regulations, the greatest potential risks for laboratorians are associated with the:
   a. improper use of disinfectants.
   b. processing of primary clinical specimens.
   c. failure to wash hands frequently.
   d. disposing of contaminated materials.

3. The CDC-NIH has issued guidelines and OSHA has issued the *Standard*. The microbiologist should know that the:
   a. guidelines duplicate the information in the *Standard*.
   b. *Standard* contains items on ergonomic safety.
   c. *Standard* is a federal regulation requiring mandatory compliance.
   d. guidelines place all biohazards into one specific BSL.

4. Encouraging laboratory workers to use safety equipment and personal protective equipment (PPE) is an important part of good laboratory practices. The most effective way to promote this use is:
   a. improvement of available equipment.
   b. education sessions on the devices.
   c. regulation and enforcement on them.
   d. promotion of fear by the instructor.

5. All health care institutions should have a written policy for:
   a. a needle recapping technique.
   b. spills of blood and body fluids.
   c. the areas in which HIV and health care practitioners can work.
   d. the disposal of used gowns.

6. The Centers for Disease Control and Prevention (CDC) has published lists of organisms and classified them in biologic safety levels (BSLs). Two organisms of concern, human immunodeficiency virus (HIV) and *Mycobacterium tuberculosis* (TB), would be dealt with at the greater security of BSL:
   a. 1
   b. 2
   c. 3
   d. 4

7. "Sharps" is a category covering needles, scalpel blades, fragile glass, and pipets. Needles are not to be recapped or bent before disposal. To avoid transmission of HBV or HIV, all sharps are to be placed in:
   a. red molded plastic boxes.
   b. cardboard boxes with liners.
   c. black polyethylene bags.
   d. open steel autoclave trays.

8. Standard Precautions include the use of gloves when appropriate:
   1. for blood and body fluids.
   2. with nonintact skin.
   3. when answering a laboratory phone.
   4. for opening laboratory doors.
   5. while training in new procedures.
   a. 1, 2, 3, 4, 5
   b. 1, 2, 5
   c. 3, 4, 5
   d. 2, 3, 4

9. Infectious droplets carrying tubercle bacilli are easily passed from a coughing patient or accidental breakage of liquid suspensions of TB. Consequently the infection rate with TB among clinical and laboratory personnel is almost eight times higher than the general population. Good safety practices when dealing with potential TB situations involve:
   1. educating and skin testing of employees.
   2. use of respirators when working.
   3. vaccination of new employees.
   4. proper directional airflow in the laboratory.
   a. 1, 2, 3, 4
   b. 2, 3, 4
   c. 1, 2, 4
   d. 2 and 4

10. When cleaning a spilled culture in the laboratory, one should wear a gown and gloves. To decontaminate the spill area which solution would be best to use?
   a. Hot water and detergent
   b. 1:10 dilution of sodium hypochlorite
   c. 50% ethyl alcohol
   d. Ethylene oxide

## CASE STUDY

A microbiologist, wearing contact lenses, failed to protect his eyes with safety glasses and had a speck of preserved fecal specimen enter his eye. He removed his contact lens, washed out the affected eye, and replaced the lens. Several hours later his eye became irritated. He again removed his contact lens and washed his eye, but this time he did not replace the lens. By the following day, his eye became very painful and he reported to Employee Health. He was quickly hospitalized with a critical eye injury.

The doctor reported that the severity of the injury may have been greatly lessened if the technologist had obtained medical assistance promptly instead of trying to treat himself and if the contact lens had not been replaced after the first washing.

### Questions

1. The technologist was working with a preserved fecal specimen. What safety items should he have been using?

2. Knowing the nature of the specimen what two types of injury would you suspect when his eye became irritated?

3. The doctor in Employee Health made some suggestions about the eye injury. What other suggestions would you make?

▶ **REFERENCES & RECOMMENDED READING**

Accident Case Histories. (1974). *Safety in the chemical laboratory.* 116–121.

Allen, J. E. (1967). An exploratory study of the attitudes of laboratory workers toward accident prevention. *Safety in the Chemical Laboratory* (3rd printing, March 1974). Reprinted from *Journal of Chemical Education,* Easton, PA: American Chemical Society.

Brown, E. M., & Simione, F. P. (Eds.). (1994). *ATCC guide to packaging and shipping of biological materials,* Rockville, MD: American Type Culture Collection.

CDC and NIH. (1993). *Biosafety in microbiological and biomedical laboratories* (3rd ed.). Washington, DC: U.S. Department of Health and Human Services.

Denys, G. A. (1992, Fall). Safe handling and management of infectious laboratory materials. *Lab O: Microbiology News & Ideas, 3,* 1–2.

Fleming, D. O., Richardson, J. H., Tulis, J. J., & Vesley, D. (Eds.). (1995). *Laboratory safety: Principles and practices.* Washington, DC: ASM Press.

Furr, A. K. (Ed.). (1990). *CRC handbook of laboratory safety* (3rd ed.). Boca Raton, FL: CRC Press.

*Healthcare environmental management system.* (Vol. 1–3). (1995). Plymouth Meeting, PA: ECRI.

Isenberg, H. D. (Ed. in Chief). Murray, P. R., Baron, E. J., Pfaller, M. A., Tenover, F. C., & Yolken, R. H. (Eds.). (1995). *Clinical microbiology procedures handbook.* Washington, DC: ASM Press.

Kubica, G. P. (1990, June 1). Your tuberculosis laboratory: Are you really safe from infection? *Clinical Microbiology Newsletter, 12.* 85–87.

McGowan, J. E., Jr., & MacLowry, J. D. (1995). Addressing regulatory issues in the clinical microbiology laboratory. In P. R. Murray, E. J. Baron, M. A. Pfaller, F. C. Tenover, & R. H. Yolken (Eds.). *Manual of clinical microbiology* (pp. 67–74). Washington, DC: ASM Press.

National Committee for Clinical Laboratory Standards. (1991). *Protection of laboratory workers from infectious disease transmitted by blood, body fluids, and tissue—Second edition: Tentative guideline.* (No. M29-T2). Villanova, PA: Author.

National Committee for Clinical Laboratory Standards. (1993). *Clinical laboratory waste management: Approved guideline, December 1993.* (No. GP5-A). Villanova, PA: Author.

National Committee for Clinical Laboratory Standards. (1994). *Clinical laboratory safety: Tentative guideline, April 1994.* (No. GP17-T). Villanova, PA: Author.

National Committee for Clinical Laboratory Standards. (1994). *Procedures for the handling and transport of diagnostic specimens and etiologic agents—Third edition: Approved standard, May 1994* (No. H5-A3). Villanova, PA: Author.

Occupational exposure to formaldehyde: Final Rule. *Fed. Reg.* Vol. 57, No. 102 (1992) (to be codified at 29 C.F.R. Part 1910).

Occupational exposures to Hazardous chemicals in laboratories: Final Rule. *Fed. Reg.* Vol. 55, No. 21 (1990) (to be codified at 29 C.F.R. Part 1910).

Phillips, G. B. (1964). Microbiological hazards in the laboratory. *Safety in the chemical laboratory,* 98–104. Reprinted from *Journal of Chemical Education* (3rd printing, March 1974). Easton, PA: American Chemical Society.

Rudman, S. V., Jarus, C., Ward, K. A., & Arnold, D. M. (1993). Safety in the student laboratory: A national survey of university-based programs. *Laboratory Medicine, 24,* 281–285.

Shapton, D. A., & Board, R. G. (Eds.). (1972). *Safety in microbiology.* (The Society for Applied Bacteriology Technical Series No. 6). London: Academic Press.

Strain, B. A., & Groschel, D. H. M. (1995). Laboratory safety and infectious waste management. In P. R. Murray, E. J. Baron, M. A. Pfaller, F. C. Tenover, & R. H. Yolken (Eds.), *Manual of clinical microbiology* (pp. 75–85). Washington, DC: ASM Press.

Use caution when substance abuse is suspected. (1995, October). [Management Q & A]. *Medical Laboratory Observer, 27,* 70.

# CHAPTER 4
# Immunologic and Molecular Techniques

Helen Viscount, PhD

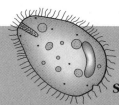

## Microbes in the News
### Southland's Burger Fans Take Tainted Meat Scare in Stride

The U.S. Department of Agriculture pressured Hudson Foods, Inc. of Rogers, Arkansas to close after hamburger patties contaminated with *Escherichia coli* 0157:H7 poisoned 16 Colorado residents. The processing plant recalled 25 million pounds of meat from the market. Nonetheless, the tainted meat scare did not appear to change the eating habits of most of the Southland's residents. Many Orange County burger fans felt confident because none of the tainted beef and beef products were sold in Southern California.

*E. coli* 0157 lives in the intestines of healthy cattle. Meat is contaminated when cattle are slaughtered. Also, cows shed the bacteria and contaminate the soil. The bacteria have been found in raw milk, roast beef, and salami. The most common food source is ground beef. Public health officials are alarmed that *E. coli* 0157 is found in raw produce—especially lettuce. They speculate that the reason is the increased use of cow manure as fertilizer. The outbreak in 1996 traced to fresh, unpasteurized apple juice produced by Odwalla Co. resulted in nationwide recall and

indefinite suspension of the production of apple juice. *E. coli* 0157:H7 isolates cultured from a previously unopened container of Odwalla apple juice had a DNA "fingerprint" pattern (restriction fragment length polymorphism) that is indistinguishable from case-related isolates.

*E. coli* 0157:H7 is diagnosed by testing stool samples. Laboratories screen samples on sorbitol-enriched MacConkey plates. *E. coli* 0157:H7 does not ferment sorbitol. Suspected colonies are confirmed by agglutination with latex-conjugated 0157 antisera. Further serotype confirmation is obtained by typing with antiserum against H7 flagellar antigen. An alternate method is the use of a direct immunofluorescent assay of 5% bleach-treated stool with 0157 lipopolysaccharide antiserum.

(*Los Angeles Times,* Orange County Edition, 23 August 1997 *MMWR 45,* 44. Noel, J., & Boedeker, E. (1997). *Enterohemorrhagic Escherichia coli: A family of emerging pathogens digestive diseases.* Basel: Karger. Public Health Fact Sheet, Massachusetts Department of Public Health, January 1997)

## KEY TERMS

Antigen
Antibody
Immunity
Serology

## LEARNING OBJECTIVES

**Upon successful completion of this chapter, the student should be able to:**

1. Discuss the features of the immune response.
2. Describe the importance of immunologic and molecular techniques in the diagnosis of infectious diseases.

3. Describe the principles of the commonly used and the more recent diagnostic procedures.
4. Enumerate the applications of the various detection techniques.

## INTRODUCTION

This chapter provides the principles and applications of immunologic and molecular techniques in the diagnosis of infectious diseases. It presents a survey of a number of methods for the detection of antigens, antibodies, and microorganisms in clinical specimens. It is divided into two parts: the first part covers immunologic aspects of diagnosis and the second part describes molecular diagnostics.

## GENERAL FEATURES OF THE IMMUNE RESPONSE

### Definition of Immunity

**Immunity** means protection from disease. Many of the mechanisms of resistance to infections are also

involved in a person's response to noninfectious substance. Hence, a more accurate definition of immunity is a reaction to harmful agents such as microbes and macromolecules like proteins (see Figure 4-1).

### The Immune System

The elements of the immune system are the molecules and cells responsible for resistance from foreign substances. Leukocytes or white blood cells (WBCs) in the bloodstream and in tissues comprise the body's basic defense mechanism. Depending on their appearance and functions, the WBCs are called monocytes (macrophages), granulocytes, and lymphocytes (see Figure 4-2).

The macrophage or reticuloendothelial system is distributed in the lymph nodes, liver, spleen, and bone marrow. The phagocytic cells in tissues are called

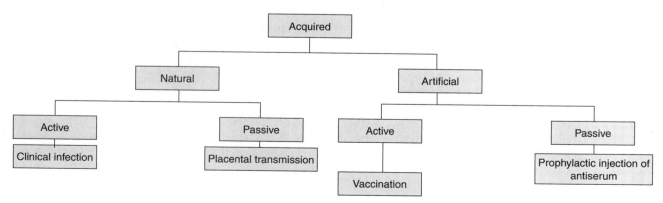

**FIGURE 4-1** Types of acquired immunity.

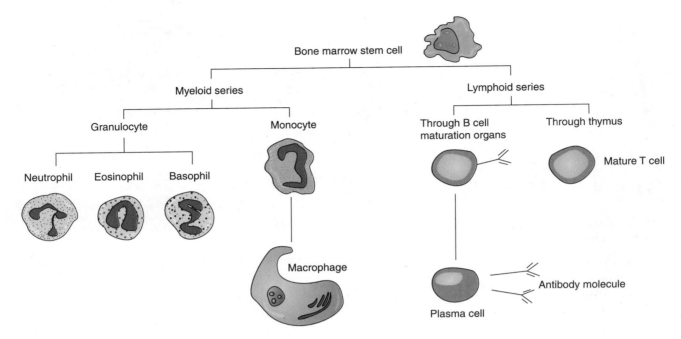

**FIGURE 4-2** Schematic of the cells of the immune system.

macrophages and those in the bloodstream are known as monocytes. These cells ingest microbes and other particulate materials harmful to the host. Macrophages collect and remove cellular debris and tissue-breakdown products.

Granulocytes contain distinctive granules in the cytoplasm. Based on the affinity of the granules with histologic dyes, three kinds of granulocytes are seen. On Wright-stained blood smears, basophils have coarse blue-black granules, eosinophils contain coarse red granules; and neutrophils contain small lavender granules in the cytoplasm. Neutrophils or polymorphonuclear cells (PMNs) are the predominant circulating WBCs. PMNs play an important role in acute inflammation and in phagocytosis.

The lymphoid system is widely distributed in the body and is mainly concentrated in lymph nodes, the spleen, and the thymus. The major cells of the lymphoid tissues are the lymphocytes, which consist of two cell types, the T and B cells.

The thymus-dependent lymphocytes or T cells originate from the bone marrow, mature in the thymus, and then circulate in the blood and lymph. T cells are functionally subdivided into three subsets. T cells that attack or lyse infected cells are called killer or cytotoxic cells. T-helper cells initiate the action of cytotoxic cells and are necessary for some antibody response. T-suppressor cells block the activity of T-helper cells. T cells regulate cell-mediated immune responses such as infections from intracellular bacteria, fungi, and viruses. T cells live for many years.

B lymphocytes live for only 1 or 2 weeks. They are thymus independent. B cells are involved in antibody-mediated immune response (humoral immunity). Tasked

with distinguishing foreign substances and thus preventing entry of harmful agents, the immune system makes proteins called **antibodies**. An antibody must discriminate among foreign and "self" molecules. Highly specific antibodies are produced against toxins and microbes. A substance that elicits antibody production against itself is known as an **antigen** or immunogen. The substance must be foreign to the individual or the body must not recognize it as "self." Usually, antigens have a molecular weight of 10,000. Most are proteins but some are complex carbohydrates.

Antibodies or immunoglobulins (Ig) are multichain glycoproteins. The basic immunoglobulin unit is a structure consisting of four polypeptide chains (see Figure 4-3). Two of the paired chain have a greater molecular weight (heavy or H chain) and the other two are light or L chain. The heavy chain is linked to the light chain by a single disulfide bond. Together, the two chains are represented as a Y-shaped molecule. Some enzymes can cleave the molecule into three pieces. Two of the pieces contain the antibody-combining site located at the amino terminal of the molecule. They are, therefore, termed the antigen-binding sites or "Fab" fragments (fragment, antigen binding). The opposite end of the heavy chain or the stem of the Y is called the "Fc" fragment (fragment, crystalline) because it has a tendency to crystallize. This third fragment mediates complement fixation, placental transport, and binding to host tissues. The antigen-binding site in the Fab fragment is a variable region that allows each immunoglobulin molecule to recognize specific antigens. The other end is a constant region; that is, the amino acid sequence is not highly variable.

Immunoglobulins are classified according to the

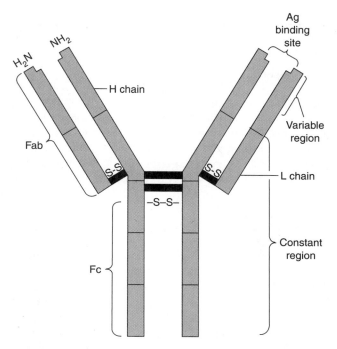

**FIGURE 4-3** Schematic diagram of immunoglobulin. Fab (antigen binding site), Fc (complement binding site), S-S (disulfide binding site).

protein composition of the heavy chain. The five classes of immunoglobulins are distinct from one another antigenically, structurally, and in their biologic properties. Plasma contains IgA, IgG, IgD, IgE, and IgM. Immunoglobulins that respond to a given antigen are composed of a heterogeneous population. The classes and distribution of immunoglobulins in plasma depend on factors such as the age and genetic makeup of the individual, the type of antigen, and the site of antibody formation.

The dominant antibody in blood is IgG. IgG promotes uptake of microorganisms by immune cells and is involved in long-term disease protection. IgM is the first antibody produced in response to infection and is involved in complement fixation and destruction of bacteria. IgA is secreted in mucous membranes. It protects the gastrointestinal and respiratory tracts from infection. IgE is associated with the allergic response and defense against parasites. IgD is a minor blood component found on the surface of some lymphocytes.

B cells have receptors on the cell surface that recognize and bind specific antigens. Activation of a B cell stimulates the proliferation of resting B cells, which are then transformed into plasma cells, the cells that make antibodies. This reaction is the primary immune response. Some of the progeny of the activated B cell become "memory cells" that remember the antigenic determinant the parent B cell was exposed to. These cells establish a reservoir of cells primed for immunoglobulin production when the same antigen reappears.

This is the secondary immune response. The antigen–antibody reaction is highly specific. An antigen promotes the production of antibody only against itself and, likewise, an antibody acts only against the antigen that promoted its development.

## SEROLOGIC DIAGNOSIS OF INFECTIOUS DISEASES

Because of the specificity of the antigen–antibody reaction, one or the other can be identified and measured if either is known. **Serology** is the study of antibodies and their reactions with antigens. These tests are valuable in establishing the etiologic agents of disease and in determining a patient's recovery from infection. The concentration of serum antibody or antibody titer changes in the course of infectious disease. To distinguish antibody levels associated with a current infection from an old one, at least two specimens are required. The first is obtained at disease onset and the second one 2 weeks later. Sera from both specimens are tested together to determine a rise in antibody titer. A fourfold rise in antibody concentration is considered significant and means that the organism being tested is the cause of infection.

## PRINCIPLES AND METHODOLOGIES OF IMMUNOLOGIC TESTS

### Agglutination

An agglutination reaction involves clumping of cellular antigens by corresponding antibodies. Soluble antigens attached to surfaces of insoluble matrices such as red blood cells (RBCs) and polystyrene latex spheres become visible as clumps when reacted with their cognate antibodies.

### Complement Fixation

Some antigen–antibody complexes have the ability to fix or combine with complement. In this procedure, an antigen or an antibody can be detected using an indicator system consisting of sensitized sheep RBCs (RBCs coated with antibodies made against them). If a serum sample is suspected of having an antibody of interest, it is heated to 56°C (to inactivate complement), serially diluted, and added to a known quantity of commercially prepared antigen and complement. The indicator system is added to the mixture. If the serum contains antibody specific to the antigen, it will form a complex with the antigen and fix complement such that no free complement remains to lyse the sensitized RBCs. A positive complement fixation test is indicated by absence of hemolysis.

## Enzyme Immunoassay (EIA)

An antibody or an antigen can be coupled to a chromogenic enzyme and the resulting complex can retain both immunologic and enzymatic activity. Several assays are available to detect and quantitate antigens and antibodies. The indirect method can be used to detect antibody (see Figure 4-4). An antigen specific for the antibody being measured is first adsorbed to a solid phase such as polystyrene beads, microtiter well plates, or tubes, and unbound antigen is washed off. Serum containing specific antibody is added, incubated, and excess antibody is removed. Then, an enzyme-labeled antispecies antibody is added and incubated. Unbound conjugate is removed by washing. The enzyme substrate is added and the reaction is terminated after the color reaction occurs. The reaction is measured spectrophotometrically.

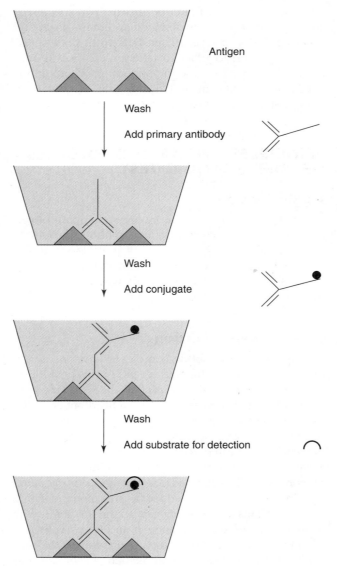

**FIGURE 4-4** Enzyme-linked immunosorbent assay.

## Immunodiffusion

Double diffusion or the Ouchterlony test is based on the principle that on diffusion of antigen and antibody through a semisolid medium, they form stable complexes. First, an agar pour plate is made. After the agar solidifies, circular wells are made in the surface. Antiserum is placed in one well and antigens are made in other wells. The plate is incubated. Lines of precipitate form where antigenic components react with homologous antibodies. Distinct precipitin lines between the wells containing antibodies and antigens are seen with indirect light. Lines of identity, partial identity, or nonidentity are possible depending on the relatedness of antibody and antigens (see Figure 4-5).

The precipitin pattern of reactions of identity develop when pure antigens are placed in wells adjacent to a centrally located homologous antibody. The lines of diffusion fuse into an arc. When different antigens are allowed to react with an unrelated antibody, the precipitin lines cross. When heterologous antigens are made to react to an antiserum, cross-reactions occur. In lines of partial identity, the antigen homologous to the antibody forms a distinct arc and the antibody will form a spur toward the cross-reacting antigen.

## Immunofluorescence

The procedure involves labeling or conjugating a fluorescent dye, such as flourescein or rhodamine, to serum proteins. These conjugates are used to detect homologous antigens in tissue sections or smear preparations. The simplest method is a direct antibody technique. A specimen containing antigen is fixed to a slide. A couple of drops of a known concentration of labeled antibody are applied to the specimen and the slide is incubated. Excess antibody is washed off. The slide is dried and examined under an ultraviolet microscope.

## Precipitation

Precipitin reactions involve binding of precipitin antibodies with soluble antigens. Where optimal proportions of antibody and antigen are reached, a precipitate forms.

## Enhanced Chemiluminescence (ECL)

Antibodies labeled with horseradish peroxidase (HRP) can be detected by the enhanced chemiluminescence reaction. Chemiluminescence is the chemical production of light. One of the most studied systems is the HRP-hydrogen peroxide catalyzed oxidation of luminol in alkaline condition. The oxidized luminol is in an excited state and decays to its ground state by a

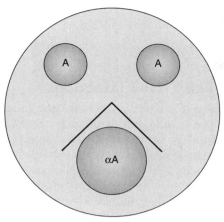

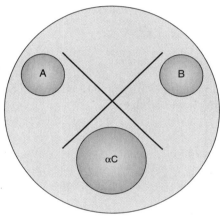

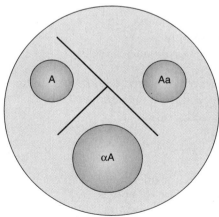

**FIGURE 4-5** Reaction patterns in immunodiffusion. A, B, Aa are antigens; αA and αC are antibodies. In (1) identical precipitin lines form between A and αA and where lines intersect, they fuse. In (2) independent lines cross between A and αC and B and αB, indicating a distinct reaction from A versus B with αC. (3) αA reacts with both A and Aa, but the lines that form do not cross completely. The spur shows shared determinants between A and Aa.

pathway that emits light. In enhanced chemiluminescence, the time of light emission is extended by oxidizing luminol in the presence of enhancers such as phenol. Maximal light emission is at 428 nm and is detected by exposure to autoradiography (x-ray) film.

## IDENTIFICATION OF BACTERIA BY IMMUNOLOGIC METHODS

Traditional techniques for the diagnosis of infectious diseases have depended on culture methods and serologic tests. The use of monoclonal antibodies has become increasingly important in the direct detection of microbial antigens in clinical samples and the identification of etiologic agents or a specific component of the agent after it has been cultured.

### Gastrointestinal and Hepatobiliary Diseases

Hepatitis A is an acute liver infection caused by a picorna virus. Diagnosis is confirmed by the presence of IgM anti-hepatitis A virus antibodies. IgGs persist for a long time and their presence signifies immunity to infection.

Hepatitis B virus (HBV) infection is transmitted by the parenteral or placental route. Individuals at risk include recipients of blood or blood products, drug addicts, and infants born to HBV-infected mothers. Serum diagnostic profiles in this infection vary according to the length and clinical outcome of the disease. Several HBV antigens and antibodies can be detected by enzyme-linked immunosorbent assay (ELISA). Viral antigen and antibody titers vary during the course of the infection.

*Salmonella* species cause enteric diseases. They can be speciated by agglutination reactions. *Salmonella typhi* is an invasive pathogen and is the only *Salmonella* species that is encapsulated. Circulating antibody against the capsular antigen is not protective but provides a marker of infection.

### Meningitis

*Haemophilus influenzae* is the most prevalent pathogen among several species of *Haemophilus*. It is a respiratory bacterium that causes pneumonia or disseminated infection. *H. influenzae* type b can be detected from the cerebrospinal fluid specimen by agglutination using anti-type b antibodies.

*Neisseria meningitidis* is a gram-negative coccus that is normally found in the pharynx. Patients deficient in some components of complement are susceptible to recurrent neisserial infection. Antibodies directed against the organism's capsular polysaccharides aid in the detection of this organism.

## Respiratory Infections

*Streptococcus pyogenes* is the most important cause of bacterial pharyngitis. It produces cytophatic proteins, O and S, that inhibit phagocytosis and subsequent killing by WBCs. Degradative enzymes such as deoxyribonucleases (DNAse), which enhance the pathogenicity of the organism, are also produced. Serologic tests for anti-streptolysin O and anti-DNAse are used to detect antibodies against this gram-positive bacterium.

*Streptococcus pneumoniae* contains a polysaccharide capsule that inhibits phagocytosis by macrophages and PMNs. Opsonization of bacteria with antibody and complement is necessary for effective phagocytosis. Agglutination reactions are used to detect the encapsulated bacteria.

*Legionella pneumophila* and related strains are intracellular parasites of macrophages. Antibodies to serogroup antigens are produced during the course of an infection and are detected by immunofluorescence.

## Wound and Tissue Infections

*Staphylococcus aureus* is perhaps the most prevalent pathogen in skin and tissue infections. The functional capability of granulocytes protects against infection against this bacterium because many antibodies produced against it by the host are not protective. Most staphylococci have capsular polysaccharides that are identified in agglutination tests.

*Pseudomonas aeruginosa* is one of the most clinically important gram-negative rods. Serotyping methods are used to distinguish *Pseudomonas* for epidemiologic purposes and vaccine investigations.

## SUMMARY

- ▶ Immunity is a reaction to harmful agents such as microbes.
- ▶ An antigen is a substance that elicits antibody production against itself.

- ▶ Serology is the study of antibodies and their reactions with antigens.

## Review Questions

1. B lymphocytes have a life span:
   a. that lasts as long as the antigen remains in the system.
   b. of one to two weeks.
   c. of several years.
   d. that is dependent upon the age of the individual.

2. The role of IgG in the immune system is:
   a. to participate in complement fixation.
   b. promotion of the uptake of microorganisms by immune cells.
   c. to cause lysis of pathogenic fungi.
   d. a and b are roles of IgG.

3. Phagocytic cells in tissues are known as:
   a. leukocytes.
   b. lymphocytes.
   c. erythrocytes.
   d. macrophages.

4. When stained with Wright's stain which of the following contain coarse red granules?
   a. Neutrophils
   b. Basophils
   c. Eosinophils
   d. Polymorphonuclear cells

5. When stained with Wright's stain which of the following contain coarse blue-black granules?
   a. Neutrophils
   b. Basophils
   c. Eosinophils
   d. Polymorphonuclear cells

6. B cells recognize and bind specific antigens with:
   a. receptors on their surface.
   b. pseudopods.
   c. pili.
   d. capsules.

7. The test that results in lines of identity, partial identity, or non-identity is the:
   a. complement fixation test.
   b. Ouchterlony test.
   c. precipitation test.
   d. immunofluorescence test.

8. The polysaccharide capsule of *Streptococcus pneumoniae* inhibits:
   a. phagocytosis by macrophages.
   b. binding of antibodies.
   c. complement fixation.
   d. release of granules from basophils.

**9.** IgA:

    a.  promotes phagocytosis of antigen by monocytes.

    b.  is the first antibody produced in response to an infection.

    c.  is the most prevalent antibody in the system.

    d.  is secreted in mucous membranes.

**10.** IgE:

    a.  is produced in response to some parasitic infections.

    b.  coats microorganisms preventing them from attaching to host tissues.

    c.  promotes phagocytosis of antigen by macrophages.

    d.  None of the above.

▶ **REFERENCES & RECOMMENDED READING**

Abbas, A., Lichtman, A., & Pober, A. (1991). Cellular and molecular immunology. In M. Wonsiewicz (Ed.). Philadelphia, PA: Saunders.

Chart, H. (Ed.). (1994). *Methods in practical laboratory bacteriology.* Boca Raton, FL: CRC Press.

Gerhardt, P., Murray, R., Wood, W., & Krieg, N. (Eds.). (1994). *Methods for general and molecular microbiology.* Washington, DC: American Society for Microbiology.

Persing, D., Smithe, T., Tenover, F., & White, T. (Eds.). (1993). *Diagnostic molecular microbiology.* Washington, DC: American Society for Microbiology.

Roitt, I., Brostoff, J., & Male, D. (1996). *Immunology* (4th ed.). London: Mosby.

Smith, A. (1985). *Principles of microbiology* (10th ed.). St. Louis: Mosby.

Steinbergh, M., Guyden, J., Calhoun, D., Staiano-Coico, L., & Coico, R. (1993). *Recombinant DNA technology.* Englewood Cliffs, NJ: PTR Prentice Hall.

Stites, D., Terr, A., & Parslow, T. (Eds.). (1994). *Basic and clinical immunology* (8th ed.). East Norwalk, CT: Appleton & Lange.

Tenover, F. (1988). Diagnostic deoxyribonucleic acid probes for infectious diseases. *Clinical Microbiology Reviews,* 1(1), 82–101.

Wistreich, G., & Lechtman, M. (1980). *Microbiology* (3rd ed.). Encino, CA: Glencoe Publishing.

# CHAPTER 5

# Quality Assurance in the Clinical Microbiology Laboratory

Kathy Nollar, MT (ASCP)

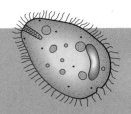

## Microbes in the News

### Resistant Germ

A staph germ that is practically impervious to the most powerful antibiotic around has shown up for the second time in the United States in a patient in New Jersey. The strain of *Staphylococcus aureus* bacteria, like the one reported in August 1997 in Michigan, showed an intermediate level of resistance to vancomycin—one step from immunity according to the U.S. Centers for Disease Control and Prevention. Doctors claim that common germs have become resistant to drugs due to the overuse of antibiotics.

(Source: *USA Today*, Monday, September 8, 1997)

**INTRODUCTION**

**COMPONENTS OF A QUALITY ASSURANCE PROGRAM IN MICROBIOLOGY**
Quality Assurance of Specimens
Quality Assurance of Media and Reagents

Quality Assurance of Equipment and Instrumentation
Quality Assurance of Methods and Procedures

**REPORTING AND USE OF QUALITY ASSURANCE DATA**
Record Retention
Trends

## KEY TERMS

In vivo
In vitro
Quality assurance

Stasis
Trends

## LEARNING OBJECTIVES

**Upon successful completion of this chapter, the student should be able to:**

1. List components of a quality assurance program.
2. Devise a plan to assess the quality of specimen collection.

3. Explain how personnel practices influence quality assurance.

# INTRODUCTION

Medical laboratory professionals do not generally work in close contact with patients. This distance can be a mixed blessing. Being *too* far removed from our patients introduces a risk. A risk of eventually finding the work dull and unrewarding and of forgetting the patients' needs and well-being. The rewards of being part of the patient care team are lost. Laboratory employees must visit a patient, draw blood specimens, or volunteer at a wound care clinic to work closely with patients. These activities bring one back to the focus of laboratory medicine. Ultimately it is the attitude toward the profession that influences the quality of the product. The quality of patient care is hard to quantitate, but not impossible to measure. This chapter discusses the tangible aspects of **quality assurance**.

## COMPONENTS OF A QUALITY ASSURANCE PROGRAM IN MICROBIOLOGY

The several components of quality assurance in microbiology include specimens, media, reagents, equipment, instrumentation, and personnel.

## Quality Assurance of Specimens

The clinical specimen is the conduit through which organisms are transferred from the patient to the laboratory. The organisms are taken from a living host to an artificial environment. It is the process in which the organisms change from **in vivo** to **in vitro**. The transfer process should be short in duration and under controlled conditions to hold the numbers and kinds of organisms in **stasis**. The quality of the specimen greatly influences the quality of the results. Concise instruction to the personnel responsible for collection is essential for consistency and accuracy in the culture process. Ideally, therapy is administered immediately after the cultures are taken. If cultures must be taken after antibiotic treatment, the results may be adversely affected. Adding antibiotics to the environment can stimulate a biochemical change. Therefore, the quality of collection is critical because recollection may not yield the same results as preantibiotic cultures. Volume and site preparation will also influence the outcome. Instructions to collection personnel, usually the nurse or physician, should include:

- How to prepare the culture site
- How to avoid contamination
- Volume recommended and the minimum required
- Labeling requirements
- Appropriate requisition form and its use

- Packaging and delivery information
- Criteria for rejection of specimens

The laboratory should provide appropriate swabs and/or containers to the submitter. This *ensures the quality* by controlling the supplies. Supplies may include mailing containers or hazardous material bags, both of which are understandably required for the protection of the delivery personnel. Information that is required on the requisition form includes:

- Patient name
- Physician(s) name(s)
- Date and time of collection
- Medical record number
- Tests to be performed
- Pertinent specimen information

## Quality Assurance of Media and Reagents

Over the years stable strains of microbiology organisms have been developed that give constant reactions. These are maintained by the American Type Culture Collection (ATCC) and are identified as ATCC strains. They are used to test the reliability of the media and reagents used in the laboratory. For example, ATCC #29213 *Staphylococcus aureus* is always coagulase positive. Every day the coagulase reagent is put into use, this organism is run first to make sure a positive reaction is obtained. Likewise an organism that is a known coagulase-negative organism is run to confirm that the reagent has not been contaminated. Only then can the identity of the *patient's* results be trusted. Laboratories purchase organisms from the collection in a lyophilized form. Freeze drying has proved an effective way to ship and hold the organisms in stasis. A rehydrated pellet or swab is streaked to a plate on arrival. A fresh culture plate is streaked out each week to keep the strain alive in the microbiology laboratory. Plates are incubated at 37°C to begin growth, then kept at room temperature to decelerate the growth so it can be used for a week. Several organisms are kept this way, the number depending on what variety of daily quality control tests. Some cultures are kept in the lyophilized state and rehydrated monthly or by lot number to be tested when shipments of reagents arrive.

Records of the quality control procedures on all tests performed are kept, reviewed by a supervisor, and retained. The length of retention time is basically dictated by the agency responsible for accrediting the laboratory. Examples of accrediting agencies are state public health departments, federal Clinical Laboratory Improvement Act (CLIA), Joint Commission of Accreditation of Healthcare Organizations (JCAHO), and the American Association of Bioanalysts (AAB).

## Quality Assurance of Equipment and Instrumentation

Most manufacturers dictate what quality assurance checks must be performed. These must be strictly adhered to, and no deviation from them or the operating procedures should be made.

All instruments require some general care such as keeping surfaces clean. A 10% bleach (sodium hypochlorite) solution works well except for metal surfaces, which will pit and rust with bleach. For metal surfaces use paper towels soaked with a disinfectant such as Amphyl (a phenol-based disinfectant). Cleaning surfaces, hoods, incubators, and other equipment is part of the daily routine in a microbiology laboratory. Cleaning is the first thing you do when you arrive and the last before you leave.

**Blood Culture Instruments.** Detecting organisms in the blood is one of the most important tests done in the clinical microbiology laboratory. Rapid detection enhances the care of the patient in critical ways. Instruments that alert the technologist to a positive reaction as soon as the criteria for positivity are met provide many advantages over visual observations and subculturing. Keeping instruments well maintained is the best insurance against trouble.

Other assessments of the instrument functionality can be done by reviewing the results it produces. Trends in the frequency and identity of organisms ensure quality as well. Periodic review of blood culture results may reveal valuable quality assurance data. Are they skin contaminants? Could there be a problem with the phlebotomy techniques? Are the physicians ordering multiple specimens on each patient? Are the multiple specimens agreeing? These are a few of the assessments that ensure quality in blood culture procurement and processing.

## Quality Assurance of Methods and Procedures

Procedure manuals are a valuable asset to the microbiology laboratory. They provide the opportunity for the full-time employee to get organized, a reference for the part-time employee, a training guide for the new employee, and a window into the quality of the lab for the inspector. The College of American Pathologists heavily emphasizes procedure manuals in their inspection guidelines. It is the documentation of a quality microbiology laboratory. Manuals should be formally updated annually and documented with a signed review by the medical director and supervisor. This constant review process enables all levels of the lab to be working as a team and provides better communication.

Certain standards must be followed in format and content of a procedure manual. The National Committee for Clinical Laboratory Standards (NCCLS) is a non-profit, education organization that provides guidelines for standards in laboratories. NCCLS publications describe laboratory procedures, bench and reference methods, and evaluation protocols. Approved standards are reviewed by the committee every 3 years. The guideline GP2-A2* is for clinical laboratory procedure manuals and is required as part of any quality laboratory.

According to the NCCLS manual, the required elements of a procedure are shown in Figure 5-1.

## REPORTING AND USE OF QUALITY ASSURANCE DATA

### Record Retention

Table 5-1 is an example of how a laboratory may correlate the various requirements for the retention of records. As technology develops, these documents will be stored electronically at reasonable cost, but now laboratories have storage problems when required to keep this much paper. The need to access this stored information occurs rarely in a laboratory where there is a dedicated effort to provide accurate and dependable results.

---

**ELEMENTS OF A PROCEDURE**

▶ Principal and/or Purpose of the Test

▶ Specimen Requirements, Patient Preparation

▶ Reagents, Standards, Controls, Media, and any Hazardous Material Identified

▶ Instrumentation including Calibration Protocols and Schedules

▶ Step-by-Step Directions

▶ Calculations

▶ Frequency and Tolerance of Controls; Corrective Actions

▶ Expected Values; Values Requiring Special Notification and Interpretation

▶ Procedure Notes

▶ Limitations of Method (e.g., interfering substances)

▶ Method Validation

▶ References

▶ Effective Date and Schedule for Review

▶ Distribution

▶ Author

**FIGURE 5-1** Elements of a procedure.

*National Committee for Clinical Laboratory Standards. Clinical laboratory technical procedure manuals—Second Edition; Approved Guideline. NCCLS document GP2-A2 (ISBN 1-56238-156-3). NCCLS, 771 East Lancaster Avenue, Villanova, PA 19085, 1992.

**Table 5–1 ▶ Time Required to Retain Documents for State and Federal Agencies**

| Procedure | State | CAP | JCAHO | RCH |
|---|---|---|---|---|
| **General Laboratory** | | | | |
| Appointment books | | | | |
| Minutes of departmental meetings | | | 2 y | 2 y |
| Procedure manuals | 2 y | 2 y after terminating procedure | 3 y | 3 y |
| | | | 6 y | life of instrument + 2 y |
| Registers of tests (chronological) PMLs of log books | 3 y | 2 y | 10 y | 10 y |
| Printouts from automated instruments *Note:* If patient, calibration, or control data are available on other types of records (handwritten or computer generated), printouts need only be retained for 90 d | 2 y for Medicare 3 y for Medical | | | 3 y |
| Equipment inspection, validation, calibration, repair and replacement records | 2 y | 2 y or while method is in use | 6 y | life of instrument + 2 y |
| Proficiency testing results | 2 y | 2 y | 6 y | 6 y |
| Quality control results | 3 y | 2 y | 6 y | 6 y |
| Test requisitions | 3 y | 2 y | 2 wk | 3 y |
| **Hematology/Coagulation/Urinalysis** | | | | |
| Blood smears (all slides) | | | | 6 mo |

CAP, College of American Pathologists; JCAHO, Joint Commission on Accreditation of Healthcare Organizations

## Trends

**Trends** are a set of a sequential values to a single test that are compared. The trend could remain constant, be inclining, or declining. They can be extremely valuable in analyzing quality. Trends point to failures in maintenance of equipment, inconsistent techniques, or reagent decay.

Tracking values over a time period provides trending data that provide a visual record, such as points on a graph. Levy-Jennings graphs are used in chemistry to track numeric trends (see Figure 5-2). Microbiology, being less numeric in reporting, is a science that must depend on less exact data to detect trending. The degree of a reaction of reagents may indicate, for example, that a reagent is weakening in its reactivity. When a reaction changes from 4+ to 3+ to 2+ progressively, it is a signal that all is not right with the testing. If a color reaction that is always bright blue changes to pale pro-gressively, that should alert the technologist to a trend that needs investigating.

External trends are data published for the physicians to examine how their treatment regimens are affecting the patient and organism population in the community. Figure 5-3 lists common isolates and the percentage of sensitivity to antibiotics they have displayed in the previous year.

Figure 5-3 gives the physicians an idea of how the treatments they are using are affecting the organism population in an area. Analyzers that perform antibiotic susceptibility testing store the reactions and compile the data. Periodically the data are published for the physicians to use. If these documents are compared from year to year, the trends of increasing resistance are demonstrated. Physicians can alter their treatment protocols accordingly.

## SUMMARY

▶ Quality assurance is a vital part of providing good care for a patient in clinical microbiology; the scope of quality assurance extends from the technical to the personnel aspects of laboratory medicine.

▶ Quality assurance provides microbiology science with structure, consistency, and reliability.

Accrediting agencies set up criteria to standardize quality from laboratory to laboratory across the country.

▶ Quality control protocols are set up for specimens, equipment, reagents, and media. The data collected from these protocols can be evaluated to ensure the quality of the testing results and the treatments that follow.

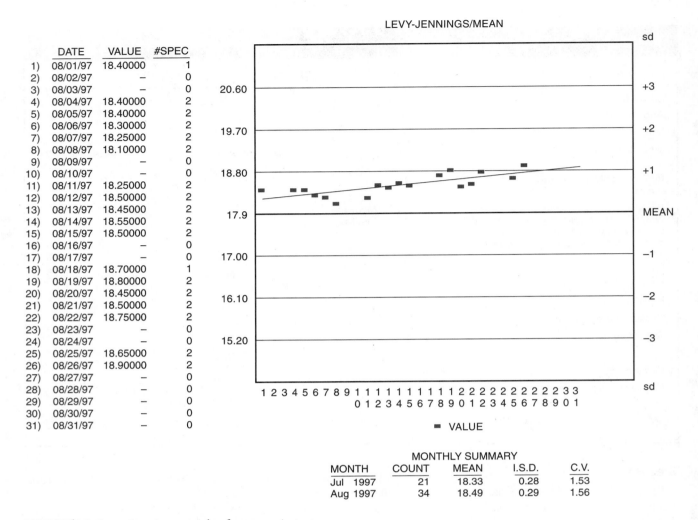

| | DATE | VALUE | #SPEC |
|---|---|---|---|
| 1) | 08/01/97 | 18.40000 | 1 |
| 2) | 08/02/97 | – | 0 |
| 3) | 08/03/97 | – | 0 |
| 4) | 08/04/97 | 18.40000 | 2 |
| 5) | 08/05/97 | 18.40000 | 2 |
| 6) | 08/06/97 | 18.30000 | 2 |
| 7) | 08/07/97 | 18.25000 | 2 |
| 8) | 08/08/97 | 18.10000 | 2 |
| 9) | 08/09/97 | – | 0 |
| 10) | 08/10/97 | – | 0 |
| 11) | 08/11/97 | 18.25000 | 2 |
| 12) | 08/12/97 | 18.50000 | 2 |
| 13) | 08/13/97 | 18.45000 | 2 |
| 14) | 08/14/97 | 18.55000 | 2 |
| 15) | 08/15/97 | 18.50000 | 2 |
| 16) | 08/16/97 | – | 0 |
| 17) | 08/17/97 | – | 0 |
| 18) | 08/18/97 | 18.70000 | 1 |
| 19) | 08/19/97 | 18.80000 | 2 |
| 20) | 08/20/97 | 18.45000 | 2 |
| 21) | 08/21/97 | 18.50000 | 2 |
| 22) | 08/22/97 | 18.75000 | 2 |
| 23) | 08/23/97 | – | 0 |
| 24) | 08/24/97 | – | 0 |
| 25) | 08/25/97 | 18.65000 | 2 |
| 26) | 08/26/97 | 18.90000 | 2 |
| 27) | 08/27/97 | – | 0 |
| 28) | 08/28/97 | – | 0 |
| 29) | 08/29/97 | – | 0 |
| 30) | 08/30/97 | – | 0 |
| 31) | 08/31/97 | – | 0 |

### MONTHLY SUMMARY

| MONTH | COUNT | MEAN | I.S.D. | C.V. |
|---|---|---|---|---|
| Jul 1997 | 21 | 18.33 | 0.28 | 1.53 |
| Aug 1997 | 34 | 18.49 | 0.29 | 1.56 |

**FIGURE 5-2** Levy-Jennings graph of a numeric test.

### % SUSCEPTIBILITY OF COMMON ORGANISMS ISOLATED 1997   compared to   % SUSCEPTIBILITY OF COMMON ORGANISMS ISOLATED 1996

| Antibotic | Group D Enterococcus | *Staphylococcus aureus* | | Antibotic | Group D Enterococcus | *Staphylococcus aureus* |
|---|---|---|---|---|---|---|
| Penicillin | 80 | 5 | | Penicillin | 90 | 10 |
| Ciprofloxacin | 35 | 60 | | Ciprofloxacin | 49 | 80 |
| Vancomycin | 89 | 90 | | Vancomycin | 100 | 98 |
| Tetracycline | 29 | 95 | | Tetracycline | 15 | 88 |
| Erythromycin | 8 | 50 | | Erythromycin | 12 | 64 |

**FIGURE 5-3** External trends for microbiology are published annually to observe changes in susceptibility of common organisms to antibiotics.

## Review Questions

1. Collection personnel need instructions on:
   a. how to prepare the culture site.
   b. packaging and delivery information.
   c. labeling requirements.
   d. all of the above.

2. Assessment of the quality of a specimen can be made by:
   a. asking for another.
   b. monitoring the span of time from collection to time of receipt.
   c. testing the specimen again.
   d. comparing it to other cultures.

3. The quality of reagents is maintained by:
   a. proper storage.
   b. using them daily.
   c. evaluating organisms of known reactions.
   d. a and c

4. Quality control of instruments:
   a. must be developed by the user.
   b. is dictated by the manufacturer.
   c. is assessed by the company's technical service representative.
   d. is of little value as long as the test results are produced.

5. A properly labeled specimen:
   a. displays the insurance information.
   b. displays the phone number of where the results go.
   c. has date and time of collection.
   d. has a PIN number.

6. Trends are:
   a. the latest in lab coat design.
   b. results showing bias.
   c. the direction of price of a test.
   d. data published for physicians to examine how treatment regimens are affecting the patient.

7. Procedure manuals are of value because:
   a. the same procedure can be followed every time tests are performed.
   b. they are a written reference for self-directed orientation.
   c. they are an organizational tool.
   d. all of the above

8. Procedure manuals must have which of the following?
   a. specimen preparation
   b. a and c
   c. step-by-step directions
   d. bound editions

9. If results of quality control tests are outside the expected values:
   a. they are acceptable if the specimen collection was done properly
   b. they are clerical errors
   c. the test must be repeated before reporting results
   d. the boss needs to be notified

## ▶ REFERENCES & RECOMMENDED READING

August, M. J., Hindler, J. A., Huber, T. W., & Sewell, D. L. (Eds.). (1990). *Quality control and quality assurance practices in clinical microbiology. Cumitech, 3A.* Washington, DC: American Society for Microbiology.

Bender, J. L. (Ed.). (1992). Clinical laboratory technical procedure manuals. *NCCLS Document GP2-A2* (12, Serial No. 10).

College of American Pathologists, Commission on Laboratory Accreditation, 5202 Old Orchard Road, Skokie, IL 60077-1034.

Isenberg, H. D. (Ed.). (1992). Instrument maintenance and quality control. In C. A. Gagne, E. Molitoris, & J. E. Baron (Eds.), *Clinical microbiology procedures handbook* (vol. 2, pp. 12.3.1–12.6.1). Washington, DC: American Society for Microbiology.

Joint Commission on Accreditation of Healthcare Organizations. *Monitoring and evaluation of pathology & medical laboratory services,* 875 North Michigan Avenue, Chicago, IL 60600-1846.

# CHAPTER 6

# Automation in the Clinical Microbiology Laboratory

Steven Mahlen, MS, M (ASCP), RM (AAM)

## Microbes in the News

### Anthrax Scare Brings Home the Threat of Biological Warfare

In February of 1998 two American men were arrested in Las Vegas, Nevada and charged with possession of the anthrax bacterium (*Bacillus anthracis*) for use as a deadly weapon. The incident made international headlines as the threat of biological terrorism seemed to materialize on American soil. Examination of vials containing the suspected weapons grade anthrax material by FBI and military experts revealed it to be a harmless anthrax vaccine. The men's attorneys said their clients were carrying anthrax vaccine for use in the testing of a device that would neutralize bacterial toxins in the human body. It is not illegal to possess bacteria, even serious pathogens, if criminal intent cannot be proven.

Although the charges against both men were dropped, one was kept in custody for violation of his parole. The man had been convicted in Ohio on wire fraud charges of illegally obtaining bubonic plague bacteria in 1997. He was sentenced to 18 months parole and was forbidden to conduct any experiments with, or obtain any infectious disease agents. He faces up to five years in prison if he is found to have violated his parole.

*Bacillus anthracis* is a gram-positive endospore-forming bacillus that causes anthrax in grazing animals including sheep, cattle, and goats. Humans can acquire the disease from inhalation of the spores ("woolsorters" disease or inhalation anthrax), through cuts or breaks in the skin (cutaneous anthrax), or from eating infected meat (gastrointestinal anthrax). Inhalation anthrax poses the greatest risk as an agent of biological weaponry for several reasons. The disease is highly lethal and is almost always fatal if treatment does not begin until symptoms are exhibited. With 100 million lethal doses per gram of anthrax material it is 100,000 times deadlier than the deadliest chemical warfare agent. The production of a stable, dry anthrax powder is low cost and does not require high technology. The material is easy to disseminate and is a silent, invisible killer.

Symptoms of anthrax begin after a 1 to 6 day incubation period and are nonspecific for inhalation anthrax. The infected individual develops a low grade fever, a dry hacking cough, and feels weak. After briefly improving, respiratory distress is followed by shock and usually death. If treatment is to be successful antibiotics such as penicillin or doxycycline, and a vaccine **must** be administered **prior** to the onset of symptoms. The antibiotics keep the patient alive while they build immunity in response to the vaccination. Anthrax can be prevented by vaccination with the FDA-licensed vaccine.

Sources:

*Time:* Catching a 48-Hour Bug. By Tamala M. Edwards. March 2, 1998 vol. 151 No. 8. Obtained on-line at:

http://www.pathfinder.com/time/magazine/1...dom/980302/nation.catching_a_48hour5.html

Information paper—Anthrax as a biological warfare agent. Obtained on-line at:

http://www.defenselink.mil/other_info/agent.html

## KEY TERMS

Chemiluminescent
Colorimetry
Chromatography
Fluorometry

Luminometer
Spectrophotometer
Turbidometry

## LEARNING OBJECTIVES

**Upon successful completion of this chapter, the student should be able to:**

1. Understand the advantages and disadvantages of automated systems for the clinical microbiology lab.

2. Understand the history of automation in the clinical microbiology lab.

3. Explain the different detection methods employed by microbiologic automated instruments.

4. Understand the different types of instrument systems available for the clinical microbiology lab.

5. Evaluate the impact that molecular biology may have in automation.

## INTRODUCTION

Clinical microbiology is, perhaps, the area of the clinical laboratory with the least amount of automation (Jorgensen, 1987). Many microbiologists, in the past, have been hesitant to adapt to automated procedures, preferring to rely on human judgment and conception (Jorgensen, 1987). However, automation has slowly crept into clinical microbiology laboratories since the 1960s, and, by now, many hospital and reference clinical microbiology laboratories have begun using automation (Woods, 1992). Automated procedures provide the capability of producing rapid, meaningful results to the clinician much faster than the old, laborious manual methods; in addition, most automated methods reduce the amount of time that the microbiology laboratory technician must spend on procedures, creating a more efficient microbiology laboratory (Woods, 1992). Automation, though, may not be for every clinical microbiology lab. One has to consider the cost of automation in this era of budget cutbacks and increasing health care cost; automated methods are, in general, more costly to perform than their manual counterparts. Automated in-

struments tend to require large initial financing. Also, one must consider whether automation is totally necessary for a particular lab; workload may not demand an automated system. A given lab should always weigh the benefits versus the disadvantages of obtaining an automated system.

Automation encompasses many different areas of clinical microbiology. Automated procedures are used to identify microorganisms and to provide antibiotic susceptibilities from both pure culture and from clinical specimens. Automated procedures are also used to measure growth of microorganisms in blood cultures and also for antigen and antibody detection. Molecular biology diagnostic methods, such as the polymerase chain reaction (PCR) and the ligase chain reaction (LCR), are also becoming automated, thus potentially providing the clinical microbiologist with some of the most rapid diagnostic tools available.

It would be difficult, if not impossible, to detail every automated instrument now on the market for use in the clinical microbiology lab; however, some of the more common instruments are discussed. The basic underlying principles of automation, which may be of more practical use for the student of microbiology, will be provided in more detail.

## HISTORY OF AUTOMATION IN CLINICAL MICROBIOLOGY

Automation has only recently come to clinical microbiology; automation, and its principles, evolved from the very first procedures in microbiology. Before the principles of automation were conceived, microbiologists used laborious methods to identify microorganisms and to determine antibiotic susceptibility patterns. These methods largely stemmed from the origins of microbiology and used test tubes and specialized agar media to perform biochemical identification tests from isolated bacterial or fungal colonies. As a natural course of evolution, paneled systems were developed to provide an easier, more efficient means of identification of clinical isolates. Paneled systems required less room and included the key biochemical tests on one tray required to identify many microorganisms. At first, paneled systems did not necessarily improve on the time required to obtain an identification of an isolate. Incubation times did not vary considerably between the manual methods and paneled systems. However, many panel systems now offer decreased incubation times; with many systems, an accurate identification is possible 4 hours after inoculation with a suspected isolate.

Automation of paneled systems was the next logical step in the history of clinical microbiology. Initially, instruments did not read biochemical test results. Rather, the microbiology technician read the biochemical results and entered them into the instrument's computer. The computer, with the aid of a large data base, would then use the biochemical results to assign a likely choice(s) for an identification.

## PRINCIPLES OF GROWTH DETECTION IN AUTOMATED INSTRUMENTS

### Antigen–Antibody Detection

Various automated immunologic detection methods are available for use in the clinical microbiology laboratory, including the enzyme immunoassay (EIA), radioimmunoassay (RIA), and the fluorescent immunoassay (FIA). All of the methods detect antigen–antibody complexes and can quantify the amount of antigen and antibody present. Many of the systems are used to detect viral antigens.

**Enzyme Immunoassay.** The EIA is a common tool for automated antigen or antibody testing; it is usually used in the form of the enzyme-linked immunosorbent assay (ELISA). One of the main advantages to using an ELISA procedure is that it uses nonisotopic labels for detecting reactions; radioactive substances are not used. Nonisotopic labels do not generate radioactive waste and usually have a long shelf life. With the ELISA, the antigen or antibody is labeled with an enzyme, such as horseradish peroxidase or alkaline phosphatase, which reacts with a substrate to produce a detectable color change. The color change, if any, is measured with a **spectrophotometer**, and compared to a reference sample.

**Radioimmunoassay.** The first automated antigen detection systems available for clinical laboratories were RIA systems (Woods, 1992). RIA is a very sensitive method that can detect minute amounts of antigen or antibody; however, the method uses radioactive labels, which creates radioactive waste. Radioactive labels also have a short shelf life. Because of these drawbacks, RIA systems have been mostly replaced by ELISA systems (Woods, 1992). RIA systems still in use test most often for hepatitis antigens and antibodies. Most RIA systems use $^{125}I$ as the radioisotope today (Pfaller, 1987). The RIA method uses the principle of competitive binding; unlabeled antibody (the patient's sample) is added to a standard concentration of a labeled antibody and unlabeled antigen. The unlabeled antibody will displace a certain amount of labeled antibody. This displaced amount of labeled antibody is equal to the amount of unlabeled antibody in the unknown sample.

**Fluorescent Immunoassay.** The FIA systems use fluorescent substrates or fluorescent-labeled antibody (such as fluorescein isothiocyanate, or FITC). Fluorescent substrates, attached to antigen, are catalytically converted to fluorescent products after antibody from the unknown sample binds to the antigen complex. The products fluoresce at specific wavelengths of light; the intensity of the fluorescence is proportional to the amount of antibody in the sample. FITC-labeled antibody has the capability to bind with proteins to form a conjugate (or complex). The conjugate then binds to antigen from the unknown sample, and the resulting fluorescence is read.

### Carbon Dioxide Detection

Detection of $CO_2$ is a method used for determining microbial growth in blood cultures. The detected $CO_2$ is the end-product (or one of the end-products) of substrate metabolism if microorganisms are present in the blood culture vial. Because cellular elements from inoculated blood (red blood cells, white blood cells, etc.) may also release $CO_2$ via metabolism, the systems detect levels of $CO_2$ above a baseline. The varying automated blood culture systems use different detection methods. Some systems use radiolabeled substrates, which are metabolized into radiolabeled $CO_2$; thus growth is detected radiometrically. Another system detects pressure changes caused by production of

$CO_2$ and other gases, or the utilization of gases. Yet another system uses a pH indicator, which changes color when metabolized $CO_2$ comes into contact with it; the color change is detected by a photometer.

## Substrate Utilization

There are a few different ways that substrate utilization by microorganisms is used in automation, including **colorimetry**, breakdown of fluorogen-labeled substrates, and detection of end-products via **chromatography** (e.g., gas-liquid chromatography [GLC] or high-performance liquid chromatography [HPLC]). Colorimetry is the detection of color changes of pH indicators after substrate utilization by a particular microbe. Typically, filters are used to absorb certain wavelengths of light, so that color changes can be easier to detect. Color changes are measured with a photometer. Colorimetry has lended itself well to automation; several automated instruments use colorimetry principles for identifying microbes. A few systems use substrates labeled with a fluorescent complex; when the substrates are metabolized, the fluorescent complexes are released, and may be detected with ultraviolet light. GLC separates the constituents of a sample, which can be the metabolic product of a microorganism or the organism itself. Often, GLC is used to identify the metabolic products of anaerobic bacteria. Anaerobes produce characteristic volatile fatty acids (such as acetic acid, butyric acid, propionic acid, and many others) or nonvolatile acids (such as pyruvic acid, lactic acid, and others) which, along with culture characteristics, often enable clinical microbiology labs to identify anaerobes faster than performing biochemical tests or other tests. GLC has also been used to analyze cellular long-chain fatty acids (mycolic acids) to rapidly identify mycobacteria from culture isolates and directly from clinical samples. In the past, this method of identifying mycobacteria was restricted almost exclusively to research labs; however, commercial systems are now available for use with clinical microbiology labs. Also, GLC can be used to identify microbial metabolites directly from clinical samples. HPLC, too, has many applications; it has been used to also identify mycobacteria by analyzing their mycolic acids.

## AUTOMATED INSTRUMENT APPLICATIONS IN CLINICAL MICROBIOLOGY

### Organism Identification/Susceptibility Testing

**Microscan.** The Microscan systems (Dade International Inc., West Sacramento, CA) include the Microscan Touchscan, Autoscan, and Autoscan Walk/Away systems. The Autoscan Walk/Away system is fully automated; it incubates, adds reagents, and interprets (and prints) results. Microscan panels consist of plastic trays containing microtubes that carry dried biochemicals and antibiotics. The panels are inoculated with a defined suspension of the isolate in question; they are then incubated. The Autoscan Walk/Away system can hold up to 96 panels at one time. The various Microscan system panels use either fluorescent markers or colorimetry for identification of microorganisms; turbidity (**turbidometry**) is used for detection of antimicrobial susceptibility or resistance. **Fluorometry** is used in the panels that detect gram-positive and gram-negative bacteria, while colorimetry is used in the *Haemophilus,* yeast, and anaerobe panels.

**Vitek.** The Vitek system (bioMérieux Vitek, Hazelwood, MO), originally designed to rapidly diagnose bacterial infections in space, utilizes colorimetric methods to determine identification of gram-positive and gram-negative bacteria, anaerobes, *Neisseria* species, *Haemophilus* species, and yeast, and turbidometric methods for antibiotic susceptibility determinations. Also, the Vitek urine card can measure growth of nine common urinary tract pathogens (including *Escherichia coli, Proteus* species, *Pseudomonas aeruginosa, Klebsiella/Enterobacter* species, and others) directly from a patient's urine specimen with turbidometric measurements. The system uses plastic cards that hold wells containing dried biochemicals and antibiotics. After pure, suspect colonies are inoculated into saline, a plastic transfer tube is attached to the card. The filler/sealer instrument will then draw, via a vacuum suction, a calibrated amount of the standardized suspension of the microorganism in question into the card through the transfer tube; then, the card is manually sealed. The sealing apparatus cuts the transfer tube flush with the card. After the urine or suspension of microorganism is suctioned into the plastic card and sealed, the card is placed in the reader/incubator. Organism identification/ susceptibility results are printed out by the system's computer in 4 to 18 hours, depending on the isolate (typically, gram-negative species such as members of the Enterobacteriaceae can be identified in 4 to 6 hours, while oxidase-positive gram-negative and some gram-positive organisms may take up to 18 hours). New software available for use with the Vitek allows tracking of resistant strains and can provide a link with the pharmacy to track antibiotic costs. See Figure 6-1 for a photo of the Vitek system.

### Blood Culture Systems

**BacT/Alert.** The BacT/Alert (Organon Teknika Corp., Durham, NC) uses colorimetry to detect $CO_2$ produced by microbes growing in the blood culture bottles. The system uses supplemented tryptic soy broth for standard aerobic and anaerobic blood cultures and supplemented brain heart infusion broth for pediatric and antimicrobial neutralizing blood cultures. The system

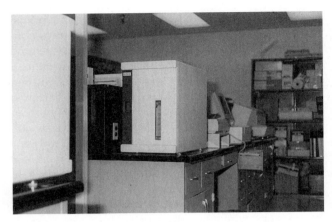

**FIGURE 6-1** Vitek system. (Courtesy of bioMérieux Vitek)

consists of an incubator, shaker, and detector. There are 11 blocks in the instrument, each of which contains 48 wells for blood culture bottles. Each blood culture bottle has a $CO_2$ sensor attached to the bottom, separated from the culture broth by a semipermeable membrane. The sensor is impregnated with water vapor and is blue to dark green colored in its normal, alkaline state. The membrane is impermeable to most substances except for $CO_2$. When an organism produces $CO_2$, the gas diffuses across the membrane and dissolves in the water vapor, creating hydrogen ions. The increase in the hydrogen ion concentration causes the sensor to become acidic, resulting in a lighter green or yellow color. There is a colorimetric detector in each well in the instrument, and each detector scans its well every 10 minutes. When the detector determines that a sensor has changed color, it flags the well as positive with a light that comes on next to the well. The bottle is then removed, and further testing is performed to identify the organism present and perform antibiotic susceptibilities, if required. Negative cultures are removed after 7 days (Thorpe et al., 1990).

**BACTEC NR-660.** The BACTEC NR-660 system (Becton Dickinson Instrument Systems, Sparks, MD) technology is based on measuring $CO_2$ by infrared spectrophotometry; it is an improvement on the radiometric method that the BACTEC 460 uses (see below). When microorganisms use the substrates present in the blood culture broth (the system uses BACTEC NR 6A (aerobic), NR 7A (anaerobic), NR8 (aerobic hypertonic), NR16 (aerobic, resin), NR17 (anaerobic, resin), and Peds Plus media), they produce $CO_2$, which has the ability to absorb infrared radiation. Thus, the system passes infrared light through the blood culture bottles; the amount of light that passes through a bottle is inversely proportional to the amount of $CO_2$ in the bottle. The system uses four different types of media. The BACTEC NR-660 is not a closed automation system. After bottles have been inoculated with blood, they are placed in a special bottle rack in an incubator/shaker (anaerobic bottles do not have to be shaken, whereas aerobic bottles should be shaken during incubation), which is located separately from the BACTEC instrument. The bottle racks are taken out of the incubator/shaker at routine intervals and placed in the BACTEC instrument to be examined for microbial growth. Growth is measured in an ionization chamber. After a set of bottles is examined, the instrument's computer will generate a report showing growth indices for each bottle; potentially positive bottles are removed and processed further. Culture bottles are held for 7 days before a negative growth result is reported.

**BACTEC 9240.** The BACTEC 9240 (Becton Dickinson Instrument Systems, Sparks, MD) is a refinement of the radiometric BACTEC system. The BACTEC 9240 detects fluorescence. When microorganisms are present in the blood culture bottle, they release $CO_2$ after metabolism of nutrients in the broth medium. The $CO_2$ reacts with dye contained in a sensor on the bottom of the bottle. The reaction modulates the amount of light absorbed by a fluorescent material in the sensor; the amount of $CO_2$ released by the microorganism corresponds to the amount of fluorescence measured by the instrument's photo detectors. Potential positive culture bottles are flagged by a light-emitting diode located next to the bottle and on the system's computer monitor; the bottles are then taken out for further work-up. One advantage of this system over the radiometric system is that bottles only need be held for 5 days before a negative result can be reported. The instrument examines bottles every 10 minutes. The system is completely self-contained. After inoculation with blood, bottles are placed in racks in a cabinet. There are six racks that hold up to 40 bottles each (up to five cabinets can be linked together for labs with particularly high work volumes); each rack is independently monitored with its own microprocessor. The racks are continuously shaken and incubated.

## Enzyme Immunoassay Systems

**ACCESS Immunoassay System.** The ACCESS Immunoassay System (Sanofi Diagnostics Pasteur, Inc., Chaska, MN) is a **chemiluminescent** EIA system designed for detecting the *Chlamydia trachomatis* lipopolysaccharide antigen. In addition, the system tests for a number of chemistry assays, toxoplasma, rubella, and other assays. For chlamydia testing, the system uses a chlamydia-specific monoclonal antibody coupled to paramagnetic particles. The treated specimen is mixed with the paramagnetic particles in a reaction vessel. If chlamydial lipopolysaccharide antigen is present in the specimen, the monoclonal antibody will bind to it. Next, a mixture of polyclonal rabbit antichlamydia antibody and alkaline phosphatase conjugated polyclonal goat anti-rabbit IgG antibody is added; this mixture will attach to the antigen captured by the monoclonal antibody/paramagnetic particles. Then, the particles with attached antigen/antibodies are separated by a magnetic field; washing removes the unbound material. Next, a chemiluminescent substrate is added, and any generated light is measured by a **luminometer**. Evaluation of the generated light indicates whether or not chlamydia is present in the sample. Reactive specimens are verified by using a blocking assay. The blocking assay uses an equine antichlamydia antibody that competes for specific epitopes on the extracted antigen; this prevents the formation of a complex with the monoclonal antibody and the primary antibody. Thus, if an original result is reactive, a verified result will have a suppressed signal. If the initial result is nonreactive, there will be little or no suppression in light signal after addition of the blocking antibody.

## Mycobacteria Identification Systems

Mycobacteria identification systems have greatly reduced the time necessary to detect mycobacteria; in many instances, organisms can be detected in 10 days or sooner, as opposed to 17 days or greater with standard culture methods (Woods, 1992). Once detection has occurred, many laboratories use biochemical tests, DNA probes, or even PCR or LCR to identify the mycobacteria present. With the current systems on the market, specimens submitted for mycobacterial analysis are concentrated and decontaminated before being placed in the systems. Automated PCR and LCR-based systems are under development for mycobacterial testing (see below).

**BACTEC TB-460.** The BACTEC TB-460 system (Becton Dickinson Instrument Systems, Sparks, MD; see Figure 6-2) is based on radiometric methods; specifically, on the measurement of $^{14}C$-labeled $CO_2$ produced by growing microorganisms. The BACTEC TB-460 blood culture bottles contain Middlebrook 7H12 broth with $^{14}C$-labeled substrates; radiolabeled $CO_2$ is the result of metabolism of these substrates. The BACTEC TB-460 is not a closed automation system. After bottles have been inoculated with the clinical specimen, they are placed in a special bottle rack in an incubator/shaker (anaerobic bottles do not have to be shaken; aerobic bottles should be shaken during incubation). The bottle racks are taken out of the incubator/ shaker at routine intervals and placed in the BACTEC instrument to be examined for microbial growth. Growth is measured in an ionization chamber. After a set of bottles is examined, the instrument's computer will generate a report showing growth indices for each bottle; positive bottles are removed and further processed. Culture bottles are held for 28 days before a negative growth result is reported. The BACTEC TB-460 can be used for susceptibility testing (Woods, 1992).

**BACTEC 9000MB.** The BACTEC 9000MB (Becton Dickinson Instrument Systems, Sparks, MD; see Figure 6-3), uses nonradiometric detection methods to detect mycobacteria. The BACTEC 9000MB uses MYCO/F medium (a modified version of Middlebrook 7H9 broth) and a fluorescent detection system (Van Griethuysen, Jansz, & Buiting, 1996). Each culture bottle has an oxygen-specific sensor consisting of a ruthenium metal complex impregnated within a silicon rubber disk; the fluorescence of a particular bottle is modulated by oxygen use by microorganisms (Van Griethuysen et al., 1996). Oxygen causes a decrease in fluorescence; thus, when microorganisms consume oxygen, fluorescence increases, and growth is detected (Van Griethuysen et al., 1996). Currently, the BACTEC 9000MB cannot be used for susceptibility testing.

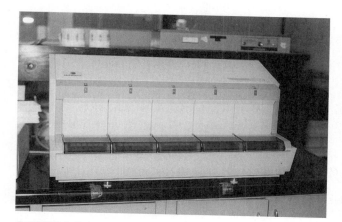

**FIGURE 6-2** BACTEC TB-460. (Courtesy Becton Dickinson Microbiology Systems)

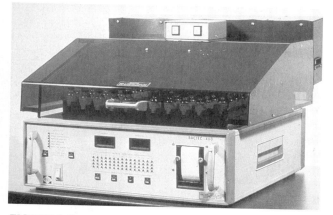

**FIGURE 6-3** BACTEC 9000MB. (Courtesy of Becton Dickinson Microbiology Systems)

## THE FUTURE OF AUTOMATION IN MICROBIOLOGY

Future automated instruments in clinical microbiology will probably concentrate on rapidly identifying microorganisms directly from clinical specimens. Molecular biology techniques, such as PCR and LCR, are already being used to detect microorganisms from clinical specimens; the efficacy of techniques like PCR or LCR in the routine clinical microbiology laboratory and in automation are being evaluated. An automated LCR-based test has surfaced, the Abbott URI*probe,* which uses Abbott LCx technology. This assay enables a clinical microbiology laboratory to detect both *Chlamydia trachomatis* and *Neisseria gonorrhoeae* from a single voided urine specimen (if so desired, URI*probe* swabs are also available to collect endocervical or male urethral specimens) from both men and women. Sensitivity of the LCx technology is well over 90% (Chernesky, Jang, et al., 1994), and automation of the procedure has enabled a very rapid turn-around time (< 1 day in most circumstances).

The cost of PCR- and LCR-based test assays may prohibit some clinical labs from performing the tests; however, the rapid, sensitive, and specific identification gained from such assays probably saves more money from avoidance of disease sequalae in some patients. Furthermore, such test assays will become more attractive to clinical labs when automated to detect members of the genus *Mycobacterium.*

## SUMMARY

- ▶ Automated instruments are able to provide rapid results for many clinical microbiology laboratories and are currently being used with increasing frequency. However, automation may not be appropriate for all clinical microbiology labs.
- ▶ Current automation procedures evolved from old, often laborious microbiologic techniques.
- ▶ There are a number of methods with which automated instruments detect the growth of microorganisms, including antigen–antibody detection, carbon dioxide detection, and substrate utilization.
- ▶ In addition to a number of different methods that automated instruments use in the clinical microbiology lab, there are a number of different microbiologic applications of automated instruments. These include organism identification/susceptibility testing, systems that monitor blood cultures, enzyme immunoassay systems, and mycobacteria identification systems.
- ▶ Future clinical microbiology automated instruments will probably focus on direct detection of microorganisms from clinical specimens. Automated molecular biology techniques are already being designed and used in this capacity.

## Review Questions

1. An automated test assay that uses antibody labeled with horseradish peroxidase:
   a. would also probably be labeled with $^{125}$I for detection.
   b. would be an example of a fluorescent immunoassay.
   c. would not be feasible for everyday use in the clinical microbiology laboratory.
   d. could be detected via a color change if the labeled antibody reacts with the proper substrate.

2. Radioimmunoassay (RIA):
   a. is rarely used now because it is so nonsensitive.
   b. has largely been replaced by ELISA.
   c. is based on FITC-labeled antigen binding to an unknown antibody and producing varying degrees of fluorescence.
   d. reagents have a very long shelf life compared to ELISA reagents.

3. Gas-liquid chromatography (GLC):
   a. may be used to rapidly identify mycolic acids of mycobacteria.
   b. detects color changes of pH indicators in a test system after microbes have broken down various test substrates.
   c. is often used to identify volatile fatty acids produced by viral specimens.
   d. is only used by research facilities to identify microorganisms.

4. Automated mycobacterial identification systems:
   a. typically use tryptic soy broth as the medium to grow mycobacteria.
   b. rarely speed the recovery time of mycobacteria from clinical specimens.
   c. usually must rely on specimen decontamination and concentration before inoculation of media.
   d. are based on antigen–antibody reactions.

5. Which of the following is NOT a characteristic of blood culture systems?
    a. Systems that measure $CO_2$ detect levels of $CO_2$ above a baseline level generated by cellular elements in blood.
    b. Blood culture systems can directly identify microorganisms from the blood culture bottle without the need for subculturing.
    c. Most of the available blood culture systems on the market use nonradiometric technology.
    d. Most of the available blood culture systems continuously shake blood culture bottles in an incubator.

6. Automated methods:
    a. are usually much cheaper to perform than manual methods.
    b. tend to increase the time it takes to report a result.
    c. should be used by every clinical microbiology laboratory, regardless of workload.
    d. tend to save technician time in the clinical microbiology laboratory.

7. PCR/LCR:
    a. may be used to identify microorganisms directly from clinical samples.
    b. are sensitive, but tend to take many days to perform.

    c. are sensitive and are less costly than most clinical laboratory tests.
    d. will probably never be of much use in the clinical laboratory.

8. Turbidometric methods:
    a. are never utilized in automation.
    b. may be used to detect color changes in media.
    c. may be used in automation to measure antibiotic susceptibilities.
    d. are the basis for blood culture automated systems.

9. Some automated enzyme immunoassay systems are designed to detect antigens from:
    a. *Chlamydia trachomatis.*
    b. *Mycobacterium tuberculosis.*
    c. *Clostridium difficile.*
    d. *Escherichia coli.*

10. Instruments that identify microorganisms (such as Aladin, Microscan, Vitek, etc.):
    a. are typically based on evaluating long-chain fatty acid profiles of organisms.
    b. are most often used to identify dimorphic fungi.
    c. are never also used for susceptibility testing.
    d. often may identify gram-positive, gram-negative, and anaerobic bacteria, and yeast.

## ▶ REFERENCES & RECOMMENDED READING

Chernesky, M. A., Lee, H., Schachter, J., Burczak, J. D., Stamm, W. E., McCormack, W. M., & Quinn, T. C. (1994). Diagnosis of *Chlamydia trachomatis* urethral infection in symptomatic and asymptomatic men by testing first-void urine in a ligase chain reaction assay. *The Journal of Infectious Diseases, 170,* 1308–1311.

Chernesky, M. A., Jang, D., Lee, H., Burczak, J. D., Hu, H., Sellors, J., Tomazic-Allen, S. J., & Mahony, J. B. (1994). Diagnosis of *Chlamydia trachomatis* infections in men and women by testing first-void urine by ligase chain reaction. *Journal of Clinical Microbiology, 32,* 2682–2685.

Jorgensen, J. H. (1987). The evolving role of automation in clinical microbiology. In J. H. Jorgensen (Ed.), *Automation in clinical microbiology* (pp. 3–4). Boca Raton, FL: CRC Press.

Morello, J. A., Leitch, C., Nitz, S., Dyke, J. W., Andruszewski, M., Maier, G., Landau, W., & Beard, M. A. (1994). Detection of bacteremia by Difco ESP blood culture system. *Journal of Clinical Microbiology, 32,* 811–818.

Pfaller, M. A. (1987). Immunoassays for measurement of antimicrobial agents in body fluids. In J. H. Jorgensen (Ed.), *Automation in clinical microbiology* (pp. 121–138). Boca Raton, FL: CRC Press.

Thorpe, T. C., Wilson, M. L., Turner, J. E., DiGuiseppi, J. L., Willert, M., Mirrett, S., & Reller, L. B. (1990). BacT/Alert: An automated colorimetric microbial detection system. *Journal of Clinical Microbiology, 28,* 1608–1612.

Van Griethuysen, A. J., Jansz, A. R., & Buiting, A. G. M. (1996). Comparison of fluorescent BACTEC 9000 MB system, Septi-Check AFB system, and Lowenstein-Jensen medium for detection of mycobacteria. *Journal of Clinical Microbiology, 34,* 2391–2394.

Woods, G. L. (1992). Automation in clinical microbiology. *American Journal of Clinical Pathology, 98 (Suppl. 1),* S22–S30.

# CHAPTER 7
# Antimicrobial Agents and Antimicrobial Susceptibility Testing

James T. Griffith, PhD, CLS (NCA) and Anne T. Rodgers, PhD, MT (ASCP)

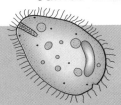

## Microbes in the News
### Possible End of the Antimicrobic Era

Treating infectious diseases with chemical substances is not something that we have been doing forever. In fact, it is a relatively new development in the history of medicine. The origins of chemotherapy for infectious diseases go back well before we knew about the existence of the offending microorganisms—at least to the time of the Ionian Greeks (the time of Pythagoras) where the assumption was that these unnatural states (infectious diseases, not explained otherwise) would be reversible by association with "natural products." The various remedies used included dirt, leaves, etc. Those notions held until the beginning of what is now referred to as modern chemotherapy, divided into three eras, the first of which existed between 1600 and 1900.

During this time, nonspecific hit-or-miss procedures, mostly involving plant and herb extracts, were used. Some of these, in fact, were quite successful and later came to be understood as the basis for specific chemical treatment of infectious diseases such as the bark of the Chinchona tree, which produces an extract later identified (circa 1820) as quinine. The root of the Ipecacuanha plant later proved to derive the ipecac alkaloid emetine. A great advance occurred, ushering in the second era of modern chemotherapy, during the period from 1900 to 1940, with the introduction of the aniline dyes and heavy metals, which were great advances over the previous substances. Even though some of them were derived

from dyes and plant extracts, they were much purer and generally more effective than their predecessors. The greatest advances in the treatment of infectious diseases have come since 1940, generally considered the start of the third era of chemotherapeutics or the antibiotic era. Original work by Greig and Smith (1917) and Gratia and Doth (1924) and the great pioneering work by Sir Alexander Fleming (1929) and others leading up to World War II provided the basis for the "discovery" of antimicrobial agents during World War II where, for a time, more deaths among the Allied Forces were attributed to infections from shrapnel bomb wounds than from bullet wounds. This resulted in a tremendous effort by the Allied Forces to discover substances that could cure, or at least minimize, the effect of these deadly infections. Those discoveries, the most important of which was Fleming's work with penicillin, ushered in the antibiotic era, and from the time after World War II to the present, we have been on a continual path discovering, manipulating, and inventing agents for these purposes. Almost from the beginning, however, problems resulting from the organisms' defense were evident and to date constitute very serious threats to the continued utility of these agents. Some authorities now contemplate the notion that the antimicrobial era may in fact be over. That notion may be a little premature, but it is no longer as wild an idea as it was only a few years ago.

INTRODUCTION

BASIC PHARMACOKINETICS OF ANTIMICROBIAL AGENTS
Cell Wall Active Agents
Cell Membrane Active Agents
Antiprotein Synthesis Agents
Antimetabolites
Nucleic Acid Active Agents

BACTERIAL RESISTANCE TO ANTIMICROBIAL AGENTS
Mechanisms of Action

SUSCEPTIBILITY TESTING TECHNIQUES
Macrodilution and Microdilution Tests
Agar Disk Diffusion Method
E-Test

SPECIAL CONSIDERATIONS IN ANTIMICROBIAL SUSCEPTIBILITY TESTING
ß-Lactamase Production
Methicillin-Resistant *Staphylococcus aureus*
Vancomycin-Resistant *Enterococcus fecalis*

# KEY TERMS

Antibiotic
Antimicrobial
Cell wall active agents

Mean inhibitory concentration (MIC)
Microbicidal

Microbistatic
Minimum bacteriocidal concentration (MBC)

# LEARNING OBJECTIVES

**Upon successful completion of this chapter, the student should be able to:**

1. Define key terms.
2. Explain how microbistatic substances help combat microbial infections.

3. Describe four ways antimicrobial agents may work against microorganisms.
4. Explain three mechanisms microorganisms may use to evade the effects of antimicrobial agents.

# INTRODUCTION

Many serious problems exist in the treatment of infectious diseases. Perhaps the greatest problem is that the offending entity (some microorganism) is in the host and, therefore, one must consider in the treatment of these agents administration routes, competing resident flora, and the general toxicity of the agents that might be used. Another problem is that the offending agents are very small and widely disseminated. As a result, one of the great treatments of medicine, surgery, is generally not an option in treating infectious disease. Another problem is that these offending microorganisms divide extremely quickly. The notion that a healthy person might otherwise be able to "outlast" the organisms does not always work. Another difficulty is that many of the offending microorganisms are similar in their biology to humans. As a result, most substances that are toxic to microorganisms are also toxic to patients. So, from the differences between medicine in public health to the limitations of the universe of possible **antimicrobial** agents, we do not have all of the weapons that we might wish.

The general philosophy used in treating infectious disease is that **microbicidal** (bactericidal, fungicidal, viricidal, etc.) agents are those substances that we discover or manipulate or manufacture that can attack something that the microorganisms have that we do not and, therefore, kill the organisms. **Microbistatic** agents are those that attack something that both the microorganism and the patient have, but somehow the microorganism needs more. Microbistatic agents only injure the organism, relying on the patient's defense reserves to finish them off. In many medical applications, however, this is not possible, for example, patients who have lymphoreticular disease, diabetes mellitus, severe debilitation, or are taking immunosuppressive

therapy. Most antimicrobial agents used today are products of secondary metabolism of other microorganisms either as they are constituted or as they have been manipulated in the pharmaceutical laboratory. These secondary metabolites include amino sugars, instead of carbohydrate metabolites, and other substances such as lactones, macrolides, polyenes, tetracyclines, and other classes or compounds. A significant number of these compounds are recovered from actinomycetes (approximately half) or fungi (approximately 20%). When secondary metabolites are constituted for chemotherapeutic use they are generally affected by a series of considerations including:

- ▶ Nature of the antimicrobial agent
- ▶ Kind of microorganism
- ▶ Temperature
- ▶ Physiologic state of microorganism
- ▶ Environmental factors

All antimicrobial agents are affected by the principles of pharmacology that affect the administration of all drugs to humans. These include the common principals of pharmacokinetics and pharmacodynamics:

1. How the agent is liberated from the form in which it is given
2. How it is absorbed in the various compartments and tissues of the patient's body
3. How it is distributed throughout the various tissue levels
4. How it is metabolized and eliminated from the body

These considerations give rise to the notion of administration, route, dose, and course, resulting in such concepts as the half-life of the agent.

# BASIC PHARMACOKINETICS OF ANTIMICROBIAL AGENTS

## Cell Wall Active Agents

Because many microorganisms (including most bacteria) have cell walls, it would be greatly advantageous to find an agent that is active against these structures. If such an agent were found, it could be used aggressively in terms of dose because it would be attacking something that the microorganisms have that hosts do not have. There are many structural differences in the limiting surfaces of microorganisms, one of the most important of which is the difference in peptidoglycan cross-link arrangement as illustrated below.

In fact, the difference between gram-positive and gram-negative cells is the basis of action for several groups of **cell wall active agents**. Penicillin and its various congenres are a prime example of agents that are effective against the cell wall. Yet resistance to these agents by microorganisms was observed as early as 1940, and by 1954, we were distinguishing "street Staph" versus "hospital Staph" as a measure of those gram-positive organisms that were likely to be sensitive to penicillin versus those that were likely to be resistant to penicillin. Another group of agents, the cephalosporins, were discovered as products of the fungal genus *Cephalosporium* in 1945 by G. Brotzu in Sardinia. Resistance continued to emerge and it was not until 1959, with the synthesis of 6-aminopenicillanic acid by Japanese scientists, that the antimicrobial era arose. Since then, we have generated a series of semisynthetic agents, that is, agents that began with the biosynthesized products of the fungal genera *Penicillium* or *Cephalosporium* and then manipulated in the pharmacologic laboratory to produce agents that were partly biosynthesized by microorganisms and partly constructed in the pharmacologic laboratory. Since the late 1950s dozens of agents, each with advantages and disadvantages in treating infectious disease, have been created. The largest group of these cell wall active agents includes substances that have a four-membered chemical ring (see Figure 7-1).

The ß-lactam ring is common to all of the so called ß-lactam agents and is the key entity in the mechanism of these agents. It is also the key to how they are defeated by microorganisms, an increasing problem. Certain subclasses of ß-lactam drugs are effective against gram-negative microorganisms and many other variations.

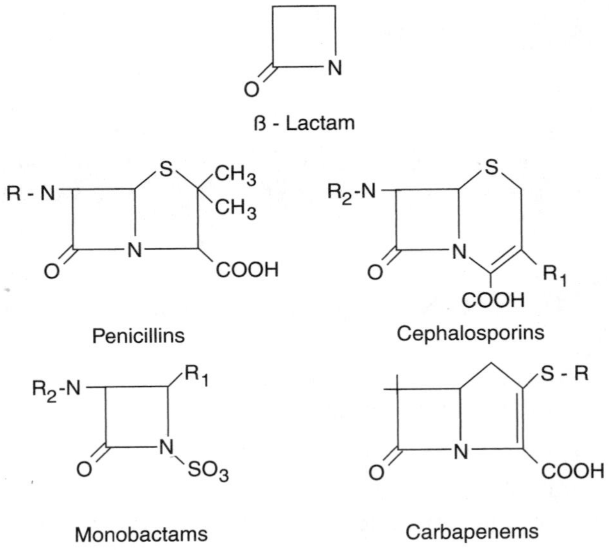

## Cell Membrane Active Agents

Attacking a microbial cell membrane is a much more difficult problem than attacking a cell wall because microbial cell membranes are similar to the corresponding structures of our own cells and, therefore, must be approached more carefully. The general categories of substances that have been used are:

**FIGURE 7-1**

1. Agents that disorganize membrane structure
   ▶ Tyrocidians and gramicidins
   ▶ Polyene antibiotics
   ▶ Polymyxins

2. Agents that alter membrane permeability
   ▶ Gramicidins
   ▶ Valinomycin
   ▶ Enniatin
   ▶ Macrotetralides
   ▶ Polyether antibiotics

3. Agents that affect membrane enzyme systems
   ▶ Oligomycin
   ▶ Antimycin
   ▶ Dicyclohexylcarbodiimide

Most of these agents are quite toxic. Although they may have specialty uses and research implications, the agents that are in most common use from this group include the polymyxins, which act with the phospholipids of the cell membrane and alter permeability and osmotic integrity. Currently the principle function of these agents is against gram-negative bacteria. They are often used outside the skin's surface (as topical agents). This is also the case with another agent from this group, bacitracin, which disrupts the membrane structure. Bacitracin is also effective against organisms outside the body, except this time principally gram-positive organisms. This substance is used in a wide variety of over-the-counter preparations. A third group of agents that are cell membrane inhibitors are principally known as antifungal agents. These polyenes act on sterols in the cell membrane and disrupt membrane structure. The most well known of these agents are amphotericin B and nystatin.

## Antiprotein Synthesis Agents

One of the central dogmas of molecular biology involves the transmission of information from DNA to desired activity in the operation of a cell. That process generally starts with transcription, whereby information is transferred from DNA to a primary transcript of messenger RNA. This is then followed by translation, which stimulates the formation of 30S and 50S ribosomal units to form a functional 70S ribosome. This process is key to producing the material (a protein or polypeptide) that was needed pursuant to the stimulus that caused the transcription and then translation. It has been possible, over the years, to discover and then manipulate agents that interfered with this process. As evolution produced increasingly complex organisms, it eventually produced organisms that conducted this process using 40S and 60S subunits, forming 80S functional ribosomes in all eucaryotes, such as ourselves. This evolution provided a selective toxicity advantage over agents that interfered with 30S, 50S, or 70S ribosomes in some way as being antimicrobial, but much less antihuman. One of the earliest of these discovered was streptomycin, characteristic of a family of agents now called the aminoglycosides (aminocyclitrols). These agents all have in common a large streptamine ring and are generally thought to be active by preventing the initiation complex formation in protein synthesis by destroying the P10 protein on the 30S subunit of microbial ribosomes.

Other agents in this category include:

Kanamycin—active on 30S ribosomes
Neomycin—active on 30S ribosomes
Amikacin—semisynthetic kanamycin derivative
Gentamycin—similar mode of action, more potent, less toxic than kanamycin
Tobramycin—very similar to gentamycin, more active against *Pseudomonas*
Spectinomycin—may be tolerated by persons allergic to ß-lactam drugs

Because of their tricyclic structure, all of these molecules depend heavily on their polarity for pharmacokinetic properties traveling throughout the body. Most of them are held in the protein-free moiety and have relatively low serum binding, which means they often have to be given at frequent intervals to remain effective. Forty to 65% of each dose in a 24-hour period is removed from the body; the rest may take up to 10 to 20 days. As a result, toxicity may eventually build up and aminoglycoside monitoring is often performed in clinical laboratories for patients receiving these drugs. The toxicity is due to the agents' direct effect on the proximal convoluted tubule after passing from the cardiovascular system through the glomerulus in the kidney.

Another important group of antiprotein synthesis agents are the tetracyclines, first discovered through a massive soil screening in 1948. The original agent, aureomycin, has been joined by doxycycline, minocycline, and several other congenres of this original material. All of these agents appear to be effective against the 30S ribosome, blocking aminoacyl-tRNA binding at the A site. These agents are generally thought to be bacteriostatic but can be bacteriocidal with higher than normally achieved cardiovascular system levels. They are effective against some gram-negative bacilli, *Mycoplasma, Chlamydia, Rickettsia.*

The tetracyclines form stable chelates with calcium, magnesium, and aluminum, and they effectively penetrate the body, including the cardiovascular system and tissues and even cancer cells. Another group of agents in this category are the linclosamides, which are thought to be active against microorganisms by the in vivo blocking of peptide bond formation on 50S ribosomes. 7-Chloro-lincomycin, or clindamycin, is one of the earliest and most well known linclosamide agents and still characterizes the group. Several of the agents in this category have been associated with pseudomembranous colitis, diarrhea, nephrotoxicity, and other adverse drug reactions, and are typically only used for serious anaerobic infections, aspiration pneumonia, and lung abscess infections. A more successful group, the macrolides, includes erythromycin, discovered in 1952 and characterized by huge lactone rings.

Macrolides are among the safest of antimicrobial agents and are the drugs of choice for several organisms that are difficult to treat, including *Corynebacterium diphtheriae,* isolated from the nasopharynx, *Mycoplasma pneumoniae, Legionella pneumophilia,* and *Bordetella pertussis.* They are often the second drug of choice for patients who are sensitive to penicillins and patients who have ß-lactamase-producing organisms. All of the macrolides are well absorbed and travel throughout the body, including the brain. Some of the newer agents have additional members on the complex ring structure that characterizes macrolides, for example, the 15-member agent released in 1992 as azithromycin and the 16-member agent spiramycin, which has activity against *Toxoplasma* and *Cryptosporidium* organisms. The macrolides are thought to interfere with protein synthesis by inhibiting the translocation of peptidyl-tRNA from the A to the P site on 50S ribosome subunits.

## Antimetabolites

Several other approaches are used for patients with infectious diseases. These include the deprivation of essential materials the microorganisms need for their metabolism. These agents are often categorized in a group called the antimetabolites and involve blocking actions on folinic acid, dihydropteroate synthetase, and others.

## Nucleic Acid Active Agents

If it were possible to find some agent that would attack, destroy, or inhibit the nucleic acids of microorganisms, such an agent would be powerful in the war on infections. This turns out to be a tricky process, however, because microbial nucleic acids are, of course, similar to our own and only some fortuitous difference would serve as the basis for action against microbial nucleic acids, but not against our own. The quinolones constitute one of these discoveries. These compounds are characteristically similar as a group to their progenitor substance, naladixic acid, first used clinically in 1962, and as such they are made up of a bicyclic moiety consisting of two six-membered rings, one with a nitrogen (quinalin) and the other with a double bond oxygen (quinone); the contraction quinalone makes sense. Divided into three major groups (carboxy quinilones, fluoro quinilones and aza quinilones) two dozen or so agents are currently available or under development. Certain of these, such as amifloxacin, penetrate tissue extremely well, unlike amino glycosides and may be effective two-route drugs. Others, such as ciprofloxacin, have high effectiveness ($MIC_{90}$) equal to 1 to 2 µg/mL against enteric bacteria, and at least one, difloxacin, has multiple group attributes. As a class, these agents appear to be effective by interfering with the normal coiling and uncoiling of bacterial DNA as it makes microbial proteins; they directly bind to gyrases and the microbial DNA.

## BACTERIAL RESISTANCE TO ANTIMICROBIAL AGENTS

### Mechanisms of Action

In 1957, Davis proposed that there were eight mechanisms of microbial resistance to antimicrobials. These have been debated, researched, and added to and are in various states of acceptance or discredit. Our problem in the clinical laboratory is that the mechanisms are varied and may not be entirely stable (therefore unpredictable) by our current appreciation of evolutionary genetics. There are several general categories by which microorganisms resist the agents that we put in their path. The first is target modification. The antibiotic, trimethoprim for example, targets an enzyme necessary for production of nucleic acid but by target modification the bacterium produces another enzyme for the same pathway, rendering the antibiotic useless. A second mechanism requires decreased requirement for the product of a target enzyme, and a third mechanism involves an alternate metabolic pathway. Reduction of target importance is a fourth mechanism and is under serious study currently. Although there are several other mechanisms of microbial resistance, these examples serve to illustrate the issue.

## SUSCEPTIBILITY TESTING TECHNIQUES

A variety of methods are used to determine the susceptibility of microorganisms to antimicrobial agents. These include broth macrodilution and microdilution tests, agar disk diffusion tests, and other protocols such as the E-test.

### Macrodilution and Microdilution Tests

These methods use **antibiotics** diluted in broth to which a standardized inoculum of the test organism is added. The dilution in which there is no visible growth is the **mean inhibitory concentration (MIC)**. If the **minimum bacteriocidal concentration (MBC)** of the antimicrobial is needed all visually negative tubes are subcultured. In this situation, the lowest dilution in which there are no viable organisms (i.e., growth on the subculture) is the MBC.

The macrodilution broth sensitivity test is performed using a series of tube dilutions for each antibiotic tested. Because of the time and cost involved in performing this test, it is not used routinely in the clinical microbiology laboratory.

A more commonly used method is the microdilution broth sensitivity test. In this case a plastic microtiter plate with dried antimicrobials in various concentrations is used. Figure 7-2 shows a microdilution plate. A measured amount of a standardized dilution of microorganisms is added to the wells of the plate and incubated. If the microorganism is able to grow in the presence of the antimicrobial at a particular dilution, a button of growth is visible. Again, as in the macrodilution test, the MIC of the organism is the dilution well in which there is no visible growth button. Microtiter plates may be used for biochemical testing as well as antimicrobial susceptibility testing and the two test systems are often combined in one microtiter plate.

### Agar Disk Diffusion Method

The standard disk diffusion method used today is the Kirby-Bauer method. It is performed using a standard media, inoculum, and paper disks that contain known amounts of antimicrobial agents. The antibiotics diffuse out into the agar at a rate unique to each antibiotic. The diffusion rate is directly related to the chemical structure. If growth of the organism is inhibited by the antibiotic, a zone of no growth appears around the disk. Zones of inhibition have been correlated with the MIC of each drug; therefore, the diameter of the zone determines whether or not the organism is sensitive (susceptible) or resistant to the particular antibiotic. Figure 7-3 shows zones of inhibition around antibiotics on a Mueller Hinton plate. Procedure 7-1 gives the standard NCCLS approved agar diffusion method based on the work of Kirby and Bauer.

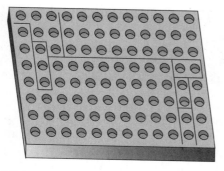

**FIGURE 7-2** Microtiter plate used for microdilution antimicrobial susceptibility testing.

**Media.** The media used is generally Mueller Hinton, but if particularly fastidious organisms such as *Neisseria gonorrhoeae, Streptococcus pneumoniae,* or *Haemophilus influenzae* must be tested, specially enriched media should be used. These include chocolate Mueller Hinton, Mueller Hinton to which 5% sheep cells have been added, and *Haemophilus* test medium (HTM). HTM is a Mueller Hinton formulation to which X and V factors have been added. In the production of these media, the pH and depth should be strictly controlled because they affect the diffusion of antibiotics into the agar.

## E-Test

The epsilometer or E-test, produced by AB Biodisk in Sweden is a relatively new test for antimicrobial sensitivity determination. It consists of a strip impregnated with graduated concentrations of antibiotic. The concentrations are marked on the strip. The inoculum for the microorganism is prepared as in the disk diffusion method and applied to the plate. The E-test disk is placed on the agar and incubated as in the disk diffusion method. Because the strip has a graduated concentration of antibiotic, the MIC can be read where the zone of inhibition crosses the strip. Although it is effective for general use, the E-test is more often used in special situations where the MIC value is desired.

## SPECIAL CONSIDERATIONS IN ANTIMICROBIAL SUSCEPTIBILITY TESTING

In several situations, determining the antibiotic sensitivity or MIC is insufficient to assess the proper treatment for a patient. These include the production of ß-lactamase by certain microorganisms, and the need for additional sensitivity testing over and above the usual protocols for methicillin-resistant *Staphylococcus aureus* (MRSA) and vancomycin-resistant *Enterococcus fecalis* (VRE).

### ß-Lactamase Production

Many clinically significant bacteria produce ß-lactamase, an enzyme that can cleave the ß-lactam ring of certain penicillin and cephalosporin drugs, making the antibiotic ineffective against the microorganism. Determining if a particular strain of bacteria is ß-lactamase positive gives immediate information as to the suitability of penicillin drugs for treatment. Many rapid tests are available that detect ß-lactamase production in a microorganism within a few minutes. One such test is the cefinase disk test (Becton Dickinson Microbiology Systems, Cockeysville, MD).

### Methicillin-Resistant *Staphylococcus aureus*

A rapid method of detecting MRSA involves using a commercially prepared medium containing oxacillin or methicillin and NaCl. The salt inhibits other gram-positive cocci and the antibiotic will inhibit the growth of staphylococci that are methicillin or oxacillin sensitive. MRSA organisms will grow well on the media. Several media manufacturers make this formulation.

### Vancomycin-Resistant *Enterococcus fecalis*

As with MRSA, selective media for the detection of VRE are available from several manufacturers. These media contain vancomycin and bile esculin. VRE will grow but non-VRE organisms will not. These media are useful for screening purposes.

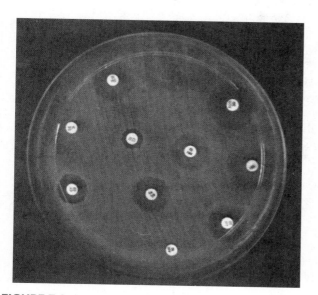

**FIGURE 7-3** Zones of inhibition in an agar diffusion sensitivity test plate.

# PROCEDURE 7-1
## Disk Susceptibility Test

### Principle:

Paper disks containing antibiotics are placed on an agar plate that has been inoculated with the test organism. The antibiotic diffuses into the agar. If the organism is sensitive to the drug, it will fail to grow up to the disk, creating a clear zone or zone of inhibition around the disk. Organisms unaffected by a particular drug will grow up to the disk.

### Equipment:

150 mm Mueller Hinton agar plates
Sterile cotton swabs
McFarland 0.5 standard
0.5-mL tubes of sterile broth (such as tryptic soy)
Sterile saline

### Method:

1. Preparation of inoculum
   Direct colony suspension method—Make a direct suspension of colonies from an 18–24-hour nonselective agar plate culture of the test organism in trypticase soy broth until it is slightly more turbid than a 0.5 McFarland standard.
   Growth method—Four to five well isolated colonies from on-selective agar culture of the test organism are touched with a loop and inoculated into 0.5 mL of tryptic soy broth and allowed to incubate until it matches or slightly exceeds the turbidity of a 0.5 McFarland standard.
2. Standardization of inoculum—The broth culture from step 1 is compared to a 0.5 McFarland standard and diluted if necessary with sterile broth or standard until the turbidity of the two tubes matches.
3. Inoculation of agar plate—A 150-mm plate must be used. Mueller Hinton agar is recommended for most organisms because it has no additives. The media and method are modified if testing fastidious organisms. To inoculate the plate, dip a sterile swab into the standardized inoculum, rotate to remove excess liquid, (i.e., "wring out" on side of tube). Swab entire plate, rotate plate 60°, swab again, and repeat once more.

4. Application of antimicrobial disks—Antimicrobial disks are applied with a commercially available dispenser and tapped gently to ensure contact with the agar surface.
5. Incubation—Plates are incubated agar side up in an ambient atmosphere at 35° to 37°C unless the organism is $CO_2$ dependent. Plates should be incubated within 15 minutes after disks are applied.
6. Measurement of inhibition zones—After 24 hours of incubation plates are examined to see if there is a lawn of growth and zones are even and circular. Zones are measured to the nearest millimeter with a caliper or ruler and recorded.
7. Interpretation—A determination of sensitive, resistant, or intermediate is made by comparing zone sizes to a table of antibiotic zone sizes supplied by the manufacturer.

### Quality Control:

1. Commercially prepared paper disks should be stored below 8°C.
2. Quality control strains of microorganisms should be used to monitor the accuracy and precision of the procedure. These may be obtained from several sources. At least one gram-negative and gram-positive organism should be tested each day that disk diffusion tests are done.
3. Complete records must be kept for each quality control strain and antimicrobial agent tested.

### Expected Results:

A confluent lawn of growth should be apparent and zones of inhibition should be circular and uniform.

### Reference:

National Committee for Clinical Laboratory Standards. (1993). *Performance standards for antimicrobial disk susceptibility tests* (5th ed.). Approved Standard M2-A5. Villanova, PA: Author.

## SUMMARY

▶ Antimicrobials are produced by a variety of microorganisms such as fungi or the actinomycetes. However, the practicality of using these as chemotherapeutic agents depends on and is affected by the nature of the agent itself, the kind of microorganism it is to be used against, the physiologic state of that microorganism, and the environment.

▶ Antimicrobials work against microorganisms in several ways. They may be cell wall active; they damage the cell wall of the organism. They may be able to disorganize, alter the permeability or affect the enzymes of the cell membrane (cell membrane active). They may be antiprotein, by altering or preventing protein synthesis in the cell. They may have antimetabolic effects or they may damage or alter the nucleic acid of the cell.

▶ There are many mechanisms by which microorganisms evade the effect of antimicrobials and thus are resistant to their effects. These include target modification and alternate metabolic pathways. Certain enzymes (e.g., ß-lactamase) produced by some microorganisms can cleave essential molecules from antimicrobials, rendering them ineffective.

▶ Several methods are available to test the effectiveness of antimicrobials against microorganisms. The most common is the agar disk diffusion method. In this method paper disks containing antibiotics are placed on an agar plate that has been inoculated with the test organism. The antibiotic diffuses into the agar. If the organism is sensitive to the drug it will fail to grow up to the disk, creating a clear zone or zone of inhibition around the disk. Organisms unaffected by a particular drug will grow up to the disk.

▶ There are special situations in which additional tests must be done to determine the best antibiotic drug to use. Some organisms produce ß-lactamase, which destroys the ß-lactam ring of the penicillins and cephalosporins. Rapid tests are available to detect ß-lactamase production, thus giving the clinician immediate information to use in choosing the appropriate antibiotic for treatment. Selective media are now available to detect MRSA and VRE in mixed cultures.

## Review Questions

1. Microbistatic substances help combat microbial infections by:
   a. killing the invading microbe so the immune system is not required.
   b. enhancing the effectiveness of another antimicrobial drug.
   c. attacking something that the microbe requires.
   d. encouraging the growth of an antagonistic microbe.

2. Which of the following affects the administration of antimicrobial drugs given to humans?
   a. The manner in which the drug is metabolized and eliminated from the body
   b. Absorption of the drug by the patient's tissues
   c. Distribution of the drug through the patient's tissues
   d. All of the above

3. It is more difficult to attack microbial cell membranes because:
   a. their cell walls serve to protect them from all classes of antimicrobial substances.
   b. of the similarities to human cell membranes.
   c. microbial cell membranes are profoundly different from human cell membranes.
   d. there are no effective drugs for this purpose.

4. Drugs like the polymyxins are used primarily as:
   a. injectable drugs.
   b. topical agents.
   c. oral preparations.
   d. veterinary medications.

5. Toxicity in the administration of the aminoglycosides is due primarily to:
   a. their effect on DNA synthesis in eucaryotic cells.
   b. their destructive nature on normal flora of the gastrointestinal tract.
   c. the inability of the patient to take other antimicrobials when taking these drugs.
   d. their buildup in the patient's system.

6. The tetracyclines:
   a. are not effectively absorbed by human tissue.
   b. effectively kill certain cancerous cells.
   c. effectively penetrate the body.
   d. Both a and c are true.

7. Macrodilution broth sensitivity tests of antimicrobial agents are:
   a. used routinely to evaluate those drugs.
   b. too expensive and time consuming to use routinely.
   c. not effective in evaluating those drugs.
   d. Both b and c are true.

8. The Kirby-Bauer method is:
   a. a standard disk diffusion method used to establish the effectiveness of antimicrobial drugs.
   b. a dosage determination method used to establish the most cost effective way to treat microbial infection.
   c. a tube dilution method used to establish the antibody titer after recovery from an infectious disease.
   d. None of the above are true.

9. Which of the following affect the choice of chemotherapeutic agents in the treatment of infectious disease?
   a. The kind of microbe causing the infection
   b. The nature of the antimicrobial agent
   c. The physiological state of the microbe; for example, does it form endospores?
   d. All of the above

10. The polyenes:
   a. are primarily used as antifungal agents.
   b. are cell membrane inhibitors.
   c. are effective antiprotozoan agents.
   d. Both a and b are true.

## ▶ REFERENCES & RECOMMENDED READING

Conte, J., & Barriere, S. (1988). *Manual of antibiotics and infectious diseases* (6th ed.). Philadelphia: Lea & Febiger.

Koneman, E. W., Allen, S. D., Janda, W. M., Schreckenberger, P. C., & Winn, W. C., Jr. (1997). *Color atlas and textbook of diagnostic microbiology* (5th ed.). Philadelphia: Lippincott-Raven Publishers.

Murray, P. R. (Ed.). (1995). *Manual of clinical microbiology* (6th ed.). Washington, DC: ASM Press.

National Committee for Clinical Laboratory Standards. (1993). *Performance standards for antimicrobial disk susceptibility tests* (5th ed.) Approved Standard M2-A5. Villanova, PA: Author.

Rakel, R. E. (Ed.). (1995). *Kohh's current therapy*. Philadelphia: Saunders.

Reese, R. E., & Betts, R. F. (1993). *Handbook of antibiotics* (2nd ed.). Boston: Little, Brown.

Ritschel, W. A. (1992). *Handbook of basic pharmacokinetics* (4th ed.). Drug Intelligence Publications.

# Part One: General Methods for Identification of Bacteria

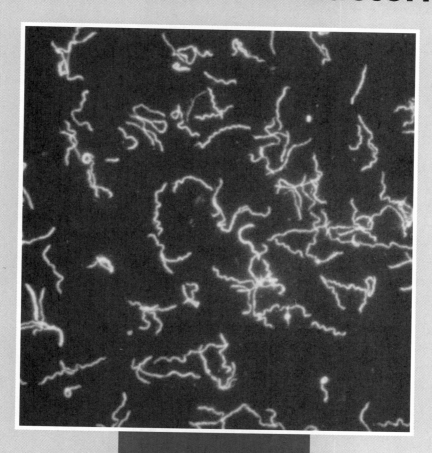

# CHAPTER 8

# Microscopic, Cultural, and Other Techniques for Bacterial Identification

Sheryl A. Whitlock, MA, MT (ASCP), BB

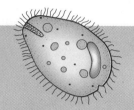

## *Microbes in the News*

Dracunculiasis is a parasitic disease caused by the filarial worm Dracunculus medinensis (Guinea worm) and is transmitted through contaminated drinking water. About 1 year after the infection occurs one or more meter-long adult female worms emerge through the skin often incapacitating the patient for up to 2 months. Although a global campaign to eradicate the disease has dramatically reduced the number of cases worldwide, occasional cases are reported in the United States. Two cases of dracunculiasis have been documented in the United States since 1995, both were imported from Sudan.

In 1995 a 9-year-old girl residing in Tennessee who had emigrated from Sudan presented at a local health clinic with a worm emerging from her left leg. She reported that another worm had emerged from her right lower leg prior to leaving Sudan. Her leg was secondarily infected and despite treatment with antibiotics required draining and a skin graft application to the wound.

In April 1997 a 31-year-old woman who emigrated to Connecticut from Sudan was diagnosed with tuberculosis. Examination and radiography of the woman revealed lung lesions suggestive of tuberculosis and a worm-like calcification in her left chest. A physical exam revealed several oval lesions on both lower legs. The woman reported that a string-like worm had emerged from her leg during the previous year. A dead and calcified Guinea worm was found in her lung.

There have been no reported cases of dracunculiasis transmitted in the United States and the risk of transmission from an active case is low. The disease can be completely prevented by keeping infected individuals from entering and contaminating the water supply. Humans are the only vertebrate host of the parasite and only the patient with the emerging worm presented any risk for transmission to others. Source: *Morbidity and Mortality Weekly Report.* March 27, 1998/ Vol. 47 / No. 11 Pages 209–211.

## KEY TERMS

| | | |
|---|---|---|
| Acid-fast stain | Decolorized | Microaerophilic |
| Acidic dye | Differential media | Mordant |
| Agar | Differential stain | Negative stains |
| Anaerobic | Dilution streaking | Primary media |
| Aseptic technique | Exudate | Primary stain |
| Basic dye | Fixing | Reducing media |
| Brownian movement | Gram negative | Selective media |
| Catalase test | Gram positive | Simple stain |
| Coagulase test | Gram stain | Smears |
| Colony | Inoculate | Special stain |
| Counterstain | Inoculum | Staining |
| Culture | Intracellularly | Streaking |
| Culture media | Isolated colonies | Universal Standards |

## LEARNING OBJECTIVES

Upon successful completion of this chapter, the student should be able to:

1. Describe and categorize bacteria by the three main types of bacterial morphology.
2. Identify and describe culture equipment and techniques for growth and identification of bacterial cultures.
3. Discuss and perform staining techniques for bacteria.
4. Outline a series of test procedures to identify a bacteria.
5. List and describe culture media for growth of various types of bacteria.

## INTRODUCTION

Microscopic and culture techniques are vital to the correct identification of bacteria in diagnostic settings. These techniques include some standard equipment, reagents, and media as well as methods that have been proven to be effective. **Aseptic technique** is a series of steps or skills that helps to reduce or eliminate contamination of cultures. This chapter focuses on methods used in the laboratory to identify bacteria. The methods include microscopic, culture, and test methods. When working with clinical specimens, laboratory workers must always remember to use **Standard standards** to protect themselves and others from accidental contamination with infectious material. When necessary, cultures should be handled under a hood to prevent accidental contamination.

## MICROSCOPIC MORPHOLOGY

Microscopic identification of bacteria requires an understanding of bacterial morphology. The three major morphologic types, cocci, bacilli, and spirochetes, may be seen in Figure 1-7. When examining the bacteria microscopically, the morphology as well as the size and arrangement should be noted. The arrangements may be in clusters, chains, or random. When cellular material is present from a clinical specimen, bacteria observed **intracellularly** should also be noted.

## MICROSCOPIC METHODS

Microscopy is used in bacteriology to examine smears made directly from clinical specimens as well as preparations made from bacterial cultures. When clinical specimens are examined for bacteria, the specimen may be a direct smear of a liquid (such as urine or cerebrospinal fluid) or an **exudate** or may be from a swab that was taken from a specific site such as a throat, wound, or discharge. The clinical specimens are most often fixed and stained for better visibility and differentiation.

### Wet Mounts

A wet mount, as implied, is a preparation where the material to be examined is suspended in a drop of liquid. The preparations may be stained or unstained.

After the liquid and material to be examined are placed on the slide, a cover slip is placed on the liquid drop. These mounts may be examined under low (10×) or high (40×) power or oil immersion objectives. In bacteriology, it is usually necessary to use high power or oil immersion due to the size of the organisms. Intensity of the light, when examining wet preps, should be low. Maximum contrast provides the best results when examining wet mounts.

A common use for wet mounts in bacteriology is to examine bacteria for motility. In this case, stain is not used because it may have a lethal effect on the bacteria. A special type of wet mount known as a hanging drop slide may also be used to determine motility. See Procedures 8-1 and 8-2 for examples of wet mount preparation for motility.

## PROCEDURE 8-1
### Wet Mount for Motility

**Principle:**

A bacterial colony is suspended in saline and observed for motility.

**Method:**

1. Place one drop of normal saline on a clean, dry slide.
2. Using aseptic technique, transfer one colony of bacteria to the drop of saline on the slide. *Note:* If using a broth culture, a drop of the broth culture is placed on the slide without saline.
3. Using the loop or needle, suspend the bacteria in the saline using a circular motion.
4. Gently place a coverslip onto the drop.
5. Examine under low power using low intensity light.
6. When the microscope is focused under low power, switch to the high power objective.
7. Examine the sample for motility. *Note:* It may be necessary to increase the intensity of the light, but a low intensity is necessary for maximum contrast of unstained preparations.
8. Motility is indicated by movement from one place on the slide to another. Vibration implies **Brownian movement** rather than motility.

## PROCEDURE 8-2
### Hanging Drop Method

**Principle:**

A drop of a broth culture of a bacteria is examined for motility.

**Method:**

1. Place some petroleum jelly around the edges of a small cover glass.
2. Using a loop, place one drop of a well-mixed broth culture in the center of the cover glass.
3. Invert a concavity slide over the drop of broth.
4. Press down gently but firmly so that the petroleum jelly sticks to the slide, but the cover glass does not break.
5. Reinvert the slide and examine microscopically.
6. Observe for motility

**Safety:**

Because the bacteria are live and potentially infectious, be certain to wear gloves and lab coat as a protective covering. Wash hands and disinfect all work surfaces on completion of the exercise.

**Expected Results:**

Motility will be present in some bacteria but not in others. Be certain to differentiate motility from Brownian movement. Motility is movement from point to point, whereas Brownian movement is vibration of the bacteria while remaining in the approximate same location.

## Stains and Stain Techniques

The process of **staining** implies that the organisms will be colored to emphasize structures or differentiate types of bacteria by their affinity for a certain type of stain. Stains are useful in the bacteriology laboratory for viewing both wet and dry preparations. The focus of this section will be staining of dry preparations.

Stains are salts made up of a positive and a negative ion. One of these ions actually lends color to the microorganisms. If the positive ion produces the color, the dye is a **basic dye**, whereas **acidic dyes** use the negative ion as their active ingredient. Basic dyes are used most frequently in bacteriology because many bacterial cell walls will have an affinity for the basic dye. Basic dyes include crystal violet and methylene blue. Acidic dyes are not as useful for staining bacteria, but will stain the background of a preparation or are used as a counterstain. An example of an acidic dye is eosin.

Stains may be divided into three major categories: **simple**, **differential**, and **special stains**. Most stains are applied to prepared **smears**. These smears are prepared either from a **culture** that has been grown in the laboratory on **culture media** or directly from an exudate or swab collected from the site of infection.

**Smear Preparation.** Smears prepared directly from an exudate or a cotton swab are applied to the slide with the swab *after* all culture plates have been prepared. If a smear is being prepared from a colony on a culture plate, some sterile water may be used to suspend the colony. This sterile water is applied with a loop. A colony of the bacteria is then transferred to the slide with a clean loop. This second loop is used to mix the bacteria and water, and the smear is allowed to air dry. **Fixing** the slide is necessary to prevent the bacteria from washing off in the staining process. The slide is usually heat fixed by passing the slide through the flame of a Bunsen burner. It is important that the slide be completely dry before heat fixing. An aerosol may be created if a wet bacterial suspension is heated. Once the smear is heat fixed and cooled, it may be stained with the chosen method.

**Simple Stains.** A simple stain is a single basic dye that is used to examine the organisms on the slide as well as their features. The most commonly used simple stains are methylene blue, crystal violet, and safranin. Simple stains are not as useful in bacteriology as other types of stains and will not be discussed further.

**Differential Stains.** Differential stains provide varying results with different types of bacteria and may be used to make distinctions. The most commonly used differential stains are the **Gram stain** and the **acid-fast stain**.

GRAM STAIN. The Gram stain divides most bacteria into two major groups: **gram positive** and **gram negative**. This differentiation is made by the bacteria's ability to bind and hold the dye crystal violet. Bacteria that bind the dye will stain a dark purple and are designated as gram-positive bacteria. Bacteria that cannot maintain the crystal violet dye will be counterstained with safranin. These bacteria appear pink in the final preparation and are known as gram-negative bacteria. Not all bacteria will stain with the Gram stain and require special staining techniques for observation.

**Steps in the Gram stain process.** A fixed smear is used to prepare a Gram stain. The first step involves the application of a **primary stain**, crystal violet. The stain is removed by rinsing with water, and the slide covered with iodine. The iodine serves as a **mordant** to make the stain appear more intense. The iodine is removed by rinsing with water, and the slide **decolorized** using acetone-alcohol. This decolorizing solution removes the crystal violet from the cells that will ultimately appear as gram-negative. The decolorizer is applied and removed quickly. The decolorizing time is dependent on the thickness of the smear. If the slide does not appear to be adequately decolorized, additional applications may be made. The final step is the addition of the **counterstain**, safranin. The counterstain will stain the cells that will be classified as gram-negative. Smears are air dried before microscopic examination.

The Gram stain will stain structures other than bacteria. If the smear is from a swab or exudate, white blood cells, red blood cells, epithelial cells, yeast, fungus, and other structures will appear stained as well as any bacteria present in the smear. Figure 8-1 summarizes the Gram stain procedure.

**Reading and interpretation of a Gram stain.** When reading a Gram stain, the slide is first focused on the low power objective. The high power objective is then put into place with focused using the fine focus adjustment knob. Only at this time can the switch to the oil immersion objective be made. All Gram stains should be read with the oil immersion objective. This enables the viewer to observe the details of the bacteria and other cells present in the preparation. The slide is then examined for presence of organisms and cells that bear clinical significance. All organisms are noted and differentiated as gram-positive (purple) or gram-negative (pink). The shape and arrangement of the organisms should be recorded. Additionally, note any other cells present as well as intracellular organisms and their Gram reaction.

ACID-FAST STAIN. Acid-fast stains are also used in the microbiology laboratory. An acid-fast stain differentiates organisms that will bind the carbolfuchsin dye. These bacteria have a waxy material, mycolic acid, in their cell walls. Organisms that commonly stain with acid-fast stains are *Mycobacterium* species including *Mycobacterium tuberculosis,* causative agent of tuberculosis, and *Mycobacterium leprae,* causative agent of leprosy. *Nocardia* species are also acid-fast.

**Acid-fast staining procedure.** Acid-fast or Ziehl-Neelsen and Kinyous stains are used in a manner similar to the Gram stain procedure. The primary stain is carbolfuchsin. This stain is applied to a heat-fixed smear and allowed to remain for the designated time period. During this time period, the slide is gently heated to enhance attachment of the stain. The slide is cooled and washed with water. A decolorizer consisting of methanol and hydrochloric acid is applied to wash the stain from cells that are not acid-fast. Finally, the slide is counterstained with methylene blue or brilliant green depending on the procedure being followed.

Acid-fast smears are read under oil immersion. The acid-fast bacteria will appear red while any bacteria that are not acid fast will be blue. Interpretations should be recorded.

**Special Stains.** Special stains are used to highlight specific parts of the microorganism. The three most important types of special stains used are capsule stains, flagella stains, and endospore stains.

Capsule stains are used to identify the presence of a capsule surrounding the microorganism. Capsular stains are **negative stains**. Negative stains actually stain the background and provide a dark background against which the colorless capsule can be seen. This type of staining is necessary because the capsules do not absorb the stain and the capsules are easily removed with the washing procedure. India ink and nigrosin are commonly used negative stains.

Endospore or spore stains differentiate the spores found in some genera of bacteria. Malachite green will stain the spore while the counterstain, safranin, will stain the remainder of the cell red or pink.

Flagella stains color the flagella that are not visible under the light microscope. A stain and a mordant are used to build up the diameters of the flagella to make them visible. Carbolfuchsin is a stain used for this purpose.

| Step | Time | Procedure | Result |
|---|---|---|---|
| 1 | one minute | Primary stain: Apply crystal violet stain (purple) ↓ Rinse slide | All bacteria stain purple 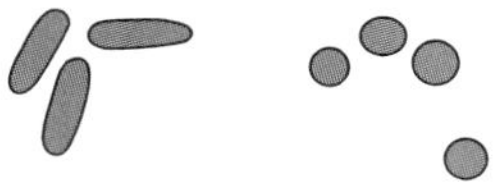 |
| 2 | one minute | Mordant: Apply Gram's iodine ↓ Rinse slide | All bacteria remain purple 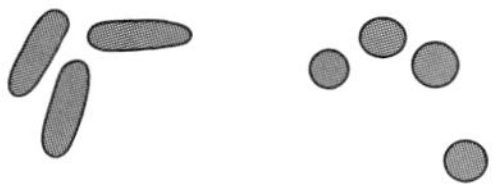 |
| 3 | three to five seconds | Decolorize: Apply alcohol ↓ Rinse slide | Purple stain is removed from gram-negative cells 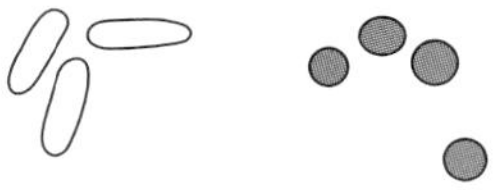 |
| 4 | one minute | Counterstain: Apply safranin stain (red) ↓ Rinse slide | Gram-negative cells appear pink-red; gram-positive cells appear purple 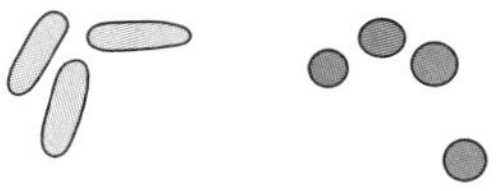 |

**FIGURE 8-1** Gram stain procedure. 1. Smear is covered with crystal violet; the dye is removed. 2. Smear is covered with iodine; the iodine is removed. 3. Smear is washed with a decolorizer; the decolorizer is washed off. 4. A counterstain is used on the smear; the stain is removed.

## PROCEDURE 8-3
### Gram Stain of a Prepared Smear

**Principle:**

A smear that has been prepared from a culture plate will be stained using the Gram stain procedure.

**Method:**

1. Heat fix a prepared smear by holding it with forceps and passing through a Bunsen burner flame two or three times.
2. When cool, place the smear on a staining rack. Flood the smear with the crystal violet stain. Allow the stain to stand for 1 minute.
3. Rinse the slide with a steady stream of water from a faucet or squeeze bottle. Tilt the slide to remove excess water.
4. Flood the slide with Gram's iodine and allow to stand for 1 minute.
5. Rinse as in step 3.
6. Holding the slide with forceps, squeeze decolorizer onto the slide until no more purple color runs off. *Note:* Do not decolorize excessively.
7. Rinse as in step 3.
8. Flood the slide with safranin for 1 minute.
9. Rinse as in step 3.
10. Remove excess water by standing slides on end. Wipe the back of the slide to remove excess stain. Allow to dry completely before reading.

**Quality Control:**

Known gram-positive and gram-negative cultures may be stained in parallel as a form of quality control. Some examples of bacteria that could be used as controls include *Staphylococcus aureus* for gram-positive and *Escherichia coli* for gram-negative.

**Expected Results:**

Organisms with an affinity for the crystal violet stain will appear purple. Those that are decolorized will stain with safranin and will appear pink.

## ASEPTIC AND PURE CULTURE TECHNIQUES

To obtain correct results from bacteriologic cultures, techniques and procedures must ensure that contamination of the culture or the workers does not occur. Aseptic technique is a series of steps that helps to do both of these things. It includes measures to protect the worker from being exposed to pathogens and those that prevent contamination of the cultures.

Aseptic technique includes proper use of equipment. Correct inoculation of media, proper transfer of bacteria from patient sources as well as from one culture media to another, and appropriate preparation of cultures for transfer are also involved.

### Use of Equipment

Equipment most commonly used for preparation and manipulation of cultures include inoculating loops and needles, Bunsen burners, and loop incinerators. This equipment is summarized in Figure 8-2.

Inoculating loops and needles are used to transfer bacteria from a plate or slant. The material may be transferred to a broth, culture plate, agar slant or deep,

or a slide. When performing these transfers, guidelines for use of nondisposable equipment include:

1. Loops and needles must be sterilized before and after use.
2. Sterilization takes place using either a Bunsen burner or a loop incinerator.
3. The wire portion of the loop or needle must be heated to red hot before and following use. This heating may be done with a Bunsen burner or incinerator. When using a Bunsen burner, the wire is heated by placing the wire into the blue portion of the flame beginning with the end closest to the handle and progressing to the end that will contact with the culture.
4. The loop must be completely cooled before touching a bacterial colony. If the loop is not cool, it will sizzle. This sizzling produces an aerosol that could prove infectious.
5. Never lay the loop or needle on the counter. This equipment should be stored in a rack and should always be sterilized before returning them to the rack after use.

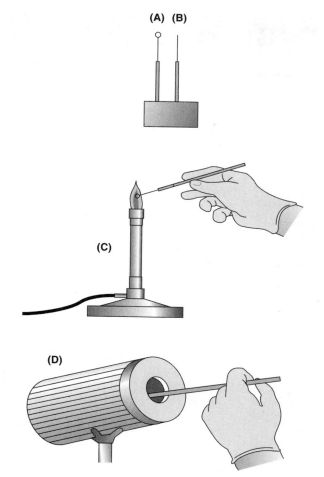

**FIGURE 8-2** Equipment for bacteriologic cultures. A. Inoculating loop. B. Inoculating needle. C. Bunsen burner. D. Loop incinerator.

Disposable loops and needles are available and are intended for a single use. They must then be discarded as a biohazard.

Bunsen burners and loop incinerators are used to sterilize nondisposable loops and needles. These items should be used with care to avoid injury. Loop incinerators are not as versatile as Bunsen burners for other uses in the laboratory.

## Artificial Media

Microorganisms may be grown outside of the host by providing the nutrients and growth factors required. The growth factors and nutrients may be derived from soy or other protein extracts. Additional substances such as blood, dyes, salts, or vitamins may be added to either enhance growth of fastidious organisms or inhibit growth of others. The media may be in the form of a liquid broth or solid or semisolid **agar**. Plates 1 through 6 provide samples of various types of media. When grown on solid agar, the microorganisms form a colony that represent the progeny of each individual bacteria in the original **inoculum**.

**Categories of Artificial Media.** Different types of artificial media are available to serve specific purposes in the clinical laboratory. A general type of nutritive media that may be used to store cultures or grow organisms that are not fastidious include nutrient agar and nutrient broth. Additional media fall into different categories. The most common types include: enriched, differential, and selective media. Table 8-1 summarizes commonly used media.

**ENRICHED MEDIA.** Enriched media has one or more added substances to increase the likelihood of growth of fastidious organisms. The added substances include blood or serum products or vitamins. Some commonly used enriched media include blood agar to which red blood cells have been added and chocolate agar to which hemoglobin has been added. Blood agar is commonly used as a **primary media** and is inoculated with the original inoculum.

**DIFFERENTIAL MEDIA.** **Differential** or indicator media is used to distinguish types of bacteria. This is accomplished by the addition of substances that will be changed as a result of metabolic activity of the bacteria. Some examples of differential media include eosin methylene blue (EMB), MacConkey's, blood agar, and mannitol salt agar (MSA).

EMB and MacConkey's media each contain substances that will indicate fermentation of sugars and the resultant change in pH. For example, on MacConkey's agar, lactose fermenters will appear as pink colonies, whereas nonfermenters will appear clear. This is due to the neutral red indicator that reacts to changes in pH. Mannitol salt agar is also differential for fermentation of mannitol and the resultant pH change that occurs will result in a color change to yellow.

Blood agar is also considered a differential media. It plays the differential role because it distinguishes bacteria that have the capability to hemolyze red blood cells. Bacteria with the capability to do this include *Streptococcus pyogenes,* the causative agent of strep throat, and *Staphylococcus aureus.*

**SELECTIVE MEDIA.** As implied, **selective media** is selective for some bacteria and inhibitory for others. This is helpful for separating mixed cultures. Some examples of selective media include EMB, MacConkey, MSA, and phenylethyl alcohol (PEA) agar. EMB and MacConkey's contain crystal violet to inhibit the growth of gram-positive organisms; PEA inhibits gram-negative organisms. Mannitol salt contains a high salt concentration that inhibits many organisms. Selective media may also be differential.

**Obtaining Culture Media.** Culture media may be either purchased in the prepared form or prepared from dehydrated media. Preparation is more economical, but

| Table 8–1 ▶ Commonly Used Bacteriologic Media | | |
|---|---|---|
| **Media** | **Contents** | **Use** |
| Bile esculin agar (BEA) | Agar base with desoxycholate and ferric citrate | Identify and isolate group D streptococcus |
| Blood agar | Soy or beef heart infusion agar base with sheep's blood | General use for growth of organisms; determination of hemolytic properties |
| Chocolate agar | Peptone base with hemoglobin | Isolate *Neisseria* and *Haemophilus* species |
| Cooked meat (CM) or chopped meat | Chopped meat particles and reducing substances | Anaerobic cultures |
| Eosin methylene blue (EMB) | Peptone base; lactose and sucrose; indicators eosin and methylene blue | Differentiate lactose fermenting organisms |
| Gram-negative broth (GN) | Broth base with glucose and mannitol; inhibitors added | Selective growth media for enteric pathogens |
| Hektoen enteric agar (HE) | Agar base with bile salts lactose, sucrose; bromthymol blue and acid fuchsin indicators | Isolate and differentiate Salmonella and Shigella |
| MacConkey agar | Peptose base with lactose; crystal violet and bile salts as inhibitors; indicator neutral red | Isolate and differentiate lactose fermenting organisms |
| Mannitol salt agar | Agar base with mannitol and 7.5% NaCl; indicator phenol red | Growth and differentiation of coagulase-positive *Staphylococcus* |
| Phenylethyl alcohol agar (PEA) | Nutrient agar with inhibitor phenylethanol | Selective growth of gram-positive cocci |
| Salmonella-Shigella agar (SS) | Peptone agar with lactose, ferric citrate and sodium citrate; inhibitors bile salts and brilliant green; indicator phenol red | Selective for *Salmonella* and *Shigella* species |
| Thayer-Martin agar (TM) | Blood agar with hemoglobin and supplement B; inhibitors | Selective for *Neisseria* species |
| Thioglycollate broth | Enriched soy broth; glucose and reducing agents | Growth of most bacteria including anaerobes and microaerophiles |
| Xylose lysine deoxycholate (XLD) | Agar with xylose, lactose, sucrose sodium deoxycholate and lysine; indicator phenol red | Selective for *Salmonella* and *Shigella* species |

time consuming, and must be done carefully to prevent contamination. Purchase of prepared culture media is more expensive, but does not require the time for preparation. You must have the ability to refrigerate the prepared media once it has been purchased.

## Culture Techniques

Techniques for preparing cultures that must be interpreted and further tested are vital to the bacteriology laboratory. These techniques include inoculating media. To **inoculate** means to transfer some of the organisms to a growth media. The organisms that are transferred are known as the inoculum.

**Inoculation of Culture Plates.** The process of inoculating culture plates is **streaking**. Streaking involves using an inoculating loop (disposable or reusable) and diluting the specimen by spreading it thinly over the surface of a plate. This process is known as **dilution streaking**. Dilution streaking is done by dividing the plate into three or four sections, known as quadrants. The first section (usually called a quadrant) is inocu-

lated with a heavy inoculum from either a swab or an inoculating loop (see Figure 8-3).

If a swab is used for the original inoculum, a loop is used for the remaining streaking. The technician must begin by flaming the loop to red hot before streaking the second quadrant. If a loop is used for the original inoculum, prior to streaking the second quadrant, the loop is heated in the Bunsen burner or incinerator, but not until red hot. Then, the loop is passed into the original inoculum two or three times with a back and forth motion. Without lifting the loop, three or four more motions are made that do not pass back into the previous quadrant. This same process is repeated either one or two more times. The effect is that the amount of bacteria in each section decreases. The desired result, after incubation, is visualized in Figure 8-4. When colonies are observed separated, they are said to be **isolated colonies**.

When handling culture plates, the plates are stored in an inverted fashion with the lid down. When a plate is being streaked, it is held in the technician's nondominant hand. The dominant hand performs the streak-

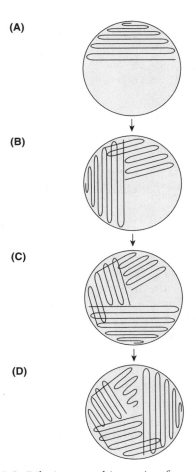

**FIGURE 8-3** Dilution streaking using four quadrants.

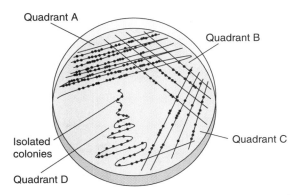

**FIGURE 8-4** Isolated colonies on a dilution streaked plate.

ing. The plate is then returned to its lid. A culture plate is never allowed to sit with the agar exposed. Contamination may occur.

To streak a urine culture, a slightly different method of streaking is used. A specific volume of urine is used. This is accomplished with a calibrated loop that will deliver 0.001 mL of urine to the plate. The loop is dipped into a well-mixed urine and streaked down the center of a plate from one end to another (see Figure 8-5). The loop is used to streak across the line that was cre-

ated by the first streak. The plate is rotated 90°, and the process repeated.

Once the culture produces colonies a calculation of the number of bacteria present may be performed. Because 0.0001 mL of urine was used to streak the plate, the number of colonies present may be multiplied by 1,000 to determine the number of bacteria per milliliter of urine.

**Inoculation of Culture Tubes and Broth.** In addition to agar plates, bacteria are sometimes cultured on agar slants or in tubes of broth or agar (deeps). Inoculation of these cultures is done with either a loop or a needle with the exception of the deep that is always inoculated with a needle. Whenever tubes are inoculated, the mouth or opening of the tube is flamed before and after the inoculation takes place. This prevents accidental contamination of the culture. See Figure 8-6 for this technique.

To inoculate a slant, the bacteria are streaked onto the slanted portion of the media (see Figure 8-7). If agar slants are being used for biochemical tests, the butt of the tube might be stabbed so that inoculum is introduced to the bottom of the tube. If this is necessary, a needle is used and pushed to the bottom of the tube before the slant is streaked.

Inoculation of an agar deep is performed in much

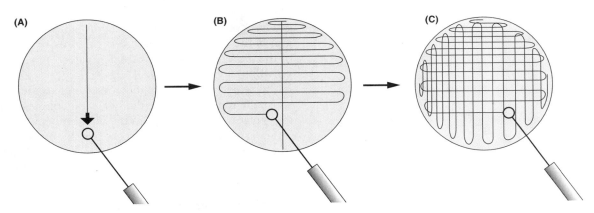

**FIGURE 8-5** Streaking pattern for a urine culture.

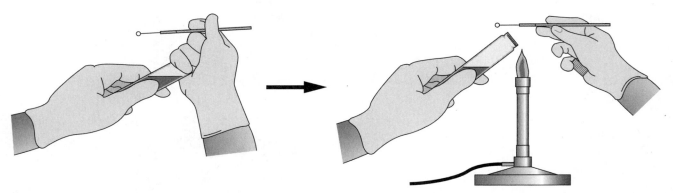

**FIGURE 8-6**  Proper method for sterilizing the opening of culture tubes.

the same way. The needle with inoculum is introduced to approximately one-half inch from the bottom of the tube and pulled straight out.

Inoculation of broth cultures is performed by introducing the inoculum from a swab, needle, or loop. The inoculum is introduced into the broth and the broth incubated. A swab may remain in the broth after the inoculation process. If this is the case, the swab may need to be broken for the cap to be placed on the tube.

**Incubation of Cultures.** After inoculation, cultures are incubated in the appropriate conditions. Agar plates are placed in baskets or racks and placed in the incubator. Broth, slants, and deeps are placed in test tube racks. Conditions for incubation will vary with the type of culture. Most cultures will be incubated at 37°C in an incubator with an established concentration of $CO_2$. Special incubation conditions are required for **anaerobic** cultures.

After incubation, cultures are read, interpreted, and further testing performed. Cultures may be refrigerated for future reference. Refrigeration may be used if it is not possible to read cultures at the end of the incubation time.

## Growth Conditions

Bacteria that are pathogenic to humans grow under conditions similar to those in the human body. The

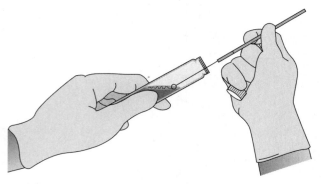

**FIGURE 8-7**  Technique for inoculating an agar slant.

factors that influence growth include physical and chemical factors. The physical factors taken into account with both culture media and environmental conditions include pH, temperature, and osmotic pressure. The chemical conditions include provision of factors for metabolism and nutritional requirements of the bacteria. These include water, oxygen, sources of carbon and nitrogen, and organic growth requirements.

**Anaerobic Culture Techniques.**  Bacteria that require anaerobic growth conditions will be cultivated using special equipment and conditions. Anaerobic bacteria require the use of **reducing media**. This media has the ability to remove dissolved oxygen to enhance the growth of the anaerobic bacteria. Examples of reducing media include enriched thioglycollate broth and cooked meat broth.

Conditions of diminished oxygen provide an anaerobic environment for growth of the cultures. This anaerobic environment may be provided by the use of a sealed anaerobic container that contains chemical substances to use the oxygen so that it is not lethal to the anaerobic bacteria. Figure 8-8A contains an anaerobic container with chemical packet, catalyst, and indicator necessary to ensure the anaerobic growth conditions. The chemical packet contains sodium bicarbonate and sodium borohydride. When water is added to the packet, hydrogen and carbon dioxide are produced. The lid of the jar contains a palladium catalyst. This catalyst combines the released hydrogen with the oxygen in the jar to form water. It condenses on the sides of the jar. The carbon dioxide generated enhances the growth of the anaerobic bacteria. An indicator is placed in the sealed jar to verify the absence of oxygen. This is usually methylene blue that will turn colorless when the oxygen is removed from the environment.

Special oxygen-free chambers may be used to cultivate and handle anaerobic cultures. These chambers contain inert gases and cultures are manipulated through glove ports (see Figure 8-8B).

**REQUIREMENTS FOR REDUCED OXYGEN CONCENTRATIONS.** The growth requirements for **microaerophilic** bacteria

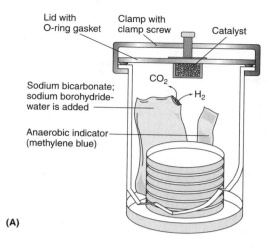

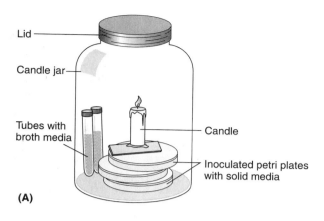

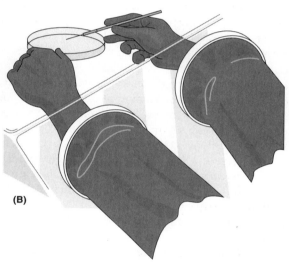

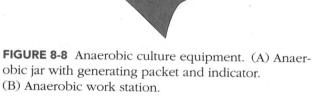

**FIGURE 8-8** Anaerobic culture equipment. (A) Anaerobic jar with generating packet and indicator. (B) Anaerobic work station.

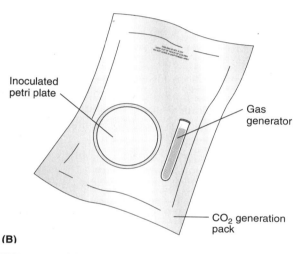

**FIGURE 8-9** (A) Candle jar;  (B) $CO_2$ gas generation pack.

are reduced oxygen conditions. This is accomplished with the use of a candle jar as seen in Figure 8-9A. The culture plates are placed in a sealed jar and a candle is lit. The candle will be extinguished when the oxygen concentration is too low to support the flame. At this point, the oxygen concentration is reduced. This same process may be accomplished with $CO_2$ incubators that allow the concentration of $CO_2$ to be adjusted or by using sealed culture packs with a $CO_2$ gas generator (see Figure 8-9B).

## Interpretation of Bacteriologic Cultures

Culture plates are interpreted by examination of the colonies formed. Colony shape, size, color, and growth pattern are observed. Changes in the media are also observed and noted. These include pitting, hemolysis, and color changes. Odors and characteristics such as swarming over the plate's surface are noted in making preliminary judgments of the bacteria present. Knowledge of normal flora at the culture site is helpful in identifying potentially pathogenic bacteria.

Colonies of different bacterial types have different characteristics. Each type of colony must be identified. This is done with stains, biochemical tests, and subculture to selective and differential media.

**Interpretation of Culture Tubes.** Broth cultures are used to promote growth, save the original organisms from a swab, and prepare suspensions of bacteria to be used for susceptibility testing. When bacteria grow in broth, there are three basic growth patterns: turbidity or cloudiness throughout the culture, sediment or growth on the bottom of the tube, or pellicle formation where the bacteria grow in one area such as on the top of the culture media. To test for gas formation, a small inverted gas tube, known as a Durham tube, may be placed in the broth. The gas formation will be indicated by bubbles in the tube.

Agar slants are inspected for growth in the same manner as plates. The growth may be heavy so that individual colonies may not be identified, or some isolated colonies may be seen. Colonies may be chosen from these slants for Gram stain or subculture. If the slant is a biochemical test for carbohydrate fermentation, it is observed for color change, gas bubble formation, and the blackening that indicates hydrogen sulfide formation. These methods of biochemical testing are of historic significance, but not routinely used in the clinical laboratory. The methods are incorporated into commercial panels for identification such as API strips.

## Pure Culture Techniques

After culture plates have been read, the bacteria to be identified may be separated. This can be done by attempting to obtain pure cultures of each. Colonies are transferred to separate growth media by choosing and "picking" a colony of each type and streaking it onto a separate plate. Once it is done and the culture incubated, the colonies should be of one morphologic type. The Gram reaction should be verified and further identification initiated.

When isolating types of bacteria, only a very small amount of inoculum is necessary. The technician should use a single colony that is touched with a sterile loop. Care should be taken not to damage the agar or touch any adjacent colonies. Once the colony has been touched, the new plate is streaked using the dilution streaking method.

## METHODS FOR BACTERIAL IDENTIFICATION

Bacterial identification is performed by using a combination of criteria. These criteria include Gram reaction, growth characteristics, and test methods. Test methods will be outlined in the following sections.

## Biochemical Tests

Biochemical tests are available for identifying specific bacteria. Probably the most important guideline for directing identification methods is the Gram reaction of the bacteria. Once the Gram reaction is determined, appropriate tests may be initiated. Some of these tests are available in multiple test systems such as the API strip while others are tests that are performed individually.

### Tests for Identification of Gram-Positive Organisms.
If the Gram reaction identifies an organism as a gram-positive cocci, specific tests may be used to distinguish *Streptococcus* from *Staphylococcus* and then individual species within the identified genus. The **catalase test** is used for this purpose. To further differentiate *Streptococcus* species, hemolysis, disk diffusion tests, and serologic antigen typing may be performed. If staphylococcal species are identified, **coagulase test** may be used to differentiate *Staphylococcus aureus* from other *Staphylococcus* species.

**CATALASE TEST.** Staphylococcal organisms produce the enzyme catalase, whereas streptococcal organisms do not. This enzyme will liberate oxygen and water from hydrogen peroxide. This test may be performed either on a slide or in a test tube.

**COAGULASE TEST.** *Staphylococcus* species should have coagulase tests performed as part of an identification profile. *S. aureus* produces the enzyme coagulase that can clot rabbit plasma. Other species of *Staphylococcus* do not produce this enzyme. This test may be performed either on a slide or in a tube.

**HEMOLYSIS ON BLOOD AGAR PLATES.** The hemolytic properties of colonies on blood agar are significant in identification of gram-positive cocci. Once the distinction between *Staphylococcus* and *Streptococcus* has been made, one may look at hemolysis to further differentiate the species. If the catalase is negative and *Streptococcus* is suspected, hemolysis will help to determine the specific species. Hemolysis can be divided into three categories: beta, alpha, and gamma. ß-Hemolysis is complete hemolysis and leaves a clear zone surrounding the colony. ß-Hemolytic streptococci include group A *Streptococcus,* the causative agent of strep throat and *S. aureus*. A further identification of group A strep may be made by using a bacitracin disk that will inhibit growth of group A strep or CAMP test that will be used to identify group B hemolytic streptococcus.

α-Hemolytic colonies are surrounded by a green zone. This indicates partial hemolysis. Most α-hemolytic streptococci are normal flora in the upper respiratory tract and represent no pathology when seen in cultures of these areas. *Streptococcus pneumoniae* will also be α-hemolytic and represent pathology. *S. pneumonia* may be identified by using an optichin disk (P disk) that will inhibit growth of the *S. pneumonia*. Disk diffusion tests are discussed in a later section. γ-Hemolysis represents no hemolysis.

If the gram-positive organism is catalase positive, the hemolytic state of the bacteria will be examined. *S. aureus* is most likely if hemolysis is seen or other *Staphylococcus* species such as *S. epidermidis* if no hemolysis is seen.

**CAMP TEST.** The CAMP test may be used to identify group B beta-hemolytic streptococci. Group B streptococci produce a substance that enhances the beta toxin produced by some strains of *S. aureus*. This test is performed by using a plate streaked down the middle with a toxin-producing strain of *S. aureus*. The questionable strep is streaked at a 90° angle to the original streak, but not touching the streak. The plate is incubated overnight and the hemolysis examined. If the ß-hemolytic strain of *Streptococcus* is group B, there will be lines of enhanced hemolysis beside the *S. aureus* streak. A positive control should always be used with this test.

**BILE SOLUBILITY TEST.** *Streptococcus pneumoniae* will autolyse when exposed to a bile salt. Use of the reagent, sodium deoxycholate, will cause a colony to flatten or disappear. This test is performed directly on a colony growing on a culture plate.

### Tests for Identification of Gram-Positive Bacilli.

Gram-positive rods may be encountered on the gram stain. *Corynebacterium* species or diphtheroids are most common. They are club shaped, not usually clinically significant and may be identified by commercial systems. *Corynebacterium diphtheriae* is the etiologic agent of diphtheria and is pathogenic. Other gram positive rods include *Listeria* species and *Bacillus* species. Some of these are pathogenic and are identified by motility tests and hemolysis results.

### Tests for Identification of Gram-Negative Organisms.

If the Gram stain indicates a negative bacilli, there are many tests to determine specificity. Commercial systems such as the API and Enterotube provide a series of tests in one easy test container. Some specific tests that are performed include oxidation-fermentation tests, indole production, oxidase tests, MR-VP (methyl red and Voges Proskauer) test, and motility to name a few. These tests are used in combination with the use of selective and differential media to determine the specific organism present.

**OXIDATION-FERMENTATION (O-F) TESTS.** Oxidation or fermentation of glucose has been used historically to differentiate bacteria in the *Enterobacteriaceae* family from those of other genera. These tests have been adapted to commercial systems and are still used. A fermenter of glucose is considered a possible candidate for *Enterobacteriaceae*. A bacterium that is not a fermenter is definitely not *Enterobacteriaceae* (see Figure 8-10).

The O-F test was historically performed by using two tubes of glucose media. One was overlaid with oil and the second was not. The results were examined after a maximum of 4 days. A fermentative organism would show a positive result in the bottom of both tubes while a nonfermenter (oxidizer) would show a positive result in the top of only the tube without the oil overlay. These tests are now incorporated into systems with multiple tests.

**SUBSTRATE FERMENTATION TESTS.** Members of *Enterobacteriaceae* are fermenters of glucose. They are further identified by determining their fermentation characteristics. Fermentation tests that are performed include lactose, sucrose, mannitol, dulcitol, adonitol, sorbitol, arabinose, raffinose, rhamnose, xylose, and melibiose. When fermentation occurs, acid formation is detected as a color change of the indicator. Gas formation is detected by the use of a Durham tube (see Figure 8-11). Historically, these fermentation tests were performed in individual tubes and a pattern of fermentation established for specific organisms. The tests are now incorporated into commercial panels with previously discussed tests.

**OXIDASE TEST.** In addition to the use of O-F media, the ability to grow on MacConkey's agar and the oxidase test are used to divide gram-negative organisms into broad categories. The oxidase test determines the presence of the enzyme cytochrome oxidase. This test uses the reagent, tetramethyl-p-phenylenediamine dihydrochloride, to test for the presence of this enzyme. This test is performed by adding the reagent directly to the colony on the plate or by placing it on the filter paper and adding the reagent. A positive reaction is indicated by a color change to blue or purple. This test is presumptive identification for *Neisseria* species and is positive for some gram-negative bacilli.

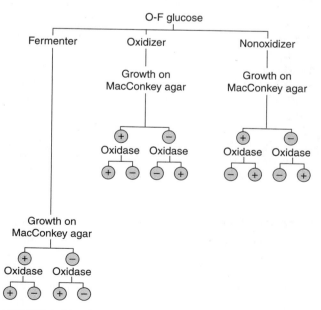

**FIGURE 8-10** Flow chart for O-F media and distinguishing gram-negative organisms.

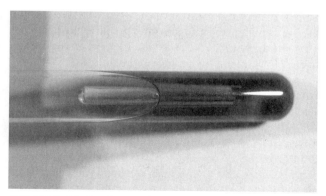

**FIGURE 8-11** Durham tube in a tube of fermentation broth.

**UREASE TEST.** Once the determination of *Enterobacteriaceae* has been made, several tests will further specify the organism. One of these is the urease test. This determination tests for the hydrolysis of urea to ammonia and water. In this process, the environment becomes alkaline and an indicator produces a pink color. *Proteus* species will yield a positive result.

**CITRATE UTILIZATION.** Gram-negative bacilli may have the ability to use citrate as their sole source of carbon. This can be determined with a culture media containing citrate and an indicator, bromthymol blue. If the citrate is utilized, the indicator will turn from green to blue. Organisms positive for this test include some species of *Enterobacter, Citrobacter, Klebsiella,* and *Yersinia.*

**DECARBOXYLATION.** The ability of an organism to decarboxylate amino acids provides a further differentiation among *Enterobacteriaceae.* Amino acids tested include lysine, arginine, and ornithine. If the amino acid is decarboxylated, the indicator, bromcresol purple, turns purple due to the alkaline nature of the media. A negative reaction will be yellow. Lysine decarboxylation occurs with *Klebsiella* and *Salmonella* species as well as *Enterobacter aerogenes, Escherichia coli,* and *Serratia marcescens.*

These tests need to be anaerobically incubated. An overlay of oil is used. They may be read up to 4 days for a positive result.

**METHYL RED AND VOGES PROSKAUER TESTS.** These two tests determine the degree of metabolism of glucose. The glucose may be metabolized to produce acidic endproducts such as acetate and formate. This can be determined with methyl red indicator producing a red color for a positive reaction. On the other hand, the metabolism may proceed to acetoin and butanediol. This latter circumstance is determined with the Voges Proskauer (VP) test.

These tests are performed using one broth that is incubated with the organism and then divided into two aliquots. One aliquot is tested with methyl red while the second is used for the VP test. *E. coli* is methyl red positive and VP negative while *Klebsiella pneumoniae* produces the opposite results.

**INDOLE TEST.** Organisms have the ability to break down the amino acid tryptophan. This breakdown produces a by-product, indole. A spot indole test is performed using 1% paradimethylaminocinnamaldehyde. The production of a purple color indicates a positive result. Some nonfermenters may require a more sensitive test. The more sensitive test uses a xylene extraction followed by addition of Kovac's reagent. Organisms that are positive for indole include *E. coli* and some *Proteus* species.

**ONPG TEST.** The ONPG test determines the presence of ß-galactosidase. A fermenter may produce slow results if it lacks the enzyme to transport the lactose across the cell membrane. This enzyme is permease. If this enzyme is missing, but the ß-galactosidase is present within the cell, fermentation can take place. The ONPG test uses the reagent, orthonitrophenyl-ß-D-galactopyranoside. When added to a bacterial suspension, this reagent will produce a yellow color if ß-galactosidase is present. Organisms that may be ONPG positive include *E. coli, Shigella sonnei,* and *Klebsiella* species.

**General Identification Tests.** Some identification tests are used both with gram-positive and gram-negative organisms. These include hydrolysis and motility tests. Although some of the previously described tests are useful in various Gram reactions and morphology, they have been placed where they prove most useful. Some tests that are useful across broad lines are described in the following sections.

**GELATIN HYDROLYSIS.** Gelatinase is produced by many organisms. Liquefaction of gelatin reagent is a positive result. Commercial systems use charcoal disks with gelatin. As the liquefaction occurs, the charcoal is released and the media darkens. Organisms producing gelatinase include *S. aureus, S. marcescens,* and *Proteus* species.

**MOTILITY TEST.** Motility tests for microorganisms have been performed in solid or semisolid agar. Many organisms are motile both at room temperature and at body temperature. Motility in these agar tubes is observed as growth out from the original stab. When an agar tube is inoculated to the bottom with a needle, bacteria will normally grow along this inoculated path. A motile organism will grow out and create a zone of growth around the original stab line.

## Disk Diffusion Tests

Filter paper disks impregnated with substances are available commercially to perform bacteriologic tests. These disks are useful for identification of two species of *Streptococcus.* Group A streptococcus will be inhibited by the substance, bacitracin. Bacitracin is impregnated onto a disk that is labeled with an "A." This disk is applied to the first quadrant of a culture plate. If a zone of inhibition is noted, the organism is group A streptococcus.

*Streptococcus pneumoniae* is inhibited by an optochin disk. This disk is labeled with a "P." The use of this disk is the same as the A disc and interpretation of the results are the same.

## Serologic Tests

Bacteria have antigens that are detectable by using specific antisera. Some bacteria that may be serologically typed are *Streptococci, Salmonella, E. coli, Shigella, Klebsiella* as well as the dimorphic fungus, *Cryptococcus.*

ß-Hemolytic *Streptococci* are serologically divided into groups by determining the cell wall carbohydrates. The possible groups include A, B, C, F, or G.

These Lancefield groups are determined by precipitin or agglutination tests.

Typing of gram-negative organisms involves different antigens: O antigens are the somatic or body antigens; H antigens are flagellar antigens; and K and Vi antigens are capsular polysaccharide antigens.

The general procedure for performing these tests includes the use of an antisera specific for the antigen being tested. This antibody may be attached to a latex particle or soluble in the antisera. The bacteria are mixed with the antibody on a slide and examined for agglutination. The presence of agglutination is a positive result; absence of agglutination is a negative result. Specific manufacturer's direction should be followed for each antisera because the observation time, volumes, and so on may vary.

## SUMMARY

▶ Microscopic morphology

1. Microscopic and cultural techniques are vital to the correct identification of bacteria in diagnostic microbiology. Microscopic identification of bacteria requires an understanding of bacterial morphology.

2. Wet mounts are a preparation where the material to be examined is suspended in a drop of fluid. A common use for wet mounts in bacteriology is to examine for bacterial motility.

3. Stains and stain techniques are used to emphasize structures or differentiate types of bacteria or other microbes. Stains are divided into three categories: simple, differential, and special stains.

▶ Aseptic and pure culture techniques are necessary to obtain correct results from any culture, technique, or procedure. Aseptic techniques prevent the contamination of bacterial cultures.

1. Use of equipment—Equipment used in the microbiology laboratory includes the inoculating loop, inoculating needle, Bunsen burner, and loop incinerator.

2. Artificial media is used to grow microorganisms outside of the host. Artificial media provides the microbe with nutrients and growth factors. The media may be liquid, semisolid, or solid.

▶ Methods for bacterial identification include Gram staining, growth characteristics, and test methods. Test methods are discussed in this section.

1. Biochemical tests are available for identifying specific bacteria. After the Gram reaction is determined the appropriate tests may be initiated.

2. Disk diffusion tests use filter paper disks impregnated with substances to differentiate various species of bacteria.

3. Serologic tests allow the differentiation of bacteria based antigens they produce.

## CASE STUDY

The microbiology technician who was reading plates at the urine culture bench encountered the following:

The blood agar plate that was to be used for a colony count was found to have a single line of very heavy growth down the center of the plate. This growth was such that colonies were indistinguishable although bacterial swarming was present surrounding the apparent line of inoculation. The remainder of the plates were streaked using the three-quadrant method.

Considering the standard method for streaking a urine culture and bacterial characteristics, in general, answer the following questions:

**Questions:**

1. Was an error made streaking the plate for colony count? If so, what was it and can the plate be used for its intended purpose?

2. What would be the next step for completing the work on this culture?

3. How should the results of this culture be reported? Why?

4. What may have caused the swarming of the bacteria?

## Review Questions

1. The media that is NOT differential is:
   a. EMB agar.
   b. MacConkey's agar.
   c. nutrient agar.
   d. mannitol salt agar.

2. A slide preparation to test for motility is a:
   a. Ziehl-Nielsen stain.
   b. Gram stain.
   c. fixed smear.
   d. wet mount.

3. A mordant:
   a. fixes the smear to the slide.
   b. makes stain more intense.
   c. decolorizes bacteria.
   d. provides acid-fast qualities.

4. In a Gram stain, the safranin serves as the:
   a. primary stain.
   b. mordant.
   c. decolorizer.
   d. counterstain.

5. *Mycobacterium tuberculosis* is suspected. A direct smear of the sputum is prepared. The correct way to stain this smear is with:
   a. Gram stain.
   b. India ink.
   c. safranin simple stain.
   d. Ziehl-Nielsen stain.

6. The bacitracin disk is used to inhibit the growth of:
   a. *Streptococcus* group A.
   b. *Streptococcus pneumoniae*.
   c. *Staphylococcus aureus*.
   d. *Staphylococcus epidermidis*.

7. Streaking a urine culture uses:
   a. four quadrants of a culture plate.
   b. a calibrated loop.
   c. a pour plate technique.
   d. confluent growth.

8. Reducing media is used for cultivation of:
   a. *Mycobacterium tuberculosis*.
   b. fungal cultures.
   c. anaerobic bacteria.
   d. spore-forming bacteria.

9. Complete hemolysis of the area surrounding a colony is known as:
   a. α-hemolysis.
   b. ß-hemolysis.
   c. δ-hemolysis.
   d. γ-hemolysis.

10. A colony that appears to be yellow and is coagulase positive most likely is:
    a. *Enterobacter aerogenes*.
    b. *Streptococcus pyogenes*.
    c. *Staphylococcus aureus*.
    d. *Staphylococcus epidermidis*.

11. Anaerobic culture techniques require the use of a system where the oxygen has been removed or utilized. When using a system of this type, the colorless strip in the jar indicates that the:
    a. oxygen has been removed.
    b. chemicals are at the proper level.
    c. incubation time is complete.
    d. jar is tightly sealed.

12. A candle jar contains conditions of:
    a. no oxygen.
    b. reduced oxygen.
    c. atmospheric levels of oxygen.
    d. 90% oxygen.

13. The reagent used to perform the catalase test is:
    a. bromthymol blue.
    b. hydrogen peroxide.
    c. Kovac's reagent.
    d. urea.

14. When performing a Gram stain, round, purple bacteria and long, pink bacteria are seen. This smear should be read as having:
    a. gram-positive cocci and gram-positive rods.
    b. gram-positive cocci and gram-negative rods.
    c. gram-negative cocci and gram-positive rods.
    d. gram-positive cocci and gram-negative spirochetes.

15. A known culture of micrococcus is Gram stained. It appears to be pink, cocci. These results are:
    a. correct.
    b. incorrect because the bacteria are not cocci.
    c. incorrect because the bacteria should appear gram-positive.
    d. incorrect because the bacteria should appear gram-negative.

## ▶ REFERENCES & RECOMMENDED READING

Finegold, S. M., & Baron, M. J. (1991). *Bailey and Scott's diagnostic microbiology*. Princeton, NJ: Mosby.

Marshall, J. (1995). *Microbiology: The clinical laboratory manual series*. Albany, NY: Delmar.

Tortora, G. J., Berdell, R. F., & Case, C. L. (1995). *Microbiology: An introduction,* (5th ed.). New York: Cummings.

Walters, N. J., Estridge, B. H., & Reynold, A. P. (1996). *Basic medical laboratory techniques* (3rd ed.). Albany, NY: Delmar.

# CHAPTER 9

## Staphylococcus and Related Aerobic Gram-Positive Cocci

Linda S. Harrison, MS, MT (ASCP)

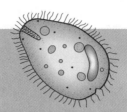

### Microbes in the News

#### Preparing for Battle Against Vancomycin Resistance

Antibiotic resistance in bacteria is a growing problem. Resistance to various antibacterial drugs has emerged with widespread use. Resistance can also spread among organisms; some traits have crossed the genus barrier. This is important because it is not uncommon for patients in tertiary care facilities to be coinfected with both **methicillin-resistant *Staphylococcus aureus*** (MRSA) and vancomycin-resistant enterococci. Vancomycin resistance in *Staphylococcus aureus* would leave physicians with few therapeutic options and minimum chance of success.

". . . Vancomycin resistance has been transferred from enterococci into *S. aureus* in the laboratory, says (Patrice) Courvalin (Pasteur Institut), "There is no barrier to expression of genes from enterococci in staphylococcus; these bacteria don't have the same ecosystem, they don't mix in nature, and that is why the transfer has been delayed. But you can confidently predict that this will occur some day. And then we're in trouble."

Source: Rowe, P. M. *The Lancet,* January 27, 1996.

## KEY TERMS

| | | |
|---|---|---|
| Catalase | *mec*A gene | Novobiocin test |
| Coagulase | Methicillin-resistant | Penicillin-binding protein |
| Coagulase-negative | *Staphylococcus aureus* | Protein A |
|    staphylococci (CNS) | (MRSA) | Scalded skin syndrome |
| Food poisoning | Normal flora | Teichoic acid |
| Impetigo | Nosocomial | Toxic shock syndrome |

## LEARNING OBJECTIVES

**Upon successful completion of this chapter, the student should be able to:**

1. Briefly describe members of *Micrococcaceae* family and list those members that are nonpathogenic, pathogenic, and opportunistic.

2. List diseases that are associated with *S. aureus*, *Staphylococcus epidermidis* and *Staphylococcus saprophyticus*.

3. Describe the toxins of *S. aureus* and their effects.

4. Differentiate *S. aureus*, coagulase-negative streptococci, *S. saprophyticus*, and micrococci by Gram stain, colony morphology, and simple laboratory tests.

5. Contrast the antimicrobic susceptibility patterns of *S. aureus*, *S. epidermidis*, and *S. saprophyticus*.

6. Discuss the historical perspectives as well as current and future implications of antimicrobial resistance in *S. aureus* with regard to nosocomial infections.

## INTRODUCTION

Although antimicrobial use has greatly contributed to lowering mortality and morbidity associated with infectious disease, many organisms develop resistance. Such organisms are thus difficult to treat and pose a greater threat to the disease outcome in the people they infect. Staphylococci, which are included in the microbiota of the skin's **normal flora**, are especially prone to developing resistance. *Staphylococcus aureus*, which intermittently colonizes humans and has the historical ability to become resistant, is an important pathogen and problematic **nosocomial** agent throughout the world. *S. aureus* is distinguished from other staphylococci by possessing coagulase, an enzyme that can clot, or coagulate, plasma. Those staphylococci that do not have this enzyme are termed **coagulase-negative staphylococci** (CNS).

Most CNS involved in human infections are *Staphylococcus epidermidis*; however, most clinical laboratories will not routinely speciate CNS because (1) they are usually easy to distinguish from *S. aureus* with simple bench-top tests, and (2) they normally do not present clinical problems different from *S. epidermidis*. Speciation can be helpful in determining isolate similarity for hospital epidemiology purposes. However, different commercial identification kits have performed with varying degrees of accuracy.

*Staphylococcus saprophyticus*, another CNS, is an important pathogen responsible for urinary tract infections (UTI). This organism generally causes problems in women and can cause disease even when low numbers of organisms are present. A simple laboratory test that indicates resistance to a **novobiocin** disk in vitro is usually sufficient to support identification of *S. saprophyticus* when a CNS is isolated from a UTI.

Staphylococci and the other organisms presented in this chapter are members of the *Micrococcaceae* family. Other members of this family include *Micrococcus*, *Stomatococcus*, and *Planococcus*. *Micrococcus* and *Stomatococcus* have been only occasionally implicated in human infections and then usually as an opportunistic pathogen in the compromised patient. Planococci are found in marine environments and have not been implicated in human infections. The ability to distinguish staphylococci from micrococci and stomatococci and perform antimicrobial susceptibilities are fundamental skills of every clinical microbiologist.

All the *Micrococcaceae* are gram-positive, having a thick peptidoglycan or murein layer. The peptidoglycan layer consists of alternating chains of polysaccharide: *N*-acetyl-D-glucosamine (NAG) and *N*-acetyl-D-muramic acid (NAM). These polysaccharides are cross-linked with short peptide chains. This forms a rigid cell wall that provides a protective barrier external to the cell membrane, making the bacteria more resistant to desiccation, heat, disinfection, and other deleterious environmental conditions. The arrangement of a thick murein layer with extensive cross-linkages, allows gram-positive organisms to retain the crystal violet/iodine complexes and resist decolorization (Baron, Peterson, & Finegold, 1994; Larsen & Mahon,1995.)

Members of the *Micrococcaceae* family are gram-positive cocci and range in diameter from 0.5 to 2.0 μm (see Table 9-1). Their division occurs in multiple planes most often resulting in pairs and clusters. This characteristic aids in distinguishing these organisms from streptococci that divide in a single plane and tend to form chains, especially when grown in broth. Micrococci and planococci will also form tetrads, which helps in identifying these less commonly isolated organisms. Refer to Color Plates 8, 9, and 10.

Most members of the *Micrococcaceae* family are **catalase**-positive organisms. Occasional strains of *S. aureus* are catalase negative, but fortunately this is quite rare. Stomatococci can be catalase positive or negative.

Colonial morphology, Gram stain, catalase and coagulase (or rapid agglutination) are the primary tests used to initially identify members of this family. Addi-

| Table 9–1 ► Commonly Isolated *Micrococcaceae* Species |
| --- |
| **Frequently associated with disease** |
| S. aureus |
| S. epidermidis |
| S. saprophyticus |
| **Occasionally associated with disease** |
| Other coagulase-negative staphylococci |
| S. haemolyticus |
| S. hominis |
| S. warneri |
| Micrococcus species |
| Stomatococcus species |

tional tests are used to differentiate micrococci and stomatococci from staphylococci. Planococci will not be covered any further in this chapter.

## Habitat and Transmission

Staphylococci and micrococci are common inhabitants of the skin and mucous membranes of humans and warm-blooded animals. Staphylococci can be nosocomially acquired and colonization of skin and nares provide a large reservoir for transmission to other hospitalized individuals. Stomatococci are common inhabitants of the human oral cavity.

These organisms are either truly pathogenic (*S. aureus, S. saprophyticus*), causing disease in otherwise healthy individuals, or opportunistic (CNS, or occasionally micrococci and stomatococci), causing problems when host defenses have been compromised. Injuries to the skin, such as trauma or burns, are predisposing factors, as are indwelling devices such as prolonged intravenous catheter lines. Chronic underlying disease or immunodeficiencies can also provide an opportunity for these organisms to breach skin and mucous membrane barriers.

## STAPHYLOCOCCUS AUREUS

*Staphylococcus aureus* is a well-documented human pathogen frequently recovered in the clinical setting.

## Organism Characteristics

Most adults, children, and many infants are intermittently colonized with *S. aureus*. Virulence factors that contribute to the pathogenicity of *S. aureus* include structural components of the cell wall, enzymes, and toxins. The cell wall of *S. aureus* is made up of a peptidoglycan interspersed with **teichoic acid** and **protein A**. Teichoic acid aids in the adherence to mucosal

membrane surfaces. Protein A can bind to the Fc portion of IgG molecules interfering with phagocytosis. Certain strains can produce extracellular capsules that aid in the colonization of indwelling medical devices, such as artificial heart valves, prosthetic joints, or intravascular lines.

Enzymes also contribute to the virulence of this organism. Catalase inactivates toxic hydrogen peroxide and increases intracellular survival. The coagulase of the bacterial cell induces the formation of fibrin from fibrinogen, which then can inhibit the movement of phagocytic cells. Hyaluronidase and lipase are thought to increase the spread of the infection through tissues. ß-Lactamases mediate resistance to certain classes of ß-lactam antimicrobials such as penicillin (Koneman et al., 1992).

## Clinical Significance

*Staphylococcus aureus* is responsible for a wide variety of infections and disease due to toxins (see Table 9-2).

Infections caused by *S. aureus* tend to be pyogenic (pus producing), and the lesions are often walled off by white blood cells. These infections can range from superficial skin infections (furuncles, boils, sties, and infectious **impetigo**) to deep-seated abscesses of hair follicles (carbuncles) and mastitis in nursing mothers. Superficial wound infections can lead to staphylococci directly invading bone or joint tissues.

Hematologic spread can also lead to deep infections of the subcutaneous tissues (cellulitis) or joints and bones (osteomyelitis). Serious systemic infections,

| Table 9–2 ► Diseases Associated with *S. aureus* |
| --- |
| **Localized infections** |
| Skin infections (folliculitis, impetigo, furuncles, carbuncles) |
| Wound infections |
| **Systemic infections** |
| Bacteremia, septicemia |
| **Organ system infections** |
| Urinary tract infections |
| Infections of bones and joints (osteomyelitis, septic arthritis) |
| Staphylococcal pneumonia |
| Endocarditis |
| **Toxin production** |
| Food poisoning |
| Scalded skin syndrome |
| Toxic shock syndrome |

such as endocarditis, are often the result of transient bacteremia induced by intravenous drug abuse or in persons with heart defects. Surgical wound complications with *S. aureus*, can lead to bacteremia, sometimes resulting in abscesses in any organ system. Staphylococcal pneumonia is a serious necrotizing process that tends to occur secondary to influenza infection, cystic fibrosis, pulmonary edema, or other trauma to the lungs.

Toxins produced by *S. aureus* cause **scalded skin syndrome** (SSS) and **toxic shock syndrome** (TSS) and are a significant cause of food poisoning. SSS is also known as Ritter's disease and generally affects children less than 5 years old. It is the result of an exfoliative toxin A and B produced at a localized infected site, such as the nasopharynx, umbilicus, or urinary tract. Phage II type *S. aureus* strains are associated with this syndrome. The exfoliative toxin produces large areas of blistered skin on the face, neck, groin, and trunk areas, giving a scalded appearance. Staphylococci are located only at the distant infected site and cannot be isolated from these exfoliated areas. Complete recovery can be expected in 3 to 5 days in most cases with treatment (antimicrobics and fluid management). If not properly treated, 1% to 10% of the cases can result in sepsis and serous fluid and electrolyte loss; the infection can be life-threatening (Waldvogel, 1995).

Toxic shock syndrome is a multisystem disease identified during the 1980s and associated with menstruating women using hyperabsorbent tampons. The tampons allowed large numbers of *S. aureus* to establish themselves in the vagina, and toxic shock syndrome toxin 1 (TSST1)-producing strains led to this disease. This syndrome is occasionally seen in men and children when they are infected with TSST1-producing *S. aureus* strains. The disease begins with fever, headache, rash, and watery diarrhea followed by severe dehydration. *S. aureus* can be recovered from vaginal discharge, blood cultures, or the localized infected site in non-tampon TSS. Medical and public awareness led to major commercial reform resulting in the removal of highly absorbent tampons from the marketplace.

**Food poisoning** caused by the toxins produced by certain *S. aureus* strains is one of the most common food-borne illnesses in the United States. The enterotoxins are produced as *S. aureus* grows in dairy or meat products stored at temperatures that are not sufficiently hot or cold. Symptoms include nausea, vomiting, followed by abdominal cramping and watery diarrhea. Onset is rapid, within 2 to 6 hours of ingestion of the enterotoxins. Management consists of monitoring fluid and electrolyte loss. Symptoms generally resolve within 8 hours and antimicrobial therapy is not required.

# PROCEDURE 9-1
## Catalase

### Principle:

Catalase is present in many bacterial cells to counteract the toxic buildup of the metabolic end-product, hydrogen peroxide. Catalase converts hydrogen peroxide into water and oxygen, creating a bubbling effect.

$$2\ H_2O_2 + \text{catalase} \rightarrow 2\ H_2O + O_2\ \text{(bubbles)}$$

### Method:

To perform the test, place a drop of 3% hydrogen peroxide onto a slide. Using an applicator stick, gently pick a colony from the primary isolation plate and add to the drop of hydrogen peroxide. Hold the stick down and observe for vigorous bubbling.

### Quality Control:

*Staphylococcus aureus*—positive
*Streptococcus pyogenes*—negative

### Expected Results:

Staphylococci will be catalase positive and produce bubbles, whereas streptococci will be catalase negative.

### Limitations:

Some organisms, along with red blood cells, possess other enzymes that can also break down hydrogen peroxide, but the reaction will not be vigorous as with catalase.

### Reference:

Koneman, E. W., Allen, S. D., Janda, W. M., Schreckenberger, P. C., & Washington, C. W., Jr. (1992). The gram-positive cocci part I: *Staphylococcus* and related organisms. *Color atlas and textbook of diagnostic microbiology* (4th ed.). Philadelphia: Lippincott.

## Cultural Characteristics and Identification

*Staphylococcus aureus* are gram-positive cocci (0.5–1.5 μm) arranged singly, in pairs, short chains, or most often in clusters. The name staphylococcus is derived from the Greek word "staphyle" meaning bunch of grapes. Organisms are facultative and will form medium to large (1–3 mm) colonies at 24 hours on sheep blood agar. Usually *S. aureus* will be ß-hemolytic, but hemolysis can vary from extensive to none. The colonies normally will be smooth and round with a butyrous consistency. Less common encapsulated strains can be convex and have a wet appearance. The colonial pigment will range from white to cream. After extended incubation, the colonies may form a golden to yellow color.

Refer to Color Plate 11 for colony morphology of *S. aureus*.

With rare exception, all staphylococci possess catalase (considered catalase positive). This enzyme will break down the hydrogen peroxide to water and oxygen, which is detected in the laboratory by bubble formation when peroxide is added to a colony (see Figure 9–1). This test is rapid and performed on colonies from the primary isolation culture. Although erythrocytes from blood agar can give a false-positive reaction, this slight bubbling caused by peroxidase can be easily distinguished from the strong reaction of a true positive. This key characteristic helps distinguish staphylococci from streptococci (which are catalase negative).

**Coagulase** is the key reaction used to distinguish *S. aureus* from *S. epidermidis* and other CNS. Coagulase can occur in a bound or free form. If an organism produces bound coagulase, or clumping factor, it will react with fibrinogen, causing clotting when mixed with plasma. The enzyme, bound coagulase, can be detected in the laboratory using a rapid slide method; rabbit plasma is mixed with selected colonies to produce coagulation. This method will detect 95% of *S. aureus* strains. If the slide method is negative, the tube method should be performed to detect extracellular or free coagulase.

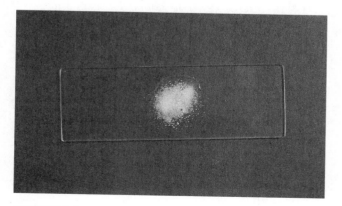

**FIGURE 9-1** Catalase reaction.

**Latex Methods.** The most common method of identifying most *S. aureus* isolates in today's clinical microbiology laboratory is by latex agglutination. A number of commercial kits are available for this purpose. Most methods use latex beads that are coated with plasma (which contains fibrinogen) and immunoglobulins of the IgG class. The fibrinogen will attach to the bound coagulase of the *S. aureus* cells causing visible agglutination. Additionally, most *S. aureus* strains have protein A as a cellular component, which will bind the Fc portion of IgG-coated latex beads causing agglutination. Latex beads in some kits have been colored to aid in visualizing agglutination.

Some MRSA strains may not possess bound coagulase and protein A, or will contain a capsule masking these substances. Commercial latex methods that use a specific antibody directed against antigens unique to MRSA have been developed to detect these isolates.

Other staphylococci may possess clumping factor, and can give a positive reaction with the slide coagulase test or a latex method; however, these are infrequently recovered from clinical sites. Another potential source of false-positive latex reactions is *S. saprophyticus* isolated from urine.

**Other Tests.** Other tests useful in identifying *S. aureus* include deoxyribonuclease (DNase) test, thermostable endonuclease test, ß-galactosidase test, and growth on Baird-Parker agar or modified P agar. These tests are used to help differentiate other coagulase-positive staphylococci from *S. aureus* (Robertson, Fox, Hancock, & Besser, 1992). The ability to ferment mannitol is another useful characteristic of *S. aureus* and is used in mannitol salt agar to screen for MRSAs from contaminated sites.

## Antibiotic Susceptibility Characteristics

**History of Penicillin Resistance.** Shortly after World War II, the recently discovered "miracle drug" penicillin became more widely available and used. It was the prototype of all subsequent ß-lactam antimicrobics; a naturally occurring substance extracted from *Penicillium* mold. By the 1950s, strains of *S. aureus* were isolated that were resistant to penicillin. They produced an enzyme that cleaves the ß-lactam ring of penicillin, which was termed penicillinase or ß-lactamase. Today most *S. aureus* stains are ß-lactamase positive and thus penicillin resistant. Newer penicillins were developed by altering the chemical structure of natural compounds. These semisynthetic, penicillinase-resistant penicillins (nafcillin, methicillin, and oxacillin) were used to treat the more resistant isolates; however, by the 1970s, resistance developed to these compounds. The MRSA have become a costly problem in hospitals and nursing homes, where antibiotic use is frequent and prolonged. Control of the morbidity and

# PROCEDURE 9-2
## Tube Coagulase

### Principle:

*S. aureus* produces coagulase, which can be detected in the laboratory to distinguish this organism from other staphylococcal species (CNS) that do not produce this enzyme (see Figure 9–2).

### Method:

1. Prepare the coagulase reagent, rabbit plasma with EDTA (BBL Microbiology Systems, Difco Laboratories), in 0.5-mL amounts in 13 × 100 mm test tubes. The prepared tubes can be refrigerated for 14 days or frozen at −20°C for several months.
2. Emulsify a fresh colony grown on nonselective media in the plasma by:
   a. Tipping the tube and rubbing the material on the side of the tube (below the fluid level).
   b. Place the tube upright in a rack, which allows the plasma to cover the inoculum.
3. Incubate the suspension for up to 4 hours at 35°C and observe for the presence of a clot, which cannot be resuspended by gentle shaking. If a clot, does not form after 4 hours, continue incubation at room temperature for up to 24 hours.

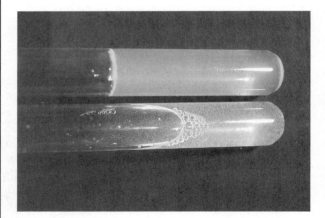

**FIGURE 9-2** Tube coagulase.

4. Staphylococcal isolates that do not form a clot by 24 hours are considered coagulase negative.

### Expected Results:

*S. aureus* should clot the plasma within 4 to 24 hours, *S. epidermidis* and other CNS will not clot the plasma even after 24 hours.

### Quality Control:

*S. aureus* ATCC 25923—positive
*S. epidermidis* ATCC 14990—negative

### Limitations:

1. Do not confuse fibrin strands with true clot formation.
2. Some *S. aureus* strains will produce enzymes capable of breaking down the plasma clot. Read all tube coagulase tests at 4 hours before continuing incubation to prevent misinterpretation.
3. Other strains of staphylococci are coagulase positive. These are animal strains and can be distinguished from *S. aureus* by a review of the patient history. *S. intermedius, S. hyicus, and S delphini* are opportunistic pathogen of animals. *S. intermedius* is part of the normal oral flora of canines and can be recovered from wounds caused by dog bites. Most are penicillin sensitive, while 95% of *S. aureus* are resistant to penicillin.

### References:

Baron, E. J., Peterson, L. R., & Finegold, S. M. (1994). *Micrococcaceae: Staphylococci, Micrococci,* and *Stomatococci, Bailey and Scott's diagnostic microbiology* (9th ed.). St. Louis: Mosby.

mortality associated with these infections depends on intelligent use of antimicrobics and strict adherence to barrier precautions, contact isolation, and proper handwashing between patients.

Although several options exist for attempting to eradicate MRSA from asymptomatic carriers, the main-

stay of anti-infective therapy rests with a single antimicrobic, vancomycin. If vancomycin-resistant MRSA strains develop (as has occurred with some strains of *Enterococcus*), treatment of patients with these infections may approach the impossible.

**MECHANISMS OF RESISTANCE AND EXPRESSION.** ß-lactamase production leading to penicillin resistance can either be intrinsic (chromosomal) or, more frequently, plasmid mediated. Hyper-ß-lactamase production can lead to "borderline" methicillin resistance, but should not be confused with true methicillin resistance, which is expressed via a different mechanism.

The MRSA strains have altered **penicillin-binding proteins** that have a decreased affinity for the antimicrobic. In other words, penicillin cannot bind onto the bacterial cell wall and, therefore, cannot inhibit cell wall synthesis. True methicillin resistance is carried on the ***mec*A gene**, and expressed in one of two ways—homoresistance and heteroresistance. Homoresistance simply means all bacterial cells (thus, all colonies) will be resistant to the drug. Heteroresistance, which is quite common, is not well understood and indicates that not all subgroups (colonies) of that population will show resistance. Actually, very few organisms will be resistant on primary isolation; however growth in the presence of a ß-lactamase-resistant penicillin, like methicillin (oxacillin is used most often in the laboratory), will select for the resistant population. Expression is unstable; if the isolate is subcultured in the absence of oxacillin several times, heteroresistant growth will return. Molecular methods, such as the polymerase chain reaction (PCR) to detect the *mec*A gene have been successful in differentiating true MRSA from borderline MRSA, but are not yet routinely used in the clinical laboratory (Kolbert, Connolly, & Persing, 1995). Some of these methods may soon be incorporated into commercial kits applicable to the clinical laboratory.

**Susceptibility Testing.** All laboratories must be able to perform accurate and timely susceptibility tests on *S. aureus*. The National Committee for Clinical Laboratory Standards (NCCLS) has issued comprehensive guidelines for susceptibility testing. A number of considerations must be observed when performing these tests. A full 24-hour incubation is required on disk diffusion tests to detect oxacillin resistance by heteroresistant populations. Detection of heteroresistant populations will also be enhanced by using salt-supplemented medium and temperatures no higher than 35°C. The use of an oxacillin screen agar is highly sensitive in this regard. This test agar might be especially useful for screening patients or confirming the accuracy of alternative methods. Borderline methicillin-resistant staphylococcal (*mec*A negative, hyper-ß-lactamase producers) isolates will not grow on this media. When oxacillin resistance is noted, report the cephalosporins as resistant regardless of in vitro results. See Chapter 7 for complete details on susceptibility testing techniques.

**Alternative Methods.** Several automated methods are available and have been widely used and evaluated for susceptibility testing of staphylococci. Results, based on turbidometric measurement, can be obtained in less than 24 hours. Other rapid methods such as the 2-hour Crystal MRSA screen test have been evaluated for detection of oxacillin resistance.

The detection of the *mec*A gene has been investigated as a rapid method for detecting oxacillin resistance, and can differentiate *mec*A-negative, hyperproducers of ß-lactamase from true MRSA having the *mec*A gene.

ß-lactamase testing can be performed on *S. aureus* isolates, although most nosocomially acquired strains will be positive. If testing is desired, induction of ß-lactamase production may be required to accurately detect the enzyme. This would be performed by picking the organism to be tested from around the oxacillin disk of a disk diffusion plate.

## *STAPHYLOCOCCUS EPIDERMIDIS* AND OTHER COAGULASE-NEGATIVE STAPHYLOCOCCI

*Staphylococcus epidermidis* is the most frequently recovered CNS species. In the past they were often considered contaminants, but their role in nosocomial infection has been well established, with increased use of indwelling devices and the growing numbers of immunosuppressed patients.

### Organism Characteristics

*Staphylococcus epidermidis* and the other CNS are natural inhabitants of skin and mucous membranes of warm-blooded animals. *S. epidermidis* is the most frequently isolated, making up 60% to 90% of the CNS recovered from clinical specimens (Archer, 1995). *S. epidermidis* strains that have an extracellular polysaccharide "slime" layer are more adherent and more likely to be associated with colonization of intravascular devices. Other CNS, such as *S. capitis* (scalp and forehead) and *S. auricularis* (ear canal), only occupy unique niches in humans, but are uncommon or rarely implicated in disease. Isolates such as *S. delphini* (dolphins), *S. felis* (cats), and *S. gallinarium* (poultry) are primarily isolated from animals and are rare human pathogens.

### Clinical Significance

*Staphylococcus epidermidis* and other CNS are implicated in human disease as opportunistic pathogens. These diseases are often associated with indwelling devices or the introduction of foreign objects. When hospital acquired they can be multiresistant, and clinicians are limited to relatively few antimicrobials. Because they are found in abundance on the skin, they often contaminate wound and improperly collected blood cultures. Therefore, determination of their role as a pathogen or contaminant can be difficult for the physician and the laboratory.

The CNS, other than *S. epidermidis*, implicated in human disease include:

- ▶ *S. haemolyticus*
- ▶ *S. hominis*
- ▶ *S. warneri*
- ▶ *S. saccharolyticus* (strict anaerobe)
- ▶ *S. schleiferi* (can give positive-coagulase reactions)
- ▶ *S. lugdunensis* (can give positive-coagulase reactions)

Table 9–3 lists infections associated with *S. epidermidis* and other CNS.

Infections caused by *S. epidermidis* are primarily hospital acquired. Most cases of nosocomial staphylococcal UTI are caused by *S. epidermidis* in patients with urinary tract complications, such as urinary stints. Community-acquired CNS are usually species other than *S. epidermidis* (Rupp & Archer, 1994).

The incidence of nosocomial bacteremia caused by *S. epidermidis* and other CNS has risen in recent years. Often the strains recovered are not related and can be the result of poor blood drawing techniques or multiple site involvement.

Infection of prosthetic heart valves is often caused by *S. epidermidis*, whereas endocarditis of native heart values is infrequently caused by *S. epidermidis*, usually involved in only 5% of these infections. Infections of other types of prosthetic devices, shunts, dialysis catheters, implants, or grafts are common with *S. epidermidis*. Ocular infections with *S. epidermidis* are common after surgery or trauma. Any time an indwelling device or foreign object is introduced, as with implants, shunts, or intravascular lines, patients are at an increased risk for *S. epidermidis* infections.

## Table 9–3 ▶ Infections* Associated with *S. epidermidis* and Other CNS

**Localized infections**
  Ocular infections (trauma, surgery)
  Wound infections (surgical and intravenous sites)
  Breast implants

**Systemic infections**
  Septicemia (nosocomial, immunosuppressed patients)
  Bacteremia (intravascular line related, vascular grafts)
  Endocarditis (prosthetic valves, pacemakers)
  Peritonitis, dialysis

**Organ system infections**
  Nosocomial urinary tract infections (catheter, stints)
  Infections of bones and joints (pins, screws, prosthetic joints)
  Cerebrospinal fluid shunt infections

*Infections are typically device or trauma related

## Cultural Characteristics and Identification

All CNS including *S. epidermidis* are facultative, catalase-positive, coagulase-negative, gram-positive cocci occurring singly, in pairs, or irregular clusters. Their size ranges from 0.5 to 1.5 μm in diameter. They will form medium to small colonies on sheep blood agar and are generally not hemolytic (see Figure 9–3).

There are over 32 species of CNS; approximately half have been involved in human infections. Although a high percentage of the CNS recovered from clinical specimens will be *S. epidermidis,* reporting of CNS as *S. epidermidis* is inappropriate unless additional testing has been performed. Most clinical laboratories simply report CNS; however, under certain circumstances a complete identification is useful as an epidemiologic tracking tool.

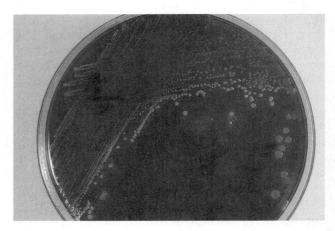

**FIGURE 9-3** Colony morphology of coagulase-negative streptococci.

**Slide and Tube Coagulase.** The slide coagulase is most useful for rapidly identifying *S. aureus*. When a slide coagulase test is negative, a tube coagulase method must be performed. The tube coagulase is read at 4 hours and must be held for 24 hours to confirm a negative result. Most clinical laboratories use a rapid method such as a latex or hemaglutination kits to quickly rule out *S. aureus*, and be able to report CNS.

**Rapid Latex Methods and Hemaglutination Methods.** The latex and hemaglutination methods described under the *S. aureus* section work well on *S. epidermidis*. Some methods might show nonspecific agglutination, and those methods with a negative control would be useful.

## Antibiotic Susceptibility Characteristics

*Staphylococcus epidermidis* and other CNS have unpredictable patterns of susceptibility. Testing should be performed on isolates recovered from clinically significant sites. Nosocomial strains are usually multiresistant and usually ß-lactamase positive, thus resistant to penicillin. A high percentage are resistant to ß-lactamase-resistant penicillins such as methicillin, oxacillin, or nafcillin.

Susceptibility testing is performed using disk dilution, broth microdilution, or an automated method. The same heteroresistance occurs in CNS as in *S. aureus* and the same precautions should be observed in testing.

## *STAPHYLOCOCCUS SAPROPHYTICUS*

### Organism Characteristics

*Staphylococcus saprophyticus* inhabits the genitourinary skin. Several protein factors aid in its attachment to uroepithelial cells causing it to establish itself as a urinary pathogen (Archer, 1995).

### Clinical Significance

This is the most frequently recovered CNS from urine in nonhospitalized patients. It generally affects sexually active women between the ages of 16 and 35 and is the second most frequent cause of uncomplicated UTIs in women, after *Escherichia coli*. It may be recovered in lower numbers than generally associated with UTI (<10$^5$ cfu/mL) caused by gram-negative enteric bacteria (Archer, 1995).

### Cultural Characteristics and Identification

*Staphylococcus saprophyticus* is a catalase-positive, gram-positive cocci, not easily distinguished from other coagulase-negative staphylococci based on Gram stain or colony morphology. It can be easily identified by its resistance to novobiocin as seen in Figure 9-4. In vitro, a few other CNS can be novobiocin resistant, but not implicated in commonly acquired UTis.

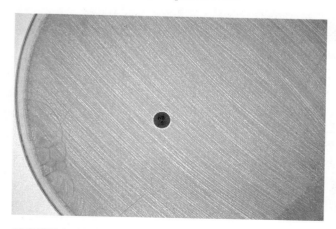

**FIGURE 9-4** Novobiocin test.

### Antibiotic Susceptibility Characteristics

*Staphylococcus saprophyticus* is generally susceptible to most antimicrobials with the exception of naladixic acid. Some resistance has been observed with the sulfonamides and nitrofurantoin (Archer, 1995).

## MICROCOCCI

### Organism Characteristics

Micrococci are saprophytic organisms, commonly found on the skin and in the environment. Often considered contaminants, they are occasionally associated with disease. There are currently nine species (Kloos & Bannerman, 1995).

### Clinical Significance

These organisms can be encountered in wound, skin, burn, and respiratory specimens. Micrococci have been associated with bacteremia, endocarditis, peritoneal dialysis peritonitis, colonization of cerebrospinal fluid shunts, and other infections associated with implantation or disruption of normal skin or mucosal barriers. It is important to be able to identify these organisms to the genus level to distinguish them from staphylococci; however, identification to species level is beyond the level of most laboratories.

### Cultural Characteristics and Identification

Micrococci are catalase-positive, coagulase-negative, gram-positive cocci. They are often pigmentated, especially *Micrococcus luteus*. The pigment will range from beige to bright yellow or orange and is often the first clue that an isolate is *Micrococcus* has been recovered. They tend to be larger (up to 2.0 μm in diameter) than staphylococci and form tetrads, when Gram stained from a broth culture (see Color Plate 12). To differentiate micrococcal isolates from other CNS use the Gram stain, colonial morphology, and one of the following tests listed in Table 9-4. The modified oxidase test is useful because it is quick and easy to perform (see Figure 9-5).

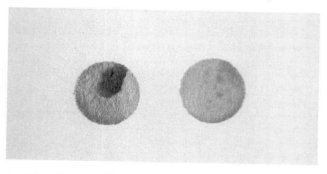

**FIGURE 9-5** Modified oxidase reaction.

## PROCEDURE 9-3
## Novobiocin Test

### Principle:

Few staphylococci are resistant to novobiocin. Of those found in humans, *S. saprophyticus* is the only one associated with UTIs.

### Methods:

Perform this test as a disk susceptibility using a 5-µg disk. See Chapter 10 for details on disk diffusion testing.

### Expected Results:

*S. saprophyticus*-resistant—<16 mm
Other CNS-susceptible—>16 mm

### Limitations:

Other CNS (*S. cohnii* and *S. xylosus*) can be novobiocin resistant, but are not likely to be recovered from a urine culture.

### Quality Control:

*S. epidermidis* ATCC 14990
*S. saprophyticus* ATCC 15305

### Reference:

Koneman, E. W., Allen, S. D., Janda, W. M., Schreckenberger, P. C., & Washington, C. W., Jr. (1992). The gram-positive cocci part I: *Staphylococcus* and related organisms, *Color atlas and textbook of diagnostic microbiology* (4th ed.). Philadelphia: J. B. Lippincott.

## Antibiotic Susceptibility Characteristics

Do not perform susceptibilities on this organism unless it is considered clinically significant. The NCCLS has not prepared disk diffusion susceptibility standards. Agar dilution studies have shown this organism to be susceptible to ß-lactams, imipenem, rifampin, and the glycopeptides, with limited activity against aminoglycosides and erythromycin (Von Eiff, Herrmann, & Peters, 1995).

## SPECIAL CONSIDERATIONS FOR IMMUNOCOMPROMISED HOSTS

Indwelling and prosthetic devices, along with the predisposing factors seen in the immunocompromised patients of intensive care units, oncology wards, neonatal nurseries, and bone marrow transplant units, make the recovery of previously considered contaminants a challenge to the clinical microbiologist. Open discussion between the clinician and laboratory personnel will aid in clinical assessment.

### Table 9–4  ▶  Differentiation of CNS from Micrococci

| Characteristic | Staphylococci | Micrococci |
|---|---|---|
| Modified oxidase reaction | − | + |
| Fermentation of glucose | + | − |
| Lysostaphin (200 µg/mL) | resistant | susceptible |
| Bacitracin (0.04 unit disk) | resistant | susceptible |
| Furazolidone (100 µg/mL) | susceptible | resistant |

## SUMMARY

▸ All member of *Micrococcaceae* family are gram-positive cocci.

▸ *S. aureus* and *S. saprophyticus* are truly pathogenic, whereas other members of this family are opportunistic, such as *S. epidermidis*, other coagulase-negative staphylococci, and occasionally micrococci and stomatococci.

▸ Staphylococci and micrococci are common inhabitants of skin and mucous membranes.

▸ Numerous infections are associated with *S. aureus*, such as skin and wound infections, bacteremia, septicemia, urinary tract infections, osteomyelitis, septic arthritis, staphylococcal pneumonia, and endocarditis.

▸ Toxigenic strains of *S. aureus* can cause food poisoning, scalded skin syndrome, and toxic shock syndrome.

▸ *S. epidermidis* and other coagulase-negative staphylococci are most often associated with infections as the result of an indwelling device or foreign object.

▸ Simple laboratory tests such as Gram stain, colony morphology, pigment, catalase, coagulase, and other easily performed tests can identify most *S. aureus*, CNS, and micrococcal isolates. In most cases further identification is not required.

▸ *S. saprophyticus* are easily distinguished from other CNS by the novobiacin test.

▸ MRSA strains are a common nosocomial agent. Their presence should be closely monitored. Development of vancomycin-resistant strains would pose a serious health threat.

## CASE STUDY 1: OSTEOMYELITIS AND SEPTIC ARTHRITIS

An 11-year old boy was admitted to the hospital because of spiking fevers. He also complained of right knee pain, and although there had been no known injury, he was active in football and enjoyed in-line skating. His mother had been giving him acetaminophen for the low-grade fever and pain for about a week.

On admission, he developed severe pain and tenderness in the right leg and a fever of 39.4°C. Radiographs were negative. Aspiration of the knee produced fluid with 3,500 leukocytes/mm³ with 86% neutrophils. A bone scan was "hot" in the distal tibia of the right leg. Bacterial cultures were ordered on blood, joint fluid, and a tibial aspirate. The next day, cream-colored colonies surrounded by a large zone of ß-hemolysis were seen on blood agar plate from all sites. Gram stain of the isolates revealed gram-positive cocci, in pairs and clusters.

### Questions:

1. What colonial and cellular morphologic features indicate a staphylococcal infection? How would you differentiate streptococci from staphylococci?

2. This patient has septic arthritis (infected joint) and osteomyelitis (bone infection) with *S. aureus*. What test would then be performed to identify this isolate as a *S. aureus*? What activities may have increased this boy's risk for infections of this type?

3. What other type(s) of infections can this organism cause?

4. What types of antimicrobial resistance can this organism exhibit? What are the mechanisms of resistance? How is resistance detected in the clinical microbiology laboratory?

## CASE STUDY 2: CATHETER-RELATED SEPSIS

A 42-year-old man had a history of leukemia that required a bone marrow transplant 6 months ago. He experienced numerous hospitalizations and required a long-term central venous catheter (right subclavian port-a-cath) for ongoing medication.

The patient had been in the hospital for a scheduled follow-up for 7 days the previous week. Four days after hospitalization, he developed fever, chills, and pain at his central line insertion site. He drove himself to the hospital where his temperature was recorded at 38.5°C. Physical examination revealed right upper extremity swelling.

Aerobic and anaerobic blood cultures were drawn into commercial vials of broth media (one set through the port-a-cath and one set via a peripheral vein), and placed into an automated blood culture instrument. Both sets of blood cultures were positive at 24 hours for gram positive cocci. The positive cultures were subcultured to nonselective media to identify the organisms.

**Questions:**

1. What is the most likely cause of this infection? Why did the positive vials have to be subcultured prior to identification? What tests will be used to identify this organism?

2. How could one determine that these isolates were the same organism?

3. Why is it significant that both sets of blood cultures were positive?

4. Vascular access catheters are frequently removed if they appear to be infected. How are catheters handled (for culture) in the microbiology laboratory?

## CASE STUDY 3: MRSA IDENTIFICATION

A 74-year-old diabetic woman was taken to the emergency room from her nursing home because of hip pain and fever. She had a long history of infected foot ulcers, which were typically treated with antimicrobics, surgical debridement, or both. Admission temperature was 101°F, and her white blood cell count was elevated at 18,000 mm³, with a predominance of neutrophils. Magnetic resonance imaging of the pelvis indicated a possible access in the inguinal area. Blood cultures and aspirates were positive with an organism with the following characteristics:

Medium-sized, nonhemolytic white colonies grew on blood and chocolate agars, with no growth on MacConkey agar. Gram stain showed gram-positive cocci in pairs and clusters. The isolate was catalase positive and negative with a commercial latex agglutination test used to differentiate *S. aureus* from the CNS. The technologist recorded a preliminary report as CNS with antimicrobic susceptibilities to follow. On the following day, susceptibilities by disk diffusion showed multiple resistance, including a heteroresistant pattern around the oxacillin disk. The technologist remembered that this patient had previously been identified as having been colonized with MRSA in axillary and groin cultures, and performed additional tests to confirm her suspicion that this was actually an MRSA isolate.

**Questions:**

1. What additional tests could be performed to prove that this was an MRSA?

2. What suggested that this might be an MRSA?

3. What was unusual about the colonial morphology (i.e., not typical of an MRSA isolate)?

4. What test would then be performed to identify this isolate as *S. aureus*?

# Review Questions

1. What Gram stain morphology does *S. aureus* have?
   a. gram-positive bacilli
   b. gram-positive cocci in clusters
   c. gram-positive coccobacilli
   d. gram-negative cocci in clusters

2. What Gram stain morphology do *Micrococcus* species have?
   a. gram-positive cocci in chains
   b. gram-positive cocci in tetrads
   c. gram-positive bacilli
   d. gram-variable cocci

3. The following might be used to identify *S. epidermidis* except:
   a. catalase reaction.
   b. coagulase reaction.
   c. Gram stain morphology.
   d. ß-lactamase reaction.

4. A blood culture from an intravenous drug abuser grows out a gram-positive coccus with the following characteristics: catalase positive, coagulase negative, multiply drug resistant. What is the most likely organism?
   a. *Staphylococcus epidermidis*
   b. *Staphylococcus aureus*
   c. *Staphylococcus saprophyticus*
   d. *Staphylococcus intermedius*

5. A young woman is seen for symptoms of a urinary tract infection. Although her urine culture only grows out 20,000 cfu/mL, it is in pure culture. The technologist uses the following tests to identify the isolate: catalase positive, coagulase negative, novobiocin resistant, naladixic acid resistant, nitrofurantoin susceptible. The organism is:
   a. coagulase-negative staphylococci.
   b. *S. aureus*.
   c. *S. epidermidis*.
   d. *S. saprophyticus*.

6. Staphylococcal food poisoning is characterized by:
   a. rapid onset—within 2–6 hours of ingestion of the enterotoxin.
   b. colonization of the GI tract by the bacterium.
   c. a 2 day–2 week incubation period.
   d. diarrhea, but no vomiting.

7. *S. epidermidis* is associated with all of the following except:
   a. wound infections.
   b. bacteremias.
   c. nosocomial urinary tract infections.
   d. toxic shock syndrome.

8. A positive blood culture shows gram-positive cocci in tetrads. The following day yellow pigmented colonies are observed. Catalase and modified oxidase reactions are both positive. What is the most likely organism?
   a. *S. epidermidis*
   b. *Stomatococcus* species
   c. *Micrococcus* species
   d. *S. aureus*

9. Detection of *mec*A in staphylococcal isolates would be useful in determining what type of antimicrobial resistance?
   a. oxacillin
   b. vancomycin
   c. novobiocin
   d. penicillin

10. A wound culture grows out gram-positive cocci with the following characteristics: ß-hemolytic colonies that are both catalase and coagulase positive. What is the most likely organism?
    a. *S. epidermidis*
    b. *S. aureus*
    c. *S. saprophyticus*
    d. *Micrococcus* species

## ▶ REFERENCES & RECOMMENDED READING

Archer, G. L. (1995). *Staphylococcus epidermidis* and other coagulase negative staphylococci. In G. L. Mandell, J. E. Bennett, & R. Dolin (Eds.). *Principal and practice of infectious disease* (4th ed., pp. 1777–1784). New York: Churchill Livingstone.

Baron, E. J., Peterson, L. R., & Finegold, S. M. (1994). *Micrococcaceae: Staphylococci, Micrococci,* and *Stomatococci, Bailey and Scott's diagnostic microbiology* (9th ed., pp. 321–332). St. Louis: Mosby.

Grant, C. E., Sewall, D. L., Pfaller, M., Bumgardner R. V., & Williams J. A. (1994). Evaluation of two commercial systems for identification of coagulase negative staphylococci to species level. *Diagnostic Microbiology & Infectious Disease, 18* (1), 1–5.

Henwick, S., Koehler, M., & Patrick, C. C. (1993). Complications of bacteremia due to *Stomatococcus mucilaginosus* in neutropenic children (Review). *Clinical Infectious Disease, 17*(4), 667–671.

Holt, J. G., Krieg, N. R., Sneath, P. H. A., Staley, J. T., & Williams, S. T. (Eds.). (1994). Gram-positive cocci. *Bergey's manual of determinative bacteriology* (9th ed., pp. 527–533). Baltimore: Williams & Wilkins.

Kaufhold, A., Reinert, R. R., & Kern, W. (1992). Bacteremia caused by *Stomatococcus mucilaginosus:* Report of seven cases and review of the literature (Review). *Infection, 20* (4):213–220.

Khatib, R., Riederer, K. M., Clark J. A., Khatib, S., Briski, L. E., & Wilson F. M. (1995). Coagulase-negative staphylococci in multiple blood culture cultures: Strain relatedness and determinants of same-strain bacteremia. *Journal of Clinical Microbiology, 33*(4), 816–820.

Kloos, W. E., & Bannerman, T. A. (1995). *Staphylococcus* and *Micrococcus.* In P. R. Murray, E. J. Baron, M. A. Pfaller, F. C. Tenover, & R. H. Yolken (Eds.). *Manual of clinical microbiology* (6th ed., pp. 282–298). Washington, DC: American Society for Microbiology.

Kloos, W. E., & George, C. G. (1991). Identification of *Staphylococcus* species and subspecies with the MicroScan Pos ID and Rapid Pos Id Panel systems. *Journal of Clinical Microbiology, 29,* 738–744.

Kloos, W. E., & Schleifer, K. H. (1975). Simplified scheme for routine identification of human *Staphylococcus* species. *Journal of Clinical Microbiology, 1,* 82–88.

Kolbert, C. P., Connolly, J. E., Lee, M. J., & Persing, D. H. (1995). Detection of the Staphylococcal *mecA* gene by chemiluminescent DNA hybridization. *Journal of Clinical Microbiology, 33*(8), 2179–2182.

Koneman, E. W., Allen, S. D., Janda, W. M., Schreckenberger, P. C., & Washington, C. W., Jr. (1992). The grampositive cocci part I: *Staphylococcus* and related organisms, *Color atlas and textbook of diagnostic microbiology* (4th ed., pp. 405–430). Philadelphia: Lippincott.

Larsen, H. S., & Mahon C. R. (1995). *Staphylococcus.* In C. R. Mahon, & G. Manuselis, Jr. (Eds.), *Diagnostic microbiology* (pp. 325–338). Philadelphia: Saunders.

Lemonick, M. D. (1994, September 13). The killers all around—revenge of the microbes. *Time Magazine,* p. 62.

Rasmussen, S. K., Overturf, G. O., Dvorak, J. A., & McLaughlin, J. C. (1996). An overnight pulsed field gel electrophoresis procedure used to investigate a clinical *Staphylococcus aureus* outbreak at a regional hospital. *Abstracts of the 96th General Meeting of the American Society for Microbiology,* C-268, p. 48.

Rhoden, D. L., & Miller, J. M. (1995). Four-year prospective study of STAPH-IDENT system and conventional method for reference identification of *Staphylococcus, Stomatococcus,* and *Micrococcus* spp. *Journal of Clinical Microbiology, 33* (1), 96–98.

Robertson, J. R., Fox, L. K., Hancock, D. D., & Besser, T. E. (1992). Evaluation of methods for differentiation of coagulase-positive staphylococci. *Journal of Clinical Microbiology, 30*(13), 3217–3219.

Rowe, P. M. (1996, January 27). Preparing for battle against vancomycin resistance. *The Lancet, 347,* p. 252.

Rupp, M. E., & Archer, G.L. (1994). Coagulase-negative staphylococci: Pathogens associated with medical progress. *Clinical Infectious Disease, 19,* 231–245.

Sherris, J. C., & Plorde, J. J. (1990). *Staphylococci.* In J. C. Sherris (Ed.), *Medical microbiology: An introduction to infectious diseases* (2nd ed., pp. 275–290). Norwalk, CT: Appleton & Lange.

Tenover, F. C., Arbeit, R., Archer, G., Biddle, J., Byrne, S., Goering, R., Hancock, G., Hebert, A., Hill, B., Hollis, R., Jarvis, W. R., Kreiswirth, B., Eisner, W., Maslow, J., McDougal, L. K., Miller, J. M., Mulligan, M., & Pfaller, M.A. (1994). Comparison of traditional and molecular methods of typing isolates of *Staphylococcus aureus. Journal of Clinical Microbiology, 32* (2), 407–415.

Von Eiff, C., Herrmann, M., & Peters, G. (1995). Antimicrobial susceptibilities of *Stomatococcus mucilaginosus* and of *Micrococcus* spp. *Antimicrobial Agents & Chemotherapy, 39*(1), 268–270.

Waldvogel, F. A. (1995). *Staphylococcus aureus* (including toxic shock syndrome). In G. L. Mandell, J. E. Bennett, & R. Dolin (Eds.) *Principal and practice of infectious disease.* (4th ed., pp. 1754–1777). New York: Churchill Livingstone.

# CHAPTER 10
## Streptococcus and Related Aerobic Gram-Positive Cocci

Helen Viscount, PhD

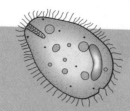

## Microbes in the News

### Flesh-Eating Bacteria in Britain and the United States

In the summer of 1994, streptomania in Britain crossed the Atlantic and struck terror in the United States. Eleven rapidly fatal illnesses in Wales and England due to a "deadly flesh eating bacteria" terrified the British. Soon, several cases in the United States caused equal fear among Americans. Tabloid headlines such as "Eaten Alive," "Killer Bug Ate My Face," and "Dither—And You Die" described the bug that destroys human flesh.

The bacterium that caught the attention of residents on both sides of the Atlantic actually is a common microorganism that causes "strep throat." The invasive form of this *Streptococcus* is transmitted by human contact and is particularly virulent—moves fast on those it infects through an open wound. The toxic chemical and enzymes this bacterium produces eat away fat and muscle at an astounding rate so that limbs may have to be amputated. If the disease is not recognized quickly, death occurs in 3 to 4 days after infection. However, it is easily treatable with antibiotics. Contrary to popular belief, this "killer strep" occurs in recurring cycles and is not a new phenomenon.

(Sources: *Time Magazine,* 20 June 1994 and *Newsweek,* 6 June 1994)

## KEY TERMS

Bacteremia
Betahemolysis
Glomerulonephritis
Lancefield antigens

Necrotizing fasciitis
Nosocomial infection
Pneumonia

Puerperal sepsis
Rheumatic fever
Strep throat

## LEARNING OBJECTIVES

**Upon successful completion of this chapter, the student should be able to:**

1. List the clinically significant streptococci and enterococci and the diseases they cause.
2. Describe the modes of transmission and habitats of the most commonly isolated species in each genera.
3. Presumptively and definitively identify each clinically significant pathogen.

4. Describe the physiologic and serologic assays used to identify these organisms.
5. Name the drug of choice for each pathogenic species.
6. Discuss the significance of emerging multiple antibiotic-resistant strains.

## INTRODUCTION

This chapter deals with the clinically significant streptococci and enterococci. For each commonly isolated species, habitat and mode of transmission are described. The principles and methodologies of the tests used in identification of each organism are described. In addition, the unique challenges presented by the compromised host are discussed.

The genus *Streptococcus* is made up of several species of gram-positive spherical or oval bacteria in pairs and chains. They are catalase negative and facultatively anaerobic. These organisms are nutritionally fastidious and require complex media for growth. Media enriched with 5% sheep blood is recommended so that the hemolytic reaction of the isolates can be identified early. The hemolytic reactions on blood agar (i.e., complete, partial or none) are usually used as a first step in categorizing streptococci and enterococci. Complete lysis of erythrocytes creates a complete clearing of the medium around the colony and is called β-hemolysis. α-Hemolysis refers to incomplete lysis of blood cells seen as greenish discoloration around streptococcal colonies. The green color is due to breakdown products of hemoglobin. Nonhemolytic or γ-hemolytic streptococci are those that have no effect on blood agar. Another characteristic of the genus *Streptococcus* is the ability to ferment glucose and carbohydrates with lactic acid as the major end-product. Furthermore, all streptococci examined so far are sensitive to vancomycin.

Streptococci constitute a major portion of the indigenous microbial flora of animals and humans. Many of the species inhabit the respiratory tract but others colonize the genital and intestinal tracts. Some species are human pathogens, notably, *Streptococcus pyogenes, Streptococcus agalactiae,* and *Streptococcus pneumoniae. S. pyogenes* causes acute pharyngitis and provokes nonsuppurative sequelae of scarlet fever, rheumatic heart disease, and glomerulonephritis. *S. agalactiae* is an etiologic agent of neonatal sepsis and meningeal infection. *S. pneumoniae* is a cause of **pneumonia** and meningitis.

*Streptococcus pyogenes* colonizes the throat of asymptomatic individuals. Streptococcal pharyngitis is spread directly or by the respiratory (droplet) route. Streptococcal sore throat (**strep throat**) is one of the most common diseases of childhood. The organism causes epidemics in military training facilities. *S. agalactiae* asymptomatically colonizes the genital and lower gastrointestinal tract of women. Exposure of newborns at birth is due to vertical transmission of the microorganism from the mother. Nosocomial colonization of the neonate is also seen in nursery settings. Cases of neonatal pneumonia, sepsis, and meningitis result from contamination of the infant. *S. pneumoniae* is exclusively a human pathogen; there are no other reservoirs of this organism in nature. *S. pneumoniae* colonizes the nasopharynx and spreads from one person to another through close contact. Day-care centers and crowded living conditions such as prisons are associated with epidemics. Pneumococcal pneumonia is associated with underlying chronic diseases such as alcoholism and diabetes.

The viridans streptococci are a heterogenous group of bacteria most of which comprise part of the normal oral flora. The viridans streptococci are the predominant cause of native valve endocarditis. *Streptococcus mutans* is implicated in initiation of dental caries in humans.

The enterococci are gram-positive cocci that occur singly, in pairs, and in chains. All members of the genus grow in media containing 6.5% NaCl and in media with 40% bile salts. Enterococci hydrolyze esculin. These bacteria are ubiquitous in the environment. In humans and other animals, enterococci inhabit the gastrointestinal and genitourinary tracts.

The most common clinically isolated enterococcal species are *Enterococcus faecalis* and *Enterococcus faecium*. Enterococci cause urinary tract infections and bacteremia. *E. faecalis* is associated with infective endocarditis. Because enterococci are part of the usual gut flora, most infections due to these organisms are endogenously acquired. Nosocomial transmissions also occur. Resistant organisms from patients or medical personnel colonize patients' gastrointestinal tracts and cause infections.

## STREPTOCOCCUS PNEUMONIAE

### Organism Characteristics

Pneumococci are commonly seen on Gram stain as lancet-shaped cocci in pairs. *S. pneumoniae* does not possess a **Lancefield antigen** but there are at least 85 antigenic types based on capsular antigens. *S. pneumoniae* is normally found in the respiratory tract. Invasion of damaged ciliated epithelia result in pneumonia. The virulence factor identified in the pathogenesis of this organism is the polysaccharide capsule, which protects the bacterium from phagocytosis. Protection against infection, then, depends on normal mucociliary barrier and functional phagocytic and T cell-independent immune response. Anticapsular antibodies opsonize encapsulated strains and confer immunity to infection. *S. pneumoniae* also has a C-polysaccharide on its cell wall, which is responsible for the reaction between the organism and acute phase proteins (C-reactive proteins) in the bloodstream of infected individuals. Bacterial autolysin acts on sites in the pneumococcal cell wall and causes the bacteria to disintegrate.

### Clinical Significance

The pneumococcus is the primary cause of community-acquired bacterial pneumonia. The incidence of pneumococcal infection increases in the elderly and in children. The bacterium is associated with many chronic infections and is a frequent cause of otitis media and bacterial meningitis in children. Two risk factors for acquiring invasive disease are lack of maternal breast-feeding and exposure to tobacco smoke. Other pneumococcal infections include sinusitis, mastoiditis, and endocarditis. Oropharyngeal carriage of pneumococci is common and makes interpretation of the significance of pneumococcus in sputum cultures difficult.

### Cultural Characteristics and Identification

The colonial appearance of pneumococci is variable depending on degree of encapsulation. On sheep blood agar, encapsulated *S. pneumoniae* appear as round α-hemolytic colonies. The heavily encapsulated strains are several millimeters in diameter, highly mucoid, and look like oil droplets. The less encapsulated strains are smaller. Older colonies are crater-like due to autolysis, but young colonies are indistinguishable from those of viridans streptococci.

The pneumococcus can be definitively identified by serologic testing of the organism's capsular polysaccharide antigen. Commercial coagglutination or latex agglutination tests are available for rapid pneumococcal identification. Presumptive tests for *S. pneumoniae* correlate well with definitive tests and are less costly. *S. pneumoniae* is susceptible to low concentrations ($\leq 5$ μg/mL) of a quinine derivative, optichin (ethyl hydrocupreine hydrochloride), that differentiates it from the viridans streptococci, which are resistant. Optichin is water soluble and diffuses readily into an agar medium. A filter paper disk impregnated with optichin is used in a diffusion test procedure. The optichin test is performed on blood agar media. Pneumococcal cells surrounding the disk are lysed due to the changes in surface tension and a zone of inhibition is produced. A zone of $\geq 14$ mm around a 6-mm disk indicates susceptibility to optichin (see Figure 10-1). If the zone of inhibition is < 14 mm, a bile solubility test or serology is performed.

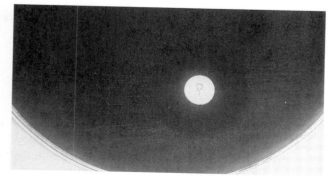

**FIGURE 10-1** Susceptibility of *S. pneumoniae* to optichin disk.

Bile salts such as sodium deoxycholate and sodium taurocholate can selectively lyse *S. pneumoniae* when added to the bacterial growth on an agar plate or in broth media. This organism has autolytic enzymes that result in the central depression or nailhead appearance characteristic of older colonies. Addition of bile salts activates the autolysins and speeds up the natural lytic phenomenon observed with pneumococcal cultures. The bile solubility test is done on a saline suspension of the organism or done directly on the agar plate. On blood agar, bile-soluble colonies disappear when drops of the deoxycholate bile reagent are placed on them. Serotyping and confirmation of pneumococcal disease can be accomplished by enzyme immunoassay or polymerase chain reaction (PCR).

## Antibiotic Susceptibility Characteristics

Pneumococci were uniformly sensitive to penicillin until 1987 when penicillin-nonsusceptible pneumococcal isolates (PNSP) emerged. PNSP is now becoming less susceptible to other antibiotics including tetracycline, erythromycin, chloramphenicol, and the cephalosporins. Because PNSPs are predominantly community acquired, the Centers for Disease Control and Prevention recommends that clinicians base their decisions on empiric antibiotic therapy for presumptive pneumococcal infection on local prevalence data.

Vaccination with multivalent pneumococcal polysaccharide vaccine protects against invasive pneumococcal disease.

## *STREPTOCOCCUS PYOGENES*

### Organism Characteristics

*Streptococcus pyogenes* form gray colonies that are approximately 0.5 mm in diameter and are surrounded by distinct zones of ß-hemolysis on sheep blood agar. The ß-hemolysis is caused by two hemolysins, streptolysin S and streptolysin O. A few strains of *S. pyogenes* produce only the oxygen labile streptolysin O, which can only be seen under anaerobic conditions. Stabbing an inoculum of bacteria into the agar displays hemolysis of colonies growing in the agar subsurface (see Color Plate 13).

The organism has a hyaluronic acid capsule that inhibits phagocytosis by polymorphonuclear cells (PMNs) and macrophages. Strains containing large quantities of M protein are highly resistant to phagocytosis by PMNs. M protein is a filamentous cell surface structure that is anchored to the cell membrane and goes through the cell wall. M protein hinders phagocytosis by inhibiting activation of the alternate complement pathway.

## Clinical Significance

The natural reservoirs for *S. pyogenes* are humans and the organism is transmitted by the respiratory route. The most common infection caused by *S. pyogenes* is pharyngitis. Individuals with the disease have severe sore throat, fever, headache, a beefy red pharynx, and anterior cervical adenopathy; those infected with strains elaborating erythrogenic toxins may develop a rash (scarlet fever). Grayish white exudate may be seen on the hyperemic tonsils of these patients. Individuals having undergone tonsillectomy experience a milder form of the disease. Although the infection is self-limiting, therapy is recommended to prevent acute rheumatic fever and other complications such as otitis media and acute sinusitis.

The nonsuppurative sequelae of *S. pyogenes* infections are **rheumatic fever** and **glomerulonephritis**. Rheumatic fever is associated with streptococcal pharyngitis, whereas glomerulonephritis is associated with pharyngeal or skin infections. Rheumatic fever is a multisystem collagen vascular disease that can cause damage to the heart valves. Glomerulonephritis is an inflammation of the renal glomeruli.

*Streptococcus pyogenes* lysogenized with a strain of temperate phages elaborate pyrogenic toxins that can cause toxic shock syndrome after initially infecting soft tissues. The symptoms are similar to staphylococcal toxic shock syndrome: hypotension, renal dysfunction, coagulopathy, and respiratory failure.

A serious but rare *S. pyogenes* infection is invasive streptococcal infection of the skin and subcutaneous tissues. **Necrotizing fasciitis** or as sometimes described by the lay media as the "flesh-eating bacterial disease" is infection that destroys muscle and fat tissue. The infection starts at a site of minor trauma or with pulmonary symptoms. The affected skin is extremely painful and swollen. Skin eventually blisters and necroses. Fever, systemic toxicity, and gas gangrene follow. Severe cases progress within hours. Without early surgical debridement, fasciotomy, or amputation and antibiotic therapy, mortality is high.

*Streptococcus pyogenes* also causes impetigo, erysipelas, wound and burn infections, bacteremia, pneumonia, and **puerperal sepsis**.

## Cultural Characteristics and Identification

*Streptococcus pyogenes* on sheep blood agar plates appear as small, compact colonies surrounded by a clear, sharply demarcated zone of ß-hemolysis. The organism's cell wall contains polysaccharide classified as the Lancefield group A antigen. To detect the cell wall antigens of streptococci, the antigen is extracted from the cell wall and solubilized. The antigen is extracted enzymatically or by using acid such as nitrous oxide or by heat (autoclaving). The extracted antigen can be detected by various methods. Lancefield used the capillary precipitin test. Other methods include coagglutination and latex agglutination. In coagglutination, the extract is allowed to react with *Staphylococcus aureus* sensitized with group-specific antisera. Streptex (Murex Diagnostics Limited, England) is a rapid latex test system for the identification of the Lancefield group of streptococci. The test uses polystyrene beads to carry the group-specific antisera that are reacted with the streptococcal antigen obtained by acid extraction. These particles agglutinate in the presence of the homologous antigen and remain in smooth suspension in the absence of the homologous antigen. The group A streptococci can be divided into serotypes based on antigenic differences in their M protein, a fibrillar molecule attached to the peptidoglycan of the cell wall and extending toward the surface.

The bacitracin test is based on the susceptibility of group A Streptococci to 0.04 U bacitracin and the resistance of other groups. Any zone of inhibition around the disk is considered a positive test. Because a small percentage of group C and G streptococcal strains are also susceptible to bacitracin, the test is performed along with the sulfamethoxazole-trimethoprim susceptibility test (1.25 µg/23.75 µg) because groups C and G streptococci are generally susceptible to this drug, whereas group A streptococci are resistant (see Figure 10-2). This test is an established presumptive test for *S. pyogenes*. Pyrrolidonyl arylamidase (PYR) hydrolysis can replace the bacitracin test for the presumptive identification of streptococcus group A. Broth containing PYR is inoculated with the organism. If PYR is hydrolyzed, free L-pyrrolidone with carboxylic acid and ß-naphthylamine is produced and is detected by the addition of the diazo dye coupler, N-N-dimethylaminocinnamaldehyde. If PYR is hydrolyzed, then a red color develops.

Serologic assays aid in confirming acute group A streptococci infection in patients with rheumatic fever or glomerulonephritis. To diagnose poststreptococcal sequelae, antistreptolysin O (ASO) and anti-DNase B (ADB) are frequently measured. Antihyaluronidase is useful in diagnosing pyoderma-associated nephritis. Direct detection of the group A antigen in throat swabs by latex agglutination is commercially available but is not as sensitive as conventional culture.

## Antibiotic Susceptibility Characteristics

Therapy is directed toward the prevention of suppurative sequelae such as rheumatic fever, sinusitis, and otitis media. The drug of choice is penicillin because of its efficacy in preventing rheumatic fever. The therapy of choice for penicillin-allergic patients is erythromycin. In areas where erythromycin-resistant *S. pyogenes* are prevalent, antimicrobial susceptibility testing should be performed.

## STREPTOCOCCUS AGALACTIAE

### Organism Characteristics

*Streptococcus agalactiae* belongs to the Lancefield antigen group B and possesses polysaccharide capsular antigens. The capsule contains sialic acid, which allows the group B streptococci to resist opsonophagocytosis by a mechanism of action is similar to that of M protein (blocks the opsonic effects of activation of the alternate pathway of complement).

### Clinical Significance

*Streptococcus agalactiae* is a major cause of pneumonia, sepsis, and meningitis in the perinatal and neonatal periods. Pregnant women become colonized and up to 70% of their infants acquire the same strain of *S. agalactiae* either in utero or during delivery. The neonate may also acquire the organism nosocomially after birth. The early onset diseases commonly seen in neonates are sepsis and pneumonia. Late onset illnesses predominantly present as **bacteremia** with meningitis. Peripartum women colonized with group B streptococci may be at risk for puerperal fever and other infections associated with gynecologic manipulations or surgery. Chronic medical conditions that predispose nonpregnant adults to group B infection include diabetes mellitus and cancer.

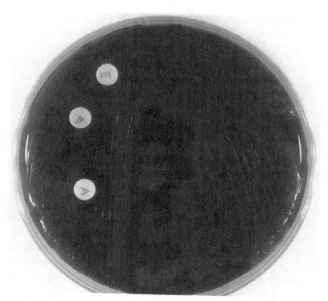

**FIGURE 10-2** Resistance of beta strep group A to sulfamethoxasole-trimethoprim.

## Cultural Characteristics and Identification

*Streptococcus agalactiae* form larger colonies and produce less distinct ß-hemolysis than *S. pyogenes*. Most of group B streptococci produce a diffusible extracellular protein called the CAMP factor that acts synergistically with the ß-lysin of most staphylococci to cause lysis of erythrocytes. CAMP is an acronym for the names of the investigators who first described the hemolytic reaction: Christie, Atkins, and Munch-Petersen. A straight streak of streptococcus perpendicular to the streak of staphylococcus on the surface of sheep blood agar and incubated in ambient air will result in an arrowhead zone of increased hemolysis in the junction into which both the lysin and the CAMP factor have diffused (see Figure 10-3). ß-lysin disks also produce a similar effect. The CAMP method identifies colonies suspected of being nonhemolytic group B streptococci and serves as a presumptive test for group B streptococci. Another presumptive test for *S. agalactiae* is hippurate hydrolysis. To perform the test, broth medium containing sodium hippurate is inoculated with the unknown organism and incubated overnight at 35°C. The cells are then centrifuged and the supernate is collected. Ferric chloride reagent is added to the supernate resulting in the formation of a precipitate. If the precipitate remains after 10 minutes, the test is positive for hippurate hydrolysis. An alternate detection method is to use ninhydrin reagent. *S. agalactiae* hydrolyzes 1% aqueous sodium hippurate to produce glycine and sodium benzoate. Glycine is then deaminated by ninhydrin, which is in turn reduced and turns into a purple color. These presumptive tests show a high degree of correlation with Lancefield grouping, which definitively identifies the organism.

Latex agglutination assays are used for the rapid diagnosis of group B streptococci. Clinical utility of latex agglutination or enzyme immunoassays are at present of questionable value as a screen for genital colonization of pregnant women because of insufficient sensitivity.

## Antibiotic Susceptibility Characteristics

Because group B streptococci are less sensitive to penicillin than that of other streptococci, infections with these organisms are treated with combinations of penicillin and an aminoglycoside.

## ENTEROCOCCI

## Organism Characteristics

The enterococci are facultative anaerobes and are made up of catalase-negative, gram-positive cocci that form pairs and chains. These organisms possess cell wall-associated glycerol teichoic acid, which is the Lancefield group D antigen. They inhabit the intestinal tract. Enterococci can grow in extreme environments such as high concentrations of bile salts and NaCl and at temperatures ranging from 10° to 45°C. They do not contain cytochrome enzymes but on occasion may appear to be catalase positive. This is due to a pseudo-catalase that is sometimes produced. Most strains are homofermentative with no gas production; lactic acid is the end-product of glucose fermentation.

## Clinical Significance

Because they are part of the normal intestinal flora, enterococci cause infections in and out of hospital environments. However, most infections occur in hospitalized patients and among those individuals undergoing hemodialysis; these types of infection are exogenously acquired. Enterococci rank as one of the most common causes of **nosocomial infections** in the United States. The risk factors include underlying disease, surgery, presence of urinary or vascular catheters, and a stay in the intensive care unit. Enterococci are increasingly important etiologic agents of disease primarily because of their resistance to antimicrobics.

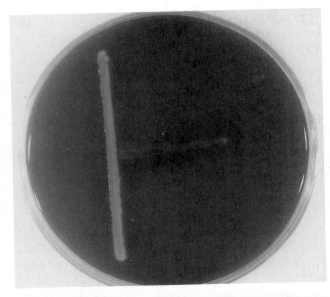

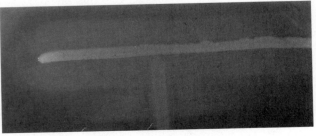

**FIGURE 10-3** CAMP test for *S. agalactiae*.

Enterococci cause opportunistic urinary tract infections and abdominal and pelvic wound infections. Bacteremia is another common cause of enterococcal infection, which can result in infective endocarditis in patients with previously damaged heart valves. *E. faecalis* is the most common organism associated with disease followed by *E. faecium*.

## Cultural Characteristics and Identification

Enterococci are nonhemolytic on 5% sheep blood agar and grow best at 35° to 37°C. To select for enterococci in clinical samples likely to have gram-negative rods, selective media containing azide such as bile-esculin azide are used for primary isolation. Other media used for the successful isolation of enterococci are Columbia nalidixic agar and phenyl ethyl alcohol agar. To definitively identify group D isolates as belonging to the genus enterococcus, the isolates must be PYR or leucine amino peptidase (LAP) positive. Alternatively, the isolates should be resistant to bile, hydrolyze esculin, and be tolerant to 6.5% sodium chloride medium (see Figure 10-4).

The bile-esculin test depends on the ability of some bacteria to hydrolyze esculin in the presence of 40% bile. Esculin is a glycosidic derivative of coumarin. In this test, esculin is incorporated to a medium containing 4% bile salts. Bacteria must survive in the presence of the

bile salts. Esculin hydrolysis results in the formation of esculetin, which reacts with ferric ions (added as ferric citrate in the medium) to form a black complex. The salt tolerance test measures the ability of the organism to grow in the presence of 6.5% sodium chloride. Heart infusion broth is a nutritional broth used to cultivate a number of bacteria. It contains 0.5% NaCl. By increasing the concentration to 6.5% NaCl, this medium becomes semiselective for the growth of enterococci.

## Antibiotic Susceptibility Characteristics

Enterococci have intrinsic as well as acquired resistance determinants to the inhibitory and bactericidal action of many antimicrobial agents. Recommended therapy for serious infections include a cell wall active agent in combination with an aminoglycoside. These combinations overcome intrinsic resistance and show synergistic effects. However, because enterococci rapidly acquire resistance to components of combination therapy, in vitro testing of isolates for resistance to synergy should be performed. Further, susceptibility testing is warranted when predominant growth of enterococci is seen in polymicrobial infections. Testing of isolates from uncomplicated urinary tract infections is optional because enterococcal isolates are susceptible to ampicillin. Nitrofurantoin is also used, but prevalence of resistance is greater. Because bacterici-

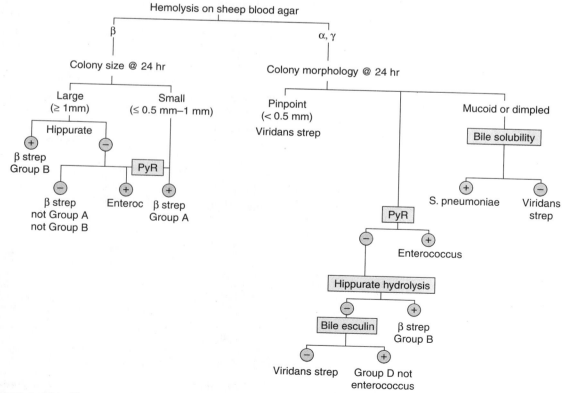

**FIGURE 10-4** Identification of streptococci and enterococci.

dal activity is not necessary for treatment of these kinds of infections, testing for resistance to component drugs in combination therapy is not indicated.

## OTHER GROUP D STREPTOCOCCI

### Organism Characteristics

Group D streptococci not enterococci are gram-positive cocci in pairs and chains, which are either α-hemolytic or nonhemolytic on sheep blood agar, catalase negative, and esculin positive but are unable to grow in 6.5% NaCl. The advent of nucleic acid hybridization techniques led to the division of group D streptococci into two separate species. Some former members of the group D species are predominant normal flora of the human gastrointestinal tract and are designated fecal streptococci or enterococci, whereas the other species that possess the group D antigen and form only a small portion of the usual enteric flora are called nonenterococci. In addition, the enterococci are more resistant to penicillin, cephalosporins, and the aminoglycosides than the nonenterococcal species.

### Clinical Significance

*Streptococcus bovis* is implicated in transient bacteremia or sepsis in newborns, whereas *S. bovis* bacteremia in adults is more often associated with infective endocarditis. Further, *S. bovis* bacteremia is associated with malignancies of the gastrointestinal tract. The organism may be isolated from the stool and blood of patients with adenocarcinoma of the colon. This organism is also implicated in meningitis.

### Cultural Characteristics and Identification

Complete characterization of species belonging to this heterogenous group can be accomplished using physiologic tests. *S. bovis* was originally characterized as a bovine bacterium that fermented arabinose, raffinose, and starch. Some strains produced mucoid colonies through glucan production from sucrose or raffinose. Commercial systems for the identification of gram-positive bacteria can be used to differentiate streptococci to the species level. One such system is the API 20Strep (BioMerieux Vitek, Hazelwood, MO). This nonautomated system is a 4-hour test strip containing 20 mini conventional biochemical tests for the group or species identification of streptococci encountered in medical bacteriology laboratories (see Figure 10-5). The strip contains cupules with dehydrated substrates for the detection of enzymatic activity, fermentation of sugars, utilization of arginine, and hydrolysis of substrates. Specifically, this commercial kit tests for possession of the enzymes pyrrolidonylarylamidase,

α-galactosidase, ß-galactosidase, ß-glucoronidase, alkaline phosphatase, leucinearylamidase, ß-glucosidase and arginine dihydrolase, production of acetoin, hydrolysis of hippurate, and fermentation of ribose, L-arabinose, mannitol, sorbitol, lactose, trehalose, inulin, raffinose, starch, and glycogen. The strip is inoculated with a suspension of bacteria of a standard turbidity and incubated aerobically at 35°C. The strip is examined for color changes by comparison with the API chart, and the results are compared to those found in the manufacturer's code book. Automated and semiautomated systems are also available that use microtiter trays or microcards to hold biochemicals, which can be read manually or by an instrument. Examples of these systems are MicroScan (Baxter MicroScan Division), Sceptor (BBL), and Vitek (bioMerieux Vitek, Inc.).

### Antibiotic Susceptibility Characteristics

Although generally susceptible to penicillin, some strains of *S. bovis* relatively resistant to penicillin may be isolated.

## VIRIDANS STREPTOCOCCI

### Organism Characteristics

The viridans streptococci possess features common to the genus *Streptococcus:* ovoid cells that form pairs and chains, nonmotile and nonsporeforming, and ferment carbohydrates with acid by-products but no gas production. They have the bacteriologic characteristics of streptococci, but they do not have the specific antigens, toxins, nor virulence of the other groups. The term *viridans* is derived from the Latin, *viridis,* denoting green. Viridans streptococci generally produce small colonies surrounded by a zone of α-hemolysis or are nonhemolytic.

### Clinical Significance

Even though their virulence is considered low, some strains can cause infection when they are pro-

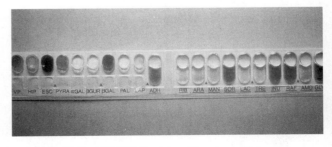

**FIGURE 10-5** API 20S for identification of gram-positive bacteria.

tected from host defenses. Viridans streptococci are often found as contaminants in blood cultures; however, their recovery may be associated with infective endocarditis in patients with damaged native valves. They are also isolated increasingly from specimens of neutropenic patients. Certain species of viridans streptococci, notably *S. mutans,* are strongly associated with dental caries. *S. anginosus* is a normal flora of the mouth and the intestinal tract. Nonetheless, it produces serious purulent infections in liver, brain, and other tissues. It is also implicated in neonatal sepsis. Except for *S. anginosus,* the viridans streptococci are nonpathogenic outside of the vascular system.

## Cultural Characteristics and Identification

Organisms classified as viridans streptococci belong to a biochemically and antigenically diverse group. Most of the strains do not have defined carbohydrate antigens in contrast to the majority of ß-hemolytic streptococci from human infections. After the isolation of α– or nonhemolytic streptococci, a presumptive identification of viridans streptococci can be made if the PYR test is negative or the optichin disk is negative (Table 10-1). To definitively identify isolates to the species level, conventional or commercial biochemical tests can be used, such as the RaPID STR System (Innovative Diagnostic Systems, L.P., Norcross, GA) (see Figure 10-6). The test panel has reaction cavities containing dehydrated reactants built into the periphery of a plastic tray, which allows for simultaneous inoculation of each cavity with a standardized inoculum. After a 4-hour incubation and addition of reagents to designated reaction cavities, color development is observed. A pattern of positive and negative

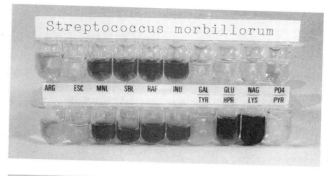

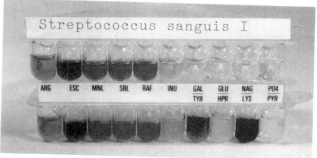

**FIGURE 10-6** RaPID STR for identification of viridans streptococci.

scores is used as a basis of identification of the unknown isolate. Reactivity patterns are compared to that of a database or a Code Compendium.

## Antibiotic Susceptibility Characteristics

The viridans streptococci are generally susceptible to low concentrations of penicillin G. Even though penicillin has been widely used for several decades,

### Table 10–1 ► Presumptive Identification of Clinically Significant Streptococci

| Organism | Hemolysis | Bacitracin (0.04 U) | SXT (23.7/1.25 µg) | CAMP | Hippurate | PYR | Bile Esculin | Growth in 65% NaCl | Optichin or Bile Solubility |
|---|---|---|---|---|---|---|---|---|---|
| *S. pyogenes* | ß | S | R | – | – | + | – | – | – |
| *S. agalactiae* | ß, γ | R | R | + | + | – | – | V | – |
| Groups C and G | ß | R/S | S | – | – | – | – | – | – |
| *Enterococcus* | ß, γ, α | R | R | – | V | + | + | + | – |
| Group D not *Enterococcus* | γ, α | R | S | – | – | – | + | – | – |
| *S. pneumoniae* | α | V | S | – | – | – | – | – | + |
| Viridans strep | α, γ | V | S | – | V | – | V | – | + |

PYR, psyrrolidonyl arylamidase

SXT, sulfamethoxasole-trimethoprim

R = Resistant

S = Susceptible

V = Variable

the susceptibility of viridans streptococci recovered from endocarditis patients has not changed. By disk diffusion testing, viridans streptococci are resistant to the aminoglycosides. However, synergy using combination of penicillin G and aminoglycosides have been shown in vitro and in experimental endocarditis. Some highly resistant strains of viridans streptococci have emerged in geographic areas where the organism is prevalent. This is due to strains that are ß-lactamase producing and are also resistant to other ß-lactam antibiotics. Other antibiotics with good in vitro activity against the viridans streptococci are clindamycin, erythromycin, tetracycline, vancomycin, and the fluoroquinolones.

## OBSCURE OR RARELY ISOLATED ORGANISMS

### Nutritionally Variant Streptococci

**Organism Characteristics.** These organisms are defined by their small size on blood agar (0.2–0.5 mm in diameter) and by their requirement for pyridoxal or thiol for growth.

**Clinical Significance.** The nutritionally variant streptococci (NVS) are usual residents of the oral cavity but are known agents of endocarditis in native and prosthetic valves. They have been isolated from patients with otitis media.

**Cultural Characteristics and Identification.** These strains are noted by their slow growth, formation of tiny colonies, and pleomorphic Gram stains. Growth on tryptose sheep blood agar must be supplemented with vitamin $B_6$ (pyridoxal or pyridoxamine), thiol compounds (cysteine), or cross-streaked with *S. aureus* (satelliting phenomenon). DNA hybridization studies indicate that there are two distinctive species, *S. adjacens* and *S. defectivus*. Both are PYR positive. They can be differentiated from one another by their carbohydrate fermentation patterns and production of beta galactosidase.

**Antibiotic Susceptibility Characteristics.** The NVS are less susceptible in vitro to penicillin than are most other streptococci. In vitro antimicrobial susceptibility testing does not correlate well with clinical outcome in endocarditis patients; therefore, it is recommended that patients with NVS endocarditis be treated with long-term combination therapy.

### Other ß-Hemolytic Streptococci

**Organism Characteristics.** Group C are common pathogens in domestic animals, birds, and guinea pigs. Groups C and G are normal flora of the oral cavity, lower gastrointestinal tract, and vagina. These streptococci form large colonies similar to group A streptococci. Some group C strains are sensitive to bacitracin and may be mistaken for group A streptococci if serologic testing is not performed on isolates from humans.

**Clinical Significance.** Groups C and G streptococci are often carried by domestic animals, but they colonize the human pharynx, gastrointestinal tract, vagina, and skin. One species of group C streptococci, *Streptococcus zooepidemicus,* causes uncommon infections in humans and has been associated with consumption of homemade cheese and unpasteurized cow's milk. Both groups C and G cause endocarditis in patients with no underlying vascular disease. The onset is acute and mortality ranges from 40% to 50%. Although groups C and G streptococci cause clinical symptoms similar to group A pharyngitis, these groups are not associated with nonsuppurative sequelae. Group C may cause severe pharyngitis followed by bacteremia and metastatic infection. Nosocomially acquired bacteremia due to these ß-hemolytic streptococci are largely associated with surgery. Groups C and G cause various cutaneous and subcutaneous infections such as cellulitis, impetigo, and wound infections. Both groups cause septic arthritis and osteomyelitis.

**Cultural Characteristics and Identification.** Group C streptococci are characteristically resistant to bacitracin but some strains are bacitracin sensitive. Thus, group C streptococci may be misidentified as group A if ß-hemolytic isolates are presumptively identified with bacitracin. Identification by antibiotic screening can be improved by using a sulfamethoxasole-trimethoprim disk to which the group C are sensitive. Groups C and G streptococci are definitively identified using a battery of physiologic and serologic tests. Latex agglutination may be used.

## SPECIAL CONSIDERATIONS FOR THE IMMUNOCOMPROMISED HOSTS

Major advances in transplantation, chemotherapy of cancer, and treatment of autoimmune conditions have resulted in an increased life span for patients who no longer succumb quickly to their primary disease. Although these patients survive defects in their host defenses arise due to therapy. For many of these individuals, infection rather than their primary illness becomes the predominant cause of morbidity and mortality. Compromised hosts are individuals with impairment of natural or acquired immunity to infection so that they are at increased risk for infectious disease.

Humans are considered compromised hosts at two stages in their lives: as neonates and as elderly people. A neonate is at risk for infection because it has an umbilicus that serves as a route of infection, a blood–cerebrospinal fluid (CSF) barrier that allows access to the meninges, and immature host defense mechanisms. The absence of IgM and IgA early in life, the lower levels of complement factors, and the incomplete functioning of phagocytic cells are critical in optimal opsonization and phagocytosis of organisms like group B streptococcus. In addition, newborns have profound defects in PMN and sometimes in monocyte chemotraction. Cellulitis caused by group A or B streptococci is common in these infants. Systemic or pulmonary infection with group B streptococci or *S. pneumoniae* can occur and can cause a high incidence of morbidity and mortality. In the elderly, there is an increased susceptibility to infections due to a degradation in the quality of the first line of defense (dryness of skin and mucous membranes), reduced vigor, increased risk for trauma, retardation of repair mechanisms, and reduction in the functioning of both the primary and secondary immune responses. Other conditions that predispose individuals to certain infectious diseases are described below.

*Streptococcus pneumoniae* and *S. agalactiae* are two of the more common etiologic agents of bacterial meningitis. The isolation of a particular species depends on the patient's age, underlying disease, and other predisposing factors. Pneumococcal meningitis is most often seen in adults and is most often associated with either distant or adjacent foci of infection. Pneumococci are the most frequent CSF isolates in head trauma patients who suffer skull fracture with resultant CSF leakage. *S. agalactiae* is a common cause of meningitis in neonates but is also seen in elderly patients. Other risk factors for group B streptococcal meningitis are diabetes mellitus, carcinoma, hepatic failure, renal failure, and corticosteroid therapy. Immune dysfunction, for reasons other than an individual's age, result in a variety of infections.

Patients with congenital immunodeficiency are prone to sudden and usually fatal infections. Individuals with Wiskott-Aldrich syndrome are especially susceptible to the development of overwhelming infections with *S. pneumoniae* and other encapsulated bacteria. Pneumococcal infections are also seen in patients with antibody or complement deficiency or with phagocyte dysfunction. These patients commonly develop acute sinusitis. This type of respiratory infection is characterized by low-grade fever, congestion, postnasal drip, and tenderness over the sinus. This infection is often associated with recurrent otitis media. In diseases like lymphoma and leukemia, and in individuals who are alcoholic or who have had splenectomy, host defenses are impaired. Chronic lymphocytic leukemia is associated with dysfunction of the humoral immune system or antibody production. Forty to 77% of patients with this disease may have extreme hypogammaglobulinemia that results in recurrent pneumococcal infections. Splenectomy enhances the risk of fulminant pneumococcal infection because the primary immunoglobulin response occurs in the spleen. For this reason, immunization with polyvalent pneumococcal vaccine is rec-

ommended for patients undergoing splenectomy. Aside from immune dysfunction, changes in patients' microbial flora also predispose them to certain infections.

Shifts in patients' endogenous flora may be due to the underlying disease, the invasive procedures performed, or the use of antimicrobics. The underlying disease, for reasons not yet fully elucidated, can result in changes in the flora colonizing a given site. The extent of illness and the administration of antimicrobic therapy further results in stronger attachment of gram-negative bacilli in the cells of the buccal mucosa and the decreased attachment of normal flora like the viridans streptococci. Iatrogenic procedures such as catheter insertions, venipuncture, parenteral nutrition, or blood transfusion predispose the immunocompromised patient to infection. Neutropenic patients, for example, are infected with organisms that are near the site where the infection develops. Bloodstream infections with vancomycin-resistant enterococci predominantly affect severely ill patients who have received extensive antibiotic treatment during a long hospitalization. Immunocompromised patients, in general, are more likely to have a persistent bloodstream infection with vancomycin-resistant enterococci. An important source of exogenous bacterial flora for a compromised host is ingestion of microorganisms. The immunocompromised host whose gut flora is suppressed by antibiotic therapy provides an excellent niche for the enhancement of colonization via outside sources. Mixed salads prepared from fresh vegetables may contain organisms ubiquitous in soil and water such as viridans streptococci and enterococci. The compromised host is particularly susceptible to infectious diseases and require extra vigilance from health care providers.

Human immunodeficiency virus (HIV) disease presents a special challenge to clinicians. Fever in HIV patients may be due to a variety of agents such as viruses, bacteria, fungi, protozoans, neoplasms, or pharmacologic effects of drugs. Bacterial infections with *S. pneumoniae* among others are common in HIV patients. Therefore, blood, sputum, and fecal cultures should be part of the fever work-up in HIV patients. Patients in the advanced state of HIV disease commonly have fever and cough. Productive cough with fever is indicative usually of pyogenic infection. One of the most common organisms in this case is *S. pneumoniae*. Pneumococcal vaccine is recommended for HIV patients at the early stage of the disease when the immune function is capable of producing protective antibodies.

Early diagnosis of infection and timely identification of the etiologic agents of serious, life-threatening infections are critical in the management of the compromised host. Molecular technologies show promise for rapid diagnostics and should be incorporated in routine clinical microbiology laboratory procedures to reduce morbidity in the compromised host.

# SUMMARY

► Streptococci comprise a large portion of the indigenous microbial flora of humans and animals.
► The most common pathogens belonging to the streptococci are *S. pyogenes, S. pneumoniae, S. agalactiae,* viridans streptococci and *Enterococcus* species.
► The hemolytic reaction of a streptococcus on sheep blood agar media is used as an initial step in categorizing streptococci and enterococci.

► ß-Hemolytic streptococci can be grouped according to their Lancefield serotype.
► The pneumococcus is a leading cause of community-acquired pneumonia.
► *S. pyogenes* is the causative agent of "strep throat."
► Enterococci are one of the most common causes of nosocomial infections in the United States.
► Advances in molecular biology are being applied to the rapid diagnosis of streptococcal and enterococcal pathogens.

## CASE STUDY 1

A 51-year-old woman presented with fever and shaking chills for 4 days. She was febrile and had marked tenderness over the right rib cage. A chest radiograph showed lesions indicative of septic pulmonary emboli. Abdominal computed tomography showed involvement of hepatic parenchyma and hepatic veins. *Streptococcus anginosus* was isolated from culture of a hepatic aspirate from the lesion and from blood cultures. *S. anginosus* is part of the normal flora of the skin and mucous membranes. Portal of entry to the patient's bloodstream was not apparent.

**Questions:**

1. Discuss how to identify to the species level viridans streptococci isolated from blood cultures.

2. Why is it important to definitively identify viridans streptococci isolated from blood cultures?

## CASE STUDY 2

A previously healthy 29-year-old man presented with high fever, swelling, and marked tenderness of the left thigh. Ultrasonography showed a hypoechoic area between the subcutaneous and muscle tissue. A clinical diagnosis of necrotizing fasciitis was suspected. Early treatment with antibiotics was indicated. A deep incision to the fascia was performed. After verification of the diagnosis, radical debridement of all necrotic tissue resolved the focus. Necrotizing fasciitis is caused by an invasive strain of *Streptococcus pyogenes*. The initial process involves inflammation and occlusion of muscle vessels followed by fascia necrosis. The necrosis spreads to subcutaneous tissue so that the swelling is observed before cutaneous signs appear. Early treatment with antimicrobics and surgical intervention are critical to preserve the patient's limb and life.

**Questions:**

1. The invasive strain of *S. pyogenes* that cause necrotizing fasciitis may cause a higher rate of more serious infection in children and in the elderly compared to the rest of the population. Explain.

2. A swab from infected tissue was sent to the laboratory for culture. What plating media should one choose to ensure the isolation of ß-streptococci?

# Review Questions

1. This microorganism is the most virulent species in the genus *Streptococcus* and is responsible for suppurative sequelae such as rheumatic fever and glomerulonephritis.
   a.  *S. pneumoniae*
   b.  *S. pyogenes*
   c.  *S. bovis*
   d.  *S. mutans*

2. Choose the most likely organism with the following characteristics and clinical significance: gram-positive cocci implicated in pneumonia of newborns and puerperal fever in postpartum females; ß-hemolytic on sheep blood agar, CAMP factor positive, hippurate hydrolysis positive.
   a.  *S. pyogenes*
   b.  *E. faecium*
   c.  *S. agalactiae*
   d.  *G. haemolysans*

3. A gram-positive coccus that is strongly associated with dental caries and belongs to a heterogeneous group of streptococci best characterizes this species.
   a.  *S. mutans*
   b.  *S. viridans*
   c.  *S. anginosus*
   d.  *S. bovis*

4. This group of organisms forms tiny colonies on blood agar, satellite around colonies of staphylococci and can cause endocarditis.
   a.  *A. viridans*
   b.  *L. garvieae*
   c.  *S. defectivus*
   d.  *G. morbillorum*

5. Emerging multiply resistant strains of this organism are becoming a major problem in the hospital environment. This bacterium grows in 6.5% NaCl and hydrolyzes esculin in the presence of bile salts.
   a.  *S. pneumoniae*
   b.  *Lactococcus* species
   c.  *S. bovis*
   d.  *E. faecalis*

6. This virulence factor acts by preventing opsonophagocytosis. It is localized in the fibrils, which are attached to the peptidoglycan of streptococcal cell wall.
   a.  M protein
   b.  Lancefield antigen
   c.  capsular polysaccharide
   d.  streptolysin S

7. Isolation of this organism from blood cultures of a patient is indicative of a possible bowel malignancy. It is bile esculin positive but does not grow in 6.5% NaCl.
   a.  *E. faecium*
   b.  *A. urinae*
   c.  *S. bovis*
   d.  *S. zooepidemicus*

8. A common cause of community-acquired pneumonia, these pathogens may appear as α-hemolytic mucoid colonies or small colonies with a crater-like center. They are optichin positive and are highly autolytic.
   a.  viridans streptococci
   b.  *S. pneumoniae*
   c.  nutritionally variant streptococci
   d.  *S. adjacens*

9. Necrotizing fasciitis is an invasive infection of muscle and fat tissues. Mortality is high unless the disease is rapidly diagnosed, the wound is surgically debrided, and antibiotic therapy instituted. The etiologic agent is:
   a.  *S. agalactiae.*
   b.  *G. morbillorum.*
   c.  group C streptococcus.
   d.  group A streptococcus.

10. A compromised host is:
   a.  more resistant than other individuals to opportunistic infections.
   b.  more susceptible than other individuals to opportunistic infections.
   c.  protected from most diseases by vaccination.
   d.  both A and C

## ▶REFERENCES & RECOMMENDED READING

Baron, S. (Ed.). (1991). *Medical microbiology* (2nd ed.). New York: Elsevier.

Coykendall, A. (1989). Classification and identification of the viridans streptococci. *Clinical Microbiology Reviews, 2* (3), 315–328.

Gillespie, S., Ullman, C., Smith, M., & Emery, V. (1994). Detection of *Streptococcus pneumoniae* in sputum samples by PCR. *Journal of Clinical Microbiology, 32* (5), 1308–1311.

Isenberg, H. (Ed. in Chief). (1994). *Clinical microbiology procedures handbook. Processing and interpretation of Upper Respiratory Tract Specimens.* Vol. 1. Washington, DC: American Society for Microbiology.

Koneman, E., Allen, S., Handa, W., Schreckenberger, P., & Winn, W. (Eds.). (1992). *Color atlas and textbook of diagnostic microbiology* (4th ed.). Philadelphia: Lippincott.

Mandell, G., Bennett, J., & Dolin, R. (Eds.). (1995). *Principles and practice of infectious diseases* (4th ed.). New York: Churchill Livingstone.

Murray, P. (Ed. in Chief). (1995). *Manual of clinical microbiology* (6th ed.). Washington, DC: ASM Press.

Peter, J. (Ed.). (1996). *Use and interpretation of tests in infectious diseases* (4th ed.). Santa Monica, CA: Specialty Laboratories.

Radstrom, P., Backman, A., Qian, N., Kragsbjerg, N., Pahlson, C., & Olcen, P. (1994). Detection of bacterial DNA in cerebrospinal fluid by an assay for simultaneous detection of *Neisseria meningitidis, Haemophilus influenzae,* and streptococci using a seminested PCR strategy. *Journal of Clinical Microbiology, 32*(11), 2738–2744.

Rubin, R., & Young, L. (Eds.). (1994). *Clinical approach to infection in the compromised host* (3rd ed.). New York: Plenum.

Sherris, J. (Ed.). (1990). *Medical microbiology* (2nd ed.). New York: Elsevier.

U.S. Department of Health and Human Services (1997). Surveillance for penicillin-nonsusceptible *Streptococcus pneumoniae*—New York City, 1995. *Morbidity and Mortality Report, 46*(14), 297–299.

Zhang, Y., Isaacman, D., Wadowsky, R., Rydquist-White, J., Post, J. C., & Ehrlich, G. (1995). Detection of *Streptococcus pneumoniae* in whole blood by PCR. *Journal of Clinical Microbiology, 33*(3) 596–601.

# CHAPTER 11

# Aerobic Gram-Positive Bacilli, Coccobacilli, and Coryneform Bacilli

Vivian Chantakrivat, MBA, MT (ASCP)

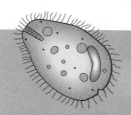

## *Microbes in the News*

### Bacterium Guards Against HIV

It's not just the stuff of bad cheese anymore! Two years ago, investigators identified the bacterium *Listeria monocytogenes*, which had fouled soft cheeses, as the cause of many cases of a flulike illness in several states. Now, researchers at the University of Pennsylvania School of Medicine in Philadelphia are trying to transform this troublesome bug into a vaccine for human immunodeficiency virus (HIV), the virus for acquired immunodeficiency virus (AIDS). Yvonne Patterson and her team began their experiment by inserting a specific HIV gene into the chromosomes of *L. monocytogenes*. They found that, when grown in culture, these genetically engineered bacteria use the information encoded by the HIV gene to manufacture one of the virus' protein products.

Paterson's team decided to immunize mice with the newly transformed bacterium suspended in a solution. After giving the animals an intramuscular injection of this vaccine, the researchers found several encouraging signs of protection. White cells called T lymphocytes taken from the mice secreted large amounts of γ-interferon, a substance thought to

keep HIV at bay, the scientists discovered. In addition, they found such mice showed long-term evidence of killer T cells against HIV. Once the *L. monocytogenes* has set up shop inside a cell, the researchers believe, the altered bacterium starts to produce the HIV protein. The cell's machinery recognizes that viral protein as foreign and escorts it to the surface of the cell—where it flags the attention of killer T cells. The researchers hope that such a process will yield protective immunity against HIV. In the event HIV does get into the bloodstream of an immunized individual, the T cells will be primed to attack, Paterson says.

*Listeria monocytogenes* can cause illness in people with impaired immune systems who eat contaminated food. Yet people with HIV appear relatively resistant to this bug. "You'd expect AIDS patients to be full of *Listeria,* but they're not," Paterson says. Still, the safety and efficacy of this approach remains to be proved, she adds.

Source: *Science News,* November 26, 1994.

## KEY TERMS

| | | |
|---|---|---|
| Anthrax | Diphtheria | Pyrazinamidase |
| CAMP test | Diphtheroid | String of pearls test |
| Cold enrichment | Erysipeloid | Sporangium |
| Coryneform | γ-bacteriophage | Emetic |

## LEARNING OBJECTIVES

**Upon successful completion of this chapter, the student should be able to:**

1. Enumerate the different genera that comprise this morphologic group.
2. Differentiate the corresponding species and their characteristics.

3. Describe the morphology and cultural requirements of the organisms.
4. Explain the clinical significance of each species.
5. Identify these important pathogens using common laboratory identification techniques.

## INTRODUCTION

This chapter discusses the clinically significant gram-positive aerobic bacilli, coccobacilli, and **coryneform** bacilli. The organisms in this group are aerobic or facultative spore-forming or nonspore-forming organisms that are widely distributed in nature and will grow well on most nonselective laboratory media. Some species in this group are primary human pathogens, some are implicated in infections acquired through handling of infected plant and animal products, some cause food poisoning, and some are contaminants and secondary invaders in compromised hosts. One obscure, rarely isolated gram-positive bacillus species is also discussed.

The more commonly isolated and clinically significant species of each genus, their cultural characteristics, the diseases and infections associated with them, and some relevant laboratory procedures including identification techniques are also included.

## BACILLUS SPECIES

These aerobic, gram-positive spore-bearing bacilli belong to the family *Bacillaceae,* which includes a highly diverse group of endospore-forming aerobic and anaerobic bacteria (see Figure 11-1). The genus *Bacillus* includes more than 50 species, some of which have uncertain taxonomic status. The organisms in this genus are aerobic or facultatively anaerobic, and gram positive or gram variable with some species losing their gram-positive reaction as the culture ages. The rods are straight, round, or square-ended and occur singly or in chains of a few to many cells long in their vegetative form. The endospore in each **sporangium** is oval,

round, or kidney-shaped, and depending on the species, the endospore is located centrally, subterminally, or terminally, and may or may not swell the sporangium. Some species under conditions of low oxygen concentration, produce a visible capsule when stained with polychrome methylene blue. Almost all species are motile, with lateral flagella. Most ferment glucose, and most are catalase positive.

Most *Bacillus* species are saprophytes and are found everywhere in nature, especially in the soil, plant, and animal products. The organisms in this genus are able to withstand extremes in environmental conditions and are capable of survival in spore form and sometimes even growth. Few species have distinctive habitats, with spore germination and spore formation dictated by availability of nutrients in nature.

Widely distributed in nature, *Bacillus* organisms are frequently found as contaminants in laboratory cultures. Because they may vary in Gram stain and other reactions, and no spores may be evident, they can be mistaken for gram-negative nonfermentative bacilli. Colonial morphology is sometimes unreliable in distinguishing these contaminants because some of these strains have very small colonies and do not exhibit the typical large flat ß-hemolytic colony. Some even show limited growth on enteric agars. Because spore formation does not occur within the time required to report a clinical isolate, two other tests may be used. One is susceptibility to vancomycin and the potassium hydroxide test in which gram-negative organisms show a viscous thread.

With the exception of *Bacillus anthracis* and *Bacillus cereus,* most *Bacillus* species have little or no pathogenic potential and rarely cause diseases in humans and animals. However, due to the resistance of the spores to many extremes in temperature, chemicals, radiation,

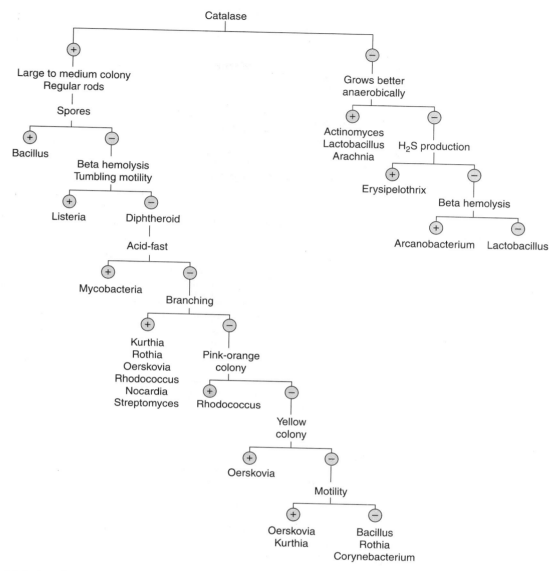

**FIGURE 11-1** Aerobic, gram-positive nonspore-forming *Bacilli* identification.

and desiccation, many species in this genus show up as tenacious contaminants in hospital operating rooms and surgical dressings, foods, and pharmaceutical products and equipment. Other species have also been implicated in cases of endocarditis, septicemia, pneumonia, meningitis, and other serious infections.

*Bacillus* species are generally susceptible to tetracycline, aminoglycosides, and chloramphenicol. Susceptibility to penicillin, ampicillin, methicillin, and cephalothin are species specific.

## Bacillus anthracis

*Bacillus anthracis,* the agent of **anthrax**, is the primary human pathogen in this genus. Cases of anthrax in the United States are most often related to hand-

ling imported wool or goat hair, animal hide, and by-products of these. Persons exposed to cattle can also contract the disease. Anthrax is not often encountered in the average hospital but in areas where industries related to cattle and animal products are found, its timely identification is crucial.

**Organism Characteristics.** *Bacillus anthracis* is a facultative, large nonmotile, square-ended, gram-positive rod with an elliptical or cylindrical central spore that does not distend the sporangium. The organisms are frequently found in long chains giving a "bamboo" appearance on primary isolation. A capsule surrounds the chains of the virulent form; avirulent forms are not encapsulated.

**Clinical Significance.** Anthrax is primarily a disease of cattle, sheep, goats, and horses. Humans contract it directly from these animals or indirectly from products made from the hide, wool, bone, or hair of these animals. Although moderately resistant to anthrax compared to these herbivores, humans are still susceptible to it in industrial and nonindustrial settings. There have been a few reports of lab-acquired infections. It is rare in the United States, with an average 2.5 cases a year in the last decade, mainly due to the development of animal and human vaccines coupled with strict hygiene and sterilization requirements for imported animal products and the increased use of synthetic alternatives to these products.

Anthrax in humans is manifest in three forms. Cutaneous anthrax (malignant pustule) is the most common form in the United States; infection is through entry of the bacilli through a cut or opening on the skin. The bacilli can be demonstrated in the discharge from the pustule.

Pulmonary anthrax or woolsorters' disease is contracted by inhaling the spores during the handling of animal hair. The bacilli are present in the sputum. Gastrointestinal anthrax is the rarest but the most severe form. Infection is by ingestion of the bacilli or spores. The organism can be isolated from the patient's stool.

**Cultural Characteristics and Identification.** The colonies are large gray white to white, opaque, and raised with a curled margin. The colonies are nonhemolytic or weakly hemolytic. The organism produces a heavy pellicle with no subsurface growth. Optimum growth temperature is 35°C. It hydrolyzes starch, the Voges-Proskauer reaction is positive, and nitrates are reduced.

A modification of the **string of pearls test** reflecting its susceptibility to penicillin has been used as a presumptive test for this species. On a Mueller-Hinton agar plate, single streaks of the suspect organism, a positive and a negative control are made. Penicillin G disks (10 U) are placed on each streak, each streak is coverslipped, and the plate is incubated at 37°C for 6 hours. *B. anthracis* growth fails on agar close to +10 U penicillin, beneath the coverslip where antibiotic concentration is less, cells of *B. anthracis* become large and spherical, occurring in chains and, as examined under the microscope, appear as a string of pearls. This is a positive test.

A suspect organism that shows the correct Gram stain and colonial morphology is nonhemolytic or weakly hemolytic, gray-white or white, nonmotile, able to produce a capsule, penicillin- and γ-**bacteriophage** susceptible is *B. anthracis*.

**Antibiotic Susceptibility Characteristics.** *Bacillus anthracis* is susceptible to penicillin, gentamicin, erythromycin, and chloramphenicol. It is usually susceptible to streptomycin but resistant to cefuroxime. Tests have shown that the infection responds to doxycycline and ciprofloxacin but not to tetracycline.

## Bacillus cereus

*Bacillus cereus* has been associated with cases of food poisoning and food-borne illnesses in the United States and Europe. It has also been isolated from wounds and implicated in some serious infections in immunocompromised patients.

**Organism Characteristics.** *Bacillus cereus* is a gram-positive rod tending to occur in chains with an elliptical or cylindrical central spore. It is morphologically similar to *B. anthracis*.

**Clinical Significance.** *Bacillus cereus* has long been implicated in food-borne illnesses caused by improper storage and handling of cooked food. There are two distinct food poisoning syndromes caused by this bacillus. The diarrheal type is characterized by abdominal pain followed by diarrhea 8 to 16 hours after ingestion of contaminated food. The **emetic** type causes nausea and vomiting 1 to 5 hours after ingestion. Both are due to the spores, which survive normal cooking temperatures, and which germinate and multiply under improper storage conditions. The reaction is due to the toxin produced by the bacillus in vivo.

*Bacillus cereus* has also been implicated in serious infections that usually affect immunocompromised hosts. Surgery and trauma patients, burn and dialysis patients, intravenous drug abusers, and patients with catheters and various prosthetic devices have proven susceptible to infection. Cases of myonecrosis after trauma or surgery have been reported as being caused by this organism, along with septicemia, pneumonia, meningitis, endocarditis, and osteomyelitis.

**Cultural Characteristics and Identification.** The colony is lavender with a slight green tinge on blood agar; the colony form varies from small, shiny and compact to one with a dull frosted-glass appearance and an undulate margin with no outgrowths, to one with rootlike, irregularly tangled or curved outgrowths that spread widely over the agar surface. It exhibits ß-hemolysis on sheep blood agar. It is catalase positive, motile, Voges-Proskauer positive, hydrolyzes starch, is resistant to penicillin and γ-bacteriophage. It does not encapsulate on bicarbonate agar, and produces hemolysin and lecithinase.

**Antibiotic Susceptibility Characteristics.** It is resistant to trimethoprim and is not susceptible to penicillin and other ß-lactam antimicrobics. It is susceptible to vancomycin, chloramphenicol, clindamycin, gentamicin, tetracycline, and sulfonamides.

## Other Bacillus Species

Several other species in this genus have been implicated in infections reported in the United States ranging from food poisoning to septicemia and meningitis. Most common are those caused by *Bacillus subtilis* and *Bacillus licheniformis*. Bacteremia, endocarditis, and respiratory infections caused by *B. subtilis* have been reported along with allergic and hypersensitivity reactions. *B. licheniformis* has been linked to cases of bacteremia, food poisoning, peritonitis, and ophthalmitis. Other species, *B. alvei, B. brevis, B. circulans, B. coagulans, B. macerans, B. pumilus, B. thuringiensis,* and *B. sphaericus* have also been incriminated with reported cases of meningitis, sepsis, wound infection, eye infection, and endocarditis.

**Antibiotic Susceptibility Characteristics.** These species are generally susceptible to tetracycline, chloramphenicol, and aminoglycosides. *B. subtilis* is susceptible to penicillin, ampicillin, and cephalothin. *B. licheniformis* is susceptible to penicillin and resistant to clindamycin.

# LISTERIA SPECIES

*Listeria* species can be found widely distributed in the environment, having been isolated from water, soil, decaying vegetable matter, animal feed, sewage, fresh and processed foods, and human and animal carriers. It has been isolated from mammals, fish, crustaceans, birds, and insects. It is a saprophyte primarily inhabiting soil and decaying vegetable matter and produces virulence factors only in an animal or human host.

*Listeria monocytogenes* was the only recognized species in this genus until after 1948 when other species were discovered. Only *L. monocytogenes* is of public health concern.

## *Listeria monocytogenes*

**Organism Characteristics.** *Listeria monocytogenes,* along with the other species of this genus, is a facultative anaerobic nonbranching, regular, short grampositive rod. It does not form spores and is motile, with peritrichous flagella. It can grow at 4°C after a few days but optimal growth is between 30° to 37°C. It is Voges-Proskauer and methyl red test positive, but negative for oxidase. It is catalase positive, hydrolizes esculin but not urea and gelatin. It is indole and H$_2$S negative, and produces acid from glucose and other sugars.

**Clinical Significance.** *Listeria* infections are often associated with food, food processing, and food production. The disease known as listeriosis can occur as an epidemic or as sporadic cases with ingestion of contaminated food being the primary mode of transmission. How the organism causes disease is not clear, but it has been shown that after contaminated food has been ingested, an invasive infection results on susceptible hosts. The organism enters the host intestinal tract and grows within the cells of the liver and spleen. The organism produces a hemolytic protein called listeriolysin, which destroys the host cells.

In pregnant women, *L. monocytogenes* causes an influenza-like illness and septicemia, which may lead to amnionitis and ultimately the infection of the unborn fetus. Some such cases have resulted in premature birth, abortion, and stillbirth. Early diagnosis can be made with blood cultures. At birth, the organism may be isolated from the placenta, blood, amniotic fluid, or meconium. Gram stain smears from these specimens are important in the diagnosis of the disease.

*Listeria monocytogenes* causes encephalitis, meningitis, or bacteremia in nonpregnant human adults. Hosts who are immunocompromised or have a predisposing condition such as AIDS, lymphoma, or transplant are highly susceptible to the disease. In neonates, it commonly presents as sepsis or meningitis. The cerebrospinal fluid (CSF) is purulent with a normal glucose and an elevated protein. The organism may or may not be apparent with Gram stain. Cultures of blood and CSF are positive only in about 70% of the cases but are the most reliable means of diagnosis.

Listeriosis is a reportable disease, with five known epidemics in the United States since 1981. Most of the cases were linked to the ingestion of contaminated dairy products and contaminated cabbage. The organism is a common contaminant of fresh and processed food, and because it can survive and multiply in refrigerator temperatures, even a small number of organisms present on the suspect food can be significant.

**Cultural Characteristics and Identification.** *Listeria monocytogenes* grows well on most laboratory media. The colonies resemble group B ß-hemolytic streptococci with small, translucent gray, smooth colonies with a narrow diffuse zone of ß-hemolysis. On Gram stain, they are gram-positive, pleomorphic rods that may palisade or appear as coccobacilli in pairs or chains. This gram-stain morphology may lead to confusion with **diphtheroids**, an over-decolorized *Haemophilus* or some species of *Streptococcus*. Observation of typical end-over-end tumbling motility under direct wet preparation can be presumptive identification. A positive catalase, Voges-Proskauer, and methyl red, with esculin hydrolysis and acid production from glucose identifies the genus *Listeria*. Speciation is important because other species of the genus are also found as contaminants but only *L. monocytogenes* is considered pathogenic. Species differentiation is by the biochemical characteristics of the organism consisting of its hemolytic property, **CAMP test** reaction, and acid production from different sugars. *L. monocytogenes* is ß-hemolytic, along with three other species but only *L. monocytogenes* is CAMP test positive and produces acid from rhamnose.

Clinical specimens from sterile sites can be plated directly on to blood agar (5% sheep) but specimens obtained from nonsterile sites, foods, and the environment need to be selectively enriched for *Listeria* species before plating. **Cold enrichment** on nonselective broth for 2 months followed by selective plating increases the likelihood of isolating the causative organism but is a slow process. More rapid methods for isolating *L. monocytogenes* have been developed due to the need for haste in investigating outbreaks, but are not 100% sensitive.

**Antibiotic Susceptibility Characteristics.** The usual regimen for treatment of listeriosis is with penicillin or ampicillin with or without an aminoglycoside. The organism is susceptible to penicillin, ampicillin, rifampin, tetracycline, erythromycin, chloramphenicol, and gentamicin. Sulfamethoxasole-trimethoprim and aminoglycosides are bacteriocidal to *L. monocytogenes;* cephalosporins are ineffective.

## ERYSIPELOTHRIX SPECIES

### Erysipelothrix rhusiopathiae

*Erysipelothrix rhusiopathiae* was the only recognized species in this genus until 1988 when another species *E. tonsillarum* was isolated from swine tonsils. *E. rhusiopathiae* is ubiquitous in the environment and nature. It is an important pathogen of animals and the humans who work with these animals. It infects swine, sheep, cattle, ducks, turkey, and even fish; human acquisition of the disease is a result of exposure to these animals and their products. It is important economically as it relates to the industries that involve these animals.

**Organism Characteristics.** *Erysipelothrix rhusiopathiae* is a facultative nonmotile, nonsporulating regular gram-positive rod. It grows on sheep blood trypticase soy agar and chocolate agar as well as selective media like calcium nutrient agar (CNA) and phenylethyl alcohol agar (PEA). Optimum growth is at 36°C with 5% to 10% $CO_2$. On primary isolation, the organism may grow as two or more distinct colony types that look different under Gram stain. The rod may appear as a small slender gram-positive bacillus or as a slender, filamentous gram-positive bacillus that tends to overdecolorize and become gram negative. It is catalase negative, and produces $H_2S$ in triple sugar iron agar (TSI) or Kligler's iron agar. It is the only $H_2S$-producing aerobic, catalase-negative, gram-positive bacillus.

**Clinical Significance.** It causes swine erysipelas and septicemia in mice. In humans, it is usually a self-limiting cellulitis on the fingers or hand called **erysipeloid** because of the similarity to erysipelas caused by streptococcus. On infection by the organism, usually through an open cut or abrasion on the skin, an elevated spreading erythematous lesion develops. The cellulitis appears 2 to 7 days after infection and can be rather painful. This is the most common form of the disease and is usually contracted by veterinarians, butchers, fish handlers, and abattoir workers.

Recently, the historically rarer form of the disease has been recorded more often. The septicemic form presents with bacteremia and skin involvement, then progresses to endocarditis, involving native valves, with or without damage. It may also involve a rarely reported complication, arthritis.

**Cultural Characteristics and Identification.** *Erysipelothrix rhusiopathiae* isolation is enhanced by incubating the blood TSI agar plates for 48 to 72 hours. After 24 hours' incubation, colonies are very small, but longer incubation yields two colony forms, one a smaller, raised smooth translucent gray colony, which stains as small and slender bacilli; the other form, a large, flat, rough gray colony yields slender filamentous bacilli. They exhibit α-hemolysis on blood agar. The organism is catalase negative, and its production of $H_2S$ on TSI or Kligler's slants is the most significant biochemical test for this species. It is positive for both lactose and N-acetyl-glucuronidase. Biochemically, it reacts the same as *E. tonsillorum* except for the latter's ability to ferment sucrose. Clinical laboratory automated identification systems like Vitek, or the API Coryne strip identify *E. rhusiopathiae* with ease.

Recently, a rapid, direct polymerase chain reaction-based test was developed to detect the organism in contaminated meat and other animal products. Serologic testing is not useful for diagnosis of *E. rhusiopathiae* infection, and no effective vaccine for either animals or humans has been developed.

**Antibiotic Susceptibility Characteristics.** The organism is susceptible to cephalothin, penicillin, and ampicillin. ß-Lactam agents and quinolones are usually effective, but the organism is resistant to aminoglycosides and sulfamethoxasole-trimethoprim. Some strains are resistant to vancomycin. Susceptibility to chloramphenicol, tetracycline, and erythromycin is variable.

## LACTOBACILLUS SPECIES

Lactobacilli are gram-positive asporogeneous rods. Most species of *Lactobacillus* are facultative anaerobes, but approximately 20% of human isolates are obligate anaerobes. *Lactobacillus* species are found in the healthy mouth, in saliva, and in plaque. They are found in the female genital tract and in the genital tract of other mammals. They are found in the intestinal tract of humans and animals, and also found in a variety of food products.

**Organism Characteristics.** On Gram stain, *Lactobacillus* species are gram-positive, asporogeneous rods. The morphology is variable, ranging from regular rods similar to the *Bacillus* species, in singles and chains, to coccobacillary and spiral forms. All species are catalase negative, and nonmotile. They reduce nitrates but do not produce indole.

**Clinical Significance.** *Lactobacillus* species are only occasionally involved in human infections. They have been isolated from blood, CSF, pleural fluid, amniotic fluid, and abscess material. Lactobacilli are usually present in large numbers in the Gram stain or culture of a healthy vagina. The organism thrives in the acid pH of the female genital tract and plays a role in protecting the female vagina from infection of the gonococcus and from bacterial vaginosis. The standard method for interpreting the Gram stain in the diagnosis of bacterial vaginosis includes the presence of the large gram-positive bacilli of the *Lactobacillus* morphotype whose presence in large numbers indicates a normal score.

**Cultural Characteristics and Identification.** The organism is a facultative or strict anaerobe, usually growing microaerophilically so anaerobic media and methods should be used in identification. The colonies of *Lactobacillus* species assume different morphology on blood agar. They can be pinpoint, smooth compact grayish white translucent colonies resembling streptococci or large, rough gray colonies. Surface growth on solid media is enhanced by 5% to 10% $CO_2$ or anaerobiasis, with optimum temperature generally 30° to 40°C. The microscopic morphology may sometimes make it difficult to distinguish the lactobacilli from streptococcus when it is found as coccobacilli in chains. Examination of the organism in thioglycollate broth will yield chains of rods. Also, the organism's resistance to vancomycin, which is unusual in gram-positive organisms will help to identify the isolate as a *Lactobacillus* species. Isolation of a chaining gram-positive rod, which is catalase negative, with small to medium gray translucent colonies that may or may not be α-hemolytic should lead one to consider *Lactobacillus* species.

**Antibiotic Susceptibility Characteristics.** The growth of lactobacilli is inhibited by penicillin, ampicillin, cephalothin, and clindamycin. In patients with endocarditis, it is recommended that aminoglycosides be given in combination with penicillin and rifampin.

# CORYNEBACTERIUM SPECIES

The corynebacteria are a group of pleomorphic, usually nonmotile gram-positive bacilli. They are tapered or slightly curved rods with rounded ends, with sides not parallel, either the end or middle is slightly wider resulting in club or cocoon shapes. The cells may be barred or segmented, are arranged singly, in pairs, or palisades of parallel cells. Some pairs form a V shape due to the incomplete separation of cells, and Chinese letter forms are seen due to uneven division during binary fission. They do not branch and are not acid-fast. The *Corynebacterium* species most likely to be encountered in the clinical lab include *C. diphtheriae*, *C. ulcerans*, *C. aquaticum*, *C. pseudodiphthericum*, *C.*

*renale, C. pseudotuberculosis, C. bovis, C. matruchotii, C. xerosis, C. jeikeium,* and *C. minutissimum.* They are found throughout nature, acting as pathogens of plants and animals. Many are part of the normal human mucous membrane and skin flora and are usually harmless saprophytes. *C. diphtheriae,* the agent of diphtheria, *C. jeikeium* (CDC JK group), and *C. urealyticum* (CDC group D2), both common causes of infection in immunocompromised hosts, are the major pathogens of humans in this genus.

## *Corynebacterium diphtheriae*

*Corynebacterium diphtheriae* causes an acute toxin-mediated infectious disease. **Diphtheria** is a contagious, febrile illness that manifests as an oropharyngeal inflammation with the formation of a pseudomembrane and subsequent heart and nerve damage. The exotoxin produced by this organism inhibits protein synthesis in heart and nerve muscle. Not all the *C. diphtheriae* produce the exotoxin. A bacteriophage carrying the gene for toxin production infects the bacteria, replicates within the bacterial genome, and does not lyse the cell (called a lysogenic infection).

**Organism Characteristics.** *Corynebacterium diphtheriae* (Klebs-Loeffler bacillus) is a facultative, nonmotile highly pleomorphic, slender gram-positive rod. It does not stain uniformly with methylene blue, but appears banded or beaded with metachromatic granules. Individual cells tend to lie parallel to each other or at acute angles to each other forming V, Y, or L shapes. This appearance is highly characteristic of this organism, but should not be used as the only means of identification because other diphtheroids and actinomycetes mimic the morphology (see Figure 11-2).

**Clinical Significance.** Diphtheria is an acute communicable disease characterized by local upper respiratory tract infection and systemic toxin effects. It presents as a sore throat, malaise, fever, headache, nausea, and a pharyngeal membrane. It can result in death from obstruction by the membrane or toxin-induced myocarditis. Some strains are not infected by the bacteriophage and are called nontoxigenic *C. diphtheriae*. They do not produce a toxin but can cause a diphtheria-like disease that is usually not as severe. Diphtheria immunization started in 1920 has almost eradicated the disease, with present occurrence limited to only a few per year as contrasted with 60,000 cases in 1932. *C. diphtheriae* also causes cutaneous diphtheria, which occurs in previously traumatized skin. The lesions become necrotic and black, occasionally forming a membrane. Both toxigenic and nontoxigenic strains have been isolated from an epidemic of cutaneous diphtheria. There are increasing reports of both toxigenic and nontoxigenic strains causing endocarditis without previous diphtheria symptoms.

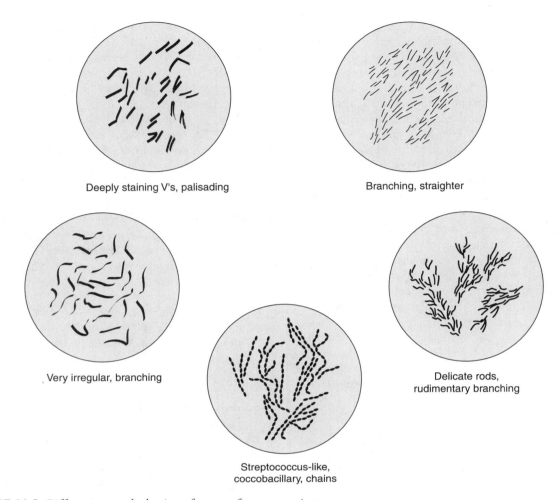

Deeply staining V's, palisading

Branching, straighter

Very irregular, branching

Streptococcus-like,
coccobacillary, chains

Delicate rods,
rudimentary branching

**FIGURE 11-2** Different morphologies of coryneform organisms.

**Cultural Characteristics and Identification.** Suspect specimens are streaked onto blood agar, a selective tellurite containing medium (Modified Tinsdale medium or cystine-tellurite agar) and a Loeffler agar slant. The growth on Loeffler's is Gram stained for demonstration of the typical morphology and metachromatic granules. Better recovery from swabs is possible by streaking on serum- or blood-containing media and subsequent subculture after 4 days. Optimum incubation temperature is 35° to 37°C with or without $CO_2$. An alternative to the use of the selective media is the placement of a fosfomycin disk after inoculation on blood agar and identification of coryneforms that grow in the surrounding zone of inhibition. Laboratory diagnosis of unsuspected diphtheria infection is difficult because the colonies of *C. diphtheriae* are not distinctive on the plates usually used to plate throat and wound cultures, and coryneforms isolated from the throat and skin are usually not reported.

There are four subtypes of *C. diphtheriae* and all form a gray-brown halo on Tinsdale medium and are **pyrazinaminidase** negative. Their colonial morphologies differ—*C. diphtheriae* subspecies *intermedius* produces small colonies, subspecies *mitis* produces larger ß-hemolytic colonies, whereas subspecies *gravis* produces larger nonhemolytic colonies.

The most useful commercial system for identification of *Corynebacterium* species and other coryneform organisms is the API Coryne System, which uses 20 biochemical tests in a strip. After 24 hours of incubation, the enzymatic results are read, with urease, sugar fermentation, and gelatin, available within 5 days. The system, though imperfect by lumping some species together, will correctly identify *C. diphtheriae*. Several automated systems like the Vitek, Minitek, and Biolog show promise but are of limited usefulness at this time due to incomplete data bases.

All *C. diphtheriae* isolates should be tested for toxigenicity because not all strains produce the exotoxin. The isolate is streaked on an Elek plate perpendicular to a filter paper strip impregnated with antitoxin. A line of precipitation forms where the toxin, if produced, meets the diffusing antitoxin (see Figure 11-3). Tissue culture methods can also be used and a definitive cytotoxic effect demonstrated. An historical test now rarely used is the guinea pig lethality test where

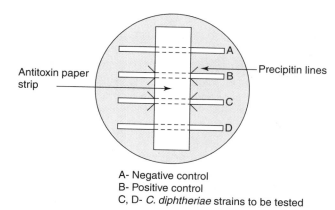

A- Negative control
B- Positive control
C, D- *C. diphtheriae* strains to be tested

**FIGURE 11-3** Elek plate toxigenicity of *C. diphtheriae.*

the toxin and test strain are injected peritoneally into the animals, with resultant death in 1 to 3 days. Polymerase chain reaction technology has also been used recently to test toxigenicity.

**Antibiotic Susceptibility Characteristics.** Immunization is the best defense against diphtheria. For patients with diphtheria, an antitoxin that is hyperimmune horse antiserum is the most important treatment. The circulating toxin is not affected by antimicrobial treatment but penicillin can be used to eliminate *C. diphtheriae* from the respiratory tract of the patient. Penicillin is also used to treat suspected carriers of the organism to stop toxin production and the spread of infection. Susceptibility testing is not necessary on clinical isolates.

## Other *Corynebacterium* Species

**Organism Characteristics.** Gram-stain morphology is typical of the genus, pleomorphic, nonspore-forming gram-positive bacilli. They are generally catalase positive, aerobic or facultative, and primarily nonmotile. They do not hydrolyze gelatin or esculin, and most of the clinically important species do not utilize lactose, xylose, and mannitol.

**Clinical Significance.** *Corynebacterium jeikeium,* the name for the Centers for Disease Control and Prevention (CDC) group JK is the most commonly isolated corynebacterial pathogen in the clinical laboratory. It has been linked with meningitis, septicemia, pneumonia, endocarditis, peritonitis, and soft tissue infections. Infections on prosthetic devices have been reported. It can be isolated from urine, but is not a cause for any disease at this site. Most common infections are nosocomial, in immunocompromised patients, patients on broad-spectrum antibiotic therapy, and those who have been in hospitals for extended periods.

*Corynebacterium urealyticum* (CDC group D2) can be found in the urine of asymptomatic patients but has been isolated in the urine of patients with urinary tract infection, cystitis, and alkali-encrusted stones. It causes bacteuria and pyelonephritis, and has been reported

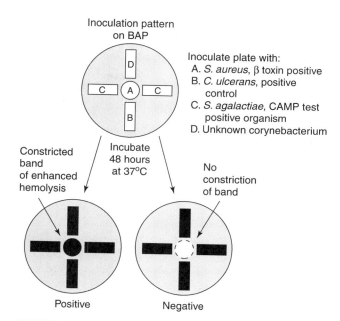

**FIGURE 11-4** Phospolipase D inhibition of CAMP test.

as a cause for nosocomial bacteremia and pneumonia. It has been isolated in wound infections and implicated in endocarditis in patients with prosthetic heart valves.

Colonization of hospitalized patients by *C. jeikeium* and *C. urealyticum* is not uncommon, with the groin and rectum being the sites most often colonized. Several other *Corynebacterium* species have been implicated in endocarditis, eye infections, tropical ulcers, graft infection, septic abscesses, and pharyngitis.

**Cultural Characteristics and Identification.** The organisms grow well on most commonly used media, and appear as opaque white or gray colonies that are nonhemolytic or α-hemolytic. Rapid biochemical tests are useful in identification of corynebacteria, along with two supplementary tests, the pyrazinamidase activity and production of enzyme phospholipase D (see Figure 11-4). Various commercial kits are available like the API 20S and the Minitek system to correctly identify the different *Corynebacterium* species.

**Antibiotic Susceptibility Characteristics.** Both *C. jeikeium* and *C. urealyticum* are resistant to a wide range of antimicrobial agents such as the aminoglycosides, penicillins, and cephalosporins. They are usually susceptible only to vancomycin, which is the drug of choice. Some newer antimicrobial agents and a combination regimen of aminoglycosides have shown some promise but long-term conclusions have yet to be drawn.

## OBSCURE OR RARELY ISOLATED SPECIES

The genus *Rothia* was created in 1967 for an organism that resembled *Nocardia* and *Actinomyces.* The only species, *Rothia dentocariosa,* is part of normal human oral flora but has been known to cause abscesses and prosthetic valve endocarditis. It can cause periodontitis and gingivitis. *Rothia* species are gram-positive filamentous bacilli that can show branching and stain evenly. This genus is considered an opportunistic pathogen. The

colonies are white, raised, and smooth at 48 hours; they become rough or globose on longer incubation. They are positive for glucose, esculin, and nitrate and are fermentative. They are catalase positive, lactose negative, and susceptible to most antimicrobial agents including aminoglycosides, cephalosporins, erythromycin, and penicillin.

## SUMMARY

▶ The *Bacillus, Listeria, Erysipelothrix, Lactobacillus,* and *Corynebacterium* species are ubiquitous inhabitants of the natural environment or normal human flora. Most are of low pathogenicity and generally cause infection and disease only after a break in the immunologic defenses of the host. They exhibit various morphologies, and grow well on commonly used nonselective media.

▶ *Bacillus* species are mostly nonpathogenic except for *B. anthracis,* the agent of anthrax, and *B. cereus,* the cause of diarrheal and emetic type food poisoning.

▶ *Listeria* infections are most commonly associated with food processing, production, and handling, causing epidemic or sporadic listeriosis, a reportable disease since 1986.

▶ *Erysipelothrix* and *Lactobacillus* species are only occasionally involved in human infections.

▶ *Corynebacterium* species, although part of the normal human mucous membrane and skin flora, include the causative agent of diphtheria, an acute, toxin-mediated infectious disease.

▶ *Rothia* is an opportunistic pathogen that may also be isolated in routine laboratory bacteriologic cultures.

## Review Questions

1. What organism is not often encountered in the average hospital except in areas where industries related to cattle are found ?
   a. *Rothia*
   b. *Lactobacillus* species
   c. *Erysipelothrix rhusiopathiae*
   d. *Bacillus anthracis*

2. An acute communicable disease, characterized by upper respiratory tract infection, and systemic toxin effects, caused by the Klebs-Loeffler bacillus is:
   a. listeriosis.
   b. syphilis.
   c. diphtheria.
   d. mononucleosis.

3. This organism resembles *Nocardia* and *Actinomyces,* an opportunistic pathogen found in the human oral cavity, which can cause abscesses and endocarditis.
   a. *Rothia dentocariosa*
   b. *Listeria monocytogenes*
   c. *Streptococcus pyogenes*
   d. *Staphylococcus aureus*

4. The localized cellulitis often on the hand, arm, or fingers of animal and animal product processors, caused by *Erysipelothrix rhusiopathiae* is:
   a. erysipelas.
   b. arthritis.
   c. erysipeloid.
   d. chancroid.

5. Primarily a disease of cattle, sheep, goat, and horses, which disease caused by a *Bacillus* species can be contracted by humans working with these animals?
   a. Listeriosis
   b. Anthrax
   c. Influenza
   d. Pericarditis

6. The *Bacillus* species that often causes food poisoning due to nondestruction of its spores by normal cooking temperatures is:
   a. *Bacillus cereus.*
   b. *Bacillus anthracis.*
   c. *Bacillus brevis.*
   d. *Bacillus pumilus.*

7. A form of anthrax characterized by a malignant pustule is:
   a. gastrointestinal anthrax.
   b. woolsorters' disease.
   c. cutaneous anthrax.
   d. emetic form.

8. A food-borne reportable disease linked to many epidemics since 1981, caused by *Listeria monocytogenes,* is
   a. diphtheria.
   b. listeriosis.
   c. cellulitis.
   d. erysipelas.

9. Frequently found in the Gram stain or culture of a healthy vagina, playing a protective role from gonococcal infection and bacterial vaginosis, which organism is occasionally involved in human infections?
   a. *Streptococcus pyogenes*
   b. *Lactobacillus acidophilus*
   c. *Staphylococcus aureus*
   d. *Bacillus subtilis*

10. The term used to denote a club-shaped bacillus or an irregularly shaped gram-positive rod is:
    a. coryneform.
    b. polymorphic.
    c. coccoid.
    d. Gram positive.

▶ **REFERENCES & RECOMMENDED READING**

Baron, J. E., & Finegold, S. M. (1990). *Diagnostic microbiology* (pp. 457–475).

Finegold, S. M., & Martin, W. J. (1982). *Diagnostic microbiology* (pp. 291–308).

Murray, P., Baron, J. E., Pfaller, M. A., Tenover, F. C., & Tolken, R. H. (1995). *Manual of clinical microbiology* (pp. 341–373).

# CHAPTER 12
## Aerobic Actinomycetes

Bardwell J. Eberly, MT (ASCP), SM

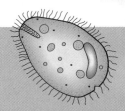

### Microbes in the News
#### "Bird Flu" Caused by Influenza A Strain H5N1

A new strain of the influenza A virus named H5N1 that usually causes disease in chickens was responsible for several deaths in humans late in 1997. Although 6 people were killed in Hong Kong, laboratory tests indicated it had not mutated into a more dangerous bug that could easily spread from person to person and cause a worldwide epidemic. Experts at the Centers for Disease Control and Prevention have not determined how the virus managed to spread from chickens to humans and that H5N1 made some people sick greatly alarmed international flu experts.

Flu virus genes are highly changeable and newly altered strains appear regularly. The new strain usually resembles the previous one and so most humans have some immunity against them. Occasionally, a new strain develops that is particularly deadly. Often they originate in birds and are spread to swine, which can host both the bird flu and human flu. The two viruses may genetically mix in the swine creat-ing a totally new flu strain for which humans have no immunity. This is what was feared had happened with H5N1 but does not seem to be the case; all of its genes are those of the bird flu. Also, this virus does not seem to be able to spread easily from person to person.

Measures taken to control the spread of the virus included slaughter of more than a million chickens in Hong Kong and blocking importation of chickens from nearby provinces in China. No new human cases of H5N1 have been reported since December 28, 1997 and no cases outside of Hong Kong have been reported. More than 100 flu surveillance laboratories worldwide have been alerted to look for evidence of H5N1 outbreaks since the incident in Hong Kong.

Source: "Studies show bird flu not a major killer." *USA Today* Health

http://ww.usatoday.com/life/health/general/lhgen017.htm Downloaded 4/6/1998

## KEY TERMS

Actinomycetoma
Cutaneous
Eumycetoma
Filamentous
Glabrous

Gomori-methenamine-silver stain
Granules
Madura foot
Mycetoma

Pulmonary
Slow growing
Subcutaneous
Tumefaction

## LEARNING OBJECTIVES

**Upon successful completion of this chapter, the student should be able to:**

1. Describe the clinical infections associated with *Nocardia, Actinomadura,* and *Rhodococcus equi.*
2. Describe the microscopic and macroscopic characteristics of *Nocardia, Actinomadura,* and *Rhodococcus equi.*

3. List the biochemical tests that can differentiate *Nocardia, Streptomyces, Actinomadura* and *Rhodococcus* species.
4. List the antimicrobial characteristics for *Nocardia, Actinomadura,* and *Rhodococcus equi.*

## INTRODUCTION

Aerobic actinomycetes were once classified as fungi due to the aerial hyphae produced. However, due to the lipid and peptidoglycan composition within the cell wall of these microorganisms, they are considered bacterial in nature. Most aerobic actinomycetes can cause infections in humans and animals. Microscopically, most aerobic actinomycetes are gram-positive, **filamentous**, branching rods. They are infrequently isolated from clinical samples. Refer to Color Plate 14.

### Habitat

These bacteria are ubiquitous in nature and can be found in soil, water, and plant material. They can be introduced into the host via aerosol exposure (dust particles), trauma (puncture through the dermal layer), or inoculation into the bloodstream (secondary seeding via the gastrointestinal tract).

### Commonly Isolated Species

The medically significant aerobic actinomycetes that cause morbidity and mortality particularly in immuno-compromised patients include *Nocardia, Actinomadura, Rhodococcus, Oerskovia, Streptomyces,* and *Tsukamurella* (McNeil & Brown, 1994; Prescott, 1991).

*Nocardia, Actinomadura,* and *Streptomyces* have been reported to be causative agents for **mycetomas**, which are localized infections involving bone and cutaneous and **subcutaneous** tissue. They are characterized by three features: swelling (**tumefaction**), draining sinuses, and **granules** (0.5 to 1 μm in diameter) (Mandell, Bennett, & Dolin, 1995). Mycetomas associated with aerobic actinomycetes are designated **actinomycetomas**, whereas mycetomas associated with fungi are designated as **eumycetomas**. Portal of entry into the host is traumatic inoculation of the organism into the skin anywhere on the body, but most frequently on the feet, legs, arms, or hands (Beaman & Beaman, 1994; Howard, Keiser, Smith, Weissfield, & Tilton, 1994).

## NOCARDIA

In 1889, Edmond Nocard, a French veterinarian, isolated an aerobic actinomycetes from granulomatous disease in cattle. It was reported as *Streptothrix farcini,* the causative agent for bovine farcy, and was later renamed as *Nocardia farcinica* by Trevisan in 1889. In 1891, Eppinger isolated the first *Nocardia* from a patient with pneumonia and brain abscess. It was not until 1896 that Blanchard formally reclassified the organism as *Nocardia asteroides* (Mandell et al., 1995; McNeil & Brown, 1994).

Several species within the genus of *Nocardia* are pathogenic to man. They include *N. asteroides* complex, *N. brasiliensis, N. transvalensis,* and *N. otitidis-caviarum.* Differentiation of species depends on the hydrolysis of casein, xanthine, tyrosine, and hypoxanthine media and resistance to lysozyme.

### Pathogenicity

Most *Nocardia* species can elicit an active inflammatory response in the host. Both polymorphonuclear leukocytes and activated lymphocytes are involved in the cellular response to the infection. Necrosis and abscess formation can be observed on hematoxylin-eosin preparations and the presence of the organism can be seen histologically on **Gomori-methenamine-silver stain** (Mandell et al., 1995). Refer to Color Plate 15.

**Pulmonary Nocardiosis.** *Nocardia* is most often isolated from **pulmonary** specimens due to inhalation of the airborne particle or aspiration of the organism into the lung. Most pulmonary nocardiosis is encountered from patients with chronic bronchitis, emphysema, asthma, or bronchiectasis.

Patients are usually systemically ill with fever, cough, and weight loss. Pleuritic chest pain often precedes or accompanies development of empyema (Mandell et al., 1995). Chronic granulomatous lesions develop, which often mimic tuberculosis or neoplastic infections. The granuloma can remain in the lungs or erode into the bloodstream, allowing the organism to invade other anatomic locations, such as the brain, meninges, kidney, liver, and spleen. Approximately 80% of the cases of primary pulmonary nocardiosis are caused by *N. asteroides*. Refer to Plates 16 and 17.

**Cutaneous Nocardiosis.** Primary **cutaneous** nocardiosis is a result of a traumatic inoculation of the organism through the skin by a thorn, splinter, puncture wound, insect bite, or animal bite (Beaman & Beaman, 1994). Several members of the medically significant *Nocardia* species may play a role in cutaneous nocardiosis but *N. brasiliensis* is the organism most often isolated from skin or ulcerated lesions from immunocompetent patients (McNeil & Brown, 1994).

**Keratitis.** This rarely reported infection occurs in both immunocompetent and immunocompromised patients, often by exogenous inoculation of the organism. For example, a person suffering a traumatic injury to the eye while wearing improperly cleansed contact lenses could develop keratitis. (Howard et al., 1994; McNeil & Brown, 1994).

## Microscopic Characteristics

Microscopically, the nocardiae appear as intertwining gram-positive filaments, approximately 0.5 to 1 μm in diameter. The filaments, which are branched and are often beaded, can fragment into bacillary and coccoid forms. One diagnostic feature of *Nocardia* is the right angle branching of the filaments (McNeil & Brown, 1994). The nocardiae appear as partially acid-fast when stained with the modified Kinyoun stain (Larone, 1995). Refer to Color Plate 18.

## Isolation

Specimens are processed in accordance with the procedures established by each laboratory. In our laboratory, clinical specimens are processed using the *N*-acetyl-L-cysteine (NALC)-sodium citrate method to rule out aerobic actinomyces. It is inoculated to enriched media (brain-heart infusion agar [BHIA]), and selective enrichment agars (modified Thayer-Martin agar, inhibitory mold agar [IMA], BHIA with chloramphenicol, cycloheximide, and gentamicin, Middlebrook 7H10).

Other enriched media such as 5% sheep blood agar or chocolate agar can be used. Inoculated plates are sealed to prevent dehydration of media. Cultures are incubated at 30°C in a non-$CO_2$ incubator for 4 weeks because the organism is **slow growing**.

## Macroscopic Characteristics

Colonies mature within 7 to 10 days on BHIA, 5% sheep blood agar, or chocolate agar. Colonies may be **glabrous**, heaped, or folded and may develop a white chalky coating. Pigmentation may vary from white to pink or orange, depending on the species (Larone, 1995). Refer to Color Plates 18 and 19.

## Cultural Identification

Biochemical tests that differentiate the major pathogenic *Nocardia* species include hydrolysis of casein, tyrosine, xanthine, and hypoxanthine, carbohydrate fermentation, and resistance to lysozyme as shown in Table 12-1. (Howard et al., 1994; McNeil & Brown, 1994; Mishra, Gordon, & Barnett, 1980; Rippon, 1988). Refer to Color Plates 21 through 24.

## Antimicrobial Characteristics

Sulfonamides and sulfamethoxazole-trimethoprim are the standard antibiotics used to treat patients with *Nocardia* infections (Mandell et al., 1995; McNeil & Brown, 1994). Response to treatment with sulfonamides is excellent with clinical improvements within 7 to 10 days following initiation of therapy (Mandell et al., 1995).

## *ACTINOMADURA*

*Actinomadura madurae* and *A. pelletieri* are clinically significant members of the genus *Actinomadura*. *A. madurae* is a soil saprophyte and *A. pelletieri* has been found only in clinical specimens. Actinomycetoma infections occurs most often in climates with alternating rainy and dry seasons, such as West Africa, Mexico, India, and Central and South America (Mandel

## Table 12–1 ▶ Identification of *Nocardia* and *Streptomyces*

| Organism | Hydrolysis of: | | | | Biochemical Reaction | | |
| --- | --- | --- | --- | --- | --- | --- | --- |
| | Casein | Tyrosine | Xanthine | Hypoxanthine | Lysozyme | Lactose | Xylose |
| *Nocardia asteroides* complex | neg | neg | neg | neg | growth | neg | neg |
| *Nocardia brasiliensis* | pos | pos | neg | ± | growth | neg | neg |
| *Nocardia otitisdis-caviarum* | neg | neg | pos | pos | growth | neg | neg |
| *Streptomyces* species | pos | pos | pos | ± | ± | ± | ± |

et al., 1995; McNeil & Brown, 1994). It is the second most common aerobic actinomycete encountered by the Centers for Disease Control and Prevention (CDC).

## Pathogenicity

*Actinomadura madurae* is the causative agent for **"madura foot"** or maduramycosis, a chronic deep subcutaneous tissue and bone infection. The most common site of infection is the foot (Mandell et al., 1995) and the etiologic agents occur in the form of granules or grains.

## Microscopic Characteristics

On Gram stain, the organism is gram positive, with fine, intertwining, branched filaments (0.5–1 μm in diameter). It is nonacid-fast, nonfragmenting, and may form a short chain of spores (Howard et al., 1994; Larone, 1995).

## Isolation

Grains or granules, if submitted, should be emulsified and inoculated to Lowenstein-Jensen medium, BACTEC 12B medium, 5% BHIA with 5% sheep blood agar, and Sabauraud's dextrose agar, Emmons. The grains (granules) are the actual colonies of the causative agent. Aspirates of the draining sinuses or pus should be processed in accordance with the method described in the isolation procedure for *Nocardia*.

## Macroscopic Characteristics

Colonies will appear waxy, heaped, folded, membraneous, or mucoid. Colonies may be white, tan, pink, orange, or red. White aerial hyphae may develop after 2 weeks of incubation on Lowenstein-Jensen medium at 37°C in $CO_2$.

## Cultural Identification

Biochemical tests that differentiate the *Actinomadura* species are seen in Table 12-2. (Howard et al., 1994; McNeil & Brown, 1994; Rippon, 1988).

## Antimicrobial Characteristics

A combination of two drugs is used to treat *Actinomadura* infections. *Actinomadura* is susceptible to streptomycin. Patients with *A. madurae* can also be treated with diaminodiphenylsulfone; *A. pelletieri* infections are treated with streptomycin and sulfamethoxazole-trimethoprim (Mandell et al., 1995).

## RHODOCOCCUS

### Pathogenicity

*Rhodococcus equi* is a soil organism that can cause respiratory illness in humans and spontaneous abortions in animals. It is rarely isolated from immunocompetent patients, but isolation from immunocompromised patients can occur (Murray, Baron, Pfaller, Tenover, & Yolken, 1995; Prescott, 1991).

### Microscopic Characteristics

*Rhodococcus* is a gram-positive coccobacillus, which can vary in appearance from long bacilli to short diphtheroid-like rods with occasional branching. Some isolates can also stain as partially acid-fast.

### Isolation

*Rhodococcus* grows on 5% sheep blood agar after 48 hours incubation at 35°C.

### Macroscopic Characteristics

Colonies appear smooth, semitransparent, and approximately 2 to 4 mm in diameter. Colonies may or may not be mucoid and may show pink to red pigmentation after several days. The cultures have a soil-like odor (Prescott, 1991).

### Cultural Identification

Isolates are typically positive for catalase and urease, negative for oxidase, do not ferment carbohydrates, and are usually nitrate positive.

### Antimicrobial Characteristics

*Rhodococcus* is susceptible to erythromycin, clindamycin, aminoglycosides, rifampin, and vancomycin.

| Table 12–2 ▶ Identification of *Actinomadura* Species | | | | | | | |
|---|---|---|---|---|---|---|---|
| | **Hydrolysis of:** | | | | **Biochemical Reaction** | | |
| **Organism** | **Casein** | **Tyrosine** | **Xanthine** | **Hypoxanthine** | **Lysozyme** | **Esculin** | **Xylose** |
| *Actinomadura madurae* | pos | pos | neg | pos | neg | pos | pos |
| *Actinomadura pelletieri* | pos | pos | neg | pos* | neg | neg | neg |
| *>75% of strains positive | | | | | | | |

## SUMMARY

▶ Aerobic actinomycetes were once classified as fungi but now are considered bacterial in nature.

▶ Common isolated species cause morbidity and mortality particularly in immunocompromised patients.

▶ Microscopically, most aerobic actinomycetes are gram-positive, filamentous, branching rods.

▶ Some of the aerobic actinomycetes may be partially acid-fast when stained by a modified Kinyoun method.

▶ These organisms grow on mycology media (Sabouraud dextrose agar) without antibiotics and on routine mycobacteriology media (Lowenstein-Jensen).

▶ Most of the aerobic actinomycetes are slow growers.

▶ The most common pathogenic aerobic actinomycetes isolated from clinical samples and reported to the CDC belongs to the genus *Nocardia*.

## CASE STUDY

A 20-year-old Mexican-American woman presented to the surgical clinic with a lump in the right popliteal fossa. She reportedly had had two resections of the lesion over a 6-year period in Mexico. Nevertheless, it continued to manifest intermittent drainage. She also complained that it became painful on exposure to cold or after prolonged standing. She had no history of trauma and a questionable history of knee injury. Physical examination revealed two scarred circumscribed subcutaneous nontender nodules, each approximately 0.5 cm in diameter, and about 3 cm apart, in the right popliteal fossa. No drainage was noted, and no masses or cysts were palpated.

Two apparent sinus tracts and a contiguous scarred area in the subcutaneous tissue of the popliteal fossa were explored. Two small nodules were noted in the mass, one of which was sectioned, revealing brown fluid, which was submitted for routine culture only. The remaining specimen was sent for pathologic examination. (Braunstein, Hicks, & Konyn, 1990)

**Questions:**

1. Given the patient's history, what diagnoses should be considered?

2. What qualities, growth characteristics, and biochemical studies will be required to identify the organism once it is isolated?

3. How is the therapeutic approach influenced by the nature of the organism?

## Review Questions

1. Which one of the following organisms are partially acid-fast when stained with the modified Kinyoun stain?
   a. *Streptomyces somaliensis*
   b. *Streptomyces griseus*
   c. *Actinomadura madurae*

2. The key to differentiate *Nocardia brasiliensis* from other *Nocardia* species is the hydrolysis of casein, tyrosine, and:
   a. failure to hydrolyze xanthine.
   b. acid-fast.
   c. failure to hydrolyze urea.
   d. ability to form aerial hyphae.

3. A kidney transplant patient developed a temperature and cough. Pulmonary x-ray showed pulmonary infiltrate. Gram-positive branching rods were observed on the Gram stain. Modified Kinyoun stain was performed. The rods were partially acid-fast. The organism grew aerobically. The etiologic agent is probably:
   a. *Actinomyces* species.
   b. *Streptomyces* species.
   c. *Nocardia* species.
   d. *Actinomadura* species.

4. The most commonly encountered pathogenic aerobic actinomycete from clinical samples is:
   a. *Streptomyces* species.
   b. *Actinomadura* species.
   c. *Nocardia* species.
   d. *Tsukamurella* species.

5. Aerobic actinomycetes:
   a. resemble fungi in that they form filaments that are 1 μm or less in diameter.
   b. may be partially acid-fast when stained by a modified Kinyoun method.
   c. colonies are usually pigmented.
   d. all of the above

6. The key biochemical to differentiate *Nocardia* species from *Actinomadura* species is:
   a. lyzozyme broth.
   b. casein hydrolysis.
   c. xylose fermentation.
   d. xanthine hydrolysis.

7. Which aerobic actinomycete is the causative agent for maduramycosis?
   a. *Nocardia asteroides* complex
   b. *Rhodococcus equi*
   c. *Tsukamurella paurometabola*
   d. none of the above

8. Which aerobic actinomycete is the causative agent for pulmonary, systemic, and cutaneous diseases, including mycetomas?
   a. *Streptomyces* species
   b. *Oerskovia* species
   c. *Rhodococcus equi*
   d. *Nocardia* species

9. The causative agents for localized infections involving bone, cutaneous, and subcutaneous tissue are:
   a. *Nocardia, Streptomyces, Actinomadura.*
   b. *Streptomyces, Oerskovia, Tsukamurella.*
   c. *Actinomadura, Rhodococcus equi, Tsukamurella.*
   d. *Nocardia, Actinomadura, Tsukamurella.*

10. The second most commonly encountered pathogenic aerobic actinomycete from clinical samples is:
    a. *Streptomyces* species.
    b. *Actinomadura* species.
    c. *Nocardia* species.
    d. *Tsukamurella* species.

## ▶ REFERENCES & RECOMMENDED READING

Beaman, B. L., & Beaman, L. (1994). Nocardia species. Host-parasitic relationships. *Clinical Microbiology Reviews, 7,* 213–264.

Braunstein, H., Hicks, L., & Konyn, C. (1990). Cutaneous nocardiosis due to *Nocardia brasiliensis. ASCP Check Sample, 33,* MB 90-3.

Harrington, R. D., Lewis, C. G., Aslanzadeh, J., Stelmach, P., & Woolfrey, A. E. (1996). *Oerskovia xanthineolytica.* Infection of a prosthetic joint: Case report and review. *Journal of Clinical Microbiology, 34,* 1821–1824.

Howard, B. J., Keiser, J. F., Smith, T. F., Weissfield, A. S., & Tilton, R. C. (1994). *Clinical and pathogenic microbiology* (2nd ed.). St. Louis: Mosby–Year Book.

Larone, D. H. (1995). *Medically important fungi: A guide to identification* (3rd ed.). Washington, DC: American Society for Microbiology Press.

Mandell, G. L., Bennett, J. E., & Dolin, R. (1995). *Principles and practice of infectious disease* (4th ed.). New York: Churchill Livingstone.

McNeil, M. M., & Brown, J. M. (1994). The medically important aerobic *Actinomycetes:* Epidemiology and microbiology. *Clinical Microbiology Reviews, 7,* 357–417.

Mishra, S. K., Gordon, R. E., & Barnett, D. A. (1980). Identification of Nocardiae and Streptomyces of medical importance. *Journal of Clinical Microbiology, 11,* 728–736.

Mossad, S. B., Tomford, J. W., Stewart, R., Ratliff, N. B., & Hall, G. S. (1995). Case report of *Streptomyces* endocarditis of a prosthetic aortic valve. *Journal of Clinical Microbiology, 33,* 3335–3337.

Murray, P. R., Baron, E. J., Pfaller, M. A., Tenover, F. C., & Yolken, R. H. (1995). *Manual of clinical microbiology* (6th ed.). Washington, DC: American Society for Microbiology Press.

Prescott, J. F. (1991). *Rhodococcus equi:* An animal and human pathogen. *Clinical Microbiology Reviews, 4,* 20–34.

Rippon, J. W. (1988). *Medical mycology* (3rd ed.). Philadelphia: Saunders.

# CHAPTER 13

## Neisseria and Other Aerobic Gram-Negative Cocci

Judith S. Heelan, PhD

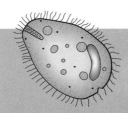

## Microbes in the News

### Bacterial Meningitis Blamed for Boy's Death

Health officials confirmed that meningitis caused by the bacterium *Neisseria meningitidis* took the life of an 8-year-old boy from Fall River, MA. Appearing well on Monday, the boy felt sick and stayed home from school on Tuesday. By Wednesday afternoon he had died.

This was the second fatal case of meningitis in this city in 1996. Meningitis is an inflammation of the lining around the brain and spinal cord. When diagnosed early, bacterial meningitis is usually curable. It is critically important to rapidly obtain cerebrospinal fluid for smear and culture when meningitis is suspected.

The bacteria that cause meningitis are spread by person-to-person contact. Transfer of saliva, kisses, coughs, sneezes, and sharing water bottles are common ways the bacteria can be transmitted.

*Providence Journal Bulletin,* June 14, 1996

---

**INTRODUCTION**

**NEISSERIA GONORRHOEAE**

Organism Characteristics

Habitat and Transmission

Specimen Collection and Transport

Clinical Significance

Cultural Characteristics and Identification

Direct Detection in Clinical Specimens

Antibiotic Susceptibility Characteristics

**NEISSERIA MENINGITIDIS**

Organism Characteristics

Habitat and Transmission

Specimen Collection and Transport

Clinical Significance

Cultural Characteristics and Identification

Direct Detection in Clinical Specimens

Antibiotic Susceptibility Characteristics

**BRANHAMELLA MORAXELLA CATARRHALIS**

Organism Characteristics

Habitat and Transmission

Specimen Collection and Transport

Clinical Significance

Cultural Characteristics and Identification

Antibiotic Susceptibility Characteristics

**OTHER NEISSERIA SPECIES**

---

## KEY TERMS

Chemiluminescent
Commensal
Dysuria
Enzyme immunoassay

Epididymitis
Nucleic acid probe
Pelvic inflammatory disease
Proctitis

Salpingitis
Tenesmus

## LEARNING OBJECTIVES

**Upon successful completion of this chapter, the student should be able to:**

1. Distinguish between the normal commensal *Neisseriae* and those species pathogenic for humans, *N. gonorrhoeae* and *N. meningitidis,* using cultural and biochemical characteristics.
2. Compare the epidemiology of *N. gonorrhoeae* and *N. meningitidis.*

3. Describe symptoms of uncomplicated gonorrhea as well as complications that may occur in men and women.
4. Appreciate the need for prompt diagnosis of meningococcal disease and institution of appropriate therapy.
5. Appreciate the fastidious nature of *Neisseriae* and environmental effects on the viability of these bacteria.

## INTRODUCTION

Medically important aerobic gram-negative cocci found in the genus *Neisseria* include *Neisseria gonorrhoeae* (the gonococcus), which causes gonorrhea, and *Neisseria meningitidis* (the meningococcus), which causes meningitis and sepsis. Other *Neisseria* species are considered to be part of the normal mucosal flora, but may occasionally be involved in human disease. *Branhamella (Moraxella) catarrhalis,* formerly known as *Neisseria catarrhalis,* will be discussed along with the *Neisseria,* because it too is a gram-negative coccus. It is frequently associated with respiratory tract infections. The other members of the genus *Branhamella* are **commensal** (usually not causing human disease) coccobacilli that colonize mucous membranes of the respiratory tract, but which cause disease in a debilitated host, and which may be associated with nosocomial infections.

The members of the genus *Neisseria,* and *Branhamella catarrhalis,* are comprised of aerobic, gram-negative diplococci; the flattened, adjacent sides of the paired cocci give them a coffee- or kidney-bean shape, as observed on gram-stained smears. They produce the enzyme cytochrome oxidase and are positive in the oxidase test. Although the nonpathogens grow readily on most routine media, the pathogens are culturally fastidious. Commensal *Neisseria* species and *Branhamella catarrhalis* can grow at room temperature; however, the pathogenic *Neisseriae* grow poorly at temperatures less than 35° to 37°C. Because of their delicate nature, clinical specimens suspected of harboring these agents should be quickly brought to the laboratory in suitable transport media.

The pathogenic *Neisseriae* are capnophilic, requiring 5% to 10% $CO_2$, and grow on enriched media in a moist environment. They are aerobic, nonmotile, and do not form spores. *Neisseria* species produce acid from carbohydrates by oxidation (an aerobic process requiring the presence of oxygen) not by fermentation (an anaerobic process not requiring the presence of oxygen).

## NEISSERIA GONORRHOEAE

*Neisseria gonorrhoeae* causes the sexually transmitted disease gonorrhea.

### Organism Characteristics

*Neisseria gonorrhoeae* is a fastidious pathogen that is highly susceptible to adverse environmental conditions, including extreme temperatures and drying. The organism is gram negative and, on Gram stain of clinical material, often appears as an intracellular diplococcus in polymorphonuclear neutrophils. Refer to Color Plate 25.

### Habitat and Transmission

*Neisseria gonorrhoeae* is always considered to be a pathogen and may infect anogenital and oropharyngeal mucous membranes, causing gonorrhea. Gonorrhea is transmitted by close contact, usually sexual, between individuals. Transmission of the bacterium appears to be more effective from men to women than from women to men. Oropharyngeal or anorectal infection is usually transmitted by means of orogenital or anogenital contact. Anogenital infections in homosexual men are due to direct inoculation during rectal intercourse. Nonsexual human transmission or fomite transmission of *N. gonorrhoeae* has not been documented (Knapp & Rice, 1995). Transmission from mothers to their infants may occur during birth, as the infant passes through the birth canal. The resulting disease, called ophthalmia neonatorum, is a serious eye infection in newborns. The incidence has declined considerably since the institution of preventive measures such as the use of silver nitrate or antibiotics (e.g., erythromycin or tetracycline) in infants' eyes at birth.

### Specimen Collection and Transport

Specimens for cultures of *N. gonorrhoeae* should be carefully obtained and planted as soon as possible.

**Clinical Specimens.**  Specimens suitable for the isolation of *N. gonorrhoeae* depend on clinical symptoms, as well as sexual practices, age, and gender. The preferred primary specimen sites are the urethra in men and the endocervix in women. Collection of an additional anorectal specimen from women increases the sensitivity of culture by 5% (Evangelista & Beilstein, 1993). Vaginal specimens are less desirable; however, they may be collected from pediatric patients, from patients with a total hysterectomy, and from those with an intact hymen. Other specimen types include the oropharynx, conjunctiva, Bartholin's gland, prostatic fluid, endometrium, blood, urine, and joint aspirate. Specimens are routinely collected on a sterile swab, consisting of Dacron or rayon on a plastic or aluminum shaft; cotton swabs on wooden shafts may contain materials toxic to the gonococci and should not be used for collection.

**Transport of Specimens.**  Immediate plating is best to ensure optimal recovery of *N. gonorrhoeae*. The ideal method to isolate the organism is for clinical specimens to be immediately inoculated onto suitable culture media, then placed in a humidified atmosphere of increased $CO_2$. Several methods are available to provide such optimal conditions. The JEMBEC plate is a rectangular polystyrene plate having a molded circular inner well that holds a $CO_2$-generating tablet, containing sodium bicarbonate and citric acid. After streaking the swab on the agar medium surface, moisture from the culture causes 5% $CO_2$ to be generated. The plate is placed in a small plastic zip-locked bag, which is incubated at 35° to 37°C. Other comparable systems include the Bio-Bag and Gono-pak systems (Becton Dickinson Microbiology Systems Cockeysville, MD), and the Isocult system (Smith-Kline Diagnostics, San Jose, CA). An alternative, although less desirable, method of collection involves use of semisolid transport media, such as Stuart's or Amie's charcoal media. Gonococci survive in these media only for a short period of time and should be delivered to the laboratory as soon as possible. Extremes of temperature, especially the cold, should be avoided.

## Clinical Significance

*Neisseria gonorrhoeae* is the causative agent of the infectious disease, gonorrhea, most commonly reported in the United States during the past 20 years, with 700,000 to 1 million cases reported per year. The gonococcus infects mucous membranes lined by nonsquamous epithelium, such as urethra and cervix, and less frequently the rectum and oropharynx (Evangelista & Beilstein, 1993). Most gonococcal infections are uncomplicated lower genital tract infections.

**Infections in Men.**  Acute urethritis is the most common clinical manifestation of gonococcal infection in men.

**URETHRITIS.**  Symptoms of urethritis include dysuria, or difficult urination, burning on urination, and a purulent discharge, following an incubation period ranging from 1 to 10 days (usually within 5 days). The discharge is initially scant but may later become profuse. In approximately 2% of cases, no symptoms occur.

**PHARYNGITIS.**  Symptomatic oropharyngeal infections may present as mild pharyngitis. Most infections are asymptomatic and resolve spontaneously within 3 months.

**ANORECTAL INFECTION.**  Symptoms of **proctitis**, which is inflammation of the rectum, include a profuse mucopurulent rectal discharge, burning, bleeding, **tenesmus** or straining, and constipation. Asymptomatic infections may occur.

**CONJUNCTIVITIS.**  Ocular infections occur rarely in adults; neonatal infection occurs in infants exposed to infected maternal secretions during birth and must be treated promptly to prevent blindness. A purulent exudate is usually present.

**Infections in Women.**  Asymptomatic infections are more common in women than men.

**CERVICITIS.**  Infection of the endocervix is the most common clinical manifestation of gonorrhea in women. Symptoms include a mucopurulent vaginal discharge, **dysuria**, bleeding, and menstrual abnormalities. In prepubescent females, vulvovaginitis may be the presenting symptom. Asymptomatic infections are often undiagnosed. When vaginal discharge is present, gonococcal infection must be differentiated from infection by *Chlamydia trachomatis* and *Trichomonas vaginalis*.

**PHARYNGITIS.**  Infection is similar to that in men.

**ANORECTAL INFECTION.**  Infection is similar to that in men but is more commonly due to contiguous spread of infection from the genital tract. The incidence of anorectal gonorrhea in women with gonococcal cervicitis has been reported to be as high as 35% to 50% (Evangelista & Beilstein, 1993).

**CYSTITIS.**  Although the gonococci do not commonly cause urinary tract infections, the acute urethral syndrome may occur. Symptoms include dysuria and frequency of urination.

**Complications of Gonococcal Infections.**  Although most cases of gonorrhea are successfully treated with appropriate antibiotics, complications may occur.

**PROSTATITIS IN MEN.**  Acute bacterial prostatitis is rare, and may be caused by a variety of bacteria, but may be caused by *N. gonorrhoeae*. Symptoms include chills and fever, frequency, or acute retention.

**EPIDIDYMITIS IN MEN.**  Inflammation of the coiled tube that receives sperm from the testes is called **epididymitis**. The condition is commonly caused by many microorganisms, including sexually transmitted pathogens. Symptoms of urethritis and urethral discharge may be present. Inflammation is common, with severe scrotal and inguinal pain.

**PELVIC INFLAMMATORY DISEASE IN WOMEN.** Endocervical infection, if left untreated, may cause an ascending infection from the lower genital tract to the fallopian tubes that may cause **pelvic inflammatory disease** (PID), resulting in **salpingitis**, or inflammation of the fallopian tubes, endometritis, peritonitis, and tubo-ovarian abscesses. Symptoms of PID include lower abdominal pain and tenderness, mucopurulent endo-cervical discharge, fever, high white blood cell count, an elevated erythrocyte sedimentation rate, and an increased C-reactive protein level. The resulting inflammation may lead to scarring and blockage of the fallopian tubes, which may lead to infertility and ectopic pregnancies. Although other microorganisms, such as *C. trachomatis* and anaerobes may cause PID, gonococci have been implicated in 10% to 70% of cases and are believed to play an important role in initial episodes of this disease (Evangelista & Beilstein, 1992; Knapp & Rice, 1995).

**DISSEMINATED GONOCOCCAL INFECTION.** Gonococcal infection may spread from the genitourinary tract to the bloodstream, particularly in untreated cases. Patients may develop symptoms of septic arthritis and dermatitis; endocarditis and meningitis are rare complications, which have a high fatality rate.

## Cultural Characteristics and Identification

Gonococci are fastidious microorganisms with complex growth requirements.

**Media.** Cultures for *N. gonorrhoeae* should always be incubated at 35° to 37°C, in a $CO_2$-enriched atmosphere. Because gonococci must frequently be isolated from body sites harboring large numbers of normal flora, the use of selective chocolate agar-based media containing various antibiotics is recommended. The culture media must be supplemented with vitamins, amino acids, iron, and other cofactors. Media must also contain starch to absorb the fatty acids that may be toxic to the gonococci. The first medium specially formulated to isolate *N. gonorrhoeae* was Thayer-Martin agar (TM), which is a chocolate agar base containing an enrichment supplement and the antibiotics colistin, which inhibits gram-negative bacilli, nystatin, which inhibits yeasts, and vancomycin, which inhibits gram-positive cocci. Modified Thayer-Martin (MTM) medium also contains trimethoprim lactate to inhibit swarming *Proteus* species, as well as colistin, nystatin, and vancomycin.

A further modification of TM medium is Martin-Lewis (ML) medium, which contains four antimicrobial agents, with a higher concentration of vancomycin to further suppress gram-positive cocci. This medium is also more inhibitory to yeasts, due to the replacement

of nystatin with anisomycin, an antifungal agent that has a longer half-life.

A selective, transparent, nonchocolate agar-based medium called New York City medium has also been used. It contains lower concentrations of antimicrobial agents. It is known that some strains of gonococci are inhibited by the concentrations of vancomycin in certain selective media. Nonselective media, such as chocolate agar, might be needed to support growth of these strains, and they should also be used for sites not normally having normal flora. Sites such as blood, joint fluids, tissue specimens, and conjunctival swabs should be cultured using both selective and nonselective media.

**Presumptive Identification.** Cultures should be examined after 24 and 48 hours of incubation. Although some variation exists, colonies of *N. gonorrhoeae* usually appear as small (0.5 mm), shiny, gray, pearly colonies and are usually visible at 24 hours. The gonococcus produces autolytic enzymes, which may destroy the cells (Baron, Peterson, & Finegold, 1994). When incubation continues beyond several days, gonococci autolyse, and the colonies become adherent and sticky. Refer to Color Plate 26.

The oxidase test detects the enzyme cytochrome oxidase, which is present in all species of *Neisseria* (see Procedure 13-1). Fresh oxidase reagent must be prepared daily. Oxidase-positive colonies should be Gram stained. *N. gonorrhoeae* will stain as a gram-negative diplococcus. The morphology will distinguish the organism from oxidase-positive gram-negative bacilli, which might grow on the media used to cultivate the gonococcus. However, oxidase-positive gram-negative diplococci growing on media selective for the gonococcus should be confirmed using definitive biochemical tests or equivalent methods. The superoxol test, similar to the catalase test, but using 30% hydrogen peroxide (superoxol), provides an additional presumptive test for the identification of *N. gonorrhoeae*. *N. gonorrhoeae* gives a strong reaction with 30% $H_2O_2$, whereas other species are negative (Baron et al., 1994). Although antimicrobial therapy may be initiated based on presumptive identification of the gonococcus, confirmation is required.

**Confirmatory Identification.** Speciation of *Neisseriae* requires further testing of oxidase-positive, gram-negative diplococci.

**BIOCHEMICAL TESTS.** *Neisseria gonorrhoeae* and other species of *Neisseria* may be differentiated by carbohydrate-utilizing tests, based on acid production from glucose, maltose, lactose, sucrose, and fructose (see Table 13-1). Traditional methods for determining acid production from these sugars relied on growth of the organism in cystine tryptic digest (CTA) agar medium containing 1% of the carbohydrate. This medium is no longer recommended because acid production by the

# PROCEDURE 13-1
## Oxidase Test

### Principle:

The enzyme cytochrome oxidase is produced by *Neisseria* species and *Branhamella catarrhalis*. This enzyme oxidizes the substrate tetramethyl-p-phenylenediamine dihydrochloride (method A) and dimethyl-p-phenylenediamine monohydrochloride (method B), forming a dark-purple end product, *indophenol*.

### Method:

Two methods are available to do the oxidase test.

A. Spot oxidase test
   1. Place a filter paper circle in a sterile Petri dish.
   2. Dispense a drop of reagent onto the filter paper.
   3. Using a sterile loop or applicator stick, remove a portion of a freshly grown colony from an agar plate and rub onto the moistened filter paper.
   4. Examine the spot for a color change.

B. Plate method
   1. Weigh out 0.1 g reagent and place in a sterile screw-capped test tube.
   2. Prepare fresh daily—add 10 mL of sterile distilled water to the tube and mix.
   3. Using a sterile pipet, add several drops of the prepared reagent to colonies on the plate.
   4. Observe the colonies for a color change.

### Quality Control:

A positive control (*Neisseria gonorrhoeae* ATCC #43069) and a negative control (*Escherichia coli* ATCC #25922) are tested on each day of use.

### Expected Results:

**Method A**  A positive reaction is indicated by the development of a dark purple color on the spot within 10 to 30 seconds. A negative reaction would give no color change.

**Method B**  Oxidase-positive colonies turn pink then purple then black. Negative colonies remain unchanged.

### Reference:

Shanahan, J. F. (Ed.). (1994). *Bailey and Scott's diagnostic microbiology* (9th ed., p. 103). St. Louis: Mosby.

Package insert—Spot-test Oxidase Reagent, Difco Laboratories, Detroit MI

---

oxidative (not fermentative) *Neisseria* species is weak, and the CTA may lack sensitivity to differentiate the organisms.

Rapid nongrowth-dependent biochemical tests have been developed. These have higher concentrations of carbohydrates to act as substrates for preformed bacterial enzymes, which increases the sensitivity of these tests to detect acid production. An example of the rapid test systems includes the API Quad-Ferm (BioMerieux Vitek, Hazelwood, MO). The RIM-*Neisseria* test (Remel Laboratories, Lenexa, KS) and the Minitek kit (Becton Dickinson, Cockeysville, MD) are alternative methods. In addition to acid production from carbohydrates, other tests may be needed to differentiate between species (see Table 13-2).

Chromogenic enzyme substrate tests, such as Gonochek II (BioMerieux Vitek), use chromogenic substrates for the detection of three bacterial enzymes. These substrates yield colored end-products when subjected to hydrolysis by specific preformed enzymes present in the bacterial cells. A limitation of these methods is the restriction to those bacteria isolated on gonococcal selective media (Knapp, 1988).

**SEROLOGIC METHODS.**  Monoclonal antibodies have been developed against the gonococcus, which can be used to confirm the identity of the isolate. A direct fluorescent antibody (DFA) test (the Syva MicroTrac *N. gonorrhoeae* culture confirmation test) uses a fluorescein-conjugated monoclonal antibody to detect the gonococcus. Bartel's *N. gonorrhoeae* DFA test (Baxter Corp., West Sacramento, CA) is a similar test.

Coagglutination methods rely on the ability of protein A in the cell wall of *Staphylococcus aureus* to bind to the Fc portion of immunoglobulin G (IgG) molecules; antibodies to *N. gonorrhoeae* can be attached to killed *S. aureus* cells. The Gonogen1 test (New Horizons Diagnostics, Columbia, MD) is based on this principle. One advantage of the coagglutination method is that it is not necessary to have a pure culture.

**NUCLEIC ACID PROBES.**  The Accuprobe *N. gonorrhoeae* culture confirmation test (GenProbe, San Diego, CA),

**Table 13–1 ▶ Differentiation of *Neisseria* Species and *Branhamella catarrhalis* by Carbohydrate Utilization**

| *Neisseria* Species | Acid Production from | | | | |
|---|---|---|---|---|---|
| | Glucose | Maltose | (ONPG) Lactose | Sucrose | Fructose |
| N. gonorrhoeae | + | – | – | – | – |
| N. meningitidis | + | + | – | – | – |
| N. cinerea | –a | – | – | – | – |
| N. mucosa | + | + | – | + | + |
| N. polysaccharea | + | + | – | – | – |
| N. flavescens | – | – | – | – | – |
| N. lactamica | + | + | + | – | – |
| N. sicca | + | + | – | + | + |
| N. elongata | – | – | – | – | – |
| N. subflava | + | + | – | v | V |
| Branhamella catarrhalis | – | – | – | – | – |

Some strains may produce a slight amount of acid in some rapid biochemical testing systems.

is used to detect rRNA sequences in the gonococcus. This test provides an alternative method for confirmation of oxidase-positive, gram-negative diplococci.

## Direct Detection in Clinical Specimens

In addition to culture, there exist rapid direct tests for *N. gonorrhoeae.*

**Enzyme Immunoassay.** The **enzyme immunoassay** (EIA) and enzyme-linked immunosorbent assay (ELISA) have been developed to detect *N. gonorrhoeae* antigen in clinical specimens, bypassing the need to culture. The gonozyme test (Abbott Laboratories, North Chicago, IL) uses antibody-coated beads to detect the presence

of gonococcal antigen in clinical specimens. This test can be used to make a presumptive diagnosis of gonococcal disease; it is of particular value in areas where culture facilities are not available, or where the viability of the organism cannot be guaranteed.

**Nucleic Acid Probe.** A **nucleic acid probe** or DNA probe is a small piece of DNA, which is complementary to a target organism's DNA. In addition to the availability of DNA probes designed for culture confirmation, probes are available to detect the rRNA of *N. gonorrhoeae* in clinical specimens. A probe assay **chemiluminescence** enhanced (PACE) test (GenProbe) uses a nonisotopic DNA probe to identify *N. gonorrhoeae* in clinical specimens. The emission of light

**Table 13–2 ▶ Other Methods to Differentiate *Neisseria* Species and *Branhamella catarrhalis***

| *Neisseria* Species | Growth on Blood Agar (35°C) | Pigment | DNase | NO₃ Reduction | Polysaccharide from Sucrose |
|---|---|---|---|---|---|
| N. gonorrhoeae | – | – | – | – | – |
| N. meningitidis | + | – | – | – | – |
| N. cinerea | + | – | – | – | – |
| N. mucosa | + | + | – | + | – |
| N. polysaccharea | + | – | – | – | + |
| N. flavescens | + | + | – | – | + |
| N. lactamica | + | – | – | – | – |
| N. sicca | + | v | – | – | – |
| N. elongata | + | – | – | – | – |
| N. subflava | + | + | – | – | v |
| Branhamella catarrhalis | + | – | + | + | – |

denotes the presence of the organism. Because the test does not allow for isolation and confirmation of the presence of the gonococcus, a presumptive diagnosis only is possible using this assay.

Because the organism is not grown in culture, neither the ELISA nor the DNA probe assays allow for the susceptibility testing of *N. gonorrhoeae.*

## Antibiotic Susceptibility Characteristics

In recent years a trend of increasing antimicrobial resistance has been observed in clinical isolates of *N. gonorrhoeae.* Neither penicillin (or ampicillin) nor tetracycline is currently considered to be a drug of choice for empiric treatment of gonococcal infections. In particular, the incidence of penicillinase-producing *N. gonorrhoeae* (PPNG) has dramatically increased in the 1980s and 1990s. Penicillinase is a member of the group of enzymes called ß-lactamases, so-called because of their ability to cleave the ß-lactam ring present in ß-lactam antibiotics, such as penicillin and ampicillin. The cefinase test (Becton Dickinson, Cockeysville, MD) is used to detect the presence of penicillinase and is described in Procedure 13-2.

Susceptibility testing of isolates of *N. gonorrhoeae* can be determined by performing the disk diffusion procedure (Kirby-Bauer method) on a medium called GC agar. Interpretive criteria for determining antimicrobial susceptibility can be found in the approved standard M2-A4 of the National Committee for Clinical Laboratory Standards (NCCLS Standards, 1993).

## NEISSERIA MENINGITIDIS

*Neisseria meningitidis* may exist in an asymptomatic carrier state or may cause life-threatening disease.

## Organism Characteristics

Meningococci appear as gram-negative diplococci both inside and outside polymorphonuclear leukocytes, especially in cerebrospinal fluid. Refer to Color Plate 27. The cells may vary in size, and may resist decolorization. The presence of a polysaccharide capsule, a virulence factor for meningococci, may sometimes be seen as a clear halo around the cells.

## Habitat and Transmission

*Neisseria meningitidis* is a normal inhabitant of the oropharynx or nasopharynx. Humans are the only natural hosts for the organism. Asymptomatic carriage of

---

# PROCEDURE 13-2
## Cefinase Test

### Principle:

Filter paper disks containing nitrocefin are intended for use in the rapid testing of isolated bacterial colonies for the production of the enzyme ß-lactamase. This enzyme hydrolyzes antimicrobial agents called ß-lactam antibiotics. Examples of such antibiotics include penicillins and cephalosporins.

### Methods:

1. Using a single disk dispenser, dispense a disk from the cartridge into an empty Petri dish or glass slide.
2. Moisten each disk with a drop of distilled water.
3. With a sterile loop or applicator stick, remove several isolated colonies from the surface of an agar plate and rub onto a disk surface.
4. Observe disk for color change and interpret reactions.

### Quality Control:

A ß-lactamase producing organism (*Staphylococcus aureus,* ATCC #29213) and a non-ß-lactamase producing organism (*Haemophilus influenzae* ATCC #10211) should be run as a positive and a negative control each day of use.

### Expected Results:

A positive reaction will show a yellow to red color change on the area where the colonies were applied (not usually over the entire disk). A negative reaction will show no color change although most bacterial strains show a positive result within 5 minutes; anaerobes may take up to 30 minutes and *S. aureus* up to 1 hour to react.

### Reference:

Package insert, Cefinase, Becton Dickinson Microbiology Systems, Cockeysville, MD.

meningococci is more common in confined persons, particularly when crowded conditions prevail, such as in military barracks. Such conditions affect both the transmission of the organism and the occurrence of actual disease. Because these organisms do not survive well outside the human host, transmission is almost always by inhalation of airborne droplets or by direct contact with contaminated respiratory secretions from infected individuals.

## Specimen Collection and Transport

Specimens for the isolation of *N. meningitidis* include normally sterile body fluids, such as cerebrospinal fluid (CSF), blood, joint fluid, pleural fluid, petechial aspirates, and biopsy specimens; less often sputum, conjunctival swabs, or nasopharyngeal swabs may be cultured. Specimens should be immediately transported to the laboratory under ambient conditions, minimizing exposure to cool temperature and drying.

## Clinical Significance

Meningococci may spread from the nasopharynx to cause meningococcal meningitis or meningococcemia. The disease ranges from sepsis with rapid recovery to a rapidly progressive fulminant disease resulting in death, as early as several hours after onset of symptoms. In milder cases meningococci may be isolated from the bloodstream, but the disease is self-limited. Classic signs of meningitis, such as confusion, headache, fever, and stiff neck may occur in only about half the patients with meningococcal meningitis; vomiting may occur, especially in children (Koneman, Allen, Janda, Schreckenberger, & Winn, 1992). Close contacts of individuals with meningococcemia must receive immediate prophylaxis to prevent disease.

Meningococcemia is often characterized by vascular changes, including a petechial or purpuric rash caused by bleeding and coagulopathies. A fulminant course resulting in the Waterhouse-Friderichsen syndrome may result in hemorrhage into the adrenal glands, as well as disseminated intravascular coagulopathy, leading to shock and, ultimately, death.

## Cultural Characteristics and Identification

The CSF and other normally sterile body fluids for culture (except blood) are collected in sterile containers; after centrifuging for 15 minutes at 1,500*g,* the supernatant fluid is removed to a sterile tube (this can be saved for further testing). The sediment is used to inoculate nonselective media and to prepare a smear for Gram stain. *N. meningitidis* is able to grow on blood agar as well as chocolate agar. A broth medium such as thioglycollate should also be inoculated; the broth should be subcultured to solid media before discarding. Plates should be incubated at 35° to 37°C, at 5% to 10% $CO_2$, and examined at 24, 48, and 72 hours. Growth of oxidase-positive, gram-negative diplococci provides presumptive evidence of meningococcal infection, but must be confirmed using methods previously described for the gonococci.

Meningococci grow more rapidly, and produce larger colonies, than gonococci. Colonies are usually smooth, round, and moist, and may be slightly tan with a greenish cast underneath (Baron et al., 1994).

Specimens from body sites having normal flora present should be inoculated to a selective medium, such as TM; blood for culture should be handled as recommended by the manufacturer of the blood culture system used in your laboratory.

Meningococci may be serologically grouped by slide agglutination methods, based on their capsular polysaccharide.

## Direct Detection in Clinical Specimens

Commercially available latex agglutination methods are available to detect meningococcal antigens in body fluids. Kits produced by Becton Dickinson Microbiology Systems (Cockeysville, MD) and Wellcome Diagnostics (Research Triangle Park, NC) contain a polyvalent antibody reagent for serogroups A, C, Y and W135 plus a reagent for serogroup B. A positive latex agglutination test for any of these antigens provides a rapid presumptive diagnosis of meningococcal infection, allowing prompt initiation of antimicrobial therapy. Because a false-positive or a false-negative reaction can occur, culture confirmation is necessary.

## Antibiotic Susceptibility Characteristics

Although there have been reports of resistance of meningococci to penicillin and tetracycline, penicillin has remained effective therapy for most cases of meningococcal infection. Chloramphenicol is recommended as an alternative agent in patients allergic to penicillin. Other newer broad-spectrum cephalosporins, including cefotaxime and ceftriaxone, are also suitable agents. Rifampin, and, more recently, ciprofloxacin, are suitable to treat potential contacts of patients with meningococcal infection, as well as to eradicate the meningococcal carrier state (Knapp & Rice, 1995).

## *BRANHAMELLA (MORAXELLA) CATARRHALIS*

The significance of *B. catarrhalis* in respiratory secretions is controversial.

## Organism Characteristics

*Branhamella catarrhalis* is currently classified in the genus *Branhamella,* based on genetic similarities with other members of this group of gram-negative coccobacilli. This species is the only one showing typical diplococcal morphology; biochemical reactions, including the production of oxidase, also resemble those of the neisseriae.

## Habitat and Transmission

It is currently believed that previous assumptions that *B. catarrhalis* was a member of the normal human oropharyngeal flora were incorrect. Although it is infrequently isolated from the oropharynges of healthy individuals, the species may be part of the normal flora in the nasopharynx, or the upper respiratory tract, rather than the oropharynx (Knapp & Rice, 1995).

## Specimen Collection and Transport

Although optimal specimens for isolation of *B. catarrhalis* from cases of sinus infections or otitis media include maxillary sinus aspirates or tympanocentesis fluid, respectively, such specimens are difficult to obtain. They involve invasive procedures, which are uncomfortable for the patient. When lower respiratory infections are suspected, sputum specimens are satisfactory.

## Clinical Significance

Prior to 1990, *B. catarrhalis* was believed to be part of the normal human upper respiratory tract flora. Frequent recovery of the organism from lower respiratory tract infections (bronchitis and bronchopneumonia) in adults, and from cases of acute sinusitis, and otitis media in children, support its pathogenic role (Doern, 1985). Infections of the maxillary sinuses, the middle ear, or bronchi may occur by means of contiguous spread from the upper respiratory tract (Knapp & Rice, 1995). *B. catarrhalis* causes a large number of lower respiratory infections in immunocompromised elderly patients with chronic obstructive pulmonary disease. Although cases of acute sinusitis associated with this organism do occur in adults, the infection is more common in children.

Patients with bronchitis caused by *B. catarrhalis* show mild respiratory distress with no fever and usually produce slight amounts of purulent sputum. In cases of pneumonia, low-grade fever and dyspnea may occur, with increasing amounts of purulent sputum. Patchy infiltrates in both lungs may be seen on x-ray. Life-threatening, systemic infections, such as meningitis, endocarditis, and bacteremia, have been shown to occur in patients who were immunosuppressed by underlying diseases, including diabetes, alcoholism, leukemias, and lymphomas. Conjunctival infections associated with this organism in neonates and in children have been documented (Knapp & Rice, 1995).

## Cultural Characteristics and Identification

Procedures for the transport of specimens, cultivation, isolation, and identification of *B. catarrhalis* are similar to those described for the gonococcus and the meningococcus. Refer to Color Plate 27. *B. catarrhalis* grows well on 5% sheep blood agar, as well as on chocolate agar. Certain strains may grow on the selective media used to isolate *N. gonorrhoeae.* On blood agar or chocolate agar, colonies appear grayish white or creamy pink, respectively. Colonies are drier in appearance, than either of the *Neisseria* species. The characteristic of being able to "push" the colony with an inoculating loop has led to the description of a "hockey puck" appearance.

Definitive methods to identify *B. catarrhalis* include those mentioned above for the gonococcus and the meningococcus. Unlike gonococcus and meningococcus, *B. catarrhalis* is asaccharolytic, does not produce acid from sugars, and is able to produce the enzyme DNase (Hughes, Pezzlo, De La Maza, & Peterson, 1987).

## Antibiotic Susceptibility Characteristics

Although penicillin was previously considered to be a suitable antimicrobial agent to treat *B. catarrhalis,* increasing numbers of penicillin-resistant strains have been reported. Most strains produce ß-lactamase enzymes (see Procedure 13-2 for the cefinase test), and should not be treated with penicillin or ampicillin. Isolates are usually susceptible to the quinolones, aminoglycosides, cephalosporins, and chloramphenicol.

## OTHER *NEISSERIA* SPECIES

*Neisseria gonorrhoeae* and *N. meningitidis* are the two species considered to be universally pathogenic for humans. Other species in this genus, previously considered to be part of the normal flora of the upper respiratory tract, have shown increasing ability to cause disease. Several of these organisms can also easily be confused with the gonococcus and the meningococcus. Characteristics used to separate these species are shown in Table 13-2.

## SUMMARY

► The general characteristics of *Neisseria* species that colonize human mucous membranes have been described.

► Specimen collection and transport for the diagnosis of gonorrhea require care and immediate attention.

► Clinical significance of infection with *N. gonorrhoeae* including the range of infection from asymptomatic to uncomplicated infection to complications in men and women are described.

► Specimen collection and transport for the diagnosis of bacterial (meningococcal) meningitis normally include sterile body fluids. Specimens should be transported under ambient conditions, minimizing exposure to cool temperature and drying.

## CASE STUDY

A previously healthy 3-month-old infant girl was seen in the Emergency Department for fever and lethargy. Her temperature was 40.5°C (105°F). She had a 1-day history of vomiting and irritability. She was noted to have muscle rigidity, a pulse of 130, respiratory rate of 45, and blood pressure 165/65. A lumbar puncture was performed and revealed purulent material showing numerous leukocytes, predominantly neutrophils on Gram stain. Bacteria were seen both intracellularly and extracellularly. CSF protein was 1200 mg/dL; the glucose level was 8 mg/dL. Several hours later the child developed a diffuse, petechial rash. Blood cultures were drawn and grew the same microorganism as was isolated from the CSF.

### Questions:

1. What is the likely diagnosis for this patient's infection? What is the infectious agent? How do you know?

2. Explain the need for prompt examination of a gram-stained smear to rapidly diagnose this infection.

3. What recommendations would you make to protect members of the patient's immediate family from developing this infection?

## Review Questions

1. The member of the genus *Neisseria* that is always considered to be pathogenic is:
   a. *N. cinerea.*
   b. *N. gonorrhoeae.*
   c. *N. meningitidis.*
   d. *N. lactamica.*

2. Which test is positive for all *Neisseriae* and *Branhamella catarrhalis*?
   a. Superoxol test
   b. Nitrate reduction
   c. Oxidase test
   d. Cefinase test

3. Which statement is correct?
   a. *N. gonorrhoeae* causes syphilis.
   b. *N. meningitidis* is also known as the gonococcus.
   c. *N. gonorrhoeae* oxidizes the sugars glucose and maltose.
   d. Gonorrhea is spread by direct contact.

4. *Branhamella catarrhalis* is a:
   a. gram-negative coccus.
   b. gram-positive coccus.
   c. gram-negative bacillus.
   d. gram-positive bacillus.

5. Selective media for the isolation of *N. gonorrhoeae* include:
   a. Thayer-Martin agar.
   b. New York City agar.
   c. modified Thayer-Martin agar.
   d. all of the above

6. *N. gonorrhoeae* is capnophilic; this means that it:
   a. is pathogenic.
   b. likes cold temperatures.
   c. requires a high concentration of $CO_2$.
   d. grows on ordinary media.

7. An enzyme that can hydrolyze antibiotics such as penicillin is:
   a. oxidase.
   b. catalase.
   c. ß-lactamase.
   d. cefinase.

8. *Branhamella catarrhalis* is apt to cause which type of infection?
   a. Gonorrhea
   b. Pneumonia
   c. Meningitis
   d. Sepsis

9. A particularly fulminant disease associated with the meningococcus is called:
   a. PID.
   b. epididymitis.
   c. Waterhouse-Friderichsen syndrome.
   d. salpingitis.

10. The following species of *Neisseria* is (are) able to produce a starchlike polysaccharide from sucrose:
    a. *N. gonorrhoeae.*
    b. *N. meningitidis.*
    c. *N. cinerea.*
    d. *N. mucosa.*

## ▶ REFERENCES & RECOMMENDED READING

Baron, E. J., Peterson, L. R., & Finegold, S. M. (1994). Aerobic gram-negative cocci (*Neisseria and Moraxella catarrhalis*). In J. F. Shanahan (Ed.). *Bailey and Scott's diagnostic microbiology,* (9th ed., pp. 353–361). St. Louis: Mosby.

Doern, G. V. (1985). *Branhamella catarrhalis:* An emerging human pathogen. *Clinical Microbiology Newsletter, 7,* 75–81.

Evangelista, A. T., & Beilstein, H. R. (1993). Laboratory diagnosis of gonorrhoea. In Abramson, C. (Coordinating Ed.). *Cumitech 4A.* Washington, DC.: American Society for Microbiology.

Hughes, B., Pezzlo, M. T., DeLaMaza, L. M., & Peterson, E. M. (1987). Rapid identification of pathogenic *Neisseria* species and *Branhamella catarrhalis. Journal of Clinical Microbiology 25,* 2223–2224.

Janda, W. M. (1994). *Neisseria* update. *Clinical Microbiology Newsletter, 8,* 21–24.

Knapp, J. S. (1988). Historical perspectives and identification of *Neisseria* and related species. *Clinical Microbiology Review, 1,* 415–431.

Knapp, J. S., & Hook, E. W. (1988). Prevalences and persistence of *Neisseria cinerea* and other *Neisseria* species in adults. *Journal of Clinical Microbiology, 26,* 896–900.

Knapp, J. S., & Rice, R. J. (1995). *Neisseria* and *Branhamella.* In P. R. Murray, E. J. Baron, M. A. Pfaller, F. C. Tenoveer, & R. H. Yolken (Eds.). *Manual of clinical microbiology* (6th ed., pp. 324–340). Washington, DC. American Society for Microbiology Press.

Koneman, E. W., Allen, S. D., Janda, W. M., Schreckenberger, P. C., & Winn, W. C., Jr. (1992). *Neisseria* species and *Moraxella catarrhalis. Color atlas and textbook of diagnostic microbiology* (4th ed., pp. 369–403). Philadelphia: Lippincott.

National Committee for Clinical Laboratory Standards. (1993). *Approved standard: Performance standards for antimicrobial disk susceptibility tests* (Document M2-A5). Villanova, PA: Author.

Wong, J. D. (1994). Pathogenic "nonpathogenic" *Neisseria* spp. *Clinical Microbiology Newsletter, 6,* 41–44.

# CHAPTER 14

# Haemophilus

Daila S. Gridley, PhD

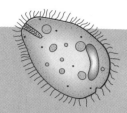

## Microbes in the News

### Conjugated *Haemophilus Influenzae* Type B Vaccines are Effective in Infants

Immunization with new conjugated vaccines against *H. influenzae* type b has proven to be extremely effective in young infants. Meningitis and other invasive infections due to the bacteria have decreased dramatically in the United States, as well as other countries in the Western Hemisphere, since the first conjugated products became available in 1988. The vaccines consist of purified *H. influenzae* type b polysaccharide conjugated to large carrier proteins such as the diphtheria and tetanus toxoids. Studies indicate that 93% to 100% of immunized infants are protected for up to 3.5 years. A decrease of 95% or more in cases of invasive *H. influenzae* infection has been noted in infants and children in the United States since these new vaccines came into routine use. The success of the vaccines present the exciting possibility of advances in immunization against other infectious agents.

## KEY TERMS

"Blood-loving"
Brazilian purpuric fever
Chancroid
Chocolate agar
Conjugated vaccine
Haemocin
Hemophilic
Hib vaccine
IgA$^1$ protease
Koch-Weeks bacillus
Latex agglutination test
Meningitis
Pfeiffer's bacillus
Pink-eye
Pneumonia
Porphyrin test
Pyogenic pathogen
Satellite phenomenon
"School-of-fish"
Stridor
"Trojan horse" mechanism
Type b polysaccharide
X factor
V factor

## LEARNING OBJECTIVES

**Upon successful completion of this chapter, the student should be able to:**

1. Define the key terms listed in the glossary.
2. List the morphologic and other pertinent characteristics of the *Haemophilus* genus.
3. Discuss the clinical significance and important virulence factors of *H. influenzae* and list laboratory tests that are useful in identification.
4. Give the drug(s) of choice for *H. influenzae* infection and explain the importance of conjugated vaccines.
5. List *Haemophilus* species other than *H. influenzae* and describe the types of infections they may be associated with.

## INTRODUCTION

The *Haemophilus* genus consists of short (approximately 0.3–0.5 × 0.5–1.5 μm), nonmotile, gram-negative rods that sometimes grow in pairs or short chains. They are typically associated with mucous membranes of the respiratory and genital tracts of humans and many vertebrate animals including pigs, sheep, and dogs. Under poor growth conditions, they may appear as long filaments; some species have a filamentous morphology regardless of their nutritional status. They are facultative anaerobes that can grow in the presence or absence of air, but prefer an aerobic environment. The genus name means "**blood-loving**" (**hemophilic**), stemming from the fact that the great majority of these organisms require one or two factors that are present in fresh blood for energy production, specifically, heme or hematin (originally called **X factor**) and nicotinamide adenine dinucleotide or NAD (originally called **V factor**). Heme is a heat-stable factor that the bacteria need for the synthesis of a cytochrome system and the catalase enzyme. NAD is heat labile and can be replaced by its phosphorylated form, NADP. All species reduce nitrates and ferment carbohydrates (albeit poorly). Transmission of the most clinically relevant species occurs from one individual to another either by the respiratory route or through sexual activity.

The most important member of the genus associated with human infections in the United States is the strain of *H. influenzae* that produces a **type b polysaccharide** capsule (*H. influenzae* type b). It is the leading cause of bacterial **meningitis** in children aged 5 months to 5 years and is also a significant agent of respiratory tract infections in both children and adults. In elderly individuals, especially those with underlying lung disease, the organisms can produce a severe **pneumonia**. The species name is somewhat unfortunate because it implies that these bacteria cause influenza ("the flu"), a respiratory tract infection that is due to the influenza virus in the *Orthomyxoviridae* family. However, the bacteria is a common secondary invader when the respiratory tract is compromised by other infectious agents such as the influenza A virus and may contribute to the severity of the illness. *H. influenzae* biotype *aegyptius* (formerly known as *H. aegyptius*) is the etiologic agent of an acute, contagious conjunctivitis. *H. ducreyi* is the cause of **chancroid**, a disease characterized by soft chancres or ulcers in the groin area. Although this species is widespread, it is especially prevalent in certain tropical areas of the world. *H. parainfluenzae*, *H. aphrophilus*, *H. paraphrophilus,* and *H. segnis* are among the normal flora of humans and are only occasionally associated with clinically relevant infection (see Tables 14-1 and 14-2).

## *HAEMOPHILUS INFLUENZAE*

### Organism Characteristics

*Haemophilus influenzae* was first isolated by Pfeiffer during the great influenza pandemic of 1892, hence it was known for a time as **Pfeiffer's bacillus**. It is a small gram-negative coccobacillus with morphologic characteristics that are similar to those of most other species in the genus. It, together with pneumococcus and meningococcus, are among the three most important **pyogenic pathogens**. The six serotypes of *H. influenzae* (a, b, c, d, e, and f) are based on the antigenic characteristics of their polysaccharide capsule (>100,000 MW).

The great majority of isolates from clinically apparent respiratory tract infections have a type b polysaccharide capsule that consists of repeated disaccharide units of ribose and ribitol phosphate (i.e., polyribose ribitol phosphate or PRP). PRP is structurally and antigenically related to the teichoic acid present in the walls of gram-positive bacteria and the polysaccharides found in the capsules of certain enteric organisms and pneumococci. The capsule is antiphagocytic, thus allowing the organisms to escape destruction by macrophages and other phagocytes. This capsular type is undoubtedly the major factor responsible for virulence (see Table 14-3). Strains producing the other

### Table 14–1 ▶ Types of Infections Commonly Associated with *Haemophilus* Species

| Species | Primary Site of Isolation | Major Types of Infections | Comments |
|---|---|---|---|
| *H. influenzae* | Nasopharynx | Meningitis, otitis media, sinusitis, pneumonia | Most cases are due to strains that produce the type b polysaccharide capsule; most common cause of meningitis in young infants; conjugated vaccines are now available |
| *H. influenzae* biogroup *aegyptius* | Conjunctiva | Purulent conjunctivitis ("pink-eye") | Highly contagious; systemic invasion has been associated with a plasmid (Brazilian purpuric fever) |
| *H. ducreyi* | Genitalia | Chancroid (soft chancre) | Most prevalent in countries with tropical climates; outbreaks occur in United States; is sexually transmitted |
| *H. parainfluenzae* | Pharynx, oral cavity | Endocarditis, urethreitis, sepsis | Most common *Haemophilus* species isolated from respiratory tract of healthy persons; clinically relevant infection is uncommon |
| *H. aphrophilus* | Pharynx, oral cavity | Endocarditis, brain abscess pneumonia | Infection may follow dental treatment or surgery; predisposing factors include rheumatic heart disease and heart valve lesions |

capsular types also cause infections (e.g., chronic bronchitis), but much less often than those with type b and they are almost always noninvasive. The other five polysaccharide types are made up of repeating units of glucose (type a), galactose (type c), hexose (type d), hexosamine (type e), and galactosamine (type f). Nonencapsulated strains (sometimes referred to as nontypeable strains) are common as part of the normal flora of the upper respiratory tract. These strains are antigenically heterogenous but can be differentiated on the basis of noncapsular characteristics.

Some of the somatic proteins are immunogenic and may play a role in the disease process, although specific mechanisms have not been identified. The organisms do not produce an exotoxin, although an extracellular toxin-like factor with the ability to stop the motility of cilia on epithelial cells of the respiratory tract has been detected. The *H. influenzae* species consists of bacteria

### Table 14–2 ▶ Differentiating Properties of Selected *Haemophilus* Species

| Species | Growth requirement X* | V† | Type a-f Capsule | ß-Hemolysis | Urease | Growth Enhanced by $CO_2$ |
|---|---|---|---|---|---|---|
| *H. influenzae* | + | + | + | – | var‡ | – |
| *H. influenzae* biotype *aegyptius* | + | + | – | – | var | – |
| *H. aphropilus* | +§ | – | – | – | – | + |
| *H. ducreyi* | + | – | – | – | – | – |
| *H. haemolyticus* | + | + | – | + | + | – |
| *H. paraphrophilus* | – | + | – | – | + | + |
| *H. parahaemolyticus* | – | + | – | + | + | + |
| *H. parainfluenzae* | – | + | – | – | – | – |
| *H. segnis* | – | + | – | – | – | – |

*X factor: heme or hematin.

†V factor: nicotinamide adenine dinucleotide (NAD).

‡A 'var' indicates variable results.

§Required on primary isolation; requirement is lost on subculturing.

## Table 14–3 ► Factors Associated with the Virulence of *H. influenzae*

| Factor | Comments |
|---|---|
| Type b capsule | Is major virulence factor; is associated with invasive disease; prevents opsonization by complement; is antiphagocytic |
| Peptidoglycan | Present in cell wall; damages vascular endothelium; damages blood–brain barrier |
| IgA protease | Degrades heavy chain of secretory IgA1; three versions synthesized |
| Exotoxin-like factor | Disrupts the beating of cilia on epithelial cells of respiratory tract |
| Lipopolysaccharide | May induce hypotension, shock, and other systemic symptoms |
| Fimbriae | Assist in adherence |
| Adhesins | Assist in adherence |

that are variable in a number of properties. The organisms have been separated into six different biotypes based on differences in biochemical reactions and other characteristics (see Table 14-4).

## Clinical Significance

*Haemophilus influenzae* is acquired after inhalation of contaminated respiratory droplets from an active case or a carrier of the organisms. After infecting the upper respiratory tract, several outcomes are possible depending on the strain of the bacteria and the age and condition of the host. Approximately 30% to 50% of children have been reported to carry the nonencapsulated strains within the nasopharynx, whereas only 2% to 3% are believed to carry those with the type b capsule. As many as seven different nontypeable strains may be carried simultaneously, although one is frequently predominant. Encapsulated strains are often

dominant, since they secrete an antibiotic known as **haemocin** that kills unencapsulated strains. Evaluation of nasopharyngeal secretions by polymerase chain reaction (PCR) techniques suggest that the incidence of *H. influenzae* (both capsulated and nonencapsulated) in specimens of this type may actually be much higher than previously thought. Statistical associations suggest that predisposition to invasive infection may be related to a cluster of genes within the major histocompatibility complex; however, socioeconomic and environmental factors undoubtedly also play important roles. Colonization rates are now dropping dramatically, probably because of the increasing use of effective immunization.

The nonencapsulated strains have been implicated in a variety of respiratory tract infections (e.g., bronchitis, sinusitis, alveolitis, and otitis media), but rarely systemic disease. Infection of the female genital tract with these organisms can lead to neonatal sepsis, which has a mortality rate of approximately 50%. They, like many other gram-negative organisms, have pili that promote attachment to mammalian cells. In addition, a family of high molecular weight nonpilus proteins, that are similar to the filamentous hemagglutinin used for attachment by *Bordetella pertussis*, have been recently characterized. It is possible that these proteins account, at least partly, for the colonization site preference (larynx, middle ear, conjunctivae, or genitalia) of different nontypeable strains.

Although infection may be subclinical, local extension of *H. influenzae* type b from the upper respiratory tract to the sinuses and middle ear can occur in both children and adults. The organisms are second only to *Streptococcus pneumoniae* as the etiologic agent of bacterial otitis media and acute sinusitis. These conditions are characterized by pain in the affected area and a redness and bulging of the tympanic membrane of the ear. They are also the most common cause of septic arthritis and cellulitis in children under the age of 2 years. Abrupt pain, fever, inflammation, and tenderness of large weight-bearing joints are seen in indi-

## Table 14–4 ► Properties of *Haemophilus influenzae* Biotypes

| Biotype | Common Sites of Infection | Indole | Urease | Ornithine Decarboxylase |
|---|---|---|---|---|
| I | Brain, blood | + | + | + |
| II | Conjunctivae, blood, ear, lower respiratory tract | + | + | – |
| III | Conjunctivae, respiratory tract | – | + | – |
| IV | Genital tract, respiratory tract | – | + | + |
| V | Ear, lower respiratory tract | + | – | + |
| VI | Upper respiratory tract | – | – | + |

A + and a – indicate that the great majority of isolates are positive or negative, respectively.

viduals with septic arthritis. Attempts to move the joints may result in severe pain. Very young children may be irritable and refuse to move the affected part of the body. The typical presentation of cellulitis is a reddish blue swelling of the cheek or periorbital region and fever. Bacteremia and subsequent infections in other sites are common. Obstructive epiglottitis (or laryngotracheitis) occurs in children on rare occasions; a few cases have also been reported in adults. It is characterized by fever, sore throat, acute respiratory distress, a bright cherry-red swollen epiglottis, and **stridor** (a high-pitched sound made during inhalation when there is laryngeal obstruction). The infection usually progresses with dramatic rapidity, resulting in prostration within 24 hours. Intubation or a tracheostomy may have to be performed in life-threatening cases to prevent suffocation. This condition is treated as a medical emergency, as are meningitis and pneumonia due to the organisms. In children and in elderly adults, especially those with chronic obstructive pulmonary disease (COPD), chronic bronchitis, or other underlying disease affecting the lungs, the organisms are a very common cause of pneumonia. The pneumonia may be relatively localized (i.e., lobar) or present as a diffuse bronchopneumonia. Airway obstruction may occur as the result of dense fibrinous exudates of polymorphonuclear cells that plug small bronchi. In general, the clinical presentation is similar to pneumococcal pneumonia.

If the organisms reach the bloodstream, they are carried to the lymph nodes and may eventually invade the meninges of the brain resulting in meningitis. It is not entirely clear how *H. influenzae* type b crosses the blood–brain barrier to reach the central nervous system (CNS). It has been noted that phagocytic cells of the monocyte-macrophage lineage can enter into the cerebrospinal fluid (CSF) compartment, that these cells can carry bacterial-sized particles into the CNS, and that *H. influenzae* type b can survive and even multiply within macrophage populations. These observations have led to the proposal that the organisms may be carried across the blood–brain barrier while sequestered within these mobile phagocytes. This mechanism of entry (dubbed as the **"Trojan horse" mechanism**) has also been proposed for several other pathogens that affect the brain. Other mechanisms, however, may also be operating. For example, the organisms possess a cell wall peptidoglycan that damages the vascular endothelium, thereby disrupting the blood–brain barrier and possibly allowing easier access.

Meningitis due to *H. influenzae* type b is a life-threatening infection in young children. Infants aged 3 months and under are protected by antibodies acquired from the mother and infection with the organisms in this age group is rare. Peak incidence of meningitis occurs between 6 months and 1 year of age, correlating with the decline in protective maternal IgG in the infant. A similar pattern of increasing incidence of infection concomitant with declining maternal antibody is seen with *Neisseria meningitidis*. Nonimmunized children over 3 to 5 years of age have naturally acquired antibodies against the PRP that makes up the type b capsule. These antibodies appear to be protective in that they enhance complement-dependent killing and phagocytosis in vitro. Approximately 95% of cases involving *H. influenzae* are due to the type b encapsulated strains. The signs and symptoms of the meningitis are very similar to those seen with other bacterial pathogens such as *N. meningitidis* and *S. pneumoniae*. There is usually a rapid onset of fever, headache, vomiting, a stiff neck, and a feeling of drowsiness. Confusion, delirium, and stupor are less common findings. Some of these signs, however, may not always be obvious in infants. Identification of the specific bacteriologic agent in the laboratory is critical because the optimal antibiotic regimen for each organism may vary. Untreated infants with *H. influenzae* type b meningitis have a very high fatality rate; rates as high as 90% have been reported in the past. Mortality in appropriately treated cases ranges from approximately 3% to 6%.

Neurologic sequelae including mental retardation, hearing loss, blindness, hydrocephaly, and convulsions occur often (approximately 30% of cases have significant neurologic problems) after recovery from *H. influenzae* type b meningitis. These complications are thought to be due to the combined effects of the microorganisms and the host's inflammatory response. Clinical trials in infants have shown that the addition of dexamethasone, an anti-inflammatory drug, to antibiotic therapy significantly reduces meningeal swelling and the incidence of hearing impairment compared to those given a placebo.

Studies of adult populations in the United States show that approximately 75% have bactericidal antibodies against *H. influenzae*. These antibodies are anticapsular, opsonic, and bactericidal in the presence of complement. Seropositive individuals have a lower incidence of clinically apparent infection. However, it appears that presence of specific serum immunoglobulins may not always be enough to prevent development of symptoms. Pneumonia and arthritis due to *H. influenzae* type b has been reported in adult patients despite preexisting anticapsular antibodies. In addition, the organisms produce a **protease** that specifically cleaves the heavy chain of **IgA1**, a property that the organisms share with *N. meningitidis* and *Neisseria gonorrhoeae*. Recent DNA cloning and sequencing studies indicate that the gene that codes for the enzyme (i.e., *iga* gene) has a similar structure in all of these species. *H. influenzae*, however, produces three different versions of the enzyme, each one breaking different peptide bonds. Nontypeable isolates can also produce three types of the protease. IgA is the major class of antibody that is found in secretions, and hence it is very important in local defense against infectious agents that enter through the respiratory, genitourinary, and intestinal tracts.

The old vaccines for *H. influenzae,* consisting of purified type b polysaccharide (**Hib vaccine**), first became available in 1985. Unfortunately, they did not induce strong protective immunity in children under the age of 18 months (i.e., the very group that most needs to be protected). The PRP, like the great majority of polysaccharides, is a T cell-independent antigen and significant secondary immune responses are not induced by booster injections. In the last few years at least three **conjugated vaccines** have become available that contain the type b polysaccharide coupled to large carrier proteins, such as the toxoid of a mutant strain of *Corynebacterium diphtheriae* (CRM$_{197}$ mutant), the toxoid of *Clostridium tetani,* and the outer membrane complex of *N. meningitidis.* These new vaccines are effective in inducing T cell-dependent immunity, that is typical of protein antigens. Immunization of young infants with conjugated Hib vaccines became standard practice in the United States by late 1990. The recommended schedule is to give two or three doses intramuscularly beginning at 2 months of age. A booster may be needed at a later time, depending on which conjugate vaccine is used. Clinical studies indicate that 93% to 100% of immunized individuals are protected and that the duration of immunity is approximately 1.5 to 3.5 years. The introduction of these new vaccines is thought to be responsible for the significant decrease in *H. influenzae* type b meningitis in the Western Hemisphere. A 95% or more decrease in the incidence of invasive infection has been reported among infants and children in the United States. These results have been so encouraging that the Public Health Service hopes to eliminate disease due to *H. influenzae* type b in children under 5 years of age by the end of 1996 (Childhood Immunization Initiative). Immunization with the DPT (diphtheria toxoid + pertussis + tetanus toxoid) can be effectively given during the same office visit. Combination vaccines consisting of conjugated Hib and all of the critical components of the DPT vaccine may soon become available (see Table 14-5). Other complex combinations (i.e., addition of inactivated poliomyelitis vaccine, hepatitis B vaccine, and others to the conjugated Hib) are currently in development. Combination vaccines would greatly simplify delivery by reducing the total number of needed childhood immunizations.

*Haemophilus influenzae* biotype *aegyptius* causes a purulent conjunctivitis that is sometimes referred to as **pink-eye**. These organisms, historically known as the **Koch-Weeks bacillus**, were first discovered in 1883 by Robert Koch in conjunctival exudates of patients in Egypt. The infection may be relatively mild, involving only the blood vessels of the eye, or very severe with lacrimation, swelling of the lids, and photophobia. The bacteria are easily transmitted and, in warmer climates, they have been implicated in epidemic conjunctivitis. A severe form of this infection, known as **Brazilian purpuric fever**, was first recognized in 1984 in Brazil (hence the name). Since then several outbreaks of the syndrome have been reported in Brazil and Australia. Eye gnats (*Chloropidae*) that feed on eye secretions and wounds have been suggested as possible vectors in mechanical transmission. Infections originating in the conjunctivae rapidly progress to purpura and systemic invasion by the organisms. All known cases of Brazilian purpuric fever have been caused by three clones of the organisms that have the ability to invade, replicate in microvascular endothelial cells, and that also exhibit a cytotoxic effect. Presence of a specific plasmid has been associated with invasiveness and severe disease. Brazilian purpuric fever is a highly lethal pediatric illness. Deaths during outbreaks have been primarily due to overwhelming endotoxemia and shock. *S. pneumoniae, Chlamydia trachomatis,* herpes simplex virus (especially type 1), and certain adenovirus serotypes are also common agents of conjunctivitis. Definitive laboratory identification of the causative agent is, therefore, very important.

| Table 14–5 ▶ Description of Conjugated Vaccines for *Haemophilus influenzae* | | | | | | |
|---|---|---|---|---|---|---|
| **Vaccine*** | **Carrier Protein** | **Immunization Schedule (mo)** | | | | |
| | | **2** | **4** | **6** | **12** | **15** |
| HbOC | *C. diphtheriae* toxoid | X | X | X | | X |
| PRP-OMP | *N. meningitidis* outer membrane protein | X | X | | X | |
| PRP-T | *C. tetani* toxoid | X | X | X | | |

*All three contain purified *H. influenzae* type b polysaccharide (polyribose ribitol phosphate, PRP).

## Cultural Characteristics and Identification

Nasopharyngeal swabs, CSF, blood, pleural fluid, sputum, and exudates from inflamed conjunctivae are among the typical specimens obtained from patients suspected of having illness due to *Haemophilus* species. Attempts to obtain direct cultures of the throat or epiglottis in cases of obstructive epiglottitis are contraindicated because the stimulation may induce a reflex reaction resulting in choking and suffocation. However, blood cultures from these patients are frequently positive. Because the organisms can lose viability rapidly, it is important to inoculate appropriate growth media as soon as possible after specimen collection. Transport media such as modified Stuart's medium or Amies' charcoal medium are frequently used. *H. influenzae* initially appear as gram-negative coccobacillary forms on direct smears of specimens and in young cultures, but exhibit great pleomorphism (i.e., elongated rods and threadlike filamentous forms) in older cultures or in nutrient-deficient media. They occasionally appear to be gram-variable, unless Gram staining is very carefully performed (because of this, they have occasionally been confused with *S. pneumoniae*). The organisms may be identified directly in clinical specimens by immunofluorescence techniques or by using specific anti-PRP serum in slide agglutination or capsule swelling (i.e., quellung) tests using type-specific antisera. *H. influenzae* taken from clinically relevant specimens frequently have a faint, refractile capsule. However, there is a strong tendency to lose the capsule on subculture, and thus the ability to type the organisms is also lost. These direct techniques can sometimes give false-negative results, if the organisms are present in small numbers. Kits that detect soluble PRP in serum and other body fluids are commercially available.

*Haemophilus* species can be isolated on **chocolate agar**, containing blood that has been heated to 80°C for 15 minutes and supplemented with factor X. Growth on chocolate agar, but not on blood agar, is strongly suggestive of *Haemophilus*. The gentle heating lyses red blood cells so that they release both X and V factors, inactivates enzymes (i.e., NADase) that could destroy factor V, and inactivates certain nonspecific substances that may inhibit growth of the organisms. The medium is often supplemented with IsoVitaleX to enhance growth. V factor is also present in many biologic fluids in addition to blood and is synthesized by certain microorganisms such as *Staphylococcus aureus* and yeast. Small, moist, transparent colonies (approximately 1 mm in diameter) usually appear after 24 to 48 hours of incubation at 37°C in an atmosphere containing 10% $CO_2$. Specimens from patients with cystic fibrosis are sometimes incubated under anaerobic conditions to prevent overgrowth by

*Pseudomonas aeruginosa*. Colonies on brain-heart infusion agar supplemented with blood have an iridescent appearance; in contrast, nonencapsulated strains lack iridescence. Variations in colony appearance have been recently associated with differences in virulence. For example, isolates producing opaque colonies tend to have more PRP and exhibit more serum resistance than those with a translucent colony phenotype.

Presumptive identification of *H. influenzae* can be made if the isolate grows only in the presence of both X and V factors. These assays can be done in several ways. Older methods use trypticase soy agar plates streaked to confluence with the organisms and overlaid with paper strips or disks containing the X and V factors. After overnight incubation, growth in areas where both factors are present is indicative of *H. influenzae* (see Figure 14-1). Reliable results, however, are not always obtained because X factor requiring isolates may retain enough of the factor from the primary medium. The **satellite phenomenon** can also be demonstrated by adding a small drop of *Staphylococcus aureus* onto the surface of a blood agar plate streaked with the unknown isolate. The *S. aureus* will lyse the red blood cells, thereby releasing factors X and V. Organisms that grow only in the vicinity of the staphyloccoccal colony are likely to be *Haemophilus*. The **porphyrin test** is more reliable than these older methods in determining the need for X factor; it is also more rapid (results can be obtained in 4 hours). The assay is designed to test for the presence of enzymes that convert δ-aminolevulinic acid

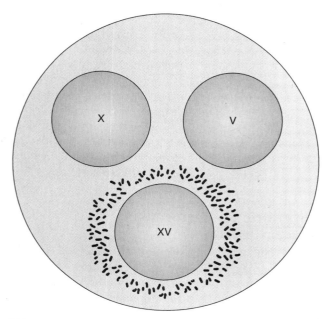

**FIGURE 14-1** Diagram of *H. influenzae* colonies around a filter paper disk impregnated with X and V factors. X, heme or hematin; V, nicotinamide adenine dinucleotide.

(ALA) into porphyrins that give off a red fluorescence that is detectable under ultraviolet light (360 nm wavelength). Species that do not require the X factor will make porphobilinogen, porphyrins, protoporphyrin IX, and heme. *H. influenzae* does not have the necessary enzymes to do this, and therefore there is no red fluorescence. Paper strips impregnated with ALA are commercially available and can be placed directly onto the medium used for primary isolation.

A number of immunologic assays have been developed for rapid detection of the free, soluble form of the type b capsular polysaccharide in CSF, serum, and urine. These assay methods include counterimmunoelectrophoresis and the **latex agglutination test**. The latter test uses latex particles sensitized with antibodies against specific antigens such as the PRP that makes up the type b capsule. The sensitized particles agglutinate when mixed with a sample containing the appropriate antigen. Although this assay is frequently used in clinical laboratories, its usefulness is somewhat controversial because of studies reporting lack of reliability. False-positive rates over 50% have been recently reported for CSF; false-negative results are also possible. Nonetheless, the test may be useful, especially when cultures are negative because of prior antimicrobial therapy. Definitive identification can also be accomplished with a battery of biochemical tests. Several rapid enzymatic biochemical kits are commercially available.

*Haemophilus influenzae* biotype *aegyptius* can be distinguished from other *H. influenzae* in the laboratory on the basis of their biochemical reactions. In addition, they tend to be more fastidious, grow more slowly, and are capable of hemagglutination. The clinical presentation together with the presence of small gram-negative coccobacilli in material taken from infected conjunctivae and typical growth on chocolate agar may be enough to establish a diagnosis. A rapid dot immunoassay using a "flow-through" cartridge has been recently developed. This test uses a monoclonal antibody that binds to a unique epitope of a 25 kDa pilin protein produced by strains that are responsible for Brazilian purpuric fever. Assays such as this may be useful in identification of children with conjunctivitis who may be candidates for prophylactic therapy.

## Antibiotic Susceptibility Characteristics

Ampicillin was the preferred antibiotic for *H. influenzae* infections for many years. However, up to 25% of the type b strains isolated in the United States are now resistant. Because ampicillin resistance is frequently due to ß-lactamase production, assays for this enzyme should be performed. The enzyme, which is virtually identical to that produced by other gram-negative bacteria such as *Escherichia coli*, can be rapidly detected in various body fluids and supernatants of cultures. Rapid filter paper disk assays (e.g., disks with nitrocefin) are available from several commercial companies. Results can sometimes be obtained within 30 minutes after applying a small amount of bacterial growth onto the disk. Strains that are ampicillin resistant by other mechanisms have been reported, but these are uncommon. Resistance to chloramphenicol (sometimes used for ampicillin-resistant mutants) can be determined in similar assays. Resistance to both of these drugs is mediated by genes carried by plasmids, and hence it is transmissible.

Ceftriaxone has now replaced ampicillin as the drug of choice for meningitis due to *H. influenzae* type b. Intravenous administration should be initiated as early as possible to minimize the risk for later neurologic complications, such as subdural empyema (localized accumulation of fluid that requires surgical drainage), intellectual impairment, and other CNS problems. Pharmacokinetic studies in adults with meningitis indicate that a single daily dose of the drug may be effective therapy. Respiratory tract infections due to this species may be treated with ampicillin, chloramphenicol, sulfamethoxazole-trimethoprim, or the newer cephalosporins. Rifampin is often given to close contacts (especially siblings who are under the age of 4 years) of patients with meningitis or those who develop signs of invasive disease, such as fever and headache. The risk for unimmunized children under the age of 4 years who are living with an index case has been estimated to be 500-fold higher than for their nonexposed counterparts. Rifampin is preferred for prophylaxis over ampicillin because it is secreted at higher levels in the saliva. Topical application of ointments and eye drops containing sulfonamides or tetracycline will usually speed recovery from most cases of conjunctivitis due to *H. influenzae* biotype *aegyptius*. Rifampin prophylaxis is effective in eliminating carriage of the organisms in children with conjunctivitis.

## OTHER *HAEMOPHILUS* SPECIES

### *H. parainfluenzae*

*Haemophilus parainfluenzae* is the only *Haemophilus* species that is routinely isolated from the respiratory tract of healthy individuals in the United States. Their prevalence is thought to be related to the fact that the bacteria have an affinity for salivary glycoproteins. These organisms are similar to *H. influenzae*, hence the species name ("para" means "like"), but can be easily differentiated because they (unlike *H. influenzae*) do not require the X factor for growth. Although usually part of the normal flora, the organisms have been isolated from a few cases of bacterial endocarditis, urethritis, and sepsis. The organisms grow in clumps and convoluted filamentous strands, which tend to break off and form abscesses distant from the original site of infection. No virulence factors have been found, but the organisms have neuraminidase activity (i.e., like the influenza A virus) and some strains may possess a capsule. Colonies on solid media usually appear grayish white to yellowish, smooth, and flat, although they may occasionally be rough and irregular. At least three biotypes can be distinguished on the basis of differences in biochemical tests.

## H. ducreyi

*Haemophilus ducreyi,* first described by Ducrey in 1889, is found only in humans. Although these bacteria are currently classified in the *Haemophilus* genus, sequence analysis of 16S ribosomal RNA from the organisms suggests that they may be more closely related to *Pasteurella* than to *Haemophilus* (note that both genera belong in the *Pasteurellaceae* family). These organisms are endemic in certain parts of the world, especially in areas with warm tropical climates. Outbreaks have also occurred in the United States and Canada. High rates of infection have long been associated with poor socioeconomic and sanitary conditions. Recent studies in the United States indicate that infection with these organisms is significantly more common among crack cocaine users, alcoholics, and those indulging in sexual activity with drug users than in the general population. Genital ulcerations due to *H. ducreyi* are thought to be underreported in the United States. This may be due, at least partly, to the clinical similarity of chancroid with other ulcerative sexually transmitted diseases and to the lack of easy laboratory confirmation.

Specific virulence factors have been difficult to identify. Although the organisms do not produce a capsule that could be classified as one of the a–f types, evidence suggests that at least some isolates possess an outer polysaccharide layer. In addition, the organisms have attachment molecules for certain epithelial cells and may have the ability to invade them. It appears also that the majority of isolates produce one or more cytotoxins that may be responsible for the development of ulcers. In vitro assays show that the organisms have a cytopathic effect on human foreskin fibroblasts after coming into direct contact with them.

*Haemophilus ducreyi* is the etiologic agent of chancroid or soft chancre, in contrast to the hard chancre seen in cases of primary syphilis. Isolation of this species from infections of the genital tract is always considered significant because it is never part of the normal flora of humans. Chancroid is a sexually transmitted disease that is characterized by ulceration, swelling, tenderness of the genitalia, and marked swelling of the lymph nodes in the groin area. After a short incubation period of approximately 2 to 5 days, the lesion begins as a small tender papule and eventually develops into a painful exudative ulcer with sharp margins. Additional lesions may develop in the surrounding area of the first ulcer as the result of autoinfection. Abscesses and rupture of greatly enlarged inguinal lymph nodes are common, especially in untreated cases. Permanent immunity does not develop after recovery from the illness.

Gram stains of material from ulcerative lesions or aspirates of enlarged regional lymph nodes show small gram-negative coccobacilli growing in chains. The appearance of the bacteria is sometimes described as a **"school-of-fish"** because the small pleomorphic rods and coccobacillary forms are often arranged in groups and chains. The organisms are often located intracellularly. Best growth is obtained at 33°C in 10% $CO_2$ on chocolate agar supplemented with IsoVitaleX and vancomycin (to inhibit proliferation of contaminating organisms). Nonetheless, growth is generally slow and it may take 7 days of incubation before colonies become visible. Supplementation of the medium with fetal calf serum is often done to enhance growth and increase the chance for successful isolation. A simplified colorimetric test using PCR has been developed and may prove to be particularly useful in countries where other laboratory methods are difficult to perform.

Erythromycin, ceftriaxone, and sulfamethoxazole-trimethoprim are used successfully to treat infections caused by *H. ducreyi* in the United States. Widespread failure, however, has been reported with the latter two drugs (especially sulfamethoxazole-trimethoprim) in several other parts of the world. Azithromycin, a new antimicrobial, appears to be exceptionally effective in the United States. Clinical studies on the efficacy of the drug are currently ongoing in several endemic countries.

## OBSCURE OR RARELY ISOLATED ORGANISMS

*Haemophilus haemolyticus* and *H. parahaemolyticus* are related organisms that produce strong ß-hemolysis on agar plates containing horse or rabbit blood. Most strains of both species produce a urease enzyme. Although both can produce catalase, *H. haemolyticus* is more consistent in this characteristic. They can be isolated from the nasopharynx of healthy individuals and, on rare occasions, from children with moderately severe respiratory tract infections. *H. parahaemolyticus* has also been associated with occasional cases of pharyngitis, endocarditis, and oral infections.

Organisms within the *Actinobacillus* genus can be isolated from humans, as well as a variety of animals. *A. actinomycetemcomitans* (briefly classified as *Haemophilus actinomycetemcomitans*) is quite different from other species within the genus in that it is urease negative and its growth is consistently enhanced by $CO_2$. The organisms also do not fit well into the *Haemo-*

*philus* genus in that they do not require either factor X or factor V for energy production and growth. The species name means "with actinomyces." Individual cells are small, short, and may be either straight or curved. Under the electron microscope, small projections or membranous "blebs" may be seen protruding out from the cells. These organisms are routinely found in the oral cavity of approximately 30% to 40% of the population in the United States. A variety of assays may be used to differentiate them from the closely related *H. aphrophilus,* including the hydrogen peroxide test (i.e., they are catalase positive). In addition, they form colonies that appear to have a star-shaped structure in the center. These organisms are frequently isolated from bone lesions ("actinomycotic lesions") and occasionally from cases of endocarditis and abscesses within the brain. Spread to these body sites is thought to be from the oral cavity through the blood circulation. The bacteria grow relatively well on a variety of basal media supplemented with blood (heated or unheated). Small, nonhemolytic, grayish white, smooth colonies form on blood agar when incubated in air containing 5% to 10% $CO_2$. There are approximately eight to ten biotypes that can be differentiated on the basis of sugar fermentation reactions. The organisms are usually susceptible to aminoglycosides, cephalosporins, and tetracyclines, but resistant to erythromycin. Resistance to penicillin and other ß-lactam antibiotics has been reported.

## SPECIAL CONSIDERATIONS FOR IMMUNOCOMPROMISED HOSTS

*Haemophilus influenzae* bacteremia can occur in immunocompromised children within the 6 months to 3 years age range without any evidence of local infection. Individuals with splenectomy or an intact but nonfunctional spleen (e.g., sickle cell anemia) are among those at greatest risk because of their poor response to polysaccharide antigens and low serum opsonizing ability. The spleen, like the lymph nodes, contains phagocytic cells that are capable of filtering out microorganisms that circulate through the bloodstream. It is also a site for generating immunologic responses (e.g., antibody production and synthesis of certain complement components). Persons with compromised spleen function are also prone to infection with *S. pneumoniae, N. meningitidis,* and various staphyloccocci.

Although associated strongly with underlying chronic lung disease, pneumonia due to *H. influenzae* in elderly adults occurs more often and is more severe in immunodeficient individuals than in those with normal immune responses. Chronic alcoholism is an additional risk factor in elderly persons.

Recent studies indicate that infants infected with human immunodeficiency virus type 1 (HIV-1) are less likely to develop high titers of antibody against the *H. influenzae* type b polysaccharide after immunization with conjugated vaccines than their noninfected counterparts. The poor response is especially striking in those who are symptomatic. These findings suggest that HIV-1 infected subjects may be more susceptible to meningitis and other types of infections due to the bacteria.

Reports from several African countries indicate that HIV-1 infected individuals with chancroid do not respond as well to drugs for *H. ducreyi* as noninfected persons. In addition, the presence of raw genital ulcers increases the risk for transmission, as well as acquiring, the virus. These latter observations are thought to account, at least partly, for the heterosexual spread of HIV-1 in countries where chancroid is common.

## SUMMARY

▶ *Haemophilus* organisms are nonmotile gram-negative rods associated with the respiratory and genital tracts of humans and animals. These organisms are referred to as "blood-loving" because they require X and/or V factors that are present in fresh blood.

▶ *H. influenzae* is a leading cause of meningitis in young children and is an important respiratory tract pathogen. The most severe infections, such as pneumonia, are due to strains that produce the type b polysaccharide capsule.

▶ *H. influenzae* biotype *aegyptius* causes pink-eye (a purulent conjunctivitis) and Brazilian purpuric fever. *H. ducreyi* infection results in chancroid (soft ulcerations in the genital area). *H. parainfluenzae* is a very common isolate from the respiratory tract of healthy individuals.

▶ *Haemophilus* species can be isolated on chocolate agar (heated blood supplemented with factor X) from specimens such as nasopharyngeal swabs, cerebrospinal fluid, blood, pleural fluid, sputum, and conjunctival exudates. Presumptive identification of *H. influenzae* can be made if the organisms grow only in the presence of both X and V factors. The porphyrin test is a reliable method for determining X factor requirement. The latex agglutination test may be used for rapid detection of soluble type b polysaccharide in cerebrospinal fluid, serum, and urine.

▶ Ceftriaxone has replaced ampicillin as the drug of choice for *H. influenzae* infection due to increasing ampicillin resistance. The original Hib vaccine for *H. influenzae,* consisting of purified type b polysaccharide, has been made signifi- cantly more effective by conjugating it to a large carrier protein such as diphtheria toxoid, tetanus toxoid, or a membrane complex from *N. menin- gitidis.*

## CASE 1: INFANT WITH MENINGITIS DUE TO *H. INFLUENZAE* TYPE B

An 8-month-old boy was brought to the emergency room by his parents because the child had suddenly become irritable and was experiencing breathing difficulty. While in the emergency room the child vomited and had a convulsion. The physician noted that the patient had a stiff neck and a fever of 39.8°C. A lumbar puncture was performed and blood was collected for culture. Laboratory analyses revealed a cloudy cerebrospinal fluid (CSF) with 25,400 white blood cells/mm³ (97% were neutrophils), an elevated level of protein of 1,421 mg/dL (normal range is approximately 15–45 mg/dL) and a low glucose concentration of 19 mg/dL (normal is approximately 40–80 mg/dL). Numerous white blood cells and small gram-negative coccobacilli were found in stained smears of the CSF (thus ruling out *S. pneumoniae* as the causative agent). A latex agglutination test performed on the sample was positive for the type b capsular polysaccharide of *H. influenzae.* Culture of the CSF on chocolate agar showed the typical colonial growth of *Haemophilus.* Blood cultures were also positive. A diagnosis of meningitis due to *H. influenzae* type b was made. The infant responded well to intravenous infusions of ceftriaxone and was discharged from the hospital the following week.

**Questions:**

1. Are the given signs and symptoms specific for meningitis due to *H. influenzae* type b?

2. What other types of specimens could have been tested?

3. Is there a vaccine that could have prevented the disease?

## CASE 2: CHANCROID IN A PROMISCUOUS DRUG ADDICT

A 28-year-old man recently returned from the Mardi Gras in New Orleans presented with ulcerative lesions on the genitalia. The ulcers were soft and painful. On questioning the patient admitted to crack cocaine addiction and prostitution in exchange for the drug. Gram stains of exudate from the lesions showed pleomorphic gram-negative rods arranged in groups and chains. Most of the organisms were intracellular. No growth was evident on IsaVitaleX-supplemented chocolate agar until after 6 days of incubation in air containing 10% $CO_2$. A diagnosis of chancroid due to *H. ducreyi* was made and the patient was treated successfully with erythromycin.

**Questions:**

1. Did the promiscuous nature of the patient increase his risk of acquiring chancroid?

2. How can *H. ducreyi* be differentiated from *H. influenzae?*

3. Is erythromycin the best antibiotic to use for *H. ducreyi?*

## Review Questions

1. Which of the following statements apply to *Haemophilus?*
   a. They are facultative anaerobes.
   b. All species require $CO_2$ for growth.
   c. All pathogenic isolates have a capsule.
   d. Some species may be part of the normal flora.

2. Chocolate agar is used for the isolation of *Haemophilus* species because it provides the organisms with:
   a. a high level of many different sugars.
   b. heme and nicotinamide adenine dinucleotide.
   c. δ-aminolevulinic acid.
   d. enzymes needed for metabolism of nutrients.

3. The primary virulence factor associated with *H. influenzae* is:
   a. a secreted exotoxin.
   b. the production of adherence factors.
   c. a very potent endotoxin.
   d. a polyribose ribitol phosphate capsule.

4. A small gram-negative coccobacillus isolated from a patient with conjunctivitis is MOST LIKELY to be:
   a. *H. parainfluenzae.*
   b. *H. aphrophilus.*
   c. *H. parahaemolyticus.*
   d. *H. influenzae* biogroup *aegyptius.*

5. The most common bacteria causing meningitis in young children aged 6 months to 3 years is:
   a. *H. influenzae* type b.
   b. *Streptococcus pneumoniae.*
   c. *H. parahaemolyticus.*
   d. *Neisseria meningitidis.*

6. Identify the correct statement regarding the new conjugated vaccines for *H. influenzae.*
   a. A protein from *H. influenzae* is conjugated to a large polysaccharide.
   b. They contain a mixture of different capsular polysaccharides.
   c. They do not induce protective immunity in children under the age of 18 months.
   d. They induce protection against *H. influenzae* infection for up to 3.5 years.

7. Which of the following is a sexually transmitted species of *Haemophilus* that causes chancroid?
   a. *H. segnis*
   b. *H. aphrophilus*
   c. *H. ducreyi*
   d. *H. paraphrophilus*

8. Identify the correct statement regarding the characteristics of *Haemophilus* species.
   a. *H. influenzae* type b is never isolated from the nasopharynx of asymptomatic children.
   b. *Haemophilus* satellites around colonies of *Staphylococcus aureus* because the staphylococci secrete V factor.
   c. Soluble type b polysaccharide is undetectable in cerebrospinal fluid, urine, and serum.
   d. Encapsulated *H. influenzae* always retains the ability to produce a capsule even when the organisms are subcultured.

## ▶ REFERENCES & RECOMMENDED READING

Ajello, G. W., Matar, G. M., Swaminathan, B., Bibb, W. F., Helsel, L. O., & Perkins, B. A. (1995). A rapid dot immunoassay for detecting the Brazilian purpuric fever clone of *Haemophilus influenzae* biogroup *aegyptius* with a "flow through" device. *Current Microbiology, 30,* 345–349.

Brenner, D. J., Mayer, L. W., Carlone, G. M., Harrison, L. H., Bibb, W. F., Brandileone, M. C., Sottnek, F. O., Irino, K., Reeves, M. W., Swenson, J. M., et al. (1988). Biochemical, genetic, and epidemiologic characterization of *Haemophilus influenzae* biogroup *aegyptius* (*Haemophilus aegyptius*) strains associated with Brazilian purpuric fever. *Journal of Clinical Microbiology, 26,* 1524–1534.

Cabellos, C., Viladrich, P. F., Verdaguer, R., Pallares, R., Linares, J., & Gudiol, F. (1995). A single daily dose of ceftriaxone for bacterial meningitis in adults: Experience with 84 patients and review of the literature. *Clinical Infectious Diseases, 20,* 1164–1168.

Chadwick, P. R., Malnick, H., & Ebizie, A. O. (1995). *Haemophilus paraphrophilus* infection: A pitfall in laboratory diagnosis. *Journal of Infection, 30,* 67–69.

Coll-Vinent, B., Suris, X., Lopez-Soto, A., Miro, J. M., & Coca, A. (1995). *Haemophilus paraphrophilus* endocarditis: Case report and review. *Clinical Infectious Diseases, 20,* 1381–1383.

Davies, J., Carlstedt, I., Nilsson, A. K., Hakansson, A., Sabharwal, H., van Alphen, L., van Ham, M., & Svanborg, C. (1995). Binding of *Haemophilus influenzae* to purified mucins from the human respiratory tract. *Infection and Immunity, 63,* 2485–2492.

DiCarlo, R. P., Armentor, B. S., & Martin, D. H. (1995). Chancroid epidemiology in New Orleans men. *Journal of Infectious Diseases, 172,* 446–452.

Doern, G. V., Jones, R. N., Gerlach, E. H., Washington, J. A., Biedenbach, D. J., Brueggemann, A., Erwin, M. E., Knapp, C., & Raymond, J. (1995). Multicenter clinical laboratory evaluation of a beta-lactamase disk assay employing a novel chromogenic cephalosporin, S1. *Journal of Clinical Microbiology, 33,* 1665–1667.

Faden, H., Duffy, L., Williams, A., Krystofik, D. A., & Wolf, J. (1995). Epidemiology of nasopharyngeal colonization with nontypeable *Haemophilus influenzae* in the first 2 years of life. *Journal of Infectious Diseases, 172,* 132–135.

Hamed, K. A., Dormitzer, P. R., Su, C. K., & Relman, D. A. (1995). *Haemophilus parainfluenzae* endocarditis: Application of a molecular approach for identification of pathogenic bacterial species. *Clinical Infectious Diseases, 19,* 677–683.

Hollyer, T. T., DeGagne, P. A., & Alfa, M. J. (1994). Characterization of the cytopathic effect of *Haemophilus ducreyi. Sexually Transmitted Diseases, 21,* 247–257.

Lagergard, T. (1995). *Haemophilus ducreyi:* Pathogenesis and protective immunity. *Trends in Microbiology, 3,* 87–92.

Miller, M. A., Meschievitz, C. K., Ballanco, G. A., & Daum, R. S. (1995). Safety and immunogenicity of PRP-T combined with DTP: Excretion of capsular polysaccharide and antibody response in the immediate post-vaccination period. *Pediatrics, 95(4),* 522–527.

Morse, S. A. (1989). Chancroid and *Haemophilus ducreyi. Clinical Microbiology Reviews, 2,* 137–157.

Murphy, T. F. & Apicella, M. A. (1987). Nontypeable *Haemophilus influenzae:* A review of clinical aspects, surface antigens, and the human immune response to infection. *Review of Infectious Diseases, 9,* 1–15.

Purven, M., Falsen, E., & Lagergard, T. (1995). Cytotoxin production in 100 strains of *Haemophilus ducreyi* from different geographical locations. *FEMS Microbiology Letters, 129,* 221–224.

Quinn, F. D., Weyant, R. S., Worley, M. J., Whit, E. H., Utt, E. A., & Ades, E. A. (1995). Human microvascular endothelial tissue culture cell model for studying pathogenesis of Brazilian purpuric fever. *Infection and Immunity, 63,* 2317–2322.

Roche, R. J. & Moxon, E. R. (1995). Phenotypic variation in *Haemophilus influenzae:* The interrelationship of colony opacity, capsule and lipopolysaccharide. *Microbial Pathogenesis, 18,* 129–140.

Rubin, L. G. (1995). Phase-variable expression of the 145-kDa surface protein of Brazilian purpuric fever case-clone strains of *Haemophilus influenzae* biogroup *aegyptius. Journal of Infectious Diseases, 171,* 713–717.

Subedar, N., & Rathore, M. H. (1995). Changing epidemiology of childhood meningitis. *Journal of the Florida Medical Association, 82,* 467–469.

Ueyama, T., Kurono, V., Shirabe, K., Takeshite, M., & Mogi, G. (1995). High incidence of *Haemophilus influenzae* in nasopharyngeal secretions and middle ear effusions as detected by PCR. *Journal of Clinical Microbiology, 33,* 1835–1838.

# CHAPTER 15

# Miscellaneous Fastidious Aerobic and Facultative Gram-Negative Bacilli and Coccobacilli

James E. Daly, MEd, MT (ASCP)

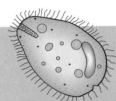

## Microbes in the News

### An old enemy reappears: Recent resurgence of pertussis

Before the development of a vaccine, pertussis or "whooping cough" was a prevalent respiratory disease of dramatic implications. Statistically, the incidence of pertussis peaked in 1934 when more than 265,000 cases were reported, and the disease caused the death of 5 in every 1,000 U.S. children. As recently as 1950, more than 120,000 cases of this condition were seen annually in the United States.

Following widespread availability of a vaccine, this number declined swiftly to a historical low of 1,010 cases in 1976. Since 1976, however, the number of pertussis victims has again begun to climb, with 1,730 cases reported in 1980, 4,162 in 1986, and nearly 5,500 in 1993. It is thought that this resurgence is due primarily to public alarm in response to reports of adverse effects of the DPT (diptheria/pertussis/tetanus) vaccine used, in which a small number of children developed encephalopathy and permanent neural damage in the late 1980s. However, epidemiologists believe that the efficacy of the vaccination far outweighs the risks, and more aggressive public education is needed to increase vaccination rates, and again put this deadly disease at bay.

## KEY TERMS

Aerobe, obligate
Capnophilic
Clue cells
Facultative anaerobe

Fusiform
Pleomorphic
Purulent
Pus

Rectal prolapse
Tropism
Ubiquitous
Undulant fever

## LEARNING OBJECTIVES

**Upon successful completion of this chapter, the student should be able to:**

1. Describe the organism characteristics of pathogens in the genera *Pasteurella, Francisella, Brucella, Bordetella, Gardnerella, Legionella, Kingella, Eikenella, Capnocytophaga,* and *Cardiobacterium.*

2. Describe the clinical significance of pathogens in the genera *Pasteurella, Francisella, Brucella, Bordetella, Gardnerella, Legionella, Kingella, Eikenella, Capnocytophaga,* and *Cardiobacterium.*

3. Describe the cultural characteristics and identification of pathogens in the genera *Pasteurella, Francisella, Brucella, Bordetella, Gardnerella, Legionella, Kingella, Eikenella, Capnocytophaga,* and *Cardiobacterium.*

4. Describe the antibiotic susceptibility characteristics of pathogens in the genera *Pasteurella, Francisella, Brucella, Bordetella, Gardnerella, Legionella, Kingella, Eikenella, Capnocytophaga,* and *Cardiobacterium.*

## INTRODUCTION

This chapter covers a wide array of gram-negative bacilli and coccobacilli that vary in their habitat and distribution. The group includes many that are **ubiquitous,** widespread in natural habitats, those found as normal resident flora in human urogenital and oropharyngeal tracts, and several that are resident flora in animals and are contracted in human infection from animal sources. The routes of transmission of these organisms are as varied as their habitats and will be covered as the organisms are described.

The organisms discussed in this chapter are relatively rare isolates of human infection, and their frequency is described throughout the text. Table 15-1 shows the most commonly isolated genera covered in this chapter and some of their identifying biochemical characteristics.

**Table 15–1** ▶ **Characteristics of Miscellaneous Gram-Negative Bacilli and Coccobacilli**

| Genus | Glucose Fermentation | Motility | Oxidase | Growth on MacConkey | Special Isolation Media |
|---|---|---|---|---|---|
| *Pasteurella* | + | + | + | v | — |
| *Francisella* | – | – | – | – | Cysteine-glucose blood agar |
| *Brucella* | – | – | + | v | Brucella agar |
| *Bordetella* | – | v | v | v | Regan-Lowe agar |
| *Legionella* | – | + | v | – | Buffered charcoal yeast agar |
| *Kingella* | + | + | + | – | — |
| *Eikenella* | – | – | + | – | — |

Key: +, positive; –, negative; v, variable reactions.

# PASTEURELLA

## Organism Characteristics

Organisms in the genus *Pasteurella* are widespread as normal flora in the respiratory and gastrointestinal tracts of many domestic and wild animals. It is estimated that they are present in 40% to 66% of domestic dogs and 70% to 100% of domestic cats. These organisms are extremely virulent, largely due to the presence of a capsule that protects the organism from the effects of phagocytosis and allows its survival.

## Clinical Significance

Because of their prevalence in animal populations, infections with species of *Pasteurella* most commonly occur as abscesses and cellulitis resulting from animal contact, predominantly cat scratches and bites. Symptoms of infection typically develop within 24 hours of the bite incident, and wounds are often extremely **purulent**, producing large amounts of **pus**. Because of the **facultative anaerobic** preferences of the organism, infection is more common in wounds that have been sutured, providing a low oxygen environment. It is recommended that all but the worst of animal bites be cleaned and left open to the air to discourage infection. The most frequently isolated species of the genus is *Pasteurella multocida*.

Human infection with *Pasteurella* species has also been seen to cause respiratory disease, especially in patients with preexisting pulmonary conditions, meningitis, and osteomyelitis. In cattle populations, it is a major cause of hemorrhagic septicemia during transport in cattle cars, known as "shipping fever."

## Cultural Characteristics and Identification

*Pasteurella* stains microscopically as a gram-negative coccobacilli. The organism has no special growth requirements and grows well on blood and chocolate agars, preferring facultative anaerobic conditions. It will not generally grow on MacConkey agar. Growth appears as small, nonhemolytic, grayish, rough or smooth colonies that often cause brownish discoloration of the media. A strong "musty" odor is often detected, due to the strong positive indole result of most species. All species are positive for glucose fermentation, and differentiation can be accomplished by ornithine decarboxylase, arginine decarboxylase, urease, indole, maltose, and xylose results. Table 15-2 shows the biochemical characteristics of the common species of *Pasteurella*.

Due to the prevalence of *P. multocida* as the most commonly isolated species of this genus, identification of this species may be simplified using certain criteria. (It has been suggested that when culturing a patient source known to be an animal bite or scratch, isolation of a gram-negative bacilli that [a] fails to grow on MacConkey agar, [b] demonstrates a positive oxidase, and [c] demonstrates a positive spot indole result, can be considered presumptive evidence of infection with *P. multocida* [Koneman, 1992].)

Another approach to identification of *Pasteurella* is based on its unique sensitivity to penicillin among gram-negative organisms. Demonstrated sensitivity to a 2-U penicillin disk using standard Kirby-Bauer methodology is considered good presumptive identification of *Pasteurella* species (see Procedure 15-1).

## Antibiotic Susceptibility Characteristics

Species of *Pasteurella* are universally susceptible to penicillin G, and this is the treatment of choice for infection. Alternate antibiotics include ampicillin, carbenicillin, tetracycline, and cephalosporins. The organism is resistant to aminoglycosides, clindamycin, and vancomycin, and demonstrates intermediate reactions to erythromycin.

**Table 15–2 ▶ Biochemical Characteristics of *Pasteurella* Species**

| Species | Indole | Urease | ODC | ADC | Maltose | Xylose |
|---|---|---|---|---|---|---|
| P. multocida | + | – | + | + | – | v |
| P. aerogenes | – | + | v | – | + | v |
| P. dagmatis | + | v | – | – | + | – |
| P. gallinarum | – | – | – | + | + | – |
| P. haemolytica | – | – | – | – | + | v |
| P. pneumotropica | + | + | + | – | + | + |

Key: +, positive; –, negative; v, variable reactions; ADC, albumin, dextrose, catalase; ODC, ornithine decarboxylase.

---

## PROCEDURE 15-1
## Penicillin Sensitivity of *Pasteurella* Species

### Principle:

*Pasteurella* species are unique among gram-negative bacteria in that they are sensitive to penicillin, whereas most other gram-negative bacteria are not. Demonstration of sensitivity to penicillin is considered a good screening test for presumptive identification of *Pasteurella* species.

### Method:

1. Prepare a suspension of suspected *Pasteurella* organism in sterile water, equal to a 0.5 McFarland turbidity standard.
2. Using a sterile cotton swab, heavily inoculate this suspension onto the surface of a Mueller-Hinton agar plate, streaking in three directions.
3. Dispense a filter paper disk of 2U penicillin onto the inoculated plate.

4. Incubate at 37°C for 24 hours and examine for evidence of inhibition of growth by the antibiotic.

### Quality Control:

A known isolate of *P. multocida* may be inoculated using the same procedure as a positive control, and *Escherichia coli* may be used to demonstrate resistance to the drug.

### Expected Results:

Any zone of inhibition around the penicillin disk is evidence of sensitivity to the antibiotic. If the isolate being tested is a gram-negative bacilli or coccobacilli, sensitivity to penicillin is considered presumptive identification of a *Pasteurella* species.

---

## FRANCISELLA

### Organism Characteristics

*Francisella* is named for Sir Edward Francis, who isolated and identified the organism in Tulare County, California in 1925. Species of the genus are widespread in nature as resident flora of animals. The organism has been isolated from approximately 100 different types of wildlife and is most commonly contracted in man from rabbits, squirrels, beavers, muskrats, and deer. Infection is most common in individuals who handle animal carcasses or skins, notably hunters, trappers, taxidermists, and forest rangers. Transmission by insect vectors such as deer flies, ticks, and mosquitoes has also been documented, as well as dog or cat bites following ingestion of the organism by the animal while eating infected rodents. Seasonal increases in infection rates are seen during hunting seasons, as handling and skinning rabbits is the most frequent source of infection.

*Francisella* is very invasive and extremely virulent, owing to the presence of a capsule. It has also been stated that the organism can penetrate intact skin; however, this characteristic is debated. It is more likely that penetration occurs through minute breaks in the skin, and as few as ten organisms have been demonstrated to cause infection when introduced subcutaneously. Infection can also be by inhalation or by animal bite.

### Clinical Significance

The primary pathogen of the genus is *Francisella tularensis*, the causative agent of the disease tularemia in both man and animals. The organism is capable of surviving within the macrophages of the reticuloendothelial system, leading to the formation of granulomas in the infected tissue. Symptoms of the disease include fever and headache, generalized lymphadenopathy, and ulceration at the site of the insect bite if contracted from a vector. Six forms of tularemia have been described: ulceroglandular, glandular, typhoidal, oculoglandular, pneumonic, and oropharyngeal. Before the availability of treatment, tularemia carried a 10% fatality rate. Currently, the disease is less than 1% fatal.

Two other species of *Francisella* cause similar disease, *F. novicidia* being a rare human pathogen, and *F. philomiragia* being a pathogen mainly in victims of near-drowning accidents and patients with chronic granulomatous disease.

### Cultural Characteristics and Identification

The specimens of choice for culturing for the diagnosis of tularemia include aspirate or exudate from granulomas of infected tissue, lymph node aspirates, or respiratory secretions. Because of the highly contagious nature of the organism, Biosafety Level 3 precautions are required when isolating and identifying the pathogen. It is for this reason that many laboratories choose to send work on suspected tularemia specimens to a reference laboratory.

Microscopically, *Francisella* appears as a tiny gram-negative coccobacilli. The tiny size and the weak staining character of this bacteria may make the bacilli nearly invisible. Growth of the organism requires media containing cystine and is well supported on commercial chocolate agar formulas containing Isovitalex, special cystine-glucose blood agar, and also on the buffered charcoal yeast extract agar used for the isolation of *Legionella* species.

*Francisella* is a **obligate aerobe**, requiring oxygen and preferring slightly increased concentrations of $CO_2$. Growth is slow, with colonies generally appearing after 2 to 4 days, sometimes requiring up to 2 weeks for visible growth. Isolates are oxidase negative and weakly positive for catalase activity. Once isolated onto media, identification of bacterial growth as *Francisella* is performed by serologic agglutination of the colonies. In addition to isolation and identification of bacterial growth, diagnosis of tularemia is also commonly accomplished by direct fluorescent staining of direct smears, or testing of acute and convalescent serums for antibodies to the organism.

## Antibiotic Susceptibility Characteristics

The drug of choice for treatment of tularemia is currently streptomycin. *Francisella* is also susceptible to aminoglycosides, tetracycline, and chloramphenicol. However, there is a higher rate of relapse with these drugs.

## *BRUCELLA*

### Organism Characteristics

The genus *Brucella* is named for David Bruce, who discovered the organism in Malta in 1887. Bruce isolated the bacteria from the liver and spleen of patients who were experiencing an unknown febrile disease. Organisms of this genus are normal resident flora in the genital and urinary tracts of many animals. Although the relationships are not always specific, the four common species of *Brucella* are most frequently associated with four types of animal. Table 15-3 shows the prevalent animal hosts of these four *Brucella* species. In addition to these hosts, the organisms are also found in buffalo, reindeer, caribou, camels, and other species.

Infections with *Brucella* species are most commonly contracted by inhalation, ingestion, or breaks in the skin in patients with close contact with host animals or animal products. Susceptible populations include those ingesting unpasteurized cow or goat milk or cheese, meat packers and butchers, farmers, veterinarians, and those involved in animal husbandry. Occasional unique outbreaks are also seen, such as that in 1983, among women using a cosmetic beauty treatment made of bovine fetal and placental tissue.

### Clinical Significance

Once introduced into the host, *Brucella* species demonstrate notable resistance to normal immune mechanisms. Phagocytosis of the organism takes place, yet the bacteria survive the normal intracellular bacteriocidal mechanisms. This allows the organism to be carried within neutrophils directly to the lymph nodes and other tissue. Infection results in the formation of granulomas in infected tissue. Symptoms develop 7 to 21 days following initial infection, and are fairly nonspecific, including fever, chills, nausea, malaise, fatigue, and lymphadenopathy. Further complications may involve the central nervous system (meningitis), gastrointestinal tract (hepatitis, cholecystitis), skeletal system (osteomyelitis), and the heart (endocarditis). Fever and other symptoms are often seen to relapse, giving rise to the common name of this infection, "**undulant fever**."

In addition to human infection, *Brucella* is an important cause of abortion, sterility, and decreased milk production in cattle, goats, and hogs. Infection with this organism is fairly uncommon in the United States, limited to 100 to 150 cases per year. This is largely due to widespread pasteurization of dairy products and vaccination of livestock.

### Cultural Characteristics and Identification

*Brucella* species are most commonly isolated from blood cultures or biopsies of reticuloendothelial tissue. As with *Francisella,* Biosafety Level 3 precautions are necessary when working with material suspected to be infected with *Brucella.*

| Table 15–3 ▶ Animal Hosts for *Brucella* Species | |
| --- | --- |
| **Species** | **Common Animal Host** |
| *B. melintensis* | Sheep and goats |
| *B. abortus* | Cattle |
| *B. suis* | Swine |
| *B. canis* | Dogs (domestic and wild) |

The organism is a tiny gram-negative coccobacilli. Counterstaining reactions may be extremely weak, making the organism nearly invisible. A modified counterstain procedure may be used to enhance the staining of *Brucella,* in which safranin staining time is increased to 3 minutes, or carbol fuschin is substituted as the counterstain.

*Brucella* is a strictly aerobic slow-growing organism on blood agar and chocolate agar. The translucent, grayish, nonhemolytic colonies grow best in 5% to 10% $CO_2$, sometimes requiring up to 3 weeks for visible colony growth. Special selective *Brucella* blood agar is recommended, and it will also grow well on the buffered charcoal yeast extract agar used for *Legionella* isolation. It will not grow on MacConkey agar.

Colonies of *Brucella* are catalase positive and oxidase positive; some species have the unique characteristic of developing positive urease results within minutes of inoculation. Biochemically, species can be differentiated by inhibition of growth with thionine and fuschin dyes, $CO_2$ requirements, hydrogen sulfide formation, and urease reaction times. Table 15-4 shows these biochemical results for the different species of *Brucella.* Diagnosis may also be made by direct fluorescent antibody stain of direct specimen smears or by serologic antibody titers. A single antibody titer ≥1:160 or a fourfold increase between the acute and convalescent serum specimens are considered presumptive diagnosis of a *Brucella* infection.

## Antibiotic Susceptibility Characteristics

Being an intracellular organism, *Brucella* is more difficult to treat successfully. The generally accepted antibiotic therapy currently used is a combination of doxycycline and rifampin, administered over 6 weeks. Also effective are tetracycline with streptomycin or rifampin with trimethoprim. Even with these regimens, up to 10% of patients experience a relapse of symptoms within 3 months following treatment.

## BORDETELLA

## Organism Characteristics

*Bordetella* species are tiny gram-negative coccobacilli. One species, *Bordetella pertussis,* is a particularly virulent human pathogen. Its virulence owes to a polysaccharide capsule that protects the organism against normal bacteriocidal processes, as well as the production of several toxins that contribute to the severity of infection. Four toxic products have been described as being produced by *B. pertussis*: filamentous hemagglutinin, pertussis toxin, adenylate cyclase, and tracheal cytotoxin. Filamentous hemagglutinin is a surface protein located on the cell wall of the organism, which facilitates adhesion of the organism onto respiratory surfaces. In addition, the microbe secretes pertussis toxin, an exotoxin that increases histamine release and enhances other aspects of inflammatory response. Adenylate cyclase is a compound that inhibits the phagocytosis of the organism. The fourth product is a tracheal cytotoxin that immobilizes the cilia of the trachea and causes tissue necrosis and airway obstruction as colonization occurs.

## Clinical Significance

In 1906, Bordet and Gengou were the first to identify *B. pertussis* as the causative agent of "whooping cough," a disease contracted by inhalation of cough droplets from an infected individual. Prior to development of a vaccine, this infection was a prevalent and devastating disease in the United States, peaking in 1934 when more than 265,000 cases were reported; the disease caused the death of 5 in every 1,000 children. Since vaccination began, the numbers dropped off swiftly, declining to a low of 1,010 cases in 1976. However, in recent years the number of cases reported have dramatically increased and the disease is again becoming a major public health concern.

Infection with *B. pertussis* in the nonimmunized host has been described to progress through three dis-

## Table 15–4 ▶ Biochemical Characteristics of *Brucella* Species

| Species | Positive Urease Reaction | H₂S Production | Inhibited by Thionine | Fuschin | CO₂ Required |
|---|---|---|---|---|---|
| B. melitensis | 2 h | + | − | − | − |
| B. abortus | 2 h | v | + | − | − |
| B. suis | 15 min | v | − | − | v |
| B. canis | 15 min | − | − | + | − |

Key: +, positive; −, negative; v, variable reactions.

tinct stages. The first, or "prodromal stage," begins following a 5- to 21-day incubation, and consists of nonspecific flulike symptoms. Late in this stage, the patient develops a cough, which becomes the hallmark of the second stage, the "paroxysmal stage." In this stage, the glottis becomes swollen and narrow, which causes frequent coughing attacks in which the patient is gasping for breath, resulting in the characteristic "whoop" or "staccato" cough. Coughing spells are frequently followed by vomiting, and occasionally patients need to be put on ventilators to assist with breathing. This stage is also marked by an increased total leukocyte count and increase in relative percentage of lymphocytes on the differential. The third, "convalescent stage" occurs over a 4-week period. Further complications of infection may also include otitis media, central nervous system involvement, and inguinal hernia or **rectal prolapse** (displacement of the rectal mucosa through the anus, due to damage to the support tissue) caused by the severity of coughing spells.

Infection of an immunized individual with *B. pertussis* results in a mild state that mimics the common cold. It is these persons who are most likely the source of outbreaks of whooping cough. The species *B. parapertussis* causes a much milder form of whooping cough, and it is postulated that this organism may in fact be a strain of *B. pertussis* that does not produce pertussis toxin and tracheal cytotoxin. A third species, *B. broncoseptica,* is mostly nonpathogenic in man, but implicated in rare cases of wound and respiratory infections.

## Cultural Characteristics and Identification

Currently, it is generally thought that the best specimen for isolation of *B. pertussis* is a wire calcium alginate or Dacron nasopharyngeal swab inserted through the nose to the nasal pharynx and left in place for 1 minute while the patient is coughing. Cotton swabs should not be used because fatty acids in the cotton fibers inhibit the growth of the organism. Transport of the swab is best on half-strength Regan-Lowe media, but other transport media may also be used. Nasopharyngeal aspiration has also been demonstrated to be an effective means of collection.

The organism stains as a tiny gram-negative coccobacilli, but a modified counterstain may be necessary to see the morphology. This modification can be an increase in the safranin staining time to 2 minutes, or substitution of carbol fuschin for the counterstain. Growth of *B. pertussis* requires special media. Two formulas have been routinely used. Bordet-Gengou agar is a potato infusion agar with 20% sheep's blood and has only a 24-hour shelf life. More recently, Regan-Lowe agar has been used successfully for isolation of the organism. This agar contains charcoal, cephalexin,

and sheep's blood and has a much improved stability. The organism will also grow on the buffered charcoal yeast extract agar used for isolation of *Legionella.*

*Bordetella pertussis* is an obligate aerobe and colonies appear as "pearls" or "drops of mercury" on the agar. Refer to Color Plate 29. Species of the genus can be differentiated by catalase and oxidase results (see Table 15-5). More commonly, direct fluorescent antibody stain of isolates is performed.

Culture of *Bordetella* can be difficult, and some studies have only demonstrated a 40% to 80% sensitivity for this method of diagnosis. Identification can also be accomplished by direct fluorescent antibody stain of nasopharyngeal smears using fluorescein-labeled rabbit antipertussis antibody. This method has shown sensitivity of nearly 100% in some studies; however, considerable experience is necessary for the proper performance and interpretation of the direct fluorescent antibody method.

## Antibiotic Susceptibility Characteristics

Erythromycin is the universal antibiotic for treatment of *Bordetella* infection. Prevention of pertussis is successfully accomplished through proper vaccination. A killed whole cell vaccine (in combination with diptheria and tetanus toxoids, the "DPT" vaccine) is given in three bimonthly doses starting at 4 weeks of age, then boosters are administered at 1 year and 6 years old.

## GARDNERELLA VAGINALIS

## Organism Characteristics

*Gardnerella vaginalis* is a **pleomorphic**, gram-negative or gram-variable coccobacilli of variable morphology. It is present as normal vaginal flora in approximately 40% to 50% of normal healthy women. Its unique cell wall structure causes adhesion to the surfaces of epithelial cells, one characteristic that aids in identification of its presence in vaginal fluids (**clue cells**).

**Table 15–5  ▶  Differentiation of *Bordetella* Species**

| Species | Catalase | Oxidase |
|---|---|---|
| B. pertussis | + | + |
| B. parapertussis | – | – |
| B. bronchoseptica | – | + |

Key: +, positive; –, negative.

## Clinical Significance

The clinical significance of *G. vaginalis* is a widely debated topic; however, strong evidence suggests that it is probably a sexually transmitted organism in part responsible for a condition known as "bacterial vaginosis," previously referred to as "nonspecific vaginosis." This condition is a polymicrobial infection, probably involving anaerobes or yeast as well as *Gardnerella*. It is a noninflammatory, asymptomatic state resulting in large volumes of thin milky vaginal discharge with a foul odor. Clinically, the condition is defined as the presence of at least 20% clue cells, plus a vaginal pH of at least 4.7, an amine odor, or production of homogeneous vaginal discharge.

In addition to bacterial vaginosis, there is increasing evidence that *G. vaginalis* also causes postpartum bacteremia and endometriosis, premature labor, and neonatal septicemia. These infections were previously unreported because the sodium polyanethol sulfonate (SPS) additives common in blood culture collection systems inhibit the growth of *Gardnerella*.

## Cultural Characteristics and Identification

*Gardnerella vaginalis* grows as clear nonhemolytic pinpoint colonies on blood agar and calcium nutrient agar. It is most effectively isolated on human blood bilayer Tween agar (HBT) or nonselective vaginosis agar (V agar). On both of these media, the organism will demonstrate ß-hemolysis due to the human blood in the agar. Isolates are catalase negative, oxidase negative, hippurate positive, and starch hydrolysis positive. Identification of *G. vaginalis* may also be performed by demonstrating sensitivity to an SPS antibiotic disc on HBT or V Agar (see Color Plate 30).

Rather than isolation and identification of *G. vaginalis,* diagnosis of vaginosis is better accomplished through direct examination of Gram stain or wet mount of the vaginal discharge, which is characteristic of the condition. This examination should demonstrate large numbers of clue cells, and the lack of the gram-positive bacilli *Lactobacillus,* normally present as resident flora of the vaginal tract.

The vaginal discharge can also be tested by adding 10% potassium hydroxide to the collected fluid. The production of a strong "fishy" odor is considered good evidence of vaginosis.

If postpartum bacteremia or neonatal septicemia is suspected, it is now being suggested that the blood culture specimen be directly planted onto agar to avoid SPS-containing blood culture media.

## Antibiotic Susceptibility Characteristics

In vitro susceptibility testing of *Gardnerella* isolates should not be performed. The universal treatment for vaginosis is metronidazole, even though *Gardnerella* demonstrates in vitro resistance to this drug. The success of this treatment supports the theory that anaerobic organisms are involved in the disease process of vaginosis.

## *LEGIONELLA*

### Organism Characteristics

*Legionella* was first identified and named in 1977 as the causative agent of a 1976 outbreak of pneumonia among American Legion convention attendees at a Philadelphia hotel. There were 182 cases of infection documented in that outbreak and 29 deaths. Currently approximately 33 species of *Legionella* are recognized. *Legionella pneumophila* is the most commonly isolated species.

*Legionella* is found worldwide in many natural habitats, particularly where standing bodies of fresh water are found, such as lakes, streams, and ponds. The organism is capable of surviving up to 1 year in water. *Legionella* are parasites of amebae; it is likely that these amebae act as reservoirs for the organism's survival in water environments.

The organism can also be found in many man-made habitats such as showerheads, whirlpools, hot tubs, water-cooling towers, and evaporative condensers of air-conditioning systems. These devices often create aerosols that can dispense *Legionella* organisms into the air where they are easily inhaled. *Legionella* tolerates both high and low temperatures easily. Killing the bacteria requires extremely high temperatures (above 70°C [158°F]) for 72 hours, or high chlorination of at least 2 parts per million.

### Clinical Significance

Since the infamous Philadelphia outbreak of 1976, retroactive studies of saved serum and tissue samples from unresolved cases have indicated previous epidemics of *Legionella* in 1947, 1957, 1965, and 1968. Epidemiology studies based on seroconversion have suggested an exposure rate of 25,000 cases per year in the United States. It is also estimated that *Legionella* is responsible for 10% to 30% of nosocomial pneumonia in some hospitals.

Infection with *Legionella* can demonstrate variable symptomatology depending on the victim's immune status and the dose of inoculum. Groups of individuals predisposed to severe *Legionella* infections include smokers, drinkers, older men, and patients with diabetes mellitus, chronic obstructive pulmonary disease, and other immunosuppressive conditions.

Infection with *Legionella* generally presents in two distinct forms. The pneumonic form is known as "Legionnaire's disease," a severe pneumonia with a high mortality rate up to 30% if not treated. The milder form of infection, "Pontiac fever," is named for a 1968 Michigan outbreak. This form is an acute, self-limiting, systemic febrile disease with symptoms similar to severe flu. Victims usually recover within 2 to 5 days and the mortality rate is very low.

## Cultural Characteristics and Identification

The specimen of choice for isolation of *Legionella* is a transtracheal aspirate or bronchial washing. Lung aspirates or biopsies are also acceptable. The organism is usually not present in sputum samples and these are generally considered unacceptable for culture.

*Legionella* species are tiny, thin, gram-negative bacilli. A modified counterstain may be required for the organism to be visible. This may be performed by increasing the safranin staining time to 2 minutes or by substituting carbol fuschin as the counterstain. This weak staining characteristic is probably the reason this organism remained unrecognized until 1977. The organism does not grow on routine laboratory media. L-Cystine and iron salts are required for growth, and buffered charcoal yeast extract agar is considered the media of choice for isolation. Growth is also optimal in ambient air rather than $CO_2$. In fact, $CO_2$ concentrations greater than 5% may actually inhibit the growth of *Legionella*. Colonies appear in 5 days, and are grayish white to blue-green, often with a yellowish or greenish fluorescent pigment. Refer to Color Plate 7.

Isolates are positive for catalase activity, negative for all carbohydrate utilizations, positive for gelatin liquefaction, and negative for nitrate and urease activity. *L. pneumophila* is positive for hippurate hydrolysis, whereas all other species are negative. Differentiation of *Legionella* species is not considered clinically necessary because all species are treated with the same antibiotic regimen.

Diagnosis may also be made by direct fluorescent antibody stain of direct smears and serologic antibody titers. A single titer of ≥1:128 or a fourfold increase between acute and convalescent specimens is considered good presumptive evidence of *Legionella* infection.

## Antibiotic Susceptibility Characteristics

Differentiation between the species of *Legionella* is not necessary because all species are treated identically. Infections are treated with intravenous erythromycin, often given concomitantly with rifampin in critical cases.

In vitro susceptibility testing is not recommended because it is not predictive of in vivo response.

## OBSCURE OR RARELY ISOLATED ORGANISMS

### Kingella

**Organism Characteristics and Clinical Significance.** *Kingella kingae* and *K. denitrificans* were first identified in the 1960s as normal flora in the human mouth and throat. *K. kingae* has been implicated in cases of bacteremia, skin lesions, endocarditis, and osteomyelitis, particularly in juvenile patients. It is thought that the organism gains entry to the bloodstream through breaks in the oropharyngeal mucosa and is carried to the specific tissues it infects. *Kingella* demonstrates specific tissue **tropism** or affinity for bone and heart tissue. Individuals with poor oral hygiene are thought to be more prone to these types of infections.

**Cultural Characteristics and Identification.** *Kingella kingae* is most commonly isolated from joint fluid, blood cultures, and skin drainage. It stains as a tiny gram-negative coccobacilli. Colonies appear on blood agar and chocolate agar after 3 to 5 days in 5% to 10% $CO_2$ as small ß-hemolytic, grayish colonies. These can sometimes have a "fried-egg" appearance with a raised center, and also sometimes can "pit" the agar. The organism does not grow on MacConkey agar. Growth is catalase negative and oxidase positive.

*Kingella denitrificans* is capable of growing on Thayer-Martin agar and is oxidase and glucose fermentation positive, making it easily confused with *Neisseria gonorrhoeae*. Differentiation between these two organisms may be accomplished with nitrate reduction testing, for which *Kingella* species are positive and *Neisseria* is negative.

*Kingella* infections are treated with ß-lactams such as penicillin, gentamycin, or chloramphenicol.

### Eikenella

**Organism Characteristics and Clinical Significance.** *Eikenella corrodens* is found as normal flora in the human mouth. Most commonly, the organism is isolated from wounds associated with human bites or "fist trauma" from fist fights. It can also be seen in meningitis, endocarditis, osteomyelitis, brain abscesses, and periodontitis, usually in immunocompromised patients. The organism probably gains access to the bloodstream through breaks in the oral mucosa. In addition, infection is seen as a result of a practice known as "skin-popping" by drug addicts, in which the needle is lubricated with saliva before being injected into the bloodstream.

**Cultural Characteristics and Identification.** *Eikenella corrodens* is a tiny gram-negative bacilli, a facultative anaerobe that grows best in high $CO_2$ concentrations and high humidity. It grows well on blood agar and chocolate agar, demonstrates a pale yellow pigment, and 40% to 50% of the colonies will "pit" the agar. Isolates also emit a characteristic "bleach-like" odor.

Identifying characteristics include positive oxidase, lysine decarboxylase, (LDC), and nitrate results, and negative catalase, urease, indole, and carbohydrate fermentation tests.

## Capnocytophaga

**Organism Characteristics and Clinical Significance.** The genus *Capnocytophaga* includes several species that are normal oropharyngeal flora in humans or animals. Table 15-6 lists the normal habitats of the most common species.

Organisms of this genus have most commonly been implicated in cases of juvenile periodontitis, and have also been known to cause sepsis, osteomyelitis and endocarditis, especially in leukemic or granulocytopenic patients. Species inhabiting the oral cavities of animals have also been implicated in animal bites, particularly from dogs. Immunosuppressed individuals seem to be more susceptible to infection with *Capnocytophaga* species than others.

**Cultural Characteristics and Identification.** *Capnocytophaga* species are **capnophilic** (preferring increased concentration of $CO_2$), gram-negative bacilli with a **fusiform** or tapered, spindle-shaped appearance. The organism grows well on blood and MacConkey agars in 48 to 72 hours. Colonies appear as opaque, nonhemolytic, yellowish colonies with "gliding" motility similar to the swarming seen with *Proteus* species.

Biochemically, species of the genus are oxidase negative, catalase negative, glucose positive, urease negative, and LDC negative. Most commercial anaerobic identification kits will identify species of *Capnocytophaga*. Some strains are ß-lactamase positive; therefore, susceptibility testing should be performed on isolates to determine appropriate therapy.

## Cardiobacterium

**Organism Characteristics and Clinical Significance.** *Cardiobacterium hominis* is the only species of this genus and is normal flora in the human mouth. The

**Table 15–6 ► Normal Habitats of Capnocytophaga Species**

| Normal flora in Human mouth | Normal flora in Animal mouth |
|---|---|
| C. ochracea | C. canimorsus |
| C. sputigena | C. cynodegmi |
| C. gingivalis | |

only type of infections associated with *C. hominis* are bacteremia and endocarditis, particularly in patients with a history of recent dental work. Incidence of infection with this organism seems to be rising over recent years, perhaps due to increased numbers of susceptible, immunosuppressed patients.

**Cultural Characteristics and Identification.** Isolation of *C. hominis* is limited to blood cultures from infected individuals. The organism is a pleomorphic gram-negative or gram-variable bacilli appearing in rosette formations. It is a facultative anaerobe that appears as round, small, opaque, α-hemolytic colonies on blood and chocolate agars in 5% to 10% $CO_2$ at 37°C in 48 hours.

Biochemically, isolates are catalase negative, oxidase positive, spot indole positive, and nitrate positive. Table 15-7 describes the carbohydrate fermentation characteristics of this species.

The treatment of choice for *Cardiobacterium* infections is penicillin.

## HB-5

**Organism Characteristics and Clinical Significance.** *HB-5* is a tiny gram-negative coccobacilli that has recently been classified and named *Pasteurella bettae*. It is found as normal flora of the genitals in both men and women. The most common types of infections seen with this organism are skin lesions and abscesses.

**Cultural Characteristics and Identification.** *Pasteurella bettae* grows as nonhemolytic colonies on blood agar in 5% to 10% $CO_2$. Isolates demonstrate negative catalase activity, a positive nitrate reductase, weakly positive indole, and variable oxidase results.

**Table 15–7 ► Carbohydrate Fermentation of C. hominis**

| Glucose | Maltose | Sorbitol | Sucrose | Lactose |
|---|---|---|---|---|
| + | + | + | + | − |

## SUMMARY

▶ *Pasteurella* species are widespread as normal flora in animals and this represents the main source of human infection.

▶ *Pasteurella* species are gram-negative coccobacilli that grow well on blood and chocolate agars, emit a strong "musty" odor due to a positive indole reaction, and can be differentiated based on ODC, ADC, urease, indole, maltose, and xylose reactivities.

▶ Gram-negative bacilli cultured from an animal bite or scratch that fail to grow on MacConkey agar and that demonstrate positive oxidase and indole results can be presumptively identified as *P. multocida*.

▶ *Francisella* species are typically contracted from contact with wild animals or their carcasses and furs.

▶ Identification of *F. tularensis,* the cause of tularemia, is best accomplished in a reference laboratory by culturing of aspirates or exudates from granulomas of infected tissues, or by serologic studies.

▶ Undulant fever, a recurrent febrile disease caused by *Brucella* species, is contracted in patients with close contact with host animals or animal products.

▶ *Brucella* species are tiny gram-negative coccobacilli that can be identified based on their urease results, inhibition by thionine and fuschin dyes, carbon dioxide requirements, and hydrogen sulfide formation.

▶ "Whooping cough" is an extremely contagious respiratory disease caused by four toxins produced by the gram-negative coccobacilli *B. pertussis.*

▶ *B. pertussis* can best be identified from a nasopharyngeal swab by either culture of the organism on Regan-Lowe or Bordet-Gengou agars, or by direct fluorescent antibody stain.

▶ *G. vaginalis* is a gram-variable coccobacilli that is often normal vaginal flora, but can also cause "bacterial vaginosis," a noninflammatory infection resulting in a foul-smelling vaginal discharge containing many "clue cells."

▶ Infection with *G. vaginalis* can be identified by the presence of "clue cells" or by isolation and identification of the organism biochemically, or by its sensitivity to SPS.

▶ *L. pneumophila* causes epidemics of pneumonia and nonpneumonic disease of variable severity, especially in patients with certain predisposing conditions.

▶ *L. pneumophila* can be isolated on buffered charcoal yeast extract agar and identified biochemically, by direct fluorescent antibody stain of direct smears, or by serologic antibody titers.

▶ *Kingella* species are gram-negative coccobacilli that are normal flora of the human mouth that can also cause infections, predominantly in bone and heart tissue.

▶ *E. corrodens* is normal flora of the mouth that can be isolated from human bite wounds, emits a bleach-like odor, and whose colonies will "pit" the agar.

▶ Species of *Capnocytophaga* are fusiform gram-negative bacilli that most commonly cause juvenile periodontitis, grow well on blood and MacConkey agars, and can be identified with most commercial identification kits.

▶ *C. hominis* is normal mouth flora that can cause endocarditis, especially in patients with recent dental work.

▶ *HB-5* is a species of *Pasteurella* that can cause skin lesions and abscesses and can be identified by catalase, indole, nitrate, and oxidase results.

---

## CASE STUDY 1

A specimen on a 3-year-old girl is received from a pediatrician's office labeled "leg wound drainage." At 48 hours, small grayish nonhemolytic colonies are observed on blood and chocolate agars. Although the colonies Gram stain as gram-negative bacilli, there is no growth on MacConkey agar. A distinct "musty" or "mushroom-like" odor is detected, and the colonies demonstrate a positive oxidase result.

### Questions:

1. Based on the information given, what organism do you suspect? What further background information would you request from the pediatrician's office to support your suspicions?

2. The cause of the "musty" odor can be determined by a spot bench test useful in identifying this organism. What test should be performed to assist in identification?

3. The suspected organism can be screened for based on sensitivity to a common antibiotic. What is the screening procedure often used?

## CASE STUDY 2

A 23-year-old man is seen in the emergency room for an infected wound on his hand. The wound is swollen, feverish, and red, and a moderate amount of pus has accumulated at the site. On questioning, the patient explains that he was involved in a fist fight at a local night club 1 week earlier. During the fight, he had hit the other man involved in the mouth and broken several of his teeth, at which time he was bitten deeply by his opponent. The wound is a result of that bite. The physician lances the wound and bacterial culture of the drainage is performed.

After 48 hours incubation in 10% $CO_2$, tiny opaque colonies with a pale yellow pigment are observed on blood agar and chocolate agar plates. The organism Gram stains as a small gram-negative bacilli. Colonies are oxidase positive and catalase negative.

**Questions:**

1.  What organism is the most likely pathogen isolated in this example? What was the source of the organism?

2.  What other common colony characteristics would be helpful in presumptively identifying this organism?

## CASE STUDY 3

A 37-year-old man was admitted to a local hospital complaining of a severe headache of several days, moderate fever, chest pain, and a productive cough. Swollen lymph nodes and a tender, enlarged liver were also noted. He is a professional furrier and trapper and had recently returned from an excursion on which he had trapped and skinned approximately 30 rabbits.

Routine sputum and blood cultures were collected and inoculated aerobically and anaerobically onto routine media (blood agar plate, MacConkey agar, and CA, MAC). Although Gram stains of both the blood and sputum seemed to demonstrate the presence of very faintly staining gram-negative coccobacilli, no growth was obtained on any of the cultures after 72 hours.

After 6 days, the chocolate agar plates from the blood culture began to grow tiny transparent colonies of the organism. These colonies were oxidase negative and weakly catalase positive. Unable to conclusively identify the organism using any of their routine methods, the laboratory sent the isolate to a reference laboratory.

While awaiting the final identification results from the reference laboratory, the patient's pneumonia condition worsened, complicated by liver failure, and he died 3 weeks following admission.

**Questions:**

1.  Given the patient's history and symptoms, what disease and organism do you suspect has infected the patient?

2.  Assuming the laboratory was aware of the patient's specific history, describe the special precautions that should have been taken when working on specimens from this patient.

3.  Why did the organism only grow on chocolate agar? Name two other types of media on which the organism will grow well.

# Review Questions

1. Of the following gram-negative organisms, which are commonly capable of growing on MacConkey agar?
   a. *Pasteurella*
   b. *Bordetella*
   c. *Legionella*
   d. None of the above

2. A suspected isolate of *Pasteurella* can be identified by its susceptibility to:
   a. gentamycin.
   b. sodium polyanethol sulfonate.
   c. penicillin.
   d. rifampin.

3. A patient develops a nonspecific disease several weeks following receiving a gift of Mexican goat cheese. A gram-negative coccobacilli is isolated from the patient's blood cultures. Based on this information, what is the most likely organism present?
   a. *Bordetella*
   b. *Kingella*
   c. *Brucella*
   d. *Legionella*

4. Even though *Gardnerella vaginalis* causes postpartum and neonatal bacteremia and septicemia, it will not be identified in blood cultures using most common systems because:
   a. the organism remains localized in the vagina and does not enter the bloodstream.
   b. *Gardnerella* does not grow on routine media such as blood and chocolate agars.
   c. *Gardnerella* is an anaerobe, and blood cultures are usually incubate aerobically only.
   d. growth of *Gardnerella* is inhibited by the sodium polyanethol sulfonate present in many blood culture collection medias.

5. *Legionella* was probably not recognized prior to 1977 because:
   a. it does not Gram stain easily, and is often invisible.
   b. it does not grow on most of the routinely used bacterial media.
   c. it did not exist prior to the Philadelphia hotel outbreak.
   d. both a and b are true.

6. Which bacterial media is best for isolation of *Legionella* species?
   a. Bordet-Gengou agar
   b. Buffered charcoal yeast extract agar
   c. Regan-Lowe agar
   d. Cysteine-glucose blood agar

7. A drug addict with visible "tracks" on his arm develops an infection among the lesions. The organism isolated is a tiny gram-negative bacilli that grows on blood agar but not MacConkey, is oxidase positive, and a majority of the colonies "pit" the agar. What is the most likely pathogen?
   a. *Eikenella corrodens*
   b. *Pasteurella multocida*
   c. *Kingella kinga*
   d. *Kingella denitrificans*

8. It is common practice for dentists to prescribe prophylactic penicillin 2 weeks prior to any dental work on patients with a history of any heart defects to avert possible endocarditis. This would most likely be to prevent infection with:
   a. *Eikenella corrodens*
   b. *Kingella kingae*
   c. *Cardiobacterium hominis*
   d. *Capnocytophaga canimorsus*

9. Which of the following are likely to result in contraction of tularemia?
   a. Trapping and skinning of wild rabbits
   b. Raising of cattle for dairy purposes
   c. Tending to herds of sheep
   d. Human bite wounds

10. Which of the following would constitute the BEST diagnosis of "bacterial vaginosis"?
    a. The isolation of a tiny gram-variable bacilli from a vaginal swab of a patient experiencing no symptoms
    b. Observation of "clue cells" in a milky white vaginal discharge emitting a "fishy" odor
    c. Isolation of a gram-negative bacilli that demonstrates resistance to sodium polyanethol sulfate from a vaginal discharge
    d. Growth of nonhemolytic colonies on "V" human blood agar

## ▶ REFERENCES & RECOMMENDED READING

Baron, E. J., Peterson L. R., & Finegold, S. M. (1994). *Bailey & Scott's diagnostic microbiology* (9th ed.). St. Louis: Mosby–Year Book.

Boyd, R. F. (1995). *Basic medical microbiology* (5th ed.). Boston: Little, Brown.

Davis, S. F., Strebel, P. M., Cochi, S. L., Zell, E. R., & Hadler, S. C. (1992). Pertussis surveillance—United States, 1989–1991. *Morbidity and Mortality Weekly Report, 41* (8), 9–11.

Farizo, K. M., Cochi, S. L., Zell, E. R., Brink, E. W., Wassilak, S. G., & Patriarca, P. A. (1992). Epidemiological features of pertussis in the United States, 1980–1989. *Clinical Infectious Diseases, 14* (3), 708–719.

Hallander, H. O., Reizenstein, E., Renemar, B., Rasmuson, G., Mardin, L., & Olin, P. (1993). Comparison of nasopharyngeal aspirates with swabs for culture of *Bordetella pertussis. Journal of Clinical Microbiology, 31* (1), 50–52.

Hillier, S. L., Lipinski, C., Briselden, A. M., & Eschenbach, D. A. (1993). Efficacy of intravaginal 0.75% metronidazole gel for the treatment of bacterial vaginosis. *Obstetrics & Gynecology, 81* (6), 963–967.

Holst, E., Rollof, J., Larsson, L., & Nielsen, J. P. (1992). Characterization and distribution of *Pasteurella* species recovered from infected humans. *Journal of Clinical Microbiology, 30* (11), 2984–2987.

Howard, B. J., Keiser, J. F., Smith, T. F., Weissfeld, A. S., & Tilton, R. C. (1994). *Clinical and pathogenic microbiology* (2nd ed.). St. Louis: Mosby–Year Book.

Joklik, W. K., Willett, H. P., Amos, D. B., & Wilfert, C. M. (Eds.). (1988). *Zinsser microbiology* (19th ed.). Norwalk, CT: Appleton & Lange.

Koneman, E. W., Allen, S. D., Janda, W. M., Schreckenberger, P. C., & Winn, W. C., Jr. (1997). *Color atlas and textbook of diagnostic microbiology* (5th ed.). Philadelphia: Lippincott-Raven Publishers.

Kristensen, B., Schonheyder, H. C., Peterslund, N. A., Rosthof, S., Clausen, N., & Frederiksen, W. (1995). *Capnocytophaga* (*Capnocytophaga ochracea* group) bacteremia in hematological patients with profound granulocytopenia. *Scandinavian Journal of Infectious Diseases, 27* (2), 153–155.

Laboratories in the hot zone. (1996, July/August). *Lab Reporter,* pp. 1, 11. Fisher Scientific Company.

Legionnaires' disease associated with cooling tower: Massachusetts, Michigan, and Rhode Island. (1993). *Morbidity & Mortality Weekly Report, 43* (27), 491–493.

Linton, D. M., Potgieter, P. D., Roditi, D., Phillips, A., Adams, B. K., Hayhurst, M., & Knobel, G. J. (1994). Fatal *Capnocytophaga canimorsus* (DF-2) septicaemia: A case report. *South African Medical Journal, 84* (12), 857–860.

Mahon, C. R., & Manuselis, G., Jr. (1995). *Textbook of diagnostic microbiology.* Philadelphia: Saunders.

Peetermans, W. E., & DeMan, F. (1995). Soins dentaires et prophylaxie de l'endocardite infectieuse [Dental care and prevention of infectious endocarditis]. *Revue Belge de Medecine Dentaire, 50* (1), 34–45.

Pertussis: United States, January 1992–June 1995. (1995). *Morbidity & Mortality Weekly Report, 44* (28), 525–529.

Ramsey, M. K., & Roberts, G. H. (1992). *Legionella pneumophila:* The organism and its implications. *Laboratory Medicine, 23* (4), 244–247.

Resurgence of pertussis: United States, 1993. (1993). *Morbidity & Mortality Weekly Report, 42* (49), 952–953.

Ryan, K. J. (Ed.). (1994). *Sherris medical microbiology: An introduction to infectious diseases* (3rd ed.). Norwalk, CT: Appleton & Lange.

Seabolt, J. P. (1994). Resurgence of pertussis. *Clinical Laboratory Science, 7* (5), 278.

Strebel, P. M., Cochi, S. L., Farizo, K. M., Payne, B. J., Hanauer, S. D., & Baughman, A. L. (1993). Pertussis in Missouri: Evaluation of nasopharyngeal sucture, direct fluorescent antibody testing, and clinical case definitions in the diagnosis of pertussis. *Clinical Infectious Diseases, 16* (2), 276–285.

U.S. Department of Health & Human Services. (1993). *Biosafety in microbiology and biomedical laboratories* (3rd ed.). Washington, DC: U.S. Government Printing Office.

Wortis, N., Strebel, P. M., Wharton, M., Bardenheier, B., & Hardy, I. R. (1996). Pertussis deaths: Report of 23 cases in the United States, 1992 and 1993. *Pediatrics, 97* (5), 607–612.

Valtonen, M., Lauhio, A., Carlson, P., Multanen, J., Sivonen, A., Vaara, M., & Lahdevirta, J. (1995). *Capnocytophaga canimorsus* septicemia: Fifth report of a cat-associated infection and five other cases. *European Journal of Clinical Microbiology & Infectious Diseases, 14* (5), 520–523.

Young, E. J. (1995). An overview of human brucellosis. *Clinical Infectious Diseases, 21* (2), 283–289.

# CHAPTER 16

# Gram-Negative Enteric Bacilli

Daila S. Gridley, PhD

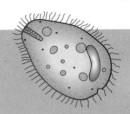

## Microbes in the News

### Plague Alert Closes Popular Areas in a National Forest

Routine checks in 1996 by health department officers in the Angeles National Forest in California led to the discovery of several ground squirrels infected with *Yersinia pestis*, the bacterium that causes plague. Although no human cases of bubonic or pneumonic plague had been reported in the county for 12 years, the United States Forest Service promptly closed three popular picnic sites in the area. The timing was especially unfortunate for vacationers because the closures came right before the long Fourth of July weekend. Sylvatic plague is endemic in the mountains and forests of California. However, the heavy rainfall in the winter of 1996 allowed more grass to grow, creating an environment in which squirrels and fleas (a vector for *Y. pestis*) thrive. The three areas remained closed to the public while health officials worked to eradicate both the squirrels and the fleas.

## KEY TERMS

Bacteremia
Bacteriocins
CLED medium
Dysentery
Enteric fever
Enteroaggregative *E. coli* (EAEC)
Enterocolitis
Enterohemorrhagic *E. coli* (EHEC)

Enteroinvasive *E. coli* (EIEC)
Enteropathogenic *E. coli* (EPEC)
Enterotoxigenic *E. coli* (ETEC)
Heat-stable exotoxin (ST)
Heat-labile exotoxin (LT)
Lipopolysaccharide
Mesenteric adenitis
MUG test
Nephropathogenic *E. coli* (NPEC)

O, K, H, and Vi antigens
Plague
R plasmids
Shiga toxin
Swarming
Typhoid fever
Verotoxin
Widal test

## LEARNING OBJECTIVES

**Upon successful completion of this chapter, the student should be able to:**

1. List the general characteristics and the antigenic properties of the *Enterobacteriaceae* family as a whole.

2. Describe distinguishing features of the presented genera and the major species of importance in human infections.

3. Correlate the various organisms with the type(s) of infection(s) they cause and describe the nature of the illness.

4. Discuss the major virulence factor(s), if known, that are associated with the organisms and discuss their importance in the disease process.

5. List and describe major laboratory tests that are used to differentiate the various organisms.

6. Discuss the appropriate treatments and preventive measures for each.

## INTRODUCTION

The *Enterobacteriaceae* consist of numerous gram-negative rods with heterogenous characteristics. In general, they are rather large, straight bacilli (0.4–0.6 × 2–4 µm) with rounded ends, although coccobacillary and filamentous forms have also been observed. Most members have peritrichous flagella and pili, multiply rapidly under anaerobic or aerobic conditions in simple media, and are able to ferment many sugars with a variety of end products that are useful in identification. Many members of the family are found free living in the environment and as natural inhabitants of the intestinal tract of humans and animals. Because of this latter characteristic, they are sometimes collectively referred to as "enteric gram-negative rods," "the enterics," or "the coliforms." The presence of enteric bacteria in water or milk is a sign of fecal contamination. The Centers for Disease Control and Prevention (CDC) has estimated that in 1 year approximately 940,000 people in the United States get sick from drinking water that is contaminated with microbes. A portion of these infections are due to members of the *Enterobacteriaceae*. Despite this large number of cases, relatively few (i.e., approximately 900/year) develop a fatal infection.

Most of the *Enterobacteriaceae* associated with humans are part of the normal flora. They do not produce disease unless they reach parts of the body they do not usually inhabit or when they produce toxins or other virulence factors. Commonly isolated genera that are usually nonpathogenic in healthy individuals are *Escherichia, Klebsiella, Enterobacter, Serratia, Proteus, Providencia,* and *Morganella.* In contrast, only the *Salmonella* and *Shigella* are considered to be overt pathogens. Nonetheless, the *Enterobacteriaceae* are the leading cause of urinary tract infections and bacteremia in the United States. Many members of the family are also implicated in a large percentage of the 7 million episodes of diarrhea that occur each year. They also account for about 80% of clinically significant gram-negative isolates and approximately one-half of all clinically significant isolates.

# General Characteristics Used in Identification

Characteristics that are common to all members of the *Enterobacteriaceae* family include the ability to ferment glucose with the production of acid, the ability to reduce nitrates to nitrites, and the lack of an oxidase enzyme. Most of the organisms have peritrichous flagella. They are facultative anaerobes or aerobes, have a complex antigenic structure, may or may not possess a capsule, and ferment many carbohydrates with a variety of end products. A battery of biochemical tests and enzyme assays are needed to differentiate among the various genera and species. Commonly available multiassay kits are now frequently used to expedite identification of isolates.

Some of these organisms produce **bacteriocins**, which are small substances that kill certain other strains of the same or similar species as the one producing them. They do not cause damage to the bacteria that synthesized them. The bacteriocins, which are under the control of genes in plasmids, have been given different names. Examples include colicins, marcescins, and pyocins that are produced by *Escherichia coli, Serratia marcescens,* and *Pseudomonas* species, respectively. Bacteriocins play a role in protecting the host from colonization by other bacteria that may be pathogenic and are also useful in epidemiologic studies.

The *Enterobacteriaceae* grow relatively rapidly on a variety of commonly used laboratory media. Colonies are usually present within 1 day of incubation at 37°C. Differential media used to help identify the organisms contain dyes (e.g., EMB agar has *e*osin-*m*ethylele *b*lue) or carbohydrates such as lactose (e.g., MacConkey agar). These media are useful in distinguishing between lactose fermenters and those that do not ferment the sugar. For example, lactose fermenters form pinkish colonies on MacConkey agar, whereas nonfermenters form colorless translucent colonies. Stool specimens are often inoculated into Kligler's iron agar (KIA) or triple sugar iron (TSI) agar slants, which are especially useful in distinguishing the salmonellae and shigellae from the other enteric bacteria. Commercially available multitest identification systems (e.g., API 20E, API Rapid E, Enterotube II, and Minitek) are inoculated with a suspension of organisms made from a single isolated colony. Some of these kits generate results in as little as 4 hours. Table 16-1 summarizes the typical reactions observed in the most commonly isolated enteric bacteria.

## Antigenic Structure

The classification of the *Enterobacteriaceae* has been difficult because the organisms represent one continuous spectrum with many shared properties and overlapping characteristics. Classification is partly based on the more than 150 somatic **O antigens**, that is, the **lipopolysaccharides** (LPS) that protrude from the bacterial cell wall. O antigens are heat stable and resistant to degradation by alcohols. Antibodies produced against them are primarily of the IgM class. Different organisms can share one or more O antigens; hence, considerable cross-reactivity exists among genera, as well as among species. Nearly all members of the family that have been tested have the 014 antigen. The lipid A portion of the LPS, when released because

## Table 16–1 ▶ Typical Reaction Patterns of Commonly Isolated *Enterobacteriaceae*

| | E. coli | Klebsiella | Enterobacter | Serratia | Proteus | Providencia | Morganella | Citrobacter | Salmonella | Shigella |
|---|---|---|---|---|---|---|---|---|---|---|
| Lactose | +* | + | + | –* | – | – | – | +/– | – | – |
| Motility | + | – | + | + | ++† | + | + | + | + | – |
| Indol | + | +/–‡ | – | – | +/– | + | + | +/– | – | +/– |
| VP | – | + | + | + | – | – | – | – | – | – |
| MR | + | – | – | – | + | + | + | + | + | + |
| Citrate | – | + | + | + | +/– | + | – | + | + | – |
| Urease | – | + | – | – | + | +/– | + | – | – | – |
| PD | – | – | – | – | + | + | + | – | – | – |
| H₂S | – | – | – | – | + | – | – | +/– | +/– | – |
| DNase | – | – | – | + | +/– | – | – | – | – | – |

*A + and – indicate that the majority of common isolates give a positive or negative reaction, respectively.

†A ++ indicates very high motility (i.e., "swarming").

‡A +/– indicates that different species within a genus often give opposite results or that members within one species are highly variable.

VP, Voges-Proskauer; MR, methyl red; PD, phenylalanine deaminase.

of antibiotic treatment or a destructive immune response, is responsible for many of the pathophysiologic effects seen in patients with septic shock (i.e., fever, hypotension, leukopenia, and disseminated intravascular coagulation).

The capsular **K antigens** are usually composed of polysaccharides, although in a few organisms they consist of protein. The more than 100 different K antigens are often associated with virulence. Some of the salmonellae contain capsular antigens that are known as **Vi antigens**.

The **H antigens** are found in the flagella. These proteins (flagellins) are susceptible to heat and alcohol.

The antigenic formula is standardized so that the O, K, and H antigens are always listed in the same order and are separated by a colon. Phase 1 flagellar antigens are expressed by lower case letters, whereas phase 2 antigens are given arabic numerals. For example, the antigenic formula for *E. coli* may be O55:K5:H21; the formula for *Salmonella typhimurium* may be O1,4,5, 12:Hi:1,2.

Although specific antibodies develop during infection with the enteric bacteria, in most cases it is doubtful that protective immunity is generated. Furthermore, because of the large number of serotypes, it is unlikely that exposure to one or a few antigenic variants would confer resistance against all other members of a particular genus or species.

Some of the antigens of the *Enterobacteriaceae* are the same or very similar to antigens of bacteria in other families. For example, certain K antigens are cross-creactive with polysaccharides found in the capsules of *Neisseria meningitidis, Haemophilus influenzae,* and *Streptococcus pneumoniae* (see Figure 16-1).

## *ESCHERICHIA*

## Organism Characteristics

*Escherichia coli* is a relatively small, straight, lactose-positive, gram-negative rod that tends to grow singly and is easily dispersed into a single-celled suspension in liquid media. It is present in large numbers in the intestinal tract of both humans and many different animals. Most infections are endogenous, that is, they are the result of the individual's own organisms rather than acquired from an outside source. There are at least five species that belong in this genus, but *E. coli* is by far the most frequently isolated. It is also the most common member of the *Enterobacteriaceae* that is associated with clinically apparent disease.

## Clinical Significance

*Escherichia coli* is often identified as the etiologic agent of urinary tract infections, diarrheal disease, sepsis, and neonatal meningitis. Individuals who are debil-

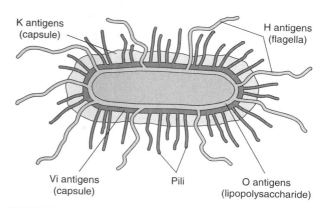

**FIGURE 16-1** Diagram showing the antigenic structure of a typical *Enterobacteriaceae*.

itated or have other predisposing factors are at much higher risk for infection than healthy persons. Table 16-2 compares the characteristics of the organisms that are associated with various disease entities in humans.

**Urinary Tract Infections.** *Escherichia coli* is an extremely common cause of urinary tract infections in young women, toddlers who are still at the diaper stage, and in hospitalized patients with indwelling catheters. The organisms may affect any part of the urinary tract, including the kidney (pyelonephritis). **Nephropathogenic *E. coli* (NPEC)** often have certain O antigens, a capsule, and a P pilus that binds to a portion of the P blood group substance. Patients experience urinary frequency, dysuria, and hematuria. Flank pain may be intense when the upper urinary tract is involved. Indwelling catheters, or other obstructions, may need to be removed in patients with urinary tract infections to facilitate recovery during antibiotic therapy.

**Diarrhea.** The *E. coli* that cause diarrhea are classified according to certain virulence factors that result in different mechanisms of disease production. Specific identification of the various isolates may be accomplished in reference laboratories, although many large medical centers now also have this capability. Infants are especially susceptible to infection with **enteropathogenic *E. coli* (EPEC)**. It is often implicated as the etiologic agent of diarrheal disease in outbreaks in nurseries. In infants the illness usually resolves in 5 to 15 days, but it may relapse. Chromosomal genes code for adherence factors that allow the organisms to bind tightly to mucosal cells of the small bowel. EPEC can sometimes invade the cells. A variety of serotypes, based on O (and occasionally H) antigens have been identified. *E. coli* with O111 and O125 antigens are often implicated as the etiologic agents. The clinical presentation includes watery diarrhea, microvilli loss, and characteristic lesions that can be visualized in biopsy specimens. The disease is usually self-limiting, but may become chronic.

**Table 16–2** ▶ **Characteristics of *E. Coli* Associated with Disease**

| Group | Type of Infection | Important Factors | Comments |
|---|---|---|---|
| Nephropathogenic *E. coli* (NPEC) | Urinary tract infections (pyelonephritis) | Capsule, P pili, hemolysin | Common in women, young children in diapers, and catheterized patients |
| Enteropathogenic *E. coli* (EPEC) | Watery diarrhea | 055, O111, O125 antigens | Common in infants; outbreaks in nurseries |
| Enterotoxigenic *E. coli* (ETEC) | "Traveler's diarrhea" | Heat-labile and heat-stable enterotoxins, pili, colonization factors | Common in travelers to endemic areas; diarrhea may be very severe if both toxins are produced |
| Enterohemorrhagic *E. coli* (EHEC) | Hemorrhagic colitis, hemolytic uremic syndrome (HUS) | O157:H7 serotype, verotoxin (Shiga-like toxin) | Associated with undercooked ground beef, raw milk, apple cider, other foods; acute renal failure; may be fatal |
| Enteroinvasive *E. coli* (EIEC) | Bloody diarrhea | Ability to penetrate epithelial cells in intestinal mucosa | Dysentery-like disease; most common in young children in developing countries |
| Enteroaggregative *E. coli* (EAEC) | Watery diarrhea | O112 antigen (possible adherence pili and "heat-stable-like" protein) | Most common in young children in developing countries; diarrhea may be acute or chronic |
| No group designation | Meningitis | K1 antigen | Most common in infants; high mortality rate; neurologic and other problems in survivors |

"Traveler's diarrhea" is frequently caused by **enterotoxigenic *E. coli* (ETEC)**. Colonization factors produced by the organisms enhance their adherence to the epithelial cells of the small intestine. Many of these organisms produce either one or two different toxins whose expression is under the control of genes found in plasmids. A **heat-labile exotoxin (LT)**, which has a molecular weight of approximately 80,000 daltons, is secreted by some strains. The LT consists of a B subunit that binds to ganglioside $G_{M1}$ present on epithelial cells of the small bowel. This binding facilitates the entry of the active A subunit (26,000 molecular weight) into the cells. The A subunit increases the cyclic adenosine monophosphate (cAMP) concentration in mammalian cells by activation of the adenylyl cyclase enzyme. The end result is the hypersecretion of water and chloride, hypermotility of the gut, and diarrhea, which usually persists for several days. The structure and mechanism of action of LT is similar to the enterotoxin of *Vibrio cholerae*. Some strains of ETEC produce a **heat-stable exotoxin (ST)**. It induces the hypersecretion of fluid by activating guanylyl cyclase, which, in turn, increases the intracellular level of cyclic guanosine monophosphate (cGMP). Organisms that produce both types of toxins generally induce more severe diarrhea than those that produce only one. In cases of severe diarrhea, antibiotic therapy, as well as measures to correct dehydration and electrolyte imbalance, may need to be initiated. However, individuals who live in countries where ETEC strains are prevalent may already have protective antibodies against the toxins. Interestingly, *E. coli* was the leading cause of diarrheal disease among U.S. troops during the Gulf War. More than 50% of the soldiers experienced at least one episode of "traveler's diarrhea."

**Enterohemorrhagic *E. coli* (EHEC)** produce a very severe form of bloody diarrhea known as hemorrhagic colitis. They are also responsible for a potentially fatal hemolytic uremic syndrome (HUS), which includes microangiopathic hemolytic anemia, thrombocytopenia, and acute renal failure. Blood transfusion and hemodialysis are often required. HUS is seen in approximately 10% of EHEC cases; most of these are in children younger than 5 years of age. The 0157:H7 serotype (discovered in 1982) is the most common EHEC isolated in the United States. It is transmitted by ingestion of undercooked ground beef, raw milk (the serotype is frequently isolated from asymptomatic dairy cattle), apple cider, and other foods. According to the CDC, at least 20,000 persons become ill and 250 die each year due to infection with this serotype of *E. coli*. Survivors of the infection may have problems in the future due to extensive urinary tract damage. **Verotoxin** (given this name because it kills Vero cells, i.e., a kidney cell line from the African Green monkey) is a major virulence factor that is produced in large amounts by the 0157:H7 serotype. The toxin can kill endothelial cells that line the inner lumen of blood vessels. Its properties are similar to those of Shiga toxin, which is produced by some strains of *Shigella dysenteriae*. Because of this, the toxin is sometimes referred to as *Shiga-like* toxin or SLT. The organisms also possess an *eae* gene that codes for "attaching and effacing" proteins that are similar to those produced by the EPEC. The combined effects of the toxin and the *eae* gene are thought to be responsible for hemorrhagic colitis. Kidney involvement (HUS) presumably occurs when the toxin is absorbed systemically. The 0157:H7 serotype has been responsible for several recent outbreaks of severe disease in which the organisms were traced to contaminated ground beef served in fast-food restaurants. Other serotypes that have been associated with this form of *E. coli* infection include O1, O26, O91, and O145.

**Enteroinvasive *E. coli* (EIEC)** invade the epithelial cells of the intestinal mucosa and produce a disease that is very similar to shigellosis, but generally milder. They are important primarily in young children living in developing countries, although travelers to these countries may also become ill. An outbreak of EIEC in the United States was traced to contaminated imported cheese. Invasive strains of *E. coli* often have the O112 antigen. **Enteroaggregative *E. coli* (EAEC)**, which are also prevalent in some developing countries, cause acute and chronic diarrheal disease with watery stools. To date, specific virulence factors in these organisms have not been well characterized, although there are reports describing adherence pili and an ST-like protein that differs from that found in ETEC.

**Meningitis.** *Escherichia coli* is an extremely common cause of meningitis in infants. The mortality rate for this infection ranges from 40% to 80% and the majority of survivors have neurologic or developmental abnormalities. Infants are likely to be exposed to the organisms during childbirth. Epidemiologic studies indicate that colonization of the maternal intestinal tract by *E. coli* with the K1 antigen increases during pregnancy. Indeed, most isolates (i.e., approximately 75%) from infants with meningitis have the K1 antigen, the sialic portion of which is similar to the capsular polysaccharide type B of *N. meningitidis*. The mechanisms by which the presence of the K1 antigen predisposes to developing meningitis are unclear. The organisms are rarely identified as the etiologic agent in adult populations with the disease and there is no association with the K1 antigen.

## Cultural Characteristics and Identification

*Escherichia coli* is a motile rod that ferments lactose. The major exceptions to this are the strains of EIEC, which are not motile and either do not ferment lactose or ferment it very slowly. On blood agar, *E. coli* forms round, smooth, convex colonies with a distinct edge. It exhibits a very characteristic iridescent "sheen" on EMB agar. More than 90% of isolates produce ß-glucuronidase, which can readily be tested for by using 4-*methylu*mbelliferyl-ß-glucuronide (MUG) as a sub-

strate. EHEC with the 0157:H7 serotype can be biochemically differentiated from other strains, e.g., they do not use sorbitol and they are negative in the **MUG test**. In addition, new selective media are now available for rapid identification of 0157:H7 isolates. For example, on Rainbow Agar 0157™ (Biolog, Inc., Hayward, CA) this serotype forms black colonies, whereas non-O157 and most nonverotoxin-producing *E. coli* produce blue, purple, violet, or red colonies. Agglutination tests using specific antisera against O, H, and K antigens can be done, but are usually performed only in reference laboratories.

## Antibiotic Susceptibility Characteristics

Antibiotic susceptibility testing is very important because there is a great variation in susceptibility patterns and multiple drug resistance occurs frequently. Resistance to drugs, which is determined by genes present in plasmids (i.e., **R plasmids**), can be readily transmitted from one organism to another. Antibiotics that generally have strong activity against *E. coli,* as well as many other enteric gram-negative rods, include the sulfonamides, ampicillin, cephalosporins, chloramphenicol, tetracyclines, and aminoglycosides. Sulfamethoxazole-trimethoprim (e.g., Bactrim, Spectra) and ciprofloxacin are usually very effective when treatment is started early. Bismuth subsalicylate or the tetracyclines may be used prophylactically to decrease the risk for travelers.

## *KLEBSIELLA-ENTEROBACTER-SERRATIA*

### Organism Characteristics

The organisms in these three genera, unlike the other commonly isolated enteric bacteria, usually produce acetyl-methyl carbinol from dextrose and hence they are positive in the Voges-Proskauer reaction. The most important species involved in human infections are *Klebsiella pneumoniae, Enterobacter aerogenes,* and *S. marcescens. K. pneumoniae* can be isolated from the respiratory tract, as well as the stool, of approximately 5% of healthy persons. *Enterobacter* can be found in the soil, dairy products, water, and sewage. It may also be present in the intestinal tract of humans and animals. *S. marcescens* is ubiquitous in the environment.

### Clinical Significance

*Klebsiella pneumoniae* is responsible for approximately 3% of all bacterial pneumonias (community and hospital acquired) in the United States. In elderly individuals with underlying problems, the disease can be very severe with hemorrhagic necrotizing consolidation of the lungs (lobar pneumonia). The sputum has sometimes been described as "currant jelly" because of its thick, reddish appearance. The infection is often fatal, if not treated promptly and aggressively. The presence of the large gelatinous capsule prevents phagocytosis of the organisms and also inhibits leukocyte migration into involved areas. *K. pneumoniae* can also cause milder forms of respiratory tract infection, most notably bronchitis or bronchopneumonia. Both *K. pneumoniae* and *Klebsiella oxytoca* may cause hospital-acquired infections. *Klebsiella ozaena* and *Klebsiella rhinoscleromatis* can also affect the upper respiratory tract. These two species are endemic in certain parts of eastern Europe, Latin America, southern Asia, and central Africa. Infections with these *Klebsiella* are rare in the United States, but are sometimes noted in immigrants from these areas. *K. ozaena* is associated with a progressive atrophy of the nasal mucosa and a mucopurulent fetid discharge. *K. rhinoscleromatis* produces a destructive granuloma of the nose and pharynx (i.e., rhinoscleroma) that can sometimes result in bony invasion and airway obstruction. *Serratia* infections are relatively common in heroin addicts. This association was first made in San Francisco during the 1970s, when the organisms were isolated from cases of endocarditis and osteomyelitis in this population. *E. aerogenes, Enterobacter agglomerans,* and *Enterobacter cloacae* generally do not cause disease in healthy individuals. *Klebsiella, Serratia,* and *Enterobacter* are significant causes of infections in immunocompromised or otherwise debilitated patients (see section on immunocompromised hosts).

## Cultural Characteristics and Identification

Rapid presumptive identification of *K. pneumoniae* can be made on the basis of its unusually large capsule, large and highly mucoid colonies, lactose fermentation,

and lack of motility. In addition, lysine carboxylase and citrate tests are usually positive. Specific capsular antigens can be determined by capsular swelling tests using antisera. Isolates from respiratory tract infections usually possess K1 and K2 antigens, whereas those from the urinary tract have K1, 8, 9, 10, and 24. More than 70 different K antigens have been identified in *Klebsiella. K. ozaenae* and *K. rhinoscleromatis* are biochemically much less active than *K. pneumoniae. E. aerogenes* is usually motile, has a capsule that is considerably smaller than that of *Klebsiella,* and forms raised, viscous colonies. It is a lactose fermenter that produces gas from glucose and gives positive results for citrate and ornithine decarboxylase. *S. marcescens* ferments lactose very slowly and is motile. It produces DNase, gelatinase, and lipase. *Serratia liquifaciens* and *Serratia rubidaea* can be differentiated from *S. marcescens* by their decarboxylation and sugar fermentation reactions. Some strains of *Serratia* produce a bright red pigment, although isolates from humans usually do not. This unusual property was used as a marker by the U.S. Army in the 1950s to evaluate population susceptibility to aerosolized bacteria. Disclosure of these experiments generated great public controversy and resulted in their termination. In addition, it has been suggested by some individuals that historical reports of "the miraculous appearance of blood" on communion wafers and other foods may be explained by growth of chromogenic strains of *Serratia.*

Table 16-3 shows the typical reaction patterns that are helpful in differentiating among the most common members of this group of organisms.

## Antibiotic Susceptibility Characteristics

Susceptibility to any particular antibiotic is unpredictable and testing should be performed. *Klebsiella* is now among the most resistant of the enteric bacteria.

| | **Klebsiella** | | **Enterobacter** | | **Serratia** |
|---|---|---|---|---|---|
| **Test** | **pneumoniae** | **oxytoca** | **aerogenes** | **cloacae** | **marcescens** |
| Indole | 0 | 99 | 0 | 0 | 1 |
| Lysine decarboxylase | 98 | 99 | 98 | 0 | 99 |
| Ornithine decarboxylase | 0 | 0 | 98 | 96 | 99 |
| Arginine dihydrolase | 0 | 0 | 0 | 97 | 0 |
| Gelatin hydrolysis (22°C) | 0 | 0 | 0 | 0 | 90 |
| Arabinose fermentation | 99 | 98 | 100 | 100 | 0 |

**Table 16–3** ▶ **Tests Used to Differentiate *Klebsiella, Enterobacter,* and *Serratia***

Each number represents the percentage of isolates giving a positive reaction (Farmer, 1995).

There are reports of isolates that are highly resistant to all common antimicrobial agents. Increasing drug resistance of *Klebsiella* in the hospital setting is attributed to acquisition of R plasmids, as well as changes in chromosomal genes. Most isolates of *Enterobacter* are resistant to ampicillin and first-generation cephalosporins. Second- and third-generation cephalosporins may be effective, although the incidence of resistance due to ß-lactamase production is relatively high. *S. marcescens* is frequently resistant to aminoglycosides and penicillins; infections have been successfully treated with third-generation cephalosporins.

## PROTEUS-PROVIDENCIA-MORGANELLA

### Organism Characteristics

These organisms are part of the normal flora of the intestinal tract. They are motile, grow on potassium cyanide (KCN) medium, ferment xylose, and deaminate phenylalanine. The motility of *Proteus* species is especially striking. *Proteus mirabilis, Proteus vulgaris, Providencia rettgeri, Providencia alcalifaciens, Providencia stuartii,* and *Morganella morganii* are the species that are isolated from human infections most often.

### Clinical Significance

*Proteus mirabilis* is a very common cause of urinary tract infections. The urease enzyme produced by the organisms (also *Morganella*) hydrolyzes urea resulting in the release of $CO_2$ and ammonia, causing the urine to become alkaline. The alkalinity of the urine promotes the formation of calculi (kidney stones). These stones may obstruct urinary flow and serve as foci of

persistent infection. Acidification of the urine is rarely accomplished in the presence of the organisms. The urease enzyme in and of itself can also contribute to renal tubule toxicity. In addition, the fimbrae that attach to uroepithelium and the highly motile nature of the organisms facilitate invasion of the urinary tract. Secreted hemolysins may also play a role in virulence. Most other members of these three genera are usually nonpathogenic in healthy individuals. However, they can produce severe disease in debilitated persons (see section on immunocompromised hosts).

### Cultural Characteristics and Identification

The identification of *Proteus* species is facilitated by their lack of lactose fermentation, production of urease, and high motility ("**swarming**"). Because of this latter characteristic, the organisms do not form discrete colonies on ordinary media and other bacteria that may be present are covered by a thin film of *Proteus*. The "swarming" is inhibited when the organisms are grown on a solid medium containing phenylethyl alcohol or on cystine-lactose-electrolyte-deficient (**CLED**) **medium**. *M. morganii*, like *Proteus* species, produces urease, whereas *Providencia* usually does not. Some isolates of *Proteus* and *Providencia* ferment lactose slowly. These and other reactions are summarized in Table 16-4.

### Antibiotic Susceptibility Characteristics

Treatment of *P. mirabilis* infection is frequently successful with penicillins. Although aminoglycosides and cephalosporins are usually effective against the other organisms in this group, resistance is becoming increas-

**Table 16–4 ▶ Tests Used to Differentiate *Proteus, Providencia,* and *Morganella***

| Test | Proteus | | Providencia | | | Morganella |
| | mirabilis | vulgaris | rettgeri | alcalifaciens | stuartii | morganii |
|---|---|---|---|---|---|---|
| Indole | 2* | 98 | 99 | 99 | 98 | 95 |
| Urease | 98 | 95 | 98 | 0 | 30 | 95 |
| Ornithine decarboxylase | 99 | 0 | 0 | 1 | 0 | 95 |
| Gelatin hydrolysis (22°C) | 90 | 91 | 0 | 0 | 0 | 0 |
| D-glucose, gas | 96 | 85 | 10 | 85 | 0 | 90 |
| D-mannitol fermentation | 0 | 0 | 100 | 2 | 10 | 0 |
| Adonitol fermentation | 0 | 0 | 100 | 5 | 98 | 0 |
| L-rhamnose fermentation | 1 | 5 | 70 | 0 | 0 | 0 |
| D-xylose fermentation | 98 | 95 | 10 | 1 | 7 | 0 |

*Each number represents the percentage of isolates giving a positive reaction (Farmer, 1995).

ingly common (especially aminoglycoside resistance in *P. rettgerii* and other indole-positive isolates). Treatment with amikacin, newer ß-lactam antibiotics, and newer quinolones is often required when aminoglycoside-resistant mutants are involved.

## *CITROBACTER*

### Organism Characteristics

*Citrobacter* (previously known as the Bethesda-Ballerup group) is present in the environment, but can also be isolated from the feces of humans and animals. They are opportunists that can infect virtually any body site, but are most often implicated in urinary tract infections and neonatal meningitis. *Citrobacter freundii* and *Citrobacter diversus* are the two most commonly isolated species from clinical specimens.

### Clinical Significance

Clinically significant infections with *Citrobacter* occur primarily in individuals with underlying diseases or other predisposing factors (see section on immunocompromised hosts).

### Cultural Characteristics and Identification

These organisms can be cultured on many of the same media as the other *Enterobacteriaceae*. They are citrate positive (hence the name), motile, ferment lactose slowly or not at all, and most isolates produce a weak urease enzyme that gives positive results in 2 days. *C. freundii* is the only species that produces $H_2S$ from sodium thiosulfate. They can be differentiated from the salmonellae by their inability to decarboxylate lysine. The antigenic structure of the organisms resembles those of the *Salmonella* and *Escherichia;* there is considerable cross-reactivity with respect to the O antigens. Some strains have the Vi antigen of *Salmonella typhi.* Table 16-5 shows the reaction patterns that are most frequently noted for the two common *Citrobacter* species.

### Antibiotic Susceptibility Characteristics

Aminoglycosides, chloramphenicol, and tetracycline are effective against most isolates. Resistant strains are frequently found in patients who have been hospitalized for extended periods of time or who have previously received antibiotic therapy. *C. freundii* and *C. diversus* usually exhibit different antibiotic susceptibility patterns. The former are frequently susceptible to carbenicillin, but not to cephalothin, whereas the latter are unaffected by carbenicillin and are sensitive to cephalothin. Overall, resistance to antibiotics is seen most frequently with *C. freundii.*

## *YERSINIA*

### Organism Characteristics

The *Yersinia* are gram-negative rods with a striking bipolar pattern of staining. Most species have animals as their natural hosts. They are usually transmitted to humans by an insect vector or by ingestion of contaminated food or water. They all possess LPS, which has endotoxin activity when released from disrupted cells. The most important species affecting humans are *Yersinia pestis, Yersinia enterocolitica,* and *Yersinia pseudotuberculosis.*

*Yersinia pestis* is the cause of **plague** (previously called the "black death" and pestilence), a devastating disease that has killed millions of people throughout history. In 14th century Europe, more than 25 million people (one-third of the population) died of the disease within a 4-year period. Rodents (mice, rats, gerbils, skunks, moles, etc.) and other animals are the primary reservoirs for the organisms. Sylvatic (wild) plague exists in at least 13 states of the western portion of the United States. Other endemic areas of the world include India, Vietnam, Africa, South America, and Mexico. In animals, the organisms produce septicemia, bacteremia, and death. The major vector is the flea (especially *Xenopsylla cheopsis* or the rat flea), a blood-sucking insect that transmits *Y. pestis* from one host to another by its bite. Human-to-human transmission is also possible via aerosols and the human flea (*Pulex irritans*).

The endotoxin of the organisms, although similar to that of other *Enterobacteriaceae,* has 50 to 100 times more potent pathophysiologic effects in the body. The endotoxin (possibly together with the murine exotoxin) is thought to be largely responsible for the bluish black skin of plague victims. Studies conducted by United States military personnel in Vietnam indicate that not all people who are infected develop the disease. Approxi-

| Table 16–5 ▶ Tests Used to Differentiate *Citrobacter* Species | | |
|---|---|---|
| **Test** | **C. freundii** | **C. diversus** |
| Indole | 33 | 99 |
| Hydrogen sulfide ($H_2S$) | 78 | 0 |
| Ornithine decarboxylase | 0 | 99 |
| Adonitol fermentation | 0 | 99 |
| Growth in potassium cyanide (KCN) | 89 | 0 |

Each number represents the percentage of isolates giving a positive reaction (Farmer, 1995).

mately 10% of close family members of patients with plague carried the organisms in the nasopharynx for long periods of time and had no history of the disease.

*Yersinia enterocolitica* and *Y. pseudotuberculosis* are found in the intestinal tract of many animals including rodents, sheep, cattle, dogs, and cats. *Y. pseudotuberculosis* can also be isolated from birds. Ingestion of materials contaminated with the feces of the animals can result in diarrhea and **mesenteric adenitis**.

## Clinical Significance

The symptoms of bubonic plague appear after an incubation period of approximately 2 to 7 days. On entry into the body, *Y. pestis* multiplies both intra- and extracellularly and is rapidly transported via the lymphatics to the lymph nodes. An intense inflammatory response occurs in the nodes, causing them to become greatly enlarged (hence the designation of "buboes" and bubonic plague). The lymph nodes, usually in the groin or axillary region, become hemorrhagic, necrotic, and painful. Systemic symptoms (i.e., vomiting and diarrhea) usually occur at the time of sepsis. Eventually, the organisms reach the blood circulation and become widely disseminated. Hemorrhagic lesions may appear in virtually all parts of the body. Meningitis and pneumonia are among the most serious complications. Disseminated intravascular coagulation, hypotension, kidney shutdown, and cardiac failure can result in death. The fatality rate is approximately 50%, if untreated.

Pneumonic plague can occur after inhalation of the organisms in respiratory droplets from a coughing patient with plague or as the result of dissemination from another site. This form of plague is highly contagious. The lungs are heavy, frothy, and filled with fluid. Patients may become cyanotic because of great breathing difficulty. Respiratory symptoms may not be apparent until the day of death. The fatality rate for untreated pneumonic plague approaches 100% within 3 days.

Most countries of the world consider plague as a quarantinable disease. Ships or airplanes arriving with known or suspected plague cases (human or animal) are disinfected. In the United States all patients suspected of having plague, either bubonic or pneumonic, are isolated for at least 72 hours while treatment proceeds. A formalin-inactivated vaccine, although not very effective, is licensed for use in persons at high risk, such as technicians working with antibiotic-resistant strains in research laboratories, public health officials engaged in field operations involving wild animals in plague-infested areas, and travelers to endemic regions. Control of sylvatic plague is done with the use of insecticides, followed by rodent extermination procedures.

Ingestion of a large number of either *Y. enterocolitica* or *Y. pseudotuberculosis* can result in inflammation and ulceration of the intestinal mucosa, especially in the ileum. After an incubation period of 5 to 10 days, fever and diarrhea (watery or bloody) may occur. The organisms may progress further to the mesenteric lymph nodes and cause mesenteric adenitis. Abdominal pain can be very severe and simulate acute appendicitis because of its location in the right lower quadrant. Some patients may develop reactive arthritis and Reiter's syndrome (urethritis and conjunctivitis), possibly as the result of an immunologic response against the organisms. These types of inflammatory conditions can also occur with other enteric bacteria, such as *Salmonella, Shigella,* and *Campylobacter.*

## Cultural Characteristics and Identification

Rapid identification of *Yersinia* is critical in patients suspected of being exposed to the plague bacillus, so that treatment can be promptly initiated. The organisms are short, plump, nonmotile gram-negative rods that exhibit bipolar staining. The bipolarity is especially striking with Wayson's stain but can also be seen with Wright-Giemsa. Definitive identification is done by immuno-fluorescence staining of specimens taken directly from the patient (i.e., aspirates of lymph nodes, blood, sputum, and cerebrospinal fluid). All materials are cultured on blood agar, MacConkey agar, and in infusion broth. Best growth is obtained at 30°C in media containing blood or tissue fluids. Growth is slow at 37°C, although blood cultures may be positive within one day. Colonies are initially gray and viscous, but become rough and irregular after passage. Biochemical tests may be done for confirmation. The organisms do not ferment lactose and exhibit little metabolic activity compared to most other *Enterobacteriaceae.* They produce catalase, but are oxidase negative. An antibody titer of 1:16 or greater in a nonimmunized individual suggests infection with *Y. pestis.* A four-fold or greater increase in the titer in early and convalescent specimens confirms the diagnosis. All clinical samples and cultures from possible cases of plague should be considered highly infectious and should be handled with great caution.

Gram staining of stool specimens, blood, or material obtained during surgical exploration are generally not helpful for *Y. enterocolitica* and *Y. pseudotuberculosis.* Samples of feces and rectal swabs are first put into buffered saline at pH 7.6 and incubated at 4°C for 2 to 4 weeks to increase the small number of organisms that may be there. This procedure, known as "cold enrichment," kills most other bacteria that are present in the intestinal tract. Subsequent inoculation of MacConkey agar and other media may then be done. Serologic assays for antibodies may show a rise in titer. However, vibrios, brucellae, and salmonellae induce cross-reactive antibodies. Typical reaction patterns of *Yersinia* species are shown in Table 16-6.

**Table 16–6** ▶ Tests Used to Differentiate *Yersinia* Species

| Test | *Y. pestis* | *Y. enterocolitica* | *Y. pseudotuberculosis* |
|---|---|---|---|
| Indole | 0 | 50 | 0 |
| Urease | 5 | 75 | 95 |
| Ornithine decarboxylase | 0 | 95 | 0 |
| Sucrose fermentation | 0 | 95 | 0 |
| D-sorbitol fermentation | 50 | 99 | 0 |
| L-arabinose fermentation | 100 | 98 | 50 |

Each number represents the percentage of isolates giving a positive reaction (Farmer, 1995).

## Antibiotic Susceptibility Characteristics

Time is critical in the treatment of plague. Streptomycin is highly effective against *Y. pestis* and is the drug of choice. For individuals who cannot tolerate streptomycin, tetracycline and kanamycin are effective alternative drugs. Drug-resistant mutants have not been isolated from natural infections in the United States. However, resistant strains have been recently reported in several countries in the Far East. The other *Yersinia* species are usually susceptible to aminoglycosides, tetracycline, chloramphenicol, sulfamethoxazole-trimethoprim, piperacillin, third-generation cephalosporins, and fluoroquinolones. Carbenicillin, ampicillin, and first-generation cephalosporins are usually ineffective. In cases of sepsis, third-generation cephalosporins or a fluoroquinalone are used, either alone or in combination with other drugs. Surgical exploration is often performed when the differential diagnosis suggests either appendicitis or mesenteric adenitis (unless there is a cluster of cases with *Yersinia* infection).

## SALMONELLA

## Organism Characteristics

Many of the salmonellae are found naturally in the intestinal tract of animals such as birds, cattle, and rodents. Some of them (e.g., *S. typhi*), however, are present primarily in humans. The members of this genus are the most common cause of diarrhea (i.e., **enterocolitis**) due to ingestion of foods contaminated by animals or animal products. Human infection has been traced to poultry, dried or frozen eggs, dairy products (especially ice cream, cheese, and custard), shellfish from contaminated waters, beef, pork, and other foods. Explosive epidemics of salmonellosis have occurred because of water contaminated with the feces of infected animals or humans. Cases of enteritis have also been linked to marijuana and other illegal drugs,

pets (e.g., turtles, cats, and dogs), and to animal dyes used in foods and cosmetics. Unidentified human carriers (especially food handlers) who are excreting the organisms in the stool are also an important reservoir for the organisms. Relatively few salmonellae are responsible for **enteric fever (typhoid fever)** and systemic disease. The total number of documented *Salmonella* infections in the United States is undoubtedly low. It is believed that only 1% to 5% of cases are actually detected and reported.

The classification of these organisms is complex. There are more than 2,000 different variants based on their O, capsular Vi, and H antigens, which may be biphasic (i.e., in phase 1 or phase 2). Unfortunately, each new serotype has been given a name, as if it were a new and separate species. Several classification schemes have been proposed over the years in attempts to simplify the nomenclature. Recent genetic analyses indicate that the DNA of virtually all isolates is identical. Because of this, it has been suggested that there should be only a single species (i.e., *S. enterica*). However, this suggestion has not gained wide acceptance. Most experts continue to refer to the clinically most significant organisms by their more familiar names, e.g., *S. typhi*, *Salmonella paratyphi* A, and *Salmonella choleraesuis*.

## Clinical Significance

The salmonellae are always considered to be pathogenic, although many subclinical infections undoubtedly occur. Enteric fever (typhoid fever), the most severe clinical manifestation of infection, is caused primarily by *S. typhi*. These organisms, as well as some of the other salmonellae, can invade nonphagocytic cells, thereby evading the host's immune defenses. In addition, unlike the nontyphoidal members of the genus, *S. typhi* are not killed by macrophages and can even multiply within them. After ingestion, the organisms that survive the acidity of the stomach reach the small intestine, infect the Peyer's patches (collections of lymphoid tissue), and enter the lymphatic system. From there they are disseminated to many parts of the body (including, again, the intestinal tract) via the peripheral blood circulation. This provokes an inflammatory response in the gallbladder, lungs, periosteum, and other organs. Focal hemorrhagic lesions may appear in the intestinal lumen and liver. The patient experiences a gradual rise in temperature, which eventually plateaus at about 39° to 40°C. The fever may persist for 4 to 8 weeks in untreated cases. Headache, bradycardia, and myalgia also occur after an incubation period of approximately 10 to 14 days. Constipation is followed by bloody diarrhea. Hepatosplenomegaly (enlargement of the liver and spleen) is present in many patients. In rare cases, a pinkish skin rash ("rose spots") appears on the abdomen and trunk during the time of the fever. *S. paratyphi* can cause a similar syndrome, but the disease is usually much milder (see Figure 16-2).

*Salmonella* can sometimes invade the bloodstream (**bacteremia**, septicemia) very early after ingestion. This results in rapid dissemination of the organisms, a spiking fever, and the formation of focal lesions in the lungs, bones, meninges, and other parts of the body. Intestinal manifestations are usually absent. The incubation time before symptoms appear is variable. In the United States, *Salmonella choleraesuis* is the one that is most often isolated from this type of infection, although other serotypes can also be involved.

The development of enterocolitis (old name is "gastroenteritis") is the most common result of infection with the salmonellae. Although virtually any of the more than 2,000 serotypes can cause this illness, *S. typhimurium* is most prevalent in the United States. Within 8 to 48 hours after ingestion, there is an abrupt onset of nausea, vomiting, headache, low-grade fever, and diarrhea. Inflammatory lesions may be present in the intestinal tract, but stool specimens have few or no leukocytes. The great majority of cases are self-limiting and resolve without treatment within 2 to 3 days. There is evidence that the diarrhea-causing *Salmonella* produce a cholera-like toxin that activates cAMP and induces production of inflammatory mediators, which may affect electrolyte and fluid transport across cell membranes. However, these serotypes are cleared fairly rapidly from the body by phagocytic cells, and therefore the illness is usually self-limiting.

After recovery, an individual may asymptomatically carry and excrete the organisms for long periods of time in the stool or, less often, in the urine. "Typhoid Mary" (i.e., Mary Mallon, a cook in Oyster Bay, NY, in the early 1900s), the first documented carrier of *S. typhi*, was responsible for several outbreaks of enteric fever and a number of deaths before she was apprehended by public health authorities for the last time and put into isolation. Approximately 3% of patients who have recovered from the disease become permanent carriers, unless properly treated. The organisms tend to persist in the gallbladder (especially in the presence of gallstones) and biliary tract, where bile provides a good culture medium for the organisms. Treatment of typhoid carriers consists of antibiotic therapy, removal of gallstones, and cholecystectomy (surgical removal of gallbladder).

An individual can experience more than one episode of salmonellosis and relapses are possible. Reinfection generally results in less severe disease. Some degree of cross-protective immunity may be generated after infection with *S. typhi* and *S. paratyphi*. The presence of secretory IgA is thought to prevent attachment of the organisms to the intestinal epithelium.

There are at least three vaccines available for *S. typhi*, none of which is routinely used in the United States. One of these is an acetone-killed suspension of the bacteria. It induces partial immunity against infection with a small dose of the organisms. Another vaccine consists of a live, attenuated strain of *S. typhi*. This is an oral preparation that confers significant protection and is used in areas where the organisms are endemic. A purified Vi polysaccharide vaccine may be useful in older children and adults. The efficacy of these vaccines ranges from 60% to 80%.

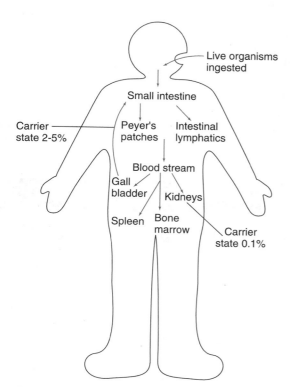

**FIGURE 16-2** Progression of *Salmonella typhi* infection in a case of typhoid fever. (Original diagram was conceived by Leonard Bullas, Ph.D., Active Emeritus Professor at Loma Linda University School of Medicine, Loma Linda, CA; reproduced with permission.)

## Cultural Characteristics and Identification

Selenite F or tetrathionate broth are enrichment media that are frequently used to increase the number of salmonellae in stool specimens. They both allow growth of the salmonellae, but they are inhibitory to most other enteric bacteria. After a 1- to 2-day incubation in an enrichment medium, other types of media can then be inoculated. Differential media such as EMB, deoxycholate, or MacConkey are frequently used. These media are somewhat inhibitory to gram-positive bacteria and will also permit rapid identification of gram-negative rods that do not ferment lactose. SS (*Salmonella-Shigella*) agar, Hektoen enteric agar, and deoxycholate-citrate agar are selective media that favor the growth of salmonellae and shigellae compared to other enteric organisms. *S. typhi,* as well as many other salmonellae, produce $H_2S$ and, thus form black colonies on media containing bismuth sulfite. The results from a series of biochemical tests and from slide agglutination assays performed on cultured organisms are used to help identify isolates (see Table 16-7).

The organisms can be recovered from the blood during the first week after infection in cases of enteric fever and bacteremia. Stool cultures are usually positive during the first week of enterocolitis and during the second to third weeks of enteric fever. Blood and stool specimens should be taken repeatedly to increase the likelihood of positive cultures. The bone marrow may give positive results when other sites are negative. This is presumably due to the fact that the organisms are capable of multiplying within the monocyte/macrophage cells of the marrow. Urine specimens may also be useful in some cases. Carriers may be identified by isolating salmonellae from specimens of duodenal drainage.

Serum agglutinins against the organisms usually appear 2 to 3 weeks after infection. However, they may exhibit some cross-reactivity with other members of the *Enterobacteriaceae.* The **Widal test** is the standard tube agglutination assay used to detect the presence of antibodies. Serum samples should be obtained 7 to 10 days apart during the course of the illness. A high ($\geq$1:160) or rising titer against certain O antigens suggests that infection with salmonellae is ongoing. In contrast, a high anti-H antibody titer suggests either past immunization or past infection (see Figure 16-3).

## Antibiotic Susceptibility Characteristics

Most *Salmonella* infections (i.e., enterocolitis) are self-limiting and do not require treatment. Neonates with diarrhea, however, are an important exception. Enteric fevers and bacteremias with focal lesions should always be treated. Ampicillin, sulfamethoxazole-trimethoprim, third-generation cephalosporins, and chloramphenicol are usually effective against most salmonellae. Antibiotic susceptibility tests, however, should be performed because isolates that are resistant to multiple drugs are becoming increasingly common. The first well-documented epidemic of multiple drug resistant bacteria occurred in Mexico in the early 1970s. There were more than 100,000 confirmed cases of typhoid fever due to *S. typhi* that was resistant to chloramphenicol, ampicillin, streptomycin, and sulfonamide. This same pattern of resistance had been previously observed in Central America, but in *Shigella dysenteriae*. It was speculated that resistance genes had been transferred from the *Shigella* to the *Salmonella*. Nontyphoidal *Salmonella* that are resistant to several antibiotics have caused outbreaks of diarrhea involving as many as 100,000 people in the United States. In Europe and

### Table 16–7  ▶  Tests Used to Differentiate Clinically Significant *Salmonella*

| Test | S. typhi | S. paratyphi A | S. choleraesuis | Most Other Serotypes |
|---|---|---|---|---|
| Citrate | 0 | 0 | 25 | 95 |
| Hydrogen sulfide | 97 | 10 | 50 | 95 |
| Lysine decarboxylase | 98 | 0 | 95 | 98 |
| Ornithine decarboxylase | 0 | 95 | 100 | 97 |
| D-glucose, gas | 0 | 99 | 95 | 96 |
| Dulcitol fermentation | 0 | 90 | 5 | 96 |
| L-arabinose fermentation | 2 | 100 | 0 | 99 |
| L-rhamnose fermentation | 0 | 100 | 100 | 95 |
| Trehalose fermentation | 100 | 100 | 0 | 99 |

Each number represents the percentage of isolates giving a positive reaction (Farmer, 1995).

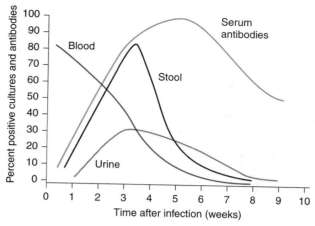

**FIGURE 16-3** Frequency of *Salmonella typhi* isolation from cultures of blood, stool, and urine during the course of typhoid fever. The rise and fall of specific serum antibodies is also shown. Incubation period is approximately one week.

Asia, there are now reports of salmonellae that produce modified ß-lactamases. Some of these organisms are treatable only with fluoroquinolones. The correct choice of an antibiotic is important because some of the drugs used in the past have been known to prolong the length of time that symptoms are present and extend the time of shedding. Fluid and electrolyte replacement should be initiated in cases of severe diarrhea. Since the introduction of effective antibiotic therapy for enteric fever, the mortality rate has dropped to about 1% or less in the United States. The rate of relapse, however, has significantly increased. This latter observation may be the result of aborted induction of cell-mediated immunity by early and highly effective treatment. A few surviving intracellular organisms may continue to multiply and cause the relapse.

## *SHIGELLA*

### Organism Characteristics

DNA hybridization studies have recently shown that the shigellae are identical to *Escherichia*. However, the majority consensus is that the name *Shigella* be retained for those isolates that can be biochemically distinguished from *E. coli*. In addition, unlike *E. coli,* these organisms are highly adapted to the intestinal tract of humans, although they may occasionally be isolated from the stool of nonhuman primates. These organisms cause a disease known as bacillary **dysentery**. They are readily transmitted from one individual to another by the four "Fs"—food, fingers, feces, and flies. In addition, the bacilli can remain viable in water supplies for up to 6 months. The number of organisms needed to induce infection is very small (i.e., several hundred to several thousand). Crowded, substandard sanitary conditions promote spread of the organisms, although outbreaks have also been reported on luxury cruise ships. Most cases of shigellosis in the United States occur in children under the age of 10 years. Prevention of infection relies partly on close regulation of water supplies, food, and milk, proper sewage disposal, and control of flies. Treatment of subclinical cases and carriers is also important. The shigellae have more than 40 somatic O antigens. The four pathogenic species are *Shigella dysenteriae* (serotype A), *Shigella flexneri* (serotype B), *Shigella boydii* (serotype C), and *Shigella sonnei* (serotype D). The latter species is the one that is isolated most often in the United States and other industrialized countries. It tends to cause relatively mild illness, whereas disease due to *S. dysenteriae* is the most severe.

### Clinical Significance

After ingestion of *Shigella* species, the organisms invade the mucosal epithelial cells (i.e., the M cells) of the large intestine and terminal ileum. They escape from the phagocytic vacuole to the cytoplasm, multiply there, and spread to other cells in the near vicinity. Microabscesses, bleeding, necrosis, and ulceration of the mucous layers leads to the formation of a "pseudomembrane." The newly formed membrane consists of the bacteria, fibrin, leukocytes, and dead cell debris. As the disease resolves, scar tissue forms in the affected areas of the intestinal wall. The organisms themselves almost never progress very far from their initial site of multiplication and bacteremia is rare. Symptoms, including severe abdominal pain and fever, appear soon after infection (i.e., usually in 1–2 days). Diarrhea is initially watery, but soon contains mucus and blood due to increasing involvement of the colon and ileum. More than 50% of cases in adults resolve in 2 to 5 days without treatment. In children and the elderly, the infection is likely to be more severe, resulting in dehydration, acidosis, and possibly death.

*Shigella dysenteriae* type 1 (seen mostly in developing countries) causes the most severe disease. In addition to the endotoxin that all shigellae have, it produces a heat-labile exotoxin that is sometimes referred to as **Shiga toxin**. This exotoxin is a protein with enzymatic activity that affects not only the gut, but also the central nervous system. It inactivates the 60S ribosomal subunit in mammalian cells, thereby inhibiting protein synthesis. Its effects on the intestinal tract result in grossly bloody diarrhea, thus resembling the verotoxin of *E. coli*. Its neurotoxic effects can lead to meningismus (pain in the meningeocortical region of the brain; excitation followed by depression of the cortex) and coma. Interestingly, infection with *Shigella flexneri* or *Shigella sonnei* induces antitoxin antibodies that are capable of neutralizing the Shiga toxin in vitro.

## Cultural Characteristics and Identification

Although these organisms are facultative anaerobes, best growth is obtained under aerobic conditions. Specimens of stool, flecks of mucus, and rectal swabs are inoculated onto differential media such as MacConkey or EMB agar and on selective media (Hektoen or SS agar). The nonmotile organisms form transparent, round colonies, do not ferment lactose, and do not produce $H_2S$. All of them, except *S. dysenteriae,* ferment mannitol. Only *S. sonnei* has the ornithine decarboxylase enzyme. Most isolates can produce acid from carbohydrates, but usually not gas. Additional biochemical tests (e.g., KIA and multitest systems) and slide agglutination tests using specific antisera are performed. Assays for serum antibodies are usually not done, although serial samples may show an increase in titer during illness. Healthy individuals often have antibodies against several *Shigella* species. Table 16-8 summarizes commonly used laboratory tests for differentiating the shigellae.

## Antibiotic Susceptibility Characteristics

Many cases of shigellosis are self-limiting. A number of antibiotics, including ciprofloxacin, ampicillin, chloramphenicol, tetracycline, and sulfamethoxazole-trimethoprim, can decrease the severity of symptoms and the period of infectivity to other individuals. The 4-fluoroquinolones (the most reliably effective drugs) have been limited by the Food and Drug Administration for use only in persons over the age of 17 years because of the potential for joint damage in younger children. In addition, multidrug resistance due to transfer of plasmids is widespread. This problem is especially serious in developing countries where *S. dysenteriae* type 1 is prevalent. Prophylactic therapy has been attempted in military personnel, but resistant strains emerge rapidly.

## OTHER *ENTEROBACTERIACEAE*

### *Edwardsiella*

The *Edwardsiella* are motile rods that produce indole, gas from glucose fermentation, $H_2S$, lysine decarboxylase, and ornithine decarboxylase. The *Edwardsiella* genus includes *E. tarda, E. hoshinae, E. ictaluri,* and other species. Human disease, usually manifested as a salmonella-like enterocolitis, is due almost exclusively to *E. tarda.* The watery diarrhea usually lasts for several days and may be accompanied by vomiting and low-grade fever. Its pathogenic properties resemble those of the salmonellae in that it can also invade through the intestinal epithelium and produce systemic disease. In rare instances it has been associated with bacteremia, liver abscesses, meningitis, sepsis, and wound infections. A good response is achieved with many of the antibiotics commonly used for other *Enterobacteriaceae.* Treatment for uncomplicated enterocolitis is usually not indicated. The 'tarda' species designation reflects the fact that these organisms do not ferment lactose and are usually negative in routine tests that are not mentioned above.

### *Hafnia*

Organisms within the *Hafnia* genus are closely related to *Enterobacter* (i.e., *Hafnia* was previously known as *Enterobacter hafnia*). *Hafnia alvei* is the only species designation. It has been found in drinking water, fish farm water, and the intestines of fish and rabbits. In addition, it has been implicated as the etiologic agent in cases of diarrhea. Human infections, however, are infrequent and are seen almost exclusively in the hospital setting. The great majority of isolates are motile, indole negative, and Voges-Proskauer reaction positive (at 22°C). The organisms produce gas from glucose fermentation, urease, and the carboxylase enzymes for lysine and ornithine, but not for arginine. More than 90% of isolates are positive in the *o*-nitrophenyl-D-galactopyranoside (ONPG) test. Susceptibility to various antibiotics is similar to that of *Enterobacter.*

## SPECIAL CONSIDERATIONS FOR IMMUNOCOMPROMISED HOSTS

Although not all hospitalized patients are immunocompromised, approximately 5% to 10% of those in acute care institutions in the United States acquire an infection that was not originally present or was not incubating at the time of admission. This translates into

| Test | Serotypes A, B, and C (*S. dysenteriae*, *S. flexneri*, and *S. boydii*) | Serotype D (*S. sonnei*) |
|---|---|---|
| Indole | 50 | 0 |
| Lactose fermentation | 0 | 2 |
| L-arabinose fermentation | 60 | 95 |
| L-rhamnose fermentation | 5 | 75 |
| Ornithine decarboxylase | 1 | 98 |
| ONPG test | 2 | 90 |

**Table 16–8** ► **Tests Used to Differentiate the *Shigellae***

Each number represents the percentage of isolates giving a positive result (Farmer, 1995).

ONPG, *o*-nitrophenyl-D-galactopyranoside. Test detects the presence of ß-galactosidase.

more than 2 million cases of nosocomial infections each year. Urinary tract infections, followed by infections of the respiratory tract (pneumonias) and surgical wounds, are the most common. Prevalent use of antibiotics in hospitals leads to the emergence of many drug-resistant strains, resulting in significant mortality and morbidity. Gram-negative rods of the *Enterobacteriaceae* family are among the most frequently identified organisms.

*Escherichia coli* remains the single most common microorganism isolated from nosocomial infections, especially those involving the urinary tract. Use of urinary catheters greatly increases the risk for infection with enteric organisms in general. *E. coli* accounts for 5% to 10% of nosocomial pneumonias and is prevalent in medical device-related, as well as sporadic bacteremias. In debilitated persons, *E. coli* can cause numerous other types of infections including sinusitis, thrombophlebitis, osteomyelitis, endocarditis, peritonitis, septic arthritis, suppurative thyroiditis, endophthalmitis, and abscesses of the brain, liver and intra-abdominal region. Epidemic infantile diarrhea due to certain serotypes of EPEC in newborn nurseries is a significant problem. Newborns are especially susceptible because they do not yet have a fully matured immune system. The infection may be exacerbated in premature infants and in those with underlying diseases (i.e., those in special care nurseries). Diarrhea in very young infants can be especially severe because they have immature homeostatic mechanisms and limited reserves of fluid and electrolytes. Otitis media, pneumonia, and bacteremia are relatively common complications. *E. coli* infection is relatively prevalent among oncology patients, especially those with persistent granulocytopenia (due to chemotherapeutic drugs and radiotherapy) and cancers of immune system cells (e.g., acute leukemias and chronic lymphocytic leukemias). Individuals with diabetes mellitus have a substantially increased incidence of *E. coli* bacteriuria.

*Klebsiella pneumoniae* accounts for approximately 8% of all bacterial nosocomial infections in the United States. The organisms are most frequently isolated from infections of the urinary tract, lower respiratory tract, biliary tract, and surgical wounds (more or less in decreasing order of frequency). Many isolates from hospitalized patients are resistant to multiple drugs and susceptibility testing is required for optimal therapy. The other *Klebsiella* species are significantly less common in nosocomial infections.

*Enterobacter* species rarely cause primary infections in healthy individuals. They frequently colonize hospitalized patients and are easily spread from one patient to another by medical personnel who do not practice appropriate aseptic techniques (e.g., handwashing). These organisms have now replaced *K. pneumoniae* as the third most common gram-negative isolate from nosocomial infections. They are often recovered from burn, wound, urinary, and respiratory tract infections.

In the 1970s *E. cloacea* and *E. agglomerans* were associated with a very large epidemic involving intravenous lines in 25 different hospitals. *E. cloacea,* however, is the predominant species within this genus.

*Serratia* has been known as an opportunistic pathogen since the 1960s. It has been demonstrated that, in the hospital setting, these organisms differ from other *Enterobacteriaceae* in that they tend to colonize the urinary and respiratory tracts of patients, rather than the gastrointestinal tract. Indeed, over the last decade or more, *S. marcesens* has become increasingly common in hospital-acquired infections in these two organ systems. An increase in the incidence of bacteremias due to the organisms has also been recently reported. Bacteremias in oncology patients have been traced to contaminated chemotherapeutic drugs that are given intravenously. Many other nosocomial cases have been associated with urinary, intraperitoneal, and intravenous catheters.

*Proteus* species are implicated in many urinary tract infections, wound infections, pneumonias, and septicemias in debilitated patients. In the past, several large outbreaks of hospital-acquired urinary tract infections due to highly drug resistant *P. rettgeri* have been reported. The major reservoir of the organisms is often the gastrointestinal tract of antibiotic-treated patients. Several studies indicate that *P. stuartii* is the most common species isolated from bacteremias in nursing home patients with indwelling catheters.

Although *Citrobacter* is a relatively uncommon isolate, it can produce severe urinary and respiratory tract disease in the hospital setting. Endocarditis and bacteremia have also been reported. In the latter case, the mortality rate is very high and the organisms are usually present as part of a mixed flora. *C. diversus* can cause meningitis and brain abscesses in neonates. Meningitic strains have been shown to express a unique protein on their outer membrane, which may be associated with virulence.

The incidence of shigellosis is increased in patients with acquired immunodeficiency syndrome (AIDS), due to the human immunodeficiency virus type-1 (HIV-1), compared to the general population. *S. flexneri* is the most commonly isolated species in the genus. The dysentery is often described as particularly severe, persistent, or both. Bacteremia, which occurs only rarely in immunocompetent adults with *Shigella,* is seen in up to 50% of persons with HIV-1 infection. HIV-infected individuals also have increased incidence of *Salmonella* infection, with *S. typhimurium,* followed by *S. enteritidis* and *S. dublin,* being the most common serotypes in the United States. In countries where *S. typhi* is prevalent, HIV infection results in increased risk for disease due to this pathogen as well. Nonspecific symptoms, such as fever, fatigue, weight loss, and anorexia may be present for several weeks before the patient seeks medical attention. Septicemia and bacteremia occur in a high percentage of cases and many organ systems may be involved in this high-risk population. Diagnosis is usually made by culturing the organisms from the blood or stool. Most isolates are susceptible to the same antibiotics that are commonly used to treat *Salmonella* infections and 2 to 3 weeks of parenteral therapy is usually effective. Recurrent *Salmonella* sep-

ticemia has been listed as an AIDS-defining condition by the CDC since 1987. Relapse of both shigellosis and salmonellosis occurs frequently after treatment and chronic therapy with a well-tolerated oral agent often needs to be initiated. Recurrence apparently results because clearance of the organisms is incomplete due to impaired cell-mediated immunity.

# SUMMARY

▶ The "enterics" consist of a large group of gram-negative rods, most of which belong in the *Enterobacteriaceae* family. Most do not cause disease in healthy individuals; some, however, are considered to be overt pathogens. Major types of infections associated with these organisms are diarrhea, urinary tract infections, and bacteremia.

▶ Classification is largely based on the antigenic structure. There are R (polysaccharides, non-specific), O (polysaccharides, highly specific), flagellar or H (protein), and capsular (K and Vi) antigens. Lipopolysaccharide (LPS, endotoxin) sticks out from the cell wall; it consists of lipid A (toxic) and the R and O antigens. LPS induces numerous pathophysiologic effects (indirectly via the induction of tumor necrosis factor-$\alpha$ and interleukin-1), including hypotension, shock, and disseminated intravascular coagulation.

▶ Pathogenic *Escherichia coli* can cause urinary tract infections, traveler's diarrhea, infantile diarrhea, hemorrhagic colitis, and hemolytic uremic syndrome, and neonatal meningitis. The organisms produce at least two enterotoxins: the heat-labile and heat-stable toxins that lead to loss of fluid from the intestinal tract. *E. coli* is the most common cause of nosocomial infections.

▶ *Klebsiella pneumoniae* can be found in the intestinal and respiratory tracts of humans. It has a large gelatinous capsule and is the cause of acute bacterial pneumonia, which can be very severe in the elderly. *Enterobacter* is very similar to *E. coli*, but can be differentiated from it on the basis of biochemical reactions. *Serratia marcescens* is an opportunist found in the environment. It produces a bright red pigment. It has been implicated in septicemia, cellulitis, and urinary tract and other types of infections.

▶ *Proteus, Providencia,* and *Morganella* are closely related opportunistic organisms that are occasionally found in the colon. *Proteus* species are unusual in that they have "swarming" motility. In addition, they produce urease, which facilitates the formation of kidney stones. *Proteus mirabilis* is the most common cause of urinary tract infections within this group.

▶ *Yersinia pestis,* a small gram-negative coccobacillus with bipolar staining, is the cause of plague. The organisms are transmitted primarily by flea bite, although aerosol transmission is possible. Bubonic plague is characterized by high fever and greatly enlarged lymph nodes ("bubos"). Pneumonic plague occurs most frequently as the result of dissemination from another site. Plague is highly contagious and death is almost certain once symptoms appear, if untreated.

▶ The genus *Salmonella* consists of a huge number of serotypes. These organisms cause three types of infections: typhoid fever, septicemia, and enterocolitis (most common clinical manifestation). *Salmonella typhi,* the cause of typhoid fever, multiplies in Peyer's patches and disseminates via the blood. Typhoid fever is characterized by early constipation and, later, bloody diarrhea. Carriers present a major obstacle in eradicating the disease.

▶ *Shigella* is highly infectious, but never invades blood circulation. The organisms are associated with crowding and unsanitary conditions. Shigellosis is a bacillary dysentery characterized by inflammation, sloughing of cells and mucus, and rectal spasms. *S. dysenteriae* can produce a potent exotoxin that has enter- and neurotoxic effects.

▶ Isolation of enteric gram-negative rods is usually accomplished with the use of differential media such as EMB and MacConkey agar. Further identification is largely based on a battery of biochemical tests including lactose, motility, indol, Voges-Proskauer, methyl red, citrate, urease, phenylalanine deaminase, and $H_2S$. Rapid identification is possible with the use of commercially available multitest identification systems. Kligler's iron agar (KIA) and triple sugar iron (TSI) agar slants are especially useful in detecting the salmonellae and shigellae.

▶ Antibiotic susceptibility testing is critical for most of these organisms because there is great variation among different isolates and drug resistance is increasingly common. Antibiotics that may be effective include sulfonamides, ampicillin, cephalosporins, chloramphenicol, tetracyclines, and aminoglycosides.

## CASE STUDY 1: SEVERE DIARRHEA DUE TO ENTEROHEMORRHAGIC *E. COLI*

A previously healthy 9-year-old boy was awakened by excruciating abdominal cramps, nausea, and copious watery diarrhea every 30 to 60 minutes. He was brought to the emergency room later that evening when it appeared that there was bright red blood in his stool. Because of the severe nature of the illness, he was admitted to the hospital. The boy had no known contact with other persons with diarrhea and no history of recent travel outside of the United States. Symptoms appeared 24 hours after eating a hamburger at the local fast-food restaurant. It was determined that the patient had an elevated white blood cell count, but no fever. Erythrocytes, but no leukocytes, were found in the stool. Edema, erythema, and exudation were observed in the wall of the ascending and transverse colon during sigmoidoscopy; ulcers and pseudomembranes were not noted. There was concern that the infection may progress to hemolytic uremic syndrome, but urine tests were repeatedly normal. Routine cultures of stool revealed no *Salmonella*, *Shigella*, *Yersinia*, or *Campylobacter* and microscopic examination for enteric ova and parasites were negative. A sorbitol-nonfermenting *E. coli*, believed to be of the O157:H7 serotype, was recovered from the stool. The serotype was later confirmed by the State Public Health Laboratory. Antibiotics and intravenous fluids were administered over the next few days. The boy's stool was negative for the *E. coli* isolate by the time he was discharged from the hospital.

**Questions:**

1. Is the consumption of hamburger significant in this case history?

2. Why does this serotype of *E. coli* produce such severe illness?

3. Can *E. coli* O157:H7 be identified by means other than serotyping?

## CASE STUDY 2: *KLEBSIELLA PNEUMONIAE* IN A CHRONIC ALCOHOLIC

A 55-year-old male transient stumbled into the emergency room of a large county medical facility. He was pale, coughing, and complaining of chest pain. "Rales," indicative of alveolar involvement, were heard on auscultation. Physical examination revealed an underweight, undernourished man with a rapid respiratory rate of 38/min, a temperature of 102.3°F, and alcohol on his breath. On questioning he admitted to "sipping" a pint of gin a day. Chest x-ray showed extensive consolidation with cavity formation in the lower right lobe of the lung. A bloody sputum was obtained by tracheal suction because the patient had difficulty in providing a specimen on his own. Numerous encapsulated gram-negative rods and a large number of neutrophils were noted. Cultures of the sputum for *Streptococcus pneumoniae*, *Mycoplasma pneumoniae*, and *Legionella pneumoniae* were negative; a heavy growth of *Klebsiella pneumoniae* was obtained. Despite high doses of broad-spectrum antibiotics, the patient's condition worsened and he was provided with a mechanical ventilator. The patient died of septicemia shortly thereafter.

**Questions:**

1. Why did antibiotic therapy in this patient fail?

2. Do other *Klebsiella* species cause respiratory tract disease?

3. Can *K. pneumoniae* be rapidly differentiated from other members of the *Enterobacteriaceae* family?

# Review Questions

1. A midstream "clean-catch" urine from an asymptomatic 30-year-old pregnant woman yields numerous motile, lactose-positive organisms that are susceptible to common antibiotics. Which organism is MOST LIKELY responsible for the infection?
   a. *Serratia marcescens*
   b. *Escherichia coli*
   c. *Klebsiella pneumoniae*
   d. *Pseudomonas aeruginosa*

2. Which of the following is a nonmotile organism with a large gelatinous capsule that can be found in the respiratory tract, as well as the intestinal tract, of healthy humans?
   a. *Escherichia coli*
   b. *Enterobacter*
   c. *Klebsiella*
   d. *Proteus*

3. A picnic feast of potato salad, chicken, and hamburgers was consumed during a family reunion on a hot summer day. Within 24 hours eight family members experienced diarrhea, fever, and abdominal pain, which lasted for 2 days. Three people were eventually hospitalized and $H_2S$-producing gram-negative bacilli were isolated from the stool. Which of the following is the MOST LIKELY organism?
   a. *Shigella dysenteriae*
   b. *Shigella sonnei*
   c. *Shigella flexneri*
   d. *Salmonella typhimurium*

4. Microscopic examination of the stool from a patient with diarrhea revealed numerous red and white blood cells and mucus. A nonmotile, gram-negative rod that failed to ferment lactose was isolated from the stool. Blood cultures were negative. Which of the following is MOST LIKELY to be the causative organism?
   a. *Escherichia coli*
   b. *Enterobacter* species
   c. *Klebsiella* species
   d. *Shigella sonnei*

5. A gold miner in the southwest who develops the symptoms of bubonic plague is determined to have had contact with a/an:
   a. rodent.
   b. arthropod.
   c. wild dog.
   d. dead bird.

6. Identify the MAJOR factor in *Yersinia pestis* that is associated with virulence, as well as the induction of protective immunity.
   a. Coagulase
   b. Lipid A
   c. V-W antigen system
   d. Fraction I

7. Which of the following organisms is MOST LIKELY to cause a watery diarrhea?
   a. Enterohemorrhagic *E. coli*
   b. Enteropathogenic *E. coli*
   c. Enteroinvasive *E. coli*
   d. *Shigella sonnei*

8. A common nosocomial pathogen with "swarming" motility is:
   a. *Enterobacter cloacae*.
   b. *Providencia stuartii*.
   c. *Proteus mirabilis*.
   d. *Serratia marcescens*.

## ▶ REFERENCES & RECOMMENDED READING

Aguilera, A., Pascual, J., Loza, E., Lopez, J., Garcia, G., Liano, F., Quereda, C., & Ortuno, J. (1995). Bacteremia with *Cedecea neteri* in a patient with systemic lupus erythematosus. *Postgraduate Medicine Journal, 71,* 179–180.

Angulo, F. J. & Swerdlow, D. L. (1995). Bacterial enteric infections in persons infected with human immunodeficiency virus. *Clinics in Infectious Disease, 21,* 884–893.

Berkowitz, F. E., & Metchock, B. (1995). Third generation cephalosporin-resistant gram-negative bacilli in the feces of hospitalized children. *Pediatric Infectious Disease Journal, 14,* 97–100.

Butler T., et al. (1991). Patterns of morbidity and mortality in typhoid fever dependent on age and gender: Review of 552 hospitalized patients with diarrhea. *Reviews of Infectious Disease, 13,* 85.

Centers for Disease Control and Prevention. (1993). Update: Multistate outbreak of *Escherichia coli* O157:H7 infections from hamburgers—western United States, 1992–1993. *Morbidity and Mortality Weekly Report, 42,* 258–263.

Devreese, K., Claeys, G., & Verschraegen, G. (1992). Septicemia with *Ewingella americana. Journal of Clinical Microbiology, 30,* 2746–2747.

Donnenberg, M., & Kaper, J. (1992). Minireview: Enteropathogenic *E. coli. Infection and Immunity, 60,* 3953.

Farmer, J. J. III. (1995). *Enterobacteriaceae,* introduction and identification. In P. R. Murray, E. J. Baron, M. A. Pfaller, J. C. Tenover, & R. H. Yolken (Eds.), *Manual of clinical microbiology* (6th ed., pp. 438–449). Washington, DC: ASM Press.

Farmer, J. J. III, et al. (1985). Biochemical identification of new species and biogroups of *Enterobacteriaceae* isolated from clinical specimens. *Journal of Clinical Microbiology, 21,* 46.

Friedland, G., & Klein, R. (1992). Tuberculosis and other bacterial infections. In V. T. DeVita, Jr., S. Hellman, & S. A. Rosenberg (Eds.), *AIDS: Etiology, diagnosis, treatment, and prevention* (3rd ed., pp. 180–193). Philadelphia: Lippincott.

Goldberg, M. B., & Sansonetti, P. J. (1993). Minireview: *Shigella* subversion of the cytoskeleton: A strategy for epithelial cell colonization. *Infection and Immunity, 61,* 4941.

Hedberg, C. W., Korlath, J. A., D'Aoust, J. Y., et al. (1992). A multistate outbreak of *Salmonella javiana* and *Salmonella oranienburg* infections due to consumption of contaminated cheese. *Journal of the American Medical Association, 268,* 3203.

Heizmann, W. R., & Michel, R. (1991). Isolation of *Ewingella americana* from a patient with conjunctivitis. *European Journal of Clinical Microbiology, and Infectious Disease, 10,* 957–959.

Hyams, K. C., Hanson, K., Wignall, F. S., Escamilla, J., & Oldfield, E. C. III. (1995). The impact of infectious diseases on the health of U.S. troops deployed to the Persian Gulf during operations Desert Shield and Desert Storm. *Clinics in Infectious Disease, 20,* 1497–1507.

Jawetz, E., Melnick, J. L., & Adelberg, E. A. (1995). *Medical microbiology,* (20th ed.). East Norwalk, CT: Appleton & Lange.

Johnson, J. R. (1991). Virulence factors in *Escherichia coli* urinary tract infection. *Clinical Microbiology Reviews, 4,* 80.

Meyer, K. S. et al. (1993). Nosocomial outbreak of *Klebsiella* infection resistant to late-generation cephalosporins. *Annals of Internal Medicine, 119,* 353.

Neu, H. C. (1992). The crisis in antibiotic resistance. *Science, 257,* 1064–1073.

News and Views: More than a simple case of food poisoning. (1995). *Laboratory Medicine, 26,* 704.

Ridell, J., Siitonen, A., Paulin, L., Lindroos, O., Korkeala, H., & Albert, M. J. (1995). Characterization of *Hafnia alvei* by biochemical tests, random amplified polymorphic DNA PCR, and partial sequencing of 16S rRNA gene. *Journal of Clinical Microbiology, 33,* 2372–2376.

Ridell, J., Siitonen, A., Paulin, L., Mattila, L., Korkeala, H., & Albert, M. J. (1994). *Hafnia alvei* in stool specimens of patients with diarrhea and healthy controls. *Journal of Clinical Microbiology, 32,* 2335–2337.

Roa, A., Castillon, M. P., Goble, M. L., Virden, R., & Garcia, J. L. (1995). New insights on the specificity of penicillin acylase. *Biochemical Biophysical Research Communication, 206,* 629–636.

Ross, V. (1990). Nosocomial infections during the age of AIDS. *ASM News, 56,* 575–578.

Schlager, T. A., Whittam, T. S., Hendley, J. O., Hollis, R. J., Pfaller, M. A., Wilson, R. A., & Stapleton, A. (1995). Comparison of expression of virulence factors by *Escherichia coli* causing cystitis and *E. coli* colonizing the periurethra of healthy girls. *Journal of Infectious Disease, 172,* 772–777.

Yogev, R., & Kozlowski, S. (1990). Peritonitis due to *Kluyvera ascorbata:* Case report and review. *Reviews in Infectious Disease, 12,* 399–402.

# CHAPTER 17

# Nonfermenting Aerobic Gram-Negative Bacilli

Daila S. Gridley, PhD

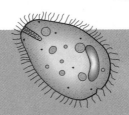

## Microbes in the News

### Septic Shock Due to *Pseudomonas Aeruginosa* in a Previously Healthy Woman

*Pseudomonas aeruginosa,* well known as a nosocomial pathogen, is being implicated with increasing frequency in apparently healthy individuals. One dramatic case is that of a 48-year-old woman who experienced a sudden attack of back pain, fever, and shock. Chest radiographs revealed pneumonia and *P. aeruginosa* was isolated from the blood and sputum. The patient recovered promptly after treatment with piperacillin, dopamine, and fluid replacement. Laboratory tests failed to reveal any immunologic deficiencies. The case is remarkable because septic shock due to this organism is very rare in immunocompetent individuals. There have been only four other previously reported cases.

## KEY TERMS

Adhesins
Alginate polysaccharide
Biofilm
Blue-green pus
Cystic fibrosis

Ecthyma gangrenosum
Elastase
Exoenzyme S
Exotoxin A
Folliculitis

Glanders
Melioidosis
Metallic sheen
Nonfermenter
O-F media

## KEY TERMS (cont.)

| | | |
|---|---|---|
| Otitis externa | Pyocyanin | Pyoverdin |
| Otitis media | Pyomelanin | Slime layer |
| Phospholipase C | Pyorubrin | Swimmer's ear |
| Polar flagellum | | |

## LEARNING OBJECTIVES

**Upon successful completion of this chapter, the student should be able to:**

1. Describe the salient features of this group of organisms as a whole.

2. List the unique features of the presented genera and the species that are of major importance in human infections.

3. Discuss known virulence factors and how they contribute to the illness.

4. Identify important tests that are used in establishing a laboratory diagnosis.

5. List the commonly used therapies and preventive procedures.

## INTRODUCTION

This chapter discusses a diverse group of motile gram-negative bacteria that are aerobic, that is, they require oxygen for growth. Many of these organisms do not ferment carbohydrates, including glucose and lactose, and hence they are referred to as **nonfermenters**. *As a group, they generally grow well on MacConkey agar, forming colorless, translucent colonies that are indicative of their inability to ferment lactose. Lactose fermenters produce pinkish red colonies on this medium.* Some of the genera discussed in this chapter produce blue, yellow, rust, and brown pigments, which are useful in identification. However, many isolates do not react in biochemical tests that are routinely performed in clinical laboratories, thereby delaying their identification because of the need for additional assays. They are widely distributed in soil, water, and vegetation, but may occasionally colonize animals and humans as part of the normal flora. *Pseudomonas,* especially *P. aeruginosa,* is the major member of the group that affects humans. Other much less common, but also important, organisms include *Acinetobacter, Flavobacterium, Alcaligenes, Moraxella,* and *Xanthomonas.* These genera represent 75% or more of all nonfermenters that are isolated from humans. With the exception of *P. aeruginosa,* they generally do not cause disease in healthy individuals. However, in debilitated persons, in hospitalized patients, or when introduced into areas of the body that are devoid of normal host defenses, severe infections may occur. Table 17-1 summarizes the differentiating characteristics of this group of organisms.

## PSEUDOMONAS

### Organism Characteristics

The morphologic characteristics of *Pseudomonas* species are similar to those of the *Enterobacteriaceae* family, except that they are slightly thinner and paler after Gram staining. They are relatively short, straight or slightly curved rods that tend to grow as individual cells. They usually have a single **polar flagellum** (refer to Color Plate 31), but they may occasionally have two or three. *P. aeruginosa* can produce one or more of four water-soluble pigments: **pyocyanin** (blue), **pyoverdin** (yellow), and occasionally **pyorubrin** (rust) and **pyomelanin** (brown). The cell walls of the organisms contain lipopolysaccharide (LPS) and pili (fimbriae) that extend outward from the surface. In some strains, individual and multiple cells are surrounded by an outer **slime layer** that has a mixed composition, but consists primarily of polysaccharide. This extracellular polysaccharide has an unusual structure with acetylation of disaccharide units that resembles components of some algae; hence, it is sometimes referred to as **alginate polysaccharide** (or alginate exopolysaccharide).

The organisms can multiply over a wide temperature range of 20° to 42°C. Their growth requirements are very simple; ammonium and $CO_2$ are sufficient as the only sources of nitrogen and carbon for most isolates. Some species can use a broad range of substances (i.e., approximately 80–100) including various amino acids, amines, alcohols, saturated and unsaturated fatty acids, or other simple organic compounds. The degradation of organic material results in inorganic

**Table 17–1 ▶ General Characteristics of Nonfermenting Aerobic Gram-Negative Bacilli**

| Family: | Pseudomonadaceae | | Neisseriaceae | | Alcaligenaceae | Cytophagaceae* |
|---|---|---|---|---|---|---|
| | **Pseudomonas** | **Xanthomonas** | **Acinetobacter** | **Moraxella** | **Alcaligenes** | **Flavobacterium** |
| Oxidase | + | – | – | + | + | + |
| Indole | – | – | – | – | – | Variable |
| Penicillin | Resistant | Resistant | Resistant | Sensitive | Resistant | Resistant |
| Polymyxin | Variable | Variable | Sensitive | Sensitive | Sensitive | Resistant |
| Pigment | Yes | No | No | No | No | Yes |
| Arginine dehydrolase | Variable | Variable | – | – | – | – |
| Flagella | Polar | Peritrichous | None | None | Peritrichous | None |

*A heterogenous group that is undergoing taxonomic revision. Most members appear to have characteristics associated most closely with the *Cytophagaceae* family.

A + or – indicates that > 90% of isolates within the genus give a positive or negative reaction, respectively.

A variable designation indicates that there is great variability among species or isolates within a species.

substances; this process is known as "mineralization." Thus, these organisms play a significant role in the balance of nature.

*Pseudomonas* species are found worldwide, primarily in the environment. They are extremely hardy organisms, surviving under conditions that would kill most other bacteria. Viable isolates have been obtained even from hot tubs with low chlorine concentrations and radioactive water from atomic piles at nuclear power plants. Their ability to survive under extremely adverse conditions is related to at least two factors: secretion of numerous enzymes that can break down potentially toxic substances and the relative impermeability of their cell wall.

There are at least 13 species of pseudomonads, which can be differentiated on the basis of growth and other characteristics (see Table 17-2). *P. aeruginosa* is found in the throat and stool of approximately 5% to 10% of healthy persons. It is by far the most common species within the genus that is isolated from human infections. Interestingly, these organisms (and some other pseudomonads) can also infect and cause disease in fish, amphibians, insects, and even plants. Approximately 17 subtypes of *P. aeruginosa* have been identified with antisera specific for various O antigens. The glycoprotein and several outer proteins of the organisms are also antigenic. In addition, different patterns of reactivity have been noted with pyocins (bacteriocins) and bacteriophages that specifically lyse *P. aeruginosa*. Molecular techniques based on rRNA and DNA homology have also been used to distinguish strains involved in outbreaks of infection.

## Clinical Significance

Immunocompetent humans generally have very good defense mechanisms against most *Pseudomonas* species. Normal serum contains C3, a major protein of the complement system, and other opsonins that enhance phagocytosis by polymorphonuclear cells and result in destruction of the bacteria. Preexisting antibody against the oligosaccharide side chain and core of the LPS and to surface glycoprotein increase the effectiveness of complement action against the organisms. Antibody against exotoxin A has also been shown to be protective. These bacteria, thus, usually do not survive for long in the blood or sites of entry into the body.

***Pseudomonas aeruginosa.*** This organism can occasionally cause disease in healthy individuals, although infections in debilitated or immunocompromised hosts are significantly more common and more serious. This species is a very important opportunistic pathogen in hospitalized patients. It is now the second most common gram-negative bacillus isolated from hospital-acquired infections (*Escherichia coli* is most common). Unfortunately, the organisms are being recognized with greater frequency in drug-resistant nosocomial infections and even in patients who appear to be immunocompetent. Because of their hardy nature and their low nutritional requirements, they are often found in hospitals and extended care facilities as contaminants in humidifier and respirator water, faucet aerators, distilled water, aerosol medications, sinks, cleaning solutions, soaps used by physicians and nurses, and even flower arrangements in rooms of patients.

**Table 17–2 ▶ Characteristics of the Most Common *Pseudomonas* Species**

| Species | rRNA Homology Group* | Fluorescence | Growth at 42°C | Gas from Nitrate | Gelatin Hydrolysis | Acid Production in O-F Media | | | Decarboxylase | | Arginine Dihydrolase |
|---|---|---|---|---|---|---|---|---|---|---|---|
| | | | | | | Glucose | Lactose | Fructose | Lysine | Ornithine | |
| P. aeruginosa | I | + | + | +/– | +/– | + | – | + | – | – | + |
| P. fluorescens | I | + | – | – | + | + | +/– | + | – | – | + |
| P. putida | I | + | – | – | – | + | +/– | + | – | – | + |
| P. alcaligenes | I | – | +/– | – | – | – | – | – | – | – | – |
| P. pseudoalcaligenes | I | – | +/– | – | – | +/– | – | + | – | – | +/– |
| P. stutzeri | I | – | + | + | – | + | – | + | – | – | – |
| P. cepacia | I | – | +/– | – | +/– | + | + | + | + | +/– | – |
| P. pickettii | I | – | +/– | + | +/– | + | +/– | + | – | – | – |
| P. pseudomaller† | I | – | + | + | + | + | + | + | – | – | + |
| P. diminuta | IV | – | +/– | – | +/– | – | – | – | – | – | – |
| P. vesicularis | IV | – | – | – | +/– | +/– | – | – | – | – | – |
| P. paucimobilis | V | – | – | – | – | + | + | + | – | – | – |
| P. putrefaciens‡ | V | – | +/– | – | + | + | – | +/– | – | + | – |

*Group III includes the *Comamonas acidovarans* and *P. facilis-delafieldii* groups that are almost never found in human infections.

†*P. mallei* is also in rRNA homology group II.

‡Recently renamed as *Shewanella putrefaciens*.

A + or – indicates that at least 90% of isolates are positive or negative, respectively.

A +/– indicates a variable reaction, depending upon the isolated strain.

O-F, oxidative-fermentative media.

In healthy individuals *P. aeruginosa* is often the cause of infections associated with injuries in which environmental contamination exists (i.e., extensive burns, deep puncture wounds, open wounds after car accidents, etc.). Infected burns and wounds may have **blue-green pus** or exudate due to production of pyocyanin and pyoverdin in various amounts by the organisms. Severe infections, as well as colonization of the intestinal tract, can be followed by bacteremia. In some of these cases, a cutaneous syndrome known as **ecthyma gangrenosum** develops. It begins as one or a few painful maculopapular skin lesions (usually on perineum, buttocks, extremities, or in the axillae) that grow larger over a period of 2 to 3 days. The center of each lesion becomes purple, then black and necrotic because of invasion and direct destruction of small arteries and veins by the organisms. The lesions are often surrounded by erythema, but contain little or no pus. A 50% to 70% mortality rate is reported in neutropenic patients with high-grade bacteremia. Osteomyelitis (inflammation of the bone) due to the organisms may occur after deep wounds and compound bone fractures. The infection may remain localized or spread throughout the marrow, cortex, and other bone components. Surgical debridement, as well as antibiotic therapy, is sometimes necessary.

*Pseudomonas aeruginosa* frequently inhabits the external auditory canal under wet or simply humid conditions. "**Swimmer's ear**" (**otitis externa**) is seen quite frequently in children who spend long summer days in swimming pools. This condition can be painful and itchy but is relatively benign and self-limiting. A "malignant" otitis externa may occur on rare occasions in elderly individuals with diabetes mellitus or in very young infants with underlying diseases. In these cases the organisms become locally invasive and penetrate through the epithelium into underlying soft tissue. The condition may be chronic, but may become life-threatening if not treated promptly. Individuals who soak in contaminated swimming pools, whirlpools, spas, and hot tubs may develop **folliculitis** (infection of hair follicles) of the skin. The rash is usually most evident in areas of the body covered by swimming suits, but may be more widespread. *P. aeruginosa* concentrations in some hot tubs have been reported to be as high as 100 million organisms per milliliter. In a 1992 report, 20 persons developed a follicular skin rash after using a whirlpool-spa containing water with a low chlorine concentration. This incident prompted the Environmental Protection Agency to more strictly enforce regulations concerning whirlpool-spas. *Pseudomonas* folliculitis can develop into severe ecthyma gangrenosa within 24 hours in immunocompromised individuals.

The organisms are frequently involved in eye infections (i.e., conjunctivitis, endophthalmitis, and keratitis), which can sometimes have devastating results. They often follow accidental or surgical trauma or after the use of contaminated contact lens solutions. In addition, the organisms can adhere to worn, extended-use soft contact lenses. In some cases of keratitis (corneal ulcer), the eye lens is destroyed within 1 to 2 days. Destructive progression of the organisms may result in the loss of the entire eye.

Meningitis and brain abscesses due to *P. aeruginosa* can occur as the result of bacteremic spread from a distant site of infection, extension from a contiguous structure such as the ear, mastoid, or paranasal sinus, or direct inoculation by means of head trauma, surgery, lumbar puncture, or other invasive procedures. The symptoms are similar to those seen in other bacterial meningitis cases with fever, headache, and confusion being common. *Pseudomonas* meningitis may be acute, subacute, or relapsing. It is seen most often in immunocompromised individuals and cancer patients.

Urinary tract infections due to *P. aeruginosa* are usually hospital acquired and iatrogenic (i.e., resulting from the activity of physicians). They can occur as the result of the organisms being introduced by urinary tract catheterization, other instrumentation, irrigating solutions, surgical procedures, and even renal transplantation. According to the Centers for Disease Control and Prevention (CDC), these organisms are now also a very common cause of urinary tract infections outside of the hospital setting (*E. coli* is number one). The clinical manifestations are usually indistinguishable from those produced by other bacteria.

The organisms have also been associated with endocarditis, especially in intravenous drug users and in patients with prosthetic heart valves. Most drug addicts with infective endocarditis are young men who do not have any specific underlying disease, although some have had rheumatic valvular disease or previous staphylococcal endocarditis. The tricuspid valve of the heart is most often involved. The diagnosis of endocarditis due to *P. aeruginosa* can often be made by positive blood cultures in the absence of extracardiac sites of infection. Poor prognostic indicators include age over 30 years and involvement of the left side of the heart. Left-sided endocarditis often requires surgery, as well as other medical treatment.

Primary pneumonia due to *P. aeruginosa* occurs mostly in patients with chronic lung disease, congestive heart failure, or both. Bacteremic pneumonia is seen primarily in individuals with malignancies involving the hematopoietic system or those who are neutropenic or granulocytopenic (see section on immunocompromised hosts) as the result of chemotherapy. Patients in intensive care units appear to be particularly susceptible. In addition, *P. aeruginosa* are now extremely common colonizers of the respiratory tract of patients with **cystic fibrosis**, an inherited disease characterized by excessive buildup of mucus in the smaller respiratory passages.

They induce an inflammatory response with subsequent decline in pulmonary function. Once established, the organisms are virtually impossible to eradicate. They form a **biofilm** of microcolonies within the bronchi. Tracheobronchitis or pneumonia due to the bacteria are often complicating factors in the management of this disease and are a highly significant cause of morbidity and death in these patients. The *P. aeruginosa* strains isolated from cystic fibrosis patients produce an alginate extracellular polysaccharide that gives them a strikingly mucoid appearance. It appears that the lung environment of these patients selects for the expression of the genes that code for this polysaccharide. At least four gene loci are thought to regulate the synthesis of the alginate. On subculture, the organisms often revert to the nonmucoid phenotype.

The various types of infections associated with *P. aeruginosa* are summarized in Table 17-3.

*Pseudomonas aeruginosa* produces a number of factors that are associated with virulence. Fimbriae and adhesion molecules (**adhesins**) are important in the early stages of infection in that they allow for attachment. The fimbriae bind to epithelial cells, whereas the adhesins appear to bind to certain disaccharides of the mucin (made up of carbohydrates) of the respiratory tract. Recent evidence, however, indicates that the organisms do not adhere well to normal intact epithelium. It has been demonstrated in animal models that adhesion is significantly enhanced when the epithelium is damaged by the influenza virus, endotracheal intubation, or irritating chemicals. The adherence properties of *P. aeruginosa* appear to vary greatly from one strain to another, possibly as the result of variations in the expression of different adhesins.

**Exotoxin A** is thought to be among the most important virulence factors once the organisms gain entry into the body. It is produced by more than 90% of *P. aeruginosa* isolated from clinical specimens and its secretion is often associated with fatal bacteremia. Experimental animal studies show that antibodies against exotoxin A are protective against an otherwise lethal challenge of exotoxin A-producing organisms. The endotoxin of the cell wall has lipid A, but it is less potent than that found in the *Enterobacteriaceae*. Nonetheless, it plays a role in the induction of fever, leukopenia, shock, and other manifestations seen in patients with *Pseudomonas* infections. An enterotoxin produced by the organisms has been shown to increase fluid secretion in the intestinal tract of experimental animals. Its role in human infection, however, is not clear.

The secretion of collagenase, lecithinase, at least two broad-spectrum proteases, as well as other enzymes, undoubtedly contribute to injury, invasion, and persistence of the organisms. The proteases are not highly toxic to cells, but they disrupt respiratory cilia. **Elastase** digests the elastin found in the lung and arterial walls,

| Table 17–3 ▶ Types of Infections Associated with *Pseudomonas aeruginosa* | |
|---|---|
| **Infections** | **Comments** |
| Burns and wounds | Seen in previously healthy individuals; wounds may be due to accidental or surgical trauma; may progress to bacteremia and other complications in the immunocompromised; infection is often accompanied with blue-green pus due to pigment production. |
| Bacteremia/septicemia | Result of progressive infection; seen primarily in immunocompromised individuals. |
| Ecthyma gangrenosum | Syndrome with painful, maculopapular skin lesions; tends to occur in association with bacteremia. |
| Osteomyelitis | Inflammation of bone; associated with deep wounds and compound fractures; may be local or spreading; may require surgical intervention. |
| Otitis externa | "Swimmer's ear" in children who spend prolonged time in swimming pools, usually self-limiting; "malignant" form seen in elderly adults with diabetes mellitus. |
| Folliculitis | Infection of skin involving hair follicles; associated with contaminated whirlpools, spas, hot tubs, and swimming pools; usually requires little or no treatment. |
| Conjunctivitis, endophthalmitis, and keratitis | Eye infections associated with accidental or surgical trauma, contaminated contact lens solutions and extended-wear soft contact lenses. |
| Pneumonia and lung abscesses | Associated with neutropenia, immunosuppression, and cytotoxic drugs; seen in patients with cancers of hematopoietic system cells, third degree burns, and cystic fibrosis. |
| Meningitis | Seen mostly in the immunocompromised; may be result of extension from other sites, lumbar puncture, or other invasive medical procedures. |
| Urinary tract infections | Very common in hospitalized patients; associated with catheters and other medical procedures; incidence of infection outside of hospital setting has been increasing and is now common. |
| Endocarditis | Seen mostly in drug addicts; occasionally seen in patients with prosthetic heart valves; left-side heart involvement may require surgery. |

resulting in hemorrhaging. **Phospholipase C** hydrolyzes phospholipids, especially those that are found in eukaryotic cell membranes. It also has hemolysin activity. Pyocyanin can undergo redox cycling under aerobic conditions resulting in the generation of superoxide and hydrogen peroxide. These unstable oxygen radicals can mediate tissue injury. Furthermore, the pyocyanin may act together with one or more proteins, also derived from the organisms, to generate a synergistic increase in oxygen radical production. Pyocyanin, elastin, and alkaline protease have immunosuppressive activities (see section on immunocompromised hosts).

The factors associated with the virulence of *P. aeruginosa* and their major biological effects are summarized in Table 17-4.

### Pseudomonas (Burkholderia) cepacia.
Infections due to *P. cepacia* (recently renamed as *Burkholderia cepacia*) occur primarily in the hospital setting, especially when massive amounts of the organisms are accidentally introduced into patients. Contaminated disinfectants, medical devices, or breakdown in proper sterilizing procedures have been implicated in outbreaks. Several cystic fibrosis centers have reported increased incidence of *P. cepacia* isolation from the lungs of their patients. In some cases there is no change in clinical status, whereas in others there is a rapid deterioration

in health. In general, the presence of these organisms signals a poor clinical prognosis. *P. cepacia* is associated with development of lung abscesses and pneumonia. Genotypic, as well as biochemical, analyses of isolates from outbreaks indicate that the organisms have marked phenotypic variability. A secreted protease, similar to the elastase produced by *P. aeruginosa*, has been recently found in culture supernatants of the organisms. Under experimental conditions the protease can induce bronchopneumonia with leukocyte infiltration into the lungs of rats. Its role in human infections has not yet been clearly defined.

### Pseudomonas (Burkholderia) pseudomallei.
*Pseudomonas pseudomallei* (recently reclassified as *Burkholderia pseudomallei*) is the cause of **melioidosis**, usually manifested as an acute pneumonia within 2 to 3 days after infection, although subacute and chronic disease is also possible. Fever, leukocytosis, and consolidation of the lungs are typical for the disease. With the development of upper lobe cavities and an afebrile state, clinical symptoms and radiologic findings may eventually resemble tuberculosis. Respiratory failure can occur rapidly and abscesses may develop in the skin, brain, myocardium, liver, bone, and other organs in severe cases. *P. pseudomallei* has a limited geographic distribution. Infections due to this species are found

**Table 17–4** ▶ **Factors Associated with the Virulence of *Pseudomonas aeruginosa***

| Virulence Factor | Biologic Activities |
|---|---|
| Fimbriae (pili) | Mediate attachment to epithelial cell surfaces |
| Adhesins | Mediate attachment to mucins of respiratory tract and other mucous membranes |
| Alginate polysaccharide | Enhances adherence to respiratory tract; increases resistance to phagocytosis; forms "biofilm" of multiple bacteria within a matrix in patients with cystic fibrosis |
| Exotoxin A | Inhibits protein synthesis by adenosine diphosphate-ribosylation (inactivates elongation factor-2, EF-2); produced by great majority of clinical isolates; correlates highly with virulence and invasiveness |
| Endotoxin (LPS) | Has lipid A; induces fever, leukopenia, and shock; is weaker than endotoxin of enteric gram-negative rods |
| **Exoenzyme S** | Adenosine diphosphate-ribosylates several proteins other than EF-2; kills cells and produces tissue damage |
| Collagenase | Breaks down collagen; participates in tissue damage and invasiveness |
| Lecithinase | Breaks down lecithin; participates in tissue damage and invasiveness |
| Proteases | Break down many different proteins; alkaline protease breaks down the IgG class of antibody and complement and inhibits activity of neutrophils and interferon-γ |
| Elastase | Degrades elastin in lungs and arterial walls; produces hemorrhaging; inhibits neutrophil function |
| Phospholipase C | Hydrolyzes phospholipids, especially those in eukaryotic cell membranes; has hemolytic activity |
| Pyocyanin | Induces production of oxygen radicals, which damage tissues; may act synergistically with another protein to induce even greater amounts of oxygen radicals; is produced by great majority of clinical isolates; is one of the pigments that produces blue-green pus |

primarily in tropical countries that lie between 20°N and 20°S latitude. It exists as a saprophyte in rice paddies, ponds, soil, and vegetable produce in the Philippines, Indonesia, Northern Australia, and Southeast Asia. In Africa the bacteria emerge from the clay layer of soil and appear in muddy, stagnant waters during the rainy season. About 150 cases of melioidosis were documented in American servicemen during the Vietnam war. These organisms can produce disease in otherwise healthy individuals, although most infected persons in endemic areas are asymptomatic. Rodents, sheep, goats, swine, horses, and other farm animals may also be infected. Human infection usually occurs through inhalation of contaminated dust or via direct contact with environmental sources. Person-to-person transmission has been documented but is extremely rare. Latent infections can be reactivated months to years later following stress or debilitating illnesses such as cancer. This delay in emergence of clinical disease has earned melioidosis the nickname of "Vietnamese time-bomb." During reactivation the organisms can be isolated from blood, urine, sputum, and pus. Untreated disease has a very high mortality rate; approximately 30% of patients die despite antibiotic therapy. *P. pseudomallei* secretes a potent toxin that blocks protein and DNA synthesis in macrophages. The organisms are able to survive and multiply within these cells, as well as in polymorphonuclear phagocytes. This characteristic may account for its persistence in the body for long periods of time. The toxin also appears to be responsible for the abscesses associated with the disease.

***Pseudomonas (Burkholderia) mallei.*** **Glanders**, a disease of horses, donkeys, and certain other mammals, is caused by *P. mallei* (recently renamed *Burkholderia mallei*). Localized pulmonary disease, which may be acute or suppurative, is the most common clinical manifestation. Glanders has been eliminated from the equine populations of the United States and Canada and, thus, human infection in these countries is almost nonexistent.

**Vaccine Development.** There is currently great interest in developing a vaccine to prevent *Pseudomonas* infection or colonization. At least two vaccines containing the cell wall of *P. aeruginosa* have been produced. However, results from clinical trials in patients with cystic fibrosis and patients in burn units have been inconclusive. In addition, side effects have been noted, especially with multiple injections of the preparations. Several newer vaccines with a lower LPS content appear to have a lower incidence of adverse reactions. A purified toxoid preparation of exotoxin A has induced high and persistent levels of antitoxin antibody in healthy human volunteers. Efforts are also being made to develop vaccines for application to mucosal surfaces to prevent colonization. Genetically attenuated mucosal pathogens have been tested as vehicles for *P. aeruginosa* genes encoding antigens that can induce protective immunity. Somewhat promising results have been obtained with passive immunization using immunoglobulin preparations. The efficacy of some of these approaches is currently being evaluated in controlled large-scale clinical trials.

## Cultural Characteristics and Identification

Gram stains of pus, sputum, skin lesions, urine, spinal fluid, blood, and other clinical specimens from patients with *Pseudomonas* infections usually show the presence of gram-negative rods, but generally do not reveal any distinguishing morphologic features. Blood agar and differential media that are commonly used for the gram-negative enteric bacilli are usually inoculated. All *Pseudomonas* species also grow well on very simple media. They are often identified easily because of their pigment production, positive oxidase and catalase reactions, motility, and ability to grow on selective media such as eosin-methylene blue (EMB) and MacConkey agar. Their isolation from wounds and sputum specimens may not always be significant, because of their prevalence in the environment. In contrast, isolation of *Pseudomonas* from a blood culture indicates serious infection.

The organisms form either flat, feathery or "ground glass" colonies on blood agar and usually exhibit strong ß-hemolysis. Extremely mucoid colonies are produced by alginate polysaccharide-producing isolates from cystic fibrosis patients. *P. aeruginosa* has a very characteristic odor that is similar to overripe grapes and areas with dense colonial growth will frequently appear pigmented due to the production of pyocyanin (blue). This pigment is especially evident on *Pseudomonas* P agar (Difco Laboratories) and Tech agar (BBL Microbiology Systems). The blue color may be masked in strains that produce the other pigments. Strains that produce pyoverdin (yellow) will fluoresce under a short-wave ultraviolet light (i.e., 254 nm wavelength as opposed to the 365 nm wavelength used in Wood's lamp). The fluorescent pigment can occasionally be seen in wounds, burns, and urine. Observation of fluorescence is enhanced by culture on *Pseudomonas* F agar (Difco Laboratories) or Flo agar (BBL Microbiology Systems). *P. fluorescens* and *P. putida* also produce fluorescent pigments. In vitro production of pigment is partly dependent on the incubation temperature and the cation content of the agar. In KIA or TSI *P. aeruginosa* produces an alkaline slant over an unchanged (red) butt. A **metallic sheen** is often observed on the slant. Its growth at 42°C helps to distinguish it from most other *Pseudomonas* species isolated from clinical specimens. Selective media, such as the cetrimide-containing Pseudosel agar (BBL Microbiology Systems), has been

developed for its isolation from contaminated specimens such as stool. Identification of *P. aeruginosa* in stool specimens is useful because colonization of the intestinal tract frequently precedes development of infection in hospitalized patients.

A very important test that is used to help distinguish *Pseudomonas*, as well as other nonfermenters, from the *Enterobacteriaceae* is performed using oxidative-fermentative **(O-F) media**. This is a low-peptone medium to which different carbohydrates (i.e., glucose, maltose, or other sugar) are added. It allows detection of acid production by organisms that metabolize weakly and for which Kligler's iron agar (KIA) and triple sugar iron (TSI) agar reactions are slow. For example, *P. aeruginosa* will produce a yellow color (due to acid) in open (aerobic) tubes, but not in mineral oil overlaid, closed (anaerobic) tubes of O-F medium containing glucose. This indicates that they are oxidative for glucose, but cannot ferment it. No color change in either tube containing O-F medium with maltose indicates that *P. aeruginosa* is nonoxidative and nonfermentative for the maltose.

*Pseudomonas cepacia* is isolated frequently from patients with cystic fibrosis, although less often than *P. aeruginosa*. It produces rough colonies with serrated edges that sometimes appear yellow or yellow-green due to nonfluorescent pigments. The organisms oxidize glucose, lactose, maltose, and mannitol. However, they can exhibit marked variability in many other biochemical tests. In one study of 100 isolates from a single hospital, the organisms could be placed into 12 groups on the basis of six enzymes, a hemolytic substance, and a yellow pigment. Genomic typing of these same isolates indicated that the majority belonged to only one strain.

Isolation of *P. pseudomallei* from clinical material occurs very rarely in the United States, but should always be considered significant. Staining with Wright's stain or methylene blue may reveal bipolar staining. The organisms will usually grow on all common media (although growth on blood agar is slow) and produce mucoid or dry wrinkled colonies similar to those of *P. cepacia* and *P. stutzeri*. Many strains are pigmented (color ranges from cream to orange) and have a putrid yeast-like odor. Three or more polar flagella can be seen with flagellar stains. Serologic tests for antibodies often need to be performed in cases of subacute or chronic melioidosis, since the organisms themselves are rarely isolated.

*Pseudomonas mallei* is the only nonmotile species. It often does not produce colonies on blood agar and fails to grow at 42°C on all media. However, grayish white colonies (eventually turning yellow) usually appear within 48 hours on brain-heart infusion agar incubated at 37°C. Pleomorphic coccal and filamentous rods that sometimes exhibit branching are seen quite frequently on Gram stains.

## Antibiotic Susceptibility Characteristics

*Pseudomonas aeruginosa* is one of the most highly resistant organisms encountered in clinical laboratories. It is sometimes referred to as being "naturally" resistant because resistance is observed before initiation of any antibiotic therapy. Infection with the organisms is never treated with a single agent because the success rate is very low. Usually a penicillin (ticarcillin, mezlocillin, or piperacillin) is used together with an aminoglycoside (gentamicin, tobramycin, or amikacin). The newer quinolones (ciprofloxacin), aztreonam, imipenem, and other third-generation cephalosporins are also active against the organisms. Antibiotic susceptibility tests, however, need to be performed because the patterns of susceptibility vary geographically. Approximately 25% of *P. aeruginosa* isolated in some institutions are now reported to be resistant to all fluoroquinolones. In addition, mutational and plasmid-mediated resistance to penicillins and aminoglycosides can emerge during treatment. Therapy of burns infected with *P. aeruginosa* consists of attempts to keep the bacterial load below $10^5$/g tissue because prevention of colonization is virtually impossible. Maintenance of a low number of organisms lowers the risk for septicemia. These procedures often involve topical application of sulfamylon cream, silver sulfadiazine cream, or soaks of silver nitrate.

Most strains of *P. cepacia* are sensitive to chloramphenicol and sulfamethoxazole-trimethoprim. Third-generation cephalosporins, such as ceftazidime, may also be effective. The organisms are resistant to ß-lactams, fluoroquinolones, and aminoglycosides.

Tetracycline, sulfamethaxazole-trimethoprim, chloramphenicol, and sulfonamides have been used successfully to treat melioidosis (*P. pseudomallei*). Parenteral or oral therapy is often given using several drugs in combination. Best results are obtained when the drugs are administered for at least 8 weeks. Treatment for 6 months to 1 year may be needed for patients with extrapulmonary suppurative lesions. The organisms are resistant to many aminoglycosides and have developed new ß-lactamases that make them resistant to broad-spectrum cephalosporins. Patients with *P. mallei* infection have been successfully treated with a tetracycline plus an aminoglycoside.

## *ACINETOBACTER*

### Organism Characteristics

*Acinetobacter* species (previously known as *Mima* and *Herella*) appear as short, plump gram-negative coccobacilli that often grow in pairs and may be intracellular. Because of these and other features, it has occasionally been confused with *Neisseria* species (*Acinetobacter* belongs in the *Neisseriaceae* family). The organisms are widely distributed in soil, water, and sewage, but may also be recovered from skin, mucous membranes, and secretions of humans. There are at least six species within the genus: *A. baumannii, A. calcoaceticus, A. haemolyticus, A. lwoffii, A. johnsonii,* and *A. junii*. Only the first four species are clinically important.

### Clinical Significance

*Acinetobacter* is isolated from clinical specimens mostly as an innocuous contaminant or colonizer. The organisms are commensals and usually do not cause disease in healthy individuals, although on occasion they have been implicated in community-acquired infections. When clinical disease develops, it is usually seen as a pneumonia in hospitalized patients who have undergone respiratory therapy procedures with contaminated equipment or solutions. Cases of urinary tract infections, infections of soft tissues, sepsis, and bacteremia have also been reported. Contaminated water in room humidifiers and vaporizers, feather pillows, and intravenous catheters have been identified as sources of *Acinetobacter* in nosocomial infections. Its similarity to *Neisseria* species has occasionally posed problems. For example, in some women with urethritis and vaginitis, *Acinetobacter* has been misidentified as *Neisseria gonorrhoeae,* whereas in a few patients with meningitis it has been mistaken for *Neisseria meningitidis*. A recent case of neonatal meningitis in a developing country ended tragically. The infant developed hydrocephalus and cerebral palsy due to an infectious agent that was identified very late in the disease process as *Acinetobacter*. A member of the medical team in charge of the case emphasized in a 1995 publication the difficulty in establishing a correct bacteriologic diagnosis in the absence of a qualified microbiologist.

### Cultural Characteristics and Identification

The organisms form gray to white colonies on blood agar and may or may not exhibit hemolysis. They form clear, colorless colonies typical of a lactose negative enteric bacteria on MacConkey agar. In fact, their growth patterns and colonial morphology often resemble those of the *Enterobacteriaceae*. However, they do not ferment carbohydrates and do not reduce nitrates to nitrites. They are oxidase negative and, thus, can be differentiated from *Neisseria*. *The clinically important species are citrate positive. A. baumannii and A. junii exhibit growth at 42°C, whereas other species do not. A. haemolyticus is the only one that hydrolyzes gelatin.*

## Antibiotic Susceptibility Characteristics

*Acinetobacter* species are frequently resistant to antimicrobial agents and control of infection can be difficult. Resistance to penicillins, cephalosporins, and chloramphenicol is common. Some isolates are also resistant to aminoglycosides. Recently reported multidrug-resistant *A. baumannii* infections in 40 patients in an intensive care unit resulted in a 25% mortality rate and extended hospitalization by more than 10 days for the survivors. Gentamicin, amikacin, tobramycin, and the newer penicillins and cephalosporins have proven to be most effective. Thus far, most species have been susceptible to carbapenems such as imipenem, but it is expected that resistance to these drugs will emerge as it has in many other organisms. Susceptibility testing must be performed to select the most appropriate therapy.

## *FLAVOBACTERIUM*

### Organism Characteristics

The *Flavobacterium* genus consists of aerobic gram-negative rods with rounded ends. They are widely distributed in nature, especially soil and water. They have been isolated from marine plants and animals, salt water, and freshwater. They are not found in humans as part of the normal flora. *F. meningosepticum* is the most common member in the genus that is associated with human infections. Other species that have been isolated from clinical specimens include *F. indologenes, F. breve, F. odoratum,* and *F. multivorum.*

### Clinical Significance

*Flavobacterium* does not produce disease in healthy persons. However, it is very common in the hospital environment. It can be recovered from saline solutions, ice machines, waterbaths, incubators, humidifiers, respiratory equipment, and indwelling catheters. Infections are usually due to *F. meningosepticum* and infants, especially those who are premature, appear to be especially susceptible. Neonatal meningitis, which has a very high fatality rate, is the major type of infection observed. Meningitis can also occur in adults, but is generally much less severe and is often the consequence of operative or other invasive procedures. No specific properties have been identified which could explain the neurotropism of this species.

### Cultural Characteristics and Identification

*Flavobacterium species grow best at temperatures between 25°C and 30°C, although isolates from clinical specimens will initially proliferate at 35°C. F. menin-*

*gosepticum* usually can be cultured from blood in cases of meningitis. Primary isolation is best accomplished on blood agar or chocolate agar. On blood agar, they form small colonies and produce a lavender-green discoloration in red blood cells within 1 day. They grow slowly, if at all on McConkey agar. *F. odoratum emits a characteristic fruity odor.* Most members of the *Flavobacterium* genus produce an intense yellow pigment. However, this is a weak property of *F. meningosepticum* unless they are cultured on nutrient agar at room temperature. The organisms are oxidase positive, catalase positive, and very weakly fermentative. Virtually all strains digest casein and hydrolyze gelatin, esculin, and DNA. Indole production can be detected when using sensitive tests. The organisms may appear to be encapsulated in clinical specimens.

## Antibiotic Susceptibility Characteristics

*Flavobacterium* species, including *F. meningosepticum,* are usually resistant to the great majority of currently used antimicrobial agents. Rifampin, sulfamethoxazole-trimethoprim and erythromycin may be of some benefit.

## *ALCALIGENES*

### Organism Characteristics

*Alcaligenes* belongs in the *Alcaligenaceae* family, same as the *Bordetella.* There are three species and two subspecies within this genus: *A. faecalis, A. xylosoxidans* subspecies *xylosoxidans, A. xylosoxidans* subspecies *denitrificans,* and *A. piechaudii.* These organisms are sometimes found as part of the normal flora in a number of different anatomic sites. They are primarily opportunists that infect only immunocompromised patients.

### Clinical Significance

*Alcaligenes* species have been isolated from numerous types of clinical specimens including blood, wounds, urine, respiratory secretions, cerebrospinal fluid, and abscesses. However, it has been most strongly linked to infections of the urinary tract and wounds, and then only occasionally. The organisms are almost never found as the sole source of infection. Renal dialysis and respirator systems in hospitals have been identified as the sources of the organisms in some cases. *A. xylosoxidans* (formerly called *Achromobacter xylosoxidans*) is the most common species in the genus that is isolated from clinically important infections. This species has also been recovered from patients with endocarditis following aortic valve replacement and keratitis after penetrating keratoplasty.

## Cultural Characteristics and Identification

Organisms within the *Alcaligenes* genus form flat, spreading, rough colonies on blood agar. The edges of the colonies often have a feathery appearance. Some strains produce α-hemolysis. They are also able to grow on MacConkey agar. The organisms are oxidase and catalase positive and motile (peritrichous flagella). In addition, an alkaline reaction is observed in citrate medium and in glucose-containing O-F medium. *The organisms are able to use acetate as the only source of carbon. A. xylosoxidans* is able to reduce nitrates to nitrites and is saccharolytic; *subspecies xylosoxidans can oxidize xylose. A faecalis is relatively inert biochemically. A. odorans* emits a sweet odor that is similar to that of fresh apple cider.

## Antibiotic Susceptibility Characteristics

Infections due to *Alcaligenes* species have been successfully treated with combinations of ticarcillin, piperacillin, azlocillin, and the newer quinolones.

## MORAXELLA

### Organism Characteristics

Organisms in the *Moraxella* genus are gram-negative coccobacilli that usually grow in pairs. They are part of the normal flora of mucous membranes in humans, as well as animals. There are at least six species within the genus. The clinically important species are *B. catarrhalis, M. atlantae, M. lacunata, M. nonliquefaciens, M. osloensis,* and *M. phenylpyruvica*. These bacteria, like *Actinobacter,* have sometimes been confused with the *Neisseria* (they belong in the *Neisseriaceae* family). Indeed, *B. catarrhalis* was previously classified as a species of *Neisseria*. More recently it went by the name of *Branhamella catarrhalis*.

### Clinical Significance

These organisms are opportunists that can cause certain types of nosocomial infections, especially those of the respiratory tract. *B. catarrhalis,* which can be part of the normal oropharyngeal flora, is being increasingly recognized as a respiratory tract pathogen. It has been implicated in pneumonia, acute and chronic bronchitis, and other types of respiratory tract infections in adults. In some cases of group A streptococcal tonsillopharyngitis, it has been identified as one of the copathogens. Bacteremia due to *B. catarrhalis* can occur secondarily to respiratory tract infections in immunocompromised as well as healthy immuno-competent individuals. It can vary in severity from self-limiting illness with fever to lethal sepsis. The total number of bacteremic cases due to the organisms is thought to be underreported, since it (like many *Neisseria* species) may be inhibited by sodium polyanethol sulfonate, a blood culture anticoagulant. It is also a cause of persistent coughing, **otitis media**, and sinusitis in children. In a recent study of pediatric patients these organisms were responsible for 8% of otitis media cases. *M. lacunata* may be isolated from the eye; occasionally it has been associated with conjunctivitis and extraocular infections, some of which have been traced to ofloxacin eye drops. In a series of unusual outbreaks of bloodstream infections at seven different hospitals, the CDC reported that *M. osloensis* was one of the agents involved. The source of contamination was determined to be a lipid-based anesthetic. The agency concluded that with the increased use of lipid-based medications (which support rapid bacterial growth at room temperature), specially strict aseptic techniques are essential. *Moraxella* species have also been isolated from infected wounds.

## Cultural Characteristics and Identification

These are relatively fastidious organisms, sometimes requiring enriched media containing blood (i.e., chocolate agar). However, most isolates will grow slowly on MacConkey agar; the major exception to this is *M. lacunata*. This species is rather unusual also in that it sometimes produces pitting in blood agar and may hydrolyze gelatin. It can also liquefy serum and, thus form depressions in Loeffler's serum agar slants. Colonies on solid media are nonpigmented. They are nonmotile, oxidase positive, and are unable to utilize carbohydrates. All species, except *M. osloensis,* grow in media containing 3% NaCl. The great majority do not grow at 42°C. Unlike the other species, *M. phenylpyruvica* produces a urease enzyme and deaminates phenylalanine.

## Antibiotic Susceptibility Characteristics

The *Moraxella* are usually susceptible to the newer penicillins. *B. catarrhalis,* however, is often resistant because of ß-lactamase production. Isolates with increased resistance to ampicillin, co-trimoxasole, and macrolides have been reported. This species, however, is susceptible to third-generation cephalosporins such as cefiximine.

# XANTHOMONAS (STENOTROPHOMONAS)

## Organism Characteristics

*Xanthomonas maltophilia,* previously known as *Pseudomonas maltophilia,* is in the *Pseudomonadaceae* family. It is a free-living gram-negative rod that is ubiquitous in the environment. It frequently colonizes the oropharynx of healthy individuals, and the significance of its isolation in respiratory tract infections cannot be immediately assumed.

## Clinical Significance

Nosocomial infections due to *X. maltophilia* are becoming increasingly common. Several clusters of hospital-based outbreaks due to the organisms have been documented. They are especially prevalent in patients who are receiving antimicrobial therapy. The organisms have been isolated from the respiratory tract, wounds, blood, urine, and skin. Bacteremias due to these agents are associated with the long-term use of plastic intravenous catheters.

## Cultural Characteristics and Identification

*Xanthomonas maltophilia* is the second most frequently isolated organism among those that are discussed in this chapter. This species oxidizes both maltose and glucose and is motile (peritrichous flagella). Isolates can be easily differentiated from *P. aeruginosa* by a negative oxidase reaction, inability to grow on cetrimide-containing media, and lack of pyoverdin production. Colonies on blood agar are rough, grayish or lavender-green, and exude an ammonia-like odor. Some strains exhibit alpha hemolysis. *They do not produce oxidase, arginine dihydrolase, ornithine decarboxylase, or any pigments, but are positive for lysine decarboxylase and gelatin hydrolysis. The majority (>80%) of isolates produce acid in O-F medium utilizing lactose, glucose, and fructose.*

## Antibiotic Susceptibility Characteristics

Sulfamethoxazole-trimethoprim is usually effective in the treatment of infections due to *X. maltophilia.* These organisms, however, tend to be resistant to many other commonly used antibiotics including cephalosporins, aminoglycosides, quinolones, imipenem, and penicillins. Their resistance to penicillins is attributed to the low permeability of their outer membranes and to production of ß-lactamases with broad-spectrum activity.

# SPECIAL CONSIDERATIONS FOR IMMUNOCOMPROMISED HOSTS

Patients with low polymorphonuclear cell (neutrophil) activity, frequently seen in acute myelogenous leukemia and chronic granulomatous disease, are highly susceptible to *P. aeruginosa* infection. Pneumonia due to the organisms can be especially severe in these immunocompromised individuals. Alveolar necrosis, infarcts, vascular invasion by the organisms, and bacteremia occur often. Individuals with leukopenia due to chemotherapy, hematologic malignancies other than myelogenous leukemia, and third degree burns also have increased susceptibility to *P. aeruginosa* infection. (Note: patients with third degree burns also exhibit functional defects in phagocytic cell populations.) Indeed, fatal infection occurs most often in patients with leukemias and lymphomas and in those with extensive burns. A 50% to 70% fatality rate has been reported in these individuals if they are neutropenic and develop bacteremia.

It is not entirely clear why *P. aeruginosa* appears to have such a high affinity for cancer patients; they are, indeed, extremely common inhabitants of the nasopharynx and gut of these individuals. Their natural resistance to various chemotherapeutic drugs used to treat malignant diseases (as well as their resistance to numerous antibiotics) is thought to be a significant factor. It is important to note also that certain substances produced by *P. aeruginosa* can lower immune responsiveness. For example, the elastase enzyme not only degrades elastin, but can also inhibit the function of neutrophils. The alkaline protease of the organisms breaks down immunoglobulins (IgG) and complement and inhibits neutrophil function. It can also inhibit the activity of interferon-γ (IFN-γ), a protein secreted by T helper lymphocytes. IFN-γ activates macrophages and augments T cytotoxic lymphocyte and natural killer cell functions.

*Pseudomonas aeruginosa* is isolated quite frequently from persons who are infected with the human immunodeficiency virus type-1 (HIV-1). The infection may be nosocomial or community acquired. Recent studies suggest that the organisms may cause a substantial proportion of sinusitis cases in this population; in individuals with acquired immunodeficiency syndrome (AIDS), the organisms are implicated in the development of pneumonia. However, *P. aeruginosa* occurs less frequently in AIDS patients compared to certain other infectious agents (e.g., *Pneumocystis carinii, Streptococcus pneumoniae, Haemophilus influenzae,* and cytomegalovirus).

Many of the isolates from immunocompromised subjects show multidrug resistance. Mechanisms of resistance that have been noted include inducible chromosomally mediated cephalosporinase, ß-lactamase production, aminoglycoside-inactivating enzymes, and changes in the bacterial cell wall. Experimental vaccines administered to high-risk subjects have provided some protection against the development of sepsis. Transfusion of granulocytes and infusion of hyperimmune gamma globulins have also been used with a moderate degree of success.

Not surprisingly, many of the other aerobic nonfermenters discussed in this chapter produce more severe infections in immunocompromised subjects than in healthy persons. For example, *Acinetobacter* species are more likely to produce sepsis, *B. cattharbalis* is more likely to cause bacteremia, and *F. meningosepticum* is more likely to cause meningitis in an individual whose immune functions are less than optimal.

## SUMMARY

▶ This group of organisms consists of aerobic, motile, gram-negative rods that often fail to ferment carbohydrates ("nonfermenters"). They are frequently found in the environment and usually do not cause disease in healthy individuals.

▶ *Pseudomonas aeruginosa,* an extremely ubiquitous and hardy organism, is the most important member of the group. It has one to three polar flagella and is oxidase positive. It produces water-soluble pigments, including pyocyanin and pyoverdin ("green pus"), exhibits ß-hemolysis, and emits a characteristic odor. These properties are useful in laboratory diagnosis.

▶ *P. aeruginosa* is very common in infected burns and wounds and can cause numerous other types of infections, including echthyma gangrenosum, otitis externa ("swimmer's ear"), folliculitis (hot tubs, spas), and urinary tract infections. The organisms frequently colonize the respiratory tract of patients with cystic fibrosis. Among the most important virulence facts are exotoxin A and a "slimy" capsule (alginate polysaccharide).

▶ *P. aeruginosa* is highly resistant to many antibiotics and carries R plasmids. Combination treatment with an aminoglycoside plus azlocillin may be effective; the fatality rate is high with septicemia.

▶ *P. mallei* and *P. pseudomallei,* found primarily in animals, can cause glanders and melioidosis, respectively. Clinical manifestations in humans are skin infections and pneumonia. Outcome can be fatal, of untreated.

▶ *Acinetobacter,* associated most commonly with pneumonia in hospitalized patients, is oxidase negative and thus can be differentiated from *Neisseria* species.

▶ Neonatal meningitis is the most common clinical manifestation of infection with *Flavobacterium,* an organism that often produces an intense yellow pigment.

▶ *Alcaligenes* species are most strongly linked to urinary tract and wound infections.

▶ *Moraxella* is implicated primarily in pneumonia and bronchitis.

▶ *Xanthomonas maltophilia* is becoming an increasingly common isolate from nosocomial infections; colonies may exhibit a lavender-green color and exude an ammonia-like odor.

## Review Questions

1. A gram-negative rod is isolated from the sputum of a 20-year-old woman with cystic fibrosis. Laboratory tests reveal that the organism is an aerobic "nonfermenter" that produces a blue pigment and is highly resistant to numerous antibiotics. Given this description, the organism is MOST LIKELY to be:
   a. *Pseudomonas aeruginosa*
   b. *Pseudomonas pseudomallei*
   c. *Pseudomonas fluorescens*
   d. *Pseudomonas putida*

2. Which of the following is an important factor in the virulence of *P. aeruginosa*?
   a. Enterotoxin
   b. Pyomelanin
   c. Exotoxin A
   d. Siderophorin

3. A factor produced by *P. aeruginosa* that can break down antibodies and complement is:
   a. pyocyanin.
   b. elastase.
   c. exoenzyme S.
   d. alkaline protease.

4. Which of the following best describes the mechanism of action of exotoxin A?
   a. It breaks down the endothelial layer of small blood vessels.
   b. It interferes with polymerase enzymes that synthesize DNA.
   c. It binds to cytoplasmic membranes and increases their permeability.
   d. It stops protein synthesis by ADP-ribosylation of elongation factor-2.

5. *Pseudomonas* species are MOST LIKELY to cause serious infection in individuals who:
   a. take care of patients with leukemia.
   b. are employed in a hospital.
   c. compete in swimming events.
   d. have a very low neutrophil count.

6. Melioidosis is caused by which of the following organisms?
   a. *Xanthomonas maltophilia*
   b. *Pseudomonas pseudomallei*
   c. *Alcaligenes xylosoxidans*
   d. *Flavobacterium meningosepticum*

7. *P. aeruginosa* infection in patients with AIDS is MOST LIKELY to be manifested as:
   a. pneumonia.
   b. folliculitis.
   c. osteomyelitis.
   d. otitis externa.

8. Glanders is caused by which of the following organisms?
   a. *Acinetobacter lwoffii*
   b. *Moraxella caterrhalis*
   c. *Moraxella lacunata*
   d. *Pseudomonas mallei*

---

## CASE STUDY 1: *PSEUDOMONAS AERUGINOSA* INFECTION IN A PATIENT WITH LEUKEMIA

A 15-year-old girl with acute lymphocytic leukemia went into remission while in the hospital. She was discharged, but was continued on long-term maintenance chemotherapy for the disease as an outpatient. Within 2 weeks she developed a slight fever and mild respiratory distress, but no other symptoms. However, her condition worsened rapidly and she returned to the hospital. At arrival her pulse rate and breathing were rapid and her temperature was 102°F. Laboratory analyses revealed that her white blood cell count was $0.3 \times 10^9$/L (significantly below normal). A combination of tobramycin and ceftazidime was initiated. Within hours, however, the patient's breathing became more labored, requiring intubation and respiratory assistance with a mechanical ventilator. Hypotension and shock due to low blood pressure were circumvented by the intravenous administration of fluids and drugs. Blood specimens taken during the first 2 days of hospitalization were positive for *P. aeruginosa*. Subsequent samples were negative. The patient improved slowly over the next few days and was eventually discharged. Chemotherapy for the leukemia was discontinued until her white blood cell count was above $1.0 \times 10^9$/L.

### Questions:

1. Does leukemia predispose to developing *P. aeruginosa* infection?

2. What are the mechanisms by which *P. aeruginosa* enters the blood circulation?

3. What types of laboratory tests were likely to be used to identify *P. aeruginosa* in the blood specimens?

## CASE STUDY 2

A 9-month-old infant who failed to develop normally due to nutritional neglect developed secondary immunodeficiency characterized by marked thymic involution (atrophy or shriveling). The child died of systemic *P. aeruginosa* infection. Clinical manifestations included pneumonia, lung abscesses, and endocarditis. Multiple gangrenous ecthymas consisting of deep ulcers, inflammation, and induration were observed on the skin of the entire body. Autopsy revealed that the lungs were hemorrhagic and had multiple abscesses with necrotizing arteritis; the heart showed dark brown verrucae at the cusps of the mitral valve. Large numbers of *P. aeruginosa* were isolated from the lungs, heart, and skin lesions on bacteriologic examination. (Based on a case described by Ohshima et al., 1991.)

**Questions:**

1. How is the poor nutritional status of the infant related to development of secondary immunodeficiency and infection with *P. aeruginosa*?

2. What is the cause of the widespread tissue destruction in the infant?

3. Is the multisystem involvement unusual for *P. aeruginosa*?

## CASE STUDY 3

A 30-year-old man with quadriplegia due to spinal cord transection was transferred to a hospital from a chronic care facility because of fever (39.9°C temperature) and increased need for ventilatory support. The patient had ulcerative skin lesions ("bed sores") and had recently been given a 10-day course of intravenous oxacillin therapy. On presentation, his breath sounds in the left hemithorax were decreased. The white blood cell count was 12.0 × $10^9$/L; the differential showed increased percentages of segmented neutrophils and bands. Chest radiography revealed partial collapse of the left lung. Radiography after bronchoscopy indicated the presence of a persistent infiltrate in the left lower lobe. *B. catarrhalis* was cultured from the blood. Sputum cultures yielded *Acinetobacter anitratus*, *Klebsiella pneumoniae*, and *Haemophilus influenzae*. The patient improved during a 10-day course of ceftazidime therapy. (Based on a case described by Ioannis et al., 1995.)

**Questions:**

1. Is bactermia due to *B. catarrhalis* unusual?

2. Which of the isolated organisms is most likely to be responsible for the pulmonary symptoms?

3. What is the significance of the elevated white blood cell count and increased percentages of neutrophils?

## ▶ REFERENCES & RECOMMENDED READING

Bennett, S. N., McNeil, M. M., Bland, L. A., Arduino, M. J., Villarino, M. E., Perrotta, D. M., Burwen, D. R., Welbel, S. F., Pegues, D. A., Stroud, L., et al. (1995). Postoperative infections traced to contamination of an intravenous anesthetic, propofol. *New England Journal of Medicine, 333*, 147–154.

Britigan, B. E., Roeder, T. L., Rasmussen, G. T., Shasby, D. M., McCormick, M. L., & Cox, C. D. (1992). Interaction of the *Pseudomonas aeruginosa* secretory products pyocyanin and pyochelina generates hydroxyl radical and causes synergistic damage to endothelial cells. Implications for *Pseudomonas*-associated tissue injury. *Journal of Clinical Investigation, 90*, 2187–2196.

Cheron, M., Abachin, E., Guerot, E., el Bez, M., & Simonet, M. (1994). Investigation of hospital-acquired infections due to *Alcaligenes denitrificans* subsp. *xylosoxydans* by DNA restriction fragment length polymorphism. *Journal of Clinical Microbiology, 32*, 1023–1026.

Coullioud, D., Van der Auwera, P., Viot, M., & Lasset, C. (1993). Prospective multicenter study of the etiology of 1051 bacteremic episodes in 782 cancer patients. *Support Care Cancer, 1*, 34–46.

Dunn, M., & Wunderink, R. G. (1995). Ventilator-associated pneumonia caused by *Pseudomonas infection. Clinics in Chest Medicine, 16*, 95–109.

Ezzedine, H., Mourad, M., Van Ossel, C., Logghe, C., Squifflet, J. P., Renault, F., Wauters, G., Gigi, J., Wilmotte, L., & Haxhe, J. J. (1994). An outbreak of *Ochrobactrum anthropi* bacteremia in five organ transplant patients. *Journal of Hospital Infection, 27*, 35–42.

Gillian, P. H. (1995). Pseudomonas and Burkholderia. In P. R. Murray, E. J. Baron, M. A. Pfaller, F. C. Tenover, & R. H. Yolken, (Eds.). *Manual of Clinical Microbiology* (6th ed., pp. 505–519). Washington, DC: ASM Press.

Ibrahim, M. (1995). Hydrocephalus and cerebral palsy due to *Acinetobacter* meningitis in a neonate. *West African Journal of Medicine, 14*, 59–60.

Ioannidis, J. P. A., Worthington, M., Griffiths, J. K., & Snydman, D. R. (1995). Spectrum and significance of bacteremia due to *Moraxella catarrhalis. Clinics in Infectious Disease, 21*, 390–397.

Ishihara, S., Takino, M., Okada, Y., & Mimura, K. (1995). Septic shock due to *Pseudomonas aeruginosa* in a previously healthy woman. *Intensive Care Medicine, 21*, 226–228.

Jones, R. N. (1992). The current and future impact of antimicrobial resistance among nosocomial bacterial pathogens. *Diagnostic Microbiology and Infectious Disease, 15*, 3S–10S.

Keller, D. W., & Breiman, R. F. (1995). Preventing bacterial respiratory tract infections among persons infected with human immunodeficiency virus. *Clinics in Infectious Disease, 21*, 877–883.

Kielhofner, M., Atmar, R. L., Hamill, R. J., Musher, D. M. (1992). Life-threatening *Pseudomonas aeruginosa* infections in patients with human immunodeficiency virus infection. *Clinics in Infectious Disease, 14*, 403–411.

Lesseva, M. I., & Hadjiski, O. G. (1995). Analysis of bacteriuria in patients with burns. *Burns, 21*, 3–6.

Lortholary, O., Fagon, J. Y., Hoi, A. B., Slama, M. A., Pierre, J., Giral, P., Rosenzweig, R., Gutmann, L., Safar, M., & Acar, J. (1995). Nosocomial acquisition of mutiresistant *Acinetobacter baumannii:* Risk factors and prognosis. *Clinics in Infectious Disease, 20*, 790–796.

Marshall, W. F., et al. (1989). *Xanthomonas maltophilia:* An emerging nosocomial pathogen. *Mayo Clinic Proceedings, 64*, 1097.

May, T. B., Shinaburger, D., Maharaj, R., Litto, J., et al. (1991). Alginate synthesis by *Pseudomonas aeruginosa:* A key pathogenic factor in chronic cystic fibrosis patients. *Clinical Microbiology Reviews, 4*, 191–206.

Ohshima, T., Nakaya, T., Saito, K., Maeda, H., & Nagano, T. (1991). Child neglect followed by marked thymic involution and fatal systemic *Pseudomonas* infection. *International Journal of Legal Medicine, 104*, 167–171.

Ouchi, K., Abe, M., Karita, M., Oguri, T., Igari, J., & Nakazawa, T. (1995). Analysis of strains of *Burkholderia (Pseudomonas) cepacia* isolated in a nosocomial outbreak by biochemical and genomic typing. *Journal of Clinical Microbiology, 33*, 2353–2357.

Prince, A. (1992). Adhesins and receptors of *Pseudomonas aeruginosa* associated with infection of the respiratory tract. *Microbial Pathogenesis, 13*, 251–260.

Rolston, K. V., & Bodey, G. P. (1992). *Pseudomonas aeruginosa* infection in cancer patients. *Cancer Investigation, 10*, 43–59.

Ti, T. Y., Tan, W. C., Chong, A. P., & Lee, E. H. (1993). Non-fatal and fatal infections caused by *Chromobacterium violaceum. Clinics in Infectious Disease, 17*, 505–507.

Weernink, A., Severin, W. P., Tjernberg, I., & Dijkshoorn, L. (1995). Pillows, an unexpected source of *Acinetobacter. Journal of Hospital Infection, 29*, 189–199.

# CHAPTER 18
## Vibrio and Other Curved Aerobic Gram-Negative Bacilli

Daila S. Gridley, PhD

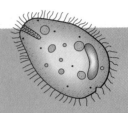

## Microbes in the News
### *Vibrio vulnificus* Warning

The Department of Health Services of Los Angeles County recently advised all health care providers in California to inform patients about the dangers of eating raw or improperly cooked seafood. Septicemia leading to shock and death due to *Vibrio vulnificus*, the most deadly of all seafood-borne organisms, has been reported in over 50% of cases occurring in the county since 1993. The majority of patients had eaten raw oysters shortly before the onset of illness. One survivor had both legs amputated to control cellulitis. Underlying conditions that were associated with high risk for severe illness included hepatitis, diabetes, and heavy alcohol consumption. Los Angeles County Department of Health Services. (1995). Physician alert: *Vibrio vulnificus*. *Public Health Letter, 18(6),* 23.

## KEY TERMS

Campy BAP medium
Cary-Blair transport medium
Cholera
Cholera toxin
Classic biotype
Comma-shaped rods

Compound O/129
Eltor biotype
"Gull-wing" morphology
Halophilic bacteria
Kanawaga-positive strains
Lophotrichous flagella

O1 serogroup
O139 serogroup
Peptic ulcer
"Rice-water" stools
Skirrow's medium
TCBS agar

## LEARNING OBJECTIVES

Upon successful completion of this chapter, the student should be able to:

1. Identify by name the major organisms that fall within this group.
2. Present the distinguishing features for each of the organisms that are important human pathogens.

3. Describe the diseases associated with each of the major human pathogens and list possible virulence factors.
4. Discuss the types of laboratory assays that are useful in identification and differentiation.
5. Identify effective treatment modalities and preventive measures.

## INTRODUCTION

The bacteria discussed in this chapter are gram-negative rods that are usually highly motile and oxidase positive, with distinctive morphologic characteristics. Individual cells have a curved, **comma-shaped rod** morphology, but sometimes may be linked end-to-end forming "S" shapes, "**gull-wings**," and spirals. Motility is mediated by means of polar flagella that vary in number. The great majority of these organisms are widely distributed in nature. Some are especially prevalent in fresh and sea waters, some are found in a variety of warm-blooded animals (both wild and domestic), and a few are present in cold-blooded animals. All genera included here have one or more species associated with diarrheal disease in humans. Some are associated with infections of wounds and cuts. Drinking contaminated water, ingesting uncooked seafood, and having direct contact with seawater are major routes of infection.

The *Vibrionaceae* family contains three genera that have one or more species associated with human disease: *Vibrio, Aeromonas,* and *Plesiomonas.* Selected characteristics of the most common isolates in these genera are presented in Table 18-1.

*Vibrio cholerae* (**O1 serogroup**) is the most notorious member of this family. Seven major pandemics of

cholera, a disease that can result in a massive loss of fluid and a high mortality rate, have been documented since the 1800s. The seventh pandemic began in 1961 and is still ongoing in Asia, the Middle East, and Africa. It arrived in Peru in 1991 and rapidly spread to all countries of South and Central America. This is the first time in nearly a century that cholera has struck with such a vengeance in the western hemisphere of the world. Millions of people have already been affected during the course of the current pandemic. In late 1992, a novel *V. cholerae* (**O139 serogroup**) appeared in southern Bangladesh and parts of India, causing large epidemics of cholera. Infections with this serogroup are rapidly spreading and there are now reports of its appearance in several developed countries. It has been suggested that the emergence of *V. cholerae* O139 may represent the beginning of the eighth cholera pandemic. Other important members of the *Vibrionaceae* that are associated with human infections include *V. parahemolyticus* and *V. vulnificus.*

*Helicobacter* and *Campylobacter* share some of the characteristics of the vibrios. *Helicobacter pylori* has now been identified as an etiologic agent of gastritis and peptic ulcer disease. These organisms are common inhabitants of the stomach, especially in older populations. *Campylobacter jejuni* is a microaerophilic organ-

| Table 18–1 ▶ Selected Characteristics of Genera in the *Vibrionaceae* Family | | | |
|---|---|---|---|
| **Characteristic** | **Vibrio** | **Aeromonas** | **Plesiomonas** |
| Cell morphology | Curved | Straight or curved | Curved |
| Flagella | Polar (1) | Polar (1 or more) | Polar (1 or more) |
| Acid from mannitol | + | + | − |
| Growth on TCBS | Yes | No | No |
| NaCl* | Yes | No | No |

A + and − indicate that the majority of isolates give a positive or negative reaction, respectively.

*Organisms either require the salt for growth or their growth is stimulated by its presence.

TCBS, thiosulfate-citrate-bile-sucrose agar.

ism found in the intestinal tract of animals. It is a frequent cause of gastroenteritis in humans throughout the world; in the United States it is now recognized as the most common agent of diarrheal disease.

# VIBRIO (CHOLERAE, PARAHEMOLYTICUS, VULNIFICUS)

## Organism Characteristics

The vibrios are curved or comma-shaped gram-negative rods that are relatively short, approximately 2 to 4 µm long. *Vibrio* species grow well on most ordinary laboratory media. Although they have a fermentative and respiratory metabolism, best growth is obtained in the presence of air. They are oxidase positive and, with the exception of *V. parahemolyticus* (which produces peritrichous flagella on solid media), they have a single polar flagellum. In addition, most of them are able to grow well at high pH (8.5–9.5), but are rapidly killed under acidic conditions. All species, except *V. cholerae* and *V. mimicus*, need NaCl for growth (i.e., they are **halophilic bacteria**). The sodium is presumably required for protein synthesis by the halophilic species. These bacteria are extremely common in many surface waters of the world, including seawater. Of the 12 species that are associated with human disease, *V. cholerae*, *V. parahemolyticus*, and *V. vulnificus* are most frequently isolated. *V. cholerae*, a nonhalophilic vibrio, is prevalent in freshwater ponds and estuaries (wide mouths of rivers leading to seas) of Asia, the Middle East, Africa, along the shores of South and North America, and parts of Europe. This species is now being seen with increasing frequency in the United States, especially in certain states that border coastal water (e.g., Florida, Texas, and Louisiana). *V. parahemolyticus*, the second most common vibrio isolated in the United States, and *V. vulnificus* are present in marine water, shellfish, other marine animals, and plankton.

Most *Vibrio* species have only a single type of heat-labile flagellar H antigen. In contrast, O antigens, based on the structure of their lipopolysaccharides, are very diverse. Isolates of *V. cholerae* are classified into groups depending on the serologic characteristics of their O antigens. Most pathogenic organisms within this species belong to the O1 serogroup, that is, they are agglutinated by antisera specific for the O1 antigen. Organisms of the O1 serogroup have been responsible for all of the cholera pandemics, as well as the great majority of epidemics. The O1 serogroup can be further divided into subgroups on the basis of three fractions of the O antigens that are designated as A, B, and C. Strains that have the AB, AC, or ABC fractions are designated as ogawa, inaba, and hikajima subgroups, respectively. *V. cholerae* O1 also consists of two biotypes, the **classic** and **eltor**. The latter biotype was first isolated in 1905 at the El Tor quarantine station in the Gulf of Suez from the dead bodies of Mecca pilgrims. The classic biotype was most prevalent until the 1960s, but has since been replaced by eltor. This phenomenon has been attributed to the fact that the eltor biotype persists longer in the environment and because it results in a higher incidence of asymptomatic carriers compared to the classic organisms. Differentiation of the two biotypes was originally based on the ability of eltor to hemolyze sheep erythrocytes. Recent pandemics, however, have been due to a nonhemolytic strain of eltor. The current pandemic is due to the eltor biotype, inaba subgroup.

## Clinical Significance

*Vibrio cholerae* is transmitted by water and food, although flies and person-to-person contact with infected individuals have also been implicated. It is estimated that only 1% to 5% of exposed persons actually develop disease. This may be due, at least in part, to the fact that the organisms are susceptible to the acidity of the stomach. Individuals who lack gastric acidity because of gastrectomy or achlorhydria due to malnutrition have a higher than expected incidence of cholera. Others at increased risk include those who are taking drugs such as cimetidine and ranitidine, that block $H_2$ receptors (stimulation of $H_2$ receptors induces gastric acid secretion). Infection in most healthy individuals requires the ingestion of very large numbers ($10^8$–$10^{10}$) of the organisms. Once they reach the small bowel (which has a more favorable alkaline pH), they penetrate through the mucous layer, adhere to microvilli of the brush border, and multiply.

The disease of cholera is largely due to the secretion of a complex enterotoxin (also known as **cholera toxin** or choleragen) that is encoded by chromosomal genes found primarily in the *V. cholerae* O1 serotype. It has been extensively studied and is the prototype for toxins that have similar mechanisms of action (e.g., the heat-labile toxin of *Escherichia coli*). This stimulates the hypersecretion of water into the intestinal lumen as the cells attempt to maintain osmotic stability. Dehydration, electrolyte imbalance, and hypotension can occur very rapidly, although the overall absorptive capability of the intestinal tract remains intact. Nontoxigenic mutants have decreased virulence and also colonize less efficiently compared to toxigenic strains. The specific role of the toxin in colonization is unclear.

The symptoms of cholera (nausea, vomiting, diarrhea, and abdominal cramps) appear after an incubation period of approximately 1 to 4 days. The characteristic **"rice-water" stools** are colorless and odorless and contain flecks of mucus, many vibrios, and epithelial cells. The mucus flecks are what give the stools the appearance of rice water. A striking feature of the disease is the huge amount of fluid loss, sometimes as much as 20 to 30 L within a 24-hour period, which leads to profound dehydration, acidosis, circulatory collapse, anuria, shock, and death. The mortality rate ranges from 25% to 50%, if untreated. The classic biotype causes more severe disease than the eltor biotype, but the eltor biotype tends to persist longer both inside and outside of the body. The organisms may be shed for 3 to 4 weeks after recovery, but chronic carriers are rare. *V. cholerae* causes disease only in humans.

It is believed that most individuals who recover from cholera develop long-term immunity to reinfection. The production of secretory IgA by submucosal lymphocytes in the intestinal tract probably plays an important role. Because currently available cholera vaccines induce only short-term protection (the World Health Organization certificate for cholera immunization is valid for 6 months), there is great interest in developing more immunogenic products. Overall, the results have been disappointing in that the degree of protection and the duration of immunity appear to be limited. Furthermore, the vaccines have not proven to be effective as control measures in the midst of epidemics. Vaccines using live attenuated strains of the *V. cholerae* O1, as well as O139, and genetically engineered versions of the cholera toxin are currently being developed. A few of these new vaccines are being tested in early clinical trials with adult volunteers.

Ingestion of raw fish or shellfish contaminated with *V. parahemolyticus* can cause acute gastroenteritis that may resemble cholera after an incubation period of 5 to 92 hours (average time is 24 hours). The infection is characterized by nausea, vomiting, abdominal cramps, and explosive diarrhea that ranges from watery to bloody in severe cases. Patients may be afebrile or have a low-grade fever. Fatty infiltration into the liver and some degree of hepatomegaly (enlargement of the liver) may be noted. Spontaneous recovery usually occurs in 1 to 4 days in otherwise healthy individuals. No enterotoxin has been identified in this species and the pathologic mechanisms are unclear, although nearly all clinical isolates are **Kanagawa-positive strains** (i.e., they produce a thermostable hemolysin). The organism is a major cause of diarrheal disease in Japan and other countries where the consumption of raw fish and other seafood is prevalent.

Infections with *V. vulnificus* most often appear as skin lesions after handling shellfish or other marine animals or after laceration with seashells. Infections of wounds may progress rapidly with swelling, erythema, pain, and development of vesicles or bullae (blister-like skin lesions filled with fluid). Sometimes this is followed by extensive tissue necrosis. Diarrhea due to *V. vulnificus* can occur after eating raw or undercooked seafood, especially oysters. Nearly all oysters that are harvested from the coastal water in the Gulf of Mexico during the warmer months of the year are infected with

the organisms; as the water cools, the infection rate drops to 5%. These observations, as well as highly publicized reports of deaths following the consumption of raw oysters, have prompted the Food and Drug Administration to consider adopting stricter regulatory limits on the seafood industry. Elderly or debilitated persons are at greatest risk for developing severe illness. Infection with the organisms can result in not only severe enteritis, but also bacteremia, septicemia, and death (see section on immunocompromised hosts).

The types of infections caused by the medically most important vibrios are summarized in Table 18-2.

## Cultural Characteristics and Identification

Stool specimens and samples from infected wounds are the usual types of specimens sent to the clinical laboratory in cases of suspected infection with *Vibrio* species. Direct Gram staining of specimens is generally not done because the characteristic morphology is rarely evident. However, the procedure may be useful when performed on samples after a 6- to 8-hour incubation period in taurocholate-peptone broth that has a pH of 8.0 to 9.0 (medium at pH 8.4 is usually used). In addition, rapidly motile vibrios may be visualized with dark-field or phase contrast microscopy. On continued in vitro passage, some vibrios (including *V. cholerae*) may become straight rods that are similar to the gram-negative enteric bacteria. Because *Vibrio* species rapidly lose viability under acidic conditions (a pH of 6.0 or less will sterilize cultures of *V. cholerae*) or in dry environments, specimens should be promptly cultured on appropriate media. **Cary-Blair transport media** and refrigeration help to ensure survival of the organisms when culturing is delayed. The vibrios do not survive for long in transport media used for most of the gram-negative enterics.

*Vibrio* species grow well on ordinary laboratory media at 37°C, including 5% sheep blood agar and MacConkey agar. They are easily differentiated from the *Enterobacteriaceae* by their production of oxidase. Indeed, the oxidase test is frequently used for early presumptive identification. However, isolates may initially be misidentified as *Pseudomonas* because this is a prevalent gram-negative rod that is also oxidase positive. *Vibrio* species form colonies that are smooth, round, and convex within 18 to 24 hours of incubation. They may appear opaque and granular when light is transmitted through them. Tests for halophilic vibrios may require media supplemented with NaCl. Inoculation of selective media for vibrios is not done routinely in the United States, due to the low incidence of positive results. However, samples from patients with a history of foreign travel, shellfish consumption, or direct contact with marine or fresh water are usually plated onto *t*hiosulfate-*c*itrate-*b*ile-*s*ucrose (**TCBS**) agar. This is the

## Table 18–2 ▶ Summary of Medically Important *Vibrio* Species

| Organism | Types of Infections | Comments |
|---|---|---|
| **COMMON** | | |
| *V. cholerae* O1 | Epidemic and pandemic gastroenteritis (cholera) | Eltor biotype, inaba serotype is the cause of the current pandemic; induces less severe illness than the classic biotype; produces cholera toxin |
| *V. cholerae* O139 | Epidemic and pandemic (?) gastroenteritis (cholera) | Newly identified serogroup (late 1992); causes severe illness similar to O1 serogroup, but previous infection with O1 is not protective; produces cholera toxin |
| Other non-O1 *V. cholerae* | Cholera-like or mild gastroenteritis; wound, ear, and other infections | Generally self-limiting illness; extraintestinal infections are rare; may produce cholera-like toxins |
| *V. parahemolyticus* | Gastroenteritis, ear infections; septicemia in debilitated persons | Associated with consumption of raw oysters and other seafood; produces a hemolysin; is the major cause of diarrhea in Japan; has been isolated from patients with acquired immunodeficiency syndrome |
| *V. vulnificus* | Wound (skin) infections, gastroenteritis; septicemia in debilitated persons | Skin lesions with vesicles and bullae; may be very painful with extensive tissue necrosis; organism is highly invasive; most cases of septicemia are associated with underlying liver disease |
| **UNCOMMON** | | |
| *V. alginolyticus* | Wound, ear, eye, and other infections | Associated with exposure to seawater |
| *V. cincinnatiensis* | Septicemia, meningitis | Has been isolated from alcoholic elderly persons |
| *V. damsela* | Infections of soft tissues | Associated with exposure to seawater |
| *V. fluvialis* | Gastroenteritis | Associated with ingestion of raw shellfish |
| *V. furnissii* | Gastroenteritis | Associated with ingestion of raw seafood |
| *V. harveyi* | Wound infections | Associated with exposure to seawater |
| *V. hollisae* | Gastroenteritis | Associated with ingestion of raw seafood |
| *V. mimicus* | Gastroenteritis | Associated with ingestion of raw seafood; possible cholera-like toxin |

most common selective medium used for cultivating stool samples in cases of suspected vibrio infection. *V. cholerae* and other species of sucrose-fermenting vibrios (including a few strains of *V. vulnificus*) form yellow colonies on TCBS agar. Those that do not ferment sucrose produce olive-green colonies. *V. cholerae* also ferments mannose, but not arabinose. In addition, this species is susceptible to **compound O/129** (2,4-diamino-6,7-diisopropylpteridine phosphate), but will grow in the presence of 6% NaCl. These latter two characteristics differentiate it from the aeromonad. Compound O/129 is commercially available in disk and powder form. Unfortunately, a high incidence of *V. cholerae* resistant to the compound is now being reported in India and southeast Asia. It is likely that resistant isolates will also appear in the United States, thus making laboratory diagnosis more difficult.

Identification of the O group to which a particular isolate belongs is important because infection with strains of *V. cholerae* O1 can cause severe illness. Slide agglutination tests using anti-O1 antiserum can be performed. Further characterization of O1 fractions can differentiate among the ogawa, inaba, and hikajuma sub-

groups. Conventional methods that are currently available do not identify *V. cholerae* O139, unless polyclonal anti-O139 antibodies are used. Several monoclonal antibody-based assays specific for this serogroup are currently in development.

Identification of *V. vulnificus* can be accomplished using conventional methodologies. However, this is considered by many to be too slow (at least 4 days), considering the rapid progression and deadly nature of the organisms. More rapid techniques, including the use of probes that target specific genetic sequences, are in development.

Pathogenic *V. parahemolyticus* produces hemolysis on Wagatsuma agar (a special blood agar). This hemolysis is known as the Kanagawa phenomenon, and thus the organisms are called Kanagawa-positive strains. The hemolysis, which is considered to be an important marker for virulent *V. parahemolyticus,* is associated with the production of hemolysins, phospholipase A, and a lysophospholipase. Reports from the western United States, Mexico, and elsewhere indicate that some isolates also produce urease (first reported in 1979). Kanagawa-negative strains can also cause gastroenteritis.

## Antibiotic Susceptibility Characteristics

Replacement of water and reconstitution of electrolyte balance are the most important aspects in the treatment of cholera. The therapy consists of oral or intravenous infusion of glucose solutions containing physiologic concentrations of sodium and chloride and high concentrations of potassium and bicarbonate. Prompt rehydration can reverse the patient's condition within a few hours and reduce the mortality rate to less than 1%. Antibiotic therapy is of lesser importance, although it can shorten the duration of the diarrhea and decrease the volume of lost fluid. In addition, fewer numbers of vibrios are excreted in the stool, thus lessening the possibility for environmental contamination. Either a 3-day regimen of tetracycline or a single dose of doxycycline (a long-acting tetracycline) is standard treatment that is usually very effective. Plasmid-mediated resistance in *V. cholerae* strains, however, has been recently reported in certain parts of Asia and Africa. Tetracycline prophylaxis has been used in areas where *V. cholerae* is endemic, but appears to have limited value in preventing spread of the disease. Recent studies indicate that the fluoroquinolones may be the best prophylactic agents. *V. cholerae,* as well as most other vibrios, are also susceptible to erythromycin, chloramphenicol, and sulfamethoxazoletrimethoprim. Antibiotic therapy, however, for diarrhea due to the majority of *Vibrio* species is often not needed and it is doubtful whether it significantly alters the course of the illness.

## *HELICOBACTER*

## Organism Characteristics

*Helicobacter* is a curved, spiral-shaped gram-negative bacillus that is prevalent in human populations worldwide. Shortly after its discovery in 1982, it was classified as a *Campylobacter.* However, differences in their flagellar characteristics and certain biochemical reactions (most notably a strong positive urease reaction) led to the creation of the *Helicobacter* genus 7 years after the discovery of the organisms. *Helicobacter* exhibits a rapid corkscrew motility that is mediated by one or more polar, sheathed flagella. The organisms apparently do not exist naturally in the environment and no animal reservoir has been documented. Spread from human-to-human appears to be highly likely, but as yet no specific routes of transmission have been identified.

*Helicobacter pylori* (formerly known as *Campylobacter pylori*) is by far the most important member of the genus. It has been estimated that one-half to one-third of the world's population harbors the organisms. In the United States, the incidence of infection is very low in early childhood, but approaches 50% and above in persons who are over the age of 50 years. In developing countries, infection occurs at an earlier age and up to 80% or more of the elderly may be infected. Once the organisms become established, it is believed that they persist in the body for years (perhaps for life). Although many cases of infection are subclinical, there is now overwhelming evidence that the organisms are a major cause of the most common type of gastritis, that is, inflammation of the stomach antrum that was previously thought to be caused by stress, chemical irritants, bile reflux, or ischemia. Certain other gastritis-associated species have been found in animals, such as dogs, ferrets, and cheetahs. *H. pylori* is also thought to play a significant role in the development of **peptic** (duodenal) **ulcers**. Approximately 4 million people in the United States suffer from this condition and new cases are diagnosed at the rate of 350,000/year. In addition, evidence indicates that the organisms may be involved in the etiology of gastric carcinomas (cancers of the stomach).

## Clinical Significance

*Helicobacter pylori*-associated gastritis and peptic ulcers are characterized by recurrent pain, bleeding, and inflammation. Nausea and anorexia are also relatively common manifestations. The organisms produce pilus-like adhesion molecules by which they attach to the intracellular junctions of mucous-secreting epithelial cells that line the gastrointestinal lumen. Recent reports indicate that the receptors on the epithelial cells are carbohydrates that contain fucose, a terminal sugar on the antigens that determine the human ABO and Lewis (Le) blood groups. Interestingly, these findings correlate with previous observations that individuals with the Le[b] and group O phenotypes are at increased risk for developing ulcers.

*Helicobacter pylori* has several mechanisms by which it can escape the acidity of the stomach. The breakdown of urea by its powerful urease enzyme results in the production of large amounts of ammonia, acting as a protective "cloud" to shield the bacteria. The production of a mucinase, together with the high motility of the organisms, allow for rapid penetration through the mucous layer to the epithelial side of the stomach where the pH is approximately 7.4 (the lumen side has a pH of 1.0–2.0). In addition, the production of a protease by the organisms modifies the mucous layer so that acids can no longer diffuse through it as readily. The organisms induce a strong inflammatory response, resulting in polymorphonuclear and mononuclear cell infiltration into the lamina propria (i.e., the connective tissue coat of mucous membranes) and subsequent damage to tissues. Injury may also be due to a cytotoxin that is similar to the α-hemolysin of *E. coli* and the adenylate cyclase of *Bordetella pertussis*. The combination of these, and possibly other, factors results in the loss of the protective mucous layer and predisposes the individual to gastritis and peptic ulcers.

Individuals who are infected with *H. pylori* produce antibodies that are specific for the organisms. The IgM isotype appears first and is followed by IgG and IgA. However, they appear to be ineffective in eliminating infection, perhaps because the bacteria reside in a relatively protected site. High titers of antibody can be routinely demonstrated in chronically infected individuals. No effective vaccine is currently available. Some investigators feel that it may be difficult to develop a vaccine for an organism that lives for decades in its host, despite the generation of a good humoral immune response against it.

Carcinomas of the stomach are by far the most common types of malignancies affecting this organ; they represent 90% to 95% of all cases. Patients with these cancers have a dismally low (<10%) chance for 5-year survival. Recent studies suggest that *H. pylori* may be a significant cofactor in the development of these neoplasms, although the supporting evidence is largely circumstantial. For example, epidemiologic data show that persons who are infected with the organisms have a six-fold higher risk for gastric carcinoma compared to noninfected individuals. Furthermore, chronic gastritis results in metaplastic and dysplastic changes in epithelial cells; these are conditions that always precede the development of these types of cancers. Most infected people, however, do not develop gastric carcinoma and it still remains to be determined whether treatment for *H. pylori* infection will result in a decrease in the incidence of these malignancies.

*Helicobacter cinnaedi* and *H. fennelliae* are much less frequently encountered than *H. pylori*. They have been isolated primarily from homosexual men with gastroenteritis, proctitis, proctocolitis, and sepsis. These two species are sexually transmitted.

## Cultural Characteristics and Identification

Laboratory identification of *H. pylori* is based partly on visualization of curved or spiraled organisms in gastric biopsy specimens that have been stained with Warthin-Starry silver or Giemsa stains. Staining with hematoxylin and eosin or Gram stain may also be done but is less likely to produce positive results. A presumptive diagnosis is often based on observation of typical cellular morphology and positive urease, oxidase, and catalase reactions. Rapid detection of urease activity (i.e., within 1–2 hours) can be performed directly on tissues or after cultivation of the organisms. In the direct assay, biopsy material is placed onto media containing urea and a color indicator. In vivo testing for urease is performed by having the patient ingest $^{13}C$- or $^{14}C$-labeled urea. Radiolabeled $CO_2$ can

be measured in the expired air ("breath test"), if urease is present.

The organisms grow best on rich media that is supplemented with blood, hemin, or charcoal to protect them from the toxic effects of hydrogen peroxide, unstable oxygen radicals, and fatty acids. Nonselective media such as *Brucella* agar with 5% sheep blood and chocolate agar and selective media such as **Skirrow's medium** (which contains vancomycin, polymyxin B, and trimethoprim) and modified Thayer-Martin agar are frequently used. Small, round, translucent, nonpigmented colonies usually appear after a 3- to 7-day incubation period at 37°C in a microaerophilic environment (5% oxygen) and a pH of 6.0 to 7.0. Successful isolation, however, may require several biopsy specimens because of the inhibitory nature of the antiseptics and antibiotics that are used during endoscopy, the irregular distribution of the organisms in the tissues, prior therapy, or contamination with other mucosal microorganisms. Several serologic assays for detection and quantitation of specific serum antibodies are available. Because antibody levels tend to persist, they are of limited value in diagnosing active infection or in monitoring the efficacy of therapy. Characteristics that are useful in differentiating among the clinically most important species of *Helicobacter* and *Campylobacter* are shown in Table 18-3.

## Antibiotic Susceptibility Characteristics

The newly gained knowledge regarding the role of *H. pylori* in gastritis and peptic ulcers is expected to revolutionize therapy for these conditions. However, as of early 1996 the Food and Drug Administration had not yet approved the use of antibiotics for either gastritis or ulcers. Bland diets, Pepto-Bismol (which contains bismuth and has long been known to decrease symptoms of "heartburn"), $H_2$-receptor blockers to decrease stomach acidity (includes antacids such as Tagamet and Zantac), and surgical removal of unresponsive ulcers are still commonly used regimens.

Results from several large clinical trials, which have only recently been completed, show that a combination of metronidazole, bismuth subsalicylate (or bismuth subcitrate), and amoxicillin (or tetracycline) is usually successful in treating *H. pylori* infection. Metronidazole is the most important agent in this treatment plan. A 14-day regimen consisting of triple drug therapy eradicates the organisms in up to 95% of patients, with subsequent resolution of disease and a greatly reduced incidence of recurrence compared to the old therapies described above. Other drug combinations are also being investigated, especially for metronidazole-resistant strains. Omeprazole appears to be very effective against most resistant isolates and

**Table 18–3** ► Characteristics of Clinically Important *Helicobacter* and *Campylobacter* Species

| Organism | Reservoir Host | Major Forms of Disease | Growth 25°C | Growth 42°C | Urease | Oxidase | Catalase | Nitrate Reduction | Hippurate Hydrolysis | Susceptibility to: Nalidixic Acid | Susceptibility to: Cephalothin |
|---|---|---|---|---|---|---|---|---|---|---|---|
| *H. pylori* | Humans | Gastritis, peptic ulcer | – | + | + | + | + | – | – | Resistant* | Susceptible* |
| *H. cinaedi* | Humans | Proctitis, enteritis | – | v | – | + | + | + | – | Susceptible | Susceptible |
| *H. fennelliae* | Humans | Proctitis, enteritis | – | – | – | + | + | – | – | Susceptible | Susceptible |
| *C. jejuni* | Birds, other animals | Gastroentritis | – | + | – | + | + | + | + | Susceptible | Resistant |
| *C. fetus* subsp. *fetus* | Cattle, sheep | Systemic infections | + | v | – | + | + | + | – | Resistant | Susceptible |
| *C. coli* | Pigs | Gastroenteritis | – | + | – | + | + | + | – | Susceptible | Resistant |

A – and + indicate that most isolates give a negative or positive result, respectively; v indicates that results are variable.
*Based on results obtained in standard assays using 30 µg/disk.

could potentially serve as a substitute for metronidazole. Interestingly, it has been noted in some of these clinical trials that persons who are treated very early with highly effective antimicrobial agents may produce only a limited amount of antibody against *H. pylori*, and thus are susceptible to reinfection.

## CAMPYLOBACTER

### Organism Characteristics

*Campylobacter* are small, curved gram-negative rods that frequently arrange themselves in "S" or "gull-wing" configurations. They are motile by means of a single polar flagellum. Their oxygen sensitivity ranges from microaerophilic to anaerobic. The organisms were classified as vibrios for several decades, largely because of these morphologic properties. However, because the organisms differ considerably from *Vibrio* in DNA base ratios, as well as in a variety of other characteristics, they were placed in a separate genus. The campylobacters have long been known to be inhabitants of the intestinal and genitourinary tracts of sheep, cattle, chickens, wild birds, dogs, and other animals. The first studies of these organisms involved their role in veterinary diseases. Human infections due to these bacteria were thought to be virtually nonexistent. However, with the development of appropriate selective media in the 1970s, *C. jejuni* became increasingly recognized as an important cause of enteritis in humans. The highest incidence of infection is in infants under the age of 1 year, adolescents, and young adults. In fact, it is a frequent cause of gastroenteritis in college students, with some campuses reporting isolation rates

from stool as high as 30%. Humans can be infected with *C. jejuni* by contact with infected animals (including sick household pets), drinking unpasteurized milk, and oral-anal sexual activity. Several outbreaks have also been traced to contaminated drinking water in rural areas and ingestion of improperly cooked poultry. In contrast to agents that cause food-borne gastroenteritis, these organisms do not multiply in food. Nonetheless, it is now estimated that *C. jejuni* is responsible for at least 2 million cases of enteritis each year in the United States; this is significantly more than what is thought to be caused by the salmonellae and shigellae combined. *C. coli* is an infrequent cause of diarrhea in humans. *C. fetus* subspecies *fetus* (formerly known as *Vibrio fetus*), a common cause of abortion in cattle and sheep, is an opportunist that usually causes severe disease only in those who are immunocompromised.

### Clinical Significance

Gastroenteritis is the most common manifestation after infection by *Campylobacter* species. *C. jejuni, C. coli, C. lari, C. upsaliensis,* and *C. hyointestinalis* have been implicated in human cases of diarrheal disease. Of these, *C. jejuni* is by far the most common isolate. The gastroenteritis due to these organisms often resembles diarrheal illness caused by *Salmonella, Shigella,* and the vibrios. Symptoms usually appear 1 to 7 days after infection. A prodrome of fever, headache, myalgia, and malaise usually precedes intestinal symptoms. Lower abdominal cramping and pain may be severe and is followed by diarrheal stools. The abdominal pain may resemble acute appendicitis when the right lower quadrant of the abdomen is affected. The diarrhea can range from watery to bloody with numerous polymorphonuclear cells. Symptoms usually persist for 3 to 5 days, although they may last for a week or two. *Campylobacter* species have lipopolysaccharides that may exhibit endotoxin activity. However, *C. jejuni* (also *C. coli* and *C. lari*) appear to possess several additional virulence factors, including a cytotoxin, an enterotoxin, and a cytotonic factor, which could contribute to their pathogenicity. The organisms also have invasive ability, as evidenced by their recovery from blood of individuals who have ingested contaminated materials. Nearly all patients stop excreting *C. jejuni* within 4 to 7 weeks after recovery, although a few become chronic carriers with continued excretion for 1 year or more. Carrier rates are considerably lower in the United States than in tropical countries. The importance of the carrier state in transmission is unclear.

*Campylobacter fetus* is different from *C. jejuni* and the other species that cause diarrheal disease in terms of clinical and epidemiologic characteristics. It is associated primarily with systemic infections although gastrointestinal disturbances are possible. The most common clinical presentation is intermittent fever without evidence of any specific organ involvement. However, the organisms may become disseminated via the blood circulation and seed various parts of the body. They appear to have a tropism for vascular sites, with thrombophlebitis being a relatively common sequela of bacteremia. Vascular necrosis may occur in patients with endocarditis, pericarditis, and heart valve infections; aortic aneurysms may also occur. Meningitis has been reported in both adults and neonates. The prognosis is especially poor in premature infants who tend to develop more complicated infections leading to death. *C. fetus* has also been isolated from numerous other types of infections including septic arthritis, lung abscesses, cholecystitis, cellulitis, osteomyelitis, and vaginosis.

## Cultural Characteristics and Identification

Clinical specimens for *Campylobacter* species should be promptly cultured. If transport to the laboratory is expected to be delayed for 2 hours or more, the material should be placed into Cary-Blair transport medium or other suitable transport media. The typical morphology of the campylobacters can be frequently seen in gram-stained smears of clinical specimens, although the staining may appear faint. Dark-field or phase microscopy of wet preparations can be used to visualize the darting motility of the organisms. A variety of selective media are available for isolation of *C. pylori* from fecal samples. Skirrow's medium, which contains three antimicrobial agents, and **Campy BAP medium**, which also has cephalothin, are among the most fre-

quently used selective media. Because many *Campylobacter* species, other than *C. jejuni,* are susceptible to cephalothin, the latter medium may not be useful for their isolation. Fecal specimens may be passed through filters with a 0.65- or 0.8-μm pore size to enhance the chance for isolation. Nonselective media are then inoculated with the filtrate. *Campylobacter* species (also *Helicobacter*) are able to move through the filter, whereas most other organisms cannot. Primary cultures for *C. jejuni* are incubated at 42°C (although the organisms will grow at lower temperatures) under microaerophilic conditions supplemented with 10% $CO_2$. Nonpigmented, grayish colonies usually appear within a few days, but longer periods of incubation may be required. Colonies on Campy BAP agar range from grayish to light pink or yellowish; they may appear slightly mucoid and elongated with a tendency to exhibit a "tailing effect" along the line of the streak. The organisms produce catalase, but not oxidase. Gas-liquid chromatography is used by a few laboratories to detect unusual fatty acids (e.g., C-19 cyclopropane fatty acid methyl ester) in the bacterial cell wall. Unlike the *Enterobacteriaceae* (and most vibrios), the campylobacters are relatively inert biochemically in that they do not oxidize or ferment carbohydrates. Inability to grow in media containing 3.5% or higher amounts of NaCl may be useful in differentiating them from halophilic organisms. The diagnosis of *C. fetus* infection is usually made by culturing blood from patients with sepsis. Up to 2 weeks of incubation may be required to obtain positive results. Table 18-3 compares the characteristics of the clinically most important *Campylobacter* species with those obtained for the species classified in the *Helicobacter* genus.

## Antibiotic Susceptibility Characteristics

Most cases of diarrheal disease due to the campylobacters are self-limiting and do not require treatment. *C. jejuni* (and most other species) is susceptible in vitro to a wide range of antibiotics including erythromycin, chloramphenicol, the tetracyclines, quinolones, aminoglycosides, nitrofurans, and clindamycin. Erythromycin is the drug of choice for treatment not only because of its efficacy, but also because of its ease of administration, low incidence of side effects, and ability to eliminate carriage within 72 hours. Cases of bacteremia are often given prolonged erythromycin treatment (i.e., for 4 weeks). Tetracycline is an alternative choice for individuals over the age of 7 years, although approximately 20% of isolates are now resistant. Systemic *C. fetus* infections require parenteral therapy and erythromycin may not be effective. Ampicillin is an alternative drug that may be used for *C. fetus,* if the isolate is susceptible to it. Most campylobacters are resistant to ampicillin and penicillin.

## AEROMONAS

### Organism Characteristics

The aeromonads are fermentative, free-living aquatic bacteria that possess a thin capsule and a single polar flagellum. They are present mostly in freshwater, but can also be isolated from saltwater-freshwater interfaces, cold-blooded animals such as fish, snakes, and frogs (for which they may be pathogenic), soil, and certain foods. The *Aeromonas hydrophila* group, consisting of *A. hydrophila*, *A. caviae*, and *A. veronii* biotype sobria, are the medically most important members of the genus. The organisms are most often associated with acute or chronic diarrhea and wound infections. Extraintestinal infections, other than at the site of a wound, occur with much lower frequency. Patients often have a recent history of drinking water contaminated with aeromonads or bathing in infected water. The incidence of human infection is highest during the months of May to November, when concentrations of the organisms are at peak levels in surface waters.

### Clinical Significance

Gastroenteritis is the most common clinical manifestation of infection with *Aeromonas* species. The disease can take a variety of forms: it can be acute and watery and accompanied by vomiting; chronic (>10 days duration); dysentery-like with blood and mucus in the stool; cholera-like with "rice-water" stools; or similar to the traveler's diarrhea usually associated with *E. coli*. Wound infections occur most frequently in the lower extremities and are manifested as a cellulitis with or without purulent drainage and fever. Cases of osteomyelitis, meningitis, and heart valve infections have been reported only rarely. It should be noted that aeromonads have been isolated from many body fluids of individuals with no indication of illness. Risk factors for developing clinically relevant infection include drinking contaminated water, reduced stomach acidity, use of antibiotics that are ineffective against *Aeromonas* species, and underlying liver or gastrointestinal disease.

### Cultural Characteristics and Identification

*Aeromonas* species from stool and other types of specimens grow readily on differential media that are used routinely for the enteric gram-negative rods. Because of this, as well as similarities in cellular and colonial morphology and in certain biochemical reactions, they may be confused with the much more commonly isolated enteric organisms. Rapid differentiation is achieved by performing an oxidase test; *Aeromonas* is positive, whereas the *Enterobacteriaceae* are negative. In addition, many aeromonads produce large zones of ß-hemolysis on 5% sheep blood agar. Trypticase soy agar supplemented with blood and ampicillin or pril-xylose-ampicillin agar may be used to select *Aeromonas* from specimens with mixed flora. Media that select for *Campylobacter* or *Salmonella* and *Shigella* are usually inhibitory. Resistance to compound O129 and inability to grow in the presence of 6% NaCl differentiates them from most of the vibrios and *Plesiomonas*.

### Antibiotic Susceptibility Characteristics

Most clinical isolates are susceptible to tetracycline, aminoglycosides, sulfamethoxazole-trimethoprim, and cefamandole. However, they are resistant to penicillin, ampicillin, cephalothin, and other ß-lactam antibiotics.

## PLESIOMONAS

### Organism Characteristics

*Plesiomonas* is an aquatic gram-negative rod that shares many of the properties of *Vibrio* and *Aeromonas* (especially *A. hydrophila*), although it may be more closely related to certain members of the *Enterobacteriaceae* family. *Plesiomonas shigelloides*, the only species in the genus, exhibits serologic cross-reactivity with *Shigella sonnei* (shigelloides means shigella-like). One of the 16 or more O groups of *P. shigelloides* bears strong antigenic resemblance to *S. sonnei*. The organisms usually produce **lophotrichous flagella**, that is, multiple, tufted polar flagella. Humans become infected by ingestion of contaminated food or water and contact with animals that are colonized with the bacteria. The organisms can cause gastrointestinal illness following the consumption of raw seafood, especially oysters and shrimp, and numerous types of opportunistic infections. Cases in the United States are often associated with recent travel to Mexico, the Caribbean, and Southeast Asia.

### Clinical Significance

The diarrheal illness associated with *P. shigelloides* is generally mild and self-limiting, following an incubation period of approximately 48 hours. However, severe illness with bloody, mucoid diarrhea and polymorphonuclear leukocytes in the stool may occur. The organisms have also been isolated from a wide variety of extraintestinal infections including cellulitis, meningitis, septicemia, perinatal bacteremia, cholecystitis, endophthalmitis, pseudoappendicitis, osteomyelitis, and septic arthritis.

## Cultural Characteristics and Identification

Isolation of *P. shigelloides* from stool specimens in patients with diarrhea is considered significant by most clinical laboratories. The organisms grow on many of the media that are commonly used for the *Enterobacteriaceae*. Typical colonies are small, convex, and transparent. Isolates can produce either pink or colorless colonies on MacConkey agar, indicating variable lactose fermentation. In contrast to the gram-negative enteric bacteria, they are oxidase positive. In addition, the organisms can be differentiated from *Vibrio* and *Aeromonas* because of their lophotrichous flagella, ability to ferment inositol, and lack of DNase and lipase. Furthermore, unlike *A. hydrophila*, they do not produce ß-hemolysis on blood agar. The organisms do not grow well on TCBS agar.

## Antibiotic Susceptibility Characteristics

Infections with *P. shigelloides* are generally not treated, unless they are very severe or the patient has a serious underlying condition. Most isolates are susceptible to aminoglycosides, cephalosporins, imipenem, ciprofloxacin, and sulfamethoxazole-trimethoprim, but resistant to penicillin, carbenicillin, ampicillin, and erythromycin. The organisms produce an inducible ß-lactamase that is similar to that of *Aeromonas*.

## CHROMOBACTERIUM

### Organism Characteristics

*Chromobacterium*, a long gram-negative rod that is sometimes slightly curved, is facultatively anaerobic. It is motile by means of a polar flagella or polar and peritrichous flagella, depending on the cultural conditions. These bacteria produce oxidase, and thus may sometimes be confused with *Pseudomonas*. *Chromobacterium violaceum*, the only species of clinical importance, is found in the soil, water, and animals. The organisms are well known in the southeastern part of the United States as an occasional cause of human infection. However, they are more commonly isolated in subtropical areas such as South America and Southeast Asia. The species name reflects the fact that isolates usually produce a violet water-insoluble pigment known as violacein, in contrast to the water-soluble pyocyanin produced by *Pseudomonas*. The bacteria synthesize the pigment by metabolizing L-tryptophan. Human infections occur most often in sites of trauma that become contaminated with soil or water and after drinking contaminated water.

## Clinical Significance

*Chromobacterium violaceum* is considered to be a very "low-grade" pathogen in that illness occurs rarely and then usually only under special circumstances. Individuals with infected wounds may develop fever, lymphadenitis, cellulitis, pustular dermatitis, and ulceration. Invasion of the bloodstream, urinary tract, and intestinal tract also has been reported, occasionally even in individuals who appear to have no underlying immunologic dysfunction. A few cases with pulmonary involvement have been initially diagnosed as tuberculosis. Infection with these organisms has a high fatality rate; approximately 50% of reported individuals have died despite treatment.

## Cultural Characteristics and Identification

*Chromobacterium violaceum* is the only violet-pigmented bacteria that produces infections in humans. The organisms can be isolated from blood, tissue exudate, or abscess fluid on many types of media including sheep blood agar, chocolate agar, trypticase soy broth, and MacConkey agar. Colonies often appear within 24 hours of incubation at 30° to 35°C, but best growth is achieved at 25°C. Although the organisms are oxidase positive, the production of violacein, which gives colonies a violet-black appearance, makes it difficult to interpret the test. Incubation under anaerobic condition suppresses pigment production so that the oxidase reaction can be more easily assessed. The weak indole reaction that is exhibited by the few nonpigmented strains is used to help differentiate them from *Aeromonas* and *Plesiomonas*. Most isolates produce hydrogen cyanide and, thus, a slight cyanide odor may be detected.

## Antibiotic Susceptibility Characteristics

*Chromobacterium violaceum* is usually susceptible to sulfamethoxazole-trimethoprim, choramphenicol, tetracycline, and gentamicin, but is resistant to most cephalosporins. Susceptibility to penicillins and other aminoglycosides is variable. Erythromycin appears to be relatively ineffective in vivo, even when in vitro assays indicate that the isolate is susceptible. A high incidence of relapse after seemingly effective treatment with this antibiotic has been reported.

## SPECIAL CONSIDERATIONS FOR IMMUNOCOMPROMISED HOSTS

Certain members of the *Vibrionaceae* family are known to produce more severe disease in immunocompromised hosts than what is usually seen in healthy individuals. For example, elderly persons, individuals receiving immunosuppressive drugs or who have underlying conditions that impair immune responsiveness, as well as those with liver disease, chronic liver failure, or hematologic disease, have significantly more severe illness due to *V. vulnificus*. Infections progress more rapidly and mortality rates as high as 50% to 60% have been reported among these high-risk populations. The elderly and infants have a naturally low stomach acidity, and thus are at increased risk for developing cholera after infection with virulent *V. cholerae*. The fact that they also have less than optimal immune responses may be an additional predisposing factor. *Aeromonas* species are more likely to cause septicemia, pneumonia, and severe gastroenteritis in immunocompromised individuals or in those with malignancies. Disease due to *P. shigelloides* is reportedly more severe in immunosuppressed patients, as evidenced by a high incidence of systemic infection.

Patients with human immunodeficiency virus type-1 (HIV-1) infection or a diagnosis of acquired immunodeficiency syndrome (AIDS) are at increased risk for severe illness due to *Campylobacter* and, to a lesser extent, *Helicobacter*. *C. jejuni, C. fetus,* and *H. pylori* are the most commonly reported species. Increased susceptibility to these organisms may be related to achlorhydria, which is seen in a subset of patients with AIDS, as well to a declining helper T-lymphocyte level. Typical manifestations in patients with *Campylobacter* infection include bloody diarrhea, abdominal cramping, and fever. Extraintestinal infections such as meningitis, septic arthritis, and endocarditis are being recognized with increasing frequency in these and other patients with depressed immunity. Newer species, such as *C. cinaedi, C. fennelliae,* and *C. hyointestinalis,* have also been identified as pathogens in these high-risk populations. Chronicity, recurrence, and bacteremia due to these organisms occur at higher rates than are expected in the general population. Antimicrobial therapy may have to be prolonged to achieve any beneficial effects. This may be a contributing factor to the increased incidence of erythromycin-resistant strains of *C. jejuni* that are isolated from patients with AIDS.

A decrease in phagocytic cell function has been associated with increased susceptibility to *C. violaceum* infection. For example, individuals with certain immunodeficiency diseases, such as chronic granulomatous disease and leukocyte glucose-6-phosphate dehydrogenase deficiency, are more likely than healthy persons to develop a high fever and bacteremia with dissemination of *C. violaceum* to many body sites. Osteomyelitis and abscesses in the liver, lungs, and abdomen are among the most common clinical manifestations.

## SUMMARY

- ▶ Vibrios are curved, comma-shaped, oxidase-positive bacteria with one polar flagella. *Vibrio cholerae* is found only in humans, is transmitted by food and water, is nonhalophilic, and grows best at high alkaline pH.
- ▶ The O1 serogroup of *V. cholerae* is the cause of cholera. There are two biotypes within this serogroup: classic (severe disease) and eltor (more persistent). The O1 serogroup secretes a powerful enterotoxin (choleragen) that leads to massive loss of fluid and electrolytes. Numerous virulence-associated genes have been identified in these organisms. Massive loss of fluid and electrolytes and "rice-water" stools are characteristic of cholera. The O139 serotype can also cause severe cholera-like disease in large populations. Other non-O1 serotypes cause only mild diarrhea and do not cause epidemics or pandemics. Replacement of fluid and reconstitution of electrolyte balance are of utmost importance in severe cases of cholera. Tetracycline is usually effective, if needed.
- ▶ *V. parahemolyticus* is transmitted by contaminated seafood and causes acute diarrhea that may resemble cholera.
- ▶ *V. vulnificus* can cause blister-like skin lesions after handling seashells and diarrhea after ingestion (raw oysters). Infection with these organisms can be highly fatal, especially in immunocompromised individuals and those with diabetes or liver disease.
- ▶ Cary-Blair transport media and TCBS agar are useful in isolation and identification of *Vibrio* species.
- ▶ *Helicobacter pylori* is a curved, spiral-shaped, rapidly motile organism with one or more polar flagella that is found in the mucous layer of the stomach (humans only). It is a major cause of gastritis, facilitates the development of peptic ulcers, and may play a role in stomach cancer. It can be identified by visualization of its characteristic morphology in stained gastric biopsy specimens and a strong positive urease reaction.

Combination therapy with metronidazole, a bismuth compound, and amoxicillin will eradicate the organisms in most people.

▶ *Campylobacter jejuni,* a curved rod arranged like "S" or "gull wings," has a single polar flagella. It is transmitted by food and water, infected animals, and oral-anal sexual activity. Most cases are seen in children and young adults. The organisms usually cause enterocolitis, but dysentery and enteric fever are possible. Most cases are self-limiting. Isolation of the organisms is done on antibiotic-containing media such as Skirrow's agar and Campy BAP and incubation at 41°C in 5% oxygen.

▶ *C. fetus,* seen mostly in immunocompromised patients and premature infants, causes bacteremia and thrombophlebitis.

▶ *Aeromonas* is a free-living aquatic organism with a single polar flagella. The *A. hydrophila* group is most important. Gastroenteritis after drinking contaminated food or bathing in contaminated waters is the most common clinical presentation. Underlying liver or gastrointestinal disease is a predisposing factor. The organisms are oxidase positive, and thus are easily differentiated from the oxidase-negative *Enterobacteriaceae.*

▶ *Plesiomonas* resembles *Aeromonas,* as well as *Shigella,* in some characteristics. It is also associated with diarrheal disease, especially after consumption of raw oysters. *P. shigelloides* is the major species.

## CASE STUDY 1: CHOLERA STRIKES DURING AIRPLANE FLIGHT

A businesswoman developed severe vomiting and diarrhea during a flight from Bangkok to Los Angeles. On landing she was examined at the airport clinic, but left against medical advice. Approximately 12 hours later she went into shock and was brought to an emergency room by concerned family members. The patient spent the next 4 days in the intensive care unit of the hospital. She had no recollection of dining in restaurants or eating seafood, except fried fish in Bangkok and sashimi on the airplane. Because of the short incubation period and lack of other in-flight cases, it seemed unlikely that the woman had become infected during the flight. Laboratory tests revealed that she had *V. cholerae,* serotype ogawa, biotype eltor in the stool. Outbreaks of cholera were reported in Bangkok and neighboring regions during the woman's visit. The patient was aware of possible dangers in drinking impure water, but not that this might give her cholera. (Based on a case reported in Los Angeles County Department of Health Services. [1994]. *Public Health Letter. 16(3),* 1.)

**Questions:**

1. Do most people become ill after consuming food or water that is contaminated with *V. cholerae?*

2. Why did the woman go into shock?

3. What is the mechanism of action of the cholera toxin?

## CASE STUDY 2: WATERY STOOL IN COLLEGE STUDENT

A 20-year-old male college student arrived in an outpatient clinic complaining of severe abdominal pain and diarrhea. He stated that the episode began approximately 5 days previously as a mild stomachache. Two or three loose bowel movements per day began shortly thereafter. Forty-eight hours before his arrival in the clinic he began experiencing intermittent pain in the right lower quadrant of the abdomen that was increasing in severity. Physical examination revealed that he had a tender abdomen, normal vital signs, and no fever. The patient had not traveled out of the United States. In addition, he denied consuming raw seafood or drinking well water. His white blood cell count, platelet count, and hematocrit were within normal limits. Further laboratory evaluation revealed a watery stool that had a slightly greenish tinge and was negative for occult blood. However, numerous white blood cells were noted on microscopic examination of the fecal specimen. Cultures on SS agar and Hektoen agar were negative. A slender, curved gram-negative rod was eventually isolated on TCBS agar and Skirrow's medium incubated at 42°C under microaerophilic conditions. The typical darting motility of *Campylobacter* was observed with dark-field microscopy. Based on these findings a diagnosis of *Campylobacter jejuni* enteritis was made. Erythromycin was prescribed and the patient recovered promptly.

### Questions:

1. What are the possible sources of infection with *C. jejuni*?

2. What are the characteristics of TCBS agar and Skirrow's medium that allowed the isolation of *C. jejuni*?

3. Is enteritis due to *C. jejuni* common in the United States?

## CASE STUDY 3: PEPTIC ULCERS IN AN EXECUTIVE

A 50-year-old male executive of a large corporation repeatedly presented with epigastric discomfort, a burning sensation in the abdominal region, and indigestion with occasional bouts of nausea and vomiting. The symptoms were more pronounced after meals and consumption of alcohol, but were partially ameliorated by Pepto-Bismol. The patient experienced pain with gentle percussion over the midepigastric region. A gastric biopsy, obtained during endoscopy, was sent to the laboratory. A positive urease test was quickly obtained by using material from the biopsy specimen and a Warthin-Starry stain revealed the presence of spiral-shaped organisms. Small round colonies appeared within a week of incubation at 37°C in a microaerophilic environment on Skirrow's agar and Thayer-Martin agar. Oxidase and catalase reactions were positive, there was no growth at 25°C or 42°C, and nitrate reduction and hippurate hydrolysis tests were negative. A diagnosis of peptic ulcer disease due to *Helicobacter pylori* was made. A regimen of metronidazole, bismuth subsalycylate, and amoxicillin was prescribed. The patient's symptoms subsided and laboratory results from follow-up visits indicated that *H. pylori* had been eradicated.

### Questions:

1. How is *H. pylori* able to survive the acidity of the stomach?

2. Are there other bacteria that can survive in the stomach?

3. Is a combination of three drugs necessary to eradicate *H. pylori*?

# Review Questions

1. Which of the following statements is correct for members of the *Vibrionaceae* family?
   a. The majority of species cause severe diarrheal illness that requires prolonged treatment with combinations of antibiotics.
   b. Kanawaga-positive organisms are nonpathogenic strains of *Vibrio parahemolyticus*.
   c. Most members are motile because they have peritrichous flagella.
   d. Because they are oxidase negative, they can be easily differentiated from members of the *Enterobacteriaceae* family.

2. A stool sample from a 46-year-old man with severe diarrhea is sent to the clinical laboratory for culture. The laboratory report indicates that the specimen contains oxidase-positive, gram-negative rods that form yellow colonies on TCBS agar and that they grow in medium containing 6% NaCl, but not in the presence of compound O/129. The organisms are MOST LIKELY to be:
   a. *Plesiomonas shigelloides*.
   b. *Helicobacter pylori*.
   c. *Vibrio cholerae*.
   d. *Campylobacter jejuni*.

3. Which of the following statements is correct regarding cholera toxin?
   a. It binds to mammalian cell DNA.
   b. It is encoded by genes on plasmids.
   c. It consists of six subunits.
   d. It is produced by all *Vibrio* species.

4. A potentially deadly organism that causes rapidly progressive and painful blister-like skin lesions is:
   a. *V. parahemolyticus*.
   b. *V. mimicus*.
   c. non-O1 *V. cholerae*.
   d. *V. vulnificus*.

5. Skirrow's medium is used for:
   a. differentiating between *Vibrio cholerae* and *Vibrio coli*.
   b. selective isolation of *Chromobacterium*.
   c. differentiating between *Aeromonas* and *Plesiomonas*.
   d. selective isolation of *Campylobacter* and *Helicobacter*.

6. The development of peptic ulcers is associated with which of the following organisms?
   a. *Helicobacter pylori*
   b. *Chromobacterium violaceum*
   c. *Campylobacter jejuni*
   d. *Aeromonas hydrophila*

7. Which of the following assays is useful is differentiating between *Campylobacter* and *Helicobacter?*
   a. Oxidase test
   b. Growth at 25°C
   c. Urease test
   d. Catalase test

8. Disease produced by *Campylobacter jejuni* most closely resembles illness due to:
   a. *Campylobacter fetus*.
   b. *Salmonella* and *Shigella*.
   c. *Vibrio harveyi*.
   d. *Vibrio vulnificus*.

## ▶ REFERENCES & RECOMMENDED READING

Bennish, M. (1994). Cholera: Pathophysiology, clinical features, and treatment. In K. Wachsmuth, P. Blake, & O. Olvsik (Eds.), *Vibrio cholerae and cholera: Molecular and global perspectives* (pp. 229–255). Washington, DC: American Society for Microbiology.

Blaser, M. J. (1996). The bacteria behind ulcers. *Scientific American.* 274(2), 104–107.

Blaser, M. J. & Parsonnet, J. (1994). Parasitism by the "slow" bacterium *Helicobacterium pylori* leads to altered gastric homeostasis and neoplasia. *Journal of Clinical Investigation.* 94(1), 4–8.

Brenden, R. A., Miller, M. A., & Janda, J. M. (1988). Clinical disease spectrum and pathogenic factors associated with *Plesiomonas shigelloides* infections in humans. *Review of Infectious Diseases, 10,* 303.

Centers for Disease Control and Prevention. (1993). Imported cholera associated with a newly described toxigenic *Vibrio cholerae* O139 strain—California. *Morbidity and Mortality Weekly Report, 42.* 501–503.

Colwell, R. R., Hasan, J. A. K., Huq, A., Loomis, L., Siebeling, R. J., Torres, M., Galvez, S., Islan, S., Tamplin, M., & Bernstein, D. (1992). Development and evaluation of a rapid, simple, sensitive, monoclonal antibody-based coagglutination test for direct detection of *Vibrio cholerae* O1. *FEMS Microbiology Letters, 97,* 215–220.

Glass, R. I., Libel, M., & Brandling, A. D. (1992). Epidemic cholera in the Americas. *Science, 256,* 1524–1525.

Gotuzzo, E., Seas, C., Echevarria, J., Carrillo, C., Mostorino, R., & Ruiz, R. (1995). Ciprofloxacin for the treatment of cholera: A randomized, double-blind, controlled clinical trial of a single daily dose in Peruvian adults. *Clinical Infectious Diseases, 20,* 1485–1490.

Hasan, J. A. K., Huq, A., Balakrish Nair, G., Garg, S., Mukhopadhyay, A. K., Loomis, L., Bernstein, D., & Colwell, R. R. (1995). Development and testing of mono-clonal antibody-based rapid immunodiagnostic test kits for direct detection of *Vibrio cholerae* O139 synonym Bengal. *Journal of Clinical Microbiology, 33,* 2935–2939.

Hirschhorn, N., & Greenough, W. B. III. (1991). Progress in oral rehydration therapy. *Scientific American, 264,* 50–56.

Los Angeles County Department of Health Services. (1994). Cholera—A reminder. *Public Health Letter, 16*(3), 1.

Los Angeles County Department of Health Services. (1995). Physician alert: *Vibrio vulnificus. Public Health Letter, 18*(6), 23.

Qadri, F., Hasan, J. A. K., Hossain, J., Chowdhury, A., Begum, Y. A., Azim, T., Loomis, L., Sack, R. B., & Albert, M. J. (1995). Evaluation of the monoclonal antibody-based kit Bengal SMART for rapid detection of *Vibrio*

*cholerae* O139 synonym Bengal in stool samples. *Journal of Clinical Microbiology, 33,* 732–734.

Summanen, P. (1993). Recent taxonomic changes for anaerobic gram-positive and selected gram-negative organisms. *Clinical Infectious Diseases, 16*(Suppl 4), S168–174.

Tacket, C. O., Losonsky, G., Nataro, J. P., Comstock, L., Michalski, J., Edelman, R., Kaper, J. B., & Levine, M. M. (1995). Initial clinical studies of CVD 112 *Vibrio cholerae* O139 live oral vaccine: Safety and efficacy against experimental challenge. *Journal of Infectious Diseases, 172,* 883–886.

Wesley, I. V., Schroeder-Tucker, L., Baetz, A. L., Dewhirst, F. E., & Paster, B. J. (1995). *Arcobacter*-specific and *Arcobacter butzleri*-specific 16S rRNA-based DNA probes. *Journal of Clinical Microbiology, 33,* 1691–1698.

# CHAPTER 19

# Gram-Negative Anaerobic Bacteria

Gloria T. Anderson, MT (ASCP), David W. Craft, PhD,
A. Christian Whelen, PhD, D (ABMM)

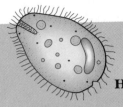

## Microbes in the News

### Hoechst-Roussel Award Lecture: "My Life and Hard Times With the Anaerobes," Dr. Sidney M. Finegold

The Hoechst-Roussel Award for 1992 was presented to Dr. Sidney M. Finegold (Professor of Medicine, Microbiology and Immunology at UCLA and Associate Chief of Staff for Research and Development at the VA Medical Center in West Los Angeles) during the 32nd Interscience Conference on Antimicrobial Agents and Chemotherapy. In an interview before his presentation, Dr. Finegold shared an overview of anaerobic infections.

The most commonly encountered anaerobic infections include periodontal disease and other dental and oral infections, with anaerobes accounting for 90% to 100%; chronic sinusitis and otitis media, over 50%; intra-abdominal **abscess**, 50% to 90%; diabetic and other infected foot ulcers, 85% to 90%; and female genital tract infections, 50% to 90%. Other common anaerobic infections are aspiration pneumonia, lung abscess, pleural empyema, pyogenic liver abscess, and osteomyelitis. Major clues to anaerobic infection include a foul-smelling discharge, tissue **necrosis**, gangrene, gas in tissues or discharges, infection associated with malignancy, infection related to the use of aminoglycosides, septic thrombophlebitis, unique morphology on Gram stain of exudate, or no growth on routine culture ("sterile pus").

The specific anaerobes most commonly encountered in clinically significant infections are from six principle genera: *Bacteroides fragilis* group (especially *B. fragilis*), pigmented *Prevotella* and *Porphyromonas; Fusobacterium nucleatum, Peptostreptococcus,* and *Clostridium perfringens, C. ramosum.* "These five organisms, or groups, taken together, account for approximately two-thirds of all anaerobes recovered from clinically significant infections involving anaerobes," Dr. Finegold observed.

"Virtually the only source of anaerobes participating in infection is the endogenous flora of mucosal surfaces of the body, and to much lesser extent, the skin. Anaerobes outnumber aerobic and facultative bacteria by a ratio of ten to one in the oral and vaginal floras and by a factor of 1000 to 1 in the colon. Normally these organisms are beneficial to us: they supply us with vitamin K, participate in bile acid recycling, and they may provide 'colonization resistance' which minimizes the likelihood of pathogenic organisms colonizing and setting up infections," Dr. Finegold said.

Excerpted from Conference Journal—Highlight Issue (sponsored by Miles Inc.), Vol. 13, No. 5, 32nd Interscience Conference on Antimicrobial Agents and Chemotherapy, October 11–14, 1992, Anaheim, CA.

*PORPHYROMONAS*
Organism Characteristics
Clinical Significance
Cultural Characteristics and
Identification
Antibiotic Susceptibility
Characteristics

*FUSOBACTERIUM*
Organism Characteristics
Clinical Significance
Cultural Characteristics and
Identification
Antibiotic Susceptibility
Characteristics

## KEY TERMS

Abscess
Aerotolerance
Capnophile

Endogenous
Facultative
Microaerophile

Necrosis
Obligate anaerobe

## LEARNING OBJECTIVES

**Upon successful completion of this chapter, the student should be able to:**

**1.** Discuss normal, anaerobic flora of humans by the four major anatomic locations.

**2.** Describe circumstances in which "normal" anaerobic flora cause disease.

**3.** Explain the three levels of identification in conventional clinical anaerobic bacteriology.

**4.** Describe common anaerobic media and primary culture strategies.

**5.** Describe the special potency disk patterns of major gram-negative anaerobes.

**6.** Based on Gram stain, colonial morphology, special potency disk pattern, determine which of the six additional level two tests are necessary for common identifications.

**7.** Solve case studies in anaerobic bacteriology.

## INTRODUCTION

Historically, infections involving anaerobes from exogenous sources have been most familiar to the medical community. Recently, **endogenous** anaerobic infections have become increasingly important. This can be attributed to improved laboratory methods that increase the recovery of anaerobic bacteria and an improved understanding of the role of anaerobes in disease. Additionally, a large proportion of the patient population is immunosuppressed (and at risk) due to malignancy, infection, trauma, hospitalization, or other predisposing conditions.

The anaerobic gram-negative bacteria are involved in a variety of infections characterized as endogenous (see Table 19-1). These bacteria are present in two-thirds of infections that involve anaerobes. Infections are usually polymicrobial and may include obligate aerobes, **facultative** microbes, or **microaerophilic** organisms. If undetected and left untreated, these infections can become serious. Proper specimen collection, transport, and processing is critical to timely

detection and correct identification of anaerobic bacteria in the clinical laboratory. A working knowledge of anaerobic bacteriology is an important skill of every clinical microbiologist.

To better understand the clinical significance of anaerobic organisms, it is important to know where they reside, how and why they cause infection or intoxication, and the types of infections they cause. Anaerobes coexist with aerobes as normal inhabitants at various sites of the human body (see Table 19-1). Facultative microorganisms use oxygen, which reduces the oxygen tension, creating an environment that allows anaerobic growth. Large numbers of anaerobes occupy niches located in the skin, the oral cavity and upper respiratory tract, the gastrointestinal tract, and the female genital tract.

This normal flora is an important component of protection against colonization and invasion by potentially pathogenic bacteria; it creates competition for the habitat. The organisms also play a role in nutrition and physiology; *Eschericha coli* and *Bacteroides* synthesize vitamin K in the gastrointestinal tract, which can be

### Table 19–1 ▶ Anatomic Locations of Typical Anaerobic Flora Found in Humans

**Oral Cavity and Upper Respiratory Tract**

| GRAM NEGATIVE | GRAM POSITIVE |
|---|---|
| Pigmented and nonpigmented *Prevotella* | *Peptostreptococcus* |
| *Porphyromonas* | *Actinomyces* |
| *Bacteroides*, especially *B. ureolyticus* group | *Propionibacterium* |
| *Fusobacterium* | *Eubacterium* |
| *Veillonella* | *Bifidobacterium* |

**Proximal Small Bowel**

| GRAM NEGATIVE | GRAM POSITIVE |
|---|---|
| Typically none | *Peptostreptococcus* |
| | *Lactobacillus* |

**Large Bowel**

| GRAM NEGATIVE | GRAM POSITIVE |
|---|---|
| *Bacteroides fragilis* group | *Peptostreptococcus* |
| *Porphyromonas* | *Clostridium* |
| *Fusobacterium* | *Eubacterium* |
| *Veillonella* | *Bifidobacterium* |
| | *Propionibacterium* |

**Female Genital Tract**

| GRAM NEGATIVE | GRAM POSITIVE |
|---|---|
| Pigmented and nonpigmented *Prevotella* | *Peptostreptococcus* |
| *Porphyromonas* | *Clostridium* |
| *Bacteroides* | *Propionibacterium* |
| | *Lactobacillus* |
| | *Eubacterium* |

**Distal Urethra**

| GRAM NEGATIVE | GRAM POSITIVE |
|---|---|
| *Prevotella* | *Propionibacterium* |
| *Fusobacterium* | *Peptostreptococcus* |

**Skin**

| GRAM NEGATIVE | GRAM POSITIVE |
|---|---|
| Typically none | *Propionibacterium* |
| | *Peptostreptococcus* |

attachment structures such as fimbriae, which allow them to adhere or invade epithelial surfaces. They can also produce toxins or enzymes that break down tissue. Finally, they may possess capsules that can inhibit or prevent phagocytosis.

Other factors that play a part in the disease process are: (1) disruption of the mucosal barrier due to surgery, trauma, or malignancy; (2) movement of anaerobic bacteria from their normal site of residence into a normally sterile site such as in aspiration pneumonia; (3) vascular disease such as diabetes mellitus; and (4) miscellaneous conditions such as cold, shock, foreign body injury, or previous infections with other microorganisms that may be exacerbated by edema and gas production.

Specimen collection and transport are critical to effective anaerobic bacteriology. Equally important is the proper incubation environment. Strategies range from large, clear, bench-top anaerobic chambers in which plates enter though air locks and are manipulated with gloved hands, to small zip-seal bags with capsule-size chemical anaerobic environment generators. Airtight jars can be used, and the appropriate atmosphere is created chemically by adding water to a commercial pouch, or by flushing the jar with anaerobic gases. Remember to always include an anaerobic indicator, commercial strips that change color when oxygen is present are most common.

The identification of anaerobes can be challenging; however, a systematic approach can facilitate the process immensely. Anaerobes normally grow more slowly than aerobes, their oxygen tolerance varies, and the enzymes they possess may take longer to produce. Patience and avoiding shortcuts in the identification process are keys to success (and also the best ways to eliminate misidentification and frustration). Table 19-2 describes the three progressive levels of identification of anaerobic bacteria typically used by clinical microbiology laboratories. Identification of genus, major groupings (*Bacteroides* are placed in two groups based on organism similarities), and sometimes species is

### Table 19–2 ▶ Levels of Anaerobe Identification That Laboratories Typically Perform

| | |
|---|---|
| Level I | Pure culture isolation; assess colonial and cellular morphology; aerotolerance testing. |
| Level II | Special potency disks and spot tests are used to presumptively identify some clinically significant anaerobes, such as differentiation of the *B. fragilis* group and identification of *Clostridium perfringens*. |
| Level III | Biochemical tests and sometimes gas-liquid chromatography are used for definitive identification of most clinically significant anaerobes. |

absorbed by the host. However, when the delicate balance is upset by trauma, malignancy, or immunodeficiency, anaerobic flora may behave as opportunistic pathogens and cause disease.

Anaerobic bacteria are able to invade and cause disease due to three major virulence factors. They possess important because this will often guide antimicrobial therapy, especially if anaerobic bacteria are visualized on direct Gram stain of patient specimens. In this chapter, we will discuss the *Bacteroides fragilis* group, *Bacteroides ureolyticus* group, *Prevotella* species (formerly in the *Bacteroides* genus), *Porphyromonas* species (formerly in the *Bacteroides* genus), and *Fusobacterium* species.

# BACTEROIDES FRAGILIS GROUP

## Group Characteristics

The *Bacteroides fragilis* group is the most important group of gram-negative anaerobic organisms because they are the most common anaerobes isolated in the clinical laboratory. They tend to be involved in serious infections and can be quite resistant to antimicrobial agents.

Presently, the *B. fragilis* group consists of 10 species: *B. caccae, B. distasonis, B. eggerthii, B. fragilis, B. merdae, B. ovatus, B. stercoris, B. thetaiotamicron, B. uniformis,* and *B. vulgatus. B. fragilis* is isolated most often in clinical specimens, followed by *B. thetaiotamicron.* These two species are considered true pathogens, whereas other species are often found in specimens contaminated with fecal material. For example, *B. ovatus* can easily be isolated from feces, but is not typically isolated from properly collected specimens. On the other hand, it may be significant if isolated from the blood of patients with polymicrobic bacteremia secondary to severe abdominal trauma or necrosis of the bowel.

## Clinical Significance

These microorganisms are predominant members of the large bowel flora. Therefore, they are most often isolated from intra-abdominal infections such as peritonitis or abdominal abscess. Infections can develop secondary to appendicitis, diverticulitis, malignancy, and bowel ischemia (inadequate blood flow) or obstruction, and following bowel surgery. Additionally, members of this group may be isolated from decubitus foot ulcers, the bloodstream, and female urogenital tract infections. It is important to note that they are usually not isolated from infections above the waist.

*Bacteroides fragilis* is the most important species of this group. It is associated with greater than 80% of intra-abdominal infections even though it comprises less than 1% of the gastrointestinal flora. The typical cell wall structure of *Bacteroides* consists of a major surface component called lipopolysaccharide (LPS). In contrast to LPS molecules of other gram-negative bacteria, the glycolipid found in *Bacteroides* has little or no endotoxin activity. This is due to the structure of the lipid A component of LPS; it lacks phosphate groups on the glucosamine residues and contains fewer fatty acids linked to the amino sugars. Most strains of *B. fragilis* are encapsulated, which renders them resistant to phagocytosis and promotes abscess formation.

## Cultural Characteristics and Identification

Members of the *B. fragilis* group are gram-negative, nonspore-forming, nonpigmented, nonmotile, obligately anaerobic bacilli (refer to Color Plate 32). Most strains are encapsulated and produce ß-lactamases. Typical isolates of the *B. fragilis* group also produce additional enzymes such as catalase, neuraminidase, DNase, hyaluronidase, gelatinase, fibrinolysin, superoxide dismutase, and heparinase.

Distinguishing characteristics of this group include microscopic and colonial morphology (refer to Color Plate 33), resistance to all three special potency antimicrobial disks (rare strains of *B. fragilis* are susceptible to colistin), growth in the presence of 20% bile, and saccharolytic metabolism.

The proper primary isolation media must be used for success isolating these organisms from clinical specimens. Strategy should include a nonselective media such as Brucella agar (vitamin K and hemin stimulate growth), selective/differential media such as *Bacteroides* bile esculin (BBE) agar and lysed (laked) blood with vancomycin and kanamycin, and an enriched broth media such as cooked meat with glucose or thioglycolate. Table 19-3 lists other recommended media for anaerobic culture. Always include an aerobic plate such a chocolate agar; it will help differentiate true anaerobes from facultative organisms (like *Haemophilus*).

Examination of the primary anaerobic culture plates should be conducted no sooner than 48 hours after inoculation and incubation in anaerobic jars or anaerobic pouches. (Exceptions include when *Clostridium perfringens* [see Chapter 20] or *B. fragilis* is suspected; blood agar plates should be examined at 24 hours. Under these circumstances, two sets of anaerobic plates should be set up and incubated in different jars or pouches. One set is opened and read at 24 hours while the other set is left undisturbed until 48 hours. Alternatively, primary anaerobic culture plates incubated in an anaerobic glove box can be examined after 24 hours.)

Although the cellular and colonial morphologies of members of the *B. fragilis* group are very similar, they do vary slightly from species to species. Cellular morphology with a Gram stain shows pale, pleomorphic, gram-negative bacilli (refer to Color Plate 32). Faint counterstaining of gram-negative anaerobes can be improved using carbol fuchsin; however, this should not be used as the initial procedure because gram-positive results

| Table 19–3 ▶ | Media* Used Primarily in the Anaerobe Laboratory for Isolation and Differentiation of Anaerobic Pathogens |
|---|---|

| Medium | Purpose and Comments |
|---|---|
| *Bacteroides* bile esculin (BBE) | Selective and differential for *Bacteroides fragilis* group |
| CDC blood agar (CDC/BA) | Enriched medium using supplemented† trypticase soy agar base with 5% sheep blood.‡ Other bases that can be used include *Brucella*, brain-heart infusion, Columbia, fastidious anaerobe agar, and Schaedler. |
| Cycloserine cefoxitin fructose agar (CCFA) | Selective media for *Clostridium difficile* (not routinely recommended) |
| Egg yolk agar (EYA) | Detection of lipase and lecithinase |
| Kanamycin-vancomycin (KV) | CDC/BA with kanamycin (inhibits most facultative gram-negative bacilli) and vancomycin (inhibits gram-positive organisms and some *Porphyromonas*). The blood may be "laked" or lysed.‡ |
| Phenylethyl alcohol (PEA) | CDC/BA with phenylethyl alcohol, which inhibits most facultative gram-negative bacilli and *Proteus* swarming. Inhibits swarming of certain clostridia. |
| Thioglycolate broth | Supplemented† broth is used for larger volume inoculation and extended incubation, which assists in the detection of slow growing organisms. |

*Prereduced, anaerobically sterilized (PRAS) media is recommended for primary isolation.

†Supplements normally include, but are not limited to, vitamin K and hemin.

‡Lysed (laked) blood enhances pigment production.

may be confused with gram-negative results. Their cells range from 0.5 to 0.8 μm × 1.5 to 9.0 μm. Cells grown in broth culture containing a fermentable carbohydrate tend to be pleomorphic, often with vacuoles (which should not be confused with spores). Some species have large swellings or long filaments, which are sometimes enhanced under suboptimal culture conditions.

Colonies on enriched primary isolation media are 2 to 3 mm in diameter, circular, convex, and gray to gray-white (refer to Color Plate 33). On selective media such as BBE, colonies are generally greater than 1 mm in diameter and black due to the hydrolysis of esculin in the media. Take care not to confuse this reaction with pigmentation (the *B. fragilis* group is nonpigmented, and pigmented organisms, such as *Porphyromonas* and some *Prevotella*, are susceptible to 20% bile). One

exception is *B. vulgatus*, which usually does not hydrolyze esculin. Keep in mind that some non-*B. fragilis* group organisms are resistant to 20% bile (i.e., *Fusobacterium mortiferum, B. splanchius, Enterococcus* species, *Enterobacteriaceae*, and some yeast). *B. fragilis* group organisms grow quickly (24 hours) on both selective and nonselective media.

Suspected anaerobes should be tested for **aerotolerance** (see Procedure 19-1). This consists of subculturing colonies to three different plates, which are incubated at 35° to 37°C anaerobically, aerobically in non-$CO_2$, and at 5% to 10% $CO_2$ (to detect **capnophiles**). All members of the *B. fragilis* group are **obligate anaerobes**, so there should be no growth on the aerotolerance plates.

Following aerotolerance testing, another Gram stain (see Procedure 19-2) is performed on colonies growing anaerobically, and isolates are plated on a Brucella blood agar plate (or another enriched medium) with special potency antimicrobial disks of kanamycin (1,000 μg), vancomycin (5 μg), and colistin (10 μg) (see Procedure 19-3). The *B. fragilis* group is resistant to all three, so the microbiologist should see growth up to the edge of all disks. (A zone of < 10 mm or growth to edge of disk is considered resistant.)

Once grouped, simple tests such as catalase and indole are used along with esculin and bile results obtained from BBE agar plate (alternatively one can use Procedures 19-4 and 19-5) to help speciate within the group. Special potency disks and spot tests do not speciate all members of the *B. fragilis* group, but they will narrow the identification to two or three possible species. Not all bile-resistant organisms are members of the *B. fragilis* group (e.g., *B. splanchnicus*). Additionally, take care not to misidentify *B. eggerthii*; it is the only member of the *B. fragilis* group that does not use sucrose. See Table 19-4 for preliminary (level I) identification and Table 19-5 for level II (group, genus, or species) identification of anaerobic gram-negative organisms. This table also serves as a guide to simple spot tests that should be performed to further identify *B. fragilis* group organisms. Commercial systems used for identification of anaerobes are based on 24- to 48-hour conventional biochemical tests (MINITEK, API 20A) or 4-hour detection of preformed enzymes (AnIDENT, RapID-ANA II, MicroScan, VITEK).

## Antibiotic Susceptibility Characteristics

Chromogenic ß-lactamase testing is performed on all gram-negative anaerobic bacilli; however, anaerobic susceptibilities are not routinely necessary on all isolates. Figure 19-1 contains a list of circumstances that may indicate a need for susceptibility testing of anaerobic isolates if specifically ordered.

Approved guidelines for standardized susceptibility

---

## PROCEDURE 19-1
### Aerotolerance Testing

**Principle:**

To establish if isolate is an obligate, facultative, or aerotolerant anaerobe.

**Method:**

1. Subculture for isolation one well isolated colony of each morphologic type from an anaerobic isolation plate to a chocolate plate in 5% to 10% $CO_2$, aerobic sheep blood agar plate (non-$CO_2$), and an anaerobic blood agar plate (anaerobic conditions) for overnight incubation at 35° to 37°C.
2. Observe plates daily for 72 hours for: no growth (obligate anaerobe), scant growth (aerotolerant anaerobe), or good growth (facultative anaerobe).

3. Once you establish isolate is an anaerobe, proceed with Gram stain, special potency disks, and simple spot tests.

**Quality Control:**

Organisms tested include *B. fragilis, Propionibacterium acnes,* and *Escherichia coli.* Testing should be verified monthly.

**Expected Results:**

*B. fragilis:* no growth on aerobic plates (obligate anaerobe)
*P. acnes:* scant growth on aerobic plates (aerotolerant)
*E. coli:* good growth on aerobic plates (facultative)

---

testing of anaerobic bacteria and interpretative values are found in Chapter 10 and in the National Committee for Clinical Laboratory Standards (NCCLS) document #M11-A3 with supplemental tables (currently M100-S7). Agar dilution is the most useful method, and most clinical laboratories use the E-test.

Antibiotic therapy combined with surgical intervention is the main approach for managing serious anaerobic infections. ß-Lactamase is produced by almost all members of the *B. fragilis* group, which makes them resistant to penicillin and many cephalosporins. However, high concentrations of some extended-spectrum penicillins (e.g., carbenicillin, piperacillin), use of ß-lactamase inhibitors, and other selected ß-lactam antibiotics (e.g., cefoxitin, imipenem) can be effective against *Bacteroides* infections. Plasmid-mediated clindamycin resistance has increased in recent years, with an average of 7% to 10% of the isolates in the United States resistant. Metronidazole is usually active against most *Bacteroides*.

*Bacteroides thetaiotamicron, B. ovatus, B. caccae,* and *B. distasonis* are generally much more resistant to antimicrobial agents than are the *B. fragilis* group. Sometimes prophylactic treatment with antibiotics is indicated when diagnostic or surgical procedures will disrupt the gastrointestinal mucosal barriers.

---

- ► Treatment failures on targeted therapy
- ► Lack of improvement on appropriate empirical therapy
- ► Recurrent infections
- ► Isolates from patients on long-term antimicrobic therapy
- ► Isolates from serious infections (e.g., central nervous system, endocarditis)
- ► Isolates from prosthetic devices
- ► Isolates from immunocompromised or debilitated patients
- ► Trending susceptibility patterns from institutional isolates
- ► Evaluating in vitro testing of new antimicrobial agents

**FIGURE 19-1** Clinical situations that may warrant anaerobe susceptibility testing.

## *BACTEROIDES UREOLYTICUS* GROUP

### Group Characteristics

The *Bacteroides ureolyticus* group is particularly important for two reasons. Certain members are responsible for deep-seated infections and they tend to be resistant to antimicrobics. Historically, the group has consisted of *B. ureolyticus, B. gracilis* and *Wolinella* species/ *Campylobacter* species. According to recent taxonomic studies, *Wolinella curva* and *W. recta* have been renamed *Campylobacter curvus* and *C. rectus.* Furthermore, "*B.*" *gracilis* is a heterogenous group of organisms with respect to bile resistance, composition of cellular fatty acids, and susceptibility pattern, and has been split into at least two different genera *Campylobacter gracilis* and *Sutterella wadsworthensis;* some

| Table 19–4 ▶ Preliminary Identification of Gram-Negative Anaerobes (Level I) | | |
|---|---|---|
| **Organisms** | **Unique Characteristics** | **Fluorescence** |
| BACILLI | | |
| *B. fragilis* group | Large (>1 mm) colonies on BBE | None |
| *B. ureolyticus* group | "Pits" the agar | None |
| *Porphyromonas* | Black/brown pigment | Red |
| *P. asaccharolyticus-endodontalis* | Black/brown pigment | Red, orange |
| *P. gingivalis* | Black/brown pigment | None |
| Pigmented *Prevotella* | Black/brown pigment | Red |
| *F. nucleatum* (presumptive) | Thin bacillus, pointed ends | None |
| *F. necrophorum* (presumptive) | Long, thin bacillus with rounded ends; umbinate colonies | Chartreuse |
| OTHER GNB | VARIOUS CHARACTERISTICS | NONE, PINK, ORANGE, YELLOW |
| COCCI | | |
| *Veillonella* | Cocci | None |

BBE, *Bacteroides* bile esculin agar; GNB, gram-negative bacilli

*B. gracilis*-related the latter of which is bile resistant and can be more resistant to antimicrobics than the *B. fragilis* group. Even though all these microorganisms are currently designated anaerobic gram-negative bacteria, the entire group are actually microaerophiles and may undergo further reclassification.

These microorganisms are normal inhabitants of the oral cavity and are associated with localized infections of the mouth. Alternatively, they may disseminate via aspiration or the bloodstream to produce infections elsewhere.

# PROCEDURE 19-2
## Modified Gram Stain

### Principle:

Same as for aerobes.

### Method:

1. Air dry smear. Fix smears by flooding the slide with absolute methanol.
2. Drain the methanol from the slide immediately and allow the smear to air dry again. Methanol fixation is preferred because bacterial cells remain intact. Heat fixation distorts cells and makes visualization of bacteria more difficult. Use methanol fixation for direct specimens and smears prepared from solid media.
3. When fixed smears are dry, flood slide with crystal violet. Add 3 to 5 drops of 5% sodium bicarbonate to each slide. This step improves the retention of crystal violet by gram-positive

anaerobes. For pale staining gram-negative organisms, confirm Gram reaction on a methanol-fixed smear using carbolfushsin as the counterstain. Do not use carbolfuchsin routinely to counterstain gram-positive organisms because it may mask crystal violet (gram-positive organisms look gram-negative).

### Quality Control:

Same as for aerobes. Methanol fixation is preferred because bacterial cells remain intact. Heat fixation distorts cells and makes visualization of bacteria more difficult. Use methanol fixation for direct specimens and smears prepared from solid media.

### Expected Results:

Same as for aerobes.

## Table 19–5 ► Key Characteristics of Typical Gram-Negative Anaerobes (Level II Identification)

| Organisms | Pigment | Kanamycin | Vancomycin | Colistin | Growth-20% Bile | F/F required | Nitrate | Indole | Catalase | Lipase | Urease |
|---|---|---|---|---|---|---|---|---|---|---|---|
| Typical GNB | – | S | R | S | S | N | – | – | – | – | – |
| B. fragilis group | | R | R | R | R | | | | | | |
| B. ureolyticus group | | | | | | Y | + | | | | +/– |
| Fusobacterium sp. | | | | | | | | + | | | |
|   F. nucleatum | | | | | | | | | | | |
|   F. necrophorum | | | | | | | | | | + | |
| Porphyromonas | + | R | S | R | | | | + | | | |
| Prevotella (pigmented) | + | R | | | | | | +/– | | | |
| Prevotella (nonpigmented) | | | R | | | | | | +/– | | |
| Veillonella | | | | | | | + | | | | |

GNB, gram-negative bacilli; F/F, formate/fumarate supplement; N, no requirement; R, resistant; S, susceptible; Y, yes, required.

---

# PROCEDURE 19-3
## Special Potency Disk Test

### Principle:

Special potency antimicrobial disks of vancomycin (5 μg), kanamycin (1,000 μg) and colistin (10 μg) help determine the Gram reaction of anaerobes and assist in preliminary grouping of anaerobic genera and species. Gram-positive organisms tend to be susceptible to vancomycin, whereas most gram-negative organisms are resistant. This is particularly useful with *Clostridium* species that stain gram-negative.

### Method:

1. Allow disk container to stabilize at room temperature before opening.
2. Subculture isolate to blood agar plate (BAP). Streak for isolation and then swab the first quadrant back and forth several times to ensure a heavy lawn of growth (similar to seeding a disk diffusion plate).
3. Place the three antibiotic disks on the first quadrant ensuring they are well separated.
4. If you have several organisms to test, it is easier to streak all the plates first, and then add the disks to them at the same time.
5. Incubate plate(s) anaerobically for 48 to 72 hours at 35° to 37°C.
6. Examine and measure the zone of inhibition around the disks.

### Quality Control:

1. Test disks by lot when initially received and weekly thereafter.
2. Suggested quality control organisms: *B. fragilis*, ATCC 25285, *C. perfringens*, ATCC 13124, and *F. necrophorum*, ATCC 25286.

### Expected Results:

1. *B. fragilis:* resistant to all three antibiotics (zone of inhibition < 10 mm).
2. *F. necrophorum:* resistant to vancomycin (zone < 10 mm); susceptible to kanamycin and colistin (zone of inhibition of ≥ 10 mm).
3. *C. perfringens:* susceptible to vancomycin and kanamycin (zone ≥ 10 mm); resistant to colistin (zone < 10 mm).

# PROCEDURE 19-4
## Esculin Hydrolysis

### Principle:

The esculin molecule is enzymatically hydrolyzed to glucose and esculetin, the latter of which reacts with iron salt (ferric ammonium citrate) to form a dark brown or black complex. Hydrogen sulfide, which is produced by several organisms, also reacts with iron to produce a black complex, and can interfere with interpretation of esculin test. Therefore, check all tubes showing darkening with ultraviolet (UV) light after the addition of the reagent. Intact esculin fluoresces white-blue under 366-nm light (negative), whereas esculetin is not fluorescent (positive).

### Method:

1. Add 5 drops of 1% ferric ammonium citrate solution to a tube of actively growing organism in peptone yeast (PY) esculin broth.
2. Observe for a dark color change without fluorescence under UV light.

### Quality Control:

Perform quality control on broth on receipt and on new lot numbers.

### Expected Results:

1. *B. fragilis:* positive; black or dark brown color development and no fluorescence under UV light (366 nm)
2. *B. vulgatis:* negative; no color development or positive fluorescence under UV light.

## Clinical Significance

*Bacteroides ureolyticus* has been recovered from infections from a variety of sources including pulmonary, head and neck, intra-abdominal, urogenital, bone, and soft tissues. *C. gracilis/S. wadsworthensis* has been recognized as an important pathogen in serious abdominal or head infections. *B. ureolyticus* is frequently isolated from superficial soft tissue or bone infections that tend to be mild. *C. gracilis/S. wadsworthensis,* in contrast, is isolated from "serious deep-seated" infections, including head and neck infections, pleuropulmonary infections, and infected sites within the abdomen and pelvis. Campylobacter species are primarily oral isolates from periodontic infections and periodontosis.

## Cultural Characteristics and Identification

Organisms of the *B. ureolyticus* group are asaccharolytic, nonpigmented, nonspore-forming, fastidious, small gram-negative bacilli that tend to "pit" anaerobic blood agar. They grow slowly on primary isolation (3–4 days), are usually inhibited by 20% bile, and require supplements for quicker growth (formate as a hydrogen donor, and fumarate [or nitrate] as a hydrogen acceptor). Special potency disk pattern is susceptible to kanamycin

and colistin and resistant to vancomycin. Other key reactions include nitrate positive and indole negative. *B. ureolyticus* and *C. gracilis/S. wadsworthensis* are nonmotile, whereas *Campylobacter* are motile. *B. ureolyticus* is urea positive, and *C. gracilis/S. wadsworthensis* and *Campylobacter* are negative. Catalase may vary for *B. ureolyticus*. On Gram stain they are thin, straight gram-negative bacilli (with the exception of *Campylobacter,* which may look thin straight, curved, or helical).

Colonies on primary isolation plates at 48 hours may be barely visible. They grow very slowly and may not be seen until 72 hours, or later. Three types of colonial morphology exist on nonselective media, all of which are translucent or transparent: (1) convex, 1 mm in diameter; (2) spreading up to 5 mm; and (3) agar pitting or corroding, also up to 5 mm in size. These latter colony types produce depressions or "pits" on the agar surface due to agarose, which resembles the corrosion of pitted sheet metal.

Special potency disk pattern for this group is the same as that of *Fusobacterium* and *Bilophila* species. They are susceptible to kanamycin and colistin and resistant to vancomycin; however, keep in mind that this group of organisms reduces nitrate and the *Fusobacterium* species do not; *Bilophila* species reduce nitrate but their colonial morphology on BBE agar is very distinct. *Fusobacterium* and *Bilophila* species do not

## PROCEDURE 19-5
### Bile Disk Test for Differentiation of Anaerobic Gram-Negative Bacilli

**Principle:**

*Bacteroides fragilis, Fusobacterium mortiferium,* and *Fusobacterium varium* are clinically significant anaerobic gram-negative bacilli that are capable of growing in the presence of 20% bile (equal to 2% oxgall). Additionally bile resistance is an important reaction in separating *B. fragilis* group from other anaerobic gram-negative bacilli (as well as in differentiating bile-resistant fusobacteria). Reactions may be interpreted on bile-containing medium, such as BBE, in 20% bile broth, or with disks impregnated with 20% bile.

**Method:**

1. Bring disk container to room temperature.
2. Subculture the anaerobic isolate on a BAP. Streak for isolation and then swab the first quadrant for confluent growth (similar to special potency disks or disk diffusion susceptibility testing).
3. Place the bile disk on the heavy inoculated area.
4. This test can be performed on the same plate as the special potency disks, as long as the disks are well separated.
5. Incubate plate(s) anaerobically for 48 to 72 hours at 35° to 37°C.
6. Examine for any zone of inhibition of growth.

**Quality Control:**

Test each lot on receipt and monthly thereafter.

**Expected Results:**

1. *B. fragilis* ATCC 25285: resistant (no zone of inhibition).
2. *P. melaninogenica* ATCC 25845: susceptible (any zone of inhibition).

require formate-fumarate supplement for growth (see Tables 19-4 and 19-5). Speciation of the members of the *B. ureolyticus* group may be important to guide proper antimicrobic therapy.

Because this group is asaccharolytic, the best way to identify them is by key tests including nitrate (see Procedure 19-6), motility, urea, special potency disks, formate-fumarate supplement (see Procedure 19-7), and supplemented with commercial identification kits.

### Antibiotic Susceptibility Characteristics

Antimicrobic susceptibility testing is problematic because *B. ureolyticus* group organisms form transparent colonies that have hazy end-points in minimum inhibitory concentration (MIC) determinations. Fortunately, they are normally susceptible to the various penicillins, cephalosporins, clindamycin, chloramphenicol, and metranidazole; however, *B. gracilis* isolates are commonly resistant to the penicillins, cephalosporins, and clindamycin.

## *PREVOTELLA*
### Organism Characteristics

Members of the new genus *Prevotella* were formerly classified under the genus *Bacteroides*. Certain members (especially the pigmented species) compose a group that are distinguished as the second most commonly isolated anaerobes- in the clinical laboratory. *Prevotella* species, particularly *P. intermedia,* can produce ß-lactamase. In circumstances such as orofacial lesions and anaerobic pleuropulmonary infections, they are more common than the *B. fragilis* group (above the waist).

Presently, 20 species (pigmented and nonpigmented) have been proposed for this genus. We will discuss only the species commonly found in human clinical material. The important pigmented *Prevotella* species are *P. corporis, P. denticola, P. intermedia, P. loescheii, P. melaninogenica,* and *P. nigrescens*; nonpigmented *Prevotella* species are *P. bivia, P. disiens,* and *P. oralis* group.

# PROCEDURE 19-6
## Nitrate Reduction Disk Test

### Principle:

Certain anaerobic bacteria are capable of reducing nitrate to nitrite, which is useful in determining the species or grouping of anaerobic organisms. Nitrite can be demonstrated by the addition of naphthylamide (reagent A) and sulfanilic acid (reagent B), which forms a red diazonium dye with nitrite. Negative results must be confirmed by metallic zinc to ensure nitrate has not been completely reduced to nitrogen gas. It is usually recommended that nitrate negative results by disk method be confirmed by nitrate broth.

### Method:

1. Inoculate organism on Brucella agar, or other nonselective anaerobic BAP.
2. Place the nitrate disk on the most heavily inoculated area.
3. Incubate anaerobically at 35° to 37°C until heavy growth occurs around the disk, normally 24 to 72 hours.
4. Remove the disk from the agar plate, and place it on a clean glass slide or Petri dish.
5. Add 1 drop each of nitrate reagents A and B. Observe for the development of a red color.
6. If no color develops within 5 minutes, add a pinch of zinc dust or zinc granules to the disk and wait 5 minutes. A true negative turns red at this time.
7. If no color develops after adding zinc, the organism reduced nitrate to nitrite (positive), and further reduced nitrite to nitrogen gas.

### Quality Control:

Check the disks and reagents when they are prepared and monthly thereafter. Facultative organisms *E. coli* ATCC 25922 and *Acinetobacter lwoffi* ATCC 43498 make convenient controls.

### Expected Results:

1. *E. coli:* positive; development of red color.
2. *A. lwoffi:* negative; no color change. After addition of zinc, red color develops.

## Clinical Significance

Many species in the genus *Prevotella* are part of the oral flora. Therefore, they tend to be isolated from infections of the oral cavity, head and neck, and lower respiratory tract. They also are involved with female urogenital tract infections (*P. bivia* and *P. disiens*). *P. melaninogenica* possesses a collagenase that may be responsible for collagen fiber destruction in gingival tissue, particularly in the periodontal ligament.

# PROCEDURE 19-7
## Formate-Fumarate Supplement

### Principle:

Slow-growing, fastidious *B. ureolyticus* group organisms are stimulated by this supplement.

### Method:

1. Slow-growing gram-negative anaerobic bacilli are subcultured to broth media containing this supplement and broth without formate-fumarate.
2. Observe turbidity within 24 hours for enhanced growth, as compared to the standard broth tube.

### Quality Control:

Set up controls in broth with and without supplement each day unknowns are tested. Set up unknowns with and without supplement also.

### Expected Results:

1. *B. ureolyticus:* positive growth enhancement; considerable turbidity develops within 24 hours (versus 3+ days without supplement).
2. *B. ureolyticus:* growth (turbidity) without supplement is slight.

## Cultural Characteristics and Identification

They are gram-negative, nonspore-forming, obligately anaerobic bacilli. Some are pigmented and some produce capsules. Pigmentation may take up to 21 days to develop. Isolates are moderately saccharolytic and some species are proteolytic as well (*P. bivia* and *P. disiens*). *P. bivia* produces an endotoxin, but it is distinct from those of aerobic gram-negative bacteria. They are fastidious, resistant to vancomycin and kanamycin and variable to colistin, and sensitive to 20% bile.

The cells of these microorganisms vary slightly from species to species, but may be described as short, coccoid, pleomorphic gram-negative coccobacilli/bacilli (refer to Color Plate 34). Young cultures may appear gram-variable. Their cell size is usually 0.3 to 0.4 μm in diameter by 0.6 to 1 μm long.

Colonies on primary isolation plates may not be detected at 48 hours because of their slow growth rate. They are fastidious, so enriched media such as lysed (laked) rabbit blood with selective antibiotics kanamycin and gentamicin works well and is reliable for rapid development of pigment for the pigmented species. The colonies on lysed (laked) blood agar with kanamycin and gentamicin will be buff to white, brown, or black. To differentiate between the pigmented and nonpigmented species in young colonies, examine under long-wave UV light (Wood's lamp). The pigmented species will fluoresce brick-red, while the nonpigmented species will not (or will fluoresce pink, orange, or yellow) (see Procedure 19-8). They are sensitive to bile so there will be no growth on the BBE agar plate. The colonies on lysed (laked) blood agar with kanamycin and gentamicin will be buff to white, brown, or black.

Aerotolerance testing will show that these microorganisms are obligate anaerobes and will not grow in air on the chocolate agar plate. They are resistant to vancomycin and kanamycin and give variable results for colistin. Do not confuse *Prevotella* with *B. fragilis* group when the disk pattern shows resistance to all three disks. The bile disk or BBE agar will differentiate between the two genera. *P. intermedia*, *P. corporis*, and *P. nigrescens* will be resistant to both vancomycin and kanamycin, but susceptible to colistin. The *P. melaninogenicus* group (*P. denticola*, *P. loeschii*, and *P. melaninogenica*) are indole negative and often resistant to all three disks. The pigmented *P. intermedia* (see Tables 19-4 and 19-5) are indole positive and lipase positive.

## Antibiotic Susceptibility Characteristics

Many pigmented organisms, particularly *P. intermedia*, commonly produce ß-lactamase antibiotics. Penicillin G can no longer be considered the drug of choice. *P. bivia* and *P. disiens* are resistant to several antimicrobics such as metronidazole and chloramphenicol, and the ß-lactamase inhibitor combinations such as ampicillin/sulbactam and ticarcillin/clavulanate are active against these organisms; clindamycin may also be effective. The broad-spectrum penicillins, cefoxitin, and other second- and third-generation cephalosporins are active against more than 95% of these strains.

More than half of the nonpigmented *Prevotella*

---

## PROCEDURE 19-8
## Fluorescence

### Principle:

Fluorescence is a result of specific molecules that absorb energy of UV light (366 nm) and become excited. Electrons will return to their original lower energy states, at which time they emit photons (energy) at a different wavelength (visible light). The presence and color of fluorescing colonies helps in the presumptive identification of certain anaerobic bacteria.

### Method:

1. Put on UV protective eyewear.
2. Expose the culture plate to the UV light source in the dark by using a UV viewing cabinet or by darkening the room.

3. Wait 10 to 15 seconds for the fluorescence to occur.
4. Note the presence and color of fluorescence.

### Quality Control:

Pigmented *Prevotella* species on anaerobic BAP serves as an excellent positive control. Verify fluorescence with each testing of an unknown.

### Expected Results:

1. *P. melaninogenica* ATCC 25845: positive; brick red fluorescence.
2. *B. fragilis* ATCC: negative; no fluorescence.

strains produce ß-lactamase. Rare strains may be resistant to clindamycin, but other antimicrobics typically used to treat anaerobic infections are effective.

## PORPHYROMONAS

### Organism Characteristics

Members of the new genus *Porphyromonas* are an important group of organisms isolated from oral infections, root canal infections, and occasionally from nonoral locations. They were formerly classified in the genus *Bacteroides*.

There are five established species: *P. asaccharolytica, P. endodontalis, P. gingivalis, P. canoris, P. circumdentaria,* and ten new or re-named members. *P. endodontalis* and *P. gingivalis* are found in the human oral cavity, whereas *P. asaccharolytica* is normally associated with the urogenital and intestinal tract. Other *Porphyromonas* species are typically isolated from animals.

### Clinical Significance

Most *Porphyromonas* strains isolated from the oral cavity are *P. gingivalis,* which has an important role in periodontal disease. *P. gingivalis* is a component of dental plaque and is the primary pathogen in experimental periodontal disease in monkeys and rats. Most of the nonoral clinical isolates from other body sites in humans are *P. asaccharolytica. P. endodontalis* is usually involved in root canal infections. Animal-associated species (*P. canoris, P. circumdentaria, P. salivosa*) are associated with animal bite infections when isolated from humans.

### Cultural Characteristics and Identification

Organisms of the genus *Porphyromonas* are obligately anaerobic, nonspore-forming, pigmented, gram-negative bacilli. Their cells are coccoid, 0.5 to 0.8 × 1.0 to 3.0 μm (refer to Color Plate 35).

One of the most distinguishing characteristics of this group of microorganisms is their unusual special-potency disk pattern; they are the only gram-negative anaerobes that are susceptible to vancomycin (disk or agar plate). They are asaccharolytic (they do not ferment glucose or other carbohydrates), sensitive to 20% bile, and indole positive; all of them are pigmented (usually fluoresce), are nonmotile, and are obligate anaerobes (no growth on the aerotolerance plates incubated under aerobic conditions).

Colonies on primary isolation plates are tan to buff and will fluoresce brick-red under long-wave UV; older colonies will be brown to black. *P. gingivalis* is pigmented, but will not fluoresce. There is no growth on selective media containing vancomycin or bile. However, reduction of vancomycin to 2 μg/mL allows for growth of most *Porphyromonas.*

The typical special-potency disk pattern of resistance to colistin and kanamycin and susceptible to vancomycin allows easy genus determination; however, species level identification requires additional tests. Commercial enzymatic determination tests such as API ZYM, Rapid ID 32A, or RapID ANA are practical approaches to identify them to that level. See Table 19-4 for preliminary identification and Table 19-5 for level II identification.

### Antibiotic Susceptibility Characteristics

Characteristics are very similar to the pigmented *Prevotella* species.

## FUSOBACTERIUM

### Organism Characteristics

*Fusobacterium* are anaerobes commonly isolated in the clinical laboratory, some of which are extremely virulent organisms. Presently, there are about 20 species in this genus. We will discuss only the most frequently isolated or the medically important organisms: *F. nucleatum, F. necrophorum, F. mortiferum,* and *F. varium.*

### Clinical Significance

Fusobacteria are involved in serious infections from various body sites, and some produce ß-lactamase enzymes. They are found in head and neck infections, brain abscesses, chronic sinusitis, liver abscess, and other intra-abdominal infections.

### Cultural Characteristics and Identification

The *Fusobacterium* species are weakly saccharolytic or nonfermentative and produce butyric acid without isobutyric or isovaleric acids. The colonial morphology of fusobacteria varies greatly. Most strains produce greening of blood agar when exposed to air due to hydrogen peroxide production, and many fluoresce chartreuse under UV light. Fusobacteria are nonspore-forming, obligately anaerobic gram-negative bacilli.

The typical special potency disk pattern of fusobacteria is resistant to vancomycin and susceptible to colistin and kanamycin. Some strains are indole, lipase, bile, or esculin positive.

Characteristic Gram stain is a thin gram-negative bacilli with pointed ends (refer to Color Plate 36). Colonies of *F. nucleatum* will be 1 to 2 mm in diameter, translucent, often with flecked appearance when viewed by transmitted light (refer to Color Plate 37). They are usually nonhemolytic (horse and rabbit blood), but may be slightly hemolytic under the area of confluent growth or even produce green discoloration of the blood agar on exposure to oxygen. There are three characteristic colonial morphologies of *F. nucleatum:* bread crumb, speckled, and smooth.

*Fusobacterium nucleatum* is an obligate anaerobe and resistant only to vancomycin. It is indole positive and lipase negative (see Table 19-5). A new species, *F. periodonticum,* is very similar in colonial and cellular morphology; however, it differs in the fermentation of galactose: *F. nucleatum* is negative and *F. periodonticum* is positive.

Colonies of *F. necrophorum* on blood agar are 1 to 2 mm in diameter, convex to umbonate often with a bumpy, ridged, or uneven surface; translucent to opaque, often with mosaic internal structures (refer to Color Plate 38). (Cells from glucose broth are 0.5–0.7 mm in diameter with swellings up to 1.8 mm.) The ends of the cells are usually rounded but may be tapered. Cell length ranges from coccoid bodies to filaments of 1.0 mm (refer to Color Plate 37). Filamentous forms with granular inclusions are common in broth, while bacilli are more common in older culture and growth on agar.

Important characteristics include the colonial and cellular morphology mentioned above, typical *Fusobacterium* special potency disk pattern, lipase production (although in *F. necrophorum* subspecies *funduliforme* is lipase negative), indole-positive reaction, and chartreuse fluorescence. See Table 19-4 for preliminary identification and Table 19-5 for level II identification.

Colonies of *F. mortiferum* on primary isolation plates are 1 to 2 mm in diameter, circular with entire, diffuse, or slightly scalloped edges, convex, slightly umbonate, and translucent. On Gram stain the cells are extremely pleomorphic gram-negative bacilli with filaments containing swollen areas, round bodies, and irregular staining. Although less common, this same type of morphology can be seen with *F. ulcerans* and *F. necrophorum.*

In addition to the morphology, distinguishing characteristics include growth in 20% bile and esculin hydrolysis with the typical *Fusobacterium* disk pattern.

## Antibiotic Susceptibility Characteristics

In general, fusobacteria are fairly susceptible to antimicrobial agents. Unfortunately, resistance to penicillins has emerged in some strains of *F. nucleatum* due to ß-lactamase production. Fusobacteria can also produce L-form colonies with in vitro exposure to cell wall-active antimicrobics. This makes interpretation of MIC end-points difficult to read. Organisms are typically susceptible to metranidazole, imipenem, ß-lactamase inhibitor combinations, and second- or third-generation cephalosporins.

## SUMMARY

- ▶ The four anatomic sites where anaerobes are found as normal flora are the oral cavity, gastrointestinal tract, female urogenital tract, and skin.
- ▶ Resident anaerobic flora can cause disease when the ecologic niche is disrupted, such as in trauma, malignancy, or immunosuppression.
- ▶ Identification of anaerobes is categorized based on information available from primary plate (level I), spot tests and special potency disks (level II), and biochemical and physiologic characteristics (level III).
- ▶ A good primary isolation strategy for anaerobes includes enriched media (i.e., Brucella agar, CDC BA), selective media (BBE, KV, etc.), and an anaerobic broth (cooked meat, cooked meat with glucose, thioglycolate supplemented with vitamin K and hemin).
- ▶ As a general rule, gram-negative anaerobes are resistant to the special potency disk vancomycin (except *Porphyromonas*), and susceptible to kanamycin and colistin (*Prevotella* are resistant to kanamycin and variable to colistin).
- ▶ The seven additional tests that are important for level II identification are indole, catalase, lipase, urease, motility, formate-fumarate, and nitrate.
- ▶ The *B. fragilis* group contains the most common, clinically important anaerobic gram-negative bacterial pathogens.
- ▶ The *B. ureolyticus* group are slow-growing organisms that tend to "pit" the agar, and whose growth is enhanced with formate-fumarate supplement.
- ▶ *Prevotella* species can be resistant to all the special potency disks, like the *B. fragilis* group; however, they are susceptible to 20% bile.
- ▶ *Porphyromonas* species are pigmented and are characteristically susceptible to vancomycin.
- ▶ *Fusobacterium* species are typically involved in infections of the head and neck, some of which are serious.

## CASE STUDY 1: YOUNG WOMAN WITH ABDOMINAL PAIN

A 25-year-old woman complained of 3 days of diffuse abdominal pain. At first she thought the pain was cramps, but she was concerned because the pain persisted and she was losing her appetite. On physical examination she was febrile to 40°C, had an accelerated heart rate (155 beats/min), and a rapid respiratory rate. She had midgastric and right lower quadrant abdominal tenderness. Blood cultures obtained on admission were positive for anaerobic, gram-negative bacilli in 48 hours, at which time the patient was taken to surgery.

**Questions:**

1. What is the most likely group of anaerobes?

2. The doctors decided to perform abdominal surgery. What types of diseases would you suspect could lead to anaerobic bacteremia?

3. What would tissue samples of the appendix probably grow on culture?

## CASE STUDY 2: ACUTE BACTERIAL CELLULITIS

A 58-year-old woman presented to the emergency department of a community hospital suffering from an acutely enlarged neck that was making it difficult for her to breathe. Onset was sudden, with no history of pharyngitis. Her condition worsened, and the doctors had to perform an emergency tracheotomy to keep her airway open. She was transported to the University Medical Center by air ambulance. On physical examination, she had massive swelling under her jaw and around her throat, most of which was bright red. There were no detectable fluid (pus) pockets to drain, so the physicians took some punch biopsies and started her on empiric antimicrobic therapy for acute cellulitis.

**Questions:**

1. What is your clinical diagnosis? Why is it important to establish that there was no previous history of sore throat?

2. Aerobic cultures grew catalase-negative, gram-positive cocci exhibiting α-hemolysis. Anaerobic cultures grew indole-positive, gram-negative bacilli with rounded ends that were resistant to vancomycin and susceptible to kanamycin, colistin, and bile. Based on the clinical diagnosis and preliminary culture results, what are the most likely presumptive identifications?

3. How does this patient's disease differ from Vincent's angina? Vincent's disease?

## Review Questions

1. Which genus consists of moderately saccharolytic, pigmented and nonpigmented, gram-negative organisms?
   a. *Prevotella*
   b. *Porphyromonas*
   c. *Bacteroides*
   d. *Veillonella*

2. Select the asaccharolytic, pigmented, nonspore-forming, gram-negative anaerobe(s) found in human infections due to animal bites.
   a. *Porphyromonas canoris*
   b. *Porphyromonas circumdentaria*
   c. *Porphyromonas salivosa*
   d. All of the above

3. Applying level II identification, which important test will help differentiate between *Porphyromonas* and *Prevotella?*
   a. Gram stain
   b. Special potency disks, especially vancomycin
   c. Fluorescence
   d. Gas-liquid chromatography

4. What wavelength is recommended when testing for fluorescence in anaerobic gram-negative pigmented organisms?
   a. Short
   b. Intermediate
   c. Long
   d. None of the above

5. Which two enzymes are produced by strains of *B. fragilis,* and are easily detected in the laboratory?
   a. Lipase, lecithinase
   b. Catalase, ß-lactamase
   c. Lecithinase, catalase
   d. ß-Lactamase, lipase

6. Which of the following media enhances the fluorescence test?
   a. Egg yolk agar
   b. Bacteroides bile esculin agar
   c. Phenylethyl alcohol
   d. Lysed (laked) blood or rabbit blood agar

7. Why is it important to ensure special potency disks have warmed to room temperature before using them?
   a. Condensation may cause a loss of potency.
   b. Results may indicate false susceptibility.
   c. Results may indicate false resistance.
   d. a and c are correct.

8. What obligate anaerobic gram-negative bacillus is described as long and thin with tapered ends, has no fluorescence, and is resistant only to vancomycin disks (susceptible to kanamycin, colistin, and 20% bile)?
   a. *Fusobacterium nucleatum*
   b. *Fusobacterium necrophorum*
   c. *Prevotella melaninogenica*
   d. *Bacteroides fragilis* group

9. Which test differentiates the *B. ureolyticus* group from *Fusobacterium* species?
   a. Growth in 20% bile
   b. Nitrate
   c. Gram stain
   d. Fluorescence

10. Special potency antimicrobial disks support level II identification of anaerobes by:
    a. grouping organisms with similar characteristics (e.g., *B. fragilis* group).
    b. supporting the Gram stain.
    c. all of the above
    d. none of the above; disk patterns are not used in level II identification.

## ▶ REFERENCES & RECOMMENDED READING

Baron, E. J., Peterson, L. R., & Finegold, S. M. (1994). *Bailey and Scott's diagnostic microbiology* (9th ed.). St. Louis: Mosby–Year Book.

*Bergey's manual of systematic bacteriology* (Vol. 1). N. R. Krieg (Ed.). Baltimore: Williams & Wilkins.

*Clinical and Infectious Diseases.* (1997) Vol. 25 Suppl. 2.

Finegold, S. M. (1992). Conference Journal—Highlight Issue (32nd Interscience Conference on Antimicrobial Agents and Chemotherapy), Vol. 13, No. 5, October 11–14, 1992, Anaheim, CA.

Finegold, S. M., Baron, E. J., & Wexler, H. M. (1992). *A clinical guide to anaerobic infections.* Belmont, CA: Star Publishing.

Finegold, S. M., Rosenblatt, J. E., Sutter, F. L., & Atterbery, H. R. (1974). *Scope monograph on anaerobic infections.* Kalamazoo, MI: Upjohn Company.

Gilligan, P. H., Shapiro, D. S., and Smiley, M. L. (1992). *Cases in medical microbiology and infectious diseases.* Washington, DC: American Society for Microbiology Press.

Mangels, J. I. (Section Ed.), (1992). Anaerobic bacteriology. In H. D. Isenberg (Chief Ed.), *Clinical microbiology procedures handbook.* Washington, DC: American Society for Microbiology Press.

Murray, P. R., Baron, E. J., Pfaller, M. A., Tenover, F. C., & Yolken, R. H. (Eds.). (1995). *Manual of clinical microbiology* (6th ed.). Washington, DC: American Society for Microbiology.

Pezzlo, M. (Sec. Ed.). (1992). Aerobic bacteriology. In H. D. Isenberg (Chief Ed.), *Clinical microbiology procedures handbook*. Washington, DC: American Society for Microbiology Press.

Summanen, P., Baron, E. J., Citron, D. M., Strong, C. A., Wexler, H. M., & Finegold, S. M. (1993). *Wadsworth anaerobic bacteriology manual* (5th ed.). Belmont, CA: Star Publishing.

Tortora, G. J., Funk, B., & Case, C. L. (1995). *Microbiology: An introduction*. Redwood City, CA: Benjamin/Cummings.

Volk, W. A., Gebhardt, B. M., Hammayskjohd, M., & Kadner, R. J. (1995). *Essentials of medical microbiology* (5th ed.). Philadelphia: Lippincott.

# CHAPTER 20
# Gram-Positive Anaerobic Bacteria

Gloria T. Anderson, MT (ASCP), David W. Craft, PhD,
A. Christian Whelan, PhD, D (ABMM)

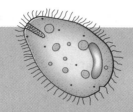

## Microbes in the News

"What can I do about acne?" is a common question among young adults today. Some of the answers are found in the study of the gram-positive anaerobic bacteria. One such bacterium, *Propionibacterium acnes,* plays a role in acne by eliciting a local inflammatory response. Leukocytes are recruited to the sebaceous follicles where the bacilli reside. During phagocytosis, a number of bacterial enzymes are released to include lipases, proteases, neuraminidases, hyaluronidases, and other hydrolytic enzymes. These precipitate the inflammatory response leading to rupture of the sebaceous follicle. The lipase also frees long-chain fatty acids in the skin that may be irritating enough to contribute to the formation of acne pustules. Acne is unrelated to the effectiveness of skin cleansing because the lesion develops within the follicles. Primary treatment is topical benzoyl peroxide and antibiotics such as erythromycin and clindamycin.

## KEY TERMS

Aerotolerant anaerobe
Diphtheroid
Exogenous infection

Obligate anaerobe
Spores
Toxins

Toxoid
Virulence

## INTRODUCTION

As seen with infections involving gram-negative anaerobic bacteria, many gram-positive anaerobic infections are polymicrobial. These organisms are, for the most part, components of the normal flora of the skin or mucosal surfaces of humans and often cause disease as opportunists, flourishing in a localized environment with decreased or no oxygen. Anaerobic gram-positive cocci and nonspore-forming bacilli may be isolated from infected sites located in close proximity to their normal habitat. They are most frequently recovered from clinical specimens taken from urogenital or oral sites, or from patients with systemic infections originating from these sites. This group of microorganisms is most likely to be recovered from abscess, body fluid, or wound specimens. Frequently they must be separated from anaerobic gram-negative bacilli or facultative organisms, even when care is taken to avoid contamination during specimen collection.

The gram-positive anaerobic spore-forming bacilli are often associated with **exogenous infections**, which involve organisms introduced from outside the body. Alternatively, disease can originate internally from a disruption of the integrity of the bowel environment due to trauma, malignancy, ischemia, or antibiotic use. The infectious disease process may result from invasive or noninvasive mechanisms. Pathogenesis for noninvasive disease often involves **virulence** factors such as **toxins**. Examples include botulism, tetanus, gastroenteritis, and antibiotic-associated pseudomembranous colitis (AAPC). Invasive disease leads to tissue destruction often mediated by histolytic enzymes and may or may not be toxin associated. Clostridial myonecrosis, or gas gangrene, is a good example of an invasive disease with a toxin component.

## ANAEROBIC, GRAM-POSITIVE COCCI AND NONSPORE-FORMING BACILLI

These organisms are usually found as normal flora of the skin and mucous membranes and may spread to adjacent sterile areas due to trauma, aspiration, or changes in the surrounding normal flora. Primary isolation media for these organisms should include a supplemented blood agar, such as Brucella blood agar, phenylethyl alcohol blood agar, and thioglycollate broth. Additional media may include modified Schaedler blood agar, brain-heart infusion agar, CDC agar, or colistin-nalidixic acid agar (see primary isolation media, Chapter 21).

In general, the anaerobic gram-positive cocci occur in pairs, tetrads, irregular masses, and chains when examined microscopically. The anaerobic gram-positive rods appear coccobacillary or pleomorphic and sometimes branched. An exception are the lactobacilli, which are normal flora in the female urethra and genital tract and commonly occur as short to long slender rods in chains. At times, some strains of anaerobic bacilli resemble cocci, particularly in gram-stained preparations of young colonies on blood agar. Likewise, some streptococci and peptostreptococci may appear rod-shaped when grown on blood agar. The anaerobic gram-positive cocci are generally susceptible to ß-lactams, including most cephalosporins and vancomycin; clindamycin and metranidazole are less active. The anaerobic gram-positive bacilli are generally susceptible to penicillin G, carbenicillin, chloramphenicol, and vancomycin. Clindamycin, erythromycin, and tetracycline are used with varying efficiencies. The most commonly isolated microorganisms are *Peptostreptococcus* species, *Propionibacterium acnes*, *Actinomyces* species, *Bifidobacterium dentium*, *Mobiluncus* species, and *Eubacterium* species (see Table 20-1).

## PEPTOSTREPTOCOCCUS

### Organism Characteristics

Gram-positive anaerobic cocci may appear under the microscope as large and coccobacillary, large and in tetrads, or small and in chains (refer to Color Plate 40).

### Clinical Significance

*Peptostreptococcus* are second only to the anaerobic gram-negative bacilli as the most commonly isolated

**Table 20–1 ► Level II Group and Species Identification of the Nonspore-Forming Anaerobic Gram-Positive Organisms**

| | Special Potency Disks | | | | | | |
|---|---|---|---|---|---|---|---|
| BACTERIA | KANAMYCIN | VANCOMYCIN | COLISTIN | SPS | CATALASE | INDOLE | NITRATE |
| **Cocci** | V | S | R | V | V | V | ± |
| P. anaerobius | R | S | R | S | – | – | – |
| P. assacharolyticus | S | S | R | R | V | + | – |
| P. magnus | | S | R | | + | – | – |
| P. micros | | S | R | | – | – | – |
| P. prevotii | | S | R | | V | – | – |
| **Bacilli*** | V | S | R | | V | V | V |
| P. acnes | S | S | R | | + | + | + |
| Actinomyces species | | S | R | | –† | – | V |
| B. dentium | | S | R | | – | – | – |
| Mobiluncus species* | | S | R | | – | – | V |
| E. lentum | S | S | R | | V | – | + |

*All the bacilli are nonmotile except *Mobiluncus*.

†Only *A. viscosus* produces catalase.

Obscure or rarely isolated organisms: *Peptococcus niger, Lactobacillus catenaforme, Rothia* species, *Eubacterium lentum*

R, resistant; S, susceptible; V, variable; SPS, sulfite polymixin sulfadiazine.

anaerobic bacteria. They are normal flora of the mouth, upper respiratory tract, skin, large intestine, and female genital tract. They are obligate anaerobes exhibiting slow growth on culture media even at 5 to 7 days. Like the anaerobic gram-negative rods, they are encountered in the clinical laboratory in blood cultures, other body fluids, and in a wide variety of wound and abscess specimens. The majority of bacteremias caused by peptostreptococci originate from the genital tract in women or contamination during venipuncture. The major pathogenic species include *P. magnus, P. assacharolyticus, P. anaerobius, P. micros,* and *P. prevotii.* Clinical symptoms may be associated with and include bone and joint infection, intra-abdominal sepsis, salpingitis, septic abortion, pleuropulmonary infection, diabetic foot ulcers, or head and neck infection.

## PROPIONIBACTERIUM ACNES

### Organism Characteristics

Gram-stained cells are often unevenly stained and appear **"diphtheroid"** due to snapping after cell division (refer to Color Plate 41).

## Clinical Significance

*Propionibacterium acnes* is the most commonly isolated gram-positive, anaerobic bacillus found in clinical specimens. They may be isolated from skin, intestinal abscesses, and subgingival plaque, and are frequently found as contaminants of blood cultures. However, they may be pathogenic if isolated from bone and joints, central nervous system, endocarditis cases, or in conjunction with indwelling devices such as shunts and prosthetic devices. This is also the bacterium associated with common "acne," or acne vulgaris (see Figure 20-1). Another species, *P. propionicus,* causes disease that is indistinguishable from actinomycosis. It may be differentiated from *P. acnes* by a negative catalase reaction.

## Cultural Characteristics

Colonies on sheep blood agar are initially small and white. On further incubation, colonies will grow larger and may turn a shade of yellow.

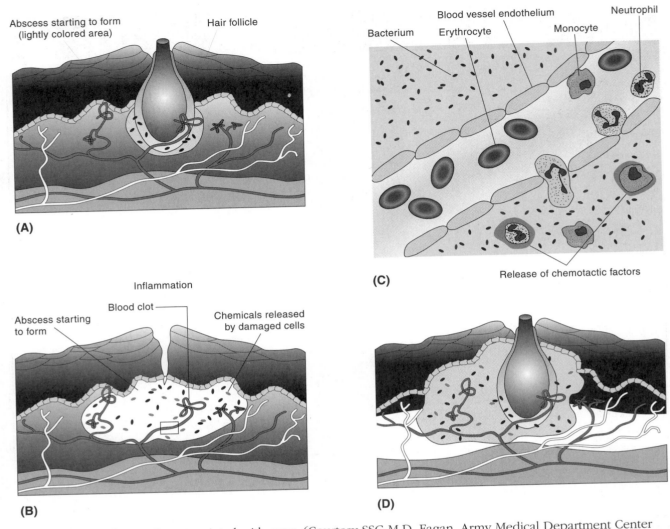

**FIGURE 20-1** Inflammation associated with acne. (Courtesy SSG M.D. Fagan, Army Medical Department Center and School)

## ACTINOMYCES

### Organism Characteristics

These infections produce a characteristic purulent discharge containing sulfur granules that appear as white, yellow, or brown granular bodies. Under the microscope, granules are actually clumps of organisms surrounded by purulent exudate. Bacterial cells often appear as diphtheroid, club-shaped, or filamentous rods with some branching (refer to Color Plate 42).

### Clinical Significance

These bacteria are normal flora of the mucous membranes (primarily the mouth and genitourinary tract) and are frequently recovered in mixed cultures. Infections occur in tissue and bone, and present as cervicofacial, pulmonary/thoracic, abdominal, or pelvic inflammatory disease in women using intrauterine devices (IUD).

Actinomycosis or "lumpy jaw" develops as a chronic granulomatous lesion that becomes suppurative and forms abscesses that drain externally (sinus tracts). The initial incubation period is 5 to 7 days. Because of the nature of the lesion, it is difficult to achieve adequate diffusion of antimicrobic within the lesion. A common risk factor is poor oral hygiene or a history of invasive dental procedure or oral trauma.

Actinomycosis occurs in other anatomic sites as well, similar to that of oral-facial disease progression. In pulmonary actinomycosis, draining sinuses can exit the chest wall and cause osteomyelitis of the ribs. Septic emboli may disseminate via the blood and become localized in organ capillary beds, especially the brain. Sinus tracts in women with IUDs may exit the abdominal wall and sometimes perforate the colon.

## Table 20–2 ▶ *Clostridium* Species and Human Disease

| Disease | Organism Association | Treatment |
|---|---|---|
| Gas gangrene (histolytic) | C. perfringens (type A), C. septicum, C. novyi type A, C. bifermentans, C. histolyticum, C. sordellii, C. sporogenes | Surgery and antimicrobics* |
| Tetanus | C. tetani | Toxoid vaccine, antitoxin |
| Botulism | C. botulinum (rare—C. butyricum and C. baratii) | Antitoxin |
| AAPC | C. difficile | Metranidazole, oral vancomycin |
| Food poisoning | C. perfringens, C. botulinum | Fluid management, antitoxin (bot) |

Other important diseases†:

C. septicum—colorectal carcinoma, bacteremia, infected wounds

C. tertium—bacteremia, neutropenia, hematologic malignancies

C. ramosum—post-traumatic intra-abdominal infection

*Antimicrobics effective in treating clostridial infections include ß-lactams, most third-generation cephalosporins, and clindamycin. The drug of choice for C. difficile and many other anaerobes is oral metranidazole (less expensive than oral vancomycin).

†Treatment will depend on concurrent therapy of associated diseases.

AAPC, antibiotic-associated pseudomembranous colitis.

## Cultural Characteristics

Colonies on primary isolation media often exhibit characteristic "molar tooth" morphology, whereas some exhibit "bread crumb" or smooth morphology.

## BIFIDOBACTERIUM DENTIUM

Another etiologic agent associated with actinomycosis and sometimes periodontal diseases is *Bifidobacterium dentium*. The organisms are found in the normal flora of the oral and genitourinary tracts and appear as gram-positive diphtheroidal forms sometimes described as bifid or "Y" forms under the microscope (refer to Color Plate 43).

## ANAEROBIC GRAM-POSITIVE SPORE-FORMING BACILLI

The medically important, anaerobic, gram-positive, spore-forming bacilli are classified in the genus *Clostridium*. These bacteria are **aerotolerant** to **obligate anaerobes** that are found in soil, dust, and water, and in the intestinal tract of humans and animals. Most infections are acquired endogenously, often by the disturbance or translocation of normal bowel flora. Infections of exogenous origin include tetanus and gas gangrene (clostridial myonecrosis); syndromes mediated by toxins include tetanus, botulism, and *Clostridium perfringens* food poisoning (see Table 20-2).

Primary isolation media used is the same as that of other anaerobic bacteria with the exception of egg yolk agar, which helps in speciating the clostridia based on proteolytic enzyme activity (refer to Color Plate 44). These enzymes include lipase indicated by a "mother of pearl" sheen on the colonies and lecithinase indicated by a white precipitate around the colony. Some species often stain gram-negative, most are motile, catalase and indole negative, kanamycin and vancomycin susceptible, and colistin resistant. The most common clinical isolates are *C. perfringens* and *C. ramosum;* the most commonly recognized pathogenic species are *C. perfringens, C. septicum, C. botulinum, C. tetani,* and *C. difficile* (see Table 20-3).

Keys to grouping and identifying clinically significant *Clostridium* species: *C. perfringens* is the most frequent clinical isolate, followed by *C. ramosum, C. septicum, C. clostridio-forme,* and *C. innocuum.* The Nagler test (see Procedure 20-1) can be used for identification of *C. perfringens, C. sordellii,* and *C. bifermentans. C. perfringens* demonstrates the most complete neutralization of the α-lecithinase in the Nagler test. It is readily differentiated from the other Nagler-positive bacteria exhibiting double zone hemolysis, boxcar-shaped cells, a positive glutamic acid decarboxylase test, and a positive reverse CAMP test (see Procedure 20-2). It is also nonmotile. *C. bifermentans* and *C. sordellii* may be distinguished by urease production, the former being urease negative and the latter almost always positive.

*Clostridium difficile* is infrequently isolated from specimens other than stool and is usually diagnosed by the

**Table 20–3** ▶ **Level II Species Identification of the Genus *Clostridium***

| Bacteria | Kanamycin | Vancomycin | Colistin | Indole | Nitrate | Catalase | Reverse CAMP |
|---|---|---|---|---|---|---|---|
| *Clostridium* species | V | V | R | V | V | – | |
| Nagler positive | | | | | | | |
| *Clostridium* species | S | S | R | V | V | – | |
| C. perfringens | S | S | R | – | V | – | + |
| C. bifermentans | S | S | R | + | – | – | – |
| C. sordellii | S | S | R | + | – | – | – |
| Nagler negative | | | | | | | |
| *Clostridium* species | V | V | R | V | V | – | |
| C. difficile | S | S | R | – | – | – | |

R, resistant; S, susceptible; V, variable

presence of a specific enterotoxin or cytotoxin by enzyme immunoassay or cytopathic effect in tissue culture.

*Clostridium tertium* and *C. histolyticum* are the most frequently encountered aerotolerant clostridia in the laboratory. Growth can be very good in air, but a Gram stain of growth from an aerobic plate will not show **spores**. Speciation of all the clinically important clostridia relies on gelatin hydrolysis and carbohydrate fermentation. As with all anaerobes, definitive identification may require submission to reference laboratories per-

forming metabolic end-product analysis by gas-liquid chromatography and/or whole cell fatty acid analysis by gas chromatography.

## *CLOSTRIDIUM PERFRINGENS*

### Organism Characteristics

The microscopic detection of gram-positive spore-forming bacilli is extremely useful for debrided tissue

---

# PROCEDURE 20-1
# The Nagler Test (modified with permission from *Bailey and Scott's Diagnostic Microbiology*, 9th ed.)

**Principle:**

The Nagler test is used to detect α-lecithinase-producing clostridia (*C. perfringens, C. baraatii, C. bifermentans, C. sordellii*) by inhibiting the lecithinase reaction with a specific antitoxin.

**Method:**

1. Swab one-half of an egg yolk agar plate with antitoxin.
2. Allow the liquid to absorb.
3. Inoculate the test organism on the antitoxin-free half, and then streak once across to the antitoxin side of the plate.
4. Incubate anaerobically for 24 to 48 hours at 37°C.

**Quality Control:**

Test a known α-lecithinase producer such as *C. perfringens* and a lecithinase producer (non-α) such as *C. limosum*.

**Interpretation:**

Both organisms produce a white, opaque halo in the medium. The opacity in the medium is dramatically decreased or obliterated in the presence of α-lecithinase antitoxin.

## PROCEDURE 20-2
### Reverse CAMP Test

The reverse CAMP test is similar to the CAMP test explained in Chapter 10. In the reverse CAMP procedure, the *Staphylococcus aureus* streak is replaced with a streak of the unknown clostridial isolate. A known group B *Streptococcus* is inoculated at right angles to the unknown, stopping just before the unknown line is reached. While some enhanced hemolysis may be observed with any *Clostridium*, only *C. perfringens* results in the characteristic arrowhead formation due to synergistic ß-hemolysis.

specimens. Blood cultures are positive in about 15% of patients. Gram-stained cells appear as large boxcar-shaped rods (2.0 × 4.0 µm) occurring singly or in chains; distinct oval subterminal spores are rarely seen.

## Clinical Significance

*Clostridium perfringens* is the most common clostridial isolate from human sources (excluding stool) and may be associated with either simple colonization or severe, life-threatening disease. Clinical syndromes include (1) gas gangrene (clostridial myonecrosis) and other soft tissue infections; (2) enterotoxin-mediated severe necrotizing disease of the small bowel; and (3) entero-toxin-mediated food poisoning. There are five toxin types, with type A associated with gas gangrene and food poisoning. Type C is associated with sporadic occurrence of small bowel necrosis, or enteritis necroticans.

Gas gangrene caused by *C. perfringens* is a life- or limb-threatening example of histotoxic clostridial disease. Introduced by surgery or trauma, the wound is contaminated by spores or live bacteria from soil or feces. Disease symptoms begin with intense pain and erythema, progressing to muscle necrosis with the presence of gas (crepitus), shock, renal failure, and death in as few as 2 days. Other histolytic clostridial soft tissue infections present as cellulitis and fasciitis. Other clostridia associated with histolytic tissue destruction are *C. septicum, C. histolyticum, C. bifermentans, C. novyi,* and *C. sordellii.* Treatment depends on an aggressive debridement of devitalized tissue (and perhaps hyperbaric oxygen) and antimicrobial therapy.

*Clostridium perfringens* gastroenteritis is the third most common cause of food poisoning in the United States. It involves type A strains (positive for lecithinase on Nagler test) and follows the ingestion of high numbers of vegetative cells in food that, on sporulation in the gut, release an enterotoxin. The symptoms appear within 12 to 15 hours and include abdominal cramps and watery diarrhea without fever, nausea, or vomiting. Food-borne gastroenteritis caused by *C. perfringens* has commonly implicated beef and poultry, especially in stews or gravies that have been warmed for a second serving. The spores, common in both raw products, that survive the initial cooking germinate and multiply during the slow cooling of these viscous, fatty products where the oxygen tension has been reduced and atmospheric oxygen cannot easily diffuse. *C. perfringens* can multiply at temperatures of 120°F. Consequently if the heating for the first or second serving is not sufficient, high numbers of vegetative cells will survive and sporulate in the gut with the ensuing symptoms of gastroenteritis. Interestingly, sporulation occurs easily in the intestine but is difficult to induce in foods and laboratory media. Treatment requires appropriate fluid management and does not require antimicrobics.

## Cultural Characteristics

After 1 day of growth, colonies produce a double zone of ß-hemolysis on blood agar and exhibit lecithinase activity on egg yolk agar. They are nonmotile but exhibit spreading on laboratory media typical of motile organisms. They are Nagler and reverse CAMP positive, lipase negative, and protease negative (refer to Color Plate 45).

## CLOSTRIDIUM BOTULINUM

### Organism Characteristics

Gram-stained cells are large and pleomorphic, with rounded ends occurring singly, or in pairs and chains, with oval subterminal spores appearing as club shaped.

### Clinical Significance

Four forms of botulism are recognized today as distinct clinical entities. Food-borne (classical) botulism is caused by the ingestion of preformed toxin in food. This occurs most frequently with improperly canned vegetables. Infant botulism is caused by the absorption of toxins produced by toxigenic organisms that colonize the intestinal tract of infants under 1 year of age.

Wound botulism, the rarest form of botulism, is caused by growth of the organism and toxin production at the site of a wound, including infections in intravenous drug users. A fourth, but not well understood type of botulism, occurs in individuals older than 12 months in whom no food or wound source is implicated.

The botulinum toxin is the most toxic biologic substance known (see Table 20-4). It acts at the myoneural junctions to inhibit the release of acetylcholine at the motor nerve terminals causing flaccid (passive) paralysis. Early symptoms appear 12 to 24 hours after ingestion, typically including weakness, dizziness, and constipation. Later signs include double vision and difficulty in swallowing or speaking. Death is usually caused by respiratory paralysis or airway obstruction. Treatment includes trivalent botulinal antitoxin and ventilatory support, and penicillin for wound botulism only.

The clinical diagnosis of botulism can be confirmed by stool culture or demonstrating toxin activity in serum, feces, gastric contents, or vomitus. The toxin neutralization test is normally performed at a reference or public health laboratory.

In 1976, infant botulism was recognized as a distinct clinical and epidemiologic entity. Infant botulism occurs in infants between 1 week and 12 months of age and results from the absorption of botulinum toxin produced by toxigenic clostridia that colonize the intestinal tract. The clinical spectrum ranges from infants who are asymptomatic carriers through those who develop various degrees of paralysis or even sudden death. Spores may be present in honey and dust, which serve as environmental sources of the agent.

Infant botulism has a broad spectrum of clinical symptoms. The main features are constipation, listlessness, lethargy, difficulty in sucking and swallowing, weak cry, pooled oral secretions, hypotonia, general muscle weakness, and loss of head control. During the 1980s, a number of studies were performed in an attempt to link sudden infant death syndrome (SIDS) to *C. botulinum*. These studies concluded that infant botulism can explain only a small number of SIDS cases in North America and Europe and is therefore not considered a significant factor in the cause of sudden death. It has also been shown that clostridial species other than *C. botulinum* can produce the botulinum toxin that causes infant botulism.

## Cultural Characteristics

They are lecithinase negative, lipase positive, and protease negative on egg yolk agar. These are the only motile clostridia.

## *CLOSTRIDIUM TETANI*

### Organism Characteristics

Gram stain reveals slender rods with rounded ends and round swollen terminal spores in a characteristic "drumstick" or "tennis racket" appearance (refer to Color Plate 46). Vegetative cells may occur in filaments.

### Clinical Significance

Tetanus is strictly toxin mediated and usually a result of a puncture wound or soil contamination of an existing wound. Like botulinum toxin, "tetanospasmin" also inhibits the release of acetylcholine. It becomes bound to gangliosides in the central nervous system, suppressing inhibitory motor neuron activity and leading to an intensified reflex response. Clinical symptoms follow an incubation period of 4 to 10 days after exposure and begin with generalized muscle stiffness followed by spasms of jaw muscles. Subsequent spasms cause clenching of the jaw ("sardonic smile"), arching of the back, extension of the extremities, and possible bone fractures. Prophylaxis includes **toxoid** as part of the diphtheria-pertussis-tetanus (DPT) shot and treatment may include antitoxin, muscle relaxants, analgesics, and sedatives.

### Cultural Characteristics

*Clostridium tetani* is an obligate anaerobe and therefore extremely difficult to culture. It is present in small quantities in the wound and relatively inactive metabolically. When culture attempts succeed, growth on blood agar exhibits a narrow zone of hemolysis. Enzymatic activity on egg yolk agar is lecithinase negative, lipase variable, and protease negative.

## *CLOSTRIDIUM DIFFICILE*

### Organism Characteristics

Gram stain of fecal material reveals many polymorphonuclear cells and gram-positive to gram-variable long thin rods with oval subterminal spores.

| Table 20–4 ▶ A Tale of Two Toxins |  |
|---|---|
| **Neurotoxins** | |
| TETANOSPASMIN | BOTULINUM |
| Lethal | Most lethal known |
| Spastic (rigid) paralysis | Flaccid (passive) paralysis |
| One toxin—tetanospasmin | Seven serologically related neurotoxins, types A through G |
| Vaccine protection: Toxoid (DPT) | Vaccine protection: Toxoid—as needed (Michigan Department of Public Health) |

## Clinical Significance

*Clostridium difficile* is the major cause of antibiotic-associated diarrhea and pseudomembranous colitis. The organism is part of the normal flora in some healthy persons and hospitalized patients and is a very important cause of nosocomial infection in hospitals and nursing homes.

Two toxins are associated with clinical symptoms: (1) an enterotoxin (toxin A) that promotes fluid secretion and destroys intestinal lining cells, and (2) cytotoxin (toxin B) that is cytopathic to the cellular cytoskeleton. Pathology is ultimately due to toxin-mediated necrosis and sloughing mucosal lining. It is induced by prolonged use of almost any antibiotic with a resulting change in the normal flora of the gastrointestinal tract. This permits the overgrowth of these relatively resistant organisms or makes the patient more susceptible to exogenous acquisition of *C. difficile*. Proliferation of the organisms with localized production of their toxins in the colon leads to disease.

Nonculture diagnostic testing for suspected toxigenic *C. difficile*-associated disease can be accomplished by commercially available test kits (see Table 20-5). Methods include enzyme immunoassay for toxins A and B and cell culture cytotoxicity assays with specific neutralization for toxin B. (For nontoxigenic strains, there are latex agglutination test kits for detection of a *C. difficile* common protein antigen.) The cytotoxicity assay and specific neutralization with antisera to toxin B is considered the "gold standard" by which the sensitivity and specificity of the immunoassays are measured.

## Cultural Characteristics

Culture is not often performed, but if so, is done on selective egg yolk media such as cycloserine-cefoxitin fructose agar and nonselective CDC-anaerobe blood agar. There is a characteristic "horse-stable" odor with no lecithinase, lipase, and protease activity. Indole, nitrate, and urease tests are also negative. Treatment includes stopping the offending antimicrobic agent, oral metranidazole, or oral vancomycin.

**Table 20–5 ► Detection of *Clostridium difficile*-Associated Toxins**

| Method | System | Capture | Detection |
|---|---|---|---|
| A. Enterotoxin (Toxin A) | | | |
| 1. Immunobinding | Membrane Cassette | Mab | E-Ab conjugate and substrate |
| 2. EIA | Microtiter | Mab | E-Ab conjugate and substrate |
| B. Cytotoxin (Toxin B) | | | |
| 1. *Tissue culture* | Cell culture tube/chamber | | *Gold standard* |
| a. Positive | | Cells | CPE |
| | | Cells + Antitoxin | No CPE |
| b. Negative | | Cells | No CPE |
| | | Cells + Antitoxin | No CPE |
| 2. Tissue culture | Microtiter | | |
| a. Positive | | Cells | CPE |
| b. Negative | | Cells | No CPE |

CPE, cytopathic effect on susceptible cells; E-Ab, enzyme-antibody; EIA, enzyme immunoassay; Mab, monoclonal antibody.

## SUMMARY

▶ Anaerobic bacteria are often normal flora of the mucous membranes and frequently recovered in mixed cultures.

▶ Many gram-positive anaerobic infections are polymicrobial, flourishing in a localized environment with decreased or no oxygen.

▶ Gram-positive anaerobes are most likely to be recovered from abscess, body fluid, or wound specimens.

▶ Gram-positive anaerobic cocci (*Peptostreptococci*) are second only to the anaerobic gram-negative bacilli as the most commonly isolated anaerobic bacteria. They are most often recovered in blood cultures.

▶ *Propionibacterium acnes* is a diphtheroid and is the most commonly isolated gram-positive, anaerobic bacillus found in clinical specimens.

▶ *Actinomycosis* species infections may produce sulfur granules that present clinically as lumpy jaw, and often exhibit molar tooth colony morphology.

▶ The gram-positive anaerobic spore-forming bacilli may arise from either exogenous infection or internal disruption of an organ system, usually the bowel.

▶ Gram-positive anaerobic spore-forming bacilli may be invasive and histotoxic or noninvasive and toxin-mediated such as botulism, tetanus, gastroenteritis, or antibiotic-associated pseudomembranous colitis.

▶ Egg yolk agar is a primary isolation media for the gram-positive, spore-forming anaerobic bacilli in which proteolytic enzyme activity, such as lipase and lecithinase, is exhibited.

▶ *Clostridium perfringens* is the most frequent clostridial isolate, exhibiting large boxcar-shaped rods on Gram stain, double zone ß-hemolysis, nonmotility, and positive Nagler and reverse CAMP tests.

▶ *C. perfringens* causes a histolytic myonecrosis (gas gangrene) and is also the third most common cause of food poisoning (gastroenteritis) in the United States.

▶ There are four clinical forms of botulism, all mediated by the botulinum toxin, the most lethal toxin known to man.

▶ Tetanus is a strictly toxin-mediated disease, usually the result of a puncture wound or soil contamination of an existing wound.

▶ *Clostridium difficile* pseudomembranous colitis may be confirmed by the presence of a specific enterotoxin or cytotoxin by enzyme immunoassay or cytopathic effect in tissue culture.

## CASE STUDY 1: ALCOHOLIC WITH CHEST PAIN

A 63-year-old man presented to the emergency room with a chief complaint of localized right chest pain. Past medical history was unremarkable. Social history included homelessness, heavy smoker, and 2 to 3 glasses (pints) of wine daily. He denied intravenous drug abuse or sexually transmitted disease. He had received a tuberculosis skin test at the "shelter," and recalled it to be negative. Physical examination revealed poor dentition. His lungs were clear, but he winced in pain on deep inspiration. He had another tuberculin skin test, with an anergy panel, and was sent to x-ray. Chest radiographs indicated a mass in the right middle lobe near the rib cage. Closer inspection of his external chest revealed a 0.5-cm lesion that drained when pressure was applied.

### Questions:

1. What organisms might cause this patient's symptoms?

2. What specimens would you send to the microbiology lab? What tests would you order?

3. Gram-positive, delicately branching, club-end bacilli were seen in large clumps on drainage and aspirate specimens. Other stains were negative. What was the most likely organism?

## CASE STUDY 2: SCHOOL TEACHER WITH FEVER

A 38-year-old female elementary school teacher went to her physician complaining of intermittent low-grade fever, weight loss over the last 6 months of 20 pounds, and abdominal discomfort. Initially she thought she had gotten the "bug that was going around," but her husband urged her to seek medical attention. A week prior to the current visit, she had a chest x-ray, purified protein derivative, urinalysis, and a stool specimen worked up for enteric or parasitic agents (including *C. difficile*), all of which were negative. Her fever was worse today, 39°C, and her doctor decided to admit her to the hospital. Admission labs were remarkable for a white cell count of 16,000 with 76% neutrophils. Blood cultures were drawn, and both anaerobic bottles were positive at 48 hours (aerobic bottles remained negative). Gram stain revealed gram-positive bacilli, and subculture produced a rapidly spreading anaerobic culture by the next day.

### Questions:

1. What gram-positive anaerobes would one expect to see in blood cultures?

2. This spore-forming organism was saccharolytic (glucose, lactose, maltose, mannose) and proteolytic (hydrolyzes gelatin). Other than esculin hydrolysis, biochemical tests were negative. Using your tables, what identification do you propose?

3. What significance do you assign to this particular species?

4. Under what circumstances would you expect *C. difficile* to cause abdominal discomfort and diarrhea? How is it diagnosed?

## Review Questions

1. Select the one best definition of an obligate anaerobe.
   a. Limited growth in room air or in 5% to 10% $CO_2$
   b. Fail to multiply in the presence of $O_2$ or in a $CO_2$ incubator
   c. Sensitive to UV light when incubated in the biosafety cabinet
   d. Grows only on pre-reduced media when incubated at 5% to 10% $CO_2$

2. The pathogenesis of gram-positive, nonspore-forming, anaerobic infections includes all of the following, EXCEPT:
   a. more than one organism at site of infection (polymicrobial).
   b. microbes often found as normal flora on the skin or mucosal membranes.
   c. always are toxin mediated.
   d. found in an environment with decreased or no $O_2$.

3. Characteristics of the *Peptostreptococcus* sp. include:
   a. gram-positive anaerobic cocci.
   b. clinical symptoms include bone infection, intra-abdominal sepsis and diabetic foot ulcers

   c. often isolated in blood or body fluid cultures.
   d. all of the above

4. The most frequently isolated gram-positive, nonspore-forming bacilli is:
   a. *Actinomyces* species.
   b. *Bifidobacterium dentium*.
   c. *Clostridium perfringens*.
   d. *Propionibacterium acnes*.

5. The most frequently isolated gram-positive spore-forming anaerobic pathogen is:
   a. *Clostridium botulinum*.
   b. *Clostridium perfringens*.
   c. *Peptostreptococcus micros*.
   d. *Clostridium difficile*.

6. Identify this isolate at level II: anaerobic gram-positive, nonspore-forming diphtheroid bacilli, nonmotile, and +/+/+ for catalase, indole, and nitrate, respectively.
   a. *Clostridium perfringens*
   b. *Actinomyces* species
   c. *Mobiluncus* species
   d. *Propionibacterium acnes*

7. Identify this isolate at level II: gram-variable bacilli, Nagler positive, and −/+/−/+ for indole, nitrate, catalase, reverse CAMP, respectively.
    a. *Clostridium perfringens*
    b. *Clostridium difficile*
    c. *Clostridium bifermentans*
    d. *Clostridium sordellii*

8. Potential reactions on egg yolk agar include:
    a. lipase.
    b. oxidase.
    c. lecithinase.
    d. a and c only.

9. The most potent biologic substance known is produced by which of the following bacteria?
    a. *Clostridium difficile*
    b. *Clostridium tetani*
    c. *Clostridium perfringens*
    d. *Clostridium botulinum*

10. *Clostridium difficile* toxins are often detected by which method?
    a. Radioimmunoassay
    b. Chromatographic procedures
    c. Cytotoxicity assay
    d. High-pressure liquid chromatography

## ▶ REFERENCES & RECOMMENDED READING

Baron, E. J., Peterson, L. R., & Finegold, S. M. (1994). *Bailey and Scott's diagnostic microbiology* (9th ed.). St. Louis: Mosby–Year Book.

Fagan, M. D., Levy, R. M., & Murray, J. M. (1996). *Inflammation associated with acne* (Lesson Plan No. SMML-19F, Anaerobic Bacteriology). Fort Sam Houston, TX: U.S. Army Medical Department Center and School.

Finegold, S. M., Baron, E. J., & Wexler, H. M. (1992). *A clinical guide to anaerobic infections.* Belmont, CA: Star Publishing.

Finegold, S. M., Rosenblatt, J. E., Sutter, V. L., & Attebery, H. R. (1974). *Scope monograph on anaerobic infections.* Kalamazoo, MI: Upjohn Company.

Gilligan, P. H., Shapiro, D. S., & Smiley, M. L. (1992). *Cases in medical microbiology and infectious diseases.* Washington, DC: American Society for Microbiology Press.

Gorbach, S. L. (1979). Other *Clostridium* species (including gas gangrene). In G. L. Mandell, R. G. Douglas, Jr., & J. E. Bennett (Eds.), *Principles and practice of infectious diseases* (pp. 1876–1885). New York: Wiley.

Hatheway, D. L. (1990). Toxigenic clostridia. *Clinical Microbiology Reviews, 3,* 66–98.

Knoop, F. C., Owens, M., & Crocker, I. C. (1993). *Clostridium difficile:* Clinical disease and diagnosis. *Clinical Microbiology Reviews, 6,* 251–265.

Koneman, E. W., Allen, S. D., Janda, W. M., Schreckenberger, P. C., & Winn, W. C. Jr. (1994). *Introduction to diagnostic microbiology.* Philadelphia: Lippincott.

Mangels, J. I. (Sec. Ed.). (1992). Anaerobic bacteriology. In H. D. Isenberg (Chief Ed.), *Clinical microbiology procedures handbook* (Vol. 1, Sec. 2). Washington, DC: American Society for Microbiology Press.

Midura, T. F. (1996). Update: Infant botulism. *Clinical Microbiology Reviews, 9,* 119–125.

Murray, P. R., Baron, E. J., Pfaller, M. A., Tenover, F. C., & Yolken, R. H. (Eds.). (1995). *Manual of clinical microbiology* (6th ed.). Washington, DC: American Society for Microbiology.

Pezzlo, M. (Sec. Ed.) (1992). Aerobic bacteriology. In H. D. Isenberg (Chief Ed.), *Clinical microbiology procedures handbook* (Vol. 1, Sec. 1). Washington, DC: American Society for Microbiology Press.

Summanen, P., Baron, E. J., Citron, D. M., Strong, C. A., Wexler, H. M., & Finegold, S. M. (1993). *Wadsworth anaerobic bacteriology manual* (5th ed.). Belmont, CA: Star Publishing.

Talaro, K., & Talaro, A. (1996). *Foundations in microbiology* (2nd ed.). Dubuque, IA: William C. Brown Publishers.

# CHAPTER 21

## Mycobacteria

Geneva M. Burch, BS, MT (ASCP, CLS, NCA), MLT (ASCP)

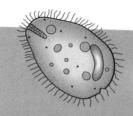

### Microbes in the News

Crohn's disease is a chronic inflammatory disorder affecting the entire alimentary tract; inflammation occurs in all layers of the intestine. Its pathogenesis is a mystery. Treatment remains nonspecific and consists predominantly of immunosuppression.

It has been suggested mycobacteria is a possible cause of the disease given that chronic enteritis in animals, termed Johne's disease, is caused by tubercule bacilli.

Source: *British Medical Journal*, March 20, 1995

**INTRODUCTION**

**GENUS CHARACTERISTICS**

**NUTRITIONAL AND GROWTH REQUIREMENTS**

**GROWTH RATE**

**COLONY APPEARANCE AND PIGMENT PRODUCTION**

**MYCOBACTERIUM TUBERCULOSIS**
Species Characteristics
Clinical Significance
Pathogenesis of Tuberculosis
Symptoms

Tuberculosis Disease Patterns
Extrapulmonary Tuberculosis
Specimen Collection
Specimen Processing
Skin Tests
Drug Therapy
Infection Control
Immunization

**MYCOBACTERIUM LEPRAE**

**MOTT—MYCOBACTERIA OTHER THAN TUBERCULOSIS**
*Mycobacterium kansasii*
*Mycobacterium gordonae*

*Mycobacterium scrofulaceum*
*Mycobacterium marinum*
*Mycobacterium avium-intracellulare* complex

**LABORATORY STUDIES**
Isolation and Culture
Staining

**IDENTIFICATION PROCESS**
Macroscopic Examination
Biochemical Testing
Indirect Method

## KEY TERMS

Acid-alcohol
Acid-fast bacillus
Bacille Calmette-Guérin
Droplet nuclei
Exudative
Ghon complex
Granuloma
Isoniazid

Kinyoun method
Lepromin
Mantoux test
Miliary tuberculosis
Nonphotochromogen
Photochromogen
Productive
Purified protein derivative

Runyon classification
Scotochromogen
Tine test
Tubercle
Tuberculin
Tween 80
Ziehl-Neelsen method

## LEARNING OBJECTIVES

**Upon successful completion of this chapter, the student should be able to:**

1. Explain the pathogenesis of tuberculosis including symptoms, stages of the disease, diagnosis, and treatment.

2. Name the most common species of the *Mycobacterium* genus and the possible infections caused by the organism.

3. Explain the procedures for identification of the *Mycobacterium* genus including rate of growth.

4. Prepare, stain, and examine a smear for the presence of *mycobacteria*.

5. List the chemotherapy used to treat mycobacterial infections.

## INTRODUCTION

The classification of bacteria includes many varieties. Each family of bacteria is different and species are unique within that family. The *Mycobacteriaceae* possess a distinction placing them in a category separate from other prokaryotes. The major difference lies in the structure of the cell wall.

The *Mycobacterium* genus includes pathogenic, opportunistic, and normal flora microorganisms. The disease-causing species are capable of producing severe illness in humans by invading a variety of body tissues and systems. Symptoms of diseases can involve the urinary, digestive, or respiratory tracts. Clinical manifestations may include diarrhea, lung complications, or skin lesions. Opportunistic members of the genus tend to invade the immunosuppressed patient. Bacteria within the genus cause diseases such as tuberculosis, leprosy, and nontuberculosis pulmonary disease. Specimen collection for isolation of the microorganism is likely from an array of body tissues including ocular, cutaneous, genital, lymphatic, nervous, and pulmonary. These diverse characteristics make the *Mycobacterium* genus clinically significant.

## GENUS CHARACTERISTICS

Microscopic examination of *Mycobacteriaceae* reveals a slightly curved or straight bacillus ranging in size from 0.2 to 0.6 μm by 1.0 to 10 μm. The bacillus may have branches, filaments, or mycelium-like growth that on smear preparation disperses into a singular arrangement. The genus is nonmotile and nonspore forming without capsules, conidia, or hyphae.

Bacterial cells contain lipids in high quantities especially in the cell wall. The lipid content includes waxes in the form of mycolic acids (fatty acids) having long, branched, carbon chains of 80 atoms or more. For this reason the organism does not react well to the Gram staining process and is therefore designated as a gram-variable bacteria. However, if the genus does react it is a weak gram-positive organism. Mycobacteria require a special staining process capable of breaking through the lipids in the cell wall to cause a reaction. The process uses acid and sometimes heat to remove this stain-resistant barrier. Because the organism does not decolorize after rinsing with an acid wash, it is designated as being acid-fast.

## NUTRITIONAL AND GROWTH REQUIREMENTS

The *Mycobacterium* genus includes obligate parasites, saprophytes, and intermediate forms differing in nutritional requirements. Saprophytes will grow on simple media with general nutritional contents; others require more complex media and supplements for growth such as living tissue. Other special needs include albumin and specific acids.

The entire genus is aerobic, which allows for a wide range of growth possibilities. The natural habitats for the organisms are soil, warm-blooded animals such as man, and cold-blooded animals including fish, turtles, frogs, and snakes. For example, *Mycobacterium phile* resides in soil, *Mycobacterium smegmatius* on humans, and *Mycobacterium marinum* on fish.

## GROWTH RATE

Species grow from slow to very slow with a time variation of from 2 days to 8 weeks of incubation at 25°C to 45°C for full growth. Convenience in classification is provided by dividing the organism into three groups depending on the requirements for rate of growth and special nutritional or temperature needs.

1. Slow growers—The grossly visible colonies are apparent only after 7 days or more. Examples are *Mycobacterium bovis, Mycobacterium kansasii,* and *Mycobacterium tuberculosis.*

2. Rapid growers—The grossly visible colonies are apparent in less than 7 days at a temperature of 25°C to 37°C. Examples are *M. phlei* and *M. smegmatis.*

3. Special growers—These organisms have special growth requirements or have not been cultured in vitro. Examples are *Mycobacterium leprae* and *Mycobacterium lapraemurine,* both requiring living tissue for growth, and *Mycobacterium thermoresistibile* requiring high temperatures.

The **Runyon classification** scheme is also useful for grouping mycobacteria according to pigment production, effect of light on pigment production, and growth time (see Table 21-1).

## COLONY APPEARANCE AND PIGMENT PRODUCTION

The *Mycobacterium* genus contains a variety of colony appearances. The surface view ranges from smooth to rough in texture with thickness from thin to a high dome. Cells of the rough strains can have filamentous branches extending from the colony and still another forms serpentine cord-like masses.

Pigment for the genus varies from buff to yellow to orange because of carotenoid pigments that usually do not diffuse. Formation of the pigment may or may not require exposure to light. Therefore, some species are photochromogenic and others are nonphotochromogenic.

## MYCOBACTERIUM TUBERCULOSIS

The name tuberculosis is a term originating in the recent annals of medical history. In about 400 BC, Hippocrates described a disease called "phthisis" (Greek for "to dry up" or "to waste"), which was a classic observation through history until the 19th century when tuberculosis was referred to as "consumption" (Latin for "consumare" meaning "to waste"). The 20th century began with tuberculosis so rampant that it was the leading cause of death in the United States (accounting for 10% of all deaths).

A German physician, Robert Koch, discovered *M. tuberculosis,* the bacteria causing tuberculosis, in 1882. It is also known as the tubercle bacillus or Koch's bacillus. Eight years later Koch prepared **tuberculin,** an extract prepared from killed tuberculosis bacilli. The extract became the basis for the tuberculin skin test used today as a diagnostic tool.

A vaccine composed of live attenuated *M. bovis,* a closely related species found in cattle, was developed in 1921. **Bacille Calmette-Guérin** (BCG) was first administered to humans in the same year and is still used in developing countries. **Purified protein derivative** (PPD), developed in 1934, provided a more reliable diagnostic tool for tuberculosis.

The discovery of streptomycin in 1944 began a pathway to the treatment and cure of the disease. By the late 1960s five additional medications were introduced and the morbidity of tuberculosis patients was greatly reduced.

Today, control and treatment of those with tuberculosis is more effective for several reasons:

▶ The causative agent is identified more often.
▶ Diagnostic tests are more accurate.
▶ The mode of transmission is better understood.
▶ Combination drug therapy has been developed.

In 1986, for the first time in three decades, the morbidity of tuberculosis increased in the United States. The surge occurred in demographic groups and geographic areas with increasing numbers of individuals

## Table 21–1 ▶ Runyon Classification of Mycobacteria other than *M. tuberculosis*

| Runyon Group | Characteristics | Organisms |
|---|---|---|
| I. Photochromogen | Colonies produce a yellow pigment when exposed to strong light. | M. kansasii<br>M. simiae<br>M. marinum<br>M. szulgai |
| II. Scotochromogen | Colonies produce a bright yellow pigment in the light or the dark. | M. scrofulaceum<br>M. gordonae<br>M. flavescens |
| III. Nonphotochromogen | Colonies do not produce intense color when exposed to light; some may produce small amounts of pale yellow pigment that does not become more intense. | M. avium-intracellulare<br>M. terrae<br>M. gastri<br>M. malmoense<br>M. haemophilum |
| IV. Rapid growers | Colonies often appear in 3–5 days; the two listed may cause disease of the skin, the eye, or multiple organ dissemination in the immunosuppressed patient. | M. fortuitum<br>M. chelonei |

with acquired immunodeficiency syndrome (AIDS). This increase in tuberculosis suggested that the spread of the virus was influencing the morbidity of those infected with both diseases.

## Species Characteristics

**Microscopic.** *Mycobacterium tuberculosis* bacilli range in size from 0.3 to 0.6 μm by 1.0 to 4.0 μm. Bacilli are slender and straight or slightly curved, occurring singly and in occasional threads. Staining may produce a granular or a beaded appearance in the organism. Like the corynebacteria, mycobacteria are often seen in palisade or in "V" and "L" positions.

**Cultural.** The tubercle bacillus is a slow grower, taking 3 to 6 weeks for colony growth to appear. Although aerobic, growth may be enhanced with a 5% to 10% increase in atmospheric $CO_2$ during incubation at 35°C. On most solid media the colonies appear dry, rough, raised, and thick with a nodular or wrinkled surface and an irregular thin margin. Some media produce a corded serpentine colony. Pigmentation may range from off white to buff to yellow, with buff being the most common.

Several nonelective solid media are available for culture of the tubercle bacillus. The organism requires complex nutrients to grow; these include egg, potato, and serum cofactors.

Because the tubercle bacillus may produce lesions in various body tissues, many types of specimens can be cultured. Some, such as sputum and voided urine, may contain large numbers of normal flora. These organisms grow faster on media than mycobacteria; therefore, available nutrients deplete quickly and the mixed culture makes detection of the tubercle bacillus nearly impossible. To prevent this occurrence specimens are treated with chemicals that destroy the contaminates prior to culturing. The tubercle bacillus, because of its cell wall structure, is more resistant than other organisms to alkalies and acids.

After treatment the sample is centrifuged to concentrate the specimen. The sediment is inoculated to culture media, incubated, and examined routinely each week for growth. A culture with negative growth is not discarded until it has been incubated for 8 weeks. Positive growth, within the 8 weeks, is reported (refer to Color Plates 47, 48, 49, 50).

## Clinical Significance

Tuberculosis is a chronic infectious disorder caused by *M. tuberculosis*. Others in the genus produce pulmonary diseases similar to tuberculosis. Clinically these diseases are not distinguishable from tuberculosis so diagnostic testing is used to differentiate the various species.

The route of entry for the tubercle bacillus, as well as the others causing pulmonary disease, is the respiratory tract. The disease is highly infectious and spread person to person, through the air, by infectious droplets called **droplet nuclei** containing organisms. These droplets are 1.0 to 5.0 μm in diameter and are produced when a person with tuberculosis of the lungs and larynx sneezes, speaks, coughs, or sings. These droplets may be inhaled by a person sharing airspace with the diseased individual. The susceptibility of the person inhaling the droplet helps determine if infection occurs. Transmission of droplets may also occur through manipulation of lesions or tissue and secretion processing in the hospital or clinical laboratory.

## Pathogenesis of Tuberculosis

Droplet nuclei are inhaled and pass down the bronchial tree and implant in a bronchiole or alveolus past the mucociliary system. The bacillus may multiply here without resistance from the host. Macrophages may slowly engulf organisms that may remain viable and multiply within the cell.

Tubercle bacilli spread through the lymphatic system to the circulatory system to the entire body. The bacilli reach body areas susceptible to developing the disease such as the kidneys, brain, bones, and apices of the lungs.

In the lungs, lesions may be produced and will be one of two types, either **exudative** or **productive**. Exudative lesions consist of a liquid exudate containing neutrophils and monocytes. The lesions are formed by acute inflammatory response. This type of lesion may heal, progress to necrosis of local tissue, or develop into a **tubercle**. The second type, or productive lesion, consists of cells without exudate, organized around the bacilli. The collection of cells and organisms is called a **granuloma**. In the center of the granuloma is a compact mass of giant cells. Surrounding this mass are epithelioid cells, lymphocytes, monocytes, and fibroblasts. Eventually the tubercle will become a **Ghon complex** having a fibrous outside and calcified inside. The organisms inside may die or survive for years.

## Symptoms

Tuberculosis is usually asymptomatic. Infected patients are recognized through a history of exposure, an abnormal chest radiograph, a positive reaction to a tuberculin skin test, and a culture positive for the bacillus.

Some patients are aware of anorexia, fatigue, irregular menses, weight loss, or low-grade fever that persists for weeks to months. Even with these symptoms, however, tuberculosis is often not the diagnosis. These same symptoms are more often attributed to emotional stress and overwork. If the disease progresses to a chronic state, coughing will progress with expectoration of bloody sputum. This can cause lung damage and the patient has a risk of death if treatment is not commenced quickly. In first infections with tuberculosis the incubation period is 4 to 6 weeks. The incubation period is from the time of exposure to the appearance of a primary lesion (see Table 21-2).

## Tuberculosis Disease Patterns

Two patterns of tuberculosis are recognized: primary and reinfection. Primary tuberculosis, with initial lesions, is the acute exudative form that spreads rapidly by way of the lymphatic system to regional nodes. Within a few days the organisms have disseminated to all parts of the body. The lesions usually heal with some residual fibrosis and scarring. The primary type occurs most frequently in children but can be seen in adults. First-time infections with primary tuberculosis will have lesions in the lower two-thirds of the lungs.

Reinfection tuberculosis is the chronic form characterized by productive lesions. Reinfection may occur due to new exogenous sources or by organisms that survive from primary tuberculosis lesions (endogenous). Lesions of this type usually begin in the apex of the lungs and progress downward.

An endogenous reinfection may occur from several months to years after a first-time infection appears to have healed. The organisms spread through the body the same as with primary tuberculosis. A general infection may occur with tubercle formation in several body organs. Because the tubercles resemble millet seeds, this distribution is called **miliary tuberculosis**.

## Extrapulmonary Tuberculosis

Because the organisms causing tuberculosis are transported throughout the body, extrapulmonary infections can occur. Bacillus infections may cause clinical dysfunction and damage to the genitourinary tract, lymph nodes in the cervical and supraclavicular areas, bones, joints, meninges, peritoneum, pericardium, larynx, brain, adrenal glands, skin, or other body organs.

## Specimen Collection

The identification of the tubercle bacillus is critical when diagnosing tuberculosis. Successful isolation of the bacillus depends on observing proper handling, proper collection, and proper processing of the specimen. All specimens should be transported to the laboratory and processed as soon as possible after collection.

The level of laboratory service for mycobacterial disease determines the amount and type of specimen processing (see Table 21-3). For this reason the possibility of mailing specimens is high for tuberculosis samples. The following four items must be considered when this occurs.

1. Each container should have a single specimen of 10 mm or less.
2. Containers must be shipped according to the regulations of the laboratory receiving the specimen.
3. Mail as early in the week as possible.
4. Refrigerate specimens immediately if mailing must be delayed.

Because mycobacterial disease can be present in any site in the body, a wide variety of clinical specimens are possible for processing and mailing. The possibilities include sputum, gastric washing, urine, cerebrospinal fluid, pleural fluid, bronchial washing, pus, endometrial scraping, bone marrow biopsy, other biopsy specimens, and various other tissues and body fluids.

Sputum collection is the most difficult to regulate because medical personnel may not be present during the process. It is important that patients be given proper and clear instructions for collecting the sputum. The patient must be told that nasopharyngeal discharge and saliva are not sputum, and therefore, not acceptable specimens for processing and diagnostic procedures. The collected specimen must be brought up from the lungs after coughing. As with any specimen only an approved container and a proper label should be used. To protect those handling the specimen the

**Table 21–2 ▶ International Classification of Tuberculosis**

Class 0—No history of tuberculosis exposure, not infected

An individual with no history of exposure and reaction to the tuberculin skin test is < 5 mm.

Class 1—Tuberculosis exposure, with no evidence of infection

An individual with a history of exposure but reaction to the Mantoux skin test is < 5 mm.

Class 2—Tuberculosis infection but no disease

An individual exhibiting a significant reaction to the Mantoux skin test (> 5 mm if exposed to a case of tuberculosis, > 10 mm if seropositive for human immunodeficiency virus) but has no radiographic evidence of tuberculosis and/or has negative bacteriologic studies.

Class 3—Tuberculosis, current disease

An individual with either M. tuberculosis-positive cultures or clinical and/or radiologic evidence of current disease.

Class 4—Tuberculosis, no current disease

An individual with a history of a previous episode of tuberculosis or abnormal but stable radiographic findings, negative bacteriologic studies, and no clinical evidence of current disease.

Class 5—Tuberculosis suspect

Diagnosis is pending awaiting results of culture or full clinical evaluation. An individual should not remain in this category for more than 3 months.

---

**Table 21–3** ▶ **Laboratory Service Levels for Mycobacterial Diseases**

| Level | Facility Type | Service Provided |
|---|---|---|
| I | Physician's office<br>Outpatient clinic<br>Small hospital | Specimen collection<br>Microscopic examination<br>Ship to level II or III for identification and susceptibility testing |
| II | Selected laboratories (private, state, county, city) | Specimen collection<br>Microscopic examination<br>*M. tuberculosis* identification<br>Susceptibility testing<br>Ship other mycobacteria to level III for identification |
| III | Reference laboratories (private, federal, state) | All procedures for level II and identification and susceptibility procedures for all *Mycobacteria* species |

---

container should be placed in a disposable water-tight plastic bag. A 3-day series of single specimens should be collected.

Children unable to produce sputum, even with aerosol inhalation, may require a gastric aspiration. Gastric contents of 50 mL should be aspirated early in the morning after the patient has fasted for 8 to 10 hours. Collection should occur while the patient is still in bed, most likely in a hospitalized situation.

Other possible methods for obtaining lung samples are fibrotic bronchoscopy with bronchial washing, bronchoalveolar lavage, and transbronchial biopsy. Sputum should be collected, in the usual manner, following a bronchoscopy because the procedure causes the patient to produce sputum for several days.

Urine specimens for mycobacterial examination should be the first morning-voided midstream clean-catch type. Multiple specimens are needed to show the presence of *Mycobacterium*. The patient should not be receiving broad-spectrum antibiotics at the time of collection because of the possibility of inhibiting the growth of *Mycobacterium* from the specimen.

Expeditious and appropriate handling of tissue and other body fluid specimens must be ensured before a physician performs an invasive procedure to obtain the specimen. Rapid transport of the specimen to the laboratory is essential. Any specimen placed in formalin for histologic examination cannot be used for culture.

## Specimen Processing

Most clinical specimens contain large amounts of nonmycobacteria contaminants; therefore, a special two-step process must be performed. The purpose of processing is to inhibit the growth of fast-growing contaminants that can overgrow the slow growing *Mycobacterium* in 18 to 48 hours. Decontaminating agents kill undesirable microorganisms and increase the survival rate and growth of *Mycobacterium*. Thick specimens will also be liquefied during the process, which breaks down organic debris such as tissue, mucus, blood, or exudate surrounding organisms. This part of

the process is called digestion. The digestion and decontamination of specimens for mycobacterial studies is possible because the genus is more refractory to harsh chemicals than other organisms due to cell wall structure.

The most widely used decontaminate for sputum is sodium hydroxide. Others are trisodium phosphate, sulfuric acid, and oxalic acid, which are used for special specimen decontamination such as having large numbers of gram-negative rods present in the sample. Four percent sodium hydroxide will digest and decontaminate sputa. If the process uses *N*-acetyl-L-cystine (NALC) or dithuthreitol, the concentration of sodium hydroxide can be lowered. Distilled water is added after the process is completed to neutralize chemical reactions. See Procedure 21-1.

## Skin Tests

*Mycobacterium tuberculosis* produces a hypersensitivity reaction in the form of tuberculin associated with immune T lymphocytes. The immune reaction can be detected by skin tests using protein antigens from filtrates of tubercle bacillus cultures (see Table 21-4). Reaction to tuberculin begins within 4 to 6 weeks after infection and persists for long periods.

If the antigen is injected into the skin of a hypersensitive individual, an inflammatory response will occur. The response is attributed to activated macrophages responding to stimulation. Along with this cellular filtration the blood vessels increase permeability. The increase causes a reddened slightly raised, hard area of induration in the skin at the site of antigen injection. The intensity of the reaction depends on individual immunity. The reaction is usually fully developed in 48 to 72 hours. Therefore, reaction areas of the skin must be examined and interpreted within this time period (see Figure 21-1).

A positive reaction indicates a past infection that may or may not be currently active or that the individual has been vaccinated for tuberculosis. The hypersensitivity reaction to tuberculosis is long lasting once

## PROCEDURE 21-1
## N-Acetyl-L-Cysteine (NALC), Sodium Hydroxide Method for Liquefication and Decontamination of Mycobacterial Sputum and Other Liquid Specimens

### Principle:

N-acetyl-L-cysteine (NALC) is the mucolytic agent used to digest the specimen. NALC also shortens the time needed to decontaminate the specimen. Using NALC allows for the use of a low concentration of sodium hydroxide, a highly toxic substance. Sodium hydroxide is the decontaminate and emulsifier necessary to liquefy the specimen.

### Method:

1. The NALC-sodium hydroxide solution used in the procedure must be prepared fresh. The mucolytic activity of NALC deteriorates on standing (18–24 hours shelf life). Determine the amount required by adding the total volumes for all specimens to be treated.
2. Perform the procedure within a biologic hood and wear gloves. Place a maximum of 10 mL of sputum, urine, or other body fluid in a sterile plastic 50-mL conical centrifuge tube and add an equal amount of NALC solution. Tighten the cap.
3. Vortex the specimen mixture for 15 seconds but not more than 20 seconds. Invert the tube to check for homogenicity. If clumps remain, vortex the tube periodically as other specimens are digesting. A small amount of NALC may be added to liquefy the mixture. Allow the specimen to stand for 15 minutes at room temperature.
4. After the 15 minutes of digestion add phosphate buffer to within 1 cm of the tube top. Close the cap tightly and invert to mix the solution and to end the digestion process. The buffer also increases the specific gravity of the solution, allowing organisms to settle as the tube is centrifuged.
5. Centrifuge the tube for 15 minutes at 2,000 to 3,000g.
6. Decant the supernatant fluid into a discard container of disinfectant, wipe the tube lip with gauze soaked in disinfectant and replace the cap.
7. Add 1 to 2 mL of sterile water or buffer solution to the test tube and shake gently to resuspend the sediment. If specimens are not being cultured immediately, 1 to 2 mL of 0.2 bovine albumin may be used in place of the water or buffer solution.
8. The resuspended sediment may be inoculated to media and smears may be prepared.

### Quality Control:

A portion of sterile sputum or urine should be treated with the entire procedure along with the patient specimen. Use sterile buffer to resuspend the sediment. Prepare smears and inoculate media with the control sediment.

### Expected Results:

If acid-fast bacilli are present in the specimen the organisms will be observed on the smears and will grow on the inoculated media.

### Reference:

Centers for Disease Control and Prevention. *Isolation and Identification of Mycobacterium tuberculosis.*

infection has occurred. To determine if the infection is current, a clinical examination, a chest x-ray, and a variety of bacteriologic studies should be performed. A negative skin reaction occurs if the individual has never been infected, if the individual is in the preallergic early stages of infection, or if the individual has advanced miliary tuberculosis.

The preferred antigen for skin testing is prepared by concentrating a filtrate from a broth culture of the tubercle bacillus. PPD is then obtained by chemical fractionation and purification of the concentrated filtrate.

Several techniques are available for tuberculin skin tests. Each detects hypersensitivity with accuracy. The most common methods are the Tine and Mantoux tests. The **Tine test** uses dried antigen on metal tines imbedded in a round plastic head. The tines are pressed against the skin for intracutaneous application of the antigen.

| Table 21–4 ▶ Tuberculin Skin Test Interpretation | |
|---|---|
| **Tine Test Induration** | **Mantoux Test Induration** |
| Negative: < 2 mm | Negative: < 5 mm |
| Doubtful: 2–4 mm, do Mantoux | Doubtful: 5–9 mm |
| Positive: 5 mm or more, do Mantoux and further clinical testing | Positive: 10 mm or more, do further clinical testing |
| Each test must be read in 48–72 h. Reading outside these times makes results unreliable. | |

Each tine unit is used once and discarded. This is the best and most convenient method for mass surveys for tuberculosis, such as school children in a particular area. The Tine test is not a quantitative evaluation.

The **Mantoux test** is an intradermal injection of the antigen PPD and is used to determine hypersensitivity. It is the most accurate skin test. A quantitatively dilute antigen aliquot of 0.1 mL is introduced via needle and syringe to an area within the epidermal layer (see Figure 21-2). Because individual needles and syringes are

necessary the Mantoux test is not advantageous for mass surveys. If an individual has a positive Tine test reaction during a mass survey, the Mantoux test is usually performed before a chest x-ray is ordered.

Once the Mantoux test has been completed the area of application should be read and interpreted in 48 to 72 hours. Strong reactions may last for several days but weak reactions will disappear after 72 hours. During the first 24 hours nonspecific reactions may occur but will not persist to 48 hours.

## Drug Therapy

A first-time infection with tuberculosis usually heals without recognition or treatment. However, if recognized the person should be hospitalized to prevent a chain of contact infections and to give treatment.

**Isoniazid** (INH), ethambutol, and rifampin are the most useful antituberculosis drugs. A combination of two is generally used to treat the patient. *M. tuberculosis* may quickly develop resistance to any one of the drugs used for treatment. Adjustment in the therapeutic regimen may be necessary if susceptibility studies demonstrate resistance to a drug used in the treatment of the patient. An antibiotic susceptibility test may be done on

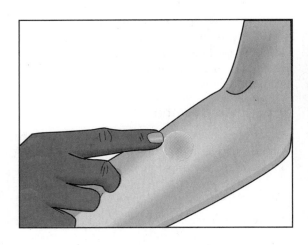
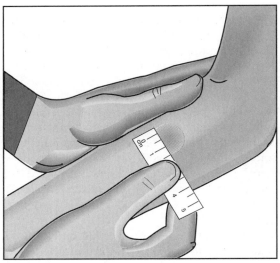

(A) **Positive reaction** for past or present infection: 10 mm or more of induration

(B) **Doubtful reaction**: 5–9 mm (In persons who are suspected to have been exposed to TB an induration of 5–9 mm is considered suspicious. Further diagnostic testing should follow.)

(C) **Negative reaction**: without induration or less than 5 mm

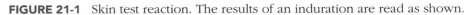

**FIGURE 21-1** Skin test reaction. The results of an induration are read as shown.

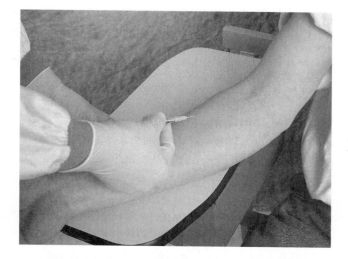

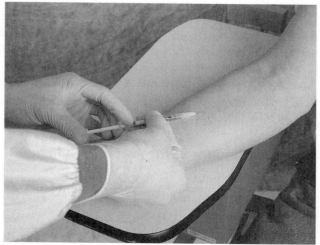

**FIGURE 21-2** Administering the Mantoux test.

initial culture of the tubercle bacillus. This testing is required if the patient's sputum remains acid-fast positive after 6 months of treatment or if a tuberculosis-negative patient receiving treatment reverts to positive cultures.

## Infection Control

Halting the spread of tuberculosis depends on an understanding of preventive measures for transmission of the bacillus. Patients infected with tuberculosis should be educated concerning the mode of transmission by direct contact and droplet nuclei. Those in close contact with infected individuals should also be informed of precautions to prevent infection. This is accomplished by medical personnel educating those involved.

## Immunization

The vaccine BCG provides some protection, but among all tuberculin-negative individuals inoculated, 80% produce a positive skin sensitivity after injection.

Protection is only partial and duration of protection is undetermined. Therefore, mass vaccination with BCG is only applicable in situations where the risk of infection and the number of tuberculin-negative contacts are both in high numbers.

## MYCOBACTERIUM LEPRAE

The *M. leprae* organism causes leprosy or Hansen's disease. The bacilli resembles *M. tuberculosis*. However, the presence of cells in high numbers and clinical symptoms make it possible, without difficulty, to distinguish the leprosy bacilli from the tubercule bacilli. Hansen's bacillus is slender, long, and appears straight or slightly curved; club-shaped cells can be seen occasionally. The rods are nonmotile and nonspore forming with heat labile capsules. A characteristic arrangement, groups of cells in a bundle like packets of cigars, appears intracellular. The Hansen bacillus can also be found in lymph spaces.

Leprosy is a chronic disease of the skin, mucous membranes, and nervous system that progresses slowly, requiring many years to develop. The disease is highly contagious but more than 95% of all individuals are resistant to infection. Those developing the disease appear to have a defect in cell-mediated immunity that is not quite understood.

If untreated, leprosy progresses to disfigurement that has generated horror and fear for centuries. Traditionally called lepers, victims were subjected throughout history to social ostracism and physical exclusion. Modern medical knowledge has produced objectivity to this problem, thereby relieving the onerous pressure from leprous patients. In the past, infected individuals were placed in leper colonies as outcasts from society. Today infected individuals remain within society functioning the same as everyone else.

Total understanding of the disease has been elusive over the centuries because the organism causing the disease is difficult to grow. The obligate intracellular bacillus has never been cultured in vitro. In recent years the organism has been cultured in the armadillo and in the foot pad of the mouse.

Diagnosis is usually made by histologic examination of material from a skin lesion or earlobe of the patient. The organism, when acid-fast stained, resembles the tubercle bacillus except that it usually lies in parallel bundles in cells of infected tissue.

A reliable serologic test, skin antigen type, has been developed using **lepromin**. The process can distinguish the three forms of the disease. Treatment consists of diapsone (DDS) and is often given in combination with rifampin. Clofazimine is also excellent but requires several months to accumulate an active concentration in patient tissues. Treatment may continue for 3 years or more. The BCG vaccine appears to afford some protection against leprosy. Patient contacts may be treated prophylactically with diapsone for three years. Refer to Chapter 32 for more information on leprosy.

## MOTT—MYCOBACTERIA OTHER THAN TUBERCULOSIS

Species other than *M. tuberculosis* and *M. leprae* cause disease.

### Mycobacterium kansasii

*Mycobacterium kansasii,* a **photochromogen**, causes pulmonary disease, especially in white emphysematous men over age 45 years. The disease cannot be distinguished from tuberculosis, but it does follow a more chronic course.

Acid-fast examination of *M. kansasii* reveals long, branched, beaded cells that are strongly reactive. Optimum growth is at 35°C in 2 to 3 weeks. Colonies of this species are smooth with a tendency to develop roughness. When the organism is grown in the dark, colonies are buff, but when exposed to light the colonies are a bright lemon yellow. However, if colonies are continuously exposed to light (2–3 weeks) ß-carotene forms crystals on the surface and bright orange pigment appears. *M. kansasii* has variable susceptibility to INH and streptomycin with moderate susceptibility to rifampin. Infections with the organism respond to conventional antituberculosis therapy but triple therapy, including rifampin, is best.

### Mycobacterium gordonae

The gordonae species of *Mycobacterium* is found in water from faucets or natural settings and in soil. The potential pathogen is a **scotochromogen** producing a deep yellow to orange pigment in the dark. If the cultures are exposed to continuous light for extended periods (2 weeks), the pigment will darken to an orange or a dark red. This characteristic aids with identification of the species. On Lowenstein-Jensen and Middlebrook 7H10 media the organism produces small scattered yellow-orange colonies in the light and dark. Growth of *M. gordonae* takes 2 to 6 weeks. *M. gordonae* is rarely associated with human diseases, but it is important to distinguish this organism from the pathogenic mycobacteria.

### Mycobacterium scrofulaceum

Slow growth is a characteristic of the scrofulaceum species. The organism produces smooth, domed to spreading, yellow colonies in the light and the dark. If exposed to continuous light the colonies produce an orange or brick red pigment. The change to brick red pigment is characteristic of the species. The species causes adenitis, bone and other infections, especially in children. *M. scrofulaceum* is often resistant to INH and para-aminosalicylate.

### Mycobacterium marinum

Also found in water, *M. marinum* is often associated with granulomatous lesions of the skin, particularly on the extremities. Infection usually occurs after abraded skin is exposed to contaminated water. The organism has been associated with infections related to home aquariums, bay water, and industrial exposures involving water. It is best known for causing swimming pool granuloma. Growth of the organism is best at 25°C to 35°C. Growth patterns correspond to the reduced skin temperature in the extremities. At 35°C there is sparse or no growth of the bacteria. Infections with this species is never associated with sputum. *M. marinum* can be distinguished from *M. kansasii* by the source of the infection and its more rapid growth at 25°C. *M. marinum* is most sensitive to amikacin and kanamycin but tetracycline is inhibitory.

### Mycobacterium avium-intracellulare Complex

The *M. avium* complex is a **nonphotochromogen** that grows slowly at 35°C producing a colony that is domed, opaque, and yellow. At 25°C a thin, transparent, lobed to smooth, buff colony will appear. This type of colony is initially the isolate from AIDS patients infected with the complex. It has been proven that the rough or opaque colony is less virulent and its cell wall is more permeable to antibiotic drugs.

The *M. avium* complex has two phonetically similar, but genetically distinct species: *M. avium* and *M. intracellulare*. These two species are most often encountered as opportunistic pathogens in patients with AIDS or other immune dysfunctions. Research has shown that 90% of all AIDS patients are infected only with *M. avium*. Non-AIDS patients have a two-thirds occurrence of infection with *M. intracellulare*.

The *M. avium* complex causes serious tuberculosis-like endobronchial lesions in non-AIDS patients and disseminated disease in the majority of AIDS patients. However, this complex can appear in clinical specimens as nonpathogens. The two-organism complex is resistant to most antituberculosis agents. Two of the newer agents, ansamycin and clofazimine, appear active against the group. Combination drug treatment with rifampin, ethambutol, and amikacin has little success in patients also having AIDS. The best treatment for these patients seems to be the use of five drugs in combination, if five drugs can be found that are active in vitro.

# LABORATORY STUDIES

## Isolation and Culture

The identification of *Mycobacteria* species cannot be determined by microscopic examination of a smear. Species identification requires the isolation and culture of the organism so that diagnostic tests can be completed (Procedure 21-2). The amount of growth should be reported as part of the process (see Table 21-5).

Mycobacteria are resistant to many of the most common antimicrobial drugs; therefore, several have been placed into media to inhibit the growth of contaminates (Table 21-6). The most commonly used drugs are penicillin derivatives, cycloheximide, trimethoprim, amphotericin B, and nalidixic acid.

There are many different groups of media available for culture of *Mycobacterium* species, which can be broken down into three basic types. The first is coagulated egg, the second is media composed of soluble nutrients and trace elements, and the third is an egg-free liquid.

Selective culture media is available for both widely used types of media. Penicillin, nalidixic acid, and RNA are added to produce Gruft's Lowenstein-Jensen media. Another modification adds cycloheximide, nalidixic acid, and lincomycin to either Lowenstein-Jensen or 7H10 to control the growth of contaminates such as fungus and nonmycobacterial organisms.

Double sets of chosen media may be incubated as one set in the dark and the other in the light and at different temperatures to separate the photochromogens from the nonphotochromogens and the slow growers from the rapid growers. All mycobacteria will grow in or on the media listed.

## Staining

The initial step in the process of identifying mycobacteria from a clinical specimen is the staining and microscopic examination of a smear for the detection

### Table 21–5 ▶ Reporting Amount of Culture Growth for Mycobacteria

| Number of colonies | Report |
|---|---|
| No colonies | Negative |
| < 50 colonies | Actual count |
| 50–100 colonies | 1+ |
| 101–200 colonies | 2+ |
| 201–500 colonies | 3+ (almost confluent growth) |
| > 500 colonies | 4+ (confluent growth) |

of **acid-fast bacillus** (AFB). The presence of acid-fast organisms provides the physician with preliminary confirmation of a diagnosis. The quantitative estimate of the number of bacilli present in the specimen assists the physician in assessing the extent of patient infection. Various studies show that 50% to 80% of pulmonary tuberculosis patients have a positive sputum smear for acid-fast bacillus. The most common methods for staining *Mycobacterium* are the **Ziehl-Neelsen method**, the **Kinyoun method**, and the various flurochromatic procedures using auramine and rhodamine stains. A process for flurochrome staining using phenolic acridine orange and methylene blue is on the increase in the clinical laboratory. The process stains the *M. avium* complex and *M. leprae* as well as *M. tuberculosis* (see Figure 21-3).

Once the smear is heat-fixed the staining process begins with a primary stain, decolorization with **acid-alcohol** (ethanol and HCl), and finally counterstaining with a contrasting color stain. Control slides with a positive and negative comparison should also be stained and observed (see Procedure 21-3).

Smears stained with fluorescing material have acid-fast bacilli that appear as bright points of light against a dark background. This type of slide is easier to read than a conventional stained smear.

### Table 21–6 ▶ Selective Mycobacteria Isolation Media Information for *Mycobacterium tuberculosis* and Other Mycobacteria

| Medium | Ingredients | Inhibitory Agents |
|---|---|---|
| Lowenstein-Jensen | Coagulated egg, defined salts, glycerol, potato, flour, RNA | Malachite green, 0.025 g/100 mL penicillin, 50 U/mL nalidixic acid, 35 µg/ml |
| Middlebrook 7H10 | Defined salts, vitamins, oleic acid, albumin, cofactors, glucose, catalase, glycerol | Malachite green, 0.025 g/100 mL cycloheximide, 360 µg/mL lincomycin, 2 µg/mL; nalidixic acid, 20 µg/mL |
| Middlebrook 7H11 | Defined salts, vitamins, oleic acid, albumin, cofactors, glucose, catalase, glycerol, casein hydrolyase | carbenicillin, 50 µg/mL amphotericin B, 10 µg/mL polymyxin B, 200 U/mL trimethoprim latate 20 µg/mL |

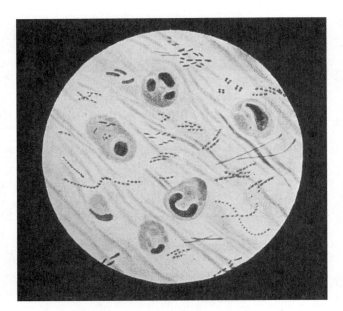

**FIGURE 21-3** *Mycobacterium tuberculosis* var. *hominis* (tubercle bacillus) from sputum. Stained by Ziehl-Neelsen technique Beaded forms. (Courtesy of Centers for Disease Control and Prevention, Atlanta, GA)

Several methods are available for reporting the results of acid-fast smear examination. Table 21-7 represents the current recommended method. The report results assist the physician's planned therapy and gives laboratory personnel information needed to prepare inocula for drug susceptibility testing.

Experience is required to gain proficiency in acid-fast microscopy. Of all specimens submitted for acid-fast testing, about 5% are positive. Some estimates state that 1 mL of sputum must contain approximately 6,000 acid-fast bacilli to have a 50% chance of finding three stained bacilli on a smear. Another source states that

10,000 acid-fast bacilli must be present to have the same chance. For this reason experience is necessary in reading acid-fast smears. Laboratories that do fewer than 15 to 20 specimens per week will have difficulty maintaining proficiency at reading smears. These laboratories should have all acid-fast smears confirmed by a laboratory that processes a higher number of specimens per week.

Examination of smears requires scanning in an orderly manner. The usual pattern is successive horizontal sweeps across the smear at a magnification of 1000×. It is recommended that 300 microscopic fields be observed before reporting a negative result. With fluorescence microscopy 30 fields at 250× should be observed before reporting.

## IDENTIFICATION PROCESS

After mycobacteria have been cultured and colonies are growing, examination as well as biochemical tests and antimicrobial susceptibility testing can be performed. By comparing the rate of growth, colony morphology, pigmentation, and biochemical test results the species can be identified (see Table 21-8).

### Macroscopic Examination

A preliminary identification of mycobacteria can be made by determining the rate of growth, growth temperature, colony texture, colony morphology, and pigmentation. The unknown organisms should be tested along with quality control organisms (see Table 21-9).

Once it has been established that the unknown is acid-fast (by staining) the organism should be subcultured to Middlebrook 7H9 broth. If the organism was originally cultured to broth then this step is not necessary. When culturing to broth use caution so that a heavy inoculum is not used. This will make slow growers appear to grow in a short time period.

Rate of growth will determine the initial category of the unknown isolate. If cultures have been examined on a routine basis during incubation this factor will be known when full growth of the colonies appears.

Mycobacteria species synthesize carotenoid in various amounts and thus produce pigments to varying degrees. The unknown can be placed in one of three Runyon classification categories on the basis of pigment production in the light or dark (see Table 21-10). Cultures should be exposed to light to observe for pigment production. Some species will produce pigment in a few hours and others will require longer exposure.

Temperature has an effect on pigment production. Certain species of *Mycobacterium* will produce a pigment in the dark, which will become darker in color when exposed to light at a lower temperature. Therefore, original culturing should include a set of media

| Table 21–7 ▶ | Method for Reporting Smears at 800x to 1000x for Acid-Fast bacilli, Recommended by CDC | |
|---|---|---|
| **Number of AFB Observed** | **Report** | |
| 0 | Negative for AFB | (–) |
| 1–2/300 fields | Number seen | (+/–) |
| 1–9/100 fields | Average number/100 fields | (1+) |
| 1–9/10 fields | Average number/10 fields | (2+) |
| 1–9/field | Average number/field | (3+) |
| > 9/field | Greater than 9/field | (4+) |

Counts of less than 3/300 fields are negative but another specimen should be processed if available. A clump of bacilli touching is counted as one cell because it is considered to be a single colony-forming unit.

## Principle:

For *Mycobacterium* species to grow in vitro specimens must be inoculated and incubated properly.

## Method:

1. Once the specimen has been processed for digestion and decontamination the sediment is inoculated to the proper media. Most laboratories use both liquid and solid media. The solid media may be a plate or a slant, with slants the most popular choice. Certain solid media are only available as a slant. Two of each of the following media should be inoculated:

   Solid media, agar base, available as a plate or a slant: Middlebrook 7H10 or 7H11.

   Solid media, egg base, available as a slant only: Lowenstein-Jensen with RNA or pyruvic acid.

   Liquid media: Middlebrook 7H9 Broth, Middlebrook 7H12 or Bactec 12B medium. Middleboook solid media has a poor recovery rate for mycobacteria, but it is excellent for colony morphology studies. Lowenstein-Jensen media is good for recovery of the acid-fast bacilli and must be used for certain diagnostic tests. Middlebrook Broth allows a positive culture to be ready for antibiotic susceptibility testing as soon as possible after the organism is identified.

2. Inoculation of media:

   Solid media, slants: Use a sterile pipet to allow 2 to 3 drops of the specimen to run down the surface of the slant.

   Solid media, plates: Use a sterile pipet to place 2 to 3 drops of the specimen on the surface of the plate. With a sterile bent glass rod spread the inoculum over the surface of the plate.

   Broth media: Use a sterile pipet to add 2 to 3 drops of the specimen to the broth.

3. Incubation:

   One set of each type of media inoculated is incubated in an atmosphere of 5% to 10% $CO_2$ with high humidity (in the dark). Tube caps should be loose for the first 2 to 3 weeks of incubation to allow entry of $CO_2$ and evaporation of excess liquid present in the tube.

   The other set of inoculated media is incubated at room temperature and wrapped in aluminum foil so that light does not enter the tubes.

4. During the 6 to 8 weeks incubation period cultures should be examined once a week for growth. Cultures with positive growth should be reported as per Table 21-5. Smears of the colonies should be made and stained to confirm that the organism growing is indeed acid-fast positive. Growth should also be evaluated for rate and amount of growth, pigmentation and colony morphology, all of which are recorded. If no growth appears by the end of 8 weeks the culture is reported as negative and discarded.

5. Interpretation: All the information gathered and reported in step 4 is used to assist in the identification of the *Mycobacteria* species.

## Quality Control:

The control sample processed with the specimen should be placed on media in the same manner as the patient sample. The cultures set up as quality control when processing and inoculating should be examined along with the other specimen cultures. All should be negative for growth.

## Expected Results:

Cultures containing mycobacteria should grow on the selective media and provide information for identification of the species.

## Reference:

Centers for Disease Control and Prevention. *Isolation and Identification of Mycobacterium tuberculosis.*

incubated at 25°C and a set at 35°C to determine this characteristic.

## Biochemical Testing

After the unknown *Mycobacterium* isolate has been categorized by the macroscopic and microscopic procedures, biochemical testing is done to give a definitive identification. Most of the biochemical tests are quantitative and based on color reactions.

The niacin (nicotinic acid) test (Procedure 21-4) reacts to oxidation-reduction occurring during metabolism. Some species of mycobacteria produce nicotinic acid and others produce niacin. These substances accumulate in the media during growth. The niacin test should be performed on cultures growing on Lowenstein-Jensen media for no less than 3 weeks and having at least 50 colonies. The procedure can be performed with reagents in a tube or by using the paper strip method.

Some acid-fast bacilli have the ability to reduce nitrate to nitrite. Reduction is influenced by the age of the colony, temperature, enzyme inhibitors, and pH. Therefore, rapid growers should be tested at 2 weeks of growth and slow growers at 3 to 4 weeks of growth. The procedure (Procedure 21-5) is available as a tube test or as paper strips.

The intracellular enzyme catalase (Procedure 21-6) is produced by some mycobacteria species. Catalase has the ability to produce water and oxygen from hydrogen peroxide. The oxygen produced is seen by the presence of bubbles in the reagent. Catalase production can be measured by two different procedures. The first is a semiquantitative method that measures the amount of enzyme activity by the height of the column of bubbles produced in the reaction. The other measures the ability of the enzyme to remain active after heat (68°C) is applied.

**Tween 80** (Procedure 21-7) is the detergent polyoxyethylene sorbitan mono-oleate. Some mycobacteria can hydrolyze this substance into oleic acid and polyoxyethylated sorbitol. Tween 80 hydrolysis will assist in separating the Runyon classification organisms into species.

Potassium tellurite is reduced by some species of mycobacteria. The rate at which the substance is reduced varies by species. Rapid growers have the ability to reduce tellurite in as little as 3 days.

The thiophene-2-carboxylic acid hydrazide (TCH) sensitivity test is used to distinguish *M. bovis* from *M. tuberculosis*. *M. bovis* is unable to grow in the presence of 2 µg/mL of TCH.

---

## PROCEDURE 21-3
## Acid-Fast Staining, Kinyoun Method, Cold Method

### Principle:

The need for heating of the slide is eliminated by adding an increased concentration of basic fuchsin and phenol to the staining process.

### Method:

1. Completely cover the slide with Kinyoun carbol fuchsin and allow to stand for 5 minutes.
2. Rinse the slide with deionized water and allow to drain.
3. Decolorize using acid alcohol continuing for 2 minutes or until no red color runs off of the slide.
4. Rinse the slide with deionized water and allow to drain.
5. Completely cover the slide with methylene blue stain and let it remain for 4 minutes.
6. Rinse the slide with deionized water and allow to air dry.
7. Examine the slide under oil immersion at 1000X for the presence of acid-fast bacilli.

### Quality Control:

Prepare control slides in advance or use commercially purchased control slide along the specimen smear.

### Expected Results:

Acid-fast positive bacilli will be small, red, slightly curved, and possibly beaded with tapered ends against a blue background. Non–acid-fast organisms will be blue.

### Reference:

Centers for Disease Control and Prevention. *Isolation and Identification of Mycobacterium tuberculosis.*

## Table 21–8 ▶ Identification Properties of *Mycobacterium* Species

| Species | Growth Rate at 37°C | 25°C* | Pigmentation Category~ | Niacin | Nitrate | Catalase-SQ | Catalase-heat | Telurite | Tween 80 | TCH |
|---|---|---|---|---|---|---|---|---|---|---|
| M. tuberculosis | S | – | N | + | + | – | – | +/– | – | – |
| M. bovis | S | – | N | – | – | – | – | +/– | – | – |
| M. africanum | S | – | N | – | – | – | – | +/– | – | + |
| M. ulcerans | – | – | N | – | – | – | – | – | – | V |
| M. marinum | +/– | M | P | +/– | – | – | + | – | – | |
| M. kansasii | S | S | P | – | + | + | + | +/– | + | – |
| M. simiae | S | | P | + | – | + | + | +/– | + | – |
| M. astiaticum | S | S | P | – | – | + | + | + | – | – |
| M. scrofulaceum | S | S | S | – | – | + | + | – | + | – |
| M. szulgai | S | S | S/P | – | + | + | + | +/– | – | – |
| M. gordonae | S | S | S | – | – | + | + | +/– | +/– | – |
| M. flavescens | M | M | S | – | + | + | + | – | + | – |
| M. xenopi | S | | S | – | – | – | + | +/– | + | – |
| M. avium | S | +/– | N | – | – | – | +/– | +/– | – | – |
| M. intracellulare | S | +/– | N | – | – | – | +/– | + | – | – |
| M. gastri | S | S | N | – | – | – | – | + | – | – |
| M. malmoense | S | S | N | – | – | – | +/– | + | + | – |
| M. haemophilum | – | S | N | – | – | – | +/– | + | + | – |
| M. shimoidei | S | | N | | | | – | – | – | – |
| M. terrae | S | S | N | – | – | – | + | – | – | – |
| M. triviale | M | S | N | – | + | + | + | – | + | – |
| M. nonchromogenicum | S | S | N | – | + | + | + | – | + | – |
| M. fortuitum | R | R | N | – | + | + | + | + | V | – |
| M. chelonae | R | R | N | V | – | + | V | V | V | – |
| M. phlei | R | R | S | + | + | + | V | V | V | – |
| M. smegmatis | R | R | N | + | + | + | + | + | + | – |
| M. vaccae | R | R | S | + | + | + | + | + | + | – |

*S, slow; M, moderate; R, rapid. ~P, photochromogen; S, scotochromogen; N, nonphotochromogen; V, variable reaction.

## Table 21–9 ▶ Quality Control Organisms

| Test | Control Positive | Negative |
|---|---|---|
| Niacin | M. tuberculosis | M. avium<br>M. smegmatis |
| Nitrate reduction | M. kansasii<br>M. tuberculosis | M. avium |
| Catalase at 68°C | M. avium | M. tuberculosis |
| Catalase quantitative | M. kansasii | M. avium |
| Tween 80 | M. kansasii | M. tuberculosis |
| Tellurite | M. avium | M. tuberculosis |
| TCH | M. bovis | M. tuberculosis |
| Acid-fast stain | M. tuberculosis | Any nonmycobacteria genus |

## Indirect Method

Plates for the indirect method are prepared in the same manner as the ones for the direct method. A growth control quadrant is also used. The indirect method uses dilutions of the specimen to inoculate the media; therefore, two sets of quadrant plates are needed. Three drops of a 1:1,000 dilution is added to one set of plates and a 1:10,000 dilution to the other. The plates should be examined at 2 and 3 weeks.

### Table 21–10 ▶ Pigment Production by Mycobacteria

| Species | Pigmentation Dark | Pigmentation Light | Colony Morphology |
| --- | --- | --- | --- |
| M. tuberculosis | buff | buff | rough |
| M. bovis | buff | buff | rough, thin, transparent |
| M. africanum | buff | buff | rough |
| M. ulcerans | buff | buff | rough |
| M. marinum | buff | buff | smooth to roughness |
| M. kansasii | buff | buff | smooth to roughness |
| M. simiae | buff | yellow | smooth |
| M. astiaticum | buff | yellow | |
| M. scrofulaceum | orange to red | yellow | smooth |
| M. szulgai | yellow at 37°C buff at 25°C | yellow to orange | smooth to rough |
| M. gordonae | orange to red | yellow to orange | smooth |
| M. flavescens | orange to red | yellow to orange | smooth |
| M. xenopi | orange to red | yellow to orange | smooth, filamentous |
| M. avium | buff | buff | smooth, thin, transparent |
| M. intracellulare | buff | buff | smooth, thin, transparent |
| M. gastri | buff | buff | smooth to roughness |
| M. malmoense | buff | buff | smooth |
| M. haemophilum | gray | gray | rough |
| M. shimoidei | buff | buff | rough |
| M. terrae | buff | buff | roughness |
| M. triviale | buff | buff | rough |
| M. nonchromogenicum | buff | buff | roughness |
| M. fortuitum | buff | buff | smooth or rough, filamentous |
| M. chelonae | buff | buff | smooth |
| M. phlei | orange to red | yellow to orange | rough |
| M. smegmatis | buff to yellow | buff to yellow | smooth or rough |
| M. vaccae | orange to red | yellow to orange | smooth |

# PROCEDURE 21-4
## Niacin Test

Niacin can be tested using paper strips or chemical reagents.

### Principle:

Niacin accumulates in the media as certain mycobacteria grow. This will occur when the enzyme that converts niacin to another metabolite is absent. The presence is measured by the production of a color.

### Method:

1. Use a culture of Lowenstein-Jensen or other egg-based media for the procedure. Add 1.0 mL of sterile distilled water to the surface of the media.
2. Place the tube in a horizontal position to allow the water to come in contact with the entire surface of the media. Use the pipet tip to lightly poke or scratch the surface of the agar.
   This will allow the water to dissolve the accumulated niacin in the media.
3. Let the tube stand for 15 to 30 minutes at room temperature. A longer time period will produce a stronger reaction.

### Paper Strip Method:

4. After the time has elapsed, the water should appear cloudy. Remove approximately 0.6 mL of the water from the tube and place in a clean 12 × 75 mm screw-cap tube.
5. Insert a niacin test strip into the tube with the arrow pointing downward, following manufacturer's directions.

6. Place the cap on tightly and incubate the tube at room temperature for 20 minutes. At intervals throughout the time period mix the tube by shaking being sure to have the liquid come in contact with the paper strip.
7. When time has expired observe the color of the liquid against a white background. A positive reaction will be yellow and a negative reaction is colorless.
8. Remove the paper strip and discard into a container with 10% NaOH to neutralize the cyanogen bromide present in the paper.
9. Negative specimens can be repeated with a fresh culture that is 3 to 4 weeks old that has been subcultured from the original.

### Quality Control:

A positive and negative control organism should be tested along with the unknown cultures. The controls are:
Positive: *M. tuberculosis*
Negative: *M. avium*

### Expected Result:

A positive reaction to niacin is yellow and a negative reaction is colorless.

### Reference:

Centers for Disease Control and Prevention. *Isolation and Identification of Mycobacterium tuberculosis*.

# SUMMARY

► Introduction
  1. The Mycobacteria includes species that are pathogens and normal flora.
► Genus Characteristics
  1. Slightly curved rods that may branch or form filaments. The cell walls of Mycobacteria contain the lipid, mycolic acid which causes the cells to gram stain poorly. They are weakly gram positive.

► Nutritional and Growth Requirements
  1. The Mycobacteria have varying nutritional requirements. The entire genus is aerobic. Natural habitats for these bacteria include the soil and a variety of warm- and cold-blooded animals.
► Growth Rate
  1. Species grow from slow to very slow taking from 2 days to 8 weeks of incubation at 25° to 45°C.
  2. The Runyon Classification scheme groups Mycobacteria according to pigment produc-

# PROCEDURE 21-5
## Nitrate Reduction

### Principle:

The presence of the enzyme nitroreductase is detected by the formation of a color after the addition of reagents. Nitrate is reduced to nitrite by the enzyme nitroreductase. If the enzyme reduces past nitrite to gas the addition of zinc dust will convert nitrate to nitrite and the nitrite will produce a color.

### Method:

1. Place 0.2 mL of sterile water in a 16 × 125 mm screw-cap tube. Use an applicator stick to emulsify two large colonies in the water. Growth should be from a 4-week-old culture on Lowenstein-Jensen media.
2. Add 2.0 mL of nitrate substrate ($NaNO_3$) to the tube and add to a 37°C water bath. Shake the tube and incubate for 2 hours. Heat will transfer to the tube and increase enzyme activity.
3. After the time expires remove the tube from the water bath and add a drop of dilute HCl.
4. Add two drops of 0.2% sulfanilamide.
5. Add two drops of *N*-naphthylethylenediamine dihydrochloride.
6. Immediately examine for the formation of a pink to red color. This is a positive reaction indicating the formation of nitrite. Therefore, the organism reduces nitrate to nitrite. A negative reaction is colorless.
7. If the reaction is negative the process must be confirmed. Add a small amount of zinc dust to the tube. The zinc will catalytically reduce nitrate to nitrite and the reaction is a true negative. If, after zinc, the color turns to red then unreduced nitrate is present. This indicates that the organism is nitroreductase negative. If there is no color change, after zinc is added, the test result should have been positive before the addition of zinc. Repeat the nitrate test.

### Quality Control:

A positive and a negative control should be done each time the nitrate test is performed. The controls are:
Positive:  *M. tuberculosis*
           *M. kansasii*
Negative:  *M. avium*

### Expected Results:

If nitrate is reduced to nitrite a pink to red color will develop after the addition of reagents. If nitrate is not reduced the reaction will be colorless and the test is negative. Negative reactions must have zinc dust added to confirm a true negative. After zinc a true negative will turn a red color and a positive reaction is colorless. Repeat the test.

### Reference:

Centers for Disease Control and Prevention. *Isolation and Identification of Mycobacterium tuberculosis.*

---

tion, the effect of light on pigment production, and growth time.

▶ Colony Appearance and Pigment Production
1. A variety of colony appearances occur in the genus *Mycobacterium*. The surface may range from smooth to rough and the colony may be thin to a high dome.
2. Pigment varies from buff to yellow to orange.

▶ Commonly Isolated Species
1. *Mycobacterium tuberculosis*—The cause of tuberculosis, an age-old disease. This bacterium was first discovered by Robert Koch.
   A. Species characteristics: Slender and straight or slightly curved rods.
   B. Cultural: A slow grower taking 3–6 weeks for colony growth to appear. Specimens can be obtained from several body sites.
   C. Clinical Significance: Tuberculosis is a chronic, infectious disorder. The respiratory tract is the route of entry.
   D. Pathogenesis of Tuberculosis: Droplet nuclei are inhaled and bacilli multiply within macrophages. Tubercle bacilli spread through the lymphatic system to the circulatory system and to the rest of the body.
   E. Symptoms: Most infected individuals are asymptomatic. Some describe a variety of symptoms that usually do not lead to diagnosis of tuberculosis. If the disease progresses to a chronic state coughing will occur producing a bloody sputum.
   F. Tuberculosis Disease Patterns
      a. Two patterns are recognized: primary and reinfection.

## PROCEDURE 21-6
## Heat Stable Catalase Test (pH 7.0, temperature 68°C)

### Principle:

The species of *Mycobacterium* can produce catalase. The enzyme can be heat stable or can be denatured by heat.

### Method:

1. Begin by preparing a 1/15 M phosphate buffer solution.

   Solution 1:
   | | |
   |---|---|
   | $Na_2HPO_4$ (anhydrous) | 9.47 g |
   | Distilled water | 1,000 mL |

   Solution 2:
   | | |
   |---|---|
   | $KH_2PO_4$ | 9.07 g |
   | Distilled water | 1,000 mL |

   Mix 61.1 mL of solution 1 with 38.9 mL of solution 2. Check to be sure the pH is 7. If it is not then adjust. Store this solution in the refrigerator.
2. Add 0.5 mL of the phosphate buffer using a sterile pipet to a sterile 16 × 125 mm screw-cap tube.
3. Incubate the tubes for exactly 20 minutes in a 68°C water bath or heating block. The temperature must remain at 68°C throughout the entire incubation period.
4. Remove the tubes after the incubation time expires and let the tubes cool to room temperature.
5. Add 0.5 mL of the Tween 80-hydrogen peroxide solution prepared in Procedure 21-7. Positive tubes will bubble and negative tubes will not bubble. Hold negative tubes for 20 minutes before reporting. Carefully observe tubes for tiny bubbles, which would be a positive reaction.

### Quality Control:

A positive and a negative control organism should be tested at the same time as the unknowns. The control organisms are:
Positive: *M. avium*
Negative: *M. tuberculosis*

### Expected Results:

A positive heat stable catalase test will produce bubbles after the reagent is added. A negative reaction will not produce bubbles after the reagent is added.

### Reference:

Centers for Disease Control and Prevention. *Isolation and Identification of Mycobacterium tuberculosis.*

---

G. Resistance
   a. The number of organisms released from productive foci, the route of spread, and host resistance determine the extent with which reinfection tuberculosis progresses.
H. Extrapulmonary Tuberculosis
   a. Extrapulmonary infections with *M. tuberculosis* can occur at almost any body site.
I. Specimen Collection
   a. Successful isolation of *M. tuberculosis* depends on proper collection and processing of the specimen.
   b. A variety of specimen types are possible with a sputum sample being most difficult to collect.

J. Specimen Processing
   a. Because most clinical specimens contain large amounts of contaminants a special two-step process must be performed to inhibit the growth of the fast-growing species.
K. Skin Tests
   a. *M. tuberculosis* produces a hypersensitivity reaction that can be detected by skin tests using filtrates of tubercle bacillus cultures.
   b. Skin tests for tuberculosis include the Tine test and the Mantoux test.
L. Drug Therapy
   a. Isoniazid, ethambutol, and rifampin are the most useful antituberculosis drugs. A combination of at least two drugs are used to help overcome resistance problems.

# PROCEDURE 21-7
## Tween 80 Hydrolysis Test

**Principle:**

Tween 80 will bind with the phenol red indicator at an acid pH. If Tween 80 is hydrolyzed it will not bind to the indicator, which will produce a pink or red color.

**Method:**

1. Prepare the Tween 80 hydrolysis substrate according to the manufacturer's package directions.
2. Inoculate the substrate with one large colony from an agar slant.
3. Incubate the unknown at 35°C.
4. Examine the unknown after 1, 5, and 10 days incubation. Look for a change in substrate color from orange to pink or red. Use an uninoculated substrate for color comparison.

**Quality Control:**

A positive and a negative control should be tested along with the unknown. The controls are:
Positive:  *M. kansasii*
Negative:  *M. tuberculosis*

**Expected Results:**

A positive Tween 80 hydrolysis reaction will be pink or red. A negative reaction will be orange.

**Reference:**

Centers for Disease Control and Prevention. *Isolation and Identification of Mycobacterium tuberculosis.*

---

M. Infection Control
- a. Patients with tuberculosis, and individuals in close contact with infected persons, should be educated on how to prevent transmission of the disease.

N. Immunization
- a. The BCG vaccine provides some protection but its duration is undetermined, making mass immunization impractical.

2. *Mycobacterium leprae*
- A. *M. leprae* causes leprosy, or Hansen's disease. It is easy to distinguish the bacterium from *M. tuberculosis.*
- B. Leprosy is a chronic disease of the skin, mucous membranes, and nervous system that progresses slowly.
- C. Diagnosis is usually by histologic examination of material from a skin lesion or earlobe of the patient. The organism is acid-fast.
- D. Treatment involves the use of diapsome, which is often used with rifampin. Treatment may continue for 3 or more years.

3. MOTT—Mycobacteria Other Than Tuberculosis
- A. *Mycobacterium avium-intracellulare* complex
  1. The two phonetically similar, but genetically distinct species, *M. avium* and *M. intracellulare,* are most often encountered in AIDS patients.
  2. *M. avium* complex causes serious tuberculosis-like endobronchial lesions in non-AIDS patients and disseminated disease in AIDS patients. The two organisms are resistant to most drugs.

▶ Laboratory Studies
1. Isolation and Culture
- A. Identification of Mycobacterium species cannot be determined by microscopic examination of a smear. Diagnostic tests must be completed.
- B. A variety of selective media are available to inhibit fast-growing contaminants.
2. Staining
- A. Staining and microscopic examination of a smear is the first step in the process of identification of Mycobacteria. The smear is examined for the presence of acid-fast bacilli.
- B. The most commonly used methods for staining are the Ziehl-Neelsen method and the Kinyoun method. Other staining methods are available.

▶ Identification Process
1. Macroscopic Examination
- A. Preliminary identification of Mycobacteria can be made by examination of the colonies. The rate of growth and pigment

production should be noted. Temperature has an effect on pigment production.

2. Biochemical Testing
   A. Biochemical testing is done to make a definitive identification of Mycobacteria.

Most of the tests used are quantitative and based on color reactions.

B. The Niacin Test and the ability to reduce nitrate to nitrite are two of the tests that are used to differentiate Mycobacteria species.

## CASE STUDY

A 32-year-old man presents with a low-grade fever, nonproductive cough, and a left upper lung lobe infiltrate 3 months after a diagnosis of AIDS. The patient's symptoms and radiograph improved, but 1 month later he was admitted with acute hepatitis. The usual antimycobacterial medications were administered but after the incident of hepatitis the medication was stopped. One year later, the same patient presented with fever, cough, and progression of his left upper lobe infiltrate. He improved after treatment for tuberculosis and 6 weeks later he was admitted with headache, fever, and a cough productive with purulent sputum.

Vital signs were: temperature, 40°C; pulse, 108 beats/min; respirations, 22/min; BP, 102/62. His general appearance was thin with minimal respiratory distress. Examination of his mouth revealed thrush and leukoplakia. A chest examination revealed bilateral inspiratory crackles over the upper lung fields.

Laboratory findings included white blood cell count, 4,800/μL; CD4 count, 5/μL. The findings in chemistry studies revealed aspartate transaminase, 50 U/L; alkaline phosphatase, 121 U/L. Bone marrow and sputum smears were positive for acid-fast bacilli. Lumbar puncture results were glucose, 43 mg/dL; protein, 50 mg/dL; white cell count, 10 cells/mm$^3$ (all lymphocytes); India ink, negative; cryptococcal antigen titer, 1:32. A chest radiograph showed bilateral infiltrates.

### Questions

1. What is the etiologic agent causing the recurrent respiratory symptoms?

2. What antimicrobial therapy would be appropriate?

## Review Questions

1. A scotochromogen:
   a. produces a yellow pigment when exposed to light.
   b. produces a yellow pigment only in the dark.
   c. does not produce a pigment in the light or the dark.
   d. produces a yellow pigment in the light or the dark.

2. Which of the following is not associated with *M. tuberculosis?*
   a. BCG
   b. DDS
   c. PPD
   d. INH

3. If more than 9 acid-fast bacilli are seen per microscopic field the report is:
   a. greater than 9/field.
   b. 9/field
   c. 9 +/field.
   d. too numerous to count.

4. The lepromatous form of leprosy is:
   a. indicated by the absence of nodules on the skin.
   b. also called tuberculoid leprosy.
   c. the third form of leprosy.
   d. none of the above.

5. A *Mycobacterium* is isolated and has the following characteristics: nonphotochromogen, produces a domed opaque yellow colony at 35°C and a transparent lobed buff colony at 25°C. The organism is most likely:
   a. *M. gordonae.*
   b. *M. avium complex.*
   c. *M. tuberculosis.*
   d. *M. kansasii.*

6. An unknown *Mycobacterium* is positive for the nitrate test, both catalase tests, Tween 80 test, and may or may not be positive for the tellurite test; all other tests are negative including TCH. The organism is most likely:
   a. *M. tuberculosis.*
   b. *M. scrofulaceum.*
   c. *M. marinum.*
   d. none of these.

## ▶ REFERENCES & RECOMMENDED READING

Abbott Laboratories. (1994). Abbott announces first treatment for AIDS-related infection, biaxin for *Mycobacterium avium* complex. *AIDS Weekly,* January, 2–4.

American Thoracic Society. (1983). Levels of laboratory services for mycobacterial diseases. *American Review of Respiratory Diseases, 128,* 1.

American Thoracic Society. (1990). *Diagnostic standards and classification of tuberculosis.* American Lung Association.

Baldwin, S., & Orme, I. (1994). The potential use of *Mycobacterium vaccae* as an adjunct to therapy of tuberculosis evaluation of activity at the immunological level. *AIDS Weekly,* December 22.

Bloch, A. B., Cauthen, G. M., Onorato, I. M., Dansbury, K. G., Kelly, G. D., Driver, C. R., & Snider, D. E. (1994). Nationwide survey of drug-resistant tuberculosis in the United States. *Journal of the American Medical Association, 271,* 665–667.

Blumberg, L. (1994). Mycobacteria other than tuberculosis. *AIDS Weekly,* July 23.

Bouza, E., Diaz-Lopez, M. D., Moreno, S., Bernaldo de Quiros, J. C. L., Vincente, T., Bererger, J. (1993). *Mycobacterium tuberculosis* bacterium infection patients with and without human immunodeficiency virus infection. *Archives of Internal Medicine, 153,* 496–501.

Boyle, E. M. Jr., Stephens, K. Jr., & Pohlman, T. H. (1994). Mycobacterium avium-intracellulare and acute abdominal pain. *Western Journal of Medicine, 161,* 415–418.

Boyles, S. (1995). Multidrug treatment needed for AIDS patients with MAC (*Mycobacterium avium* complex). *AIDS Weekly,* July 15.

Columbia University. (1996). International Classification of Tuberculosis. www./cpmc.columbia.edu/tbccp/i-classt. html.

Difco Laboratories. (1996). *Difco manual of microbiology* (9th ed.). Detroit: Difco.

Edelstein, H. (1994). *Mycobacterium marinum* skin infections: Report of 31 cases and review of the literature. *Archives of Internal Medicine, 154,* 1359–1366.

Freidman, L. N. (Ed). (1994). *Tuberculosis: Current concepts and treatment.* Ann Arbor, MI: CRC Press.

Goldsmith, M. F. (1992). Surgeons say cutting out some TB and MOTT may be the answer in multidrug-resistant infections. (tuberculosis, mycobacterium other than tuberculosis). *Journal of the American Medical Association, 268,* 3178–3180.

Herold, C. D., Fitzgerald, R. L., & Herald, D. A. (1995). Mycobacterial detection and speciation by fatty alcohol profiles with gas chromatography-mass spectrometry. *AIDS Weekly,* July 19.

Holt, J. G., Krieg, N. R., Sneath, P. H. A., Stanley, J. T., & Williams, S. T. (1994). *Bergey's manual of determinative microbiology* (9th ed.). Baltimore: Williams & Wilkins.

Jakeman, P. (1995). Risk of relapse in multibacillary leprosy. *The Lancet, 334,* 4–6.

Jereb, J. A., Klevens, M., Privett, T. D., Smith, P. J., Crawford, J. T., Sharp, V. L., Davis, B. J., Jarvis, W. R., & Dooley, S. W. (1995). Tuberculosis in health care workers at a hospital with an outbreak of multidrug-resistant *Mycobacterium tuberculosis. Archives of Internal Medicine, 155,* 854–860.

Leburn, L. E. F., Poveda, J. D., Vincent-Levy-Frebault, V. (1992). Evaluation of nonradioactive DNA probes for identification of mycobacteria. *Journal of Clinical Microbiology, 30,* 2476.

Petty, T. L. (1992). Treatment strategies in the prevention of tuberculosis. *Western Journal of Medicine, 157,* 463.

Pohl, A. D., & Keim, A. C. (1993). Screening respiratory specimens for mycobacteria culture. *Journal of the American Medical Association, 269,* 857.

Qiao, C., Fukui, J., Takegaki, Y., Ueda, S., & Yano, I. (1994). Serotype identification of *Mycobacterium avium* complex on the analysis of surface glycopeptido-lipid antigen. *AIDS Weekly,* November 20.

Singleton, P., & Sainsbury, D. (1993). *Dictionary of microbiology and molecular biology* (2nd ed.). New York: Wiley.

Smithwick, R. W. (1994). *The working mycobacteriology laboratory.* Ann Arbor, MI: CRC Press.

Stanford, J. L., Nye, P. M., Rook, G. A. W., et al. (1981). A preliminary investigation of the responsiveness or otherwise of patients and staff of a leprosy hospital to groups of shared or specific antigens of mycobacteria. *Leprosy Review, 52,* 321–327.

Stewart, G. (1994). Nontuberculosis mycobacterial infections of the head and neck. *Journal of the American Medical Association, 272,* 1636–1638.

Strong, B. E., Kubica, G. P. U.S. Department of Health and Human Services, Public Health Service, & Centers for Disease Control and Prevention. (1995). *Isolation and identification of Mycobacterium tuberculosis.* HHS Publication No. (CDC) 81-8390.

U.S. Department of Health and Human Services & Centers for Disease Control and Prevention. (1992). Tuberculosis transmission in a state correctional institution—California, 1990–1991. *Morbidity and Mortality Weekly Report, 41,* 92730.

U.S. Department of Human Services & Centers for Disease Control and Prevention. (1993). Outbreak of multidrug-resistant tuberculosis at a hospital—New York City. *Morbidity and Mortality Weekly Report, 42,* 427–430.

U.S. Department of Health and Human Services & Centers for Disease Control and Prevention. (1995). Screening for tuberculosis and tuberculosis infection in high risk groups. *Morbidity and Mortality Weekly Report, 39,* 1–5.

U.S. Department of Health and Human Services & Centers for Disease Control and Prevention. (1995). The use of preventive therapy for tuberculosis infection in the United States. *Morbidity and Mortality Weekly Report, 39,* 6–8.

# CHAPTER 22

## Spirochetes

Lisa Shimeld, MS

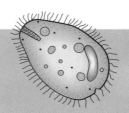

### Microbes in the News

#### Sewer Workers at Risk for Leptospirosis

A study was conducted by G. De Serres and colleagues on 76 of the 101 municipal sewer workers (75%) of Quebec City to compare the prevalence of antibodies in their serum against *Leptospira* and hepatitis A virus (HAV) to controls. Each of the 76 sewer workers was matched to two controls of the same age and gender. The subjects' serum was tested for five serovars of *Leptospira interrogans* and HAV.

The results showed that although the sewer workers had a significantly higher prevalence of antibodies against *Leptospira* than the controls (12% versus 2%), antibodies against HAV were not significantly different (54% versus 49%). The researchers concluded that though the sewer workers are at risk for leptospirosis, HAV no longer poses a serious threat. They recommend vaccination of sewer workers for leptospirosis and caution that the possibility of future HAV outbreaks be taken into consideration before deciding against HAV vaccination.

Source: De Serres, G., et al. (1995, August). Need for vaccination of sewer workers against leptospirosis and hepatitis A. *British Journal of Industrial Medicine, 52,* 505–507.

*Note:* This article was downloaded from the Internet.

*Note:* This journal was formally called *Occupational and Industrial Medicine* but according to the Crafton Hills College library it changed to the above title in 1994 with volume 51.

## KEY TERMS

Automated reagin test (ART)
Axial filaments
Barbour-Stoenner-Kelley
    (BSK) broth
Bell's palsy
Caratae

Chancre
Congenital syphilis
Direct fluorescent-antibody
    test for *T. pallidum* (DFA-TP)
Early Lyme disease (acute
    Lyme disease)

Ellinghausen, McCullough,
    Johnson, and Harris
    (EMJH) media
Endemic relapsing fever
Epidemic relapsing fever
Erythema migrans

## KEY TERMS (cont.)

Fletcher's media
Fluorescent treponemal antibody absorption (FTA-ABS)
Gumma
Hepatosplenomegaly
Hyperkeratoses
Interstitial keratitis
Late Lyme disease (chronic Lyme disease)
Latent stage syphilis
Leptospiremic
Leptospiruric
Lyme disease
Lyme meningitis

Macroscopic slide agglutination test
Maculopapular rash
Microhemagglutination test for antibody to *T. pallidium* (MHA-Tp)
Mucocutaneous relapse
Neurosyphilis
Nontreponemal tests
Nonvenereal endemic syphilis
Osteochondritis
Periplasmic flagella
Pinta
Primary stage syphilis

Rapid plasma reagin (RPR)
Relapsing fever
Secondary stage syphilis
Serous exudate
Sexually transmitted disease (STD)
Tertiary stage syphilis
Treponemal tests
Venereal Disease Research Laboratory (VDRL)
Venereal syphilis
Yaws
Zoonosis

## LEARNING OBJECTIVES

Upon successful completion of this chapter, the student should be able to:

1. Define the key terms.
2. List the characteristics of *Treponema*, *Borrelia*, and *Leptospira*.
3. List and discuss the human diseases (and characteristics of those diseases) caused by spirochetes.
4. List and explain the tests used to diagnose human diseases caused by spirochetes.
5. Indicate the antibiotics that are used to treat human diseases caused by spirochetes.

## INTRODUCTION

The spirochetes are long, slender, gram-negative, helically shaped cells. They have caused disease in humans since prehistoric times and were first described in the 1600s in tooth scrapings taken by Anton van Leeuwenhoek. The spirochetes can be distinguished from other bacteria by their distinctive morphologic features and unique method of motility. Two or more flagella-like organelles called **axial filaments** (or **periplasmic flagella**) wrap around the cell and are enclosed inside of an outer sheath located within the periplasmic space in the cell wall. One end of each axial filament is attached to a pole of the cell. Rotation of the axial filaments causes the cell to move in a corkscrew-like fashion in the opposite direction. This method of motility is especially efficient for moving through liquids such as water and lymph fluid.

The spirochetes are members of the order Spirochaetales and those species that are human pathogens are contained in two families: Spirochaetaceae and Leptospiraceae. Family *Spirochaetaceae* includes the genera *Treponema*, *Borrelia*, *Cristispira*, and *Spirochaeta* while family *Leptospiraceae* includes only the genus *Lep-*

*tospira*. Species that are human pathogens are in the genera *Treponema*, *Borrelia*, and *Leptospira*.

Spirochetes are distinguished on the basis of morphology, number of axial filaments, and biochemical and metabolic activity. Species in the genus *Treponema* are slender and tightly coiled, whereas *Borrelia* species are slightly thicker and are more loosely coiled (see Figure 22-1). The ends of *Leptospira* cells are hooked. The slender cells of *Treponema* and *Leptospira* are difficult to visualize using light microscopy and conventional staining techniques such as Gram staining. Many species are viewed by dark-field, immunofluorescent, or electron microscopy, or are stained by processes such as silver staining that effectively increase their diameter making it possible to view them by light microscopy. *Borrelia* species are seen easily by Giemsa or Wright staining of blood smears collected during the bacteremic phase of the disease.

### Habitat and Transmission

In nature, many species of spirochetes are found free living as saprophytes in a variety of environments including contaminated water, sewage, soil, and decay-

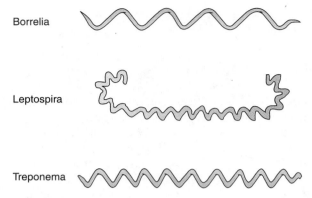

**FIGURE 22-1** Spirochetes.

ing matter. Other species are pathogenic in humans and animals, whereas a few are normal flora.

*Treponema* species are host associated and are found in the oral cavity, gastrointestinal tract, and the genitals of animals and humans. *Treponema pallidium* subspecies have no reservoirs in nature. Treponemal species that are pathogenic for humans are transmitted by direct contact, sexual or otherwise, or by transplacental transfer. *Borrelia* species are transmitted by arthropod vectors and *Leptospira* species are transmitted to humans who are bitten by an infected animal or who come into contact with water contaminated by animal urine.

## TREPONEMA

*Bergey's Manual of Systematic Bacteriology* (vol. 1) recognizes 13 species in the genus *Treponema*. Of these, 10 species are anaerobic, whereas the other three are probably microaerophilic or aerobic. *T. pallidium,* a significant sexually transmitted pathogen in humans, prefers 1.5% to 3.0% oxygen concentration. Some of the major characteristics of the four species of *Treponema* that are human pathogens are listed in Table 22-1. Other treponemal species may play an as of yet undefined role in some human skin ulcers, periodontal disease, and diarrheal illnesses (Howard, 1994). Syphilis (acquired and congenital) is the only treponemal disease discussed in detail in this chapter.

## Organism Characteristics

**Treponema pallidium.** Three subspecies of *T. pallidium* are recognized in Bergey's *Manual*. They are *T. pallidium* subspecies *pallidium*, *T. pallidium* subspecies *pertenue*, *T. pallidium* subspecies *endemicum*. All three are isolated from humans and have no reservoirs in nature. The three subspecies are indistinguishable by morphology and serologic testing. They are, however, distinguished by the manifestations of the diseases that they cause. The average size of the tightly

coiled cells of *Treponema* varies from 0.13 to 0.15 μm in diameter and 10 to 13 μm in length. Three axial filaments are inserted into each end of the cell.

Many feel that *T. pallidium* subspecies *pallidium* and *T. pallidium* subspecies *pertenue* are variants causing different degrees of virulence and clinical symptoms rather than true subspecies. This idea is supported by the 100% DNA/DNA homology that exists between the two. Insufficient numbers of *T. pallidium endemicum* and *T. carateum* have been collected to determine DNA homology between them and the others.

All three subspecies of *T. pallidium* cause disease in humans. *T. pallidium* subspecies *pallidium* is the cause of **venereal** (acquired) and **congenital syphilis**, diseases with cosmopolitan distribution. *T. pallidium* subspecies *pertenue* causes a disease known as **yaws**, that is most often seen in tropical areas. The disease caused by *T. pallidium* subspecies *endemicum* is restricted to the Middle East, Africa, Southeast Asia, and Yugoslavia and is called **nonvenereal endemic syphilis**. Some characteristics of the diseases caused by each *T. pallidium* subspecies and *T. carateum* are listed in Table 22-1.

**Treponema carateum.** *Treponema carateum* is the cause of **pinta** or **caratae**, a disease that is transmitted by contact with lesions that occur during the primary stage. Pinta is the Spanish word for "spotted" and refers to the altered skin pigmentation and **hyperkeratoses** that characterize the secondary and tertiary stages. This disease usually occurs in tropical areas such as Mexico, Central America, parts of subtropical South America, the West Indies and Cuba (*Bergey's,* vol. 1).

## Clinical Significance

Syphilis remains a significant problem in the United States with over 81,000 cases (all stages) reported in 1994 (Centers for Disease Control and Prevention, 1994). The number of new syphilis cases in the United States has been fairly stable since dropping with the introduction of antibiotics in the late 1940s as illustrated in Figure 22-2. Most especially, there has been a decline in the incidence of syphilis in the male homosexual population due primarily to behavior modification in response to acquired immunodeficiency syndrome (AIDS) (Reese & Betts, 1991).

Although syphilis is occasionally spread by nongenital contact (such as an oral lesion), it is most often a **sexually transmitted disease** and is transmitted by direct sexual contact with an individual who has active primary or secondary lesions. Transplacental transmission causing congenital syphilis can occur during the first 3 years (approximately) of infection. Transmission of syphilis by fomites is unlikely because the treponemes are unable to survive for long when separated from the warm, moist environment provided by the host.

The spirochetes enter the body through breaks or abrasions in the skin, or between epithelial cells of the

**Table 22–1 ► Characteristics of Pathogenic Treponemes**

| | Treponema pallidium | | | |
| | Subspecies pallidium | Subspecies pertenue | Subspecies endemicum | T. carateum |
|---|---|---|---|---|
| Disease caused | Syphilis | Yaws | Endemic syphilis | Pinta (caratae) |
| Site of entry | Genitalia and other | Exposed skin | Skin and oral mucosa | Exposed skin |
| Incubation | 10–90 d (usually 3 wk) | 10–90 d (usually 3 wk) | 3 wk | 3–60 d (usually 2–3 wk) |
| Primary lesions | Yes | Yes | Uncommon | Yes |
| Congenital transmission | Yes | No | No | No |
| Causes systemic infection | Yes | No | No | No |
| Usually restricted to cutaneous lesions | No | Yes | Yes | Yes |
| Sexually transmitted | Yes | No | No | No |
| Cosmopolitan distribution | Yes | No | No | No |
| Restricted to tropical countries | No | Yes | No | Yes |
| Restricted to Middle East, Africa, Southeast Asia, and Yugoslavia. | No | No | Yes | No |

mucous membranes. After a 10- to 90-day incubation period (3 weeks is average) the **primary stage** of **syphilis** develops and is characterized by the development of one or more local lesions called **chancres** on the genitals, anus, or mouth. A **serous exudate** is formed in the center of the chancre that is rich in spirochetes and highly infectious. The chancres are the site of spirochete multiplication. Humoral antibodies are usually not detectable until 1 to 4 weeks after the chancre forms. Serologic testing conducted during the primary stage is positive approximately 80% of the time (Reese, 1991).

There is little initial tissue reaction to multiplication of the spirochetes within the lesions due probably to the

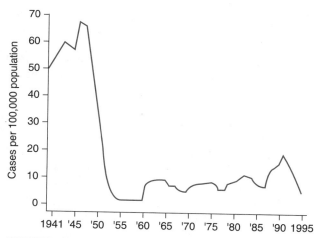

**FIGURE 22-2** Incidence and distribution of primary and secondary syphilis in the United States. (From Centers for Disease Control and Prevention. [1994]. (From Summary of notifiable diseases, *Morbidity and Mortality Weekly Report, 42* [52])

lack of endotoxin and exotoxin production by the treponemes. The chancres are indurated and are painless or slightly tender. They may go undetected, especially in female genitalia. Healing of the chancre occurs without treatment in 3 to 8 weeks. For reasons unknown at this time, the disease remains silent for the next 2 to 10 weeks. During this time dissemination of the spirochetes is taking place and a generalized, **maculopapular rash** develops marking the **secondary stage** of **syphilis**. The rash is commonly seen on the palms, soles, oral mucosa, and genitals (refer to Color Plate 51).

Dry lesions that occur on the external skin during secondary syphilis do not contain many spirochetes and are generally not contagious (Reese, 1991). The shallow, painless lesions of the mucous membranes do contain spirochetes and are highly contagious. Other symptoms indicative of systemic infection are fever, malaise, swollen lymph nodes, and patchy hair loss. These symptoms may persist for several weeks and may relapse, or, in mild cases go unnoticed. Approximately 25% of patients will develop what is called **mucocutaneous relapse** during the first year of infection. Serologic testing done during the secondary stage of syphilis is almost always positive.

The symptoms of secondary syphilis subside after a few weeks and the patient enters the **latent stage** of **syphilis**. Although no symptoms are exhibited during this period, serologic tests (treponemal tests) for syphilis are positive. After about 2 to 4 years the patient is usually no longer infectious and most cases do not progress any further, even without treatment.

Approximately one-half of those patients not receiving treatment enter the **tertiary stage** of **syphilis** usually at least 10 years after entering latency. Tertiary syphilis develops in about one-third of those persons who are originally infected. The tertiary stage of syphilis occurs after a period of latency that can last from several months to more than 40 years. Reactivation of the treponemes is due to an upset in the balance between the host and the parasite. This change may be due to declining acquired resistance in the host. Persons with tertiary syphilis are not infectious by direct contact and transplacental infection causing congenital syphilis is rare.

Although the treponemes are not extremely antigenic, most tertiary symptoms are probably due to cell-mediated immune reactions. Clinical manifestations of tertiary syphilis are numerous and include devastating lesions consisting of rubbery masses of tissue known as **gummas** (refer to Color Plate 52). These gummas rarely contain spirochetes and are not infectious. They develop on many internal organs and sometimes on the external skin as well. The treponemal cells also invade the central nervous system (CNS) (**neurosyphilis**), cardiovascular system, the eye, other internal organs, and the skin. Ultimately this damage can result in a loss of motor control, brain damage, blindness, seizures, and eventually, dementia.

Congenital syphilis occurs on transplacental transfer of *T. pallidium* subspecies *pallidium* from an infected mother to the fetus and usually does not take place until 18 weeks after gestation. The amount of damage to the fetus depends on the stage of syphilis in the mother (transplacental transfer occurs during primary and secondary syphilis) and the infectious dose. If the fetus receives a large infectious dose then miscarriage or stillbirth is likely to occur.

Because of the transplacental transfer that initiates congenital syphilis, no primary symptoms are seen. The infant with early congenital syphilis may present symptoms at birth, or more likely, at several weeks to up to 2 years of age. Possible symptoms include extensive cutaneous lesions, mucous membrane lesions that cause a mucoid discharge, **osteochondritis** of the long bones, anemia, **hepatosplenomegaly**, and possibly CNS disease. Late congenital syphilis involves damage to a variety of tissues and may not appear until after the child is 2 years of age. **Interstitial keratitis**, eighth nerve deafness, interfered development of the second teeth, perforation of the nasal septum, and cutaneous gummas are characteristic of late congenital syphilis.

## Cultural Characteristics and Identification

**Procedures and Principles.** Treponemes are not cultivable on artificial media and so far have only been successfully grown by intratesticular inoculation of rabbits or inoculation into the footpads of mice. These techniques and most of the serologic tests mentioned here are outside of the realm of the clinical microbiology laboratory and are usually performed by laboratories specializing in testing for STDs.

**DIRECT MICROSCOPIC EXAMINATION.** Direct examinations for motile spirochetes using dark-field microscopy or **direct fluorescent-antibody test for *T. pallidium* (DFA-TP)** of specimens obtained from primary or secondary lesions of the genitals are performed in the clinical microbiology laboratory. Examination of oral lesions is not recommended because they sometimes contain nonpathogenic spirochetes that can be mistaken for *Treponema*. The DFA-TP technique is preferred over dark-field examination of oral and rectal specimens because it detects and differentiates pathogenic treponemes from nonpathogenic treponemes.

Specimens for dark-field examination are collected by first cleaning the surface of the lesion to be tested with saline (Larsen, Hunter, & Kraus, 1990). The lesion is then gently rubbed with gauze until a serous exudate appears. Care must be taken to avoid excessive bleeding because erythrocytes can interfere with the examination. Using gauze, wipe away the first of the fluid then collect a drop by touching a glass slide to the lesion. Add a drop of saline to the slide if necessary and cover with a coverslip. Examine immediately for the presence of motile spirochetes. Extreme care should be taken while collecting and examining the specimen because the fluid is highly infectious.

Although syphilis is characterized by the numerous clinical manifestations that were discussed in the previous section, the disease is subclinical for much of its course. Each stage of syphilis has its particular testing requirements. Although direct microscopic examination of lesion material permits the most definitive diagnosis of syphilis, this is not always possible. It is necessary for the clinician to rely on a variety of seroimmunologic tests (serologic) in addition to direct observations. All genital lesions should be sampled because the syphilitic chancre may resemble the lesions seen in chancroid and herpes.

**NONTREPONEMAL TESTS.** Seroimmunologic tests may either be treponemal or nontreponemal. A reagin antibody (IgG) produced against a lipoidal agent seen in treponemal infection is the basis of **nontreponemal tests** such as **Venereal Disease Research Laboratory (VDRL)**, **rapid plasma reagin (RPR)**, and **automated reagin test (ART)**. Although nontreponemal tests are usually less expensive and easier to perform than are treponemal tests some pitfalls are associated with them. The most significant of these problems is that they may yield false-positive results (except for the VDRL test) in patients with a variety of acute and chronic conditions. These include pregnancy, mycoplasmal pneumonia, autoimmune diseases, intravenous drug use, collagen vascular disease, acute viral or bacterial infection, and leprosy. Recent consumption of alcohol can also alter the test results. The results of these tests are often quantitated and reported as the highest twofold dilution of serum yielding a positive reaction. A drop in titer occurs after effective treatment of syphilis.

TREPONEMAL TESTS. **Treponemal tests** such as **fluorescent treponemal antibody absorption** (**FTA-ABS**) and **microhemagglutination test for antibody to *T. pallidum*** (**MHA-Tp**) directly detect the antibodies produced by the body in response to the spirochetes. These tests are used to confirm reactive nontreponemal test results, especially in patients who do not exhibit any clinical symptoms. Cerebrospinal fluid assays are used to assist in the diagnosis of acquired and congenital syphilis.

For these reasons, the diagnosis of syphilis is based on a combination of factors including the observation of a suggestive clinical syndrome, direct observation of spirochetes in lesions, nontreponemal tests, and confirmation with more specific and sensitive treponemal tests. Serologic testing should be conducted at 3 and 6 months after treatment, and every 6 months thereafter until the titer stabilizes or disappears.

## Antibiotic Susceptibility Characteristics

Because treponemes are not cultivatable on artificial media, it is not possible to conduct the usual antibiotic susceptibility tests. Penicillin G is the drug of choice for treatment of all stages of acquired and congenital syphilis. The preparation used (benzathine, aqueous procaine, or aqueous crystalline), the dosage, and the length of treatment depend on the stage and the symptoms. Doxycycline, tetracycline, or erythromycin can be used in the penicillin allergic, nonpregnant patient.

## BORRELIA

Several species of *Borrelia* are pathogenic in humans and are vectored by lice or ticks. *Borrelia burgdorferi* causes **Lyme disease**, or Lyme borreliosis, a tick-vectored disease with cosmopolitan distribution. First recognized in 1975 in the town of Old Lyme, Connecticut, Lyme disease is now the most common tick-borne disease in the United States and has been reported in 46 of the 50 states (see Figure 22-3). According to the Centers for Disease Control and Prevention (CDC), 13,043 cases were reported in the United States in 1994 (see Figure 22-4). The disease is endemic in the Northeast and Midwest, especially in Connecticut, Massachusetts, Rhode Island, New Jersey, New York, Wisconsin, Minnesota, and northern California (CDC Lyme disease pamphlet).

*Borrelia burgdorferi* was first isolated from an *Ixodes* tick in 1982 by Dr. Willy Burgdorfer who also related the bacterium to Lyme disease. Two species of *Ixodes* transmit Lyme disease in the United States.

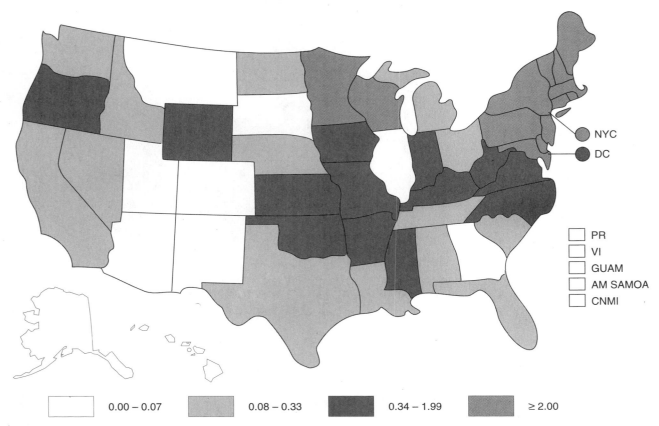

NYC
DC

☐ PR
☐ VI
☐ GUAM
☐ AM SAMOA
☐ CNMI

☐ 0.00 – 0.07    ▢ 0.08 – 0.33    ■ 0.34 – 1.99    ▨ ≥ 2.00

**FIGURE 22-3** Lyme disease distribution in the United States. (From Centers for Disease Control and Prevention. [1994]. Summary of notifiable diseases, *Morbidity and Mortality Weekly Report, 43* [53], 38)

*Ixodes scapularis* (formally *I. dammini*), the deer tick, is seen in the Northeast and Midwest, whereas *I. pacificus,* or the western black-legged tick, is common in the western states (see Figure 22-5). Two additional tick species have been identified in parts of Europe and Asia (refer to Color Plate 53).

**Relapsing fever** is a disease caused by over 15 species of *Borrelia* and also has cosmopolitan distribution. The louse-borne variety of relapsing fever, or **epidemic relapsing fever**, is seen in all parts of the world except the United States, and is caused by *Borrelia recurrentis*. Epidemic relapsing fever is vectored by the louse, *Pediculus humanus*. The tick-borne variety of the disease is known as **endemic relapsing fever**. It has cosmopolitan distribution, including the United States, where it is seen primarily in the western and Rocky Mountain states. The three species causing endemic relapsing fever in the United States are *B. parkeri, B. hermsii,* and *B. turicatae* (Table 22-2). Although the three species have close DNA homology they are distinguished on the basis of their vector associations. Only Lyme disease is discussed in detail in this chapter.

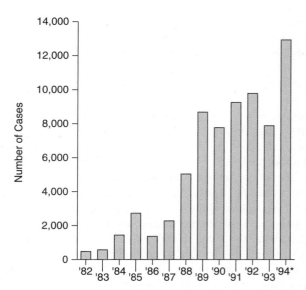

**FIGURE 22-4** Number of Lyme disease cases in the United States from 1982–1994. (From the Lyme disease pamphlet published by the Centers for Disease Control and Prevention, Atlanta, GA)

## Organism Characteristics

According to *Bergey's Manual, Borrelia* are helical cells that vary in size from 0.2 to 0.5 μm in diameter and 3 to 20 μm in length. The cells have from 3 to 10 loose coils, and 15 to 20 axial filaments (refer to Color Plate 54). They are actively motile and exhibit frequent reversal of direction.

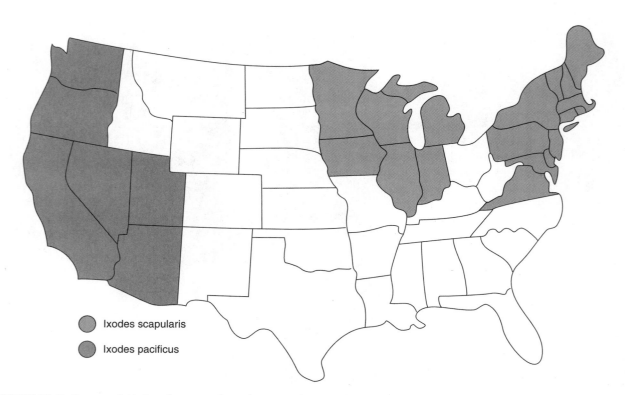

**FIGURE 22-5** Geographic distribution of *Ixodes scapularis* and *Ixodes pacificus* in the United States. (From the Lyme disease pamphlet published by the Centers for Disease Control and Prevention, Atlanta, GA)

| Table 22–2 ▶ Characteristics of *Borrelia* Species Causing Tick-Borne Endemic Relapsing Fever in the United States | | | |
|---|---|---|---|
| **Species** | **Vector** | **Hosts** | **Distribution** |
| *B. parkeri* | *Ornithodoros parkeri* | Rodents and humans | Western United States |
| *B. hermsii* | *Ornithodoros hermsi* | Rodents and humans | Western United States and Canada |
| *B. turicatae* | *Ornithodoros turicatae* | Rodents and humans | Western United States and Mexico |

## Clinical Significance

Lyme disease begins with the bite of an infected *Ixodes* tick. These ticks usually feed on and acquire *Borrelia* bacteria from infected wild animals such as the white-footed mouse, deer, and birds, but will feed on humans when the opportunity arises. It is most often the tiny nymph stage (< 2 mm) of *Ixodes* that feeds on and infects humans with *B. burgdorferi*. The ticks search for hosts on the tips of grasses and shrubs and are picked up by animals or humans that brush against the vegetation. There is no evidence that suggests Lyme disease is transmitted from person to person or directly to humans by wild or domestic animals. Although the disease can be transmitted by adult ticks they are larger and are more likely to be detected and removed before they can transmit the bacterium. The adult ticks are more active during the cooler months of the year making contact with humans less likely at that time. Anyone who frequents wooded, brushy, and grassy areas should be aware of the risk of contracting Lyme disease. The 2-year life cycle of *Ixodes* is illustrated in Figure 22-6.

**Early** or **acute Lyme disease** is characterized by one or more of the following symptoms: headache, fatigue, chills and fever, myalgia and joint pain, swollen lymph nodes, and a skin rash called **erythema migrans** (refer to Color Plate 55). Erythema migrans is a circular, red rash that appears 3 days to 1 month after the tick bite occurs. One or more expanding patches may develop, and their centers often clear resulting in a "bull's-eye" appearance. These patches can occur in many locations, and because the ticks often crawl into parts of the body covered with hair such as the scalp and the groin, they may go unnoticed. Other rashes that are due to an allergic reaction to tick saliva on the skin may also occur but usually do not expand, and disappear within a few days. Antibodies are frequently not detectable in the patient with early Lyme disease.

The often devastating symptoms of **late** or **chronic Lyme disease** may not appear for weeks, months, or years, after the tick bite occurs. Arthritis of one or more of the large bone joints is common and usually appears as brief bouts of pain and swelling. Nervous system abnormalities include numbness and pain in the arms or legs and **Bell's palsy**. **Lyme meningitis** can occur when *B. burgdorferi* invades the nervous system and usually occurs within the first few months of infection (Pachner, 1995). Thinning of the skin on the hands and feet is also seen in some cases of late Lyme disease. Antibodies are usually present in chronic Lyme disease but at this time a truly accurate test is not available. No vaccine is presently available for the prevention of Lyme disease.

## Cultural Characteristics and Identification

**Procedures and Principles.** All species of *Borrelia* are morphologically identical and cannot be distinguished by microscopy. Because *B. burgdorferi* is so rarely present in observable quantities in the blood of patients with Lyme disease, direct examination of their blood is not a reliable means of diagnosis. Serologic tests are also unreliable due to antigenic shifts that occur in *Borrelia* during the course of the disease. *Borrelia* species causing relapsing fever are usually present and can be observed in Giemsa or Wright's stained, thick or thin blood preparations that are examined by bright-field microscopy. It is not uncommon for relapsing fever to be diagnosed in the clinical

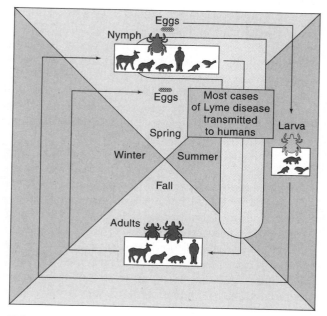

**FIGURE 22-6** Life cycle of Lyme disease ticks.

microbiology laboratory during a differential blood count (Howard, Keiser, Smith, Weissfeld, & Tilton, 1994). Wet preparations made of blood and sterile saline are examined by dark-field microscopy. Rapidly motile *Borrelia* cells can usually be observed in preparations of peripheral blood collected during the febrile stages of relapsing fever.

Unlike the treponemes, *Borrelia* can be cultivated in vitro but have complex nutritional requirements. They are microaerophilic and grow best between 30°C and 35°C, in **Barbour-Stoenner-Kelley (BSK) broth**, a complex, enriched medium (Baron, Chang, & Howard 1994). Although possible, cultivation is difficult and unreliable, and is not usually performed in the clinical microbiology laboratory. *Borrelia* is extremely sensitive to chemical and physical agents of control. Although birds and rodents are the primary reservoir hosts of *Borrelia*, domestic and other wild animals may serve as reservoirs as well. Isogai and associates (1994) describe Lyme disease causing *Borrelia* spirochetes in the skin lesions, brain, heart, kidneys, and liver of foxes in Japan.

## Antibiotic Susceptibility Characteristics

Several antibiotics, including tetracycline and erythromycin, are effective for the treatment of Lyme disease. The specific antibiotic and course of treatment depends on a number of factors including allergic history, age of the patient, stage of the disease, and conditions such as pregnancy. Early Lyme disease usually responds well to antibiotic treatment, but the response of chronic Lyme disease to treatment is variable. If untreated for many years, the damage to the nervous system and the joints may require a prolonged period for repair after elimination of the infection. Some cases do not respond to antibiotics.

## *LEPTOSPIRA*

Leptospirosis is an acute, febrile **zoonosis** with cosmopolitan distribution that is caused by many of the about 180 serovars of *Leptospira interrogans*. The three most commonly implicated of these serovars are *L. interrogans* subspecies *canicola, pomona,* and *icterohaemorrhagiae*. Many animals, domestic and wild, are reservoirs of *L. interrogans* but in the United States the organism is most often transmitted to humans by dogs and domestic livestock such as cattle, swine, and horses (see Table 22-3). Rodents associated with human habitation are also important in transmission of the disease.

## Organism Characteristics

*Leptospira* is described in Bergey's Manual as flexible, helical rods 0.1 μm in diameter and 6 to 12 μm in length. These thin cells are gram-negative and motile. A single axial filament is inserted at each end of the cell. They are obligate aerobes that grow best between 28°C and 30°C. The cells are not visible by bright-field microscopy but can be observed with dark-field and phase-contrast microscopy methods. Hooked ends are characteristic of *Leptospira*. *Leptospira* is sensitive to physical and chemical means of control and is susceptible to chlorine concentrations used to treat drinking water.

## Clinical Significance

The disease caused in humans by *L. interrogans* ranges from subclinical to severe, depending on several factors including the portal of entry, the infecting serovar, the infectious dose, and host condition. Subclinical cases are often misdiagnosed as meningitis or fever of unknown origin. In more severe cases the three organ systems that are most often involved are the CNS, kidneys, and liver.

*Leptospira* is harbored in the renal tubes of many animals and is shed in their urine. Human infection occurs on direct or indirect contact with water contaminated by infected animal urine, through drinking, or by other contact such as swimming, or by handling infected animals. The leptospires can survive in moist soil for at least 2 weeks, and up to several months to even years in water. The bacteria gain entry to the human body through the mucous membranes of the eye or the mouth, the genital tract, or abraded skin. Human-to-human transmission is rare.

After infection occurs, the incubation period lasts from approximately 1 to 2 weeks, and in clinical cases leads to the **leptospiremic**, or acute phase. Symptoms include fever (102°–106°F), chills, severe headache, malaise, and myalgia. Anorexia, nausea, and vomiting are common, and occasional severe cases experience jaundice. This phase of the disease usually lasts from 4 to 8 days. Leptospires can be detected in the blood and spinal fluid of patients for about 1 week after the onset of symptoms, and in their urine for several months after that time (*Bergey's Manual,* vol 1.).

| Table 22–3 ▶ Common Animal Reservoirs of the Three Serovars of *Leptospira interrogans* Seen Most Often in the United States | |
|---|---|
| **Serovar of L. interrogans** | **Animal Reservoirs** |
| canicola | Cattle and swine |
| pomona | Dogs, cattle, horses, swine |
| icterohaemorrhagiae | Dogs, cattle, swine, rats |

The **leptospiruric**, or immune phase, begins at about the second week of the disease. Patient symptoms are variable. Recurrence of the fever lasting from 1 to 2 days is possible. By this time the leptospires have been eliminated from most of the body except maybe from the eyes, kidneys, and possibly the brain. In excess of 90% of human leptospirosis cases are self-limiting with recovery occurring in about 2 to 3 weeks. Severe cases may take several months for complete recovery. Renal failure is the most common cause of death in the 5% to 30% of untreated patients who experience jaundice.

Immunity to leptospirosis is serovar specific and is permanent. An important component of leptospirosis prevention is rodent control. A vaccine for dogs is required in the United States and one for cattle is available as well. A heat-killed vaccine for humans is available and is recommended for persons at high risk. This includes ranchers, veterinarians, and sewer workers.

## Cultural Characteristics and Identification

*Leptospira* is easier to cultivate than are the other genera of spirochetes. The type of specimen collected for isolation and cultivation depends on the phase of the disease. The bacteria are found in the blood and cerebrospinal fluid of infected persons during the first week of infection and in their urine for several months thereafter. Although urine samples are collected by clean-catch or catheterization they are often contaminated with other organisms. This problem is in part overcome with the use of selective media. Cultures are incubated at 30°C in tubes of **Fletcher's media** or **Ellinghausen, McCullough, Johnson and Harris (EMJH) media** in the dark for up to 6 weeks. The spirochetes grow beneath the surface of the media. Cultures are examined once a week by dark-field microscopy for at least 10 weeks. Look for cells with hooked ends, exhibiting corkscrew-like motility.

Immunoserologic blood tests are most often used to diagnose leptospirosis. Antibodies appear in the blood of infected persons 1 to 2 weeks after development of the first symptoms. The highest levels can be detected during recovery and may persist for years. The **macroscopic slide agglutination test** using formalinized serogroup-specific organisms as antigens is a useful, rapid screening method (Baron, 1994). Appassakij and colleagues report that an immunofluorescent antibody test that they evaluated was moderately sensitive and specific.

## Antibiotic Susceptibility Characteristics

Antibiotic therapy is effective only if it is begun early in the infection with *Leptospira*. Penicillin or tetracycline may be helpful in modifying the disease but only if started no later than the fourth day of illness (Baron, Peterson, & Finegold, 1994).

## SPECIAL CONSIDERATIONS FOR IMMUNOCOMPROMISED HOSTS

### Syphilis in HIV-Positive and AIDS Patients

Syphilis and human immunodeficiency virus (HIV) interact at several levels. Initially, the genital lesions experienced during syphilis can enhance transmission of HIV, and once infected with the virus the course and treatment of syphilis may be altered. Occasionally, HIV-positive and AIDS patients coinfected with syphilis fail to exhibit serologic reactivity (to syphilis) so diagnosis must be made on the basis of treponemes in biopsied suspicious skin lesions. In most cases, however, nontreponemal titers are significantly higher in HIV-infected patients than in non-HIV infected patients. The treatment of syphilis in HIV-positive and AIDS patients is often less effective than in the non-HIV-infected patients and requires the administration of higher doses of benzathine penicillin G. The response to this chemotherapy is typically slower than in non-HIV infected patients.

## SUMMARY

▶ Spirochetes have axial filaments that cause them to move in a corkscrew-like fashion.
▶ Spirochetes are members of the order Spirochaetales. Those that are human pathogens are in two families: Spirochaetaceae and Leptospiraceae. Pathogenic species are in the genera *Treponema, Borrelia,* and *Leptospira.*
▶ The genus *Treponema* has 13 species; some are anaerobic, others use oxygen.
▶ The three subspecies of *T. pallidum—pallidum, pertenue,* and *endemicum*—cause disease in humans.
▶ *Treponema carateum* causes pinta, a disease that is transmitted by contact with lesions, altered skin pigmentation, and hyperkeratoses.
▶ Syphilis, usually an STD, is still a significant problem in the United States. After a 10- to 90-day incubation period, the primary stage is characterized by one or more chancres, which heal without treatment in 3 to 8 weeks. A macu-

lopapular rash develops during the secondary stage. During the latent stage, symptoms subside. After 2 to 4 years the patient is usually no longer infectious.

▶ Congenital syphilis occurs on transplacental transfer of organisms from an infected mother to her fetus.

▶ Treponemes are not cultivatible on artificial media and must be grown in rabbits or in the footpads of mice.

▶ Nontreponemal tests for syphilis include Venereal Disease Research Laboratory (VDRL), rapid plasma reagin (RPR), Wasserman, and automated reagin test (ART). False-positive reactions are a problem with nontreponemal tests.

▶ Treponemal tests include fluorescent treponemal antibody absorption (FTA-ABS) and micro-hemagglutination test for antibody to *T. pallidum* (MHA-Tp). Penicillin G is the drug of choice for treatment of treponemal infection.

▶ *Borella burgdorferi* causes Lyme disease in humans and is vectored by the *Ixodes* tick. It is the most common tick-borne disease in the United States.

▶ Ticks become infected from wild animals such as the white-footed mouse, deer, and birds. The tick has a 2-year life cycle. Early Lyme disease is characterized by several flu-like symptoms and erythema migrans. Late Lyme disease may appear weeks, months, or years later.

▶ Several antibiotics including tetracycline and erythomycin are effective for the treatment of Lyme disease.

▶ Leptospirosis is a zoonosis that is caused by *Leptospira interrogans*. The organism is harbored in the renal tubes of many animals and is shed in their urine. Humans are infected by contact with this urine or water that is contaminated with infected urine. *Leptospira* is easier to cultivate than other spirochetes. Antibiotics are only effective if treatment begins early.

▶ Syphilis and HIV interact at several levels. The treatment for these patients is often less effective than in non-HIV-infected individuals.

## CASE STUDY: RELAPSING FEVER

Eleven days after returning from a camping trip to the North Rim of the Grand Canyon (June 21, 1990), a 61-year-old man from California developed fever, chills, headache, myalgias, and drenching sweats. These symptoms lasted for 2 days. Over the next 2 weeks he experienced three febrile relapses and was finally hospitalized. A physical examination and a variety of laboratory tests were performed but were nondiagnostic. While in the hospital the patient experienced a fourth episode of fever during which time a peripheral blood sample was obtained and examined. Spirochetes were observed and relapsing fever was diagnosed. The patient was unable to recall a tick bite. He was treated with tetracycline and recovered.

After investigation of the cabin in which he stayed, and phone and mail surveys of over 10,000 other Grand Canyon visitors (from nine states, Canada, and Germany), 14 other cases (4 laboratory confirmed, 10 clinically defined) of relapsing fever were confirmed. The cabins were sprayed with an acaricide and structural changes were made to deter rodents from nesting in and around the buildings.

From: *Morbidity and Mortality Weekly Report*. (1991). *40* (18), 296–297.

### Questions:

1. What is the most likely cause of this infection?

2. What three species cause endemic relapsing fever in the United States?

3. What is the vector of epidemic relapsing fever?

# Review Questions

1. Which of the following techniques would be most appropriate for the diagnosis of Lyme disease?
   a. Examination of a Giemsa-stained, thick blood preparation
   b. Cultivation of cerebrospinal fluid on Barbour-Stoenner-Kelley broth
   c. The microhemagglutination test
   d. There is no reliable test for Lyme disease at this time.

2. A 9-year-old boy is admitted to the hospital after two bouts of fever (105°F), headache, myalgias, right upper quadrant pain, and chills. What is the most probable diagnosis and the likely drug of choice?
   a. Lyme disease, tetracycline
   b. Congenital syphilis, penicillin G
   c. Relapsing fever, penicillin G
   d. Pinta, erythromycin

3. Which of the following techniques is most appropriate for the identification of spirochetes in genital chancres?
   a. Bright-field examination of a Gram stain made from the serous exudate obtained from the chancre
   b. Dark-field examination for motile spirochetes
   c. Direct fluorescent examination for motile spirochetes
   d. Either b or c

4. Infection of domestic animals with which of the following can result in significant economic losses?
   a. *Leptospira interrogans*
   b. *Leptospira biflexa*
   c. *Borrelia recurrentis*
   d. *Borrelia burgdorferi*

5. The successful treatment of syphilis is indicated by:
   a. the elimination of all skin rashes.
   b. a reduction or elimination of the titer.
   c. an increase in the titer.
   d. a negative nontreponemal reaction.

6. *Treponema* species are transmitted to humans by which of the following?
   a. Transplacental transfer
   b. Sexual contact
   c. Direct contact
   d. All of the above

7. The development of a maculopapular rash is characteristic of:
   a. leptospirosis.
   b. primary syphilis.
   c. secondary syphilis.
   d. tertiary syphilis.

8. A pregnant woman is being treated with doxycycline for a spirochete infection. She is admitted to the hospital with headache and muscle pain and is going into labor in the first week of her seventh month of pregnancy. The above are characteristic of:
   a. the Yaws reaction.
   b. tertiary syphilis.
   c. borreliosis.
   d. an allergic reaction to the antibiotic.

9. Another name for the "bull's-eye" rash that is characteristic of Lyme disease is:
   a. the "migrating rash."
   b. the Jarisch-Herxheimer reaction.
   c. a macopapular rash.
   d. erythema migrans.

10. Which of the following could result in a false-positive reaction for syphilis using a nontreponemal test?
    a. An acute viral infection
    b. Pregnancy
    c. Mycoplasmal pneumonia
    d. All of the above

## ▶ REFERENCES & RECOMMENDED READING

Anderson, K. N. (Ed.). (1994). *Mosby's medical, nursing, and allied health Dictionary,* (4th ed.). St. Louis: Mosby.

Appassakji, J., Silpapojakul, K., Wansit, R., & Woodtayakorn, J. (1995). Evaluation of the immunofluorescent antibody test for the diagnosis of human leptospirosis. *American Journal of Tropical Medicine and Hygiene, 52* (4), 340–343.

Baron, E., Chang, R. S., Howard, D. H., Miller, J. N., & Turner, J. A. (1994). *Medical microbiology: A short course.* New York: Wiley-Liss.

Baron, E., Peterson, L. R., & Finegold, S. M. (1994). *Bailey and Scott's diagnostic microbiology* (9th ed.). St. Louis: Mosby.

Centers for Disease Control and Prevention. (1994). Summary of notifiable diseases, 1991. *Morbidity and Mortality* Weekly Report, *42* (52).

Dai, B. (1992). Advances in research on leptospira and human leptospirosis in China. *Chinese Medical Sciences Journal, 7* (4), 239–243.

Daniel, E., Beyene, H., & Tessema, T. (1992). Relapsing fever in children—Demographic, social and clinical features. *Ethiopian Medical Journal, 30* (4), 207–214.

DeSerres, G., Levesque, B., Higgins, R., Major, M., Laliberte, D., Boulianne, N., & Duval, B. (1995). Need for vaccination of sewer workers against leptospirosis and hepatitis A. *Occupational and Environmental Medicine, 52* (8), 505–507.

Dohahue, J. M., Smith, B. J., Poonacha, K. B., Donahue, J. K., & Rigsby, C. L. (1995). Prevalence and serovars of leptospira involved in equine abortions in central Kentucky during the 1991–1993 foaling seasons. *Journal Veterinary Diagnostic Investigation, 7* (1), 87–91.

Hoffman, J. C., Stichtenoth, D. O., Zeider, H., Follmann, M., Brandis, A., Stanek, G., & Wollenhaupt, J. (1995). Lyme disease in a 74-year-old forest owner with symptoms of dermatomyositis. *Arthritis Rheumatism, 38,* (8), 1157–1160.

Howard, B. J., Keiser, J. F., Smith, T. F., Weissfeld, A. S., & Tilton, R. C. (1994). *Clinical and pathogenic microbiology* (2nd ed.). St. Louis: Mosby.

Isogai, E., Isogai, H., Kawabata, H., Masuzawa, T., Yanagihara, Y., Kimura, K., Sakai, T., Azuma, Y., Fujii, N., & Ohno, S. (1994). Lyme disease spirochetes in a wild fox (*Vulpes vulpes schrencki*) and in ticks. *Journal of Wildlife Disease, 30* (3), 439–444.

Jaret, P. (1991, January). The disease detectives. *National Geographic Magazine,* 114–140.

Jethwa, H. S., Schmitz, J. L., Dallabetta, G., Behets, F., Hoffman, I., Hamilton, I., Lule, G., Cohen, M., & Folds, J. D. (1995). *Journal of Clinical Microbiology, 33* (1), 180–183.

Larsen, S. A., Hunter, E. F., & Kraus, S. J. (1990). *A manual of tests for syphilis.* Washington, DC: American Public Health Association.

Noel, R. K. (Ed.). (1984). *Bergey's manual of systematic bacteriology: Vol. 1.* Baltimore: Williams & Wilkins.

Pachner, A. R. (1995). Early disseminated Lyme disease: Lyme meningitis. *American Journal of Medicine 98* (4A), 30S–37S.

Petchclai, B., Hiranras, S., Kunakorn, M., Potha, U., & Liemsiwan, C. (1992). Enzyme-linked immunosorbent assay for leptospirosis immunoglobulin M specific antibody using surface antigen from a pathogenic *Leptospira*: A comparison with indirect hemagglutination and microagglutination tests. *Journal of the Medical Association of Thailand, 75* (Suppl. 1), 203–208.

Reese, R. E., & Betts, R. F. (Eds.). (1991). *A practical approach to infectious diseases* (3rd ed.). Boston: Little, Brown.

Spach, D. H., Liles, W. C., Campbell, G. L., Quick, R. E., Anderson, D. E. Jr., & Fritsche, T. R. (1993). Tick-borne diseases in the United States. *New England Journal of Medicine, 320* (13), 936–947.

Teglia, O. F., Battagliotti, C., Villavicencio, R. L., & Cunha, B. A. (1995). Leptospiral pneumonia. *Chest, 108* (3), 874–875.

Tortora, G. J., Funke, B. R., & Case, C. L. (1995). *Microbiology: An introduction.* Redwood City, CA: Benjamin/ Cummings.

Turgeon, M. L. (1996). *Immunology and serology in laboratory medicine.* St. Louis: Mosby.

# CHAPTER 23
# Chlamydia, Mycoplasma, and Rickettsia

James D. Kettering, PhD, Daila S. Gridley, PhD

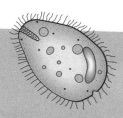

## Microbes in the News

### A Role for Mycoplasma in AIDS?

*Mycoplasma penetrans* has received much attention as a possible cofactor in the development of acquired immunodeficiency syndrome (AIDS). This is partly due to its relatively high incidence of patients with the disease. Additional supporting data include the ability of mycoplasmas to act as potent stimulators of lymphocyte proliferation, thereby possibly inducing the multiplication of human immunodeficiency virus type-1 (HIV-1), and their ability to enhance the lethal effects of the virus on cells. If proven to be true, it may be that treatment for mycoplasma could delay the onset of AIDS or may decrease the severity of symptoms. However, a number of other factors such as the strain of the virus and the age of the infected individual undoubtedly also play important roles in the large variability seen in clinical latency following HIV-1 infection.

## KEY TERMS

ATP-energy parasites
Atypical pneumonia
Cholesterol
Cold-agglutinin syndrome
Elementary body
"Fried egg" colony
Gimenez stain
Group-reactive antigen

Inclusion bodies
Inclusion conjunctivitis
  LGV-TRIC
Nongonococcal urethritis
  (NGU)
Phagosome
Psittacosis
Reticulate body

Rickettsemia
Superantigen
T strains
Trachoma
TWAR strain
Unit membrane
Weil-Felix Reaction
Zoonoses

## LEARNING OBJECTIVES

**Upon successful completion of this chapter, the student should be able to:**

1. Identify the major human pathogens found in the *Chlamydia* and *Mycoplasma* genera and *Rickettsiaceae* family and discuss their distinguishing characteristics.
2. Outline the intracellular life cycle of *Chlamydia*.
3. Discuss the clinical relevance and the diseases associated with each of the major organisms.
4. Describe the critical laboratory assays used for isolation and identification of the *Chlamydia, Mycoplasma,* and *Rickettsia*.
5. List the drugs of choice for each of the major pathogens and discuss preventative measures as appropriate.

## INTRODUCTION

*Chlamydiae* and *Rickettsiae* are bacteria that are obligate intracellular parasites. That is a feature similar to the growth requirement of viruses, but these two groups of organisms possess features of true bacteria that viruses do not, such as cell walls and RNA and DNA. *Chlamydiae* are viewed as gram-negative bacteria that lack mechanisms for the production of metabolic energy and cannot synthesize adenosine triphosphate (ATP). Once in their intracellular location, the host cell furnishes the energy-rich intermediates needed for chlamydial growth. *Chlamydia trachomatis, Chlamydia psittaci,* and *Chlamydia pneumoniae* produce a large variety of human diseases.

*Rickettsiae* are small bacteria that are transmitted to humans by arthropod (insect) vectors, except for the agent causing Q fever. Rickettsial diseases (except for Q fever and ehrlichiosis) typically present with fever, rashes, and vasculitis. The two main human disease groups caused by these organisms include typhus and spotted fevers.

There are several species in the genus of cell wall-free bacteria known as *Mycoplasma*. In humans, three are of primary importance. *Mycoplasma pneumoniae* causes pneumonia and has been associated with joint and other infections. *Mycoplasma hominis* may cause postpartum fever and has been found to be present in mixed bacterial populations in fallopian tube infections. *Ureaplasma urealyticum* may cause nongonococcal urethritis in men and is associated with lung disease in premature infants. Other members of the genus *Mycoplasma* are pathogens of the respiratory and urogenital tracts and joints of animals.

## CHLAMYDIA

Chlamydia is the most common sexually transmitted disease (STD) in the United States today, infecting over 4 million people each year. It has reached epidemic proportions and it is thought to infect one-fourth to one-third of all sexually active college students. If left untreated, which happens often because most cases are asymptomatic, chlamydia can cause infertility in men and women. Direct contact of mucous membranes during sexual activity, causing the exchange of bodily fluids, allows efficient transmission of the organism. Mothers can transmit to their babies during childbirth, and many of these infants suffer from eye infections and potentially fatal form of pneumonia. It is possible to contract this disease repeatedly because prior infection appears not to ensure immunity against future exposures. High-risk groups include white men, aged 15 to 24, people with multiple partners, and women using contraceptives or intrauterine devices (IUDs). It is possible to control the disease using a combination of diagnostic procedures, antimicrobials, barrier protection, and education.

### Organism Characteristics

The family *Chlamydiacea* has one genus (*Chlamydia*), with three species (*C. trachomatis, C. psittaci,* and *C. pneumoniae*). *Chlamydia* are obligate intracellular parasites of eukaryotic host cells, contain both DNA and RNA (compare: virus characteristics), multiply by binary fission, and are susceptible to several kinds of antibiotics. The cell wall is similar to that found in gram-negative bacteria. The organisms contain ribosomes, allowing for direct protein synthesis. Chlamydiae are unable to store or produce ATP. Their obligate intracellular parasitism is, therefore, based on being an **ATP-energy parasite**.

*Chlamydia psittaci* and *C. pneumoniae* are resistant to sulfonamides, and infected host cells do not contain an iodine-staining glycogen inclusion body. *C. trachomatis* is sensitive to sulfonamides, and its infected host cell contains an iodine-staining glycogen inclusion. *C. trachomatis* and *C. pneumoniae* are found only in human hosts, whereas most strains of *C. psittaci* can be found in numerous avian and mammalian species. Humans are accidental hosts for *C. psittaci* infections.

All chlamydia have a **group-reactive antigen** detectable in the supernatants of host cell lysates. It appears to be a heat-stable lipoprotein-carbohydrate complex, and antibodies to this antigen may be detected by complement fixation tests or assays using fluorescent antibody procedures.

The intracellular development cycle is unique in bacteriology. The infectious particle is called an **elementary body** (EB) (see Figure 23-1), which measures about 0.3 µm in diameter. This attaches to the host cell surface receptor sites, and the EB is taken into the host cell by phagocytic action. In the host cell cytoplasm, the EB is enclosed in a vacuole (**phagosome**) (see Figure 23-1). Within 6 to 8 hours, the EB reorganizes into a larger (0.8–1.5 µm) form called a **reticulate body** (RB) (refer to Color Plate 56 and Figure 23-1) or initial body. The EB divides within this area by binary fission over a 24-hour period. The growth cycle ends when the RB condenses and matures into new EBs. The inclusion ruptures and releases 300 to 1,000 new EBs. The growth cycle duration is about 48 hours, and the effect of chlamydial infection is host cell death (see Figure 23-1).

## Clinical Significance

*Chlamydia trachomatis* has long been recognized as the etiologic cause of lymphogranuloma venereum, **trachoma,** and **inclusion conjunctivitis (LGV-TRIC)**. It is now also recognized as a major cause of **nongonococcal urethritis (NGU)**, epididymitis, cervicitis, and pelvic inflammatory disease (PID).

*Chlamydia trachomatis* infections can be divided on an epidemiologic basis into three categories: classic trachoma (reservoir-chronic ocular infections; transmission-fingers, fomites, flies); sexually transmitted genital infections (LGV, rare in developed countries; non-LGV constitutes the majority of recognized *C. trachomatis* infections in developed countries); and perinatal infant eye and respiratory infections acquired from the mother's chronically infected cervix. It has been estimated that about 10% of pregnant women in the United States carry chlamydia in their cervices at parturition. The risk of neonatal infection constitutes a major public health problem.

Trachoma (chronic follicular keratoconjunctivitis) is the leading cause of preventable blindness globally. It has been estimated that more than 400 million cases of trachoma exist currently and some 20 million people

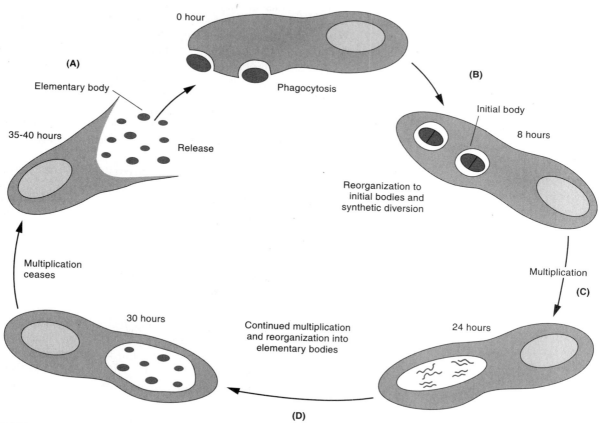

**FIGURE 23-1** Life cycle of chlamydia. (A) Elementary body (EB) of chlamydia attaches to host cell. (B) EB is enclosed in phagosome. (C) EB reorganizes into a larger reticulate body (RB). (D) RB condenses and matures into new EBs. The cell ruptures and releases many infectious elementary bodies.

have become blinded. Following an abrupt onset, infiltrating polymorphonuclear lymphocytes and macrophages form necrotic follicles. Secondary bacterial infections lead to corneal ulcers. Serotypes A-C are primarily involved in these infections. Inclusion conjunctivitis has been documented in 10% to 15% of newborn infants and represents a significantly less serious infection. Serotypes D-K are related to these cases.

Lymphogranuloma venereum is the only *C. trachomatis* infection that produces multisystem involvement and constitutional manifestations. It is endemic in Asia, Africa, and South America, with approximately 500 cases per year reported in the United States. In the first stage 2 to 6 weeks following exposure, lymphadenopathy occurs and buboes form. The second stage is characterized by systemic symptoms (fever, chills, headache, myalgia). The third stage represents complications that arise in about 5% of infected men. This is evidenced as a progress ulceration and infiltrative involvement of the penis, urethra, or scrotum. Serotypes $L_1$-$L_3$ are involved here.

Other genital infections are related to serotypes D-K. In NGU, *C. trachomatis* can be isolated from 30% to 50% of men with this disease. This is about twice as frequently as gonococcus (GC) involvement, and about 20% of men with urethral GC have concurrent *C. trachomatis* urethral infection. It has been estimated that more than 50% of NGU is due to *C. trachomatis*. Diagnosis of NGU requires documentation of leukocyte exudate (15 or more per high power field in urine sediment) as well as exclusion of urethral GC by Gram stain and culture. Epididymitis is common in men under age 35, and cervicitis infections often escape detection. The organism is isolated from the cervix of 30% to 60% of women with GC infection. In addition to inclusion conjunctivitis of the newborn, interstitial pneumonia may occur in infants. This can develop gradually, over a 1- to 3-month period.

*Chlamydia psittaci* causes **psittacosis** (parrot fever, ornithosis). It is a highly infectious disease of birds, and transmission to humans is rare. It occurs by inhalation of dried feces, although *C. psittaci* may be present in blood, tissues, excreta, and feathers of infected birds. Human infections feature a 7- to 15-day incubation period, with chills, high fever, and a persistent unproductive cough.

*Chlamydia pneumoniae* (**TWAR strain**) is the cause of approximately 20% of community-acquired pneumonia in young people. Seroprevalence studies show that 30% to 60% of the U.S. population have antibodies. The disease is relatively mild and is clinically indistinguishable from infection caused by *M. pneumoniae*. The mild **atypical pneumonia** usually presents a clinical picture of bronchitis and pharyngitis.

## Cultural Characteristics and Identification

Specimen collection is critical for positive test results. It should contain host cell epithelial scrapings to increase the isolation possibility. Ideally, the sample should be taken at bedside, placed in transport media, and delivered to the laboratory immediately.

Although isolation represents the "gold standard" test for chlamydia, technical problems exist that may adversely affect the recovery of the organism. Relatively few laboratories offer cell culture diagnosis.

Direct fluorescent antibody (DFA) staining methods use monoclonal antibodies to either the outer membrane proteins or lipopolysaccharides of *C. trachomatis*. These are conjugated to fluorescein isothiocyanate and require an experienced technician and a fluorescent microscope to detect the EBs in smears of clinical material. One widely used system is the MicroTrak DFA (Syva Co, San Jose, CA). It is reported that DFAs achieve at least a 90% sensitivity compared to culture evaluations of symptomatic men and high-risk women. The sensitivity of DFA is lower in populations with asymptomatic infections, probably due to fewer inclusion-forming units in patient specimens.

Antigen can also be detected by enzyme-linked immunosorbent assays (ELISAs). Several companies have kits commercially available. One (Chlamydiazyme—Abbot Laboratories, North Chicago, IL) has reported 79% sensitivity in men with urethritis and 90% in high-risk women. Samples from asymptomatic men are detected at about 50% sensitivity. A direct antigen detection procedure using an RNA-directed DNA probe conjugated to a chemiluminescent marker (PACE, Gen-Probe, San Diego, CA) is available, with a sensitivity that appears to be close to that of DFA. It is important to remember that in low-prevalence populations, culture remains that test of choice.

Serologic testing has limited value for diagnosis of urogenital infections in adults because most are seropositive. Complement fixation and immunofluorescence tests may be used. Negative serology can reliably exclude chlamydia infection.

## Antibiotic Susceptibility Characteristics

The first choice treatment has been doxycycline, with erythromycin being recommended for pregnant women and infants. The second choice has been erythromycin, with amoxicillin for pregnant women and sulfisoxazole for infants. The advent of azithromycin has put chlamydia management on an even footing with other STDs, such as gonorrhea and syphilis, with regard to single-dose treatment.

# MYCOPLASMA

## Organism Characteristics

Mycoplasmas are bacteria that belong in the class known as *Mollicutes.* They are the smallest free-living organisms found in nature and can replicate in cell-free media under both aerobic and anaerobic conditions. They are found worldwide in many different animals, including cattle (bovine pleuropneumonia), sheep, goats, swine, poultry, mice, rats, and dogs. Infections of certain plants (corn and aster) are also possible. At least 15 species have been isolated from humans. The organisms are highly pleomorphic, ranging in size from very small (125 to 150 nm) to elongated vesicle-like forms. They can pass through filters with a 450-nm pore size, as do the chlamydiae, and possess a relatively small genome, having DNA with a molecular weight of only $5 \times 10^5$ kDa. They are unable to synthesize precursor molecules needed to make peptidoglycan, and hence lack a rigid cell wall, a property that renders them resistant to cell wall-inhibiting drugs. In this respect, these organisms resemble the L forms that can arise from many different types of well-characterized bacteria. However, unlike L forms, mycoplasmas never revert to a walled state. In addition, they bear no antigenic or genetic relationship with the L forms. Mycoplasmas have a flexible, triple-layered "**unit membrane**" that contains a sterol, and thus is relatively hardy, surviving even in high temperature springs and acid outflows of mining wastes. They incorporate large amounts of lipids, including **cholesterol**, sphingomyelin, and phosphatidylglycerol into their cell membranes. The cholesterol, a fatty substance ($C_{27}H_{45}OH$) that is present in all animal fats and oils, as well as many of the other lipids, is obtained from the host. Some lipids, however, may be made de novo by the organisms. They are the only prokaryotes to possess cholesterol. Reproduction is thought to occur by budding, fragmentation, and/or binary fission. The distinguishing characteristics of mycoplasmas are summarized in Table 23-1.

Although there are six genera of mycoplasmas based on their cholesterol requirement and habitat, only two contain members that are pathogenic for humans: *Mycoplasma* and *Ureaplasma.* They are well-known for chronic respiratory, joint, and genitourinary tract disease. *M. pneumoniae,* a cause of atypical pneumonia in young persons, is the most important member of the group. Other important members include *M. hominis,* associated with postpartum fever and fallopian tube infections, *M. genitalium,* which may cause urethral infections, and *U. urealyticum,* a cause of NGU and lung disease in premature infants. In addition, *M. penetrans,* a new species that has been isolated from patients with AIDS, has been suggested as a possible cofactor in the progression of the disease. Transmission of the organisms occurs by inhalation of contaminated respiratory droplets or through sexual activity. Some mycoplasmas, however, are part of the normal flora of the respiratory and genitourinary tracts, especially in women.

## Clinical Significance

*Mycoplasma pneumoniae* is a relatively common and important cause of primary atypical pneumonia, usually a mild pneumonia with an insidious onset and a relatively long recovery period. Patients often remain ambulatory; hence, the disease is sometimes referred to as walking pneumonia. In addition, it occurs primarily in young people within the age range of 5 to 20 years, whereas classic pneumonia is seen most often in the elderly. It has been estimated that *M. pneumoniae,* together with *Chlamydia* species, probably account for more than 40% of these pneumonias in children. *M. pneumoniae* alone is responsible for approximately 15% to 20% of all cases of pneumonia. The organisms are transmitted from one individual to another via respiratory secretions. Infection may be subclinical, cause only pharyngitis, or may result in a pneumonia that ranges from mild (the usual case) to severe. The incubation period is usually 1 to 3 weeks followed by symptoms that include (often lasting for 8–10 days) sore throat, nonproductive cough, and headache. In severe cases, the cough may become paroxysmal with blood-streaked sputum and chest pain. Bronchitis and

---

**Table 23–1 ▶ Selected Characteristics of the Mycoplasmas**

- ▶ Smallest organisms capable of reproduction on cell-free media
- ▶ Smallest reproductive forms are 125–250 nm in diameter
- ▶ Cells are highly pleomorphic and flexible
- ▶ Lack a rigid cell wall; have a triple-layered "unit membrane" that contains sterols
- ▶ Are the only prokaryotes to possess cholesterol
- ▶ Completely resistant to penicillin and other cell wall-inhibiting agents
- ▶ Do not revert to, or originate from, bacterial parental forms
- ▶ Often form "fried egg" colonies on appropriate solid media
- ▶ Have high affinity for mammalian cell membranes
- ▶ Some appear to possess **superantigens** that trigger massive secretion of proinflammatory cytokines
- ▶ Some are normal inhabitants of genitourinary tract (especially women)
- ▶ Some are common in nature; can survive in high-temperature springs and acid outflows of mining wastes
- ▶ Originally referred to as PPLOs (pleuropneumonia-like organisms)

bronchiolitis occur frequently and there may be plugs of mucus and pus that block bronchioles, causing collapse of some alveoli and compensatory expansion of others. An unusual feature is that the alveoli tend to decrease in size because their walls swell inward and there is no intra-alveolar buildup of fluid. Chest x-rays often show dramatic consolidation of the lungs. Hematoxylin and eosin stains of lung biopsies show widespread inflammation of the lung parenchyma and thickening of alveolar walls. Inflammatory exudates consist primarily of mononuclear cells and erythrocytes. Recovery is slow, usually proceeding over a period of 1 to 4 weeks. The mortality rate is extremely low (< 0.1%), with cardiac failure most often implicated as the immediate cause of death. Bullous myringitis (i.e., infection of the tympanic membrane and auditory meatus of the ear), characterized by serous and hemorrhagic blebs, occurs occasionally.

*Mycoplasma pneumoniae* has a strong affinity for mammalian cell membranes, as do other mycoplasmas. The organisms possess an adhesin protein by which they attach to a receptor present on the surface of epithelial cells within the respiratory tract. One epithelial cell may have many of these bacteria attached to it. The organisms are not invasive and remain extracellular. The mechanisms responsible for tissue damage are largely unknown. Cell-mediated immune responses, as well as antibodies that block adherence of the organisms to mucosal surfaces or inhibit their growth, are associated with resistance to infection.

Immunologic responses, however, may contribute to disease manifestations by inducing inflammation or cell infiltration and destruction of tissues. Infection with *M. pneumoniae* may cause **cold-agglutinin syndrome**, a condition characterized by very high serum titers of agglutinating IgM antibodies that react best at temperatures below 37°C (usually 4°–32°C). Cold agglutinin titers may be in the thousands or millions. The IgM is often directed against the I antigen of the Ii blood group system found on erythrocytes, although it may be anti-i or anti-Pr. This is an interesting phenomenon, especially because the I antigen has not been found on the organisms. Neurologic problems (mono- and polyneuritis) and arthritis have been well documented in a proportion of individuals following infection with the organisms. The clinical presentations associated with this species, as well as other mycoplasmas isolated from humans, are summarized in Table 23-2.

*Mycoplasma hominis* can be isolated from the genital tract of many asymptomatic individuals (30%–70% of women and 1%–5% of men). In sexually promiscuous individuals, rates of infection are approximately 90% and 20% for women and men, respectively. The evidence for a role in clinically apparent illness is largely indirect. The organisms are most strongly associated with salpingitis (infection of the uterine tubes) and tubo-ovarian abscesses. In addition, they have been isolated from the upper urinary tract of about 10% of women with pyelonephritis and the blood of approximately the same percentage of women with postabortal or postpartum fever. They have been occasionally found in joint fluid of patients with arthritis.

*Mycoplasma penetrans* is a new species that has been recently isolated from the urogenital tract of patients with AIDS. It may appear as an elongated flask-shaped organism with two compartments or filamentous and branching with blebs. It contains granules, some of which may be ribosomal structures. Although the identity of specific target cells in vivo is unclear, likely candidates are epithelial cells of the urinary, genital, and/or intesti-

| Table 23–2 ▶ Mycoplasmas Associated with Humans | |
| --- | --- |
| **Organism** | **Clinical Significance** |
| M. pneumoniae | Atypical pneumonia ("walking pneumonia"); is most common in young people<br>Classic pneumonia in elderly<br>Associated with adult respiratory distress syndrome (ARDS)<br>Associated with development of cold-agglutinin syndrome<br>Possible contributing factor in autoimmune demyelinative neuropathies<br>Possible factor in development of erythema multiforme (Stevens-Johnson syndrome) |
| M. hominis | Often isolated from genital tract of asymptomatic persons (especially women)<br>Possible cause of uterine tube infections and tubo-ovarian abscesses<br>Occasionally isolated from upper urinary tract of women with pyelonephritis |
| M. genitalium | Isolated occasionally from cases of nongonococcal urethritis<br>Possible contributing factor in development of polyarthritis |
| M. penetrans | Frequently isolated from patients with AIDS<br>Possible cofactor in development of AIDS |
| M. fermentans | Implicated in flu-like symptoms that rapidly progress to ARDS or systemic disease |
| M. salivarium | (Normal oropharyngeal flora) |
| M. orale | (Normal oropharyngeal flora) |
| U. urealyticum | Prevalent in genital tract of sexually active asymptomatic persons<br>Possible cause of nongonococcal urethritis<br>Possible cause of lung disease in premature infants<br>Possible role in spontaneous preterm labor and delivery<br>Possible role in reproductive failure continues to be unresolved |

nal tracts. Extensive invasion and intracellular multiplication may be responsible for subsequent death of host cells. Cytopathic effects can be noted as early as 24 hours after invagination by some cell types, whereas 2 to 5 days may be required for others.

*Ureaplasma urealyticum* is prevalent in the genital tract of sexually active asymptomatic men (5%–20%) and females (40%–80%). The organisms have been implicated in a variety of human illnesses, but a direct linkage has been difficult to prove in most instances. The organisms appear to be a probable cause of NGU in some men, although *C. trachomatis* is the etiologic agent in the majority of these cases. They may also be a cause of lung disease in premature infants of low birth weight who become infected during birth. Pharyngeal colonization with these organisms, as well as other genital mycoplasmas, is a relatively common occurrence in infants during the first few days after birth. Their importance in newborn infections, however, is debatable. Cervical colonization combined with midterm infection of the amniotic cavity and high titers of antibody against the organisms can occur in asymptomatic pregnant women. However, recent evidence suggests that the risk for spontaneous preterm labor and delivery and other complications is increased (even fatal deaths have been reported) under these conditions. The possible role of *U. ureaplasma* in sterility has long been debated and remains unresolved.

There are currently no approved vaccines available for any of the mycoplasmas. Several experimental preparations of killed *M. pneumoniae* have exacerbated the illness following subsequent infection with the organisms. Experimental genetically engineered vaccines are under investigation. An especially intriguing procedure is the use of a "gene gun" to inject mycoplasmal DNA incorporated into plasmids coated with gold or heavy tungsten particles into muscle. The technique has induced protective humoral and cellular immunity against *Mycoplasma* species in rodents.

## Cultural Characteristics and Identification

Typical specimens in cases of suspected mycoplasmal infection include sputum, throat swabs, urethral and genital secretions, and inflammatory exudates. The organisms are very difficult to identify in direct smears because of their small size, great pleomorphism, and poor staining with aniline dyes. Their morphology varies considerably depending on the examination technique and the medium used for cultivation. For example, in fluid media ring-shaped, bacillary, or spiral forms can be seen, whereas on solid media they usually appear as protoplasmic masses of ill-defined shape. Mycoplasmas generally require complex media for growth because of their limited biosynthetic capability. Many will grow in heart infusion peptone broth containing 2% agar that has been supplemented with 30% human ascitic fluid or serum from animals such as horses or rabbits. After an incubation period of 2 to 4 days at 37°C, Giemsa stains of centrifuged sediment will yield typical pleomorphic structures. Most species form characteristic **"fried egg" colonies** on solid media. A dense center due to organisms superficially embedded in the agar, as well as heaped up on top, surrounded by a thin peripheral area of growth give the colonies the appearance of fried eggs. The minute, round colonies (20–500 μm diameter) can seen with a hand lens on biphasic (broth over agar) medium after a 2 to 6 day incubation period. **T strains** (i.e., *U. urealyticum*) form very tiny colonies, usually not exceeding 20 to 30 μm in diameter.

The majority of *Mycoplasma* species use glucose as a source of energy, whereas *Ureaplasma* requires 10% urea for growth. *M. genitalium* is very difficult to culture. Its presence in specimens from some patients with NGU is largely based on positive results in the polymerase chain reaction (PCR) and in assays using molecular probes.

Cold agglutinins against human group O erythrocytes appear in approximately one-half of untreated individuals with *M. pneumoniae*. A titer of 1:64 or greater supports a diagnosis of mycoplasma infection. A rapid (< 1 hour) and relatively simple procedure for detecting serum antibodies against *M. pneumoniae* is now available from Seradyn (Indianapolis, IN, Color Vue™-*Mycoplasma pneumoniae*). All necessary reagents and appropriate controls can be ordered in kit form. The test uses high-density particles sensitized with a highly purified lipid antigen of the organisms. The sensitized particles cause passive agglutination in the presence of specific antibodies.

## Antibiotic Susceptibility Characteristics

Mycoplasmas are completely resistant to drugs such as penicillin that inhibit cell wall formation. Most are also resistant to cephalosporins and vancomycin. The drugs of choice for mycoplasmal pneumonia are the tetracyclines and erythromycins. Antibiotic therapy does not eradicate the organisms, but does produce some degree of clinical improvement. Clarithromycin has been recently shown to be as effective and safe as erythromycin for children over the age of 2 years. Pyelonephritis due to *M. hominis* has been successfully treated with doxycycline (a tetracycline). *M. penetrans* may require administration of one of the quinolones such as ciprofloxacin or levofloxacin. *M. fermentans* appears to be more susceptible to azithromycin to erythromycin. *U. urealitycum* may be resistant to tetracycline.

## Special Considerations for Immunocompromised Hosts

Several mycoplasmas have been recently isolated from patients with AIDS, including *M. penetrans, M. fermentans,* and *M. pirum.* A significantly higher than expected incidence of antimycoplasmal antibodies has also been reported in individuals who are seropositive for HIV-1. The correlation between mycoplasmal infection and infection with HIV-1 is especially strong in homosexual and bisexual populations. Because of these and other findings, a number of investigators have proposed that infection with *Mycoplasma* species, especially *M. penetrans,* may accelerate progression to a diagnosis of AIDS and/or enhance some of the symptoms associated with the disease. Supporting evidence for these contentions also comes from studies showing that mycoplasmas can promote the cytopathic effects of HIV-1, are potent immunomodulators capable of activating both T and B lymphocytes, possess superantigens, and can induce massive secretion of tumor necrosis factor-$\alpha$ (TNF-$\alpha$), interleukin-1 (IL-1), and other proinflammatory cytokines. Most recently, studies suggest that mycoplasmal membranes may play a direct role in the regulation of HIV-1 transcription. The increased prevalence of *M. penetrans* infection together with Kaposi's sarcoma (an angioproliferative disease) in homosexual patients with AIDs led to the suggestion some years ago that the mycoplasma might be the etiologic agent of the sarcoma. More recent studies, however, indicate that a newly discovered herpesvirus (known as human herpesvirus-8 or Kaposi's sarcoma-associated virus) is a likely factor in the development of the malignancy.

## *RICKETTSIA*

### Organism Characteristics

*Rickettsia* species have changed the history of mankind, during wars and natural disasters. The family (Rickettsiaceae) was named after Dr. Howard Ricketts, who worked with Rocky Mountain spotted fever (RMSF) and who died of typhus in 1910. The four genera in the family are *Rickettsia, Coxiella, Rochalimea,* and *Ehrlichia.*

All genera (except *Rochalimea*) are obligate intracellular parasites. They are highly fastidious, small gram-negative pleomorphic bacilli, ranging in size from 0.3 to 0.6 by 0.8 to 2 μm. These include mites, ticks, lice, and fleas. The reservoirs are warm-blooded hosts, including humans.

Their distribution is worldwide, with RMSF (1,000 cases per year), Q fever, murine typhus, and ehrlichiosis being present in the United States.

The organisms possess DNA and RNA. They contain ribosomes, allowing protein production, and have cell walls similar to other gram-negative bacteria. As such, they are susceptible to lysis by lysozyme. They divide by binary fission, and in cell culture, the generation time is 8 to 10 hours at 34°C. They stain poorly with Gram stain, appear blue with Giemsa's stain, and with Macchiavello's stain, they appear red in contrast to the surrounding blue-staining cytoplasm. **Gimenez stain** can be used to examine clinical material, and the organisms appear reddish black.

Rickettsiae lose their biologic properties when they are stored at 0°C or incubated for several hours at 36°C. This is due to the loss of nicotinamide adenine dinucleotide (NAD). Subsequent restoration of NAD will allow metabolism to resume. Typhus rickettsiae grow in the cytoplasm of host cells, while those of the spotted fever group grow in the nucleus. Coxiellae only grow in cytoplasmic vacuoles.

Rickettsial growth is enhanced in the presence of sulfa drugs, and diseases are more severe when these drugs are present. Tetracyclines will inhibit the growth of the organisms and can be therapeutically effective.

In general, rickettsiae are quickly destroyed by heat, drying, and bacteriocidal chemicals. Although the organisms generally die quickly when stored at ambient temperature, dried feces of infected lice may remain infective for months at room temperature. Two major antigens exist. One is an ether-soluble group specific (capsular) antigen and the other is type-specific (cell wall).

Laboratory diagnosis, in most cases, depends on the demonstration of specific antibodies in serum specimens and an increase in antibody titer as the disease progresses. Although DFA can demonstrate antigen in tissue specimens, few laboratories offer this service.

Rickettsiae share antigens with other bacteria. The antigens shared with *Proteus* form the basis of the Weil-Felix agglutination test. *Proteus vulgaris* strains OX-19, OX-2, and OC-K are used. The standard **Weil-Felix reactions** are shown in Table 23-3. The test is limited

| Table 23–3 ▶ Weil-Felix Agglutination Reaction | | | |
|---|---|---|---|
| Disease | OX-19 | OX-2 | OX-K |
| Murine typhus (endemic) | 4+ | 1+ | 0 |
| Scrub typhus | 0 | 0 | 4+ |
| Rocky Mountain spotted fever | 4+ | + | 0 |
| Q Fever | 0 | 0 | 0 |
| Erhlichiosis | 0 | 0 | 0 |

by many false-positive results, but it is convenient and can be performed in any laboratory.

## Clinical Significance

The pathology of rickettsial infection begins when organisms multiply in endothelial cells of small blood vessels at the site of the vector's blood meal and inoculation. They disseminate, and the symptoms include fever (due to the thrombosis of small vessels rupture and necrosis), rash (vascular lesions in the skin), and typhus nodules (aggregation of lymphocytes, polymorphonuclear cells, and macrophages in the brain, heart, kidney, and skin). **Rickettsemia** occurs in humans during the febrile period of all diseases.

Many infections are **zoonoses**, diseases of animals transmitted to man. The vectors include the human body louse (reservoir—humans), lice, flea and ticks (rats, rabbit, dogs), and mites (house mouse, wild rodents). Human infections are usually accidental breaks in the chain. The typhus group includes:

1. Epidemic typhus (Old World typhus) is caused by *R. prowazekii*. Humans are the reservoir and the human body louse (*Pediculus humanus*) is the vector. Louse feces containing rickettsia is scratched into breaks in the skin. Symptoms include rash on the trunk, 104°F fever, chills, malaise, vomiting, stupor, and delirium. Mortality rates may reach 30%.
2. Brill-Zinsser disease (benign-typhus) is a reactivation of an old typhus infection, resulting from a latent infection of *R. prowazekii,* which may last for years in lymph nodes. A variety of events (stress, cortisone, malnutrition) may trigger the emergence, and the disease is milder than that seen in epidemic typhus.
3. Endemic typhus (murine typhus) is caused by *R. typhi*. Rodents are the reservoir, and fleas are the vectors. The disease presentation is similar to epidemic typhus, with a lower mortality rate (5%). It can be found in the southeastern United States, Mexico, South America, Africa, and Southern Europe.

The spotted fever group includes:

1. Rocky Mountain spotted fever (RMSF—New World fever) is caused by *R. rickettsii*. The reservoir includes rodents, rabbits, birds, and dogs, and disease is transmitted by a tick bite. The organism may be passed from tick to tick, transovariantly. RMSF represents one of the most important arthropod-borne infectious diseases in the United States. Symptoms include a rash of severe necrotic foci, headache, fever, chills, and gastrointestinal symptoms. Cutaneous lesions on the palms and soles are a distinctive feature of the disease. The mortality rate is about 3% to 5%.
2. Rickettsial pox (Russian vesicular rickettosis) is caused by *R. akari,* with the house mouse serving as the reservoir. The mouse mite serves as the vector. There is a rash and the disease is relatively mild. It is seen sporadically in the United States (180 cases per year), in Russia, Korea, and South Africa.

The scrub typhus group is caused by *R. tsutsugamushi*. Small mild rodents and birds are the reservoir, and disease is transmitted by the chigger-mite. There is an eschar lesion at the site of the bite, sudden illness, fever, and rash. Mortality may reach 40%. Areas include Japan, Southeast Asia, and the Southwest Pacific.

Q fever (Q = query—Queensland, Australia) is caused by *Coxiella burnetti*. This organism stains gram-positive and enters the host cell in a phagosome, where it remains without lysosomal digestion. It exhibits phase variations, is resistant to drying and pasteurization. Cattle, sheep, goats, and small mammals are the reservoir, and disease is usually transmitted by a tick bite. However, human infection frequently occurs by inhalation of an infected aerosol. Q fever exhibits no rash or local lesions. There is an abrupt headache, chills, fever, and visceral involvement. It may resemble an influenza infection. The organisms are present in urine, sputum, and blood. The illness may last for months.

Trench fever is caused by *Rochalimaea quintana*. It is located extracellularly and can be cultivated on cell-free media. Humans are the reservoir, and the vector is the body louse. There is a roseolar rash, with headache, sweating, and fever. Relapses occur routinely.

Ehrlichiosis is caused by *Ehrlichia chaffeensis* in the southern United States and by *Ehrlichia canis*. Ticks are the vector, and the disease is similar to RMSF. The rash is usually absent. The organisms infect circulating leukocytes, and diagnosis is confirmed by observing **inclusion bodies** in white blood cells.

## Cultural Characteristics and Identification

Isolation of rickettsiae is technically difficult and is of limited usefulness in diagnosis. Whole blood may be inoculated into guinea pigs, mice, embryonated eggs, or tissue culture. The risk of laboratory-acquired infection is extremely high; therefore, isolation should not be performed by most laboratories.

The least specific, but most widely used test in the United States is the Weil-Felix reaction (see above). False-positive tests continue to be a problem. Commercial suppliers produce kits that contain all necessary antigens and control sera. It must be considered a presumptive test only.

Detection of complement fixing antibodies can be done. Q fever is routinely diagnosed by this method and group-reactive soluble antigens are available to test for the typhus group and the spotted fever group. The tests are usually performed by reference laboratories.

Biopsy specimens of skin tissue from a rash can be stained directly with a specific immunofluorescent reagent. It can provide a diagnosis of RMSF only a few days after symptoms have appeared. These tests are usually done by state public health laboratories.

Enzyme immunoassay tests are among the most sensitive tests to diagnose rickettsial diseases, especially if IgM is sought. The assays do require large amounts of antigen to be used in the tests.

## Antibiotic Susceptibility Characteristics

Tetracyclines and chloramphenicol are effective if treatment is started early. These are given orally and continued for 3 to 4 days past the fever drop. In severely ill patients, the initial treatment may have to be given intravenously. Some fluoroquinolones (ciprofloxacin) are effective in spotted fevers. *Sulfonamides* enhance the disease and are *contraindicated*. Antibiotics appear to be bacteriostatic, and final elimination of the organisms from the body is dependent on the patient's immune system.

## SUMMARY

- ▶ Chlamydia is the most common sexually transmitted disease in the United States, infecting several million people each year.
- ▶ *Chlamydiae* have a unique growth cycle, involving elementary bodies, phagosomes, and reticulate bodies.
- ▶ *C. trachomatis* causes trachoma, inclusion conjunctivitis, lymphogranuloma venereum, nongonococcal urethritis, and pelvic inflammatory disease.
- ▶ *C. psittaci* infections in humans are rare, involving the upper respiratory tract, while *C. pneumoniae* (TWAR) is the cause of approximately 20% of community-acquired pneumonia in young people.
- ▶ Elementary bodies are most often detected today with an ELISA assay.
- ▶ Mycoplasmas are highly pleomorphic bacteria that are found in nature, animals, plants, and humans. They are the smallest free-living organisms that do not require cells for multiplication.
- ▶ *M. pneumoniae* is an important cause of primary atypical pneumonia ("walking" pneumonia) in young people. It is also associated with other types of clinical manifestations including bullous myringitis, adult respiratory distress syndrome (ARDS), cold-agglutinin syndrome, and erythema multiforme (Stevens-Johnson syndrome).
- ▶ *M. hominis* can be isolated from the genital tract of many healthy individuals, but has been implicated in infections such as salpingitis and tubo-ovarian abscesses. *M. genitalium* and *U. urealyticum* are possible causes of nongonococal urethritis (NGU). *M. fermentans* may cause flu-like symptoms and ARDS. *M. salivarium* and *M. orale* are normal flora of the oral cavity. *M. penetrans,* a relatively new species, has been found primarily in patients with AIDS.
- ▶ Sputum, throat swabs, urethral and genital secretions, and inflammatory exudates are typical specimens sent to the clinical laboratory for culture of mycoplasmas. Complement fixation, hemagglutination inhibition, counterimmunoelectrophoresis, and indirect immunofluorescence methods are also available for laboratory diagnosis.
- ▶ Tetracyclines and erythromycins are the drugs of choice for mycoplasma infections.
- ▶ Rickettsia are small bacteria that are mostly obligate intracellular parasites, transferred to humans by insect vectors.
- ▶ Tetracyclines or chloramphenicol inhibit the growth of rickettsiae and can be therapeutically effective.
- ▶ Cross reactions of rickettsial antibodies with specific strains of *Proteus vulgaris* antigens has been the traditional method of diagnosing rickettsial diseases, although fluorescent antibody tests and ELISAs are currently more effective.
- ▶ The typhus groups of diseases include epidemic typhus, murine typhus, and scrub typhus. The spotted fever group of diseases include Rocky Mountain spotted fever, rickettsial pox, and others found worldwide. *Coxiella burnetti* causes Q fever and is spread by airborne fomites; *Ehrlichia chaffeensis* causes ehrlichiosis and is transmitted by a tick.

## CASE STUDY: PRIMARY ATYPICAL PNEUMONIA IN A CHILD

A 12-year-old girl was admitted with fever, a persistent nonproductive cough, and night sweats; she appeared mildly dyspneic. Four weeks previously, the patient had been well. During the course of illness, she experienced episodic pain in the subscapular region and shoulder. On admission her vital signs were: temperature, 38.5°C; pulse 98/min; respirations, 29/min; and blood pressure, 125/65 mm Hg. Other laboratory tests indicated a leukocyte count of $6.3 \times 10^9$/L, white blood cell populations within normal limits, an increased blood sedimentation rate, and a high value for C-reactive protein. Chest radiographs showed bilateral lower lobe involvement. Blood cultures were negative and routine cultures of bronchial washings revealed no pathogens. An immunoblot for anti-I IgM was strongly positive and a complement fixation assay gave a serum antibody titer of >1:512 using *M. pneumoniae* antigen. Oral erythromycin and intravenous cefuroxime were administered. The patient turned afebrile within 2 days; improvement was slow, but uneventful. She was discharged from the hospital 5 days after admission.

**Questions:**

1. What does the strong positive for IgM antibodies suggest?

2. Is a slow recovery typical for pneumonia due to *M. pneumoniae*?

3. Is the patient immune to *M. pneumoniae* after this episode of illness?

## Review Questions

1. *Chlamydia trachomatis* is implicated in all of the following disease states, EXCEPT:
   a. mucopurulent cervicitis.
   b. lymphogranuloma venereum.
   c. nongonococcal urethritis.
   d. persistent unproductive cough.

2. An adequate specimen for chlamydial isolation and identification should contain:
   a. T helper lymphocytes.
   b. polymorphonuclear leukocytes.
   c. monocytes/macrophages.
   d. epithelial cells.

3. Which of the following is NOT associated with *Chlamydia trachomatis?*
   a. Intraphagosome growth
   b. Iodine-negative intracytoplasmic inclusions
   c. Obligate intracellular procaryote, which is culturable in McCoy cells
   d. Susceptible to doxycycline and erythromycin

4. Which of the following are the smallest microbes capable of cell-free reproduction?
   a. *Mycoplasma* species
   b. *Rickettsia* species
   c. *Chlamydia* species
   d. Viruses

5. Cold agglutinins that frequently appear following infection with *Mycoplasma pneumoniae* belong to which class of antibody?
   a. IgG
   b. IgA
   c. IgM
   d. IgD

6. Which of the following organisms is MOST LIKELY to cause atypical pneumonia in a child?
   a. *Mycoplasma pneumoniae*
   b. *Mycoplasma hominis*
   c. *Mycoplasma salivarium*
   d. *Mycoplasma orale*

7. Which of the following rickettsia can be cultivated on a cell-free medium?
   a. *R. prowazekii*
   b. *R. quintana*
   c. *R. akari*
   d. *C. burnettii*

**8.** A patient presenting with a generalized papulovesicular rash, eschars, and a comment of association with wild rodents and *mite* bites is suspect of having:

a. Rocky Mountain spotted fever
b. Ehrlichiosis
c. Trench fever
d. Scrub typhus

**9.** The organism *Coxiella burnetti* is the causative agent of:

a. murine typhus.
b. Q fever.
c. Rocky Mountain spotted fever.
d. Rickettsialpox.

▶ **REFERENCES & RECOMMENDED READING**

Barnes, R. C. (1989). Laboratory diagnosis of human chlamydial infections. *Clinical Microbiology Reviews, 2,* 119.

Barry, M. A., Lai, W. C., & Johnston, S. A. (1995). Protection against mycoplasma infection using expression-library immunization. *Nature, 377,* 632–635.

Block, S., Hedrick, J., Hammerschlag, M. R., Cassell, G. H., & Craft, J. C. (1995). *Mycoplasma pneumoniae* and *Chlamydia pneumoniae* in pediatric community-acquired pneumonia: Comparative efficacy and safety of clarithromycin vs erythromycin ethylsuccinate. *Pediatric Infectious Disease Journal, 14,* 471–447.

Check, W. A. (1996). Choosing the best Chlamydia trap. *CAP Today, 10*(12), 1.

Clyde, W. A., Kenny, G. E., & Schacter, J. (1984). *Cumitech 19: Laboratory diagnosis of chlamydial and mycoplasmal infections.* Washington, DC: American Society for Microbiology.

Cole, B. C., & Atkin, C. L. (1991). The *Mycoplasma arthritidis* T-cell mitogen, MAM: A model superantigen. *Immunology Today, 12,* 271–276.

Fraiz, J., & Jones, B. R. (1988). Chlamydial infections. *Annual Review of Medicine, 39,* 357.

Giron, J. A., Lange, M., & Baseman, J. B. (1996). Adherence, fibronectin binding, and induction of cytoskeleton reorganization in cultured human cells by *Mycoplasma penetrans. Infection and Immunity, 64,* 197–208.

Goulet, M., Dular, R., Tully, J. G., Billowes, G., & Kasatiya, S. (1995). Isolation of *Mycoplasma pneumoniae* from the human urogenital tract. *Journal of Clinical Microbiology, 33,* 2823–2825.

Grau, O., Slizewicz, B., Tuppin, P., Launay, V., Bourgeois, E., Sagot, N., Moynier, M., Lafeuillade, A., Bachelez, H., Clauvel, J.-P., Blanchard, A., Bahraoui, E., & Montagnier, L. (1995). Association of *Mycoplasma penetrans* with human immunodeficiency virus infection. *Journal of Infectious Disease, 172,* 672–681.

Hammerschlag, M. R. (1995). Atypical pneumonias in children. *Advances in Pediatric Infectious Diseases, 10,* 1–39.

Hayes, M. M., Foo, H. H., Timinetsky, J., & Lo, S.-C. (1995). In vitro antibiotic susceptibility testing of clinical isolates of *Mycoplasma penetrans* from patients with AIDS. *Antimicrobial Agents and Chemotherapy, 39,* 1386–1387.

Hechemy, K. E. (1979). Laboratory diagnosis of Rocky Mountain spotted fever. *New England Journal of Medicine, 300,* 859.

Horowitz, S., Mazor, M., Romero, R., Horowitz, J., & Glezerman, M. (1995). Infection of the amniotic cavity with *Ureaplasma urealyticum* in the midtrimester of pregnancy. *Journal of Reproductive Medicine, 40,* 375–379.

Kotb, M. (1995). Bacterial pyrogenic exotoxins as superantigens. *Clinical Microbiology Reviews, 8,* 411–426.

Lai, W. C., Bennett, M., Johnston, S. A., Barry, M. A., & Pakes S. P. (1995). Protection against *Mycoplasma pulmonis* infection by genetic vaccination. *DNA and Cell Biology, 14,* 743–751.

Lo, S.-C. (1992). Mycoplasma and AIDS. In: J. Maniloff, R.Nn McElhaney, L. R. Finch, & J. B. Baseman (Eds.), *Mycoplasmas: Molecular biology and pathogenesis* (pp. 525–545). Washington, DC: ASM.

Lo, S.-C., Hayes, M. M., Tully, J. G., Wang, R. Y.-H., Kotani, H., Pierce, P. F., Rose, D. L., & Shih, J. W.-K. *Mycoplasma penetrans* sp. nov. From the urogenital tract of patients with AIDS. *International Journal of Systematic Bacteriology, 42,* 357–364.

McDade, J. E. (1990). Ehrlichosis: A disease of animals and humans. *Journal of Infectious Disease, 161,* 609.

McDade, J. E. (1991). Rickettsiae. In: A. Balows, W. J. Hausler, K. L. Hermann, H. D. Isenberg, & H. J. Shadomy (Eds.), *Manual of clinical microbiology* (5th ed., 1036–1044). Washington, DC: American Society for Microbiology.

Mundy, L. M., Auwaerter, P. G., Oldach, D., Warner, M. L., Burton, A., Vance, E., Gaydos, C. A., Joseph, J. M., Gopalan, R., Moore, R. D., et al. (1995). Community-acquired pneumonia: Impact of immune status. *American Journal of Respiratory and Critical Care Medicine, 152,* 1309–1315.

Nir-Paz, R., Israel, S., Honigman, A., & Kahane, I. (1995). Mycoplasmas regulate HIV-LTR-dependent gene expression. *FEMS Microbiology Letters, 128,* 63–68.

Razin, S. (1994). DNA probes and PCR in diagnosis of mycoplasma infections. *Molecular and Cellular Probes, 8,* 497–511.

Schacter, J. (1991). Chlamydiae. In: A. Balows, W. J. Hausler, K. L. Hermann, H. D. Isenberg, & H. J. Shadomy (Eds.), *Manual of clinical microbiology* (5th ed., pp. 1045–1054). Washington, DC: American Society for Microbiology.

Sexton, D. J., et al. (1991). Spotted fever group rickettsial infections in Australia. *Reviews in Infectious Disease, 13,* 876.

Thacker, W. L., Talkington, D. F. (1995). Comparison of two rapid commercial tests with complement fixation for serologic diagnosis of *Mycoplasma pneumoniae* infections. *Journal of Clinical Microbiology, 33,* 1212–1214.

Voelker, L. L., Weaver, K. E., Ehle, L. J., & Washburn, L. R. (1995). Association of lysogenic bacteriophage MAV1 with virulence of *Mycoplasma arthritidis. Infection and Immunity, 63,* 4016–4023.

Wang, R. Y. H., Shih J. W. K., Grandinetti, T., et al. (1992). High frequency of antibodies to *Mycoplasma penetrans* in HIV-infected patients. *Lancet, 340,* 1312–1316.

# Part Two:
# Isolation and Interpretation of Bacteria from Clinical Specimens

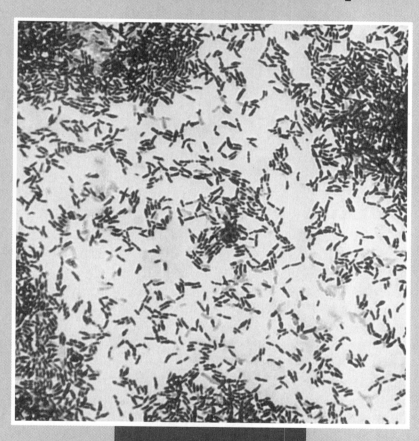

# CHAPTER 24
# Processing and Interpretation of Cultures from Clinical Specimens

Susan M. Barber, BS, MT (ASCP), SM

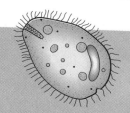

## Microbes in the News

*Escherichia coli* O157:H7 has been in the headlines over the last several years as an important pathogen responsible for outbreaks of enteric disease after consumption of undercooked beef contaminated with the organism. In January 1993, in Washington state, there was a large outbreak, mostly in children, with typical acute, bloody diarrhea. Many of these children developed hemolytic uremic syndrome, in which the renal capillaries collapse, and kidney function is severely impaired. This complication is most severe in young children and the elderly. An even more serious complication, usually affecting young adults, is thrombotic thrombocytopenic purpura, in which multiple platelet aggregates interfere with the function of many organ systems. This is frequently rapidly fatal. The disease symptoms associated with this organism are the result of toxins known as Shiga-like toxins or verotoxins.

One positive result of these outbreaks is that many laboratories have modified their procedures for stool culture such that *E. coli* O157:H7 will be sought from all stool specimens, or at least from bloody diarrhea specimens (see Figure 24-1). Unfortunately, several other serotypes of this organism can cause similar disease, and these may not be detected by the methods that detect O157:H7. In 1994, in Montana, there was a small outbreak of bloody diarrhea which was found to be due to *E. coli* O104:H21, which produces toxins similar to those produced by O157:H7. Several other serotypes have also been associated with bloody diarrhea.

Microbiologists are continuing to search for rapid, practical, accurate methods for detection and identification of these other serotypes of *E. coli*. Already, commercial kits are available for the detection of the toxin itself in the stool specimen.

## KEY TERMS

Anaerobic culture
Antibodies
Aseptically
ß-hemolysis
Bright-field microscope
cfu (colony forming units)
Clinical specimen
Colonize (colonization)
Commensals
Conventional
Cost effective
Dark-field microscope
Definitive identification

Descriptive identification
Endemic
Exogenously
Facultative
Fluorescent microscope
Hematogenously
Inflammatory cells
Macroscopic
Microaerophilic
Mucoid
Nonlactose fermenter
Normal flora
Palisades

Pathogenic
Patient population
Pleomorphic
Polymorphonuclear leuko-
    cytes (PMNs)
Presumptive identification
Pure culture
Rapid screening methods
Reference laboratory
Selective media
Sputum
Subculture

## LEARNING OBJECTIVES

**Upon successful completion of this chapter, the student should be able to:**

1. Describe the common types of direct examinations used for various clinical specimens.

2. Understand the utility of different culture protocols.

3. Describe types of resident flora found in various parts of the body.

4. Understand the difference between presumptive and definitive identification and their applications.

5. Describe the process of interpreting cultures from various clinical specimens.

## INTRODUCTION

It is essential that laboratories have defined procedures outlining the handling of various types of specimens, both for routine and special testing. This chapter covers the factors that must be considered in establish-

ing these procedures. In addition, this chapter reviews basic guidelines for defining the extent of identifying and reporting isolates from different specimen types.

## MICROSCOPIC EXAMINATION OF SPECIMENS

### Usefulness of Microscopic Examination

Direct microscopic examination of **clinical specimens** can be an extremely valuable adjunct to culture. A correctly performed microscopic examination of a properly collected specimen can provide the physician with the first clue to the etiology of an infectious disease (see Figure 24-2). Depending on the type of staining performed, results are available in a few minutes to a few hours after the specimen is received in the laboratory. Bacterial cultures generally require at least 12 to 18 hours of incubation before any preliminary results are available. Physicians can often prescribe antibiotic treatment based on the results of the microscopic examinations one or more days earlier than would be possible if they waited for the culture results (refer to Color Plates 57 and 58).

Microscopic examinations are also relatively simple

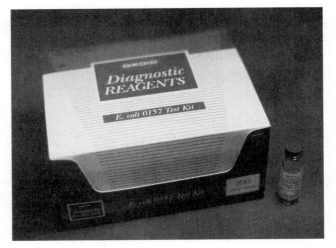

**FIGURE 24-1** A latex agglutination kit and antiserum reagent are two products that may be used in identification of *E. coli* O157 from stool specimens.

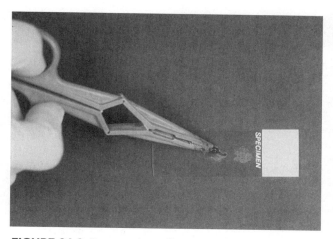

**FIGURE 24-2** Preparation of a smear for direct examination of a tissue specimen.

to perform. Most do not require expensive or elaborate equipment, and most require only a few simple, readily available reagents. Although some expertise is required for reading and interpretation, microscopic examinations are relatively straightforward. Compared to culture, microscopic examinations are very **cost effective**. The results of microscopic examinations, however, generally must be confirmed by culture.

## Types of Direct Microscopic Examination

Many simple procedures can be applied to a clinical specimen to allow direct microscopic detection of various types of organisms.

**Wet Mount.** A wet mount (see Chapter 11) is prepared by emulsifying the specimen in saline, placing a drop on a slide, and adding a coverslip. It is then examined with a **bright-field microscope** under reduced light. This technique is often performed on vaginal secretions and will allow detection of yeast, the protozoan *Trichomonas,* and clue cells. Clue cells are vaginal epithelial cells that are almost or completely covered with small, **pleomorphic** bacilli. They are associated with bacterial vaginosis, a condition in which the vaginal flora is abnormally altered.

**Dark-Field Examination.** The dark-field examination is similar to the wet mount, except that it requires the use of a **dark-field microscope**. Historically, this technique was used on preparations of genital lesion exudates to diagnose syphilis. The causative agent, *Treponema pallidum,* is a motile spirochete that can be detected by this method (refer to Color Plate 59). These organisms, however, are extremely susceptible to environmental conditions and do not survive long outside of the host. This, along with the lack of availability of dark-field microscopes in many laboratories, has made this technique less popular than it was in the

past. Today, syphilis is most often diagnosed with blood tests that detect an immune response to the infection.

**Gram Stain.** The Gram stain is the most frequently performed direct microscopic examination in the clinical laboratory. For most types of specimens, a Gram stain should automatically be performed and reported as part of the culture. Bacteria will stain either gram-positive (purple) or gram-negative (pink to red) depending on the chemical composition of their cell walls (see Chapter 11). Additionally, patient cells present in the specimen will be detected on a Gram smear. **Polymorphonuclear leukocytes (PMNs)** (refer to Color Plate 57) are **inflammatory cells** whose presence usually indicates that the specimen was collected from an area where an infection or some other inflammatory process is present. Squamous epithelial cells (refer to Color Plate 60) are normal host cells that line mucous membranes and other surfaces. It is possible to assess the "quality" of a specimen by comparing the relative numbers of PMNs and epithelial cells. Specimens with a high ratio of PMNs to epithelial cells were probably collected from a true area of infection, and all bacteria isolated from these specimens could be considered significant. Specimens with a low ratio of PMNs to epithelial cells are more likely to contain contaminants, and it is much more difficult to interpret the significance of isolated organisms.

When reading Gram stains of clinical specimens, the quantities of all bacteria seen should be reported, as well as their Gram stain reaction and arrangement ("few gram-positive cocci in pairs"). PMNs, epithelial cells, and other patient cells (red blood cells, mononuclear cells, etc.) should also be noted and quantitated.

**Acid-Fast Stains.** The acid-fast stains (see Chapter 11) are used for the detection of the organisms in the *Mycobacterium* genus. The chemical structure of these organisms' cell walls allows them to retain certain stains even when rinsed with acid solutions. These organisms can take several weeks to grow in culture and are not readily detected by Gram stain. In recent years, many strains of *Mycobacterium tuberculosis* have become resistant to numerous antibiotics, and are therefore difficult to treat. Early detection, as made possible by performing an acid fast stain of **sputum** or other specimens, can help ensure that patients infected with these organisms are put on antibiotic therapy as soon as possible.

There are several variations of the acid-fast stain. The classic Ziehl-Neelsen method requires that the slide be heated while staining. A modification of this is the cold Kinyoun acid-fast stain. Another method, the auramine-rhodamine stain, uses a fluorescent stain and is read using a **fluorescent microscope**. This offers the advantage that the slides can be read at a lower magnification and are therefore less time consuming to read than Ziehl-Neelsen or Kinyoun stains.

## Table 24–1 ▶ Common Bacteriologic Primary Plating Media

| Medium | Additives, Inhibitors, Etc. | Purpose, Comments |
|---|---|---|
| BAP (blood agar plate) TSA, Brucella, or beef heart infusion base | 5% sheep blood | General all-purpose medium, good for isolation of most pathogens. Sheep blood allows for differentiation of hemolysis. |
| BBE (Bacteroides bile esculin) | Bile salts, gentamicin, ferric ammonium citrate, hemin | Selective for *Bacteroides* species; esculin hydrolysis indicated by ferric ammonium citrate. |
| BCYE (buffered charcoal yeast extract) | Yeast extract, charcoal, L-cystine, ferric pyrophosphate, α-ketoglutarate. Some formulations supplemented with vancomycin, colistin, anisomycin, cefamandole | Selects for and supports growth of nutritionally fastidious *Legionella* species. |
| Bismuth sulfite | Dextrose, brilliant green, bismuth sulfite, ferrous sulfate | Brilliant green and bismuth sulfite inhibit gram positives and *Enterobacteriaceae* other than *Salmonella typhi* and other *Salmonella* species; $H_2S$ production indicated by ferrous sulfate. |
| Campy BAP | Brucella base with 5% sheep blood; contains vancomycin, trimethoprim, polymyxin B, amphotericin B, cephalothin | Antibiotics select for enteropathogenic *Campylobacter* species. |
| CCFA (cycloserine-cefoxitin-fructose-egg yolk agar) | Cycloserine, cefoxitin, fructose, egg yolk, neutral red | Selects for *Clostridium difficile*; neutral red indicates fructose fermentation; egg yolk indicates lecithinase and lipase reactions. |
| CDC anaerobic blood agar | 5% sheep blood, hemin, L-cystine, vitamin $K_1$ | Supports growth of anaerobes. |
| Chocolate agar | 2% hemoglobin or IsoVitaleX (BBL) | Enriched for isolation of nutritionally fastidious species such as *Haemophilus* species, *Neisseria gonorrhoeae*. |
| CIN (cefsulodin-igrasin-novobiocin agar) | Cefsulodin, irgasan, novobiocin, mannitol, bile salts, neutral red, crystal violet | Selects for *Yersinia* species; mannitol fermentation indicated by neutral red. |
| Columbia CNA blood agar | Columbia agar base with 5% sheep blood, plus colistin and nalidixic acid | Inhibits gram-negative organisms; selects for gram-positive organisms. |
| Cystine-tellurite blood agar | 5% sheep blood, potassium tellurite | For isolation of *Corynebacterium diphtheriae*; potassium tellurite reduction indicated by black colonies. |
| Eosin methylene blue | Lactose, sucrose, eosin, methylene blue | Differentiates lactose/sucrose fermenters. Levine modification has only lactose. |
| GN broth (gram-negative broth) | Sodium citrate, sodium descoycholate | Selects and enriches for *Salmonella, Shigella* species. |
| Hektoen enteric | Bile salts, lactose, sucrose, salicin, ferrous ammonium citrate, bromthymol blue, acid fuchsin | Bile salts select for *Enterobacteriaceae*; fermentation of sugars indicated by bromthymol blue and acid fuchsin; $H_2S$ production indicated by ferrous ammonium citrate. |
| LKV (laked blood-kanamycin-vancomycin) | Brucella base with laked blood, kanamycin, vancomycin, vitamin $K_1$ | Selects for *Bacteroides* species. |
| MacConkey | Bile salts, crystal violet, lactose, neutral red | Inhibitors select for gram-negative organisms. Neutral red indicates lactose fermentation. |
| MacConkey-sorbitol | Bile salts, crystal violet, sorbitol, neutral red | Inhibitors select for gram-negative organisms. Neutral red indicates sorbitol fermentation. Good for isolation of *Escherichia coli* O157 from stools. |
| Martin Lewis | GC agar base with vancomycin, colistin, anisomycin, trimethoprim | Selective for pathogenic *Neisseria* species. |
| New York City | GC agar base with vancomycin, colistin, amphotericin, trimethoprim | Selective for pathogenic *Neisseria* species; also may allow some *Mycoplasma* species to grow |
| PEA | PEA (phenylethyl alcohol) | Inhibits gram-negative organisms. Useful for isolation of aerobic and anaerobic gram-positive organisms. |
| Salmonella Shigella | Lactose, ferric citrate, sodium citrate, neutral red, brilliant green, bile salt | Brilliant green and bile salts select for *Salmonella* and *Shigella* species. Neutral red indicates lactose fermentation; $H_2S$ production indicated by ferrous citrate. |
| Selenite broth | Selenium salts | Selects and enriches for *Salmonella* species. |
| TCBS (thiosulfate-citrate-bile-salts) | Bile salts, sucrose, ferric citrate, sodium thiosulfate, bromthymol blue | Selects for *Vibrio* species, sucrose fermentation indicated by bromthymol blue indicator. |
| Thayer-Martin | GC agar base with hemoglobin; contains vancomycin, colistin, nystatin, trimethoprim | Selective for pathogenic *Neisseria* species. |
| Thioglycollate broth | Thioglycollate, agar | Oxygen potential reduced by thioglycollate and agar to allow growth of anaerobes as well as aerobes, microaerophiles. |

### Table 24–2 ▶ Sample Guide to Appropriate Primary Plating Media

| | BAP | CHOC | MAC or EMB | PEA or CNA | Thai or other broth | Anaer. plates: BBA or CDC, LKV, PEA | Anaer. broth: Thio or CMC | SS, HE, XLD (two) | Other |
|---|---|---|---|---|---|---|---|---|---|
| Abscess, pus, wound, tissue | X | X | X | X | X | X | X | | Anaerobes if deep wound, abscess, tissue; not on superficial wounds |
| Joint fluid | X | X | | | X | | | | Anaerobes may be appropriate in some cases. |
| CSF | X | X | | | X | | | | |
| Urine | X | | X | | | | | | Plant quantitatively |
| Other body fluids | X | X | X | X | X | X | X | | Specific body fluids may vary in what is appropriate. |
| Catheter tips | X | | | | X | | | | Roll tip across BAP to get colony count. |
| Ear | X | X | X | X | X | | | | |
| Eye | X | X | | | X | | | | |
| Genital | X | X | X | X | | | | | Also set TM or other selective medium for pathogenic *Neisseria* species; surgical specimens (uterus, fallopian tubes) need anaerobes. |
| Stool, colostomy contents, etc. | | | X | X | | | | X | Add Campy BAP or other selective medium to isolate *Campylobacter* species; Add MacConkey-sorbitol for detection of *E. coli* O157. |
| Respiratory (tracheal, sputum, bronchial, etc.) | X | X | X | X | | | | | Surgical specimens (sinus, etc.) need anaerobes. Throat does not need MAC/EMB, and does not need CHOC unless *N. gonorrhoeae* requested. |

X, medium recommended for that specimen site.

BAP, blood agar plate; CHOC, chocolate agar plate; MAC, MacConkey agar plate; EMB, eosin methylene blue plate; PEA, phenylethyl alcohol agar plate; CNA, Columbia colistin-nalidixic acid agar; Thio, thioglycollate broth; BBA, Brucella blood agar; CDC, CDC blood agar; LKV, laked kanamycin-vancomycin blood agar; CMC, chopped meat carbohydrate broth; SS, Salmonella-Shigella agar; HE, Hektoen enteric agar; XLD, xylose-lysine desoxycholate agar.

**Modified Acid-Fast Stain.** The modified acid-fast stain is a variation of the Ziehl-Neelsen or Kinyoun acid-fast stain; it uses a slightly weaker decolorizer. This stain is useful for detecting *Nocardia* and related species, which may be present in a variety of specimens.

**Fluorescent Antibody Stains.** Fluorescent antibody stains consist of a fluorescent dye that is bound to specific **antibodies** against a particular organism. When applied to smears of clinical specimens, the antibodies bind to the target organism present in the specimen, causing the organism to fluoresce when examined with a fluorescent microscope. There are many commercial fluorescent antibody stains available for the direct microscopic detection of various organisms, including *Legionella pneumophila*, *Bordetella pertussis*, *Streptococcus pyogenes*, and *Neisseria gonorrhoeae*.

## CONSIDERATIONS IN CHOOSING A CULTURE PROTOCOL

Many factors should be considered in choosing a culture protocol. It would be completely impractical to use every type of plating medium and all incubation conditions for every specimen. Culture protocols are established by each laboratory and are tailored to meet the needs of the patients and physicians using the laboratory's services. There are several common principles, however, that all laboratories use in determining how to culture each specimen. See Tables 24-1 and 24-2 for a description of common media and some suggested culture protocols.

## Type of Specimen

The main consideration in choosing a culture protocol is the type of specimen submitted. Each part of the body harbors different resident flora and can be infected by different potential pathogens. Culture protocols must be established with these factors in mind.

**Presence or Absence of Normal Flora.** Many parts of the body harbor a population of **normal flora**, which may interfere with the culture unless **selective media** are used. Sites such as blood, cerebrospinal fluid (CSF), deep body fluids, deep tissues, internal organs, and the like are normally sterile, so any organisms present could be significant. It is therefore not necessary to inoculate selective media from these sites because there is no normal flora to "screen out." Conversely, stool specimens contain numerous normal flora, and the aim of the stool culture is to isolate and identify only those organisms that may be causing disease. Highly selective media and techniques are therefore required for stool cultures. Other specimens, such as those from the respiratory tract, urogenital tract, eyes, and ears, are sometimes contaminated by normal flora and so require some selective media. Refer to the section entitled "Resident and Normal Flora" for a further description of the types of normal flora found in various anatomic sites.

**Anaerobic Bacteria.** In choosing a culture protocol, it is also necessary to evaluate the type of specimen to determine whether it is appropriate for **anaerobic culture**. Anaerobic bacteria are part of the normal flora in many areas of the body and cause infection when they invade adjacent areas. Specimens from normally sterile areas should be cultured for anaerobes. Specimens with normal anaerobic flora (gastrointestinal, genitourinary, skin, upper respiratory tract, eye, ear, nose) are generally not appropriate for anaerobic culture.

**Fastidious Organisms.** Some infections are caused by particularly fastidious organisms, which have special nutritional or environmental requirements. For this reason, the culture protocols for specimens that may harbor these organisms should be designed to meet these organisms' special needs.

## History and Clinical Status of the Patient

In addition to the type of specimen collected, it is necessary to consider the clinical status or medical condition of the patient when choosing a culture protocol. Patients with prosthetic devices such as artificial heart valves, for example, may harbor organisms not normally sought in patients without these devices. Patients who lack a normal immune system can become infected by organisms not normally considered pathogenic. Patients who have traveled to areas **endemic** for certain pathogens may be infected with agents not normally sought in the testing laboratory. Patients with unusual dietary habits may develop disease due to organisms not nor-

mally sought in standard culture protocols. For all of these reasons, it is essential that the clinician communicate any relevant patient information or special requests to the laboratory when specimens are submitted for culture. The culture protocol can then be adjusted to allow detection of all possible pathogens.

## Patient Population

Each laboratory serves a different and unique sector of the population. A large inner-city public hospital laboratory will have a vastly different **patient population** than a small private laboratory located in a retirement community. Laboratories must adjust their culture protocols to best serve the types of patients seen in their facility. For example, a laboratory that serves a large college-age population should have a complete set of procedures for the isolation of agents of sexually transmitted diseases (STDs). Laboratories serving populations with a low prevalence of STDs can have more limited protocols for these agents and may even choose to send such requests to a **reference laboratory**.

## Cost

Cost is a consideration in all aspects of laboratory work. In choosing the culture protocol, it is prudent to use the least expensive procedures that will still give acceptable results. Continual evaluation of products from different manufacturers may help keep the cost of media and supplies as low as feasible. Similarly, ongoing reevaluation of culture protocols may identify areas where cost can be reduced.

# RESIDENT AND NORMAL FLORA

The healthy human body is host to a large and varied population of normal flora. Under ordinary circumstances, these bacteria live within and on the body in harmony with each other and with the host. Trauma, malignancy, chemical imbalances, immune disorders, stress, and other factors can cause these **commensals** to invade areas they usually do not invade or to cause disease in their usual sites, where they normally do no harm. It is important, therefore, to know what these normal flora organisms are and where they are usually found. When one of these agents is isolated, it is necessary to evaluate the patient's condition, the method used to collect the specimen, and the results of other laboratory tests to determine the significance of the isolate.

## Respiratory Tract

Many species are frequently present in varying numbers in the upper respiratory tract of a healthy host. The most frequently isolated of these are the nonhemolytic streptococci, staphylococci and micrococci, nonpathogenic *Neisseria* species, diphtheroids, and lactobacilli. Many more species can **colonize** the respiratory tract—they may be present in healthy hosts, but can cause disease, such as pneumonia, when various factors lower the host's resistance. Some of the more frequently isolated members of this group are the α- and ß-hemolytic streptococci, *Streptococcus pneumoniae, Staphylococcus aureus, Corynebacterium diphtheriae, Neisseria meningitidis, Haemophilus, Moraxella catarrhalis, Klebsiella, Pseudomonas,* and anaerobic bacteria.

## Urinary Tract

The epithelial cells of the healthy urinary tract below the bladder host a large number of resident flora. α-Hemolytic and nonhemolytic streptococci, lactobacilli, diphtheroids, nonpathogenic *Neisseria* species, coagulase-negative staphylococci, and anaerobes all may be found. Some other species, such as enteric gram-negative rods, *Enterococcus,* and nonfermentative gram-negative rods may occasionally be present in small numbers without causing disease.

## Genital Tract

The mixed epithelial cells lining the healthy human genital tract are colonized by various organisms that ordinarily do no harm and may even prevent adherence and colonization by pathogens. The genital tract of postmenopausal women and young girls is colonized primarily by staphylococci and diphtheroids. Menstruating-age women harbor a population of lactobacilli, staphylococci, enterococci, enteric gram-negative rods, and anaerobes. Various streptococci, including group B ß-hemolytic *Streptococcus,* may also be present in the normal female genital tract. This is significant because this organism can be transmitted to a newborn on passage through the vagina, resulting in severe neonatal disease. The penis and vulva are generally colonized by a mixed population of gram-positive flora.

## Gastrointestinal Tract

The normal gastrointestinal tract has a vast population of resident flora. There is a predominance of anaerobes, along with mixed enteric gram-negative rods, nonfermentative gram-negative rods such as *Pseudomonas,* coagulase-negative staphylococci, enterococci, and streptococci. This population of normal flora plays an extremely important protective role. When antibiotic therapy or other factors upset the healthy ecology of the gastrointestinal tract, the patient is at risk to develop a severe disease known as pseudomembranous colitis. This disease occurs when *Clostridium difficile,* an organism that is normally present in small numbers, multiplies and produces toxin. The normal flora of a healthy gastrointestinal tract, however, ordinarily keeps the numbers of *C. difficile* down.

## Skin

The healthy human skin is colonized by a number of species. Diphtheroids, α-hemolytic and nonhemolytic streptococci, coagulase-negative staphylococci, lactobacilli, and other gram-positive rods, small numbers of enteric gram-negative rods, and anaerobes are all present. These organisms can contaminate various types of specimens if the skin is not properly decontaminated before the specimen is collected. CSF, joint aspirates, abscesses, and other specimens collected by using a syringe and needle all may be contaminated by skin flora during collection. Eye and ear specimens also may contain small numbers of these organisms under normal circumstances.

# PRESUMPTIVE AND DEFINITIVE IDENTIFICATION

Just as a microbiology laboratory must be able to accurately identify isolated organisms, they also need criteria to determine when a complete identification is appropriate. It would be wasting the laboratory's resources and be of no benefit to the patient if every type of organism from every type of specimen was fully identified. In fact, if every isolate were fully identified and reported, it would imply that the laboratory feels these isolates are significant, and the physician may then treat the patient with antibiotics when in fact no infection is present. Procedures defining the extent of work-up of different types of isolates from various specimen types are therefore essential.

## Use of Presumptive Identification

An identification is considered **presumptive identification** when all of the confirmatory tests have not been performed, but the identification is most likely correct based on all available data. In many circumstances, this is all that is required. Isolates from specimens containing mixed flora can usually be reported with presumptive identifications, as long as serious pathogens have been ruled out. Presumptive identifications often suffice when a confirmed identification is not required to direct antibiotic therapy. Presumptive identification is also appropriate when the presumed isolate is much more prevalent in the patient population than other related organisms with which it may be confused.

## Use of Definitive Identification

In certain circumstances, it is necessary to completely identify an isolate. **Definitive identification** is necessary when a **pure culture** of an organism is iso-

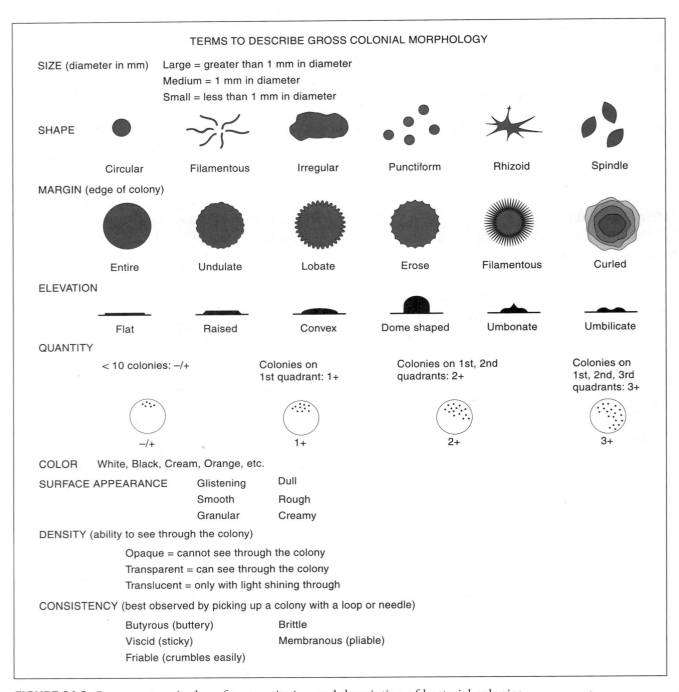

**FIGURE 24-3** Common terminology for quantitation and description of bacterial colonies.

lated from a normally sterile site, such as blood or CSF. Definitive identification is also appropriate when antibiotic therapy may vary based on the identification. For example, pure cultures of gram-negative rods in the *Enterobacteriaceae* group are usually fully identified when isolated from urine cultures. Additionally, certain specific organisms, which are much more **pathogenic** than related organisms with which they may be confused, should be fully identified. Some examples of this are *S. aureus,* which is usually much more pathogenic than other *Staphylococcus* species, and *Pseudomonas*

*aeruginosa,* which is much more significant than many of the organisms that it resembles.

## INTERPRETATION OF CULTURES FROM CLINICAL SITES ("READING PLATES")

Aerobic cultures should have an initial reading after overnight (12–24 hours) incubation at 35°C. Using bright illumination, carefully examine each culture plate and note the different colony types present. Distinctive odors should also be noted. Use standard terms to describe the numbers and appearance of each colony type (see Figure 24-3). Careful, complete documentation of initial colony appearance is very important, as some colonies change over time, and initial characteristics may aid in identification.

In addition to colony shape, size, and so on, it is important to note the presence or absence of growth on various selective media and the organisms' reactions of differential media. For example, if a colony resembling an enteric gram-negative rod is growing on the blood agar plate, knowledge of its ability to grow on MacConkey agar will help in determining if it is a member of the *Enterobacteriaceae* or not. Additionally, colonies that do grow on MacConkey agar can be differentiated by their ability or lack of ability to ferment lactose.

The extent of work-up of each colony type should be based on the type of specimen collected, the direct Gram stain result, and the numbers and types of colony types noted. Criteria stating when anaerobic bacteria should be sought must also be defined. Each laboratory must establish a set procedure defining which types of organisms should be further identified from each specimen type. Below are some suggested general guidelines. Refer to Tables 24-3 through 24-13 for help in identification of each organism group, as indicated below in the discussion of various specimen types.

## Blood

Many systems and methods are available for performing blood cultures. Most blood culture systems are broth-based, in which an aliquot of blood is **aseptically** inoculated into a vessel containing liquid growth medium. **Conventional** blood cultures (refer to Color Plate 68) require manual observation of the bottles for **macroscopic** evidence of bacterial growth. Some of these macroscopic changes that can be detected are turbidity, hemolysis of the blood, bubbles, bulging of the septum in the stopper (indicative of gas production), and visible colonies growing in the medium. Automated and semiautomated systems (see Figure 24-4) use instrumentation to detect changes in pH, gas pressure, carbon dioxide production, or other measurable indicators of growth. Once growth has been detected in a broth-based blood culture vessel, it is necessary to perform a Gram stain to get a general idea of the type of organism present. The positive culture is then **subcultured** to media appropriate for that type of organism, and the isolated can be identified.

Other blood culture systems are not broth-based. The Isolator system uses a lysing agent that breaks open the cellular elements in the blood specimen, releasing intracellular organisms. A concentrate of lysed cells and organisms is then planted directly on

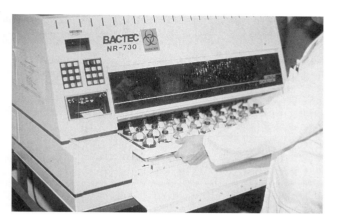

**FIGURE 24-4** The Bactec NR730 instrument detects growth by measuring carbon dioxide produced by bacteria growing in the broth.

culture plates. This system has the advantage of allowing isolated colonies to grow one or more days sooner than is possible with broth-based systems. It is also helpful for isolating obligately intracellular organisms such as *Brucella*. These organisms are not found free in the bloodstream, but within individual blood cells.

Regardless of the blood culture system used, all isolates must initially be considered potential pathogens. It is possible that inadequate decontamination of the skin could result in introduction of skin flora into the blood culture system (see Figure 24-5). Blood cultures can therefore contain "contaminants." However, the types of organisms that are usually contaminants (skin flora) are also known to cause subacute bacterial endocarditis, a type of heart valve infection that is diagnosed by blood culture. Therefore, it is usually recommended that all isolates from blood be completely identified. The clinical status of the patient and other factors must be considered when determining the significance of these "contaminant" organisms in positive blood cultures.

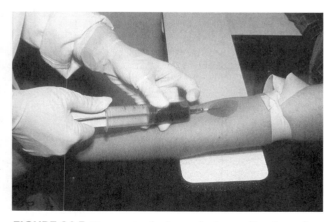

**FIGURE 24-5** Proper technique during collection of blood cultures is essential to prevent introduction of skin flora into the specimen. (Courtesy Scripps Clinic)

**Table 24–3** ▶ **Characteristics of Clinically Significant *Staphylococcus* Species**

| | Tube Coagulase | Slide Coagulase | Protein A Staphaurex | Thermo-nuclease | PYR | ODC | Urease | Novoblocin Resistance | Polymyxin B 300 U Rest. | Trehalose/ Mannitol |
|---|---|---|---|---|---|---|---|---|---|---|
| S. aureus | + | + | +* | + | – | – | +/– | – | + | + |
| S. epidermidis | – | – | – | – | – | +/– | + | – | + | – |
| S. haemolyticus | – | – | – | – | + | – | – | – | – | + |
| S. lugdunensis | – | +/– | – | – | + | + | +/– | – | +/– | + |
| S. schleiferi | – | + | – | + | + | – | – | – | – | + |
| S. saprophyticus | – | – | +/– | – | – | – | + | + | – | +/– |
| S. intermedius | + | +/– | +/– | + | + | – | + | – | – | + |
| S. hyicus | +/– | – | +/– | + | – | – | +/– | – | + | + |

*Methicillin-resistant *Staphylococcus aureus* may be negative.

Shaded boxes indicate key reactions.

PYR, pyrrolidonyl-ß-naphthylamide hydrolysis; ODC, ornithine decarboxylase.

## Other Normally Sterile Sites

Specimens such as CSF, deep body fluids, deep tissues, and internal organs, if collected properly, do not contain "normal flora," and any organism isolated from these sites should generally be completely identified. There are circumstances, however, in which some of these specimens may become contaminated with normal flora from adjacent areas, and presumptive identification will suffice. In cases of obvious contamination, such as a peritoneal fluid from a patient with a ruptured bowel, it is appropriate to use **descriptive identifica-tions**, in which a general description of each colony type is given: "enteric gram-negative rod," "α-hemolytic streptococcus," and so on. Also, as with positive blood cultures, inadequate skin decontamination prior to collection of these "sterile" specimens can result in the introduction of skin flora into these specimens. If there are small numbers of several different normal flora species isolated, a descriptive identification is usually sufficient. Regardless of the numbers and types of contaminants, however, it is important to always rule out pathogens such as *S. aureus* and *P. aeruginosa* from these sites.

**Table 24–4** ▶ **Characteristics of *Streptococcus* and Related Groups**

| | Chains | Pairs | Tetrads | PYR | 6.5% NaCl | Vancomycin Resistance | LAP | Gas from Glucose |
|---|---|---|---|---|---|---|---|---|
| *Streptococcus* | + | + | – | –* | – | – | + | – |
| *Enterococcus* | + | + | – | + | + | – | + | – |
| *Lactococcus* | + | + | – | –* | +/– | – | + | – |
| *Aerococcus* | – | + | + | + | + | – | – | – |
| *Gemella* | + | + | + | + | – | – | +/– | – |
| *Pediococcus* | – | + | + | – | +/– | + | + | – |
| *Leuconostoc* | + | + | – | – | +/– | + | – | + |

*Exceptions occur.

Shaded boxes indicate key reactions.

PYR, pyrrolidonyl ß-naphthylamide hydrolysis; LAP, leucine aminopeptidase.

## Table 24–5 ▶ Characteristics of ß-Hemolytic *Streptococcus* Species

| | Lancefield Group | Voges-Proskauer | PYR | CAMP Test | Hippurate Hydrolysis | A Disk Susceptibility | SXT Susceptibility |
|---|---|---|---|---|---|---|---|
| *S. pyogenes* | A | – | + | – | – | + | – |
| *S. agalactiae* | B | – | – | + | + | – | + |
| *S. equi*<br>*S. equisimilis*<br>*S. zooepidemicus* | C | – | – | – | – | +/– | + |
| *S. anginosus* | A,C,F,G or none | + | – | – | – | +/– | + |

Shaded boxes indicate key reactions.

PYR, pyrrolidonyl-ß-naphthylamide hydrolysis; SXT, sulfamethoxazole-trimethoprim.

## Respiratory Tract

Cultures from the respiratory tract can be very difficult to interpret. These specimen are not easily collected without introducing contamination from adjacent areas (see Figure 24-6). Furthermore, the contaminating organisms are often of a type that may sometimes be considered pathogenic from these types of specimens. For specimens from the lower respiratory tract, evaluation of the specimen by examining the direct Gram stain can sometimes help determine the "quality" of the specimen and therefore the potential significance of the isolates.

**Throat.** Throat cultures are the most straightforward of the respiratory tract cultures. The most significant bacterial pathogen of the throat is *S. pyogenes,* which appears on a blood agar plate as a small, convex, translucent, whitish colony surrounded by a clear zone of **ß-hemolysis** (refer to Color Plate 62). All ß-hemolytic colonies on throat cultures should be checked to rule out *S. pyogenes.* Prompt diagnosis and treatment of streptococcal pharyngitis is essential to prevent the very severe delayed sequelae that can occur following infections with this organism. Some of the other species of ß-streptococci have been reported in patients with pharyngitis, but it is unclear what role they play in disease.

Another significant cause of pharyngitis in selected patient populations is *N. gonorrhoeae.* This organism requires selective media such as Thayer-Martin or Martin-Lewis to be isolated from the normal throat flora. Colonies of this organism are small to medium sized, flat, gray to tan, translucent, and buttery to slightly rubbery (refer to Color Plate 63). Colonies of this type growing on the selective media should be further identified to rule out *N. gonorrhoeae.* A related organism, *N. meningitidis,* may also be carried in the throat, and its colonies are very similar. It is sometimes important to identify patients who are "carriers" of *N. meningitidis,* because they can become involved in outbreaks of meningitis. The organism does not contribute to pharyngitis, however. *N. gonorrhoeae* and *N. meningitidis* can be distinguished by biochemical tests.

Occasionally, a physician will request that the lab examine a throat culture for other possible pathogens. *C. diphtheriae* can cause pharyngitis. This organism produces colonies that are small, opaque white or gray (refer to Color Plate 64). They are catalase positive, and Gram stain reveals gram-positive rods with a "club" shape, and individual cells aligned parallel to each other, in **palisades**. Further tests are needed to confirm their identification.

**Nasopharynx.** Nasopharyngeal specimens are usually submitted primarily to rule out the causative agent of pertussis, *B. pertussis.* This organism is highly susceptible to toxic by-products found in the specimen or

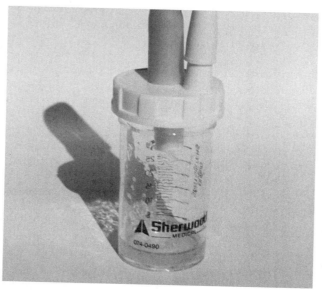

**FIGURE 24-6** Specimens such as this bronchial washing are often contaminated by normal flora from the mouth and throat.

**Table 24–6** ▶ **Characteristics of α-Hemolytic and Nonhemolytic Streptococci**

| | Optichin Susceptibility | Bile Solubility | Bile Esculin | Growth in 6.5% NaCl | PYR | Satellitism | CAMP Test |
|---|---|---|---|---|---|---|---|
| *S. pneumoniae* | + | + | – | – | – | – | – |
| *S. bovis* | – | – | + | – | – | – | – |
| *S. agalactiae* | – | – | + | +/– | – | – | + |
| *Viridans streptococci* | – | – | –* | – | – | – | – |
| *Nutritionally variant Streptococci* | – | – | – | – | + | + | – |

*Exceptions occur.

Shaded boxes indicate key reactions.

PYR, pyrrolidonyl-ß-naphthylamide hydrolysis.

produced by other organisms in culture, and requires special media that help to neutralize this toxicity. Bordet-Gengou, Regan-Lowe, and buffered charcoal yeast extract agar are all media that have been used for the cultivation of this organism. After several days of incubation, colonies are tiny, shiny round "half pearls" or "mercury droplets." Gram stain demonstrates tiny, pale gram-negative coccobacilli. Fluorescent antibody stains can be used to confirm the identification.

**Expectorated Sputum, Bronchial Washings, Endotracheal Aspirates.** These specimens are very difficult to collect without introducing contamination from the upper respiratory tract. Hence, their culture results are often the most difficult to interpret of any culture type. A specimen with a direct Gram stain indicating large numbers of PMNs, however, was probably collected appropriately, and has a good chance of growing large numbers of a significant pathogen.

α-Hemolytic streptococci-type colonies should be examined closely for the characteristic "checker" or "dimpled" appearance typical of *S. pneumoniae*. A filter paper disk containing the substance optochin ("P" disk) is often placed on the first quadrant of the blood agar plate on all lower respiratory tract specimens (see Color Plate 65). *S. pneumoniae* is inhibited by this substance and will demonstrate a zone of inhibition around the disk. All colonies suggestive of *S. pneumoniae* should be tested further to rule out or confirm the identification.

Clear to translucent, moist colonies with a "mousy" or musky odor growing on chocolate agar but not on blood agar should be Gram stained (refer to Color Plate 66). These characteristics are suggestive of *Haemophilus influenzae*, which will appear as tiny, pale gram-negative coccobacilli on the Gram stain. Several methods are available to confirm or rule out this organism.

The pathogenic *Neisseria*, *N. meningitidis* and *N. gonorrhoeae*, are also possible pathogens from these types of specimens. These colonies generally grow best on chocolate agar, although *N. meningitidis* may also grow on blood agar. They are moist, translucent tan to gray, with a buttery to rubbery texture (refer to Color Plate 63).

Another potential pathogen, *M. catarrhalis*, has hard, sticky colonies, which tend to slide across the agar when touched by a loop ("hockey puck" colonies). This is very similar to the colonial morphology of the many nonpathogenic *Neisseria* species that are often found in respiratory tract specimens (refer to Color Plate 67). If there is heavy growth of this type of colony from a specimen with a suspicious direct Gram stain, the "hockey puck" colonies should be further tested to rule out *M. catarrhalis*.

Small to medium sized, opaque, creamy white to yellow, ß-hemolytic colonies growing on blood agar are suggestive of *S. aureus*. This organism must be differentiated from the other staphylococci, which are generally considered to be contaminants from these types of specimens.

Gram-negative enteric rods will grow as large, gray or whitish, creamy moist colonies on blood agar. Some (*Klebsiella* and related species) may have very large **mucoid** colonies. The gram-negative enteric rods will also grow on MacConkey agar and other media that are selective for gram-negative organisms. Small numbers of these organisms may represent contamination or **colonization**, but if there is heavy or predominant growth, they should be fully identified.

*Legionella* species are always significant when isolated from clinical specimens, but they require special media for growth and isolation. The colonies appear in 3 to 5 days on buffered charcoal yeast extract agar, and are flat, whitish gray with a bluish purple opalescence or iridescence (refer to Color Plate 68). They will not grow when subcultured to blood agar plate. All colonies resembling *Legionella* should be Gram stained and further tested. Identification can be confirmed with fluorescent antibody stains or by a reference laboratory.

# Table 24–7 ▶ Characteristics of *Neisseria* Species and *Moraxella catarrhalis*

| | Pigment | Growth on Selective Media | Growth on Nutrient Agar 35°C | Growth on Chocolate agar 22°C | Glucose | Maltose | Sucrose | Lactose (ONPG) | DNASE | Nitrate→Nitrite | Catalase | Tributyrin |
|---|---|---|---|---|---|---|---|---|---|---|---|---|
| N. gonorrhoeae | – | +* | – | – | + | – | – | – | – | – | + | – |
| N. meningitidis | – | + | + | – | + | + | – | – | – | – | + | – |
| N. lactamica | – | + | + | V | + | + | – | + | – | – | + | – |
| N. cinerea | – | –* | + | – | V | – | – | – | V | – | + | – |
| Other Nonpathogenic Neisseria species | V | V | + | V | V | – | V | V | – | V | + | – |
| M. catarrhalis | – | – | + | V | – | – | – | – | + | + | + | + |
| Kingella species | – | V | – | – | + | – | – | – | – | + | – | – |

*Exceptions occur; V, variable.

| Table 24–8 ▶ Differentiation of Gram-Negative Cocci Isolated on Selective Media | | | |
|---|---|---|---|
| | ß-Galactosidase | γ-Glutamylaminopeptidase | Prolylaminopeptidase* |
| N. gonorrhoeae | – | – | + |
| N. meningitidis | – | + | – |
| N. lactamica | + | – | – |
| M. catarrhalis | – | – | – |

*N. cinerea, Kingella denitrificans: may be isolated on selective media, may be positive for prolyaminopeptidase.

Some other potential pathogens that may be isolated from these respiratory tract specimens are ß-hemolytic streptococci and *Corynebacterium pseudodiphtheriticum*. The latter organism, although not frequently encountered, can be significant, and should be sought if large numbers of suspicious organisms are seen on direct microscopic examination of the specimen. These organisms produce small, whitish, nonhemolytic colonies on blood agar. Of the ß-hemolytic streptococci, *S. pyogenes* is the most significant, and should be identified if present in large numbers.

**Transtracheal Aspirates, Lung Aspirates, Open Lung Biopsies.** These specimens are collected by surgical procedures or other invasive techniques that bypass the upper respiratory tract, preventing contamination by normal flora. Generally, all organisms isolated from these specimens should be identified as potential pathogens. Additionally, since there is no contamination from normal flora, anaerobes should be sought, because they are common causes of aspiration pneumonia.

## Urinary Tract

Like cultures from the respiratory tract, urine cultures can be difficult to interpret. Urines must be planted quantitatively, with a 0.001-mL calibrated inoculation loop being the most common method of plating. Colony counts of each type of organism isolated are calculated, and identifications may or may not be indicated, based on the colony counts and number of different isolates present. Urinary tract infection in an otherwise healthy host is usually demonstrated by isolating more than 100,000 **colony-forming units (cfu)** of a single type of urinary tract pathogen per milliliter of specimen. Patients with indwelling catheters or other abnormal conditions of the urinary tract may have polymicrobic infections. In these patients, multiple isolates should be identified if they are present at levels exceeding 100,000 cfu/mL. Additionally, young, sexually active women may have symptomatic urinary tract infection with as few as 100 cfu/mL of a single

isolate. Specimens collected via catheterization or nephrostomy are often considered indicative of urinary tract infection with lower colony counts than are considered significant from midstream urine specimens. It is critical that each laboratory have defined criteria to determine how extensive the work-up should be, based on how the specimen was collected and the numbers and types of organisms isolated. Equally important is good communication between the ordering physician and the laboratory regarding any unusual circumstances that would affect the interpretation of the culture.

The most frequent causes of urinary tract infection are members of the *Enterobacteriaceae* (especially *E. coli*), *Enterococcus, S. aureus, Staphylococcus saprophyticus,* certain *Corynebacterium* species, and nonfermentative gram-negative bacilli.

In addition to culture, many laboratories have adopted **rapid screening methods** for evaluating urine specimens submitted for culture. There are various methods available, with different principles, advantages, and disadvantages. Many detect either large numbers of bacteria as well as large numbers of PMNs, a good indicator of urinary tract infection. Specimens that test positive by these rapid screening methods are then cultured by standard methods, so that the causative agent can be identified.

## Wounds, Abscesses, Soft Tissue Infections

A wide variety of organisms can be responsible for various wound infections. Usually, the organisms gain entrance to an otherwise sterile area by trauma, surgery, or a disease process that weakens the host's physical defenses. Frequently, the causative agent is one that is normal flora in an adjacent area, or it may be introduced **exogenously** from outside the body. Organisms can also be spread **hematogenously** from another site and cause infection in a formerly healthy area.

Proper collection techniques are important if culture results are to be meaningful. Because these infections

# Table 24-9 ▶ Characteristics of Common, Clinically Significant Enterobacteriaceae

| | Indole | Methyl Red | VP | Citrate | H₂S | Urease | PDA | LDC | Arginine dihydrolase | ODC | Motility | Gelatin | KCN | Malonate | D-Glucose, Gas | Lactose Fermentation | Sucrose Fermentation | D-Mannitol Fermentation | Dulcitol Fermentation | Adonitol Fermentation | D-Sorbitol Fermentation | L-Arabinose Fermentation | Raffinose Fermentation | L-Rhamnose Fermentation | D-Xylose Fermentation | Melibiose Fermentation | DNAse | ONPG |
|---|---|---|---|---|---|---|---|---|---|---|---|---|---|---|---|---|---|---|---|---|---|---|---|---|---|---|---|---|
| Escherichia coli | 98 | 99 | 0 | 1 | 1 | 1 | 0 | 90 | 17 | 65 | 95 | 0 | 3 | 0 | 95 | 95 | 50 | 98 | 60 | 5 | 94 | 99 | 50 | 80 | 95 | 75 | 0 | 95 |
| Shigella A,B,C, | 50 | 100 | 0 | 0 | 0 | 0 | 0 | 0 | 5 | 1 | 0 | 0 | 0 | 0 | 2 | 0 | 1 | 93 | 2 | 0 | 30 | 60 | 50 | 5 | 2 | 50 | 0 | 2 |
| Shigella sonnei | 0 | 100 | 0 | 0 | 0 | 0 | 0 | 0 | 2 | 98 | 0 | 0 | 0 | 0 | 0 | 2 | 0 | 99 | 0 | 0 | 2 | 95 | 3 | 75 | 2 | 25 | 0 | 90 |
| Salmonella typhi | 0 | 100 | 0 | 0 | 97 | 0 | 0 | 98 | 3 | 0 | 97 | 0 | 0 | 0 | 0 | 1 | 0 | 100 | 0 | 0 | 99 | 2 | 0 | 0 | 82 | 100 | 0 | 0 |
| Salmonella para A | 0 | 100 | 0 | 0 | 10 | 0 | 0 | 0 | 15 | 95 | 95 | 0 | 0 | 0 | 99 | 0 | 0 | 100 | 90 | 0 | 95 | 100 | 0 | 100 | 0 | 95 | 0 | 0 |
| Salmonella species, most | 1 | 100 | 0 | 95 | 95 | 1 | 0 | 98 | 70 | 97 | 95 | 0 | 0 | 15 | 96 | 1 | 1 | 100 | 96 | 0 | 95 | 99 | 2 | 95 | 97 | 95 | 0 | 0 |
| Citrobacter freundii | 5 | 100 | 0 | 95 | 80 | 70 | 0 | 0 | 65 | 20 | 95 | 0 | 96 | 15 | 96 | 50 | 1 | 100 | 96 | 0 | 85 | 99 | 95 | 95 | 97 | 95 | 2 | 95 |
| Citrobacter diversus | 99 | 100 | 0 | 99 | 0 | 75 | 0 | 0 | 65 | 99 | 95 | 0 | 96 | 90 | 95 | 50 | 30 | 99 | 55 | 98 | 98 | 100 | 30 | 99 | 99 | 50 | 2 | 96 |
| Edwardsiella tarda | 99 | 100 | 0 | 1 | 100 | 0 | 0 | 100 | 0 | 100 | 98 | 0 | 0 | 90 | 98 | 0 | 0 | 0 | 50 | 98 | 0 | 0 | 0 | 0 | 0 | 0 | 0 | 0 |
| Klebsiella pneumoniae | 0 | 10 | 98 | 98 | 0 | 95 | 0 | 98 | 0 | 0 | 0 | 0 | 98 | 93 | 98 | 98 | 99 | 99 | 30 | 90 | 99 | 99 | 99 | 99 | 99 | 75 | 0 | 99 |
| Klebsiella oxytoca | 99 | 20 | 95 | 95 | 0 | 90 | 1 | 99 | 0 | 0 | 0 | 0 | 97 | 98 | 97 | 98 | 100 | 99 | 55 | 99 | 99 | 98 | 100 | 99 | 99 | 50 | 0 | 99 |
| Enterobacter aerogenes | 0 | 5 | 98 | 95 | 0 | 2 | 0 | 98 | 0 | 98 | 97 | 0 | 98 | 95 | 100 | 95 | 100 | 100 | 5 | 98 | 99 | 100 | 100 | 100 | 100 | 99 | 0 | 100 |
| Enterobacter cloacae | 0 | 5 | 100 | 93 | 0 | 65 | 0 | 0 | 97 | 96 | 95 | 0 | 98 | 75 | 100 | 98 | 100 | 100 | 15 | 95 | 95 | 96 | 99 | 99 | 99 | 99 | 0 | 100 |
| Enterobacter agglomerans | 20 | 50 | 70 | 50 | 0 | 20 | 20 | 0 | 0 | 0 | 85 | 2 | 35 | 65 | 20 | 75 | 100 | 100 | 25 | 7 | 95 | 97 | 85 | 92 | 99 | 90 | 0 | 99 |
| Hafnia alvei | 0 | 40 | 85 | 10 | 0 | 4 | 0 | 100 | 6 | 98 | 85 | 0 | 95 | 50 | 98 | 5 | 10 | 99 | 0 | 0 | 30 | 30 | 0 | 85 | 93 | 50 | 0 | 90 |
| Serratia marcescens | 1 | 20 | 98 | 98 | 0 | 15 | 0 | 99 | 0 | 98 | 97 | 90 | 95 | 3 | 98 | 5 | 99 | 99 | 0 | 40 | 0 | 2 | 5 | 0 | 0 | 0 | 90 | 90 |
| Serratia liquifaciens | 1 | 93 | 93 | 90 | 0 | 3 | 1 | 99 | 0 | 95 | 95 | 90 | 95 | 2 | 55 | 50 | 99 | 99 | 0 | 5 | 99 | 2 | 0 | 7 | 0 | 0 | 95 | 95 |
| Proteus mirabilis | 2 | 97 | 50 | 65 | 98 | 98 | 98 | 0 | 0 | 0 | 95 | 90 | 90 | 2 | 75 | 0 | 10 | 0 | 0 | 5 | 95 | 85 | 15 | 100 | 75 | 0 | 93 | 95 |
| Proteus vulgaris | 98 | 95 | 0 | 15 | 98 | 98 | 99 | 0 | 0 | 0 | 95 | 91 | 98 | 0 | 85 | 15 | 98 | 0 | 0 | 0 | 0 | 1 | 1 | 98 | 0 | 0 | 0 | 93 |
| Providencia rettgeri | 99 | 93 | 0 | 95 | 0 | 98 | 98 | 0 | 0 | 0 | 95 | 0 | 99 | 0 | 10 | 0 | 15 | 0 | 0 | 0 | 1 | 1 | 5 | 95 | 93 | 0 | 1 | 0 |
| Providencia stuartii | 98 | 100 | 0 | 95 | 0 | 30 | 95 | 0 | 0 | 0 | 85 | 0 | 95 | 0 | 5 | 50 | 100 | 0 | 0 | 100 | 1 | 5 | 0 | 10 | 0 | 0 | 5 | 1 |
| Providencia alcalfaciens | 99 | 99 | 0 | 98 | 0 | 0 | 98 | 0 | 0 | 0 | 96 | 0 | 90 | 0 | 85 | 15 | 2 | 0 | 98 | 5 | 1 | 7 | 7 | 0 | 7 | 0 | 10 | 5 |
| Morganella morganii | 98 | 97 | 0 | 0 | 0 | 98 | 95 | 0 | 0 | 98 | 95 | 0 | 98 | 0 | 90 | 0 | 2 | 0 | 0 | 1 | 1 | 1 | 1 | 0 | 0 | 0 | 1 | 1 |
| Yersinia enterocolitica | 50 | 97 | 2 | 0 | 0 | 98 | 0 | 0 | 0 | 95 | 0 | 2 | 0 | 0 | 5 | 5 | 95 | 98 | 0 | 0 | 99 | 1 | 5 | 70 | 20 | 5 | 5 | 5 |
| Yersinia pestis | 0 | 80 | 0 | 0 | 5 | 5 | 0 | 0 | 0 | 0 | 0 | 0 | 0 | 0 | 0 | 0 | 0 | 0 | 0 | 50 | 100 | 90 | 1 | 70 | 20 | 0 | 0 | 50 |
| Yersinia pseudotuberc. | 0 | 100 | 0 | 0 | 0 | 95 | 0 | 0 | 95 | 0 | 0 | 0 | 0 | 0 | 0 | 0 | 0 | 100 | 0 | 50 | 50 | 70 | 15 | 90 | 70 | 0 | 70 | 70 |

Numbers in boxes refer to percent positive. Abbreviations: VP, Voges-Proskauer; H₂S, hydrogen sulfide production; PDA, phenylalanine deaminase; LDC, lysine decarboxylase; ODC, ornithine decarboxylase; KCN, growth in potassium cyanide broth; ONPG, β-galactosidase.

| Table 24–10 ▶ | Nonfermentative Gram-Negative Bacilli (excluding unusual bacilli) |
| --- | --- |

**GLUCOSE OXIDIZED, MACCONKEY POSITIVE, OXIDASE POSITIVE**

| | |
| --- | --- |
| Agrobacterium | Methylobacterium |
| Alcaligenes | Ochrobacterium |
| EF-4b | Pseudomonas |
| EO2 | Psychrobacter |
| EO3 | Shewanella |
| Flavobacterium | Sphingobacterium |

**GLUCOSE OXIDIZED, MACCONKEY POSITIVE, OXIDASE NEGATIVE**

| | |
| --- | --- |
| Acinetobacter | Pseudomonas |
| Chryseomonas | Xanthomonas |
| Flavimonas | |

**GLUCOSE OXIDIZED, MACCONKEY NEGATIVE, OXIDASE POSITIVE**

| | |
| --- | --- |
| EF-4b | IIh |
| EO2 | IIi |
| Flavobacterium | Pseudomonas |
| IIe | Sphingobacterium |

**GLUCOSE OXIDIZED, MACCONKEY NEGATIVE, OXIDASE NEGATIVE**

IIe

Pseudomonas

**GLUCOSE NOT OXIDIZED, MACCONKEY POSITIVE, OXIDASE POSITIVE**

| | |
| --- | --- |
| Alcaligenes | M6 |
| Comamonas | Moraxella |
| Flavobacterium | Oligella |
| Ivc-2 | Psychrobacter |
| M5 | Shewanella |

**GLUCOSE NOT OXIDIZED, MACCONKEY POSITIVE, OXIDASE NEGATIVE**

Acinetobacter

Xanthomonas

**GLUCOSE NOT OXIDIZED, MACCONKEY NEGATIVE, OXIDASE POSITIVE**

| | |
| --- | --- |
| Eikenella | Oligella |
| M6 | Pseudomonas |
| Moraxella | Weeksella |

**GLUCOSE NOT OXIDIZED, MACCONKEY NEGATIVE, OXIDASE NEGATIVE**

Unusual gram-negative rods only

can occur anywhere in the body, there is often an area nearby with a large population of normal flora, some of which would be considered pathogenic if isolated from a wound. Adequate skin decontamination before aspiration of infected material will avoid introduction of these contaminants into the specimen.

One additional consideration when culturing wounds or abscesses is requests for unusual organisms or those with special nutritional or environmental requirements (e.g., anaerobes). Again, it is important for the physician to communicate these requests to the laboratory so that appropriate steps can be taken to allow cultivation of these organisms.

The most common causes of these infections are *S. aureus* (refer to Color Plate 69), ß-hemolytic streptococci, *P. aeruginosa* (refer to Color Plate 70), enteric gram-negative rods, nonfermentative gram-negative rods, *Enterococcus,* and anaerobes.

## Genital Tract

The most common genital tract pathogen isolated from genital bacterial cultures is *N. gonorrhoeae,* the causative agent of gonorrhea. All colonies growing on appropriate selective media (modified Thayer-Martin, Martin-Lewis, etc.) should be investigated, and all gram-negative diplococci should be identified. Although *N. gonorrhoeae* is much more common in genital specimens, *N. meningitidis,* which can grow on the selective media, is also considered a pathogen from genital sites.

In both sexes, the external genitalia are susceptible to infection by the same types of organisms that cause skin and wound infections elsewhere in the body. Genital cultures from female patients should also be screened for *Listeria, S. aureus,* and group B streptococci. Another organism, *Gardnerella vaginalis,* is associated with a syndrome known as bacterial vaginosis (see the section on wet mounts in this chapter). This is best diagnosed by demonstrating the presence of clue cells, squamous epithelial cells covered with small gram-negative rods. Detection of this organism in culture does not correlate well with disease.

A less common agent that can cause genital tract infection is *Haemophilus ducreyi.* It requires special media and techniques for isolation and identification.

## Gastrointestinal Tract

Infections of the gastrointestinal tract are most often diagnosed by performing stool cultures. Because the lower gastrointestinal tract, and hence the stool, contains an enormous population of normal flora, highly selective media and techniques must be used to allow the growth and isolation of the relatively few pathogens found in these specimens.

*Salmonella* and *Shigella* are the classic causes of gastrointestinal disease. Both appear as **nonlactose**

## Table 24–11 ▶ Selected Characteristics of *Vibrio* and Related Species

|  | *Vibrio* | *Aeromonas* | *Plesiomonas* |
|---|---|---|---|
| Susceptibility to 10 µg O129 | +/– | – | +/– |
| Susceptibility to 150 µg O129 | + | – | + |
| Growth on TCBS | + | – | + |
| Requires or is enhanced by NaCl | + | – | – |
| Gas from glucose | +/– | +/– | – |
| ß-hemolysis | +/– | +/– | – |

**fermenters** on differential media (refer to Color Plate 71). On those media containing appropriate indicators, *Salmonella* colonies will appear black, due to the production of hydrogen sulfide. Colonies resembling *Salmonella* and/or *Shigella* should be subjected to further testing.

*Campylobacter* species also cause gastrointestinal disease, even more frequently than *Salmonella* and *Shigella* in many areas. These **microaerophilic** organisms grow more slowly than most normal flora in the stool, and so require a highly selective medium and incubation conditions. It is recommended that the selective media for *Campylobacter* be incubated at 42°C, which allows the pathogen to grow, but inhibits many of the normal flora. All colonies isolated on the selective media for *Campylobacter* should be investigated.

Verotoxin-producing *E. coli*, such as *E. coli* O157:H7, are also a significant cause of gastrointestinal disease. Rarely, the disease can progress from bloody diarrhea to multiorgan involvement, and even death. The most practical way of screening for these organisms is to use a differential medium that demonstrates sorbitol fermentation. *E. coli* O157:H7 does not ferment sorbitol, and most commensals do; therefore, nonsorbitol fermenters should be investigated. This approach is easy to incorporate into routine stool culture protocols, but has the drawback that other, albeit less common serotypes of verotoxin-producing *E. coli* will not be detected. Methods are available for screening stool specimens for the actual verotoxin rather than attempting to isolate the toxin-producing organism.

Other agents of gastrointestinal disease that should be sought in certain circumstances are *Yersinia, Aeromonas, Plesiomonas,* and *Vibrio*. There are special selective media available for *Yersinia* and *Vibrio,* although all of these isolates, if present in large numbers, may be isolated from routine stool cultures. These organisms are generally nonlactose fermenters, and because nonlactose fermenters are investigated to rule out the more common *Salmonella* and *Shigella,* the screening procedures can be designed so that these organisms will also be detected.

In addition to the above pathogens, *S. aureus,* if isolated in large numbers, can be considered pathogenic, so cultures should be checked for the presence of this organism. *C. difficile*, like verotoxin-producing *E. coli*, can cause severe gastrointestinal disease due to production of a toxin. Although it is possible to isolate this anaerobic organism from a stool culture using selective media incubated anaerobically, it is much more meaningful to test for the presence of *C. difficile* toxin in the stool specimen.

### Anaerobes

Anaerobic bacteria can cause infection in many parts of the body, and appropriate specimens should routinely be cultured for isolation of these organisms. Most blood culture systems have an anaerobic bottle available, so no special processing techniques are required. Deep body fluids, tissues, surgically collected specimens, deep wounds, abscesses, and similar specimens should be transported in suitable devices that maintain

## Table 24–12 ▶ Characteristics of *Campylobacter* Species

|  | Catalase | Hippurate | Nitrate to Nitrite | Susceptibility to Nalidixic Acid | Susceptibility to Cephalothin | Growth at 25°C | Growth at 42°C |
|---|---|---|---|---|---|---|---|
| *C. jejuni jejuni* | + | + | + | S | R | – | + |
| *C. coli* | + | – | + | S | R | – | + |
| *C. fetus fetus* | + | – | + | R | S | + | – |

R, resistant; S, susceptible.

**Table 24–13** ▶ **Selected Characteristics of *Haemophilus* Species**

| | Requires "V" | ALA→Porphrins (does not require "X") | Urease | Indole | Glucose | Lactose | ß-Hemolysis |
|---|---|---|---|---|---|---|---|
| H. influenzae | + | – | +/– | +/– | + | – | – |
| H. parainfluenzae | + | + | +/– | +/– | + | – | – |
| H. haemolyticus | + | – | + | +/– | + | – | + |
| H. aphrophilus | – | + | – | – | + | + | – |
| H. paraphrophilus | + | + | – | – | + | + | – |
| H. segnis | + | + | – | – | + | – | – |
| H. influenzae biotype aegyptius | + | – | + | – | + | – | – |
| H. ducreyi | – | – | – | – | +/– | – | – |
| H. parahemolyticus | + | + | + | – | + | – | + |
| H. paraphrohaemolyticus | + | + | + | – | + | – | + |

Shaded boxes indicate key reactions.

viability of these anaerobic flora. If this is not possible, these specimens should be processed immediately on receipt in the laboratory. The culture protocol for isolation of anaerobes should include a rich, nonselective medium, as well as selective media (see Tables 24-1 and 24-2). It is very important that media for cultivation of anaerobes be as fresh as possible, or some of the more sensitive anaerobes may be inhibited by toxic products that form when the media sits in "room air" for extended periods of time.

Various methods are available for providing an anaerobic environment suitable for incubation of the inoculated culture plates. Airtight jars, containing a disposable gas-generating system, may be placed in a regular incubator. These jars come in various sizes to accommodate different numbers of plates. Disposable pouch systems, based on the same principles, are also available for incubation of small numbers of plates (see Figure 24-7). It is also possible to use an airtight jar hooked up to an evacuation-replacement system. Through vents in the lid, a jar containing plates to be incubated is evacuated, and the air replaced with the appropriate anaerobic gas mixture. All of the above systems are convenient and easy to use; work-ups can be performed on the regular benchtops, as long as the plates are returned to anaerobe jars or pouches very quickly. The only drawback to these systems is that the cultures should not be examined before 48 hours of incubation because many anaerobes are very sensitive to exposure to oxygen during this time.

Anaerobe chambers or glove boxes, self-contained systems attached to a supply of anaerobic gas, offer the freedom to look at the cultures as early and as frequently as desired, without fear of exposing the cultures to oxygen. Specimens and supplies are taken in and out of the chamber or glove box via a "transfer module," which is flushed and replaced with anaerobic gas before taking the items into the anaerobic environment. The hands and arms are placed in sleeves with an airtight cuff, and the space around the arm below the cuff is filled with anaerobic gas. Once placed inside the chamber or glove box, the specimens are in a totally anaerobic environment throughout all of the steps of the culture (see Figure 24-8). Chambers and glove boxes are, however, expensive, and they take up a fair amount of space.

Because many infections involving anaerobes are polymicrobic, these cultures are often very "messy,"

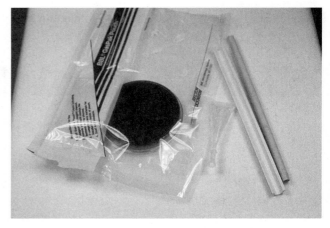

**FIGURE 24-7** One type of anaerobic pouch system.

with several different colony types isolated. It is important to examine the plates closely, perform Gram stains, and subculture each colony type to both anaerobic and aerobic media to determine whether the isolate is a true anaerobe, or just **facultative**. Once an isolate is shown to be an anaerobe, further tests can be done to reach a definitive identification. As with aerobic cultures, criteria must be established to define the extent of work-up of each anaerobe isolated from various sites.

## REPORTING CULTURE RESULTS

One of the responsibilities of the laboratory is to help educate the medical staff, all of whom may not be fluent in the diagnosis of infectious diseases. It does no good for a laboratory to have an extensive and careful set of procedures for isolation and identification of significant pathogens, unless an equally well-designed system for reporting those results is used. It would be irresponsible for the laboratory to include in every report the identifications of organisms that are not considered significant for that site. Doing so would imply that the laboratory feels the isolates are significant and may result in inappropriate antibiotic therapy. When reporting the presence of isolates of unknown significance, the laboratory may choose to include a comment indicating that this organism may represent contamination. Other organisms, such as *N. gonorrhoeae*, which are always considered significant, need no such qualification.

In addition to clarity and appropriateness, promptness is essential to good laboratory reporting. "Positive" cultures containing isolates that may turn out to be poten-

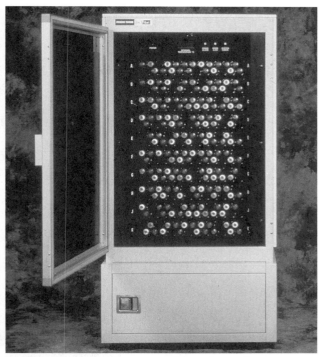

**FIGURE 24-8** Reading anaerobic cultures in an anaerobic chamber.

tial pathogens should have preliminary reports sent immediately so that the physician can start antibiotic therapy. Reports should be updated as new information becomes available and when a culture is complete. Significant isolates, and isolates from normally sterile sites, should be reported immediately by telephone. A laboratory-hospital computer system is helpful in communicating results promptly and accurately.

## Table 24–14 ▶ Selected Characteristics of Common Corynebacteria

|  | Catalase | ß-Hemolysis | Nitrate* | Urease | Dextrose | Maltose | Sucrose | Motility |
|---|---|---|---|---|---|---|---|---|
| C. diphtheriae | + | V | +* | – | + | + | – | – |
| C. ulcerans | + | + | – | + | + | + | – | – |
| C. pseudodiphtheriticum | + | – | + | + | – | – | – | – |
| C. pseudotuberculosis | + | + | V | + | + | + | – | – |
| C. xerosis | + | – | + | – | + | V | + | – |
| C. jeikeium | + | – | – | – | V | V | – | – |
| Group D2 | + | – | – | + | – | – | – | – |
| Actinomyces pyogenes | – | + | – | – | + | + | V | – |
| Arcanobacterium haemolyticum | – | + | – | – | + | + | V | – |
| Oerskovia species | + | – | V | V | + | + | + | + |

*Nitrate refers to reduction of nitrate to nitrite.

## SUMMARY

▶ Direct microscopic examination of clinical specimens, with or without the use of various stains, can help establish a preliminary diagnosis of an infectious process.

▶ Factors such as type of specimen, presence or absence of normal flora (including anaerobes), clinical status of the patient, population of patients using the laboratory's services, and cost must all be considered when deciding how to inoculate a culture from a specific specimen.

▶ The respiratory tract, urinary tract, genital tract, gastrointestinal tract, and skin all harbor a resident population of normal flora. These organisms must be considered when performing cultures from these sites. They are capable of causing disease under certain circumstances, both in their usual sites as well as by invading adjacent areas.

▶ Various types of clinical specimens can contain a large number of different pathogens. When reading cultures, the technologist must consider the type of specimen and look for colonies representative of the types of organisms that are significant from that type of specimen.

▶ Colonial and microscopic morphology, ability to grow on selective media, reactions on differential media, and the results of various biochemical tests are all used to identify bacteria isolated in culture.

## CASE STUDY

A 91-year-old male diabetic resident of a nursing home presented with a high fever, altered mental status, and severe soft tissue destruction at the site of what had been a minor skin lesion on his face. Two other patients in the nursing home had similar tissue destruction, one at the site of a surgical wound and one with no known prior wound or infection. During the same time period at the nursing home, three other patients had manifested various symptoms that could not be explained by their past medical histories, such as renal failure, hypotension, rash, and shock. One had died.

These patients suffered from invasive *Streptococcus pyogenes* disease (see Figure 24-9). Diabetes, old age, residence in nursing homes, and other underlying medical problems are all risk factors for this disease, which has an overall case fatality rate of 10% to 20%. It is possible to develop this disease without having a history of past streptococcal infection.

Invasive streptococcal disease is diagnosed by isolating *S. pyogenes* from a normally sterile site. Culture protocols must be designed such that this organism will be isolated, identified, and promptly reported.

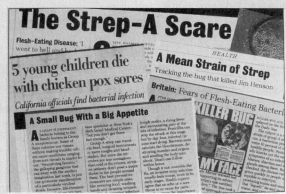

**FIGURE 24-9** *Streptococcus pyogenes*, also known as group A *Streptococcus*, has received a lot of media attention in recent years.

### Questions:

1. What is the most common infection caused by *S. pyogenes*? How is it diagnosed?

2. Describe some of the other severe diseases that can result following infection with this organism.

3. Describe techniques that can be used to identify *S. pyogenes* in the laboratory.

# Review Questions

1. Direct microscopic examination of clinical specimens offer the advantage of having results available much earlier than culture. What is one of the disadvantages of direct microscopic examination?
   a. It requires costly equipment and reagents.
   b. The procedures are extremely complicated.
   c. The results must be confirmed by culture.
   d. Most physicians want to wait for culture results to begin antibiotic therapy.

2. A gram-stained smear of an abscess specimen revealed numerous squamous epithelial cells, very few PMNs, numerous gram-negative rods, and numerous gram-positive and gram-negative cocci. Which is correct?
   a. The specimen was probably not collected properly because there are so few PMNs.
   b. The specimen was probably collected properly, as indicated by the numerous epithelial cells present.
   c. The specimen was probably collected properly, as indicated by the numerous bacteria present.
   d. The specimen was probably not collected properly, as indicated by the numerous bacteria present.

3. One suggested protocol for cerebrospinal fluid (CSF) culture includes blood agar, chocolate agar, and thioglycollate broth. Why does not this protocol include selective media such as MacConkey or Columbia colistin-nalidixic acid?
   a. Because cost containment is essential, and CSF cultures are not significant enough to justify using so many plates
   b. Because selective media may inhibit the large numbers of commensals normally found in the CSF
   c. Because CSF does not ordinarily have normal flora, so there is no need to "select" for other types of organisms
   d. Because the aim of the CSF culture is to isolate and identify only the types of organisms, which will grow on blood agar, chocolate agar, and in thioglycollate broth

4. What type of information about the patient should the physician communicate to the laboratory when submitting specimens for culture?
   a. Presence of prosthetic devices
   b. Immunocompromised status
   c. Travel to areas with different endemic diseases
   d. All of the above

5. Which of the following is NOT true about normal flora?
   a. The healthy human body has a large population of normal flora in various sites.
   b. Normal flora usually causes a lot of trouble for the host, in the various sites in which they live.
   c. Factors such as stress or immune disorders can upset the balance of normal flora.
   d. Whenever they are isolated in culture, a number of factors must be considered to determine their significance.

6. Which of the following is correct regarding presumptive and definitive identification?
   a. A good microbiology laboratory will send presumptive identifications initially, followed by definitive identifications, on all colony types isolated from all specimen types.
   b. A presumptive identification is usually adequate when a skin contaminant-type organism is isolated from a normally sterile site, such as blood.
   c. Common pathogens such as *Staphylococcus aureus* and *Pseudomonas aeruginosa* are so frequently isolated that presumptive identification is sufficient.
   d. Each laboratory needs to specify its own procedures defining when different types of isolates should be presumptively or definitively identified.

7. Which of the following is NOT a means of detecting growth from any type of blood culture system?
   a. Presence of PMNs in a Gram smear
   b. Turbidity
   c. Visible colonies in broth or on an agar plate
   d. Bulging of the septum in the bottle's stopper

8. Which of the following is true of throat cultures?
   a. All species of ß-hemolytic streptococci are known to cause severe pharyngitis.
   b. *Neisseria gonorrhoeae,* which can cause pharyngitis, requires special selective media for isolation from throat specimens.
   c. *Neisseria meningitidis,* which can cause pharyngitis, requires special selective media for isolation from throat specimens.
   d. *Corynebacterium diphtheriae,* a less common cause of pharyngitis, can be identified based solely on colonial and microscopic morphology.

9. Which of the following is NOT true of wound/abscess/soft tissue infections?
   a. These infections are usually only caused by *Staphylococcus aureus.*
   b. Trauma or surgery can inadvertently introduce normal flora into previously sterile areas, resulting in infection.
   c. It is possible for organisms to spread to a previously sterile area via the bloodstream, resulting in infection.
   d. The causative agents of these infections are frequently normal flora in an adjacent area.

10. Which of the following is NOT true about reporting results?
    a. Positive blood cultures should be reported immediately by telephone.
    b. One of the reasons for sending preliminary reports is to allow for prompt antibiotic therapy of an infection.
    c. Because most doctors have had training in infectious diseases, the laboratory can assume that all physicians fully understand all culture results and their significance.
    d. Each laboratory needs to have well defined rules for how to report the results of various types of cultures.

## ▶ REFERENCES & RECOMMENDED READING

Baron, E. J. & Finegold, S. M. (1990). *Diagnostic microbiology.* St. Louis: Mosby.

Isenberg, H. D. (Ed.). (1992). *Clinical microbiology procedures handbook.* Washington, DC: American Society of Microbiology.

It's Not Just O157! (1996). *The stool pigeon.* Cincinnati, OH: Meridian Diagnostics.

Konemann, E. W., Allen, S. D., Janda, W. M., Schreckenberger, P. C., & Winn, W. C. (1992). *Color atlas and textbook of diagnostic microbiology.* Philadelphia: Lippincott.

Murray, P. R. (Ed.)(1995). *Manual of clinical microbiology.* Washington: ASM Press.

# CHAPTER 25
# Cerebrospinal Fluid and Other Body Fluids

Diane K. Tamanaha, MS, MT (ASCP)

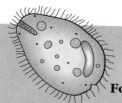

## Microbes in the News
### For all the Hysteria, 'Mad Cow Disease' Remains a Mystery

"**Mad Cow Disease**," also known as bovine spongiform encephalopathy (BSE), appeared in cows in Great Britain in 1985 and broke out in epidemic numbers there the following year. Although other herds in Europe have had cases of BSE, no cases have appeared in the United States

In 1990, BSE was noticed to be similar to Creutzfeldt-Jakob disease (CJD), a fatal infection, which occurs in humans (one in a million people per year). Other animal species have similar illnesses. It is possible that British cows were infected by eating feed supplemented with rendered sheep meat.

In 1996, there was speculation that there might be a link between BSE and 10 people in Britain who became ill. CJD has previously been spread from infected corneal transplants or hormone injections. Scientists are debating on whether a bacterium or a **prion** protein causes CJD.

Source: Article downloaded from the Internet. "For All the Hysteria, 'Mad Cow Disease' Remains a Mystery," Copyright 1996 Nando.net, Associated Press, Washington, 30 March 1996.

## KEY TERMS

Acute meningitis
Amnionitis
Amniotic fluid
Blood–brain barrier
Central nervous system (CNS)
Cerebrospinal fluid (CSF)
Cerebrospinal fluid shunts
Chorioamnionitis
Chronic ambulatory peritoneal dialysis (CAPD)
Chronic meningitis
Cryptococcal antigen
Direct antigen detection test (DADT)
Empyema
India ink stain
Lumbar puncture
Mad cow disease
Meningitis
Parapneumonic effusion
Pericardial fluid
Pericarditis
Peritoneal fluid
Peritonitis
Pleural fluid
Prion
Septic arthritis
Synovial fluid
Synovitis
Tenosynovitis

## LEARNING OBJECTIVES

**Upon successful completion of this chapter, the student should be able to:**

1. Describe the collection, handling, and processing of cerebrospinal fluid (CSF) and other body fluids.
2. List the common pathogens isolated in CSF and other body fluids.

3. Describe the changes to CSF during infections of the central nervous system (CNS).
4. Discuss how CSF and other body fluid infections are acquired.
5. Describe the common clinical symptoms associated with CNS infections.

## INTRODUCTION

**Cerebrospinal fluid (CSF)** and other sterile body fluids are important samples received in the clinical laboratory. Infections from sterile body fluids, especially from CSF, are potentially life-threatening and require rapid diagnosis and treatment. Neurologic sequelae (hearing loss, visual problems, learning disabilities, mental retardation, and other mental and motor abnormalities) from CSF infections may occur. As many as 10% to 50% of those infected may experience some residual effects, which may improve with time; however 14% to 30% suffer permanent effects (Gorbach, Bartlett, & Blacklow, 1992; Saez-Llorens & McCracken, 1990; Schlossberg, 1990; Vetter & Johnson, 1995). Therefore, rapid and appropriate microbiologic examination is critical in the clinical laboratory. Positive findings should be communicated to the physician immediately so that appropriate antimicrobial therapy may be initiated.

### Cerebrospinal Fluid

The CSF is most commonly collected to diagnose **meningitis**. Other infective processes may also produce positive cultures in CSF. These include infections occurring from anatomic defects due to trauma or surgical complications, **central nervous system (CNS)** abscesses, encephalitis, thrombosis of infected venous sinuses, bacteremia, pneumonia, pharyngitis, endocarditis, otitis media, mastoiditis, sinusitis, and others (Murray et al., 1995; Ray, Wasilauskas, & Zabransky, 1982). Table 25-1 lists the normal parameters of CSF fluid.

Infections of CSF are caused by a variety of pathogens, including bacteria, viruses, fungi, and parasites. The infecting agent varies according to the type and site of CNS infection, age, environment, underlying diseases, and other host factors. The majority of the CSF infections in the United States (70%–95%) occur in children under 5 years of age and especially among the newborn (Baron & Finegold, 1990; Wispelwey, Tunkel, & Scheld, 1990). Trauma or neurosurgery is associated with gram-negative rod and staphylococcus infections (Gorbach et al., 1992). Brain abscesses are associated with chronic sinusitis or otitis media and may involve anaerobes and polymicrobic infections (Mandell, Ben-

nett, & Dolin, 1995; Schlossberg, 1990). Pneumococcal meningitis can be found with CSF leakage (Kaufman, Tunkel, Pryor, & Dacey, 1990). The risk of developing CSF infections is increased with alcoholism, splenectomy, diabetes mellitus, prosthetic devices, immunosuppression, and other conditions (Baron & Finegold, 1990; Mahon & Manuselis, 1995).

### Other Body Fluids

Common sterile body fluids sent to the microbiology laboratory include **amniotic fluid**, **pericardial fluid**, **peritoneal fluid** [ascitic fluid, paracentesis and **chronic ambulatory peritoneal dialysis (CAPD)**], **pleural fluid** (thoracentesis fluid and **empyema** fluid), and **synovial fluid** (joint fluid). Organisms encountered in these fluids usually involve infections of the adjacent organs and tissues (e.g., endocarditis, bacterial arthritis, pneumonia). Complications to sterile body fluid and tissue infections include latent CNS infections.

## BASIC ANATOMY OF THE SYSTEM

### Central Nervous System

The CNS is composed of the brain, spinal cord, and corresponding nerves. The scalp, skeletal system, meninges, and the **blood–brain barrier** help to protect the CNS from infections (Gorbach et al., 1992). The blood–brain barrier controls the passage of various blood components into the CSF and is composed of the epithelium of the choroid plexus and the endothelium of the capillaries.

The brain and spinal cord are enclosed by three membranes known as the meninges. Starting from the brain going outward, the meninges are the pia mater, the arachnoid mater (pia and arachnoid collectively are called the leptomeninges), and the dura mater. CSF occupies the subarachnoid space between the pia mater and the arachnoid. The subdural space lies between the arachnoid and the dura mater. The epidural space is between the dura mater and the skull. Figure 25-1 shows the major components of the brain.

Approximately 70% to 85% of CSF is produced by

| Table 25–1 ▶ Normal Parameters of Cerebrospinal Fluid | | |
|---|---|---|
| **CSF Parameters** | **Adults** | **Newborn** |
| Appearance | Clear, colorless | Clear, colorless |
| Total protein | 15–50 mg/dL | 15–170 mg/dL |
| Glucose | 40–80 mg/dL (CSF glucose to serum ratio of 0.6) | 30–120 mg/dL |
| Leukocyte count | ≤ 5–10 WBC/μL (majority lymphocytes, followed by monocytes, then neutrophils | 0–30 WBC/μL (majority monocytes) |
| WBC, white blood cells | | |

secretion and ultrafiltration in the choroid plexus located in the third and fourth ventricles of the brain. Diffusion across the meninges accounts for the remainder of the production. CSF enters the subarachnoid space via the cisterna magna, supplying nutrients and cushioning the brain. CSF is reabsorbed by the arachnoid villi, with a small amount diffusing directly across the meninges. In adults, the total volume of CSF ranges from 90 to 150 mL and in newborns, 10 to 60 mL. Approximately 400

to 600 mL is formed and recirculated each day (Gray & Fedorko, 1991; Krieg & Kjeldsberg, 1991; Mahon & Manuselis, 1995; Mandell et al., 1995).

## Other Body Fluids

Sterile body fluids are obtained from their corresponding anatomic site. Amniotic fluid bathes the fetus inside the amniotic sac of pregnant women. Its func-

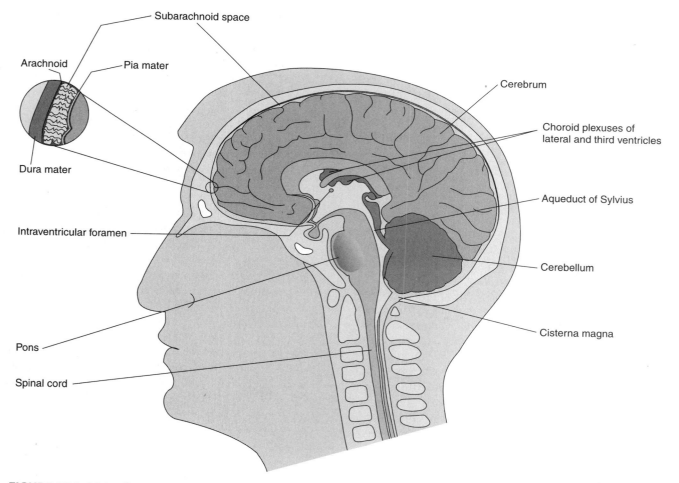

**FIGURE 25-1** Major features of the CNS. Arrows indicate the flow of CSF. Shaded area indicates the subarachnoid space.

tions are to allow for fetal protection, movement, and growth and to maintain temperature and biochemical homeostasis. Pericardial fluid occupies the pericardial cavity found between the membranes surrounding the heart. Peritoneal fluid is found in the peritoneal cavity, a space between the two layers of the peritoneum, which surrounds the surface of the abdomen and pelvis. Peritoneal fluid also includes CAPD. Fluid is injected into the peritoneal cavity and removed along with the body's waste products for those with renal disease. Pleural fluid is found in the pleural cavity between the two membranes of the pleura, which encloses the lungs. Synovial fluid may be obtained from any joint in the body. Except for amniotic fluid, these fluids are generally ultrafiltrates of plasma. Synovial fluid also has hyaluronate, a mucopolysaccharide secreted by the synovial cells. The fluids support, lubricate, and allow exchange of nutrients and waste products to the surrounding tissue (Kjeldsberg & Knight, 1986; Krieg & Kjeldsberg, 1991).

The pericardial, peritoneal, and pleural cavities are not true cavities. The membranes are very close together and separated by a small amount of fluid under normal circumstances. Infection, disease, or injury generally causes the accumulation of fluid in the cavity, called an effusion. Pericardial, peritoneal, or pleural effusions are divided into transudates and exudates. Transudates are generally due to a systemic disease such as congestive heart failure, renal failure, and cirrhosis. Exudates usually involve the membrane surfaces, such as in inflammation, malignancies, or infections, and are usually the specimens sent for microbiologic analysis (Baron & Finegold, 1990; Kjeldsberg & Knight, 1986).

## RESIDENT FLORA

The CSF and other sterile body fluids do not have normal flora. Any organism isolated from sterile body fluids is either a potential pathogen or a contaminant. Contamination of the sample may occur from normal skin flora such as *Staphylococcus epidermidis, Corynebacterium* species, *Propionibacterium acnes,* and *Micrococcus* species (Howard et al., 1994; Ray et al., 1982). Appropriate disinfection, collection, and processing procedures are essential to reduce the incidence of contaminants. "Skin contaminants" may be a true pathogen in the infection and may confuse the diagnosis. The physician must base the diagnosis not only on the culture results, but also on the patient's clinical signs and symptoms, history, and other diagnostic studies.

## SPECIMEN TYPES AND COLLECTION

### Specimen Collection

Basic collection principles of CSF and sterile body fluids (Baron & Finegold, 1990; Howard, Keiser, Smith, Weissfeld, & Tilton, 1994; Pezzlo, 1992) include:

1. Collect specimens before antimicrobial therapy is started.
2. Use sterile technique to avoid contamination by cutaneous flora.
3. Obtain adequate quantities of sample. The larger the volume the better.
4. Use swabs only as a last resort. The quantity of organisms in the sample may be low so a large volume of fluid is preferred. Inadequate sampling may cause negative smears and cultures. Also anaerobes are readily exposed to air with the use of swabs unless immediately placed into special anaerobic transport devices.
5. Transfer specimens obtained by needle aspiration into a sterile tube or other suitable closed sterile collection system according to the laboratory's established policy (e.g., blood culture bottle, sterile vacutainer tube, anaerobe transport medium).
6. Homogenize small clots, which may form in some fluids, except if fungi are suspected.
7. Avoid anticoagulant due to the inhibiting properties to some organisms. If an anticoagulant must be used, use heparin.
8. Transport to the laboratory immediately. Keep at room temperature if bacterial studies are requested. (Only requests for viral studies may be refrigerated or frozen before receipt in the laboratory.)

Collection site preparation for CSF and sterile body fluids requires the disinfection of the skin to minimize cutaneous flora contamination. The preparation is the same procedure used when collecting a blood culture. The site is cleansed with isopropyl alcohol and 2% tincture of iodine. Table 25-2 lists collection guidelines.

Cerebrospinal fluid can be obtained by subdural tap, ventricular aspiration or **lumbar puncture**. Lumbar puncture is the usual method (Koneman, Allen, Janda, Schreckenburger, & Winn, 1992). A needle is inserted into the subarachnoid space in the lumbar spine. The fluid is collected into three or more sterile tubes [tube 1: chemistry, tube 2: microbiology (or use cloudiest tube), tube 3: hematology, extra tube(s): additional studies] (see Figure 25-2).

### Specimen Processing

Sterile body fluids, especially CSF, should be processed as soon as possible. Neutrophils may lyse because the

## Table 25–2 ▸ Sterile Body Fluid Specimen Collection Guidelines

| Specimen | Minimum Volume* | Transport and Storage | Comments |
| --- | --- | --- | --- |
| CSF | Bacteria: ≥ 1 mL<br>Viral: ≥1 mL<br>Fungi: ≥ 2 mL<br>Mycobacterial: ≥ 2 mL | ASAP to lab at room temperature in sterile screw-capped tube. If viral only: send on ice within 15 min. Process immediately. | Obtain blood cultures also. |
| Amniotic fluid | ≥ 1 mL | ASAP to lab in anaerobic transport system or sterile screw-capped tube within 15 min. | Aspirate via amniocentesis, cesarean-section, or intrauterine catheter. |
| Pericardial fluid | ≥ 1 mL | ASAP to lab in anaerobic transport system or sterile screw-capped tube within 15 min. | Via percutaneous needle aspiration or surgery. Submit as much fluid as possible. May inoculate directly into blood culture bottles also. |
| Peritoneal fluid | ≥ 1 mL | ASAP to lab in anaerobic transport system or sterile screw-capped tube within 15 min. | Via percutaneous needle aspiration or surgery. Submit as much fluid as possible. |
| Pleural fluid | ≥ 1 mL | ASAP to lab in anaerobic transport system or sterile screw-capped tube within 15 min. | Via percutaneous needle aspiration or surgery. Submit as much fluid as possible. |
| Synovial fluid | ≥ 1 mL | ASAP to lab in anaerobic transport system or sterile screw-capped tube within 15 min. | Via percutaneous needle aspiration or surgery. Submit as much fluid as possible. May inoculate directly into blood culture bottles also. |

*The larger the volume the better, especially for fungal and mycobacterium cultures where the number of organisms is low.

CSF is hypotonic. After 1 hour at room temperature, cell counts may decrease by 32% and after 2 hours by 50% (Gray & Fedorko, 1992). Fastidious organisms such as *Streptococcus pneumoniae, Neisseria meningitidis,* or *Haemophilus influenzae* may not survive a long delay or variations in temperature. Pneumococci easily autolyse, and meningococci are susceptible to cold temperatures.

The concentration of bacteria is often low in sterile body fluids. If there are adequate amounts of sample

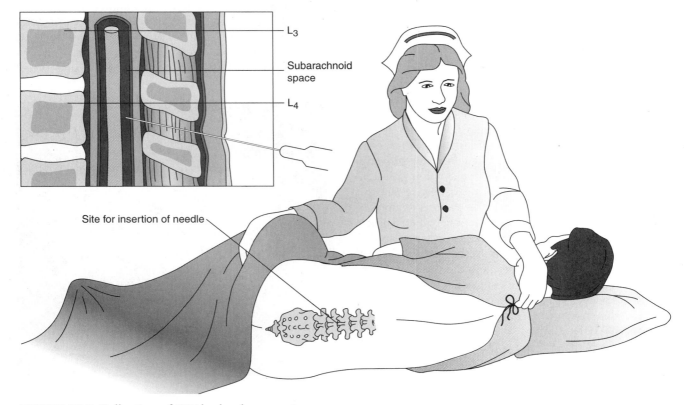

FIGURE 25-2 Collection of CSF by lumbar puncture.

(≥ 1 mL), the specimen should be concentrated for optimal recovery of organisms. Purulent body fluids may be inoculated directly (Baron & Finegold, 1990). Specimens are centrifuged at least 15 minutes at 1,500g (or 2,500g) (Howard et al., 1994; Murray, Baron, Pfaller, Tenover, & Yolken, 1995; Pezzlo, 1992). The supernatant is decanted into a sterile tube and saved for possible additional studies and may be refrigerated or frozen if not used immediately. The remaining fluid (approximately 0.5 mL) and sediment is mixed well by vortex or with a sterile pipet and used for smear and culture preparation (Baron & Finegold, 1990; Pezzlo, 1992).

Cytocentrifugation is a preferred alternative method for concentrating body fluid samples for smear preparation. The bacterial yield and cellular morphology may be superior to conventional centrifugation (Mahon & Manuselis, 1995).

Filtration is another method for concentrating the specimen. It can be used when large quantities of body fluids are received (i.e., CAPD). However, it is not practical for very viscous or clotted fluids. In a study comparing the filtration method to the centrifugation method, it was found that the two methods provided equivalent results for antimicrobial-free CSF. With antibiotic-supplemented CSF, the membrane filtration method was not as effective as the centrifugation method (Gray & Fedorko, 1992 ).

Unless fungal culture is requested, clotted body fluids should be homogenized or ground to release any trapped bacteria. Grinding may destroy fungal elements so clots should be cut into small pieces or teased apart and placed directly onto the media (Baron & Finegold, 1990; Pezzlo, 1992).

A Gram stain is prepared to determine the presence of organisms and leukocytes in the fluid. The sensitivity of the Gram stain for untreated bacterial meningitis ranges from 60% to 90%. If treated, it decreases to 40% to 60% (Mandell et al., 1995; Tunkel & Scheld, 1995). Care must be taken to avoid calling false positives on the smear, such as nonviable bacteria contaminating the lumbar puncture kit, slides, or staining solution (Baron & Finegold, 1990; Krieg & Kjeldsberg, 1991).

Acridine orange, a fluorochrome stain, is examined under low and high dry magnification, which allows for a faster examination and greater sensitivity than the Gram stain. Positive smears must be restained with Gram stain to verify and determine the Gram reaction of the organism. Prior decolorization of the acridine orange is not necessary. Because of the additional steps needed, this method is not widely used (Krieg & Kjeldsberg, 1991).

Infections of the CNS may often produce changes in the CSF, such as an increase in leukocytes, an increase in protein, and a decrease in glucose. A predominating neutrophilic differential usually indicates a bacterial or amebic infection, or early viral, fungal, or mycobacterial infection. Mononuclear leukocytes predominating are associated with viral, fungal, and mycobacterial infections (Gorbach et al., 1992). About 10% of acute bacterial meningitis may have a predominance of lymphocytes, especially with gram-negative bacilli in neonates and with listerial infections (Mandell et al., 1995). If a cloudy CSF reveals a predominance of neutrophils with no organisms seen, meningococci and pneumococci may be suspect (Schlossberg, 1990). Table 25-3 shows characteristic CSF changes with various types of infections.

Other STAT smears include **India ink stain** or nigrosin stain for encapsulated *Cryptococcus neoformans,* KOH or calcofluor white stain for fungal elements, acid-fast or auramine-rhodamine stains for mycobacteria, and wet preps for ameba. The sensitivity of the India ink stain is 25% to 50% and false positives may occur with inflammatory mononuclear cells, red blood cells, and other cells in the fluid (Gorbach et al., 1992; Krieg & Kjeldsberg, 1991; Schlossberg, 1990) (see Figure 25-3).

**Direct antigen detection tests (DADT)** can be performed on the CSF supernatant for rapid detection of commonly encountered organisms in CSF. It is an important supplement to Gram stain and culture, but is not a replacement. Currently, the most common techniques are based on latex agglutination and co-agglutination of antigen-antibody reactions. Enzyme immunoassay methods are available, but only in Europe and it cannot be performed on a STAT basis because it takes several hours to complete.

Commercial tests are available for the most commonly isolated pathogens, *H. influenzae* type b, *S. pneumoniae, N. meningitidis* serogroup A, C, Y, W-135, and group B streptococcus. These assays detect

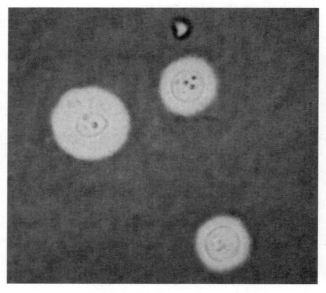

**FIGURE 25-3** India ink stain demonstrating the capsule of cryptococcus neoformans.

| Table 25–3 ▶ Changes in CSF Produced by CNS Infections | | | | |
|---|---|---|---|---|
| **Infection** | **Leukocytes** | **Cell Type** | **Protein** | **Glucose** |
| Bacterial meningitis | Increased (100–100,000) | PMN* | Increased | Decreased |
| Viral meningitis | Increased (20–2,000) | Lymphocytes† Monocytes | Normal to slightly increased | Normal |
| Mycobacterial meningitis | Increased (20–2,000) | Lymphocytes† Monocytes | Increased | Decreased |
| Fungal meningitis | Increased (20–2,000) | Lymphocytes† | Increased | Normal to decreased |
| Parasitic meningitis | Normal to increased (0–200) | Lymphocytes and/or eosinophils PMNs | Usually increased | Normal to decreased |
| Neurosyphilis | Increased (100–750) | Lymphocytes | Increased | Normal to decreased |
| CNS abscess‡ | Normal to increased (5–500) | PMN Monocytes | Increased | Normal to decreased |
| CSF shunt | Normal to increased (0–2,600) | PMN | Increased | Normal to decreased |

*Lymphocytic in newborns and in *Listeria* infections PMNs early in the illness

†PMNs early in the illness

‡Lumbar puncture not recommended for brain abscesses

PMN, polymorphonuclear leukocytes

the polysaccharide antigen in the cell of group B streptococcus and the antigens located in the capsule of the other three organisms. Antigens may be detected several days after initiation of therapy. In addition to CSF, urine or serum may be used. Serum is the least preferred specimen because of its interfering substances. Nonspecific reactions may occur with rheumatoid factor, blood, and a high protein concentration. The sensitivity of DADT is variable depending on which method and studies are examined. These are the sensitivity ranges based on several studies on CSF specimens:

▶ 66% to 100% for *H. influenzae* type b
▶ 33% to 93% for *N. meningitidis*
▶ 59% to 100% for *S. pneumoniae*
▶ 62% to 100% for group B streptococcus (Gray & Fedorko, 1992)

Direct antigen tests are also available for **cryptococcal antigen**. This test is preferred over the traditional India ink examination because of its high sensitivity and specificity.

Other miscellaneous tests for CSF include lactate dehydrogenase (LDH), lactic acid, and limulus amebocyte lysate (LAL) assay. LDH is used to differentiate between a bacterial and viral CNS infection. Higher LDH levels are found in bacterial infections. Lactic acid is also used to differentiate between a bacterial and viral meningitis. Both the LDH and lactic acid assays have poor sensitivities and specificities. The LAL assay is used to detect endotoxin caused by gram-negative organisms and is highly sensitive. It does not differentiate between the gram-negative organisms and may not be useful due to the availability of Gram stain and direct antigen testing (Kjeldsberg & Knight, 1986; Mahon & Manuselis, 1995).

## Suggested Plating (Bacteriology)

Body fluid sediment is used for the bacterial culture unless the specimen was not concentrated, in which case the whole sample is used. See Table 25-4 for the suggested culture plating of the various body fluids. Additional media may be inoculated depending on the smear result and request from the physician. Anaerobic organisms are rarely isolated from CSF, so anaerobic media is generally not inoculated unless they are suspected on the Gram stain (Baron & Finegold, 1990; Pezzlo, 1992). Use of direct inoculation of certain body fluids into blood culture bottles has recently been recommended (Howard et al., 1994; Murray et al., 1995; Pezzlo, 1992).

## OPPORTUNISTIC AND PATHOGENIC BACTERIA

### Cerebrospinal Fluid

Infection of the CSF can be manifested as various forms of meningitis, encephalitis, meningoencephalitis, CNS abscesses, and **CSF shunt** infections. Meningitis is an inflammation of the meninges, specifically the leptomeninges and subarachnoid space, and is usually bacterial in origin. Meningitis can be divided into **acute**

**Table 25–4 ▶ Suggested Plating (Bacteriology)**

| Specimen | BAP | Choc | Mac | Ana | Thio | Bc |
|---|---|---|---|---|---|---|
| CSF | X | X | | | X | |
| Amniotic fluid | X | X | X | X | X | |
| Pericardial fluid | X | X | X | X | X | |
| Peritoneal fluid | X | X | X | X | X | X (CAPD) |
| Pleural fluid | X | X | X | X | X | |
| Synovial fluid | X | X | X | X | X | X |

Ana, anaerobe media; BAP, blood agar; Bc, blood culture media; Choc, chocolate agar; Mac, MacConkey agar; Thio, thioglycollate broth

to subacute **meningitis** (onset of symptoms from several hours to several days) and **chronic meningitis** (symptoms for at least 4 weeks). Approximately 25,000 cases of meningitis occur annually in the United States. This equates to about 3.0 cases per 100,000 population (Wispelwey et al., 1990). Encephalitis is an inflammation of the brain and is more commonly associated with viral infections. Meningoencephalitis is usually of viral or parasitic origin and is an inflammation of both the brain and the surrounding meninges.

Viral infections are commonly due to enteroviruses (80%–85%), mumps, herpes simplex, arboviruses, lymphocytic choriomeningitis virus, and human immunodeficiency virus (Mandell et al., 1995). Infections with rabies, adenoviruses, rhinoviruses, and echoviruses are rare (Gorbach et al., 1992; Kjeldsberg & Knight, 1986). Fungal, mycobacterial, parasitic, and treponemal infections are rare compared to bacterial infections and are usually seen in immunocompromised persons or in endemic areas. Some of the fungi causing meningitis include *C. neoformans, Candida* species, *Histoplasma capsulatum, Coccidioides immitis,* zygomycetes, and *Aspergillus* species. Parasites such as *Entamoeba histolytica, Naegleria,* and *Acanthomoeba* may cause brain abscesses or meningoencephalitis (Kjeldsberg & Knight, 1986; Ray et al., 1982). Other rare organisms include *Brucella, Toxoplasma, Nocardia,* and *Echinococcus.*

Purulent meningitis is the accumulation of organisms and leukocytes to impart a cloudy or turbid appearance in the CSF. A cloudy CSF is usually bacterial in origin. Aseptic meningitis describes a condition with meningitis symptoms and negative CSF findings for which a cause is not apparent. Often the culture is not aseptic, but due to viruses, fungi, parasites, or certain bacteria (Mahon & Manuselis, 1995 ).

**Acute Meningitis.** The most frequent isolates of acute bacterial meningitis are *H. influenzae, N. meningitidis,* and *S. pneumoniae,* which collectively account for over 80% of the reported cases in the United States (Mandell et al., 1995; Wispelwey et al., 1990). According to two large studies done on bacterial meningitis in 1978–1981 and 1986, the incidence

rate for *H. influenzae* was 45% to 48.3%, for *N. meningitidis,* 14% to 19.6%, and for *S. pneumoniae,* 13.3% to 18% (Schlech et al., 1985; Wenger et al., 1990). *H. influenzae* mainly infects children. Neonates are primarily infected by maternal vaginal flora such as *Escherichia coli* and other gram-negative rods, *Streptococcus agalactiae* (group B streptococcus), *Listeria monocytogenes,* and other streptococci (Gorbach et al., 1992; Saez-Llorens & McCracken, 1990). The main pathogens for older children and adults are *N. meningitidis* and *S. pneumoniae* and for the elderly, *S. pneumoniae* (Murray et al., 1995; Wispelwey et al., 1990). Table 25-5 lists the common pathogens according to age.

**H. INFLUENZAE.** *H. influenzae* is a gram-negative pleomorphic bacillus that causes meningitis, epiglottiditis, pneumonia, septicemia, and arthritis (refer to Color Plate 72). Greater than 80% of *H. influenzae* infections occur in children less than 2 years of age (Saez-Llorens & McCracken, 1990; Wispelwey et al., 1990). Only a small percentage (1%–4%) of *H. influenzae* are found in adults and infection is often due to the presence of an underlying condition as the cause. *H. influenzae* type b was the most common cause of meningitis in children until the introduction of vaccination (Centers for Disease Control and Prevention [CDC], 1995). Infants less than 6 months of age are initially protected by the antibodies acquired from the mother. Thereafter, children are susceptible to infection until vaccinated or until they naturally produce their own antibodies at 5 to 6 years of age (Baron & Finegold, 1990; Mahon & Manuselis, 1995). In 1985 the first *H. influenzae* type b vaccine was released in the United States for children 2 years of age or older. This was a polysaccharide vaccine that had poor immunogenicity in infants (Gorbach et al., 1992; Vetter & Johnson, 1995). A new conjugate vaccine was introduced in 1988 for children starting at age 18 months. In 1990, this vaccine was later approved for use in 2-month-old infants (CDC, 1994; Vetter & Johnson, 1995). Since the use of the conjugate vaccine, the incidence of invasive *H. influenzae* type b has decreased by at least 95% in

| Neonates | Children | Older Children to Adults | Elderly Adults |
|---|---|---|---|
| *S. agalactiae* | *H. influenzae* type b | *N. meningitidis* | *S. pneumoniae* |
| *E. coli* | *N. meningitidis* | *S. pneumoniae* | *N. meningitidis* |
| *L. monocytogenes* | *S. pneumoniae* | Viruses | *L. monocytogenes* |
| *Citrobacter diversus* | Viruses | *H. influenzae* | *S. agalactiae* |
| *Klebsiella pneumoniae* | | Other gram-negative bacilli | *Staphylococcus aureus* |
| *Salmonella* | | Streptococci | *Enterobacteriaceae* |
| *Serratia* | | Staphylococci | *F. meningosepticum* |
| *Enterobacter* | | *L. monocytogenes* | *Pseudomonas aeruginosa* |
| *Pseudomonas* | | | *E. coli* |
| *Proteus* | | | *H. influenzae* |
| *S. pneumoniae* | | | |
| *S. aureus* | | | |
| Anaerobes | | | |
| Viruses | | | |
| Enterococci | | | |
| Nontypable | | | |
| *H. influenzae* | | | |
| *Flavobacterium meningosepticum* | | | |

Table 25–5 ▶ Pathogens of Acute Meningitis

infants and children (see Figure 25-4) (CDC, 1995). It is no longer the most frequent cause of meningitis in children and has been surpassed by the pneumococcus (Spellerberg & Tuomanen, 1994). It is believed that the *H. influenzae* vaccine also helped to decrease the incidence of disease among unvaccinated individuals by decreasing the carriage rate in the nasopharynx, thereby reducing the exposure to *H. influenzae* (CDC,

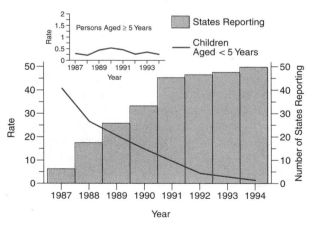

**FIGURE 25-4** Incidence rate of invasive *Haemophilus influenzae* (Hi) among children less than 5 years and over 5 years and the number of states reporting Hi surveillance data in 1987–1994. (Centers for Disease Control and Prevention [1995])

1994). *H. influenzae* type b now occurs primarily in unvaccinated or undervaccinated children (CDC, 1995).

**N. MENINGITIDIS.** *N. meningitidis* is a gram-negative, coffee bean-shaped diplococcus normally found in the oropharynx (refer to Color Plate 73). It is found most frequently in children and young adults. It is endemic and sometimes epidemic in certain developing countries, such as the meningitis belt of sub-Saharan Africa. Occasional outbreaks occur in the United States, associated with crowded conditions (military, schools, college dormitories), lack of immunization, and complement deficiencies (Baron & Finegold, 1990; Vetter & Johnson, 1995). A polysaccharide vaccine is available for serogroups A, C, Y, and W-135 as a single dose. Serogroups A, B, and C account for greater than 90% of all cases with serogroup B the most common in the United States. Group A is the most common in epidemics (Mahon & Manuselis, 1995; Vetter & Johnson, 1995).

**S. PNEUMONIAE.** *S. pneumoniae* is a gram-positive, lancet-shaped diplococcus usually occurring in pairs. Since the advent of the *H. influenzae* type b vaccine it is now the most frequent cause of childhood meningitis (Spellerberg & Tuomanen, 1994). *S. pneumoniae* is associated with pneumonia and otitis media. It is most commonly isolated in adults, especially among the elderly who are immunocompromised (alcoholism, pneumonia, liver disease, malignancy, sickle cell disease, nephrotic syndrome) in some way. The first commercially available vaccine for 14 serotypes was available in 1977 and the present vaccine for 23 serotypes appeared in 1983 (Vetter & Johnson, 1995; Wispelwey et al., 1990).

**S. AGALACTIAE.** *S. agalactiae*, also known as group B streptococcus, is a gram-positive coccus, most commonly isolated in neonatal meningitis. It can be found in the genital tract of 15% to 40% of asymptomatic women. Occasionally it is isolated in elderly adults usually with an underlying disease such as diabetes, malignancy, alcoholism, and others (Mandell et al., 1995).

**L. MONOCYTOGENES.** *L. monocytogenes* is a gram-positive bacillus that is often confused with *S. agalactiae* on culture because of similar gross morphology characteristics. It is most often found in neonates and the elderly with predisposing disease factors. *Listeria* accounts for a small percentage of cases, but has a high mortality rate of 22% to 29%. Coleslaw, raw vegetables, milk, and cheese have been associated with *Listeria* outbreaks (Mandell et al., 1995).

**OTHER BACTERIAL PATHOGENS.** Other bacterial pathogens include *Staphylococcus aureus, E. coli* and other gram-negative bacilli, and other streptococci and anaerobic organisms. Gram-negative rods are more commonly found in nosocomially acquired CNS infections in adults in comparison to pneumococcus, which is found in community-acquired infections (Durand et al., 1993). Other organisms, such as *Mycoplasma tuberculosis, Treponema pallidum* (neurosyphilis), and *Borrelia burgdorferi* (Lyme borreliosis) may be isolated. Most of these pathogens are more commonly found in chronic meningitis than in the acute stage and are associated with an underlying disease state that predisposes the individual to the particular organism (Gorbach et al., 1992).

**POLYMICROBIC INFECTIONS.** Approximately 1% of bacterial meningitis cases are mixed infections. Most common organisms are a mixture of *Enterobacteriaceae* (*Klebsiella, Enterobacter*), *Pseudomonas, S. aureus,* and obligate anaerobes (*Bacteroides, Clostridium, Peptostreptococcus*). Mixed infections are mainly nosocomially acquired infections in adults with predisposing factors including CSF fistulae, carcinomas, contiguous sites of infections, recent neurosurgery, and trauma (Chokephaibulkit & Leo, 1995; Gorbach et al., 1992; Wispelwey et al., 1990).

**Chronic Meningitis.** Chronic meningitis is less common than acute meningitis and often occurs in persons who are immunocompromised. Laboratory confirmation is frequently difficult because cultures may often be negative. The patient's history, physical examination, and signs and symptoms may sometimes help with the diagnosis. The pathogens of chronic meningitis include *M. tuberculosis,* various fungi such as *C. neoformans, C. immitis, H. capsulatum,* or *Blastomyces dermatitidis,* spirochetes such as *T. pallidum* or

*B. burgdorferi, Brucella melitensis,* and parasites such as *Toxoplasma gondii* or *Echinococcus granulosus* (Baron & Finegold, 1990; Mahon & Manuselis, 1995; Mandell et al., 1995). The following pathogens are associated with chronic meningitis:

- ► *M. tuberculosis* and other mycobacteria
- ► Fungi
    - *C. neoformans*
    - *C. immitis*
    - *H. capsulatum*
    - *B. dermatitidis*
    - *Candida*
    - *Sporothrix*
    - Other miscellaneous fungi
- ► *Actinomyces*
- ► *Nocardia*
- ► Spirochetes
    - *T. pallidum*
    - *B. burgdorferi*
    - *Borrelia recurrentis*
    - *Leptospira interrogens*
- ► *Brucella*
- ► *Franciella*
- ► *Salmonella*
- ► *L. monocytogenes*
- ► *Staphylococci*
- ► *Citrobacter*
- ► *N. meningitidis*
- ► Parasites
    - *Toxoplasma*
    - *Paragonimus*
    - *Trichinella*

## Other Body Fluids

**Amniotic Fluid.** Amniotic fluid infections may be associated with **amnionitis, chorioamnionitis,** intra-amniotic infections, or intrapartum infections. Amnionitis is an inflammation of the amnion. Chorioamnionitis is an inflammation of the fetal membrane. Normal vaginal flora may cause amniotic fluid infections and the major pathogen is *S. agalactiae.* Other agents include gram-negative rods, other streptococci, *Listeria,* and anaerobes. *Toxoplasma* and viral infections such as herpes simplex and cytomegalovirus have been known to cause infections. Infections may also be polymicrobic with both aerobic and anaerobic organisms (Kjeldsberg & Knight, 1986; Pezzlo, 1992; Sweet & Gibbs, 1990). Pathogenic agents include:

- ► *S. agalactiae*
- ► α-Hemolytic streptococci
- ► Enterococci
- ► *S. pyogenes*
- ► *L. monocytogenes*
- ► *Gardnerella vaginalis*

- ▶ *E. coli*
- ▶ *K. pneumoniae*
- ▶ *N. gonorrhoeae*
- ▶ HB-5
- ▶ *H. influenzae*
- ▶ *Haemophilus parainfluenzae*
- ▶ *Caponocytophaga* species
- ▶ Anaerobes
    - *Bacteroides*
    - *Peptococcus*
    - *Peptostreptococcus*
    - *Clostridium*
- ▶ Viruses
- ▶ *Toxoplasma*

**Pericardial Fluid.** Infections of the pericardial fluid are associated with bacteremia, endocarditis, myocarditis, and **pericarditis**. Pericarditis is usually viral in origin. The predominating viruses are the enteroviruses of coxsackie group B and echovirus type 8. Bacterial organisms that cause pericarditis include methacillin-resistant *S. aureus* (MRSA), non-group A streptococci, gram-negative bacilli, *B. melitensis*, *Salmonella* species, *Neisseria* species, *H. influenzae*, *Legionella pneumophilia*, *Francisella tularensis*, and anaerobes. Tuberculosis pericarditis is uncommon except in patients with acquired immunodeficiency syndrome (AIDS). Fungi include *Histoplasma*, *Candida*, *Cryptococcus*, *Aspergillus*, and *Coccidioides*. Other rare organisms such as *Toxoplasma*, *Borrelia*, and *Babesia*, have been known to cause infection. *S. aureus*, *H. influenzae*, and *N. meningitidis* are the most common bacterial isolates in children. Bacteremia and endocarditis may be associated with anaerobes such as *Bacteroides*, *Peptostreptococcus*, *Fusobacterium*, *Clostridium*, and *Propionibacterium* (Baron & Finegold, 1990; Gorbach et al., 1992; Howard et al., 1994; Lorrell & Braunwald, 1992). Pathogens of pericardial fluid include:

- ▶ Viruses
- ▶ Anaerobes
    - *Bacteroides*
    - *Fusobacterium nucleatum*
    - *Clostridium*
    - *Propionibacterium*
    - *Peptostreptococcus*
- ▶ *Mycoplasma pneumoniae*
- ▶ *Chlamydia*
- ▶ *M. tuberculosis*
- ▶ *S. aureus*
- ▶ *Enterobacteriaceae* and other gram-negative bacilli
- ▶ Streptococci
- ▶ *Borrelia*
- ▶ *Babesia*
- ▶ Fungi
    - *C. immitis*

- *Aspergillus*
- *Candida*
- *C. neoformans*
- *Histoplasma*
- ▶ Parasites
    - *E. histolytica*
    - *Toxoplasma*

**Peritoneal Fluid.** **Peritonitis** is an inflammation of the peritoneum. Secondary bacterial peritonitis can arise from the contamination of the peritoneal cavity from a perforation of the gastrointestinal tract. Common isolates of peritoneal fluid are usually abdominal flora such as gram-negative rods and anaerobes. The majority (75%) are usually of mixed infections. Primary bacterial peritonitis is most often found in infants and children, individuals with cirrhosis, and children with nephrotic syndrome. It is usually caused by *S. pneumoniae* and gram-negative bacilli, especially *E. coli*. Anaerobes are rarely found in primary peritonitis and infections are usually not polymicrobic, but from a single organism. Usually a polymicrobic aerobic and anaerobic infection is seen with intra-abdominal abscesses. Tuberculosis peritonitis is very rare and is usually found in those with pulmonary tuberculosis (Baron & Finegold, 1990; Gorbach et al., 1992; Kjeldsberg & Knight, 1986). Pathogens in peritoneal fluid include:

- ▶ Anaerobes
    - *Bacteroides*, usually *fragilis*
    - *Clostridium*
    - *Peptostreptococcus*
    - *Fusobacterium*
- ▶ *S. pneumoniae*
- ▶ Streptococci
- ▶ Enterococci
- ▶ *S. aureus*
- ▶ *S. epidermidis*
- ▶ *Corynebacterium*
- ▶ *E. coli*
- ▶ *Klebsiella*
- ▶ *Proteus*
- ▶ *P. aeruginosa*
- ▶ Other gram-negative rods
- ▶ *Neisseria gonorrhoeae*
- ▶ *Chlamydia*
- ▶ *M. tuberculosis*
- ▶ Fungi
    - *Candida*
    - *C. immitis*

**Pleural Fluid.** Pleural fluid isolates are usually of respiratory origin. **Parapneumonic effusions** are associated with bacterial pneumonia or lung abscesses. Viral or mycoplasma pneumonia may cause small pleural effusions. If the fluid is purulent it is known as empyema (pleural pus). Prior to the introduction of antibiotics, *S. pneumoniae* was the predominant organism, followed by group A streptococcus and *S. aureus*. Most infections were due to community acquired pneumonia. Today, anaerobes (11%–76% recovery rate) are common pathogens in empyema. The more common isolates are *Bacteroides, Peptostreptococcus,* and *Fusobacterium. S. aureus* is commonly associated with thoracic surgery or empyema in infants. Other organisms that have been recovered in pleural fluid include those associated with lower respiratory tract infections. *Legionella, Salmonella, Listeria,* streptococci, *Eikenella,* and other organisms have been recovered. Infections caused by viruses, *M. pneumoniae* or *Chlamydia pneumoniae* are rare unless coinfected with a bacterial pathogen. Mixed infections are common (Bartlett, 1988; Gorbach et al., 1992; Kjeldsberg & Knight, 1986) (refer to Color Plate 74). Pathogens of pleural fluid include:

▶ *S. aureus*
▶ *S. pneumoniae*
▶ Other streptococci
▶ *H. influenzae*
▶ *P. aeruginosa*
▶ *E. coli* and other *Enterobacteriaceae*
▶ *Eikenella*
▶ *L. monocytogenes*
▶ Anaerobes
  *F. nucleatum*
  *Bacteroides melanogenicus*
  *B. fragilis*
  *Clostridium*
▶ *M. tuberculosis* and other mycobacteria
▶ Viruses
▶ *M. pneumoniae*
▶ *Legionella*
▶ Fungi
▶ *Actinomyces*
▶ *Nocardia*
▶ Parasites
▶ *E. histolytica*
▶ *Echinococcus*

**Synovial Fluid.** Infections of synovial fluid are associated with **septic arthritis** and are usually bacterial in origin, but may be caused by viral, fungal, and mycobacterial pathogens. The most common pathogen of nongonococcal bacterial arthritis is *S. aureus* (60%), followed by streptococci, then gram-negative bacilli such as *E. coli* and *P. aeruginosa* (refer to Color Plate 75). In neonates, *S. aureus* and gram-negative rods are commonly isolated in hospital-acquired infections, whereas streptococci are more commonly found in community-acquired infections. *H. influenzae* is common in young children. In adolescents to young adults, *N. gonorrhoeae*

is commonly isolated, followed by *S. aureus* (refer to Color Plate 76). In the elderly, *S. aureus* and a variety of other bacteria are most commonly isolated. *S. epidermidis* accounts for the majority of prosthetic joint infections, followed by *S. aureus,* often in mixed infections with anaerobes. *B. burgdorferi* is sometimes isolated in those with Lyme borreliosis. Mycobacterial and fungal organisms are seen more often in a HIV infected person (Baron & Finegold, 1990; Goldenberg & Reed, 1985; Gorbach et al., 1992; Kjeldsberg & Knight, 1986). Pathogens of synovial fluid include:

▶ *S. aureus*
▶ *S. epidermidis*
▶ Other coagulase-negative staphylococci
▶ *Corynebacterium*
▶ *N. gonorrhoeae*
▶ *M. tuberculosis*
▶ *S. pneumoniae*
▶ Other streptococci
▶ *H. influenzae*
▶ Anaerobes
  *B. fragilis*
  *Prevotella*
  *Fusobacterium*
  *Propionibacterium*
  Anaerobic cocci
▶ *Actinomyces*
▶ Gram-negative bacilli
▶ Viruses
▶ Fungi
▶ *B. burgdorferi*
▶ *Brucella*
▶ *Salmonella*

## BACTERIAL DISEASES

### Cerebrospinal Fluid

**Pathogenesis.** Infections of the CNS may be acquired by the following mechanisms: by hematogenous spread and penetration of the blood–brain barrier, by contiguous spread from an adjacent area, and by direct penetration due to trauma or surgery (Howard et al., 1994; Mahon & Manuselis, 1995). Hematogenous spread is most commonly caused by bacterial, fungal and parasitic infections found in pneumonia, abscesses, endocarditis, etc. (Ray et al., 1982; Woods et al., 1993). Contiguous spread can occur through a respiratory or auditory route (otitis media, mastoiditis, sinusitis), via a neural route (sheaths of cranial or spinal nerves), or as a skin or bone infection that extends directly into the CNS (Mahon & Manuselis, 1995; Ray et al., 1982). The neural route is primarily due to viral infections (rabies, herpes simplex, varicella zoster, and polioviruses) (Woods et al., 1993). Skull fractures or defects, whether caused by trauma or surgery, may allow organisms to enter via an opening between the CNS and the surrounding area (Kaufman et al., 1990; Ray et al., 1982).

The pathogenesis of meningitis is not clearly understood but through various studies this is thought to be the general sequence of events: mucosal (nasopharyngeal) colonization → systemic invasion (bacteremia) → meningeal invasion → bacterial replication → subarachnoid infection → release of toxic bacterial components → immunomodulation → shock (Gray & Fedorko, 1992; Mandell et al., 1995; Spellerberg & Tuomanen, 1994; Tunkel & Scheld, 1993). Mucosal colonization in the nasopharynx and oropharynx may be aided by fimbriae or pili on the bacterium that allow it to attach to the mucosal cells.

The organism invades the bloodstream to create a bacteremia. The mechanism of entry is not well understood. It could involve either a direct invasion into the bloodstream via a junction breakdown between epithelial cells (probable entry for *H. influenzae*) or by passive entry through phagocytosis (probable entry for *N. meningitidis*). Nasopharyngeal epithelial cells may phagocytize the organism, then penetrate the subepithelial tissue to enter the bloodstream. Bacterial capsules may inhibit complement facilitated phagocytosis by leukocytes to allow for replication in the bloodstream. Those with complement deficiencies are more prone to *N. meningitidis* infections (Gray & Fedorko, 1992; Mandell et al., 1995; Spellerberg & Tuomanen, 1994; Tunkel & Scheld, 1993).

Entry into the CNS is uncertain as well. The concentration of organisms, the age of the host and a sustained bacteremia may be factors in meningeal invasion. Once inside the CNS, the organism multiplies freely. Because of the blood–brain barrier, the CSF is virtually sterile of phagocytic cells, complement, and immunoglobulins. As the bacteria replicate, inflammation of the meninges occurs by the presence of toxic components (teichoic acid, endotoxins) in the cell wall of the bacteria. The cell wall components stimulate the brain cells (astrocytes) and cerebral capillary endothelium to produce cytokine interleukin-1, tumor necrosis factor, and other factors that attract leukocytes, initiate the inflammatory response, and initiate the breakdown of the blood–brain barrier (Gray & Fedorko, 1992; Mandell et al., 1995; Spellerberg & Tuomanen, 1994; Tunkel & Scheld, 1993).

The leukocytes continue to penetrate into the CSF and release proteolytic products, which affect the vascular endothelium and choroid plexus epithelium, increasing the permeability of the blood–brain barrier. Further alterations occur, leading to brain edema, an increase in intracranial pressure, a decrease in cerebral blood flow, and cerebral infarction, and eventually progressing to brain damage and death (Gray & Fedorko, 1992; Mandell et al., 1995; Saez-Llorens & McCracken, 1990; Spellerberg & Tuomanen, 1994; Tunkel & Scheld, 1993).

Despite antibiotic treatment, immunomodulation may continue to occur even though organisms are not recoverable. Antibiotics that destroy the organism's cell wall cause the continued release of the toxic components. Use of adjunctive therapy with dexamethasone and other corticosteroids reduces the intensity of the immune response (Mandell et al., 1995; Spellerberg & Tuomanen, 1994; Tunkel & Scheld, 1993).

**Clinical Presentation.** Infections of the CNS may present with classic symptoms such as headache, fever, confusion, coma, focal deficits, and nuchal rigidity or signs and symptoms may be minimal or nonspecific. Clinical presentations may overlap within the various CNS infections and may depend on the severity and location of the infection, infectious agent, duration of the infection, age, and immunity-disease state of the individual. Symptoms of brain abscesses are associated with the mass exerting pressure on the surrounding tissue. Symptoms in neonates and young infants may be subtle and difficult to recognize. They may have fever, vomiting, diarrhea, temperature instability (hypothermia, hyperthermia), respiratory distress, listlessness, irritability, poor feeding, weak suck, lethargy, jaundice, high-pitched crying, seizures, poor muscle tone, abdominal distention, and a bulging fontanella. The elderly may have no fever, variable signs and symptoms, and other infections such as bronchitis, pneumonia, or sinusitis (Gorbach et al., 1992; Mandell et al., 1995; Saez-Llorens & McCracken, 1990; Tunkel & Scheld, 1995).

Meningococcal and pneumococcal infections may present with a maculopapular, purpuric, or an asymmetrical petechial rash. *S. aureus* may show symmetrical petechial lesions in the extremities. *Listeria* infections are associated with seizures and focal deficits (Mandell et al., 1995; Schlossberg, 1990; Tunkel & Scheld, 1995).

**Prion Diseases.** "Mad cow disease" has been in the news recently and so will be discussed here even though it is not a bacterial disease. This disease is part of the prion diseases that also includes Creutzfeldt-Jakob disease (CJD), kuru, and Gerstmann-Straussler-Scheinker syndrome, and fatal familial insomnia in humans. Other terminologies used for prion diseases are subacute transmissible spongiform encephalopathies, transmissible neurodegenerative disease, and unconventional slow virus disease. Four other prion diseases are found in animals—scrapie in sheep and goats, transmissible mink encephalopathy in mink, chronic wasting disease in mule deer and elk, and bovine spongiform encephalopathy (BSE), also known as "mad cow disease" in cattle, captive exotic ungulates, and domestic cats (Mandell et al., 1995; Murray et al., 1995; Schlossberg, 1990).

Prions are slow infectious agents confined to the CNS. Incubation periods range from a few months to several decades prior to clinical illness, which eventually progresses to death. Prions are distinct from viruses and viroids and are extremely resistant to substances that normally destroy viruses. A major component of the particle is made up of a protein, PrP, which polymerizes into rods ("prion protein") similar to amyloid found in Alzheimer's disease (Mandell et al., 1995; Murray et al., 1995; Schlossberg, 1990).

The characteristic features of prion diseases are the spongioform degeneration (vacuolization) of neurons, the increase in fibrous astrocytes, and the presence of amyloid plaques in the brain. Depending on the prion disease, brain function is impaired and may lead to loss of memory, loss of coordination, walking difficulties, visual impairment, dementia, convulsions, and other problems (Mandell et al., 1995; Murray et al., 1995; Schlossberg, 1990).

Prion disease has not been contagious or communicable but is transmissible and may be inherited. Transmission from man to animal has been documented. Transmission from animal to man through ingestion of infected meat is speculated. Ritualistic cannibalism, which occurred in the highlanders of Papua New Guinea, was the mode of spread for kuru. CJD has been transmitted by the transplantation of corneas, injections of human growth hormone, and by the implantation of cerebral electrodes (Mandell et al., 1995; Schlossberg, 1990).

The PrP protein can be found in CSF, but its presence is not diagnostic. Diagnosis is made by the examination of brain tissue, found along with the typical clinical presentations (Mandell et al., 1995; Murray et al., 1995).

## Amniotic Fluid

**Pathogenesis.** Bacterial invasion of amniotic fluid may occur with premature delivery, prolonged labor, and premature rupture of membranes. Premature rupture of membranes may actually be a cause rather than a result of infection. Occasionally infections may occur via a hematogenous or transplacental route or after placement of a cervical cerclage, after amniocentesis or after intrauterine transfusion (Kjeldsberg & Knight, 1986; Sweet & Gibbs, 1990).

**Clinical Presentation.** The majority of the clinical manifestations when noticed are already late signs. Symptoms include maternal and fetal tachycardia, maternal fever, uterine tenderness, irritability, leukocytosis, and foul-smelling amniotic fluid or vaginal discharge (Kjeldsberg & Knight, 1986; Sweet & Gibbs, 1990).

## Pericardial Fluid

**Pathogenesis.** Prior to the introduction of antibiotics, bacterial pericarditis was primarily due to a complication of pneumococcal pneumonia or empyema and pleuropulmonary disease. Usually pericardial infections are associated with predisposing factors such as a preexisting pericardial effusion, AIDS, lymphoma, leukemia, and other immunosuppressive states. Pericarditis may occur from a contiguous spread from a postoperative infection following thoracic surgery or trauma, endocarditis infection, extension from a subdiaphragmatic abscess, and bacteremic hematogenous spread. Children develop bacterial pericarditis in association with pharyngitis, pneumonia, meningitis, otitis media, impetigo, endocarditis, and bacterial arthritis (Gorbach et al., 1992; Lorrell & Braunwald, 1992).

**Clinical Presentation.** Common clinical features are high fevers, shaking chills, nightsweats, dyspnea, and tachycardia. Chest pain is usually absent. Pericardial friction rub is present in less than half the cases. Cardiac tamponade may develop. The presence of the pericarditis may be obscured by an underlying infection such as pneumonia or mediastinitis (Gorbach et al., 1992; Lorrell & Braunwald, 1992).

## Peritoneal Fluid

**Pathogenesis.** Peritoneal infections mainly arise from a perforation of the gastrointestinal tract by trauma or surgery or by a disease, with subsequent contamination of abdominal flora. This is known as secondary peritonitis (Gorbach et al., 1992; Howard et al., 1994).

Less than 1% of bacterial infections occur from primary peritonitis. Infections occur without any apparent abdominal perforation. Hematogenous spread is thought to be the cause of infections. A source of infection could be the transfer of organism from pelvic inflammatory disease in sexually active women. Contiguous spread may occur from abdominal infections (Baron & Finegold, 1990; Gorbach et al., 1992).

Intra-abdominal abscesses in the peritoneal cavity may arise from trauma or spontaneous gastrointestinal perforation, disruption of an anastomosis in gastrointestinal tract surgery, or from a hematogenous or lymphatic spread (Gorbach et al., 1992).

**Clinical Presentation.** Peritonitis may cause localized or general abdominal pain, muscle rigidity, rebound tenderness, and muscle guarding. Fever and a progressive tachycardia may be present. The abdomen may be distended and there may be a decrease in bowel sounds. Generally primary bacterial peritonitis symptoms are less acute than that of secondary peritonitis (Gorbach et al., 1992).

Symptoms vary with the source and location of intra-abdominal abscesses. Localized pain, tenderness, and an abdominal mass may be present. There may be diarrhea, low-grade fever, anorexia, general malaise, and weakness. Gastrointestinal bleeding may be present with progressive organ failure (Gorbach et al., 1992).

## Pleural Fluid

**Pathogenesis.** Bacterial pleural fluid infections, which result in empyema, occur as complications to pneumonia or lung abscess. Direct spread to a parapneumonic effusion is the usual route.

**Clinical Presentation.** Fever, cough, sputum production, dyspnea, and pleurisy, and pleuritic pain are common symptoms. There may be a putrid discharge of empyema fluid or sputum. Usually there is pleural fluid accumulation with dull and reduced breath sounds on the affected side of the lung. Concurrent pneumonia or lung abscess is common (Bartlett, 1988; Gorbach et al., 1992).

## Synovial Fluid

**Pathogenesis.** Synovial infections are usually by hematogenous spread due to the highly vascular synovial membrane with no limiting basement membrane. Infection of the bone, injection of corticosteroids, insertion of a prosthesis, penetrating wound, or arthroscopy may also contribute to infections. Individuals with rheumatoid arthritis are prone to joint infections. The majority of those who develop nongonococcal bacterial arthritis have some predisposing factor such as cancer, diabetes, chronic liver disease, or any other chronic joint disease. Gonococcal arthritis is associated with disseminated gonococcal infection, found more commonly in young women. Young children develop synovial infections in association with pneumonia or meningitis (Baron & Finegold, 1990; Goldenberg & Reed, 1985; Gorbach et al., 1992; Kjeldsberg & Knight, 1986).

**Clinical Presentation.** The sudden onset of an acute monoarticular arthritis is a common symptom. The knee is the most common site affected, followed by the hip, ankle, wrist, shoulder, and elbow. More than one joint is affected in 15% to 20% of cases. Joints may be swollen, red, warm, and tender. Motion in the joint may be decreased and a low-grade fever may be present. Approximately 50% have positive blood cultures. In disseminated gonococcal infections, migratory polyarthralgia is common. Fever, skin lesions, **synovitis**, and **tenosynovitis** may occur (Goldenberg & Reed, 1985; Gorbach et al., 1992).

## SUMMARY

▶ CSF and other sterile body fluid infections should be handled expediently because such infections may be potentially life-threatening.

▶ Appropriate collection, handling, and processing techniques are essential when working with sterile body fluids. Care must be taken to avoid contamination with normal skin flora, which may confuse the diagnosis.

▶ CSF is most commonly used to diagnose acute meningitis, but it can also be used for chronic meningitis and CSF shunt infection. It is not usually recommended for CNS abscesses because of the risk of cerebral herniation occurring during collection.

▶ The most common pathogens of acute bacterial meningitis are *H. influenzae, N. meningitidis,* and *S. pneumoniae.*

▶ Other sterile body fluids include amniotic fluid, pericardial fluid, peritoneal fluid, pleural fluid, and synovial fluid.

▶ Infections of other sterile body fluids are usually related to the flora and corresponding infection of the adjacent tissue, and to any underlying disease and the immune status of the host.

▶ CSF and other sterile body infections are usually acquired through hematogenous spread, contiguous spread from an adjacent infected area, and by direct penetration through trauma or surgery.

▶ The clinical signs and symptoms of CNS infections may often overlap or be minimal to absent.

## Review Questions

1. What are the three most common pathogens of acute meningitis?
   a. *S. pneumoniae, S. agalactiae, H. influenzae*
   b. *S. aureus, L. monocytogenes, H. influenzae*
   c. *S. pneumoniae, H. influenzae, N. meningitidis*
   d. *N. meningitidis, S. pneumoniae, L. monocytogenes*

2. CSF taken from a febrile 1-day-old infant showed gram-positive cocci in singles, pairs, and chains. The most likely organism would be:
   a. *S. agalactiae.*
   b. *L. monocytogenes.*
   c. *S. pneumoniae.*
   d. *S. aureus.*

3. CSF taken from an elderly diabetic woman had an increased protein level, a low glucose level, 1,000 PMNs/μL, and no organisms seen on the Gram stain. The most likely organism would be:
   a. *H. influenzae.*
   b. *M. tuberculosis.*
   c. *C. neoformans.*
   d. *S. pneumoniae.*

4. Complications of pneumonia include:
   a. pericarditis.
   b. amnionitis.
   c. empyema.
   d. both a and c.

5. Body fluid infections arise from:
   a. otitis media.
   b. bacteremia.
   c. trauma due to accidents or surgery.
   d. all of the above.

6. Which statement below is FALSE concerning the collection of sterile body fluid samples?
   a. Clean the collection area well with disinfectant and use sterile collection technique.
   b. Obtain at least 1 mL or more of fluid. The larger the volume the better.
   c. Collect sample prior to administration of antibiotics.
   d. Avoid anticoagulant due to its inhibiting properties to some organisms. If an anticoagulant must be used, use EDTA.

7. An elderly man with fever, cough, and dyspnea was seen in the emergency room. The patient was diagnosed with pneumonia. Purulent pleural fluid was collected and sent to the laboratory. The Gram stain showed gram-negative pleomorphic rods. What is the most likely organism?
   a. *Bacteroides*
   b. *E. coli*
   c. *Haemophilus*
   d. *Salmonella*

8. Which of the following statements is FALSE concerning clinical symptoms of CNS infections?
   a. Symptoms may include headache, fever, lethargy, and seizures.
   b. Symmetrical petechial rash is seen in *Haemophilus* infections.
   c. Symptoms may include nausea, vomiting, and diarrhea.
   d. Elderly may have no fever and variable signs and symptoms.

## CASE STUDY

A 9-year-old girl was seen in the emergency room following the sudden onset of a seizure. Her temperature on admission was 107°F. Her CBC showed an increase in leukocytes and platelets. She was given Ativan for the seizures and Tylenol, cool mist, and ice packs for the fever. The patient had a ventriculoperitoneal (VP) shunt in place and a prior history of a brain tumor. Four days prior to admission, the patient experienced headaches associated with anorexia. The patient's condition worsened and she was given vecuronium, mannitol, and Decadron and was also treated with prophylactic antibiotic therapy. Blood and catheterized urine specimens were obtained prior to the administration of antibiotics. CSF obtained via her VP shunt showed a clear "ruddy-brown" colored fluid with a cell count of 88 leukocytes/μL and 4 red blood cells/μL, a glucose of < 20 mg/dL, and a total protein of > 300 mg/dL. Both blood and CSF cultures were positive for *Streptococcus pneumoniae*. Despite initiation of antibiotic therapy, the patient died 2 days later.

### Questions:

1. What is the most probable diagnosis for this patient and why?

2. What is the most probable cause of her condition?

3. Why was the patient given Decadron (dexamethasone) in addition to the antibiotic?

9. A 65-year-old man visited his physician complaining of a headache increasing in severity, nausea, vomiting, and changes in mood for the past month. What course of action should be taken?

a. Send him home; patient probably has a viral infection.

b. Perform a computed tomography scan immediately to rule out a CNS abscess.

c. Collect CSF immediately to rule out chronic meningitis.

d. Treat and obtain CSF immediately; patient has acute meningitis.

10. Which statement is FALSE concerning the pathogenesis of meningitis?

a. Bacterial capsules probably aid in the colonization and invasion into the CNS.

b. *H. influenzae* and *N. meningitidis* attach to mucosal cells via frimbiae and pili.

c. Once inside the CNS, the organisms must overcome the abundant white blood cells, complement, and antibodies in the CSF.

d. Teichoic acid and endotoxin in the bacteria cell wall causes inflammation of the meninges.

# ▶ REFERENCES & RECOMMENDED READING

Baron, E. J., & Finegold, S. M. (1990). *Bailey and Scott's diagnostic microbiology* (8th ed.). St. Louis: Mosby.

Bartlett, J. G. (1988). Bacterial infections of the pleural space. *Seminars in Respiratory Infections, 3*(4), 309–321.

Centers for Disease Control and Prevention. (1995). Progress toward elimination of *Haemophilus influenzae* type b disease among infants and children—United States, 1993–1994. *Morbidity and Mortality Weekly Report, 44*(29), 545–550.

Centers for Disease Control and Prevention. (1994). Progress toward elimination of *Haemophilus influenzae* type B disease among infants and children—United States, 1987–1993. *Morbidity and Mortality Weekly Report, 43*(8), 144–148.

Durand, M. I., Calderwood, S. B., Weber, D. J., Miller, S. I., Southwick, F. S., Caviness, V. S. Jr., & Swartz, M. N. (1993). Acute bacterial meningitis in adults. *New England Journal of Medicine, 328*(1), 21–28.

Goldenberg, D. L., & Reed, J. I. (1985). Bacterial arthritis. *New England Journal of Medicine, 312*(12), 764–771.

Gorbach, S. L., Bartlett, J. G., & Blacklow, N. R. (Eds.). (1992). *Infectious disease*. Philadelphia: Saunders.

Gray, L. D., & Fedorko, D. P. (1992). Laboratory diagnosis of bacterial meningitis. *Clinical Microbiology Reviews, 5*(2), 130–145.

Howard, B. J., Keiser J. F., Smith, T. F., Weissfeld, A. S., & Tilton, R. C. (1994). *Clinical and pathogenic microbiology* (2nd ed.). St. Louis: Mosby.

Kaufman, B. A., Tunkel, A. R., Pryor, J. C, & Dacey, R. G. Jr. (1990). Meningitis in the neurosurgical patient. *Infectious Disease Clinics of North America, 4*(4), 677–701.

Kjeldsberg, C. R., & Knight, J. A. (1986). *Body fluids, laboratory examination of amniotic, cerebrospinal, seminal, serous & synovial fluids, a textbook atlas* (2nd ed.). Chicago: American Society of Clinical Pathologists Press.

Koneman, E. G., Allen, S. D., Janda, W. M., Schreckenburger, P. C., & Winn, W. C. Jr. (1992). *Color atlas & textbook of diagnostic microbiology* (4th ed.). Philadelphia: Lippincott.

Krieg, A. F., & Kjeldsberg, C. R. (1991) Cerebrospinal fluid and other body fluids. In J. B. Henry (Ed.), *Clinical diagnosis & management by laboratory methods* (18th ed., pp. 445–473). Philadelphia: Saunders.

Lorrell, H., & Braunwald, E. (1992) Pericardial disease. In E. Braunwald (Ed.), *Heart disease, a textbook of cardiovascular medicine* (4th ed., pp. 1465–1516). Philadelphia: Saunders.

Mahon, C. R., & Manuselis, G. Jr. (1995). *Textbook of diagnostic microbiology*. Philadelphia: Saunders.

Mandell, G. L., Bennett, J. E., & Dolin, R. (Eds.). (1995). *Mandell, Douglas and Bennett's principles and practice of infectious diseases* (4th ed.). New York: Churchill Livingstone.

Murray, P. R., Baron, E. J., Pfaller, M. A., Tenover, F. C., & Yolken, R. H. (Eds.). (1995). *Manual of clinical microbiology* (6th ed.). Washington, DC: American Society for Microbiology.

Pezzlo, M. (Section Ed.). (1992). Aerobic bacteriology. In H. D. Isenberg (Ed. in Chief), *Clinical microbiology procedures handbook* (pp. 1.1.1–1.18.37). Washington, DC: American Society for Microbiology.

Ray, C. G., Wasilauskas, B., & Zabransky, R. (1982). In L. R. McCarthy (Ed.), *Cumitech 14, Laboratory diagnosis of central nervous system infections*. Washington, DC: American Society for Microbiology.

Saez-Llorens, X., & McCracken, G. H. Jr. (1990). Bacterial meningitis in neonates and children. *Infectious Disease Clinics of North America, 4*(4), 623–644.

Schlech, W. F. III, Ward, J. I., Band, J. D., Hightower, A., Fraser, D. W., & Broome, C. V. (1985). Bacterial meningitis in the United States, 1978 through 1981. The national meningitis surveillance study. *Journal of the American Medical Association, 253*(12), 1749–1754.

Schlossberg, D. (Ed.). (1990). *Infections of the central nervous system*. New York: Springer-Verlag.

Spellerberg, B., & Tuomanen, E. I. (1994). The pathophysiology of pneumococcal meningitis. *Annals of Medicine, 26*(6), 411–418.

Sweet, R. L., & Gibbs, R. S. (1990). Intraamniotic infection (intrauterine infection in late pregnancy). In C. L. Brown (Ed.), *Infectious diseases of the female genital tract.* (2nd ed., pp. 337–347). Baltimore: Williams & Wilkins.

Tunkel, A. R., & Scheld, W. M. (1995). Acute bacterial meningitis. *Lancet, 346,* 1675–1680.

Tunkel, A. R., & Scheld, W. M. (1993). Pathogenesis and pathophysiology of bacterial meningitis. *Clinical Microbiology Reviews, 6*(2), 118–136.

Vetter, R. T., & Johnson, G. M. (1995). Vaccination update. Hib, hepatitis, polio, varicella, influenza, pneumococcal and meningococcal disease. *Vaccines, 98*(5), 141–150.

Wenger, J. D., Hightower, A. W., Facklam, R. R., Gaventa, S., Broome, C. V., & the Bacterial Meningitis Study Group. (1990). Bacterial meningitis in the United States, 1986: Report of a multistate surveillance study. *Journal of Infectious Disease 162*(12), 1316–1323.

Wispelwey, B., Tunkel, A. R., & Scheld, W. M. (1990). Bacterial meningitis in Adults. *Infectious Disease Clinics of North America, 4*(4), 645–659.

Woods, G. L., Gutierrez, Y., Walker, D. H., Purtilo, D. T., & Shanley, J. D. (1993). *Diagnostic pathology of infectious diseases*. Philadelphia: Lea & Febiger.

# CHAPTER 26

# Blood Cultures

James O. Murray, SM (AAM), CLS (NCA), MS

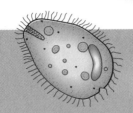

## Microbes in the News

### Less Microbiology is Best

For the past several years, the microbiology laboratory has encountered numerous changes and challenges to fundamental assumptions. Time-honored procedures are being reviewed, modified, or even discarded.

Frank Koontz, PhD, says, "Once CLIA started to breathe fire out of its cave, we started to ask whether we could justify what we were doing, especially when we were always getting the same results" from multiple samples. Michael Wilson, M.D., says that people are focusing on doing testing in a way that makes clinical sense as well as microbiologic sense by improving the quality and utilization of specimens.

L. Barth Reller, M.D., has been instrumental in evaluating a number of blood culture issues, such as sample volume, atmosphere of incubation, and the dilution of blood in broth. Looking at the relative yield from blood cultures, it was found that low-volume blood cultures with less than 10 mL per venipuncture were inadequate for detecting bacteremia. The yield was clearly better with 20 or 30 mL per puncture. So, drawing two or three large-volume specimens is just as good at diagnosing bacteremia as was the old way of drawing four to six small-volume specimens, and the laboratory's workload is reduced without sacrificing sensitivity.

For years it was thought that at least three blood cultures over 2 or 3 days were needed to diagnose bacterial endocarditis. Recent studies have revealed that the colonization of the endocardial tissue seeds a continuous bacteremia. As a result, if one culture is positive, all will be positive; and, according to Dr. Weinstein, "the diagnosis of infective endocarditis can be made with only one blood culture in a patient with a compatible clinical syndrome and with an echocardiogram showing appropriate lesions on a heart valve."

Adapted from Check, W. A. (1997). *CAP Today,* *11*(1), 21–29.

## KEY TERMS

Bacteremia
Biphasic
Blind subculture
Blood culture

Clinically significant
False-negative
Fungemia
Infective endocarditis

Positive culture
Sepsis and septicemia
Terminal subculture

## LEARNING OBJECTIVES

**Upon successful completion of this chapter, the student should be able to:**

1. Discuss the clinical patterns associated with how microbes cause bloodstream infections.
2. Define terms associated with bloodstream infections and blood culture, such as bacteremia, septicemia, infective endocarditis, biphasic, blind subculture, and continuous monitoring.
3. State the basic characteristics of blood culture media, including additives and environment.
4. State the blood culture collection technique, including collection site preparation, volume to collect, and number and timing of specimens.
5. Discuss blood culture specimen processing when using both manual and instrument methods.
6. Discuss the detection and processing of positive specimens including visible signs, subculture media, and microscopic examinations.
7. State the predominant etiologic agents of bacteremia and fungemia, and discuss special factors associated with the microbes.

## INTRODUCTION

The presence of bacteria or fungi in the bloodstream is often an indication of severe infection. Over 200,000 cases of bloodstream infections occur annually in the United States, with mortality rates ranging from 20% to 50% (Reimer, Wilson, & Weinstein, 1997). Patients with infections in the bloodstream often have an existing illness that may permit entry of microbes into the blood or may compromise the host defenses. Many of these infections occur in severely debilitated or immunocompromised patients, and infections in these patients are frequently caused by unusual pathogens whose recovery from blood requires special techniques. Also the incidence of primary nosocomial (hospital-acquired) bloodstream infections has risen greatly over the past couple of decades, due largely to the high-technology health care used today.

The diagnosis of bloodstream infections usually involves **blood cultures**, the laboratory cultivation of the bacteria or fungi in a sample of blood that has been inoculated into culture broth. Although it might seem simple to cultivate the bacteria or fungi in a blood sample, this specimen presents a complex challenge. Most of the bloodstream pathogens are relatively common and straightforward to cultivate and recover, but several of the possible pathogens present rather complex require-

ments. Some of the microbes have special nutritional or environmental requirements, and several factors are involved in determining the technique and quantity of blood to collect. Processing blood cultures is typically labor intensive and often requires several days.

Interpretation of results is also complicated. Although it varies somewhat with the mixture of patient types, usually about 10% to 12% of the specimens produce **positive cultures**, meaning that bacteria or fungi are recovered. Depending on collection and handling techniques, from 1% to 5% of the positive cultures are of contaminants, microbes that are present, but not causing the infection. All of this presents a challenge to the laboratory and medical staff in determining blood culture instruments, methods, techniques, and interpretation.

In this chapter, the nature of bloodstream infections, how and when to collect specimens, the cultivation and recovery of the bacteria present, and screening methods for rapid or presumptive identification of the bacteria pathogens will be addressed. Only when all these factors are adequately considered will the likelihood of diagnostic success be high. The reference by Reimer, Wilson, and Weinstein (1997) as well as that by Dunne, Nolte, and Wilson (1997) and that by Baron, Peterson, and Finegold (1994) should be consulted for further details and background.

## BASIC ANATOMY OF THE BLOOD AND LYMPHATIC CIRCULATORY SYSTEMS

Blood and lymphatic fluids circulate throughout the body through the arteries, veins, capillaries, and lymphatic vessels. The fluids carry blood cells, nutrients, various chemicals including defensive components, and smaller cells to practically all areas of the body. Due to the presence of capillaries and other vessels throughout almost all parts of the body, blood and lymphatic fluid would naturally have the occasion of coming in contact with sites of localized infection and areas where normal flora have entered the capillaries.

The inner lining of heart muscle and heart valve tissue is an endothelium called the endocardium. It can become inflamed and infected when bacteria colonize on the endothelial surfaces of heart valves and become entrapped in fibrin of blood clots. Bacteria are more likely to adhere to the endocardium or heart valve that is defective or has been previously damaged by disease that leaves its surface somewhat rough.

## RESIDENT FLORA

There are no true resident microbial flora of the bloodstream; however, when small numbers of various microbes such as normal skin or mouth flora enter the blood on occasion, they are quickly removed by host defense mechanisms. The most common resident flora of the skin are *Staphylococcus epidermidis* and other coagulase-negative staphylococci, *Corynebacterium* species, and the anaerobe *Propionibacterium acne*. The most common resident flora of the mouth are α-hemolytic streptococci.

The normal flora of the skin are common contaminants of blood cultures, usually because of inadequate skin disinfection at the time of specimen collection. However, the increasing incidence of nosocomial or true infections caused by normally nonvirulent resident bacteria flora causes difficulty in interpreting the significance of growth of such bacteria.

## GENERAL CONCEPTS OF BLOODSTREAM INFECTIONS

As a site of localized infection spreads, it often intrudes on capillaries and small vessels where the microorganisms can enter the blood or lymphatic fluid. Tissues such as the lungs and intestine are highly vascularized with blood capillaries. As such, they present relatively easy entry points into the blood system for bacteria that are somewhat invasive. Any infection that invades the tissues presents an increased possibility of bloodstream infection.

Once in the bloodstream, bacteria may continue to multiply and release toxins, or the may be deposited in a major organ or tissue and cause an abscess or inflammation. Microbes in the bloodstream are usually removed (cleared) by the normal host defenses. Most microorganisms that enter the bloodstream will be removed by the fixed macrophages in the liver and spleen, although bacterial capsules and other virulence factors may delay clearance. Usually clearance will occur within minutes to a few hours. However, some microbes may survive, and possibly flourish, if the normal host defenses are inadequate. Large numbers of bacteria released into the bloodstream at the same time may overwhelm the phagocytes and various chemical defenses of the blood, thus leading to the circulation of infectious bacteria.

## Clinical Patterns of Bloodstream Infections

**Bacteremia** refers to the presence of viable bacteria circulating in the blood, and **fungemia** refers to the presence of fungi in the bloodstream. The implication is that any microbe in the bloodstream that has not been removed by the body's defenses probably represents an infectious disease state such as pneumonia, intravascular infection, or localized abscess. In actuality, the bacteria are usually present only transiently or temporarily for every bacterial infection except endocarditis or severe intravascular infection.

The terms **sepsis** or **septicemia** are typically used to indicate clinical evidence of a *systemic* response to the bacteremia. Primary signs and symptoms include hyperventilation, fever, and chills. Serious complications of sepsis include hypotension (septic shock), adult respiratory distress syndrome (ARDS), bleeding due to disseminated intravascular coagulation (DIC), and hemorrhagic and ulcerative skin lesions (e.g., petechiae and purpura).

Bacteremia may be classified into three categories.

1. *Transient bacteremia* is the entry into the bloodstream of small numbers of microbes that cross the normally protective cutaneous or mucosal barriers during activities such as instrument probing of colonized mucosal surfaces, drainage of a minor abscess, or even during simple activities such as vigorous brushing of the teeth. This is normally short-term and of little significance except in patients with underlying heart valve disease, and most patients usually exhibit little, if any, signs and symptoms

2. *Intermittent bacteremia* is the entry of microorganisms into the bloodstream from an extravascular site (i.e., an established focus of infection outside the blood and lymphatic vessels), although the site may not be readily identified (see Figure 26-1). This type of bacteremia is most notably from pneumonia, meningitis,

osteomyelitis, peritonitis, subcutaneous soft tissue infection, and undrained abscess.

Because bacteria from these infections may enter the bloodstream in "showers" and in low numbers as they are released from the site of infection, the symptoms may be apparent only during periods immediately following the entry into the bloodstream. Symptoms often disappear on clearance of the microorganisms from the bloodstream, and repeated blood cultures may be necessary to recover the bacteria. For patients with intermittent bacteremia, approximately 75% to 80% of blood cultures obtained in a series of several cultures are positive.

3. *Continuous bacteremia* is the entry of microbes from an intravascular focal site of infection so that microbes are consistently present in the bloodstream. In the case of **infective endocarditis**, small numbers of bacteria colonize on rough endothelial tissue, valves, or indwelling catheters, and the endothelium becomes inflamed and continuously sheds low numbers of bacteria into the blood (see Figure 26-2).

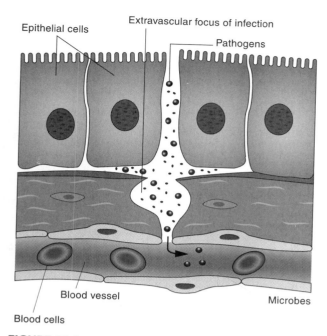

**FIGURE 26-1** Entry of microbes into bloodstream from extravascular site.

## Brief Introduction to Major Pathogens

Bloodstream infections are caused by perhaps the most widely varied microbial pathogens of all specimen types. Not only is this variety a result of the different nature of infections occurring in anatomically diverse areas of the body, but also as a result of today's high-technology health care. Today's patients with positive blood cultures may have a community-acquired

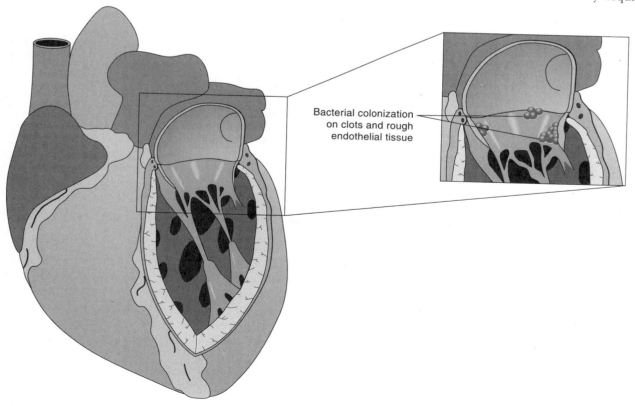

**FIGURE 26-2** Infective endocarditis.

initial infection in nonvascular tissue that has progressed to bacteremia, or the patient's defensive mechanisms may be severely compromised after having undergone trauma or major surgery, or the patient may be immunocompromised as a result of acquired immunodeficiency syndrome (AIDS), organ transplant, or cancer. Many of the intermittent and continuous bacteremias are from nosocomial causes where the entry of the bacteria is often from a focus of infection that is a medical device, which may be indwelling or implanted.

The more frequently recovered bloodstream pathogens include *Staphylococcus aureus, Escherichia coli, S. epidermidis* (and other coagulase-negative staphylococci), *Enterococcus, Pseudomonas aeruginosa, Streptococcus pneumoniae,* and anaerobes such as *Bacteroides, Peptostreptococcus,* and *Clostridium.* A characteristic of blood cultures from severely debilitated patients and immunocompromised patients is that they often grow unusual bacterial pathogens such as various *Pseudomonas* species, *Mycobacterium* species, and otherwise rarely isolated nonfermentative gram-negative bacilli, as well as fungi such as *Candida* species, and *Cryptococcus neoformans.*

The microbes listed above represent a wide variety of morphologic, nutritional, and environmental types. This variety creates the need to use culture media and environments that will fulfill the needs of as many of the likely pathogens as possible.

## SPECIMEN COLLECTION

### Introduction

Success of blood culture depends on the laboratorians' and physicians' understanding the many variables affecting the blood culture procedure. Because the numbers of bacteria may be low, the volume of blood collected is very significant. Due to the nature of the infecting microbes, special media, additives, or environment are needed for certain organisms. The thoroughness of skin disinfection affects the potential of normal flora contamination, thus significantly affecting the culture interpretation. Each of these factors produces the possible need for variations in specimen collection, processing, media, and environment. The techniques and culture media have the potential of being crucial to the outcome of the specimen.

Blood culture systems include those that are manual, semiautomated, and fully automated. The choice of one type over another is usually based on several factors, such as the number of specimens cultured per day, the type of patient population served, and the laboratory's resources. The type of blood culture system used determines many of the specifics of specimen collection and the laboratory's processing protocol.

## Culture Media

An important aspect of culturing the etiologic agents of bacteremia is that of selecting culture media with the appropriate characteristics. Depending on manufacturer, blood culture bottles contain between 30 and 100 mL of culture medium, with pediatric versions having 10 to 25 mL of broth. Media typically used to culture aerobic microorganisms contains soybean-casein digest broth (such as tryptic or trypticase soy broth), brain-heart infusion broth, Brucella broth, or supplemented peptone broth. Typical media for recovery of anaerobes are Columbia broth, thiol, or thioglycollate broth. This latter group is considered anaerobic because each contains reducing agents such as cysteine and other sulfhydryl compounds, which produce low redox potentials (Eh). Many of the unvented bottles of the "aerobic" broth have sufficiently low redox potentials that they support the growth of anaerobes (see Table 26-1).

Almost all media are bottled with vacuum and added $CO_2$. A few types of aerobic bottles will require venting after inoculation to increase the oxygen concentration. Transient venting is accomplished with a sterile, cotton-plugged needle inserted through the rubber stopper that has been disinfected with alcohol or iodine solution. The "anaerobic" bottles will usually contain $CO_2$ and nitrogen, and these should not be vented. Agitation of aerobic bottles during incubation increases microbial recovery by increasing oxygen concentration within the broth. Agitation of anaerobic bottles is not detrimental because they contain no oxygen.

Most blood culture broth contains one or more supplements. Sodium polyanetholsulfonate (SPS) is included in most broth in a concentration of 0.025% to 0.05%. SPS serves as an anticoagulant, inactivates certain antibiotics, interferes with phagocytosis, and inhibits complement. Anticoagulation and these other effects are needed because many bacteria do not survive well within a clot or in the presence of these host defenses. However, SPS is inhibitory to some bacteria such as *Neisseria gonorrhoeae, Neisseria meningitidis, Gardnerella vaginalis,* and *Peptostreptococcus anaerobius.* The addition of 1.2% gelatin to the blood culture broth may help counteract the SPS, but it may decrease the recovery of certain other organisms.

It cannot be assumed that these media are all equivalent for recovering microbial pathogens from blood. For example, thioglycollate and thiol broths are not suitable for recovery of *Pseudomonas* and yeasts. Many laboratories will use more than one type of media in an effort to increase the likelihood of recovering a wide variety of pathogens.

To improve the recovery of bacteria that have been damaged by antimicrobial agents, some manufacturers provide bottles containing antibiotic-removing resins. However, for most types of bacteria, recovery is not

## Table 26–1 ▶ Blood Culture Media Characteristics

| System and Bottle Type | Broth vol (mL) | Broth Base | Inoculum vol (mL) | Blood: Broth Ratio | Anticoag.* Conc. (%) |
|---|---|---|---|---|---|
| BBL Septi-Check | 70 | SCD | 10 | 1:7 | |
| Septi-Check with Resins | 70 | SCD | 10 | 1:7 | |
| BacT/Alert | | | | | |
| Aerobic† | 40 | SCD | 10 | 1:4 | 0.035 |
| Anaerobic | 40 | SCD | 10 | 1:4 | 0.035 |
| Pedi-BacT† | 20 | BHI | 4 | 1:5 | 0.020 |
| FAN (aerobic/anaerobic) | 40 | BHI | 10 | 1:4 | 0.050 |
| BACTEC Nonradiometric | | | | | |
| 6A (aerobic) | 30 | SCD | 5 | 1:6 | 0.035 |
| 7A (anaerobic) | 30 | SCD | 5 | 1:6 | 0.035 |
| Peds Plus (aerobic) | 20 | SCD | 4 | 1:5 | 0.025 |
| Plus 26 (aerobic with resins) | 25 | SCD | 10 | 1:2.5 | 0.050 |
| Plus 27 (anaerobic with resins) | 25 | SCD | 10 | 1:2.5 | 0.050 |
| BACTEC 9000 series (fluorescent) | | | | | |
| Aerobic/F | 40 | SCD | 5 | 1:8 | 0.025 |
| Anaerobic/F | 40 | SCD | 5 | 1:8 | 0.025 |
| Plus aerobic/F | 25 | SCD | 10 | 1:2.5 | 0.050 |
| Plus anaerobic/F | 25 | SCD | 10 | 1:2.5 | 0.050 |
| Peds Plus/F | 40 | SCD | 0.5-3 | 1:80-1:13 | 0.025 |
| Myco/F-Sputa | | | | | |
| ESP Culture System II | | | | | |
| Aerobic 80A† | 80 | SCP | 10 | 1:8 | 0.006 |
| Anaerobic 80N† | 80 | PP | 10 | 1:8 | 0.070‡ |
| EZ DRAW 40A† | 40 | SCP | 5 | 1:8 | 0.006 |
| EZ DRAW 40N† | 40 | PP | 5 | 1:8 | 0.070‡ |

*All use sodium polyanetholsulfonate (SPS) except those marked ‡ which use trisodium citrate (TSC).

†Require venting; however, ESP bottles are transiently vented when adapters are placed, separate venting not required.

BHI, brain-heart infusion; PP, proteose peptone; SCD, soybean casein digest; SCP, soybean casein peptone.

improved over that provided by media containing SPS. Because these media may improve recovery of specific pathogens, their use may be appropriate under certain circumstances. Although not widely used, hypertonic media containing 10% to 20% sucrose are sometimes used to improve the recovery of cell wall-deficient bacteria or microorganisms that have been damaged, either by host defense mechanisms or antimicrobial agents.

## Collection Technique

Although each type of blood culture system may use a different technique for collecting the blood samples, most will use some variation of a needle and syringe, vacutainer-type double-needle, or tubing with a needle on each end.

Because many patients will be undergoing the admin-

istration of intravenous (IV) fluids and medications, some consideration must be made of the dilution of the bacteria by the presence of the extra fluids. Blood should generally not be taken from the IV catheter port nor from the arm receiving the IV fluid because of the dilution as well as possible inhibition of bacteria by the medications. In addition, there is greater likelihood of picking up contamination from the IV catheter port or colonization on the catheter tip.

Due to the risk of contact with bloodborne pathogens when collecting, transporting, processing, and disposing blood culture specimens, Standard (Universal) Precautions must be observed. Although the risks are greatest from needle stick injuries, one must be alert to other exposures, such as from leaks and spills. The Centers for Disease Control and Prevention (CDC, 1988) as well as the Occupational Safety and Health Administration (OSHA, 1991) and the National Committee for

Clinical Laboratory Standards (NCCLS, 1991) have published guidelines for minimizing the risk of exposure.

**Collection Site Preparation.** Some bloodstream infections may be caused by microorganisms that are normal flora of the skin. Because it is difficult to differentiate between the role of contaminant and pathogen, it is extremely important to reduce contamination of blood cultures to a minimum. This is partially accomplished by meticulously disinfecting the skin. The most commonly recommended is a two-step disinfection process using alcohol and iodine (see Figure 26-3). The true disinfection occurs during the iodine phase rather than during the alcohol phase. Some manufacturers state that iodine may cause deterioration of the bottle's rubber stopper.

**Volume of Blood to Collect.** With each venipuncture and at each collection time, collect between 10 and 30 mL of blood from adult patients (1–5 mL from pediatrics), and divide it equally between two bottles of broth. The actual amount to collect depends on the type of blood culture system used in your laboratory (see Table 26-1).

Whatever the volume of blood collected, the ratio of blood to broth should be between 1:5 (20% of final volume) and 1:10 (10% of the final volume or 1 part of blood to 9 parts of broth). This adequately dilutes antimicrobics and other inhibitory factors and helps prevent clotting; however, avoid ratios less than 1:5 because this does not provide adequate dilution.

Do not assume that the amount of vacuum in the bottle will pull the correct amount of blood into the bottle when the patient's sample is collected. If a needle and syringe is being used to add blood to the bottle, be ready to withdraw the needle when the appropriate amount of blood has entered the bottle.

**Number and Timing of Samples.** Two or three blood culture sets should be collected from each patient, and these should be drawn from at least two different body sites. Multiple bottles filled from one venipuncture at one collection time are usually considered to be one blood culture set. In the case of bacteremia, it is important to collect more than one blood culture set per patient so that adequate volume is obtained. Blood collected from two sites is helpful in determining whether the isolate recovered is a contaminant or is a **clinically significant** pathogen. Nearly all episodes of bacteremia and fungemia can be detected when three blood cultures are drawn, so it is rarely useful to routinely collect more than three blood cultures. About 95% to 100% of blood cultures from infective endocarditis are positive when at least one culture is positive.

Whenever possible, blood cultures should be collected prior to administration of antimicrobial agents so as to eliminate the interference and inhibitory effect of the antimicrobic on the microbes. In patients with intermittent bacteremia, fever and chills often occur about 1 hour after the influx of bacteria into the bloodstream. Because bacteria are rapidly cleared from the blood, ideally, the best opportunity to collect the pathogens is immediately before or during the fever spike.

Research has shown that in actual practice, multiple blood cultures that are drawn simultaneously yield similar microbial recovery as those collected at various time intervals over 24 hours. Thus, it is more practical to collect multiple blood cultures simultaneously before administration of antimicrobial agents than to try to time the collection for the maximum presence of the bacteria.

1. Palpate to locate the vein.
2. Apply 70% isopropyl or ethyl alcohol for about 30 seconds as a general cleanser of the venipuncture site to remove oils from the skin surface and ports.
3. Apply either 10% povidone-iodine or 2% tincture of iodine for 1 to 2 minutes. Begin at the intended puncture site and move outward in concentric circles to a diameter of about 1.5 to 2 inches. (For patients who are sensitive to iodine, disinfect with a double application of 70% alcohol, leaving the alcohol on the skin for at least 1 minute and permitting the area to dry before venipuncture.)
4. Disinfect the bottle stopper by swabbing with alcohol or iodine solution, and allow it to set for 1 minute.
5. Do not touch the disinfected venipuncture site again unless the finger of the glove has been disinfected.
6. Perform the venipuncture using a needle and syringe or transfer set. Use a new needle if the vein is missed. Follow manufacturer's instructions.
7. Collect 20 to 30 mL of blood (adults) divided into two bottles, unless manufacturer specifies otherwise.
   ▶ Do not change needles between bottles.
   ▶ If a syringe is used, be careful not to allow the bottle's vacuum to pull all the blood into the first bottle.
   ▶ Mix by inverting the bottles to avoid clotting.
8. Cleanse the site with 70% alcohol to remove the remaining iodine.
9. Immediately transport the bottles to the laboratory without refrigeration.

**FIGURE 26-3** Collection site preparation and blood collection steps.

**Anaerobes.** During the past few years most hospitals have experienced a decline in the proportion of anaerobic bacteremias and the simultaneous increase of aerobes such as *Pseudomonas* species, yeast, and fastidious aerobic bacteria. The frequency of anaerobic bacteremia is now low enough in many hospitals that many laboratories have replaced the traditional anaerobic media with a second aerobic bottle to increase the likelihood of recovering the predominant pathogens. Based on local experience, some hospitals still need to routinely inoculate anaerobic media and leave it unvented.

## Pediatric Specimens

Whenever possible, the venipuncture technique used for blood cultures in adults is also used for children. However, because of the difficulty of obtaining blood by venipuncture from peripheral veins in small children, blood from central venous catheters or bone marrow aspirate may be used. Because of increased contamination and the limited volume of blood obtained by heel stick, that method is not recommended except as a last resort.

Neonates and infants who have bacteremia are usually quite ill and need rapid treatment. Acutely ill infants usually yield more than 10 colony-forming units (cfu) of bacteria per milliliter of blood so that even small amounts of blood should be adequate. This usually suggests that bacteria are sufficiently numerous to be isolated from even one specimen, so routinely delaying antibiotic treatment to obtain multiple cultures over time is not worthwhile as long as the volume of blood cultured is adequate.

Because infants and young children have significantly less volume of blood than older children and adults, it is not safe to take large samples from them. Most manufacturers provide pediatric size bottles, so that 1 to 5 mL is typically collected and inoculated into a reduced amount of broth to maintain the 1:10 ratio. Because culturing less than 1.0 mL of blood may miss substantial numbers of pathogens in children, it seems a reasonable goal to obtain 1 to 2 mL in neonates, 2 to 3 mL in infants (1 month to 2 years old), 3 to 5 mL in children, and 10 to 20 mL in adolescents.

Anaerobic bacteria are seldom found in infants and children. Common aerobic pathogens of infants and children, such as *Candida, Neisseria,* and *Pseudomonas,* fail to grow in anaerobic media. Therefore, anaerobic media should be used only in selected cases, such as peritonitis or fasciitis, and in cases when an optimal amount of blood for aerobic culture has been obtained.

## Intravascular Lines

The increased use of intravascular lines for administration of fluids and medication and for physiologic monitoring has led to increased incidence of nosocomial bloodstream infections. These lines have been used for obtaining blood samples, especially from patients with limited peripheral venous access; however, there seems to be a higher false-positive rate for blood collected from the lines. This is probably because of colonization of the lines after a few days, greater manipulation of the lines to collect the specimen, and difficulty in cleansing the sampling port on the lines. Thus, it is recommended that routine blood cultures not be collected from intravascular catheters unless venipuncture is impractical.

**Culturing a Catheter Tip.** The diagnosis of catheter-associated bloodstream infections is most accurately performed by quantitative means. In some cases, a section of the IV catheter or its tip is cultured to determine whether or not it is colonized with bacteria. The number of colony-forming units of bacteria directly relates to whether it is the source of infection. The catheter is removed from the patient after carefully disinfecting the skin around the catheter. A short section of a portion of the catheter that had been beneath the skin is aseptically cut off, dropped into a sterile container without liquid, and transported to the laboratory. Using sterile forceps, this section of catheter is rolled across the surface of an agar plate. After overnight incubation the colonies are counted. A culture with five or more colonies suggests that the catheter is serving as the source of infection (Dunne et al., 1997) (see Figure 26-4).

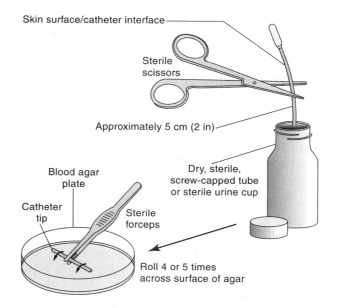

**FIGURE 26-4** Culturing a catheter tip.

## SPECIMEN PROCESSING

### General Procedures

Processing methods include conventional manual broth-based systems, agar-broth biphasic techniques, lysis-centrifugation, resins for antimicrobial removal, and various broth-based instrument systems. Because physicians can usually begin reasonably accurate therapy as soon as they know whether or not the patient has bacteremia, simply detecting growth in the specimen provides a significant piece of information.

Whatever the method used, all specimens must be properly identified. Although most of the automated systems use bar codes, the technician must ensure that all information is correct for both the laboratory information system and the instrument's data management system.

One factor affecting microbe recovery is the speed of processing. Survival of the pathogen may be affected by a delay in incubation or being placed on the instrument. This is usually not a problem in laboratories with three shifts, but it certainly may be in laboratories that are staffed for only 1 to 1.5 shifts. Die-off of bacteria may occur in specimens that are not processed (placed on the instrument) within about 8 or 9 hours of collection. Blood cultures collected when the laboratory is not receiving specimens should be incubated to permit the pathogens to begin growing. These bottles should be examined for macroscopic evidence of growth before being placed in an automated instrument.

Recent studies have shown that more than 98% of clinically significant isolates have been detected by continuous monitoring instruments within 5 days, and by conventional broth cultures within 7 days (Gibb and Karn, 1997; Levi, Sarode, Seno, Gialanella, & McKitrick, 1997; Murray, 1985). Conventional broth cultures will need to be subcultured after about a day of incubation, but no terminal subcultures are needed for either conventional or continuous monitoring systems.

### Manual Methods

**Traditional and Biphasic Broth.** Conventional broth bottles contain either 45 mL or 90 mL of broth to which 5 or 10 mL of blood, respectively, are added to achieve a 1:10 ratio. For laboratories performing anaerobic blood cultures, one bottle is usually vented to produce an aerobic environment and the second bottle is left unvented to provide better anaerobic conditions.

In efforts to speed the recovery of microbes that have difficulty growing in liquid media and to provide colonies on which identification and antimicrobic susceptibility tests can be performed, **biphasic** media were introduced. This media incorporates a slab of agar into the bottle along with the broth, thus the term "biphasic." With appropriately shaped devices, there can be more than one slab of agar media, thus providing the opportunity for selective and differential media. Having special media inoculated from the very earliest opportunity provides a presumptive identification at approximately the same time as detection of initial growth.

For hospitals using a manual blood culture method, the Septi-Chek (Septi-Chek Becton Dickinson, Sparks, Maryland) is a widely used example of a biphasic system (see Figure 26-5). It consists of a bottle with 70 mL of trypicase soy or Columbia broth, plus SPS and $CO_2$ (see Table 26-1 ) and an attachable enclosed agar-coated slide. The plastic slide (paddle) contains three agar media—chocolate agar, MacConkey agar, and malt agar, which are suitable for the subculture of bacterial and fungal growth in the broth. Pediatric size Septi-Chek bottles containing 20 mL of broth and a 70 mL bottle of soybean-casein digest broth with resins are also available.

In the laboratory, the agar slide is attached to the "aerobic" bottle by opening the bottle of broth and screwing the agar slide attachment into place. Because the bottle must be opened when the slide is attached, it is best to perform this manipulation in the biosafety cabinet to reduce the likelihood of contaminants entering the broth. The second bottle may be left unopened and without a slide to increase the likelihood of recovering an anaerobic bacterium, or it may be treated as a second aerobic bottle.

The bottle to which the agar slide is attached is tilted past the horizontal allowing the liquid to flood the slide

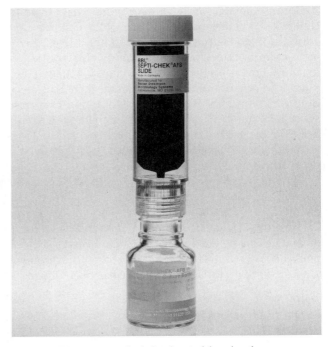

**FIGURE 26-5** Septi-Chek biphasic blood culture system. (Courtesy of Becton Dickinson Microbiology Systems)

chamber and inoculate the agar. The bottle is then returned to the upright position for incubation. Both bottles are incubated for 7 days at 35°C. The aerobic bottle should be tilted at least twice during the first 2 days, then once per day thereafter. Continuous agitation of the broth using a shaker or rotator for the first 48 hours seems to enhance recovery of aerobic bacteria. In conventional broth bottles other than Septi-Chek, agar paddles will not be incorporated, so a subculture of the broth to agar plates should be performed after 6 to 18 hours of incubation.

The primary advantages to this system are that certain bacteria are predominantly detected on the agar rather than in the broth, and colonies of the microorganisms are available for testing at an early time. All this combines to provide a system that serves well for laboratories that do not have the quantity of blood culture specimens to justify an automated system.

**Lysis-Centrifugation System.** The Wampole Isolator system (Wampole Isolator System, Wampole Laboratories, Cranbury, NJ) uses inoculation of the concentrated specimen directly onto agar media in an attempt to provide positive identification results sooner than with conventional or instrument methods (see Figure 26-6). Colonies, which can be examined by Gram stain and undergo biochemical tests, are available at the time of detection of a positive blood culture.

The procedure begins by collecting about 10 mL of blood in a tube containing chemicals that lyse the blood cells while leaving the microbial cells intact. The specimen is then centrifuged within 8 hours and, after disinfecting the top of the tube, a special device is used to insert a special cap through the rubber stopper. The technician then aseptically draws off the supernate,

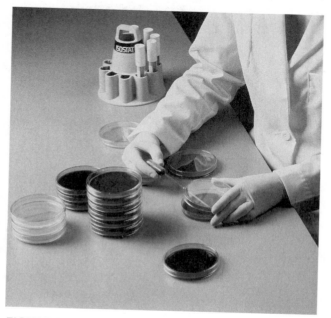

**FIGURE 26-6** Isostat lysis-centrifugation system. (Courtesy of Wampole Laboratories)

mixes the sediment, and draws up the sediment. The sediment is inoculated directly onto various agar media, which can be chosen and incubated for optimal growth of the microbes of interest.

Because there is increased likelihood of introducing a contaminant during the manipulation to insert the special cap through the rubber stopper, specimen processing should take place in a biosafety cabinet and there should be strict attention to aseptic technique.

Currently, the Isolator system is used primarily for the recovery of fungi from blood specimens. Several comparison studies have indicated the system has had good results in the recovery of fungi and mycobacteria, although producing lower overall rates of recovery of several types of bacteria.

## Blood Culture Instruments

The increase in blood culture workload and the decreasing laboratory resources of the last several years have led to an emphasis on efficiency. Part of the answer to this challenge has been the development of automated blood culture systems. Most of the current models provide for the complete handling of the incubation, continuous monitoring of microbial growth, and reporting of the blood cultures results.

These instruments generally consist of a basic system unit that houses the detector system and electronics, a vial-handling unit with incubator, and a data management system. By providing nonlabor-intensive monitoring of the vial around the clock, and by limiting the technologist to working with only positive blood cultures, the automated instruments provide for efficient use of laboratory resources in laboratories having sufficient quantity of blood culture specimens.

Specimens are incubated for 5 days on all of these instruments, and there is no need for daily visual examination of broth, blind subcultures, or terminal subcultures. In each case, the instrument will signal that a bottle is positive, whereupon the technician removes the bottle and performs a Gram stain and subcultures to provide colonies for biochemical and antimicrobic susceptibility testing.

**BACTEC Infrared Systems.** The BACTEC NR (nonradiometric) systems (Becton Fluorescent 9000 series, Becton Dickinson, Sparks, Maryland), such as model NR-860, measure $CO_2$ released from microbial metabolism into the headspace (gas above the broth medium in the sealed bottle) of the blood culture bottle. The amount of $CO_2$ in the gas is directly proportional to the metabolism of select components in the medium. A positive culture is based on $CO_2$ exceeding a threshold level or a change between two consecutive readings.

Periodically during the incubation period, the bottles are sampled for $CO_2$ production. A pair of needles are inserted through the rubber septum of each bottle, and the gas in the blood culture bottle is sampled by pulling some of the headspace gas out of the bottle and into the detector unit through one needle while fresh gas enters the bottle through the second needle. When the gas is exposed to infrared light, visible light emitted from $CO_2$ is absorbed by a photodiode that produces a voltage signal proportional to the $CO_2$ concentration in the bottle. The voltage is then converted to a growth value, which is a number representing the measured $CO_2$ produced in the bottle.

For positive cultures, growth values are dependent on the media type, the organism, the number of colony-forming units in the specimen at the time of collection and the number of hours of incubation prior to testing. A majority of vials produce growth values that rise sharply and exceed the threshold within the first several hours of incubation. However, for slow-growing organisms, a change of growth values between two consecutive readings is used to determine positivity.

A variety of media for bacteria and fungi are available for use with the BACTEC NR system and are described in Table 26-1. The nonradiometric system and the improved media have been evaluated extensively and these reports indicate that it is a good system for detection of bacteremia.

**BACTEC Fluorescence Systems.** The BACTEC Fluorescent 9000 Series (9120, 9240) (Becton Dickinson Blood Culture Systems) is an automated, noninvasive system that continually and simultaneously monitors agitates, and incubates up to 240 test vials at one time (see Figure 26-7). A barcode on the bottle is scanned as the inoculated bottles are placed into incubation blocks that rock back and forth to mix the culture.

A fluorescence sensor bonded to the inside of the bottle reacts with $CO_2$, thus modulating the amount of light that is absorbed by the sensor. The instrument's photodetectors measure the level of fluorescence every 10 minutes, and this fluorescence corresponds to the amount of $CO_2$ released by the microorganisms. The measurement is interpreted by the system's prepro-

grammed positivity parameters, and the operator is alerted to positive cultures by visual and audible alarms. Because detection is external to the bottle, the potential for cross-contamination of bottles during repeated aspirations is eliminated.

A variety of media for bacteria and fungi available for use with this system are described in Table 26-1. The media for this system appear to recover the pathogenic bacteria well, and there are fewer contaminants (false-positives) than with the invasive systems, thus making this a very good system for detecting bacteremia and fungemia.

**BacT/Alert.** The BacT/Alert System (Organon Teknika Blood Culture System, Teknica Corp., Durham, Carolina) is based on the detection of $CO_2$ by a colorimetric sensor built into the bottom of each bottle (see Figure 26-8). The base of the bottle contains an ion-selective membrane that allows $CO_2$ produced in the medium to diffuse across the membrane into a sensor solution containing an acid-base color indicator (see Figure 26-9). The change in color from green to yellow (basic to acidic) is directly proportional to the amount of $CO_2$ present in the culture.

The colorimetric detector consists of a red light-emitting diode, which shines its light on the sensor every 10 minutes, and a red light-absorbing photodiode that produces a voltage signal proportional to the intensity of the reflected light. The voltage signals are converted into reflectance units (RFUs), and these RFUs

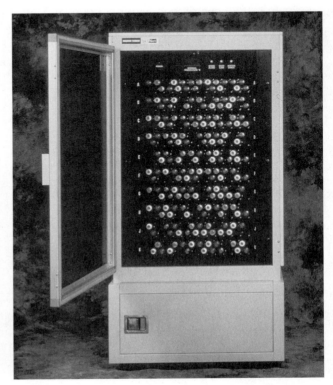

**FIGURE 26-8** BacT/Alert blood culture system. (Courtesy of Organon Teknika Corporation)

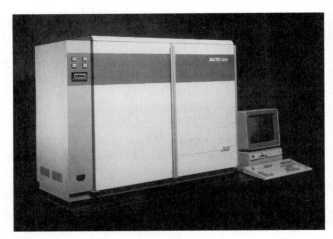

**FIGURE 26-7** BACTEC 9240 blood culture instrument. (Courtesy of Becton Dickinson Microbiology Systems)

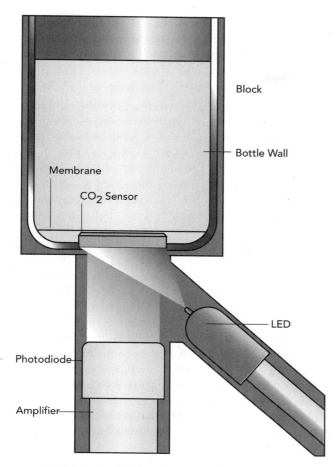

**FIGURE 26-9** BacT/Alert detector. (Courtesy of Organon Teknika Corporation)

and metabolism of microorganisms results in production and/or consumption of gases such as $O_2$, $CO_2$, $H_2$, and $N_2$. Before the inoculated blood culture bottles are placed into the instrument's incubator module, a disposable connector containing a recessed needle is placed onto each bottle. The connector needle penetrates the bottle stopper and connects bottle headspace to the sensor probe (see Figure 26-10).

Pressure-sensitive transducers regularly monitor changes in gas pressure, and positive specimens are determined by changes in gas pressure that are plotted against time to yield curves similar to those described for BacT/Alert. The data management system keeps track of the location and status of each bottle, and it indicates the detection of a positive bottle with an indicator light and audible alarm.

Average time to detection of a cross-section of typical organisms is about 18 hours for aerobes and 38 hours for anaerobes, and ESP has been shown to detect about 78% of probable pathogens within 24 hours and 96% within 48 hours (Welby, Keller, & Storch, 1995). The media for this system (see Table 26-1) recover the pathogens well, thus making this a good system for detecting bacteremia.

are plotted against time so that a growth curve is determined for each bottle. The concentration of $CO_2$ in each bottle is compared with itself over time, rather than against a fixed threshold, as in the BACTEC system. Thus, the specimen analysis is based on the rate of change of $CO_2$ (an indication of metabolism) in each bottle.

Bottles are flagged as positive based on one of three criteria: (1) an initial reading that exceeds an arbitrary threshold, (2) a sustained linear increase in $CO_2$ production, or (3) an increased rate of $CO_2$ production. Average detection time is about 15 to 20 hours. A variety of media for bacteria and fungi available for use with this system are described in Table 26-1. The media for this system appear to recover the pathogenic bacteria well, and there are fewer contaminants (false positives) than with the invasive systems. Because of performance characteristics, the duration of incubation can be limited to 5 days, and there is no need for routine terminal subculture.

**ESP Culture System II.** The ESP Culture System II (AccuMed International, Inc., Ann Arbor, MI) detects microbial growth by monitoring bottles for pressure changes in the headspace of a sealed bottle. Growth

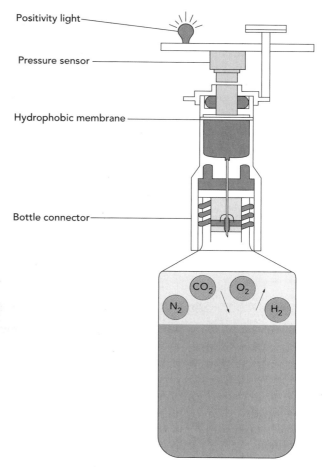

**FIGURE 26-10** ESP Culture System II bottle connector.

## Processing of Positive Blood Cultures

**Determination of Positive Blood Cultures.** Early detection of bacteremia or fungemia by an instrument or in conventional broth cultures is especially useful in establishing accurate treatment in a timely manner. The continuous monitoring system alerts the technician as soon as a positive culture is detected, and then stores the data in the system's computer for future reference.

Conventional broth and lysis-centrifugation methods require subcultures and at least daily visual examination of the culture bottles or agar plates to determine the positive specimens. For conventional broth methods, a Gram stain and blind subculture of the broth should be performed after 6 to 18 hours of incubation (also see presumptive testing below). A **blind subculture** is one in which the blood is subcultured to agar media even in the absence of visible evidence of microbial growth in the broth. The purpose is to gain early detection and colonies that can be further tested. There is no need for blind subculture of the unvented bottle, as the anaerobic bacteria tend to be adequately detected by visual means. Bottles should be incubated for 7 days, but there is no need for a **terminal subculture**, which is a subculture performed at the end of the incubation period, even without visible evidence of growth.

Bottles are examined daily for visible signs of growth (see Table 26-2). Bottles that are subcultured and examined in this manner will usually lead to detectable growth in about 2 to 3 days. Occasionally. there will be a **false-negative** specimen on an instrument. These specimens truly have bacteria in them, but the instrument failed to detect its growth. Periodic visual examination of the bottles before discarding them may reveal one of the visible signs of growth, in which case a blind subculture should be performed.

Immediately on seeing macroscopic evidence of growth, the bottles should be subcultured (see Table 26-3). Culture on agar plates is used for full identification and antimicrobic susceptibility testing. Agar plate culture is usually accomplished using blood agar plates and supplemented chocolate agar plates. In many cases, anaerobic bacteria will grow in the aerobic bottles, so anaerobic plates should be inoculated if anaerobes are suspected. For specimens with anaerobic bottles, inoculate the anaerobic plates indicated. If fastidious pathogens are suspected, use appropriate special media in addition to the routine agar media.

**Presumptive Testing.** Immediately on being alerted that the blood culture bottle is positive, aseptically remove a small aliquot of mixed broth from the bottle, spread a few drops onto a blood agar plate and a chocolate agar plate, and smear two or three drops on a microscope slide. Perform the Gram stain on this slide and fully describe the bacterial morphology observed because this may greatly assist in the presumptive identification and the selection of antimicrobics. Based on the Gram stain morphology, additional agar plate media can be inoculated as indicated in Table 26-3. The Gram stain, which has a sensitivity of about $10^5$ cfu, is one of the most common and reliable tests that will provide the physician with initial information on which to base antibiotic therapy.

If no organisms are observed with the Gram stain, yet the instrument recorded a positive signal, the acridine orange stain is a good follow-up. This stain, which uses the ultraviolet light microscope for viewing, is sensitive enough to detect $10^3$ to $10^4$ cfu/mL and reveals those that stain very lightly. Because of this sensitivity, some laboratories may use it instead of the 24-hour blind subcultures.

After staining, some rapid biochemical tests may be performed, which may lead to a tentative or presumptive identification. Begin this procedure by centrifuging 10 mL of well-mixed blood culture broth, first slowly for 5 to 10 minutes to remove the red blood cells, then at 1,500$g$ for 15 minutes to obtain a pellet of organisms to test. If a "washed" pellet is needed, then resuspend the sediment in fresh broth or saline. A small drop of this pellet can be used to perform spot tests such as the oxidase, indole with paracinnamaldehyde, tube coagulase, or bile esculin, and it can be used to inoculate a test kit such as Vitek, Microscan, or API, although these may not be approved methods (Buck and Romero, 1997; Waites, Brookings, Moser, McKinnon, & Van Pelt, 1997).

---

### Table 26–2 ▶ Visible Signs of Growth and Associated Organisms

| Microscopic Morphology | Associated Microorganisms |
|---|---|
| Hemolysis | streptococci, staphylococci, clostridia, *Listeria*, *Bacillus* species |
| Turbidity | aerobic gram-negative bacilli, staphylococci, *Bacteroides* species |
| Gas formation | aerobic gram-negative bacilli, anaerobes |
| Pellicle formation | *Pseudomonas* species, *Bacillus* species, yeast |
| Clotting | *Staphylococcus aureus* |
| Visible colonies, "puffballs" | staphylococci, streptococci |

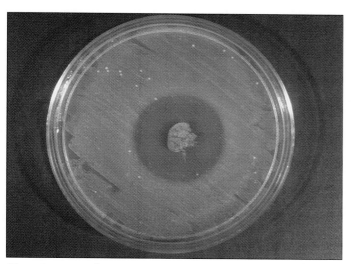

**Plate 1** *Penicillium notatum* inhibiting *S. epidermidis* growth.

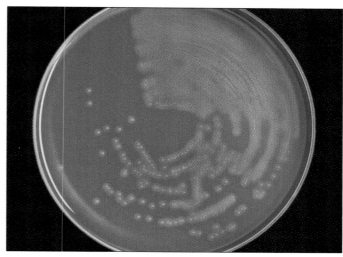

**Plate 2** Blood agar. (Courtesy of Becton Dickinson Microbiology Systems, Sparks, MD).

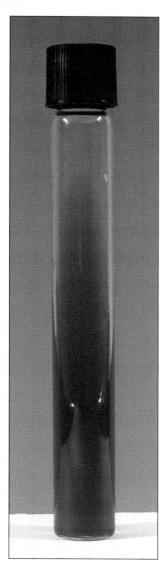

**Plate 3** Simmons citrate agar.

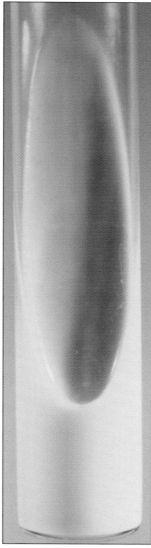

**Plate 4** Lowenstein Jensen agar.

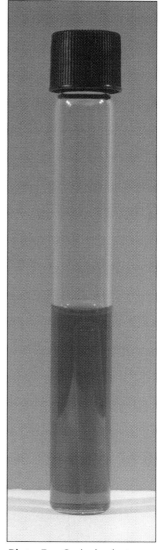

**Plate 5** Carbohydrate fermentation broth.

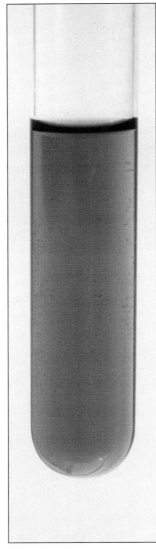

**Plate 6**    Decarboxylation broth.

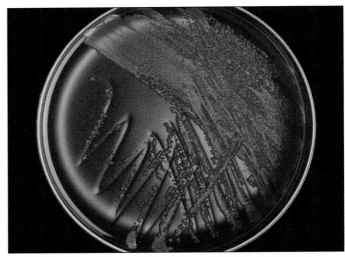

**Plate 7**    Buffered charcoal yeast extract agar (BCYE). This plate is of *Legionella pneumophila*. (Courtesy of Becton Dickinson Microbiology Systems, Sparks, MD).

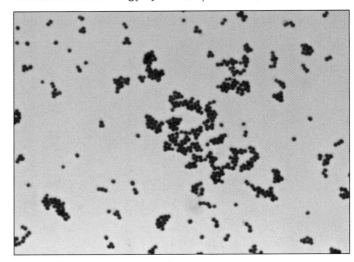

**Plate 8**    Gram stain, staphylococci.

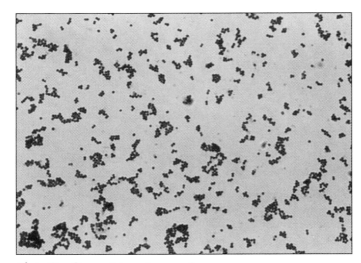

**Plate 9**    Gram stain, micrococci.

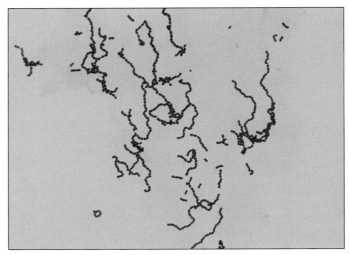

**Plate 10**    Gram stain, streptococci.

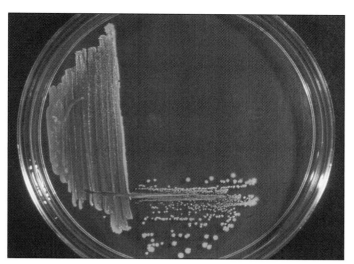

**Plate 11** Colony morphology of *Staphylococcus aureus*.

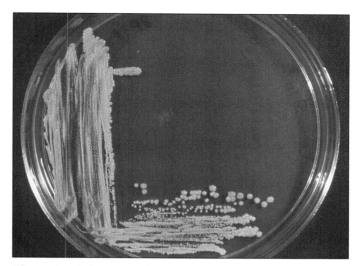

**Plate 12** Colony morphology of *Micrococcus* species.

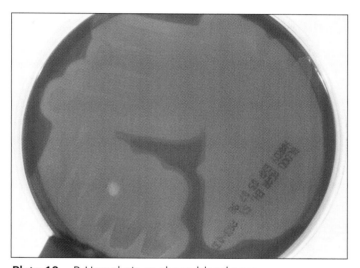

**Plate 13** B-Hemolysis on sheep blood agar.

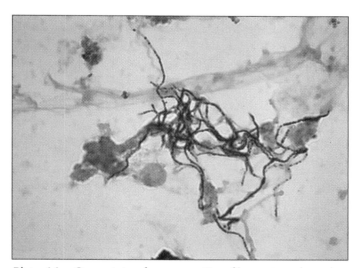

**Plate 14** Gram stain of gram-positive, filamentous, branching rods from expectorated sputum.

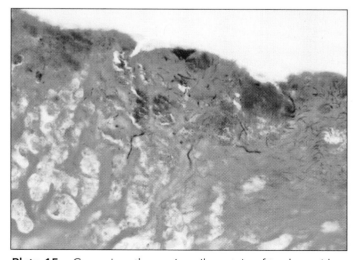

**Plate 15** Gomori methenamine-silver stain of trachea with filamentous rods.

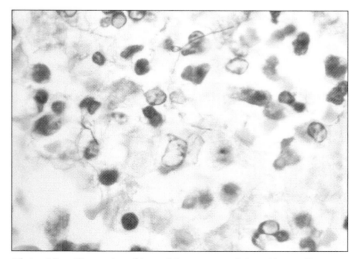

**Plate 16** Fite stain of lung biopsy containing *Nocardia* species.

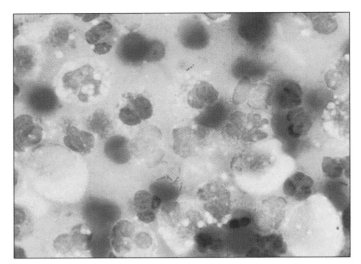

**Plate 17**    Wright stain from cytospin on cerebral spinal fluid with filamentous rods.

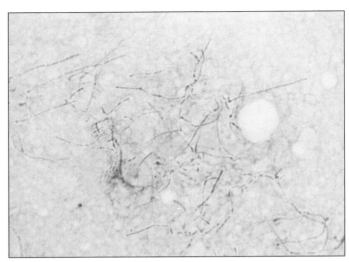

**Plate 18**    Modified Kinyoun stain of tissue biopsy containing *Nocardia* species.

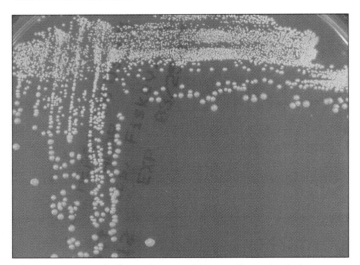

**Plate 19**    Dry, chalky colonies of *Nocardia* on brain heart infusion agar.

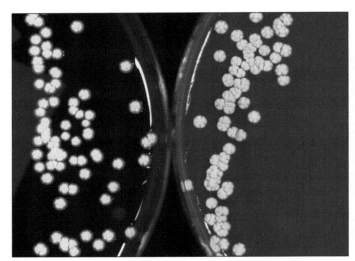

**Plate 20**    Colonial morphology of *Nocardia asteroides* on 5% sheep blood agar and chocolate agar.

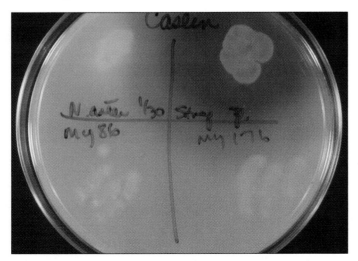

**Plate 21**    Casein agar inoculated with positive control (*streptomyces*), negative control (*Nocardia asteroides*), and tested isolate.

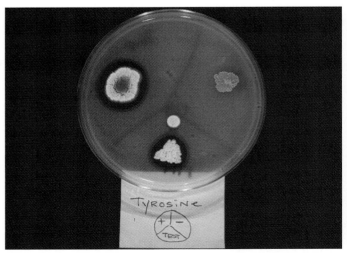

**Plate 22**    Tyrosine agar inoculated with positive control (S*treptomyces*), negative control (*Nocardia asteroides*), and tested isolate.

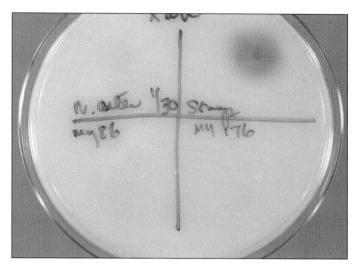

**Plate 23** Xanthine agar inoculated with positive control (*Streptomyces*), negative control (*Nocardia asteroides*), and tested isolate.

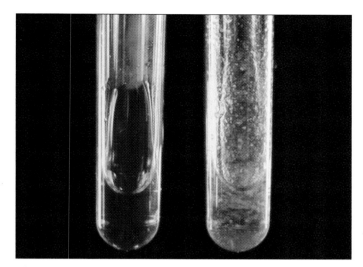

**Plate 24** Lysozyme broth: Tube #1 – no growth (isolate susceptible to lyzozyme; Tube #2 – growth present (isolate resistant to lyzozyme).

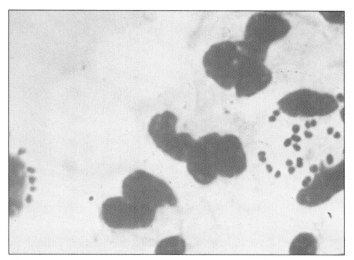

**Plate 25** Gram stain smear from male urethral discharge, showing intracellular and extracellular gram negative diplococci, morphologically resembling *Neisseria gonorrhoeae*.

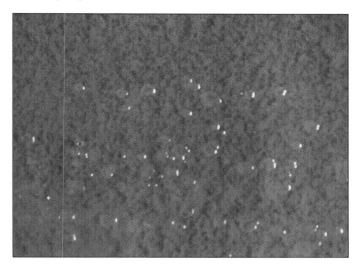

**Plate 26** *Neisseria gonorrhoeae* on chocolate agar, showing small, pearly, opalescent colonies.

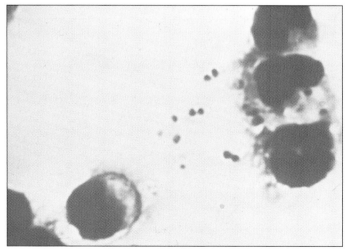

**Plate 27** Gram stain smear of cerebrospinal fluid sediment showing intracellular and extracellular gram-negative diplococci, morphologically resembling *Neisseria meningitidis*.

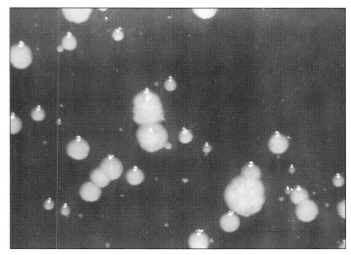

**Plate 28** *Branhamella catarrhalis* on nutrient agar, showing small, circular, grayish-white colonies with irregular margins.

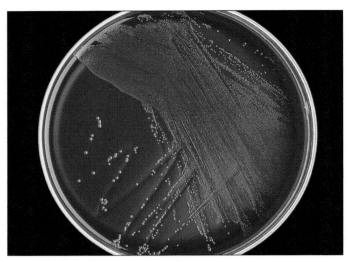

**Plate 29**   *Bordetella pertussis* on Regan-Lowe charcoal agar. (Courtesy of Becton Dickinson Microbiology Systems, Sparks, MD)

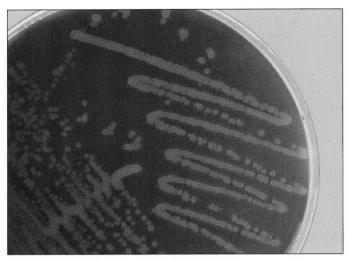

**Plate 30**   *Gardnerella vaginalis* on HBT. (Courtesy of Remel Inc.).

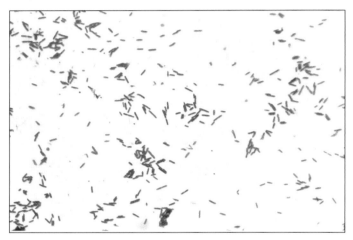

**Plate 31**   Morphological characteristics of Pseudomonas species. These aerobic nonfermenters are relatively thin gram-negative rods that may resemble the enteric bacilli (Enterobacteriaceae) on gram stains. They usually have one polar flagellum, but may occasionally have two or three. Special stains are needed to visualize the flagella.

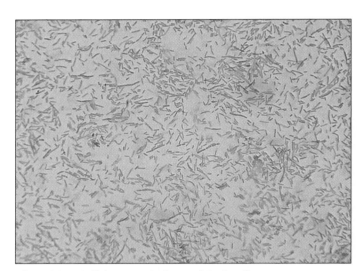

**Plate 32**   Cellular morphology of *B. fragilis.*

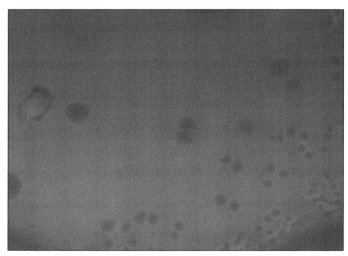

**Plate 33**   Colonial morpholgy of *B. fragilis.*

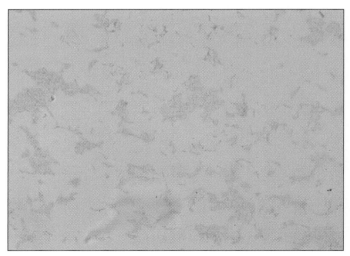

**Plate 34**   Cellular morphology of Prevotella.

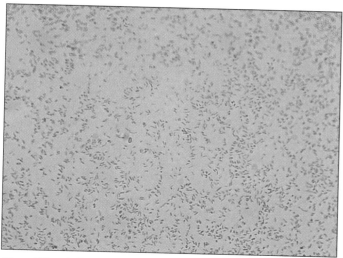

**Plate 35** Cellular morphology of *Porphyromonas*.

**Plate 36** Cellular morphology of *Fusobacterium nucleatum*.

**Plate 37** Colonial morphology of *Fusobacterium nucleatum*.

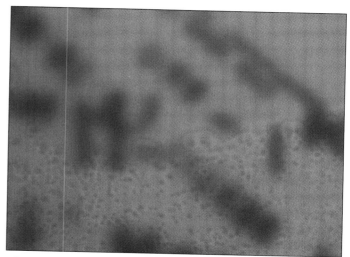

**Plate 38** Colonial morphology of *Fusobacterium necrophorum*.

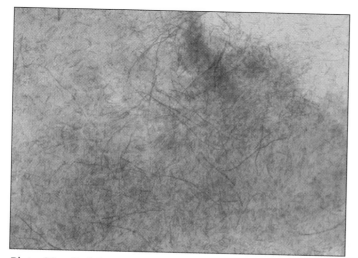

**Plate 39** Cellular morphology of *Fusobacterium necrophorum*.

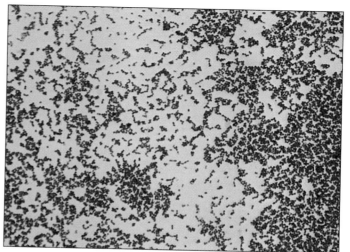

**Plate 40** Gram stain of *Peptostreptococcus anaerobius*, large coccobacillary cells that usually form chains.

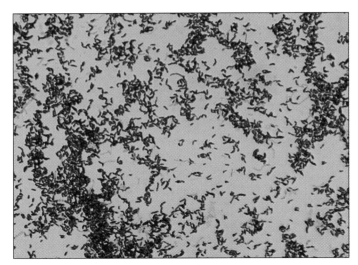

**Plate 41**   Gram stain of *Propionibacterium acnes.* Note pleomorphic, branching gram positive bacilli.

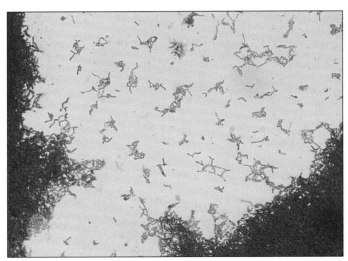

**Plate 42**   Gram stain of *Actinomyces viscosus,* note branching.

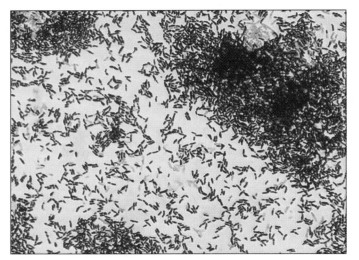

**Plate 43**   Gram stain of Bifidobacterium species, note pleomorphic bacilli with bifurcated ends.

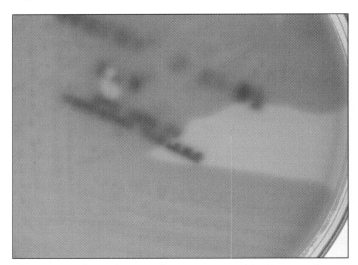

**Plate 44**   *Clostridium perfringens* on modified egg yolk agar.

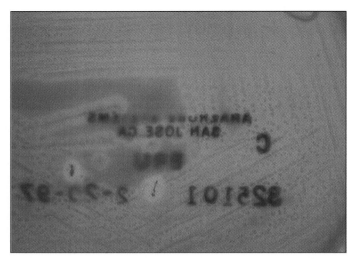

**Plate 45**   Blood culture positive for *Clostridium perfringens,* note hemolysis.

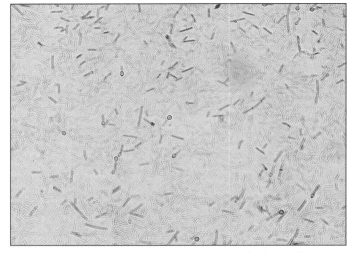

**Plate 46**   *Clostridium tetani.* Gram stain of culture shows large gram-positive bacilli, some with terminal spores.

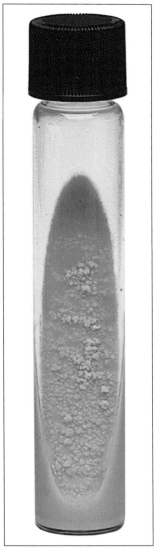

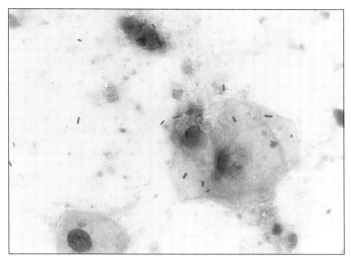

**Plate 48** Ziehl-Neelsen stain of *M. tuberculosis.*

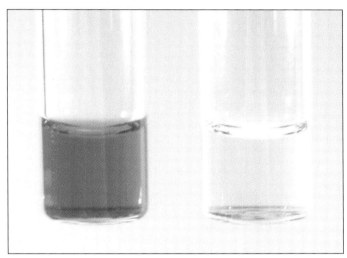

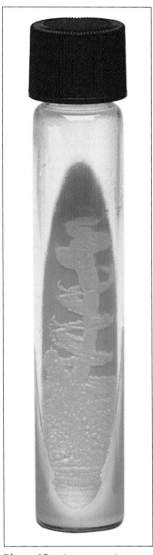

**Plate 47** Colony morphology of *M. tuberculosis* on Lowenstein Jensen media. *(Courtesy Remel Inc).*

**Plate 50** Nitrate test. Examples of (A) positive and (B) negative reactions.

**Plate 49** Lowenstein Jensen with *Mycobacterium avium.* (Courtesy Remel Inc.)

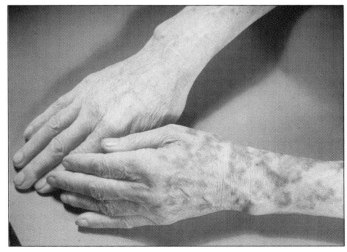

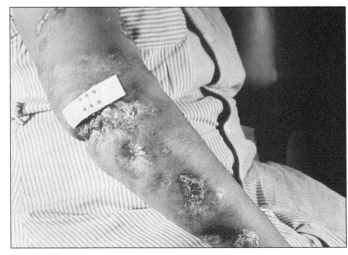

**Plate 51** Benign late syphilis. (Courtesy AFIP, slide #58-13602-14).

**Plate 52** Syphilis, tertiary. (Courtesy AFIP, slide #58-13966-8).

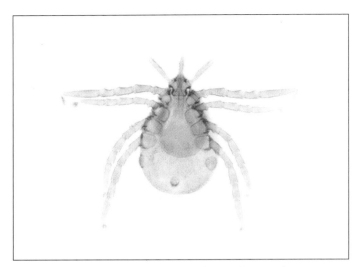

**Plate 53**    Engorged *Ixodes scapularis* tick (nymph).

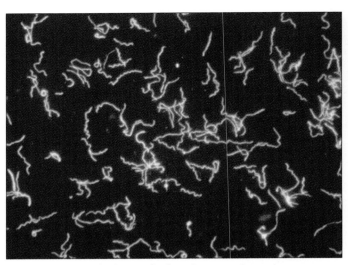

**Plate 54**    *Borrelia burgedorferi*, the spirochete that causes Lyme disease.

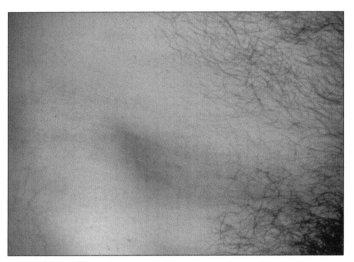

**Plate 55**    Erythema migans, the skin rash seen in many cases of early Lyme disease. (Courtesy Lyme Disease Foundation/Berger).

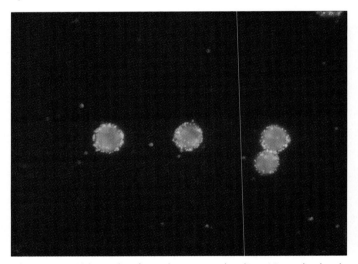

**Plate 56**    Chlamydia, free elementary bodies. Note the bodies attached to cells are close to the reticulum stage. (Courtesy BION Enterprises, Ltd., Park Ridge, IL).

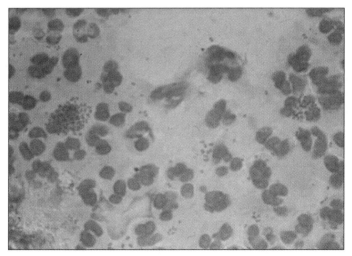

**Plate 57**    Gram stained smear of urethral discharge. Note large number of polymorphonuclear leukocytes and kidney bean-shaped gram-negative diplococci. This is presumptive evidence for gonorrhoea.

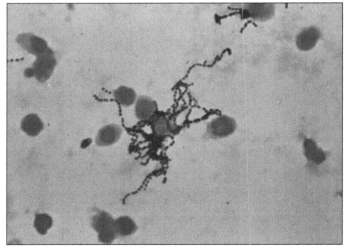

**Plate 58**    Gram stained smear of pus containing gram-positive cocci in chains, typical of Streptococcus.

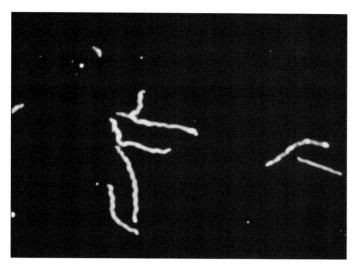

**Plate 59** Dark-field microscope preparation positive for the spirochete *Treponema pallidum.*

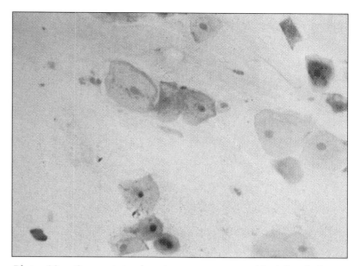

**Plate 60** Gram stain showing squamous epitheial cells in an improperly collected sputum specimen. (Courtesy of Scripps Clinic).

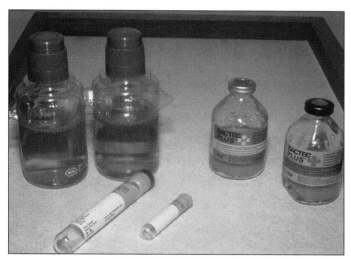

**Plate 61** Conventional blood culture broth bottles for use in the BACTEC semi-automated NR730 instrument and Isolator tubes. (Courtesy of Scripps Clinic).

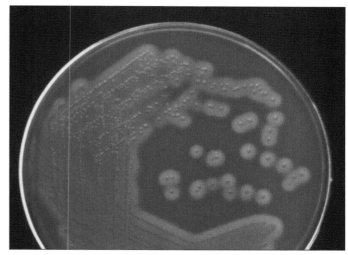

**Plate 62** *Streptococcus pyogenes* on sheep blood agar.

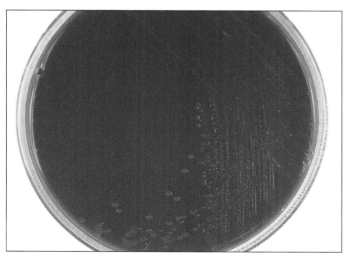

**Plate 63** *Neisseria gonorrhoeae* on modified Thayer-Martin agar.

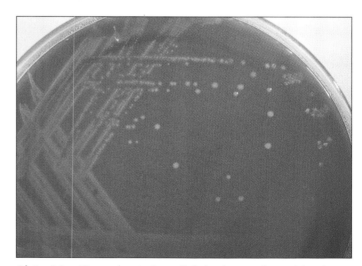

**Plate 64** *Corynebacterium diphtheriae* on sheep blood agar.

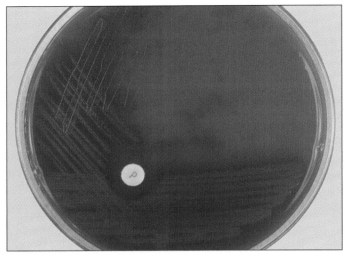

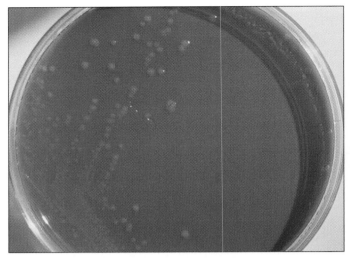

**Plate 65** *Streptococcus pneumoniae* on sheep blood agar, showing susceptibility to the "P" disc.

**Plate 66** Haemophilus on chocolate agar.

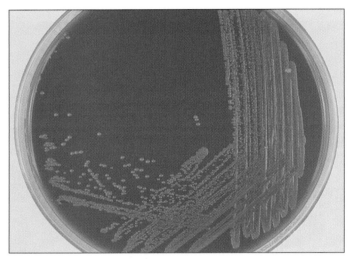

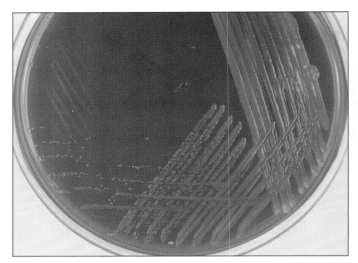

**Plate 67** *Branhamella catarrhalis* on chocolate agar.

**Plate 68** Legionella on buffered charcoal yeast extract agar.

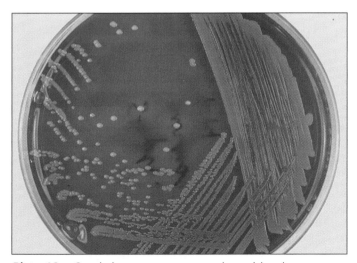

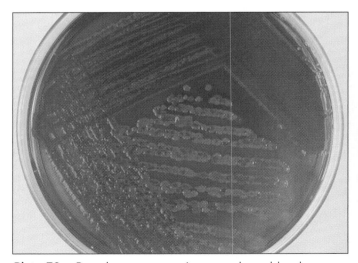

**Plate 69** *Staphylococcus aureus* on sheep blood agar.

**Plate 70** *Pseudomonas aeruginosa* on sheep blood agar.

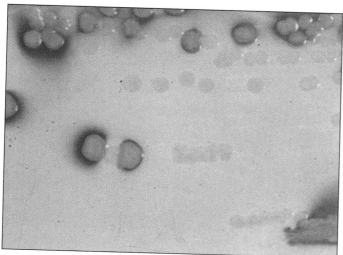

**Plate 71** On MacConkey agar, pale pink non-lactose fermenters are easy to differentiate from normal stool flora, which usually produce dark pink lactose positive colonies.

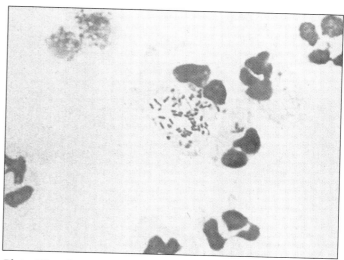

**Plate 72** Gram stain showing intracellular *Haemophilus influenzae* in cerebrospinal fluid.

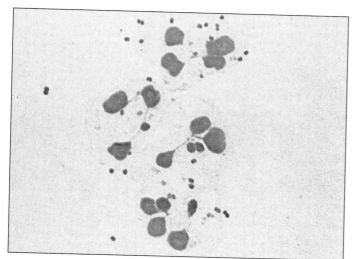

**Plate 73** Gram stain of *Neisseria meningitidis* in cerebrospinal fluid.

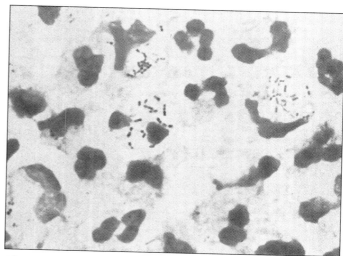

**Plate 74** Gram stain of mixed gram-negative and gram-positive bacteria in pleural fluid.

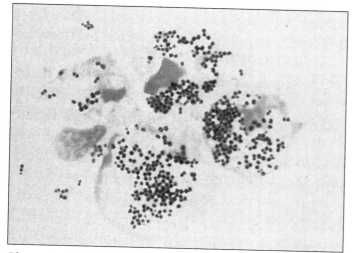

**Plate 75** Gram stain of *Staphylococcus aureus* in synovial fluid.

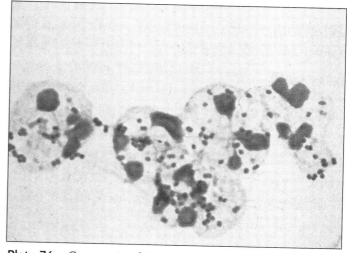

**Plate 76** Gram stain of *Neisseria gonorrhoeae* in synovial fluid.

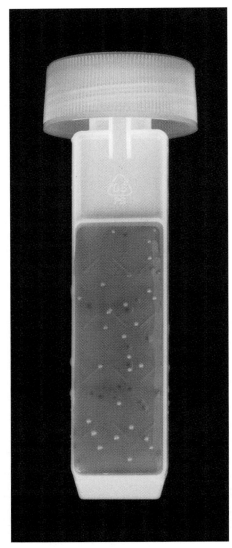

**Plate 77**    CLED

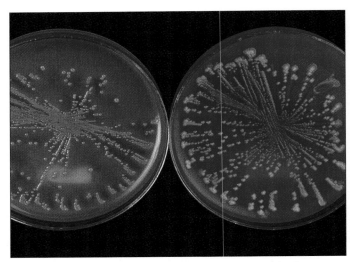

**Plate 78**    Results of a positive CCMS urine streaked onto MacConkey agar  and sheep blood agar plates. The patient had > 105 cfu/ml of E. coli.

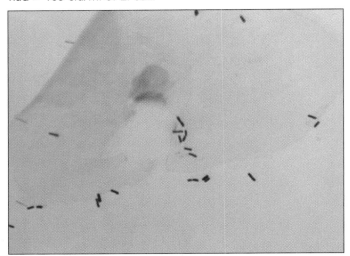

**Plate 79**    Gram-stained smear of vaginal secretions from a healthy adult, showing large numbers of lactobacilli.

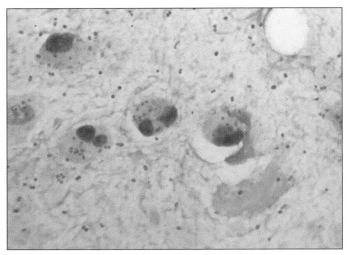

**Plate 80**    Gram-stained smear from male urethral discharge, showing intracellular and extracellular gram-negative diplococci, morphologically resembling *Neisseria gonorrhoeae.*

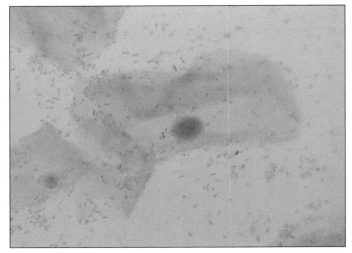

**Plate 81**    Gram stained smear of vaginal discharge from a patient with bacterial vaginosis (BV), showing squamous epithelial cells, covered by large numbers of tiny gram-variable bacterial cells, morphologically resembling *Gardnerella vaginalis.*

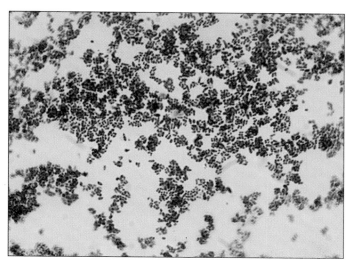

**Plate 82**  Gram stain of Corynebacterium from culture.

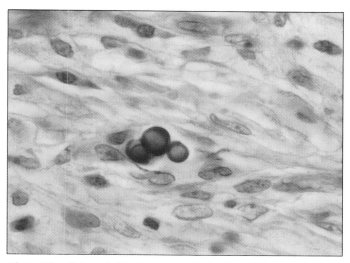

**Plate 83**  Sclerotic bodies in tissue from patient with chromoblastomycosis.

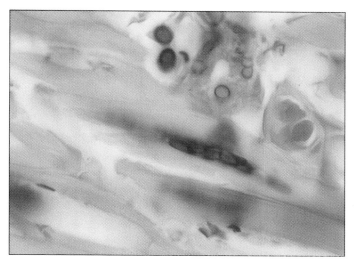

**Plate 84**  Photomicrograph of wood splinter containing dematiaceous fungi removed from patient with cystic chromomycocis.

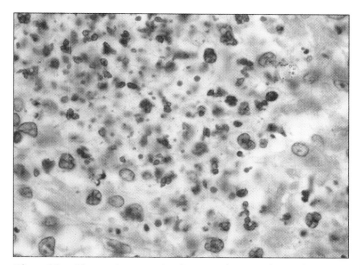

**Plate 85**  Photomicrograph of yeast of *Sporothrix schenckii* in tissue from patient with sporotrichosis.

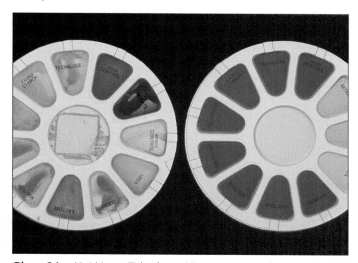

**Plate 86**  Uni-Yeast-Tek plate. (Courtesy Remel, Inc.).

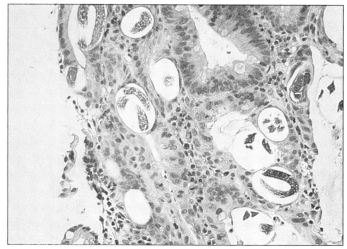

**Plate 87**  Rhabditiform larvae of *Strongyloides stercoralis* in lung tissue.

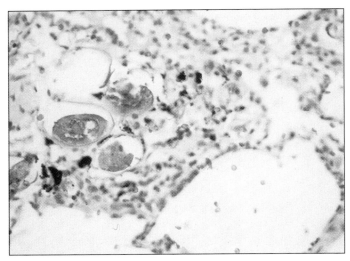

**Plate 88**   *Paragonimus westermani* ova in lung tissue.

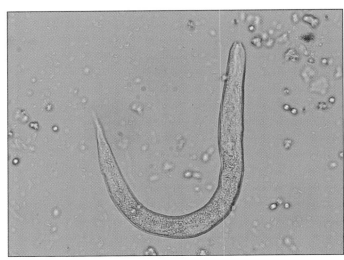

**Plate 89**   *Strongyloides stercoralis* in lung tissue.

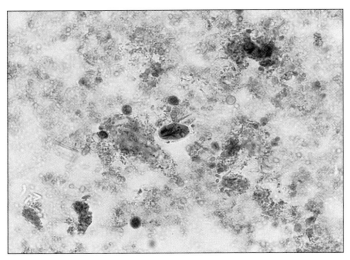

**Plate 90**   Giardia lamblia cyst at 10X.

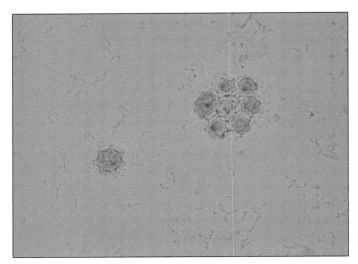

**Plate 91**   Double-walled cysts of Acanthamoeba species. Cultivated on a non-nutrient agar plates precoated with bacteria. The cysts are characterized by a wrinkled outer wall (ectocyst) and a polygonal, stellate, oval or even round inner wall (endocyst).

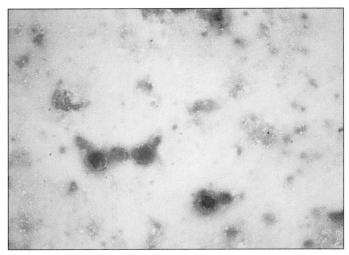

**Plate 92**   Periodic-acid Schiff (PAS) stain of lung tissue with double-walled cysts of Acanthamoeba species.

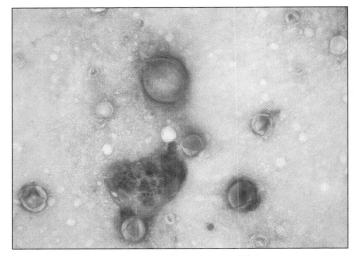

**Plate 93**   Periodic-acid Schiff (PAS) stain of lung tissue with double-walled cysts of Acanthamoeba species at 100X.

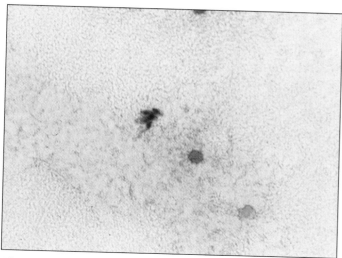

**Plate 94** Giemsa stain of promastigote stage of Leishmania species from NNN media at 10X (low power objective).

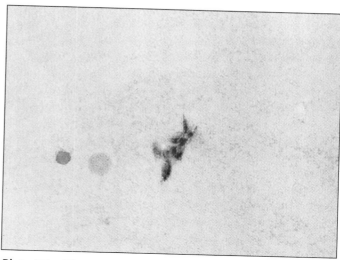

**Plate 95** Giemsa stain of promastigote stage of Leishmania species from NNN media at 100X (low power objective).

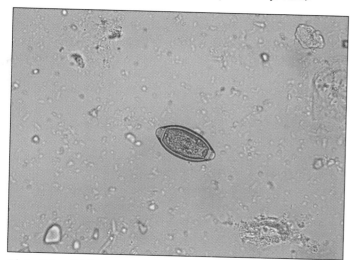

**Plate 96** *Trichuris trichiura* ova.

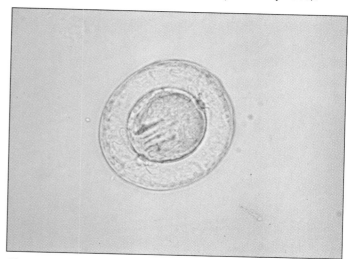

**Plate 97** *Hymenolepis nana* ova at 40X.

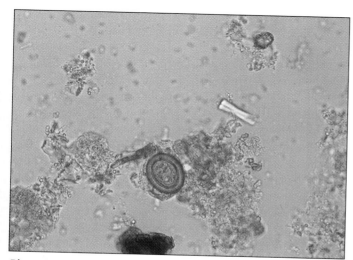

**Plate 98** Taenia species ova at 40X.

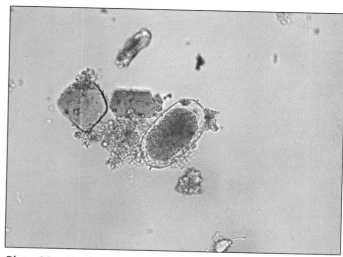

**Plate 99** Hookworm ova at 40X.

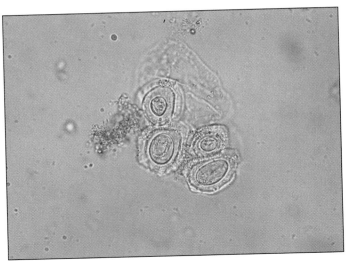

**Plate 100**  Vegetative cell in fecal preparation.

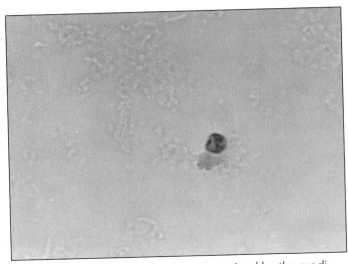

**Plate 101**  *Cryptosporidium parvum* stained by the modified acid-fast method.

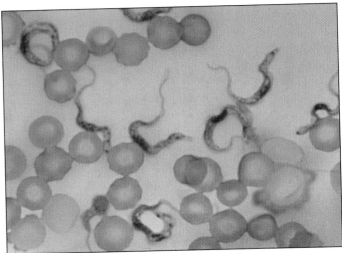

**Plate 102**  *Trypanosoma brucei gambiense* tryptomasigote in blood.

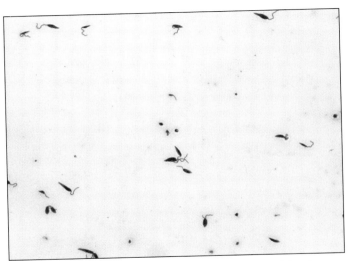

**Plate 103**  Amastigotes and tryptomastigotes in blood.

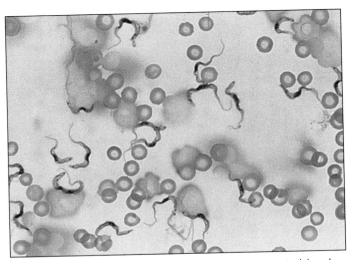

**Plate 104**  *Trypanosoma cruzi*, a tryptomastigote in blood.

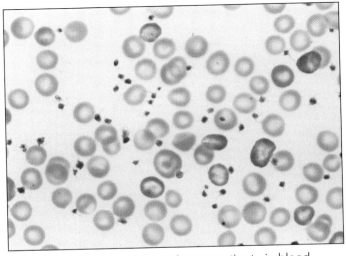

**Plate 105**  *Trypanosoma cruzi*, an amastigote in blood.

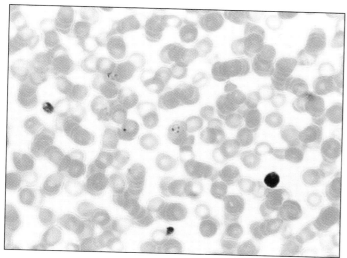

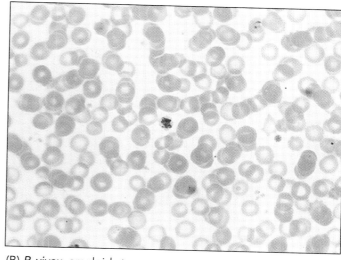

**Plate 106** Stages of life cycles of Plasmodium. (A) *P. vivax*, ring stage.

(B) *P. vivax*, ameloid stage.

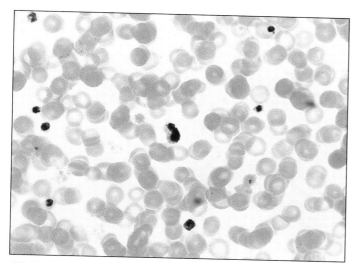

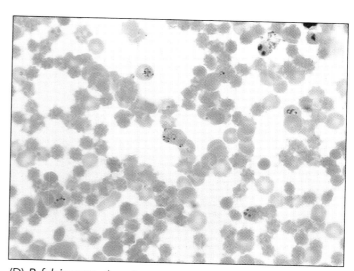

(C) *P. vivax*, schizonts.

(D) *P. falciparum*, ring stage.

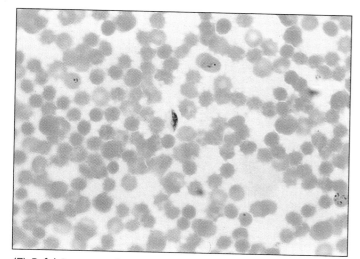

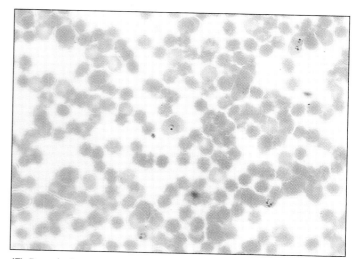

(E) *P. falciparum*, schizonts.

(F) *P. malariae*, ring stage.

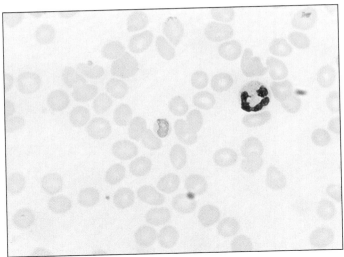

**Plate 106**    Stages of life cycles of Plasmodium. (G) *P. malariae*, banded schizonts.

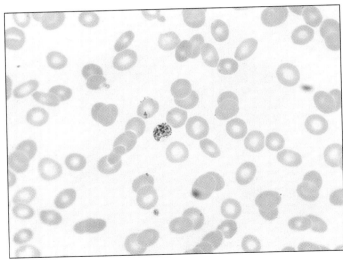

(H) *P. malariae*, gametocytes.

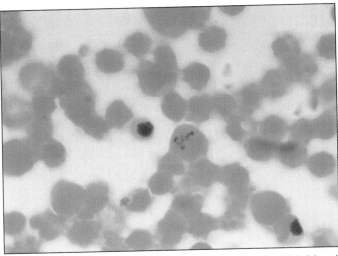

**Plate 107**    Plasmodium species, a trophozoite in thick blood smear.

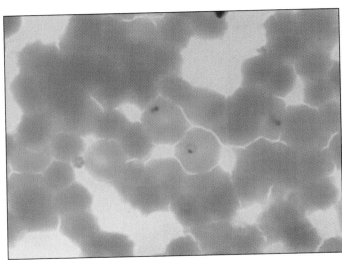

**Plate 108**    Plasmodium species, a trophozoite in thick blood smear.

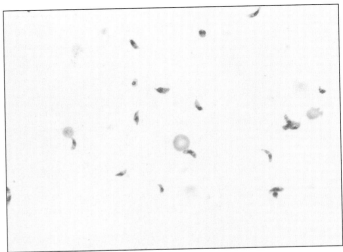

**Plate 109**    *Toxoplasmia gondii*, a trophozoite in (A) blood smear.

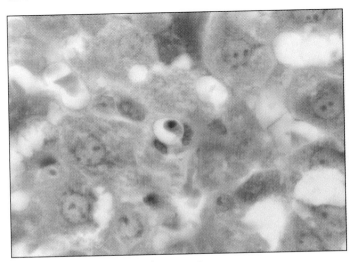

*Toxoplasmia gondii* in (B) liver section.

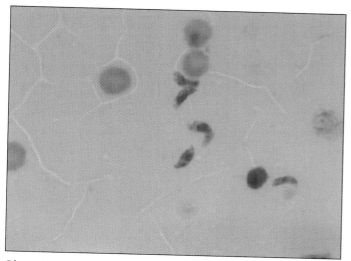

**Plate 110** *Toxoplasmia gondii*, blood smear trophozoite.

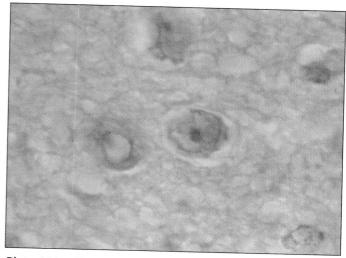

**Plate 111** *Toxoplama gondii*, an oocyst in tissue section.

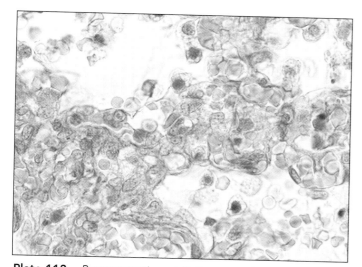

**Plate 112** *Pneumocystis carinii*, tissue section.

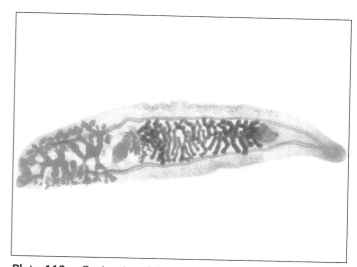

**Plate 113** *C. sinesis*, adult worm.

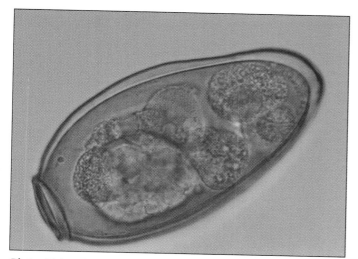

**Plate 114** *Paragonimus westermani*, egg at 40X.

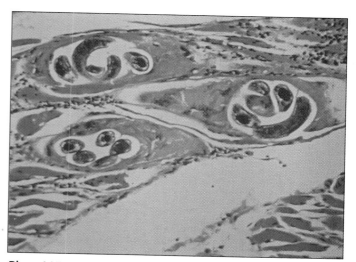

**Plate 115** Muscle biopsy of *Trichinella spiralis*. A single-coiled *Trichinella spiralis* larva in striated muscle at 300X. (Courtesy the Armed Forces Institute of Pathology (AFIP)).

**Plates 116-120**    Blood smears of Wuchereria bancrofti and Brugia malayi microfilariae (See plates 116-120).

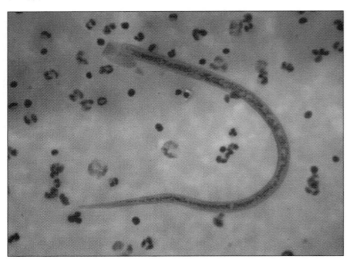

**Plate 116**    *Brugia malayi* microfilaria from peripheral blood via Knott's concentration method, stained with Delafield's hematoxylin at 350X. (Courtesy of the Armed Forces Institute of Pathology (AFIP)).

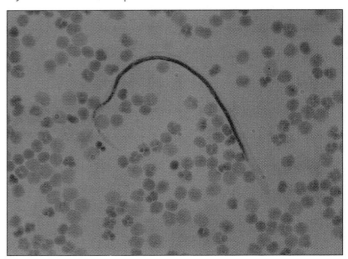

**Plate 117**    *Brugia malayi* microfilaria, anterior portion.

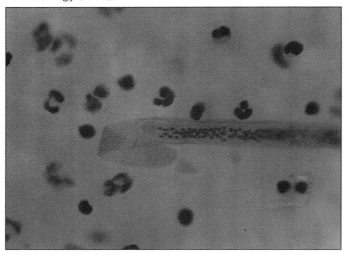

**Plate 118**    *Brugia malayi* microfilaria, posterior portion.

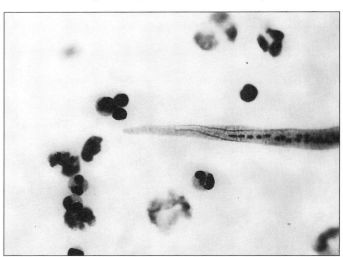

**Plate 119**    *Wuchereria bancrofti* microfilarias, anterior portion stained with Giemsa at 1,080X. (Courtesy of the Armed Forces Institute of Pathology (AFIP)).

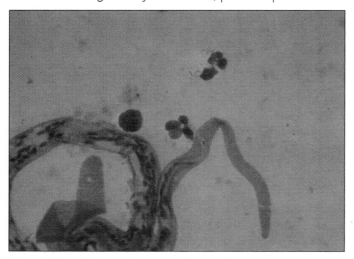

**Plate 120**    *Wuchereria bancrofti* microfilarias, posterior portion stained with Giemsa at 1,080X. (Courtesy of the Armed Forces Institute of Pathology (AFIP)).

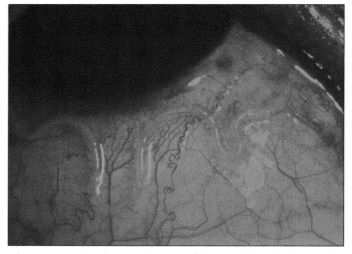

**Plate 121**    Ocular *Loa loa* microfilaria. Adult *L. loa* beneath the eye conjunctiva. (Courtesy of the Armed Forces Institute of Pathology (AFIP)).

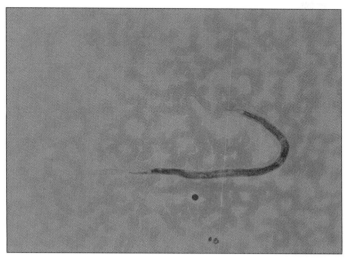

**Plate 122** Anterior portion of *L. loa* microfilaria, thin blood smear. (Courtesy of the Armed Forces Institute of Pathology (AFIP)).

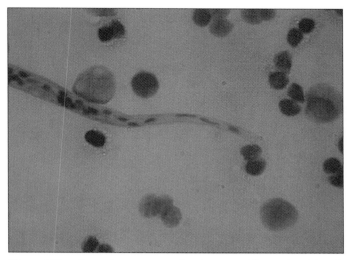

**Plate 123** Posterior portion of *L. loa* microfilaria, thin blood smear.

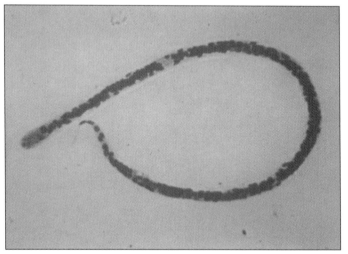

**Plate 124** *Onchocerca volvulus* microfilaria in blood and tissue sections. (Courtesy of the Armed Forces Institute of Pathology (AFIP)). Adult Onchocerca volvulus, onchocercal nodule with cross section of adult female worms at 56X.

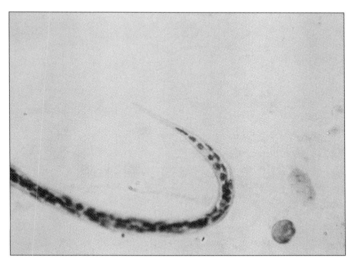

**Plate 125** Onchocercal nodule containing microfilaria at 1,080X. (Courtesy of the Armed Forces Institute of Pathology (AFIP)).

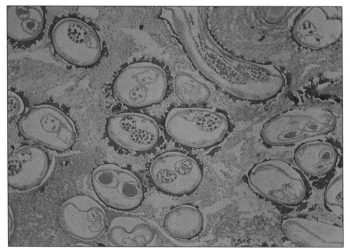

**Plate 126** *Onchocerca volvulus* microfilaria, anterior portion.

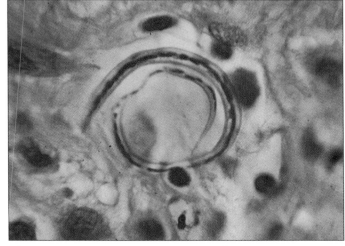

**Plate 127** *Onchocerca volvulus* microfilaria, posterior portion.

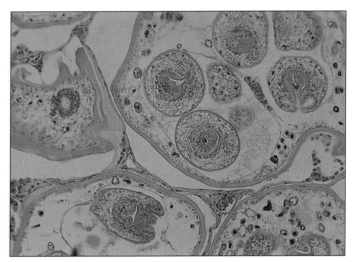

**Plate 128**   Liver biopsy showing *Echinococcus granulosus* isolated scolices at 440X. (Courtesy of the Armed Forces Institute of Pathology (AFIP)).

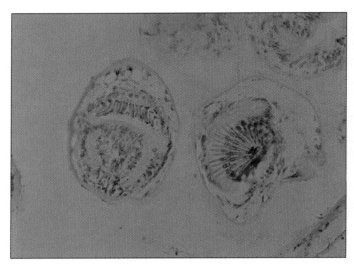

**Plate 129**   *Echinococcus granulosus* alveolar cyst. (Courtesy of the Armed Forces Institute of Pathology (AFIP)).

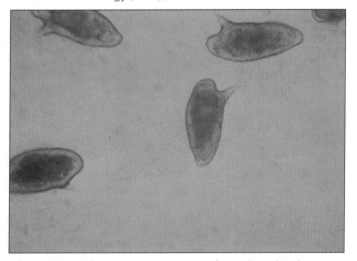

**Plate 130**   Schistosoma species ova from clinical isolates and biopsy. (Courtesy of the Armed Forces Institute of Pathology (AFIP)).

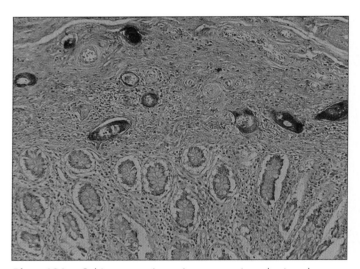

**Plate 131**   *Schistosoma japonicum* eggs in colonic submucosa at 87X. (Courtesy of the Armed Forces Institute of Pathology (AFIP)).

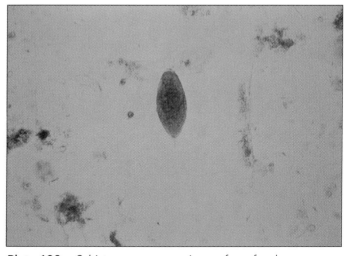

**Plate 132**   *Schistosoma mansoni* eggs from fecal prep.

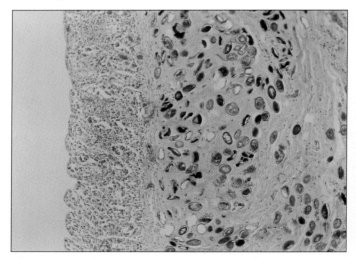

**Plate 133**   *Schistosoma haematobium* ova from tissue sample.

| Organism Type Seen on Gram Stain | Blood Agar | Chocolate Agar | MacConkey or EMB | Anaerobic Blood Agar | Anaerobic PEA or CNA |
|---|---|---|---|---|---|
| Blind subculture | X | X | | | |
| Gram-positive cocci and bacilli | X | | | Optional | |
| Gram-negative cocci and bacilli | X | X | X | X | X |
| Fungal elements seen† | X | X | | X | |
| Instrument signal positive, but Gram stain negative‡ | X | X | | X | |

**Table 26–3 ▶ Subculture Media for Positive Blood Cultures***

*Incubate all media at least 48 hours; blood and chocolate at 35°C in 5% $CO_2$; and MAC/EMB at 35°C without increased $CO_2$; anaerobic media in anaerobic environment with 5% $CO_2$.

†Add fungal medium (e.g., Sabarouds agar) and incubate at 30°C.

‡Inoculate thioglycollate broth also.

CNA, colistin nalidixic acid agar; EMB, eosin methylene blue agar; PEA, phenylethyl alcohol agar.

**Reports.** Once bacteria have been detected in the specimen, act immediately to inform the physician, keeping records of the date and time of notification as well as the name of the individual to whom the report is given. For instrument systems, the report should not wait for the results of the subculture. Provide all significant information, including the Gram stain morphology, which bottles were positive, and any results of presumptive testing. Follow all verbal reports with electronic or paper reports for the patient's chart.

For negative specimens, reports should be made at 24 and 48 hours, and at the end of incubation (5 or 7 days). Negative reports should state "No growth after __ days (or hours)."

## MICROBIAL PATHOGENS

Sources of bacteremia and fungemia are most commonly the respirator, genitourinary, and intestinal tracts. About 10% to 12% of blood cultures are positive, and the most common bloodstream pathogens are *S. aureus*, coagulase-negative staphylococci, and *E. coli* (see Table 26–4). *Enterococcus* species, yeast, *S. pneumoniae, P. aeruginosa, Klebsiella pneumoniae,* anaerobes, and miscellaneous gram-negative bacilli and streptococci make up most of the remainder.

A key change over the last 20 years is the increase in the incidence of clinically significant coagulase-negative staphylococci. This has created significant difficulties in interpretation of results because the majority represent contamination rather than bacteremia or endocarditis. The gram-positive bacilli such as *Bacillus, Corynebacterium,* and *Propionibacterium* species are almost always contaminants. The α- (viridans) streptococci are contaminants about 50% of the time. Distinguishing pathogens from contaminants is a chal-

lenge, but the presence of only a single positive blood culture out of three or more raises suspicion that the positive culture represents contamination.

Another significant change in recent years is the decline in frequency of bacteremia caused by anaerobes, down from about 15% to about 4%. This has led many laboratories to discontinue inoculating an anaerobic bottle in favor of inoculating a second aerobic bottle, which helps increase recovery of the more frequent aerobic pathogens such as fungi and *Pseudomonas*

**Table 26–4 ▶ Clinically Significant Isolates from Positive Blood Cultures (1995–1997)***

| | |
|---|---|
| *Staphylococcus aureus* | 24% |
| Coagulase negative staphylococci | 15% |
| *Escherichia coli* | 11% |
| *Enterococcus* species | 9% |
| Yeast (mostly *Candida albicans*) | 8% |
| *Streptococcus pneumoniae* | 7% |
| *Pseudomonas aeruginosa* | 6% |
| *Klebsiella pneumoniae* | 4% |
| α-Streptococci | 4% |
| Anaerobes† | 4% |
| *Enterobacter* species | 4% |
| *Acinetobacter* species | 2% |
| ß-Streptococci | 2% |
| Other | 1% |

*Composite of several studies in five sites during 1995 through 1997 having 37,125 blood cultures of which 3,799 (10.2%) were positive. (Bacteria judged to be contaminants have been omitted.)

†Primarily *Bacteroides, Fusobacterium, Peptostreptococcus* species.

species. However, the nature of the infection may still suggest that anaerobic culture is appropriate, such as with intra-abdominal and genitourinary tract infections where anaerobes account for a higher percentage of the isolates. Overall, the predominant anaerobic isolates are *Bacteroides* species, with the *B. fragilis* group making up most of these; and *Fusobacterium, Prevotella, Porphyromonas, Peptostreptococcus,* and *Clostridium* accounting for most of the rest.

A characteristic of blood cultures from severely debilitated patients and immunocompromised patients is that they often grow unusual bacterial pathogens such as various *Pseudomonas* species, *Mycobacterium* species, and otherwise rarely isolated nonfermentative gram-negative bacilli, as well as fungi such as *Candida* species, and *C. neoformans*.

The etiologic agents of bacteremia and fungemia in children are similar to those in adults except there are increased percentages of *S. pneumoniae* and *N. meningitidis* and decreased percentage of anaerobes; *Haemophilus influenzae* bacteremia has almost vanished as a result of the immunization program.

Mortality from bloodstream infections ranges from about 20% to 50%. Streptococcal bacteremia tends to have low mortality rate (about 15%), whereas enterococcal bacteremia is moderately high (about 45%). Fungemia and gram-negative bacilli bacteremia (especially *P. aeruginosa*) caused death in up to 60% to 70% of the cases.

## Infective Endocarditis

Because bacteria are continuously discharged from the endocardial vegetation in cases of infective endocarditis, these patients will produce a high percentage of positive blood cultures. The first blood culture will be positive in about 90% of the cases (depending on the type of organism present) and one of the first two blood cultures will be positive in about 99% of the cases. Fewer than 5% of infective endocarditis cases will have negative blood cultures, most of which are due to prior antibiotic therapy.

Infectious endocarditis is caused by many different microbes, but the most prevalent are streptococci, enterococci, and staphylococci (see Table 26-5). In acute endocarditis affecting native valves, *S. aureus* accounts for about 60% of cases, with the remainder being caused by streptococci and aerobic gram-negative bacilli. About 60% of the cases of subacute endocarditis of native valves are due to α-hemolytic and nonhemolytic streptococci, with enterococci, coagulase-negative staphylococci, and fastidious gram-negative bacilli causing the remainder. These fastidious organisms include the HACEK group (haemophilus, actinobacillus, cardiobacterium, eikenella, kingella).

*Staphylococcus aureus* causes about 75% of the endocarditis among intravenous drug users, with enterococci, streptococci, fungi, and gram-negative bacilli accounting for most of the other cases. Prosthetic valve endocarditis is primarily caused by coagulase-negative staphylococci, followed by *S. aureus,* α-hemolytic streptococci, and enterococci.

## Special Microorganisms and Special Concerns

Certain organisms that cause bacteremia and infective endocarditis are difficult to isolate by standard culture techniques. Prolonged incubation and specialized media are often necessary to recover these organisms. The use of fluorescent stains, enzyme-linked immunosorbent assay, and nucleic acid amplification procedures have made it much easier and quicker to identify the microbes, which are difficult to culture.

Most aerobic blood culture broth provide good recovery of *Candida albicans* within 5 to 7 days, although the BacT/Alert FAN and BACTEC Myco/F lytic bottles perform better than most others. However, lysis-centrifugation performs better for most other fungi, such as *C. neoformans, Histoplasma capsulatum,* and other dimorphic fungi where the sediment is inoculated directly onto appropriate solid media. These media should usually be incubated at 22° to 30°C for 4 weeks before being discarded as negative.

*Mycobacterium tuberculosis, Mycobacterium avium* complex, and occasionally other species of mycobacteria are frequent causes of bloodstream infection in patients infected with human immunodeficiency virus. These microbes are also occasional pathogens in patients with various other immunosuppressive conditions. There are several BACTEC media, especially the Myco/F-Sputa and 13A bottles, which provide good results with mean time to detection of about 13 days for *M. avium* and about 23 days for *M. tuberculosis*. An alternative with similar detection time is to inoculate sediment from lysis-centrifugation tubes onto Lowenstein-Jensen and Middlebrook 7H11 media.

Blood cultures for *Brucella* species have traditionally been performed in either biphasic (e.g., Septi-

## Table 26-5 ▶ Primary Etiologic Agents of Infective Endocarditis

Viridans streptococci

Coagulase-negative staphylococci

*Staphylococcus aureus*

*Enterococcus* species

*Streptococcus bovis*

Enterobacteriaceae

Fastidious gram-negative bacilli

Fungi

Chek) or broth-only media incubated for 30 days with blind subcultures every 4 or 5 days. In recent years the lysis-centrifugation method has proven to be good and BACTEC even better in sensitivity (70% versus near-100%, respectively) and speed (mean time to recovery of about 3 days) (Yagupsky, Peled, Press, Abramson, & Abu-Rashid, 1997).

Nutritionally deficient streptococci, which require vitamin B$_6$ and thiol-containing compounds grow adequately in routine culture broth. However, blood agar plates used for subculture must be supplemented with

pyridoxal, or a "staph streak" must be performed on the agar plate, which is then observed for satellite colonies around the staph streak.

*Leptospira* species may be recovered during the first week of illness by inoculating 1 to 3 drops of blood into Fletcher's medium, then incubating in the dark at 28° to 30°C for 4 to 6 weeks. Examine a drop of broth weekly using a dark-field or phase-contrast microscope.

Culture of *Francisella tulerensis* requires the addition of L-cysteine and dextrose, although the diagnosis is usually made by serologic tests.

## SUMMARY

▶ Bacteremia is defined as the presence of viable bacteria circulating in the bloodstream.
▶ Bacteremia may be classified as transient, intermittent, or continuous, and this is associated with volume and frequency of specimen collection.
▶ A variety of aerobic, anaerobic, and fungal media are available for various systems. Soybean-casein digest broth containing SPS and having an enriched CO$_2$ atmosphere is the most common formulation.
▶ Adequate venipuncture site cleansing with alcohol and iodine accompanied by good aseptic technique is needed to keep contamination to a minimum.
▶ Collect at least 20 mL of blood per collection time and divide it between two culture bottles to achieve a 1:5 to 1:10 ratio.
▶ Collect two or three sets of blood cultures near simultaneously or within a 24-hour period. Incu-

bation of the broth in an anaerobic environment is not necessary because of the low likelihood of anaerobes being the pathogen.
▶ Continuous monitoring systems provide good recovery of most microbes in a minimal time period. Blind subcultures and terminal subcultures are unnecessary. Five days of incubation is adequate.
▶ For conventional broth systems, perform a Gram stain and a blind subculture at 6 to 18 hours, but terminal subcultures at the end of 7 days of incubation is unnecessary.
▶ For all positive blood cultures, immediately perform a Gram stain and subculture to appropriate media. Report results immediately.
▶ Predominant etiologic agents of bacteremia are *Staphylococcus aureus,* coagulase-negative staphylococci, and *Escherichia coli.* The most frequent causes of infective endocarditis are viridans streptococci, coagulase-negative staphylococci, and *S. aureus.*

## Review Questions

1. The presence of viable bacteria in the bloodstream is referred to as:
   a. bacteruria.
   b. bacteremia.
   c. septicemia.
   d. sepsis.

2. The type of bacteremia that occurs when bacteria periodically enter the bloodstream from an established abscess is:
   a. transient.
   b. continuous.
   c. intermittent.
   d. infective endocarditis.

3. A blood culture medium that would NOT be appropriate for the recovery of aerobic bacteria would be:
   a. soybean casein digest broth with 0.05% SPS.
   b. Brucella broth with 5% CO$_2$ gaseous atmosphere.
   c. brain-heart infusion broth with 0.025% SPS.
   d. thioglycollate broth with 5% carbon dioxide.

4. Which of the following is most significant in recovering clinically significant isolates from blood cultures?
   a. Scrub the venipuncture site with alcohol and iodine compounds.
   b. Include one anaerobic bottle in each set.
   c. Agitate the broth while incubating.
   d. Collect four or five specimens over a 24-hour period.

5. The BACTEC fluorescent system and the BacT/Alert blood culture system detect bacterial growth in the bottle by:
   a. turbidity and hemolysis.
   b. growth on agar media.
   c. carbon dioxide production detected by a photodetector.
   d. volume of carbon dioxide or nitrogen or another gas produced by the bacteria.

6. A conventional broth blood culture system has incubated for 12 hours since it was collected. Which of the following procedures should be performed at this time (nothing except incubation has been performed up to this time)?
   a. Gram stain only
   b. Gram stain and blind subculture
   c. Only inspect for visible signs of growth
   d. Continue to incubate for testing later

7. Which of the following are two of the most predominant etiologic agents of bacteremia?
   a. *Pseudomonas aeruginosa* and *Candida albicans*
   b. *Bacteroides fragilis* and *Staphylococcus aureus*
   c. Coagulase-negative staphylococci and *Streptococcus pneumoniae*
   d. *Staphylococcus aureus* and *Escherichia coli*

8. One blood culture set was collected from each of the patient's arms. At 24 hours, one bottle of each set produced growth of a gram-positive coccus in clusters. Which of the following is the best interpretation?
   a. This bacterium is probably a clinically significant isolate.
   b. This bacterium is probably a contaminant.
   c. Consider this bacterium a contaminant if it is *Staphylococcus epidermidis*.
   d. Consider this bacterium a contaminant if it is any of the normal skin flora.

9. For optimal recovery of bacteria from blood cultures from an adult, collect _____.
   a. 5 mL of blood per bottle of broth
   b. 5 to 10 mL of blood and divide it between two culture bottles
   c. 20 to 30 mL of blood and divide it between two culture bottles
   d. 20 mL of blood per bottle of broth

## CASE STUDY 1: AN INFLAMED THUMB

Mr. Smith, a 42-year-old construction worker, cut his thumb while demolishing part of a building. By the next day the area around the cut was red and the thumb was sore, but he endured the pain as he worked all day. By evening, the thumb was swollen and throbbing, with some yellowish white material oozing out, and he noticed red streaks going up the inside of his forearm. He suddenly began to have a shaking chill and felt queasy, so his wife drove him to the hospital emergency room. On arrival at the emergency room his temperature had reached 39.7°C. He was flushed and appeared ill, with a pulse of 125 and a blood pressure of 100/60, compared to his usual of 145/85.

Blood cultures were drawn, and Mr. Smith was started on intravenous fluids and antibiotics. After about 8 hours of incubation, there was a positive blood culture signal on the instrument, and medium-large cocci in small groups and single were seen on the Gram stain. By morning he was not improved. Methicillin resistance was determined and the antibiotic was changed in the evening. By the next morning he was somewhat better, and his subsequent recovery over the next few days was uneventful.

**Questions:**

1. What were the most likely causes of the symptoms presented at the emergency room?

2. Describe how the blood culture specimens should have been collected (when to collect, how much blood, etc.).

3. What is the most likely presumptive identification of the pathogen, and what rapid tests could have been used to identify this organism?

## CASE STUDY 2: ENDOCARDITIS CHALLENGE

A 35-year-old woman with a history of childhood rheumatic fever underwent excessive dental work without antimicrobial prophylaxis. About 2 weeks later she was examined in a neighborhood clinic because of fatigue, various muscle and joint aches, nonproductive cough, and low-grade fever. A radiograph of her chest did not reveal the etiology of these signs and symptoms, and tests for rheumatoid arthritis and tuberculosis were negative. About 10 mL of blood drawn from her right arm and inoculated into an aerobic blood culture bottle resulted in the recovery of a few colonies of what appeared to be a staphylococcus skin contaminant.

About 3 weeks after the original examination, she returned with the same signs and symptoms as previously. Repeat examination demonstrated the original findings plus an enlarged heart, bilateral pleural effusions, and weight loss. At this time the patient was admitted to the hospital having a temperature of 38.1°C and small "splinter hemorrhage" on one finger. A cardiac examination showed rapid heart rate and heart murmur. An echocardiogram demonstrated mitral valve regurgitation. Each of five sets of blood cultures taken over 24 hours from each arm was positive with α-hemolytic, gram-positive cocci.

### Questions:

1. Why was there clinical evidence of endocarditis in the original episode, but not "positive" blood cultures? (What should have been done differently during the original examination to recover and identify the agent of possible endocarditis?)

2. What role did the dental work play in causing the endocarditis.

3. What is the most likely microbial pathogen causing this problem?

---

10. One of the reasons most blood culture media contain sodium polyanetholsulfonate (SPS) is because that chemical:

    a. enhances anaerobiosis.

    b. inhibits growth of coagulase-negative staphylococci.

    c. enhances growth of gram-negative cocci.

    d. inactivates certain antimicrobics.

## ▶ REFERENCES & RECOMMENDED READING

Baron, E. J., Peterson, L. R., Finegold, S. M. (1994). *Bailey & Scott's diagnostic microbiology* (9th ed.). St. Louis: Mosby.

Bryant, J. K., Strand, C. L. (1987). Reliability of blood cultures collected from intravascular catheters vs venipuncture. *American Journal of Clinical Pathology, 88,* 113–116.

Buck, L., & Romero, S. (1997). Direct ID and susceptibilities from blood culture bottles [Abstract]. *Abstracts of the 97th General Meeting of the American Society for Microbiology.* Washington, DC: American Society for Microbiology, C-439, p. 196.

Centers for Disease Control and Prevention. (1988). Update: Universal precautions for prevention of transmission of HIV, HBV, and other BBP in healthcare settings. *Morbidity and Mortality Weekly Report, 37,* 377.

Check, W. A. (1997). Less becomes best in microbiology. *CAP Today, 11*(1), 21–29.

Doern, G. V. (1994, March). In M. L. Wilson (Ed.). *Clinics in Laboratory Medicine: Blood Cultures, 14*(1), 136–138.

Dunne, W. J. Jr., Nolte, F. S., & Wilson, M. L. (1997). *Blood cultures III, CUMITECH 1B,* Coordinating ed., J. A. Hindler. Washington, DC: American Society for Microbiology.

Fuller, D., et al. (1997). Comparison of BACTEC Myco/F lytic medium to Wampole Isolator for the recovery of yeast and fungi in blood [Abstract]. *Abstracts of the 97th General Meeting of the American Society for Microbiology.* Washington, DC: American Society for Microbiology, C-231, p. 160.

Gibb, A. B., & Karn, E. (1997). Limited yield from the fifth day of incubation of BacT/Alert blood cultures [Abstract]. *Abstracts of the 97th General Meeting of the American Society for Microbiology.* Washington, DC: American Society for Microbiology, C-424, p. 194.

Henderson, D. K. (1995). Bacteremia due to percutaneous intravascular devices. In G. L. Mandell, J. E. Bennett, & R. Dolin (Eds.), *Principles and practice of infectious diseases* (4th ed., pp. 2587–2599). New York: Churchill Livingstone.

Isenberg, H. D. (Ed.). (1992). *Clinical microbiology procedures handbook* (pp. 1.7.1–1.7.11, 12.5.1–12.5.19). Washington, DC: American Society for Microbiology.

Koneman, E. W., Allen, S. D., Janda, W. M., Schrekenberger, P. C., Washington, C. W. Jr. (1997). *Color atlas and textbook of diagnostic microbiology* (5th ed.). Philadelphia: Lippincott-Raven.

Larchmer, A. W. (1993). Intravascular infection. In M. Schaechter, G. Medoff, & B. I. Eisenstein, *Microbial disease* (2nd ed., pp. 779–790). Baltimore: Williams & Wilkins.

Levi, M. H., Sarode, R., Seno, R., Gialanella, P., & McKitrick, J. C. (1997). Five vs seven day blood culture protocol using BACTEC 9240 [Abstract]. *Abstracts of the 97th General Meeting of the American Society for Microbiology.* Washington, DC: American Society for Microbiology, C-425, p. 194.

Li, J., Plorde, J. J., & Carlson, L. G. (1994). Effects of volume and periodicity on blood cultures. *Journal of Clinical Microbiology, 32,* 2829–2831.

Miller, J. M. (1996). *A guide to specimen management in clinical microbiology.* Washington, DC: ASM Press.

Murray, P. R. (1985). Determination of the optimal incubation period of blood culture broths for the detection of clinically significant septicemia. *Journal of Clinical Microbiology, 85,* 481–485.

National Committee for Laboratory Standards. (1991). Protection of lab workers from infectious disease transmitted by blood and tissue. *Tentative guideline.* (Document M29-T2). Villanova, PA: Author.

Occupational Safety and Health Administration. (1991). Occupational exposure to bloodborne pathogens. Occupational Safety and Health Act, 29 CFR 1910.1030.

Pezzlo, M. (1994, May 23). *Automated blood culture systems.* Paper presented at ASM Workshop: Instrumentation in Clinical Microbiology, American Society for Microbiology, Las Vegas.

Reimer, L. G., Wilson, M. L., & Weinstein, M. P. (1997). Update on detection of bacteremia and fungemia. *Clinical Microbiology Reviews, 10,* 444–465.

Shanson, D. C. (1990). Blood culture technique: Current controversies. *Journal of Antimicrobics and Chemotherapy, 25* (Suppl. C), 17–29.

Shapiro, D. S. et al., (1992). Brief report: *Chlamydia psittaci* endocarditis diagnosed by blood culture. *New England Journal of Medicine,* 1192–1195.

Trudel, R. R., Griffith, J. T., & Schleicher, L. H. (1995). Bacteremia. In C. R. Mahon & G. Manuselis, Jr., *Textbook of diagnostic microbiology* (pp. 935–947). Philadelphia: Saunders.

Waite, R. T., & Woods, G. L. (1997). Comparison of BACTEC Myco/F lytic medium to the Wampole Isolator for the recovery of fungi in blood [Abstract]. *Abstracts of the 97th General Meeting of the American Society for Microbiology.* Washington, DC: American Society for Microbiology, C-229. p. 160.

Waites, K. B., Brookings, E. S., Moser, S. A., McKinnon, M. L., & Van Pelt, L. (1997). Direct bacterial identification from positive BacT/Alert blood culture specimens using MicroScan overnight and rapid panels [Abstract]. *Abstracts of the 97th General Meeting of the American Society for Microbiology.* Washington, DC: American Society for Microbiology, C-429, p. 195.

Welby, P. L., Keller, D. S. & Storch, G. A. (1995). Comparison of Automated Difco ESP Blood Culture System with Biphasic BBL Septi-Chek System for detection of bloodstream infections in pediatric patients. *Journal of Clinical Microbiology, 33,* 1084–1088.

Wilson, M. L., Weinstein, M. P., & Reller, L. B. (1994, March). Automated blood culture systems. In M. L. Wilson (Ed.). *Clinics in Laboratory Medicine: Blood Cultures 14*(1), 149–169.

Woods, G. L., & Washington, J. A. (1995). The clinician and the microbiology laboratory. In G. L. Mandell, J. E. Bennett, & R. Dolin (Eds.), *Principles and practice of infectious diseases* (4th ed., pp. 169–199). New York: Churchill Livingstone.

Yagupsky, P., Peled, N., Press, J., Abramson, O., & Abu-Rashid, M. (1997). Comparison of BACTEC 9240 Peds Plus medium and Isolator 1.5 microbial tubes for detection of *Brucella melitensis* from blood cultures. *Journal of Clinical Microbiology, 14,* 1382–1384.

Young, L. S. (1995). Sepsis syndrome. In G. L. Mandell, J. E. Bennett, & R. Dolin (Eds.), *Principles and practice of infectious diseases* (4th ed., pp. 690–705). New York: Churchill Livingstone.

# CHAPTER 27
# The Respiratory Tract

Mark Shapiro, MS (ASCP), MS

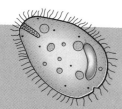

## Microbes in the News
### European Truck Drivers Develop Legionnaires' Disease

Two English long distance truck, or lorry, drivers became ill with Legionella infections in March, 1998 after staying at the same lorry park in northern Spain. The drivers both took showers at the same lorry park, then slept overnight in the cabins of their trucks. Legionella pneumophila serogroup 1 was cultured from sputum of one of the men, whose illness was confirmed as Legionnaires' disease. The other man was diagnosed serologically on the basis of a single high titre and without radiological evidence of pneumonia. Five other cases of Legionella infections in long distance truck drivers who had traveled through Belgium, France, Italy, the Netherlands, Spain, and Slovenia were reported in 1994 and 1997. In these cases all were said to have slept in the cabins of their trucks,

but took showers at lorry parks, petrol stations, or at the center to which their goods were delivered.

Sporadic cases and outbreaks of Legionella have been associated with showers in hotels and camp sites in many European countries, with at least 50 cases being reported in 1993 by The European Surveillance Scheme for Travel Associated Legionnaires' Disease. Camp site shower rooms in particular may be subject to intermittent water supplies, variable demand, fluctuations in hot and cold water temperatures, and poor maintenance.

(Source: Eurosurveillance Weekly, April 9, 1998. Reported by the European Surveillance Scheme for Travel Associated Legionnaires' Disease, PHLS Communicable Disease Surveillance Centre).

## KEY TERMS

ß lactamase
Colonization

Normal flora
Nosocomial infection

Pneumonia
Systemic infection

## LEARNING OBJECTIVES

**Upon successful completion of this chapter, the student should be able to:**

1. Discuss the anatomy of the respiratory system.
2. List the organisms encountered in the respiratory system.
3. List the organisms that cause potentially serious respiratory tract infections and describe their characteristics.
4. Indicate how specimens should be collected from the upper and lower respiratory tracts and the appropriate media for plating those samples.
5. Discuss the methods used to diagnose upper and lower respiratory tract infections.

## INTRODUCTION

The respiratory tract is a complex of interconnecting passageways by which the body acquires oxygen and removes carbon dioxide. The respiratory tract is essentially an open canal to the outside, via the oral and nasal cavities. Through these orifices we inhale air that contains oxygen, but also may contain various microbial flora that are potentially infectious. The body has a number of mechanical and chemical defense mechanisms that help protect against potential pathogens.

The respiratory tract is divided into the upper and lower respiratory tracts. The upper respiratory tract, which consists of the oropharynx and nasopharynx, is heavily colonized by indigenous **normal flora**. The lower respiratory tract, which consists of the trachea, the lungs, bronchi, bronchioles, and alveoli, is normally sterile.

The upper and lower respiratory tracts are discussed separately because of their differences.

## ORGANISMS ENCOUNTERED IN THE RESPIRATORY TRACT

The organisms considered normal respiratory flora include:

▶ α-Hemolytic streptococci not pneumococcus
▶ Nonhemolytic streptococci (γ streptococcus)
▶ *Staphylococcus* species, coagulase-negative
▶ *Neisseria* species not *N. meningitidis,* not *gonorrhoeae*
▶ *Haemophilus* species not *influenzae, parainfluenzae*
▶ Diphtheroids not *Corynebacterium diphtheriae*
▶ *Micrococcus* species
▶ *Veillonella* species
▶ Spirochetes
▶ Lactobacillus
▶ Yeast (low numbers)

These organisms colonize the upper respiratory tract. They are found in relatively equal numbers in cul-

ture. Typically, α-Hemolytic streptococci (*Streptococcus viridans* grow), *Neisseria* species, nonhemolytic coagulase-negative staphylococci, and diphtheroids are the most commonly seen organisms on aerobic media.

Organisms that cause infection of the respiratory tract are listed below in two groups, potential pathogens and pathogens.

### Potential Pathogens

▶ β-Hemolytic streptococcus
▶ *Haemophilus influenzae*
▶ *Haemophilus parainfluenzae*
▶ *Streptococcus pneumoniae*
▶ *Staphylococcus aureus*
▶ *Neisseria meningitidis*
▶ α-Hemolytic streptococcus
▶ Yeast (*Candida albicans*)
▶ Yeast (other)
▶ *Enterobacteriaceae*
▶ *Pseudomonas* species
▶ Nonlactose fermentation gram-negative rods other
▶ *Moraxella catarrhalis*
▶ *Pasteurella* species
▶ Filamentous fungi
▶ *Bacteroides* species
▶ Peptostreptococci
▶ *Mycoplasma* species
▶ Herpes simplex
▶ *Actinomyces* species
▶ *Mycobacterium* species

### Pathogens

▶ *Streptococcus pyogenes* (β streptococcus group A)
▶ *Corynebacterium diphtheriae*
▶ *Neisseria gonorrhoeae*
▶ *Mycobacterium tuberculosis*
▶ *Nocardia species*
▶ *Bordetella pertussis*
▶ *Brucella* species
▶ *Bacillus anthracis*
▶ *Yersinia pestis*

▶ *Legionella* species
▶ *Mycoplasma pneumoniae*
▶ *Chlamydia* species
▶ *Pneumocystis carinii*
▶ *Histoplasma capsulatum*
▶ *Coccidioides immitis*
▶ *Cryptococcus neoformans*
▶ *Blastomyces dermatitidis*
▶ Viruses (respiratory syncytial virus [RSV] adenovirus, enterovirus, herpesvirus, influenza, parainfluenza and rhinoviruses)

The organisms considered potential pathogens are those that may be isolated, especially in low numbers, from a "normal" patient without symptoms without causing disease. These organisms are merely colonizing the patient. Under certain conditions, these colonizing organisms can cause disease. The reason these bacteria become pathogens is not always clear. Some possible causes are an underlying disease such as cancer or human immunodeficiency virus (HIV), therapy that causes a lower immune response, severe inflammation from allergies, smoking, or contact with a person with a virulent strain.

Organisms listed as pathogens such as *C. diphtheriae*, *Mycobacterium tuberculosis*, *Neisseria gonorrhoeae*, and *Streptococcus pyogenes* are never present in a healthy person. Their presence is synonymous with disease.

## ANATOMY OF THE RESPIRATORY TRACT

The respiratory tract is a continuous system whose major function is respiration, which is the intake of fresh oxygen and the removal of carbon dioxide from the body. The system's outer openings are the nose and mouth. Air passes in and out the oral and nasal passages, and through the nasal and oral pharynx. Immediately adjacent to these areas are nasal sinuses, the frontal and sphenoid sinuses (see Figures 27-1, 27-2, and 27-3). From the pharynx, air moves down past the epiglottis and larynx into the trachea. The trachea then divides into bronchi, which extend to the right and left lungs, which consist of a number of lobes. As the bronchi penetrate the substance of the lungs, they further divide into bronchioles and alveoli, which are the functional areas of gas exchange where blood from capillaries exchanges carbon dioxide for oxygen. This oxygen is then carried via the red blood cells to the tissues where cellular exchange occurs.

## THE UPPER RESPIRATORY TRACT

The upper respiratory tract is inhabited by many microorganisms considered normal flora. These organisms play a role in protecting their environment from **colonization** and infection by opportunistic pathogens. When specimens from the upper respiratory tract are collected, invariably this normal flora is present in addition to the potential pathogens. In the following sections, we discuss methods to collect, transport, culture, isolate, and identify these pathogens from a mixed culture.

This chapter focuses on the isolation and cultivation of the following organisms: *Streptococcus pyogenes*, *Corynebacterium diphtheriae*, *Neisseria gonorrhoeae*, and *Bordetella pertussis*. When isolated in high numbers, organisms such as *N. meningitidis*, *S. aureus*, *S. pneumoniae*, and *H. influenzae* may be colonizing the host and should be reported, especially in a nursing home or hospital setting. *H. influenzae* causes disease of the epiglottis and obstruction of the airways, but is usually not a primary cause of upper respiratory disease.

Additionally, a number of viruses cause pharyngitis and rhinitis—respiratory syncytial virus (RSV), rhinovirus, adenovirus influenza and parainfluenza viruses, and others. Although significant, they are not covered in this chapter.

## Streptococcal Pharyngitis

Respiratory specimens often are collected for the diagnosis of streptococcal pharyngitis. The primary pathogen for streptococcal pharyngitis is *S. pyogenes* (group A streptococci). *S. pyogenes* infection can lead to poststreptococcal infections including rheumatic fever and glomerulonephritis. Before the actual specimen collection, the patient's identity should be verified. In a hospital setting the patient's wristband should be checked. Specimen labels (bar code labels) can be prioritized on the floor and affixed to the specimen. Once collected, the bar code can be scanned on the floor, which would enter the time of collection in the system. Specimens should be collected using a Dacron swab-holding media system such as Culturette brand or an equivalent. The specimen should be collected by first depressing the tongue with a tongue depressor, and then passing the swab back and forth across the most inflamed, ulcerated areas of the tonsils, and posterior pharynx. Care must be taken to avoid the lips, cheeks, tongue, and uvula because contact would only increase the amount of oral flora present on the culture media, making isolation of the potential pathogen more difficult.

Once the specimen is obtained, the swab should be placed fully back into the culture system, breaking the ampule to place the swab in contact with the holding media. The culture system should be fully labeled with:

Patient's name
Hospital, Social Security, or other identifying number
Time and date collected
Physician's name
Initials of the collector

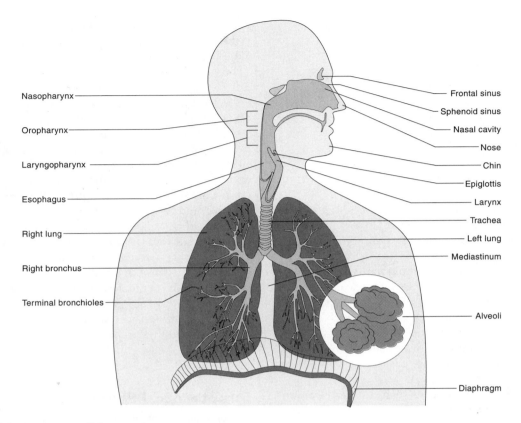

**FIGURE 27-1** Structures of the respiratory system.

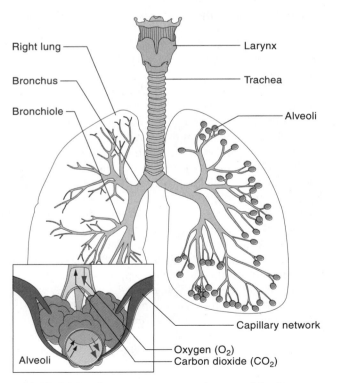

**FIGURE 27-2** The respiratory mechanism. The bronchioles and alveoli are areas of gas exchange where blood from the capillaries exchanges carbon dioxide for oxygen.

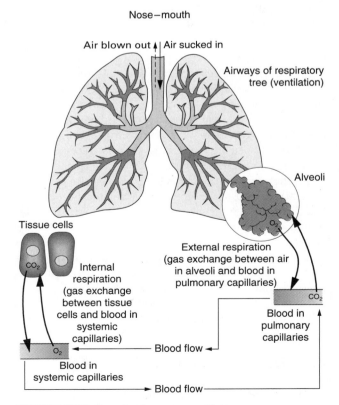

**FIGURE 27-3** Respiration vs. ventilation.

The specimen should be transported to the laboratory for culture as soon as possible, although *S. pyogenes* will remain viable up to 24 hours in holding media. Specimens should not be refrigerated in transit.

**Specimen Integrity.** The results obtained from cultures or antigen testing depend on the quality of the specimen. On the specimen's arrival in the lab, it should be checked for factors that could affect the quality of results:

- ▶ Specimen name and requisition do not match
- ▶ Specimen may be obtained from incorrect patient
- ▶ Specimen received on dry swab (ampule not cracked)
- ▶ Specimen received refrigerated
- ▶ Specimen transmit time is too long
- ▶ Specimen received on calcium alginate swab
- ▶ Specimen received unlabeled

**Specimen Inoculation.** Inoculation of all specimens is performed under a laminar flow hood (biohazard hood). This precaution is necessary to prevent any aerosols from contaminating the environment. Personnel should also wear latex gloves as an additional safeguard.

If the culture is just for the isolation of *S. pyogenes* (streptococcus screen), which is by far the most common cause of bacterial pharyngitis, trypticase soy agar with 5% sheep blood (blood agar plate [BAP]) incubated in either carbon dioxide or an anaerobic environment is appropriate. Selective trypticase soy agar with 5% sheep blood (SSA) containing chemicals such as sulfamethoxazole-trimethoprim (SXT), colistin, crystal violet incubated either in a carbon dioxide or anaerobic environment may also be used. The carbon dioxide atmosphere improves the organism's growth while anaerobiosis increases the degree of hemolysis.

Many laboratories use SSA in a carbon dioxide atmosphere with agar stabs to reduce oxygen tension created at these points, which increases hemolysis. The use of selective media greatly reduces the growth of normal flora and many contaminants, while allowing ß-streptococcus group A and group B to grow as well as *Corynebacterium haemolyticum* (*Arcanobacterium haemolyticum*). The use of a selective media greatly increases the sensitivity of this procedure.

Today, there are many shorter, less cumbersome variations of the Lancefield extraction procedure, taking as little as 10 minutes to perform. The Lancefield tests identify ß-streptococcus groups A, B, C, D, F, G. To perform, inoculate extraction fluid, incubate 10 minutes in a 35°C warmed reagent and serum mixture. Place 1 drop of sera on the slide, and add 1 drop of incubated extraction on the slide. Rock for up to 2 minutes and examine for agglutination. Using this protocol,

*S. pyogenes* can be identified within 24 hours. Susceptibility testing is not commonly performed on *S. pyogenes* from the upper respiratory tract (which is universally sensitive to penicillin).

## *Corynebacterium diphtheriae*

This bacterium can cause a severe **systemic infection**, as well as a pharyngitis-like disease. Systemic disease begins in the upper respiratory tract and in most cases is caused by a toxin-producing strain of *C. diphtheriae*. The diphtheriae bacilli grow in host tissue and produce exotoxin, which is absorbed into the body, resulting in systemic disease. The bacteria multiply rapidly in the mucous membranes and produce the grayish pseudomembrane, which may cover the pharynx, larynx, and tonsils. In young children, if the larynx and trachea are covered by the membrane, complete obstruction of the air passage may occur. Fortunately this is not common in the United States, but when it occurs it has nearly a 10% mortality rate. *C. diphtheriae* can also cause disease of the skin. In other parts of the world, *C. diphtheriae* is more prevalent and if international events occur in the United States (e.g., the Olympics), medical personnel must be alert to its presence.

Specimens are collected from the throat and nasopharyngeal and cutaneous areas when skin involvement is suspected. Collection is with a rayon or Dacron-tipped swab. Care should be taken to swab all areas of the throat, especially inflamed ones. Collection by nasopharyngeal specimens is performed using a minitipped collection kit. Pass the swab up the nose gently, passing into each nasal canal. If any firm resistance is encountered, withdraw the swab. *Do not* force the swab. The swabs are then placed back into the holders, in contact with holding media. In some cases an ampule needs to be crushed. *C. diphtheriae* is not a truly fastidious organism and will remain viable for 24 to 48 hours at room temperature when in contact with the holding media.

Media is chosen for the selective isolation and presumptive identification of *C. diphtheriae*.

*Media*
trypticase agar with 5% sheep blood
cystine-tellurite
modified Tinsdale
Loeffler's slants

Media formulations and storage requirements should be available from the media supplier, as well as certification of its meeting NCCLS guidelines for quality control. Media that warrants inhouse quality control is noted in the NCCLS guidelines. Each laboratory should have a set of procedure manuals and NCCLS manuals to follow.

## Gonococcal Pharyngitis

Gonococcal disease of the upper respiratory tract is usually limited to cases of pharyngitis. The disease, although not common, has been more prevalent in recent years. To properly isolate the pathogenic organism from the mixed flora found in the oral cavity, use selective media and nonselective media. Because of this requirement, the physician must specifically order a culture of the throat for isolation of *N. gonorrhoeae.*

As in all collection procedures, swabs are collected from inflamed areas of the pharynx, posterior pharynx, and tonsils. *N. gonorrhoeae* is a very fastidious organism and should, when possible, be transferred immediately to the proper transport media. There are several commonly available systems: Jembec, Trangrow, Bio Bag, and others. These systems produce adequate carbon dioxide for survival at room temperature of the organism on a Thayer-Martin type media.

Transport in a standard Ames, Stuart swab system is not recommended without added activated charcoal. Even these systems are of limited use and maintain validity for only 8 hours. Under no circumstances should these cultures be transported or stored at refrigerator temperatures. Transportation should be at room temperature.

Once in the laboratory, the specimens must be checked for proper specimen identification and the use of a proper transport system. Properly label all media to be inoculated.

For the isolation of *N. gonorrhoeae,* media must be truly selective and contain proper nutritional elements for the growth of this fastidious organism. Media such as modified Thayer-Martin, Martin-Lewis, and New York City are commonly used. These organisms require hemin from hemoglobin (X factor) and nicotinamide adenine dinucleotide (NAD), derived from yeast or potato extract, also known as V factor. Chocolate agar meets both requirements, and with the addition of antibiotics such as vancomycin, colistin, neomycin, and others in various concentrations, can become a selective media for the isolation of *N. gonorrhoeae.*

Once the transport systems arrive in the laboratory, it can be appropriate in some cases to further streak plates for isolation. Jenbec and Trangrow media are usually simply inoculated at 35° to 37°C for up to 72 hours in a 3% to 7% carbon dioxide atmosphere. Plates are incubated for 3 days with approximately 5% carbon dioxide concentration in a humid atmosphere. Plates are checked daily for colonies resembling *N. gonorrhoeae.* Colonies are small, gray-white, translucent, convex, with complete margins by 48 hours of incubation. Colonies may be sticky, dry, or even mucoid. In some cases more than one colonial variation may occur in one culture creating two different colony sizes. This may make the technologist apprehensive concerning the purity of these isolates.

Identification is based on colonial morphology, Gram stain characteristics, and biochemical and antigenic and even DNA testing. The organism is preliminarily tested for positive reaction with the oxidase test. Organisms are tested for their biochemical reactions to dextrose, maltose, sucrose, lactose, and ONPG (ortho-nitro-phenyl-ß-galactosidase) using the CTA sugars (cystine trypticase agar). *N. gonorrhoeae* produces acid in only glucose. This method needs to incubate at least 24 hours and is sensitive to technique differences. Newer methods are enzymatic in nature, and a heavy inoculum is needed. Various commercial systems are available such as HNID and Quad Firm, which only take 4 hours.

All laboratories should perform ß-lactamase testing for gonococcal sensitivity to penicillin. Most physicians are presently using ceftriaxone for treatment of *N. gonorrhoeae,* and there are at present no resistant strains. Where susceptibilities are ordered and/or needed, the NCCLS procedure must be carefully adhered to, using specific media and criteria.

## Bordetella Pertussis

Another disease of the upper respiratory system is whooping cough, or pertussis. This disease will, in many cases, cause a severe cough that has resulted in the name whooping cough. The typical cough is not always present and the diagnosis may be difficult. In many ways this illness is typical of some viral infections of the respiratory tract.

Whooping cough is usually caused by *B. pertussis,* a fastidious, weakly staining gram-negative coccobacillus. The organism may possess a capsule in virulent strains. *Bordetella* is found adhering to the ciliated epithelial cells of mucosal membranes. It produces cytoxins, endotoxins that have effects in the system. Less frequently other species of *Bordetella* can cause the disease including *B. parapertussis* and *B. bronchiseptica.*

The specimen of choice is either nasopharyngeal washings or nasopharyngeal swabs. Dacron or calcium alginate minitipped swabs should be used. Do not use rayon or cotton-tipped swabs for collection. (Rayon and cotton contain fatty acids, which are inhibitory to *B. pertussis.*) Cough plates may be used with Bordet-Gengou agar plates, but the recovery ratio is greater from nasopharyngeal swabs or washings.

When specimens cannot be directly plated onto growth media, transport is best using a media-based transport. Two such systems are Jones-Kendrich media or Regan-Lowe media, both of which may be supplemented with antibiotics such as cephalexin to reduce normal flora. The organisms will remain viable for a number of days in transit, which makes these agars suitable for today's central laboratory situations.

Once in the laboratory, the specimen is checked for proper patient identification and specimen integrity. Culturing is performed under a biohazard hood. The media used is Bordet-Gengou agar (BG), a potato infusion agar with 10% glycerol and 20% sheep blood. Bordet-Gengou agar is made up into plates, usually on the day of use, and only has a shelf-life of several days. Both Jones-Kendrich and Regan-Lowe media have an extended shelf-life of approximately 2 months. These media are commercially available.

These media are usually supplemented with antibiotics such as cephalexin or methicillin to reduce the normal flora present for better recovery. Once plates are inoculated and streaked for isolation, they are incubated at 35°C, preferably in a noncarbon dioxide incubator. The plates should be incubated in a humid atmosphere for up to 7 to 10 days.

Colonies are described as looking like a bisegmented pearl, dew drops, or mercury droplets. These colonies are raised, smooth with an entire edge transparent and glistening, and about 1 mm in size. They can also be mucoid and tenacious in nature, with a small hazy zone of hemolysis. Colonies appear at 48 to 72 hours of incubation. Plates should be checked daily using light with a magnifying lens or stereoscope.

Typical colonies should be Gram stained. *B. pertussis* are small coccobacilli that stain weakly gram negative. Staining may be enhanced by increased time in safranin or using Kinyoun carbolfuchsin. Some preliminary test results for identification of *B. pertussis* are catalase positive, oxidase positive, motility negative, urease negative, and growth on BAP negative.

Definitive identification is based on serologic methods. These organisms are relatively inert. Serologic identification uses either a fluorescence-labeled polyclonal antisera or agglutination with a polyvalent pertussis antiserum.

Specimens collected for complete throat cultures are obtained in the same manner as those for acute pharyngitis. Specimen transport and accessing is as previously stated for streptococcus group A. The media used also may be the same with the addition of chocolate agar, which is necessary for the growth of *H. influenzae, N. meningitidis,* and *C. albicans.* The use of Thayer-Martin will enhance the recovery of *N. meningitidis,* as well as *N. gonorrhoeae,* while inhibiting most other flora.

## IDENTIFICATION OF POTENTIAL PATHOGENS

Plates must be examined to differentiate normal respiratory flora from their closely related pathogenic relatives. First, differentiate between coagulase-negative staphylococci and coagulase-positive staphylococci (*S. aureus*), which are potentially pathogenic. Differentiate the colonial morphology of normal flora when compared to potentially pathogenic colonies, which may be mixed into the streaks of confluent growth.

*Staphylococcus aureus* colonies are usually creamy white or golden in color, smooth, convex, and entire. These colonies may be ß-hemolytic or nonhemolytic and are 2 to 3 mm in size. *Staphylococcus* colonies are catalase positive, which separates them from *Streptococcus* species. *S. aureus* is coagulase positive, usually by both slide and the tube coagulase tests. There are numerous species of coagulase-negative staphylococci of which the most common species is *Staphylococcus epidermidis*. This group is usually part of the normal flora.

*Streptococcus pneumoniae* can be differentiated into 82 antigenic types by the Neufield-Quelling reaction, which visualizes the swelling of the polysaccharide capsule found around the organisms. This procedure is no longer commonly performed; its merits are nonepidermitologic. *S. pneumoniae* is usually differentiated from α-streptococcus (*S. viridans*) by the bile solubility test and its sensitivity to the optochin disk. Colony morphology is quite varied considering the number of antigenic types. Variations exist from flat, concave, convex, and moist, to even mucoid. Colonies may be 1 to 2 mm in size having green α-hemolyses around them. Colonies of *S. pneumoniae* in contact with 10% desoxycholate (bile solution) dissolve (lyse); a zone of inhibitors around an optochin disk of 16 mm or greater is positive for *S. pneumoniae.* Further testing can be performed by biochemical panels, as well as antigenic studies.

*Haemophilus influenzae* requires, in addition to carbon dioxide for growth, added factors (traditionally known as X factor—heat-stable material found associated with hemoglobin; V factor—heat-labile coenzyme I [NAD]) found in chocolate agar, but not in BAP. *Haemophilus* will also grow as very tiny pinpoint colonies as satellites around staphylococci on BAP, which is one of its characteristics. *H. influenzae* Gram stains as small coccobacilli. The colonies on chocolate agar are transparent. These colonies are flat and usually moist in appearance with a musty odor, and seem, in many cases, to pick up the chocolate color of the media. The colony's texture, when picked, is soft and smooth. Identification is by either utilization of XV factors as growth differentiation test (whereby growth only will occur in the presence of both the X and V factors) and it is nonhemolytic on horse blood agar. Biochemical enzymatic tests such as the HNId system by Microscan are also used to identify *Haemophilus.*

*Neisseria meningitidis* in low numbers is usually not significant when isolated from throat swabs mixed with normal flora. When found as the predominant isolate, and in high numbers, or when from nasopharyngeal specimens, its identification is significant. This organism Gram stains as gram-negative diplococci and is coffee bean in appearance. The common wall (axis) of connection between the two portions of the diplococci is longer than the wall perpendicular to that common wall. This is significant, especially for reports from cerebrospinal fluid (CSF) where results may be acted on as if they are definitive in nature. Organisms such as

*M. catarrhalis* and others can give the appearance of gram-negative diplococci at times when they are truly gram-negative coccal rods, but the axis between the two coccal rods is shorter than either of its perpendicular sides.

*Neisseria meningitidis* requires carbon dioxide and enriched media such as chocolate agar for good growth, although they will grow on BAP. When grown on chocolate agar or modified Thayer-Martin, colonies are small and round, shiny and gray with a bluish tinge and are nonhemolytic on BAP. Initial identification is based on Gram stain appearance as coffee bean diplococci, a positive cytochrome oxidase reaction, and their colonial appearance.

Definitive identification has traditionally been based on biochemical methods such as CTA sugars (cystine trypticase agar with 1% sugars added), testing for the production of acid. This is a very consistent method when care is taken. In preparation of the inoculum, one must be very sure of having a pure culture, to make a thick emulsion in tripticase soy broth, boil and cool CTAs, as indicated by the manufacturers, and heavily inoculate the sugars just below the surface with a sterile Pasteur pipet. Mix the inoculum into the agar with a sterile loop no deeper than ¼ inch. Close the tops tightly and incubate up to 48 hours. Biochemical tests are also performed today by rapid enzymatic systems manufactured by a number of companies. In addition, serologic systems such as coagglutination, latex agglutination, DNA probe, and even polymerase chain reaction have been developed. Latex and coagglutination tests are suitable for stat testing of CSF and other body fluids. Finding *N. meningitidis* from nasopharyngeal specimens only shows the presence of a carrier state. If isolated from a person who has recently been in contact with one diagnosed with meningitis, it can be important and antibiotic prophylaxis may be in order.

*Moraxella catarrhalis* is not truly part of the normal flora and must be differentiated from such flora. Although it has not been well documented as a source of systemic infections, some evidence does point to varied systemic infections, especially in the elderly. These organisms grow well on either BAP or chocolate agar incubated in carbon dioxide for up to 48 hours. The Gram stain appearance is gram-negative coccal rods which, at times, mimic *Neisseria* species. They are cytochrome oxidase positive and their colonies are raised, gray white, shiny, usually dry, and somewhat larger than *Neisseria* species. The organism is $NO_3$ positive, asaccharolytic, DNase positive, and usually produce β-lactamase. There is a rapid disk screening test for an immediate result (the hydrolysis of tributyrin) as well as a more definitive 4-hour rapid enzymatic test available.

β-Hemolytic streptococcus, not group A, as noted, is not normal flora of the respiratory tract, but is not documented as a causative agent of some systemic infections. When testing for group A β-streptococci documentation of the isolation of β-streptococci, not group A, may be valuable to the clinician.

Candidiasis, also known as thrush, can be significant in immunosuppressed patients, patients with acquired immunodeficiency syndrome, and in patients in whom overtreatment with antibiotics has drastically reduced the normal flora.

The use of antibiotic therapy for organisms of the upper respiratory tract is usually limited. Nasal isolates of *S. aureus* need to be tested for antibiotic resistance. *S. pneumoniae*, formerly susceptible to penicillin, is now becoming increasingly resistant. Testing for its relative resistance by the oxicillin disk method is important.

The examination of plates set up for complete throat and nasal cultures can be more difficult than examining plates for a particular pathogen causing acute pharyngitis. Each lab must set guidelines as to which organisms are to be considered significant, from which sites, and at what quantitation in relationship to the normal flora.

## THE LOWER RESPIRATORY TRACT

The respiratory tract below the larynx is considered the lower respiratory tract, and is normally sterile unless an infectious process is progressing. Specimens from these areas, at times, are contaminated with normal flora gained while passing through the upper respiratory system. This is especially true of expectorated sputum specimens, which are the least invasive, but the most easily contaminated. Other specimens from the lower respiratory tract include trachael aspirates, bronchial washings, bronchial alveolar lavage fluid, protected bronchial brush, bronchial biopsy, transtracheal aspirates, lung aspirates, and lung biopsy specimens. The more invasive of these procedures are usually not contaminated by oral flora.

Infections of the lower respiratory tract are either acute or chronic and are caused by a wide range of organisms including viruses, bacteria, fungi, mycoplasma, and even protozoa. The discussion centers on the most common organisms isolated from respiratory specimens in the typical bacteriology laboratory of a community hospital.

### Acute Infections

Viral infections are most common in young children up to the age of 5 years. Organisms such as RSV, influenza, parainfluenza, and adenoviruses are typically found as primary invaders of this patient group. In addition to causing acute **pneumonia**, they predispose these children to a group of secondary bacterial pathogens that include *H. influenzae, S. pneumoniae, S. aureus,* and even *M. catarrhalis.*

In young adults *Mycoplasma pneumoniae* and *Chlamydia,* in addition to viruses, are a major causative agent of acute pneumonias. Once again, secondary bacterial pathogens such as *S. pneumoniae, S. aureus, B. streptococcus, M. catarrhalis,* and *H. influenzae* are common isolates of postviral infections. In addition, today there are increased numbers of immunocompromised patients due to chemotherapy, transplant protocols, as well as HIV infections. One must also be aware of parasites and fungal causative agents of acute pneumoniae. *S. pneumoniae* is the most common cause of community-acquired acute bacterial pneumonia, and, especially, is found to be most prevalent in the elderly population.

*Aspiration pneumonia* may be initiated during unconsciousness due to alcohol or drug abuse, seizures, or even when under anesthesia, and can be a major cause of hospital-acquired (nosocomial) pneumonia. It can be a mixed infection due to the aspiration of organisms from the upper respiratory tract. Aspiration community-acquired pneumonia can be caused by anaerobic isolates such as pigmented gram-negative rods, *Prevotella, Porphyromonas* species (formerly members of the pigmented *Bacteroides*), *Fusobacterium* species, microaerophilic viridans streptococci, *S. aureus,* Enterobacteriaciae (*Klebsiella pneumoniae*), and *Pseudomonas* species.

*Nosocomial pneumonias* are primarily caused by gram-negative rods, *Pseudomonas, S. aureus, Acinetobacter* species, *M. catarrhalis* and *H. influenzae,* and *S. pneumoniae,* in descending order of prevalence. *M. catarrhalis* is prevalent in the very old and young. Nosocomial pneumonia can also result from the use of inhalation therapy equipment, which has either been inadvertently contaminated or incompletely cleaned. Common isolates in these cases are *P. aeruginosa, S. aureus, K. pneumoniae, Acinetobacter* species, and *Enterobacter* species.

Acute pneumonia has many causes and diagnosis may be quite difficult for the physician. Therefore, the quality of the specimen, as well as specimen handling and processing, are important. **Nosocomial infections** increase the patient's stay in the hospital and, therefore, are one cause of increased hospital cost.

## Chronic Infections

There are fewer causative agents of chronic disease of the lower respiratory tract. The primary organisms are *M. tuberculosis, Mycobacterium* species such as *M. avium-interacellulase, Nocardia* and *Actinomyces,* and systemic fungi such as *C. immites, B. dermatitidis, H. capulatum, C. neoformans,* and even *Aspergellus* species. The isolation, cultivation, and identification of these organisms are covered elsewhere in this text. Once collected, specimens should be submitted with specific orders for fungal culture, acid-fast culture (*Mycobacterium*), and so forth. The cultivation of these pathogens is specific and is not part of a routine microbiology department.

**Specimen Examination.** Specimens examined for diagnosis of lower respiratory infection, range from noninvasive to very invasive. Expectorated sputum specimens, although the easiest to obtain and least invasive, usually are the most difficult to interpret due to the large numbers of oral flora. It is possible to reduce the contamination and to improve the chance for the evaluation of a reasonably good specimen if a few simple precautions are followed.

The patient should be instructed to rinse his mouth out and gargle with water before obtaining an early morning deeply coughed sputum specimen. The specimen should be collected and transported to the laboratory in a sterile cup within 1 hour of collection.

When specimens that resemble saliva are received in the laboratory, a notation should be made. All sputum specimens should be examined microscopically to evaluate their quality, in addition to the normal Gram stain report indicating the microbial flora present. The following methods are used for this evaluation.

Microscopic evaluations are made by comparing the number of neutrophilic white blood cells (WBCs) with the number of squamous epithelial cells. Generally speaking, specimens with high numbers of WBCs and low numbers of epithelial cells are satisfactory, whereas specimens with high numbers of squamous epithelial cells and low numbers of neutrophilic WBCs are unsatisfactory. More specifically, a method described by Geckler and colleagues recommends that specimens with greater or equal to 25 epithelial cells per low power field, not be cultured. Another procedure evaluates 10 to 20 fields under low power. This system evaluates the specimen on a graduated scale of WBCs to epithelial cells, and then grades the specimens from −3 to +3 on the basis of the relative numbers of neutrophils to squamous epithelial cells. Any of these systems must be "qualified" when considering patients who do not produce WBCs due to disease or disease therapy. Notations should also be made when ciliated epithelial cells are present, which is an indication of a lower respiratory specimen. When a specimen does not meet the criteria as sputum, recommendations vary as to how to handle a request for a new specimen.

When patients such as neonates are unable to produce a sputum specimen, their specimens are collected by introducing a mild vaporized chloride solution, which induces the patient to cough. The specimens are usually satisfactory for most needs, and are usually not heavily contaminated.

Tracheastoma and endotracheal aspirates are often colonized within 24 to 48 hours of their introduction. The interpretation of results from these specimens is therefore always in question, although aspiration pneumonia can occur.

Obtaining bronchial wash specimens is another relatively noninvasive procedure. A relatively small volume of sterile physiologic saline is introduced into the bronchia and then removed. This procedure results in a specimen that usually has reduced oral flora, but is far from devoid of this normal flora.

Bronchealveolar lavage (BAL) obtained by bronchoscopy is considered "relatively invasive." This method was developed in the 1930s and is relatively safe. These deeper specimens have been useful in identifying fungal isolates, as well as pneumocystic infections. Many physicians use quantitative BAL, as well as quantitative bronchial brush specimens to better define the causative agents of an infectious process.

Quantitative bronchial brush specimens are obtained via a double-lumen protected catheter brush. A brush capable of collecting from 0.01 to 0.001 mL is protected within the inner lumen and then advanced into areas of purest material and withdrawn into the inner lumen or tube, and then the inner tube is withdrawn through the outer lumen. The brush is cut and dropped usually into a small vial containing 1 mL Ringer's solution, sterile broth, or physiologic sterile saline. The specimen is delivered to the lab where it is vortexed and possibly further diluted, and quantitative cultures are performed. This method is usually devoid of contaminating oral flora, and the method is considered acceptable for anaerobic work-up.

Transtracheal aspirates and lung biopsy specimens are among the most invasive procedures and should be reserved for very few situations. Transtracheal aspirates are particularly significant when one is concerned with a deep anaerobic infectious process, and other, less invasive procedures have not yielded conclusive information. Biopsy specimens need to be reserved for undiagnosed life-threatening situations. Further information may be found in Bartlett, Brewer, and Ryan (1978).

All specimens must be examined for specimen integrity and positive specimen identification. Specimen labels must exactly correlate to the requisition or computer information. One must pay particular attention to the patient's hospital number, full name, and date of birth. Time of specimen collection and time of receipt into the laboratory are of particular importance, as well as quality and quantity of specimen. Many specimens from the lower respiratory tract are processed for fungus and acid-fast bacilli, as well as routine tests, and need adequate specimen volume to attain a significant result.

The processing of all specimens is performed under a laminar flow biohazard hood, which is usually certified yearly. Expectorated sputum and tracheal specimens are inoculated onto trypticase soy agar with 5% sheep blood agar, chocolate agar, and MacConkey agar. Particular attention is placed on using the most purulent flecks of a specimen. A sterile swab is used to transfer specimens to the media, spreading the specimen out in an area equivalent to one-eighth of the plate and then streaking for isolation. A relatively thin smear with thick and thin areas is made by using a swab and rolling out the sputum using a firm hand. The frosted end of the slide should be fully labeled with a pencil or special marker that does not come off in the process. The smear should *not* be made using a second slide to prepare a thin film as in hematology. Once again, the most purulent portion of the specimen equivalent to what was used for the isolation of the media must be used for the Gram stain smear. Information attained from the Gram stain smear can be most important to an early diagnosis. The smear is used for evaluation of the quality of the specimen, confirms the significance of an isolate, may even provide information of organisms that are not able to grow out on our routine media, and, in general provides the physician with preliminary results such as gram-negative enteric rods, lancet-shaped gram-positive diplococci, gram-negative coccal rods, gram-positive cocci pairs and chains. This Gram stain information may allow the physician to provide necessary imperative treatment.

The BAP and chocolate agar are incubated at 35°C in a carbon dioxide incubator and the MacConkey is incubated in a noncarbon dioxide incubator. Carbon dioxide enhances the growth of most bacteria and is needed by fastidious isolates for proper growth. Plates are read after approximately 16 to 20 hours (overnight).

# SUMMARY

▶ The respiratory tract is a complex of interconnecting passageways through which the body acquires oxygen and removes carbon dioxide. It is divided into the upper and lower tracts.

▶ The upper respiratory tract is heavily colonized with normal flora; the lower respiratory tract is normally sterile.

▶ A wide variety of microorganisms colonize the upper respiratory tract. Some of these organisms are pathogens; others are potential pathogens.

▶ The nasal and oral orifices are the outer openings of the respiratory tract. Air enters through them and moves through the pharynx, the larynx, the trachea, the bronchi, and into alveoli.

▶ Normal flora of the upper respiratory tract help prevent colonization and infection by opportunistic pathogens.

▶ *Streptococcus pyogenes* is the primary cause of streptococcal pharyngitis. Care must always be taken in the collection and transport of respiratory specimens.

▶ Respiratory specimens may be inoculated onto a variety of media, a procedure performed under a laminar flow hood. Specimens are often incubated in the presence of carbon dioxide.

▶ *Corynebacterium diphtheriae* causes systemic infections as well as pharyngitis-like disease. Systemic symptoms are caused by the production of a toxin.

▶ Gonococcal disease of the upper respiratory tract is usually limited to pharyngitis. This organism may be difficult to diagnose due to the heavy normal flora population of the upper respiratory tract.

▶ *Bordetella pertussis* causes pertussis, or whooping cough. Some symptoms of the disease are similar to some viral diseases of the respiratory tract.

▶ After incubation, plates must be examined to differentiate respiratory flora from pathogenic species.

▶ Pathogens of the respiratory tract include *Staphylococcus aureus, Streptococcus pneumoniae, Haemophilus influenzae, Neisseria meningitidis, Moraxella catarrhalis,* and others.

▶ The lower respiratory tract is normally sterile, but sometimes specimens are contaminated with normal flora from the upper respiratory tract. Infections of the lower respiratory tract are acute or chronic and are caused by a variety of microbes.

▶ Viral infections are most common in young children up to 5 years of age.

▶ Acute infections of the lower respiratory tract include community-acquired acute bacterial pneumonia, aspiration pneumonia, nosocomial pneumonia, and others.

▶ A variety of specimen types are used to diagnose these diseases.

## Review Questions

1. One of the most common problems associated with the collection of samples for the diagnosis of upper respiratory tract infections is that:
   a. most of the collection techniques are invasive in nature.
   b. a wide variety of normal flora accompanies the sample.
   c. none of the media available for the plating of the specimens are selective.
   d. those samples must reach the laboratory within 1 hour to remain viable.
   e. most of the infectious agents are viral and cannot be diagnosed in the average hospital microbiology laboratory.

2. Which of the following would be reason to reject a sample collected for diagnosis of streptococcal pharyngitis?
   a. The sample is unlabeled.
   b. The specimen was refrigerated.
   c. The specimen transit time was in excess of 24 hours.
   d. The specimen was received on a dry swab.
   e. All of the above.

3. Cystine-tellurite blood agar is especially useful in the diagnosis of infection with *Corynebacterium diphtheriae* because:
   a. the growth of all normal flora is inhibited on this media.
   b. the bacterium produces a characteristic pigment when grown on this media.
   c. a carbon dioxide incubator is not required for incubation when this media is used.

   d. colony morphology of the organism is more diagnostic on this media.
   e. a more accurate Gram stain can be obtained from colonies grown on this media.

4. The specimen of choice for the diagnosis of whooping cough is a:
   a. nasal pharyngeal wash or swab.
   b. lung biopsy.
   c. throat culture.
   d. sputum sample.
   e. bronchial biopsy.

5. Colonies of *Staphylococcus* can easily be differentiated from colonies of *Streptococcus* by a(n):
   a. acid-fast stain.
   b. catalase test.
   c. nitrate reduction test.
   d. All of the above
   e. Only a and b

6. Respiratory tract samples that are suspected to contain *Neisseria gonorrhoeae* should only be transported in a standard Ames system if:
   a. they will be plated within 1 hour of collection.
   b. Gram staining is not indicated.
   c. activated charcoal is added.
   d. X factor is added.
   e. they will be incubated in the presence of carbon dioxide.

7. *Neisseria gonorrhoeae* should always be tested for sensitivity to:
   a. tetracycline.
   b. cephalosporin.
   c. penicillin.
   d. silver nitrate.
   e. oxygen.

**8.** Methicillin-resistant *Staphylococcus aureus* is not sensitive to:

a. penicillin.

b. the semisynthetic penicillin.

c. cephalosporins.

d. All of the above

e. only b and c

**9.** When grown on chocolate agar incubated in carbon dioxide *Moraxella catarrhalis* may sometimes be confused with:

a. Haemophilus influenzae.

b. the coagulase-negative staphylococci.

e. *Bordetella pertussis.*

d. *Corynebacterium* species.

e. *Streptococcus pyogenes.*

**10.** Which of the following specimen collection techniques should be reserved for very few situations . . . and why?

a. Lung biopsies—they are very invasive.

b. Transtrachael aspirates—they are very invasive.

c. Throat swabs—they are heavily contaminated with normal flora.

d. Nasal swabs—they are difficult to transport.

e. Both a and b

## ▶ REFERENCES & RECOMMENDED READING

Bannatyne, R. M., Clausen, C., & McCarthy, L. R. (1979). In I. B. Duncan (Ed.), *Cumitech 10. Laboratory diagnosis of upper respiratory tract infections.* Washington, DC: American Society for Microbiology.

Bartlett, J. G., Brewer, N. S., & Ryan, J. J. (1978). In J. A. Washington, II (Ed.)., *Cumitech 7. Laboratory diagnosis of lower respiratory tract infections.* Washington, DC: American Society for Microbiology.

Bartlett, J. G., Ryan, K. J., Smith, T. F., & Wilson, W. R. (1987). In J. A. Washington, II (Ed.) *Cumitech 7A. Laboratory diagnosis of lower respiratory tract infections.* Washington, DC: American Society for Microbiology.

Clyde, W. A., Jr., Kenny, G. E., & Schacter, J. (1984). In W. L. Drew (Ed.)., *Cumitech 19. Laboratory diagnosis of chlamydial and mycoplasmal infections.* Washington, DC: American Society for Microbiology.

Forbes, B. A., & Granato, P. A. (1997). Processing specimens for bacteria. In *Manual of clinical microbiology* (6th ed., pp. 274–276). Washington DC: American Society for Microbiology.

Geckler, D.W., Gremillion, D.H., and McAllister, C.K. (1977). Microscopic and Bacteriological Comparison of Paired Sputa and Transtracheal Aspirate: *J Clin Microbiol,* 6:396–7.

Gilchrist, M. J. R. (1990). Laboratory diagnosis of pertussis. *Clinical Microbiology Newsletter, 12,* 49–53.

Gilchrist, M. J. R. (1991). Bordetella. In I. A. Balows, W. J. Hausler, Jr., K. L. Herrmann, H. D. Isenberg, & H. J. Shadomy (Eds.). *Manual of clinical microbiology* (5th ed., pp. 471–477). Washington, DC: American Society for Microbiology.

Greenberg, S. B., & Krilov, L. R. (1986). In W. L. Drews & S. J. Rubin (Eds.)., *Cumitech 21. Laboratory diagnosis of viral respiratory disease.* Washington, DC: American Society for Microbiology.

Herwaldt, L. A. , & Wenzel, R. P. (1997). Dynamics of hospitalacquired infections. In *Manual of clinical microbiology* (6th ed., pp. 169–176). Washington, DC: American Society for Microbiology.

Hoppe, J. E. (1988). Methods for isolation of *Bordetella pertussis* from patients with whooping cough. *European Journal of Clinical Microbiology and Infectious Disease, 7,* 616–620.

Joklik, W. K., & Smith, D. T. (1972). Bacterial morphology and ultrastructure. In *Zinsser microbiology* (15th ed., pp. 26–45). New York: Meredith Corporation.

Joklik, W. K., & Smith, D. T. (1972). *Corynebacterium diphtheriae.* In *Zinsser microbiology* (15th ed., pp. 430–437). New York: Meredith Corporation.

# CHAPTER 28
## Ear, Eye, and Sinus Tracts

Lynn L. Russell, MA, CLS (NCA)

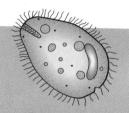

## Microbes in the News

The Food and Drug Administration has recently approved a new laser system that can be used in a doctor's office for patients with chronic ear infections. This device is an alternative to surgery for children 6 years and older to open the tympanic membrane and drain infected fluid. The laser system requires only local anesthesia on the patient.

From the April/May 1997 issue of *MediZine Guidebook*, p. 3, MediZine, Inc., Minneapolis.

## KEY TERMS

Aspiration
Blepharitis
Conjunctivitis
Keratitis
Mastoiditis
Otitis media
Paranasal sinuses
Tympanocentesis

## LEARNING OBJECTIVES

Upon completion of this chapter, the student should be able to:

1. Locate in a diagram the anatomic areas of the human ear, eye, and sinus tracts.
2. Demonstrate the processing of proper specimens to appropriate culture media and smears.
3. Distinguish resident flora from pathogenic microbes in the ear, eye, and sinus tracts.
4. Identify microbial diseases in ear, eye, and sinus tracts.

## INTRODUCTION

This chapter covers three important areas of the head and the organisms that infect them. The ear and the eye, described as the guardians of the body, are significant because unchecked infections can quickly cause loss of hearing, speech, balance, and sight. Sinusitis is a common complaint. The complications of the infections of the sinus tracts, however, can be a serious health problem.

After review of the anatomy of each system, we will focus on the microorganisms encountered in the ear, eye, and **paranasal sinuses**. The various clinical disease states and laboratory tests are presented in detail.

## BASIC ANATOMY OF THE EAR, EYE, AND SINUS TRACTS

### Ear

The ear has two functions—the perception of sound and the perception of motion and position. Figure 28-1 indicates the three anatomic areas of the human ear. The bacteria of the external auditory canal usually mirror the flora of the skin. The middle and inner ears are usually sterile. Note the eardrum (tympanic membrane) and the narrow twisting ear canal between the external and internal ear.

Infection is usually kept from reaching the middle ear by the tympanic membrane. Infection can spread upward from the pharynx by way of the eustachian tube. Pus may be liberated here under pressure and, if it cannot drain, it makes the tympanic membrane bulge, causing pain and possibly a rupture. When an infection has reached the middle ear it may go into the mastoid cavities inside the mastoid process of the temporal bone. If pus forms here and cannot escape, the otologist (physician specializing in diseases of the ear) may find it necessary to surgically establish a drain. This is a difficult procedure due to the delicate auditory structures, important blood vessels, and the proximity of the brain to the area.

In the internal ear there is the osseous labyrinth, which is a series of bony canals in three parts. Fitted to each twist and turn is a delicate membrane called the membranous labyrinth. There is fluid between the bone and the membrane (perilymph) and another fluid inside the membrane (endolymph). Because perception of both sound and position depend on these fluids, they are significant in both functions of the inner ear.

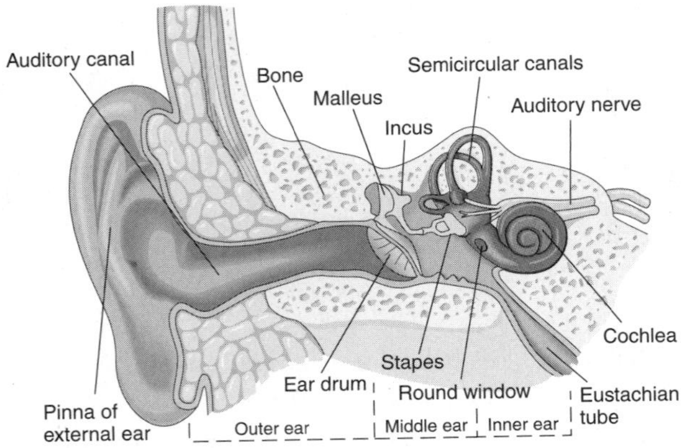

### Eye

The organ of sight is considered the most complicated sense organ of the body. As seen in Figures 28-2 and 28-3 the eye is housed in the orbital cavity. Spherical in shape, it is a hollow globe formed by three layers

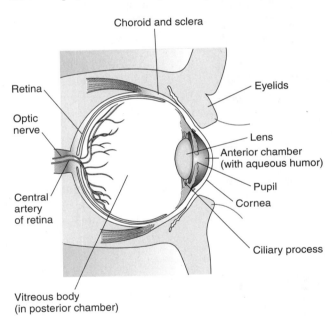

**FIGURE 28-2A** Structures of the eye.

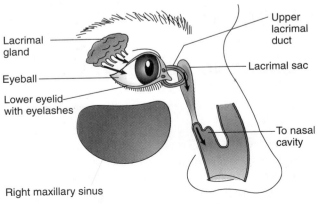

**FIGURE 28-2B** Accessory organs of the eye.

**FIGURE 28-1** Anatomic areas of the ear shown in cross section.

enclosing fluid contents. The outside layer is the sclera, which is continuous with the cornea. The middle layer includes the choroid, ciliary body, and iris. The inner or third layer is the retina.

**Accessory Organs.** Accessory organs of the eye include the eyelids, conjunctiva, and lacrimal glands and ducts. Anterior to the eye are two thin movable folds, the eyelids. Attached to the open edges of the eyelids are the eyelashes. Covering the inner surface of the eyelids and the exposed surface of the cornea and sclera is the mucous membrane known as the conjunctiva. This mucous membrane lubricates the surfaces it covers.

At the superior lateral part of the orbit is the lacrimal gland, which secretes tears. Ducts leading from the gland lead tears to the eye. They are drained from the eye through the nasolacrimal duct, which extends into the nasal cavity.

The two chambers of the globe of the eye each have fluid. The fluid (aqueous humor) in the smaller and anterior chamber has the ability to clear small amounts of bacteria. A larger amount of fluid is in the posterior chamber. This substance is gelatinous and named vitreous humor. Light is refracted through these two fluids and the lens on its way to the retina.

## Sinus Tracts

The sinuses are air-filled, mucous-lined cavities found in certain bones of the head. The accessory sinuses of the nose are contained in the maxillae, the ethmoid, the frontal, and the sphenoid bones. Note the placement and drainage of the maxillary sinuses, the ethmoidal sinuses, the frontal sinuses, and the sphenoid sinuses in Figures 28-3 and 28-4.

The openings of each of the sinuses are at points in the space that permit free drainage with the exception of the maxillary sinus. The opening into the nose is at a higher level than the bottom of the sinus. Fluid must be pushed against gravity to drain and this is accom-

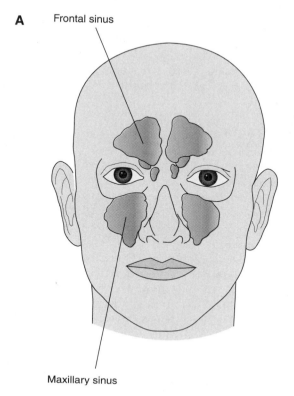

A

Frontal sinus

Maxillary sinus

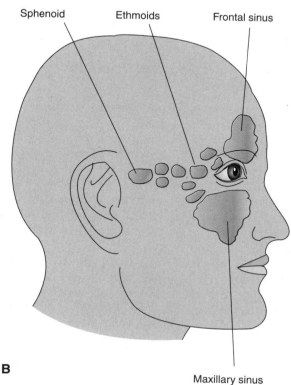

B

Sphenoid    Ethmoids    Frontal sinus

Maxillary sinus

**FIGURE 28-3** Paranasal sinuses. (A) Anterior view. (B) Lateral view.

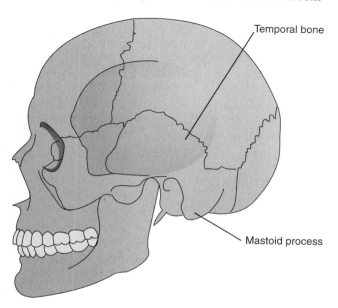

Temporal bone

Mastoid process

**FIGURE 28-4** Mastoid process.

plished by the ciliated epithelium lining the cavity. This special lining usually frees the maxillary sinuses of secretions and inhaled particles.

The functions of the sinuses are not clearly understood. Openings into these sinuses from the nose are small. Tissue that is continuous with the mucous membrane of the nose lines the openings and the sinuses. Inflammation in the nose may cause inflammation of the sinuses. If the inflammation and infection are severe, the resulting swelling could close the openings of the sinuses. Drugs may have to be given to shrink the tissues sufficiently for drainage to occur. Surgical intervention may be the next step if infection persists.

## RESIDENT FLORA

### Ear

A wide variety of microorganisms are encountered in specimens from the ear. In newborns there is a high correlation between ear canal microbiology and the mother's vaginal microflora at birth. Later in life the external ear usually reflects the person's skin flora (see Chapter 32) although *Streptococcus pneumoniae* and gram-negative rods, including *Pseudomonas aeruginosa* may be recovered here more frequently than other skin sites.

The middle and inner ears may be involved during generalized disease, or they may be affected only locally by *Staphylococcus aureus, S. pneumoniae, Streptococcus pyogenes, P. aeruginosa, Haemophilus influenzae,* and other microbes. There is an increasing incidence of penicillin- and ampicillin-resistant middle ear pathogens (Rodriguez, Schwartz, & Thorne, 1995).

### Eye

Although there is a constant supply of tears washing the eye, the healthy eye may harbor a number of skin organisms. Coagulase-negative staphylococci are the most frequently found bacteria in the eye, followed by diphtheroids. Other indigenous, though rare, microbes of the conjunctiva include viridans streptococcus, *H. influenzae, Branhamella catarrhalis, Propionibacterium acnes,* pneumococci, *Neisseria* species, *Peptostreptococcus* species, *Candida albicans,* and other yeasts.

For newborns who required phototherapy in the hospital and wore protective eye patches, problems with infection arose. Physicians noticed a high rate of pus formation in the eye and clinical **conjunctivitis**. A warning for proper eye care and better eye protection methods was given to the medical personnel caring for the neonates (Fok, Wong, & Cheng, 1995).

Disposable contact lenses, either extended or daily wear, cause changes to the normal ocular flora. They seem to provide a more favorable environment for potential pathogens. The edge of the eyelid was implicated more than the conjunctiva in this change, which occurred over several months. It has been suggested that contact lenses lower the defense mechanisms (tears, host defense) of the eye. Other studies have shown that eye closure during a full night of sleep promotes the growth of normal eye flora. This information has an impact on those who have extended-wear lenses or eye surgery (Ramachandran et al., 1995).

### Sinus Tracts

The arrangement of the sinuses makes them vulnerable to infection by the organisms normally in the upper respiratory tract. Commonly this group of organisms includes *S. pneumoniae, H. influenzae* other than group B, *Neisseria* species, *B. catarrhalis,* anaerobes, aerobic streptococci, and occasionally gram-negative rods or *S. aureus.*

Acute sinus infection is the result of viral upper respiratory tract infection, allergy, deviated nasal septum, or nasal polyps. The infection may resolve by itself or persist and become chronic. Treatment includes drainage, antimicrobial therapy, or surgical correction. The infection may spread to other tissues with consequences: inflammation around the eye, possibly with bacteremia, and in young children, brain abscesses and meningitis.

## SPECIMEN TYPES AND COLLECTION

### Proper Collection and Transport of Specimens

**Ear.** No special patient preparation is required for a culture and smear of the ear. The type of specimen preferred is exudate. An alternate specimen is scrapings of the ear canal. **Tympanocentesis** is not justified except in neonates and when antibiotic treatment fails. Middle ear **blepharitis** or ventilations are uncomfortable to obtain and have questionable reliability. The exudate material and drainage from a tympanic perforation may both be cultured in the manner described below.

For the inner ear, and an intact eardrum, clean the ear canal with a soap solution, and collect fluid by syringe. For a ruptured eardrum, collect the fluid on a flexible shaft sterile swab using an auditory speculum, which provides a "sterile tunnel." The transport to the laboratory is by sterile tube with swab transport medium or in an anaerobic system. Several commercially available systems can be used for anaerobic transport. The specimen should be delayed no more than 2 hours at room temperature. For physician's orders of multiple specimens the maximum would be one per day from the same source.

For the outer ear, use a moistened sterile swab to remove any debris or crust from the ear canal. Use two new sterile swabs to obtain a sample by firmly rotating each swab in the outer canal. These two swabs are transported in swab transport medium. The same guidelines for delay and repeat specimens apply. An air-dried smear on a glass slide, a KOH preparation, and culture to appropriate media occur in the laboratory.

For tympanocentesis fluid, clean the external ear canal with a mild soap solution. Using an **aspiration** technique, the physician will obtain the fluid by needle and syringe through the eardrum. The specimen should be transferred to a sterile tube or anaerobic transport vial before transport to the laboratory. An alternate method would be a capped syringe without a needle. (Safety precautions should be observed when removing the needle; see Chapter 3.) A summary for specimen collection of the ear is shown in Table 28-1.

**Eye.** Most specimens from the eye are collected by an ophthalmologist (a physician specializing in conditions of the eye), and before medications are given. The type of specimen preferred in suspected conjunctivitis is a pair of sterile swabs moistened with sterile saline or broth and touched to the involved area of the eye. One swab is inoculated onto appropriate plated media at the bedside or as soon as possible. The second swab would be used to make a smear or two. Examination of the smears would be by Gram stain or direct fluorescent antibody (DFA) stain.

For corneal infections, initially culture the conjunctiva and tissue above. Next, topical anesthetic is applied to anesthetize the cornea. The physician then scrapes the edge of the corneal ulcer with a sterile platinum Kimura spatula. The scrapings are used to prepare slides and to make direct cultures on appropriate plated media immediately. Organisms are better detected from scrapings than from swabs.

Ideally both eyes should be cultured separately to help in identifying which organisms are pathogens, and as quality control. Due to the continual washing of the eyes, collecting a large amount of inoculum is suggested.

Concretions (solid masses formed in the cavity) obtained from the lacrimal canal should be transported to the laboratory in anaerobic conditions. In the case of penetrating wounds of the eye, the specimen should be treated as a wound.

For viral and chlamydial specimens, the samples should be obtained before topical anesthetics are applied. In the case of the viral cultures, do not use calcium alginate swabs for specimen collection; use Dacron swabs or cotton swabs with nonwood shafts. When collecting chlamydial samples, do not use cotton swabs; use calcium alginate swabs. The caution on the type of collection material (cotton versus synthetic) is given because that would provide the best environment for the expected organisms on their way from the site of

**Table 28-1 ▶ Specimens of the Human Ear**

| Types of Cultures | Collection Notes | Reporting Results |
|---|---|---|
| Outer ear | After clearing debris, use sterile swabs in outer canal. Put in transport media. Do not delay more than 2 h at room temperature. Do not take more than one specimen from this source per day. Make air-dried slides, with one swab, KOH prep, and culture appropriate media with second swab. | 1. Telephone positive reports to the attending doctor as soon as possible. 2. Report smear results in detail. |
| Inner ear<br>  Intact tympanum | Clean the ear canal with mild soap solution. Physician collects fluid by needle and syringe. Transport to laboratory in anaerobic state. | 3. Report the culture results in terms of numbers and identification of organism(s). |
|   Ruptured tympanum | Use auditory speculum. Collect fluid on sterile swab Transport in anaerobic state (closed tube). Do not delay (see above). Take single sample daily. | 4. Comment on resident flora or contamination on the cultures. |
| Tympanocentesis fluid | Clean the external ear canal with mild soap solution. Physician obtains fluid with needle and syringe through eardrum. Transport to laboratory anaerobically (capped syringe). | |

Observe safety precautions when using needles.

infection to the culture media. A summary of specimen collection for the eye is shown in Table 28-2.

**Sinus Tracts.** Proper specimens are difficult to obtain. With sinus cultures, the assistance of an otolaryngologist ( a physician specializing in conditions of the ears and throat) may be needed. The specialist would obtain material from the sinus by needle aspirate from the maxillary, frontal, or other sinuses. The contents of the syringe are put into an anaerobic transport system or sent in a capped syringe. A needle aspirate is the only adequate specimen for proper laboratory diagnosis. The specimen should be Gram stained and cultured aerobically and anaerobically. Cultures from the mastoid sinuses are generally collected on swabs during surgery, although actual bone samples are preferred. These mastoid sinus specimens should be transported in anaerobic containers (commercially available).

Other specimens, such as swabs of the nose or nasal washings for sinus cultures, should be rejected by the microbiology laboratory. The reason for the rejection is that they are more reflective of the resident flora of the nose than of the causative agent(s) of the sinusitis. A summary for specimen collection of the sinus tracts is shown in Table 28-3.

## Smears and Stains

**Ear.** One of the swabs brought to the laboratory is for making a smear on a clean slide. Direct microscopic examination by Gram stain is recommended. This is an initial step in the identification and differentiation of

organisms from the infected ear. A separate swab should be used for plating media.

**Eye.** Specimen material should be used to prepare smears on clean slides. Smears should be appropriately fixed and then submitted to Gram, acid-fast, or Giemsa staining. There are specialized staining techniques for specific organism groups.

Direct antigen tests may be used for the detection of some organisms. Chlamydia may be visualized with a fluorescent antibody staining procedure. These techniques and immunoelectron microscopy are used to rapidly identify viral agents.

For conjunctival scrapings, Gram stains are used as well as Giemsa and fluorescent antibody techniques. When reading the Gram stain, the microbiologist should be aware of the normal flora of the conjunctiva. One example where Gram stains are significant is in differentiating bacterial conjunctivitis (with many polymorphonuclear white blood cells [PMNs]) and viral infections (where the predominant white blood cells [WBCs] are lymphocytes and monocytes). The Giemsa stain can be used to:

▶ Characterize the type of inflammatory cell response
▶ Determine the status of conjunctival epithelium cells
▶ Determine chlamydial intracytoplasmic inclusions

There are references with specific descriptions and photographs to aid in interpreting stained smears.

| Table 28–2 ▶ Specimens of the Human Eye | | |
|---|---|---|
| **Type of Culture** | **Collection Notes (For exudates, scrapings and fluids inoculation at bedside is ideal.)** | **Reporting Results** |
| Anaerobic | Use anaerobic transport, or inoculate media immediately. | 1. Telephone positive reports to the attending physician as soon as possible. |
| Bacterial | Inoculate media directly with ocular scrapings. Incubate at 35°C in 5–10% $CO_2$. Smears should accompany culture. (Swabs are rolled on the slide to make the smears.) | 2. Report the smear results in detail (relative numbers, cells seen, location of organisms in or out of cells). |
| Chlamydial | Use calcium alginate swabs. Make slides for Giemsa stain. | |
| Fungal | Inoculate media directly with ocular scrapings. Make slides. Keep plates at room temperature if there is a delay in delivery to the laboratory. | |
| Mycobacterial | Inoculate media directly with ocular scrapings. | 3. Report the culture results in terms of numbers and identification of organism(s). |
| Parasitic | Use special media to detect *Acanthamoeba* species. | |
| Viral | Use Dacron or cotton swabs with nonwood shafts. | 4. Comment on resident flora or contamination on the cultures. |

| Table 28-3 ▶ Specimens of Sinus Tracts | | |
|---|---|---|
| Type of Culture | Collection Notes | Reporting Results |
| Sinus (paranasal) | Physician obtains by needle aspiration. Transport carefully to laboratory in an anaerobic state (stoppered tube or capped syringe). | 1. Telephone positive reports to the attending physician as soon as possible. |
| | Specimen is Gram stained. For maxillary sinus examine for fungus with calcofluor white, periodic acid-Schiff stain, or methenamine silver stain. | 2. Report smear results in detail. |
| | Additional specimens may be fungal cultures of purulent material, blood cultures, and biopsied necrotic tissue. | 3. Report the culture results in terms of numbers and identification of organism(s). |
| Sinus (mastoid) | Physician obtains bone specimens during surgery, or as second choice, material on swabs. | |
| | Transport carefully to laboratory in an anaerobic state (commercially available tubes). Makes smears and put on media. Examine for bacteria and fungus as above. | 4. Comment on resident flora or contamination on the culture. |
| Observe safety precautions when using needles. | | |

When staining corneal scrapings, the Gram stain and Giemsa stain are the primary ones used. Here the Giemsa stain identifies fungal elements, provides better morphologic detail of bacteria, and puts the *Acanthamoeba* in shades of blue. If *Acanthamoeba* is suspected, a direct wet mount preparation should be examined, and a trichrome stain used. However, the most sensitive method for this parasite is the special culture described below the list of media for eye cultures. Other stains can be used for corneal scrapings. One of these is the Gomori methenamine silver stain for fungal elements. Periodic acid-Schiff (PAS) stain and carbolfuchsin can also be used. The latter is helpful when *Mycobacterium, Nocardia, Actinomyces,* or *Arachnia* is suspected. For intraocular fluid (that aspirated from either chamber of the eyeball), Gram stain, Giemsa stain, and the others mentioned in the previous paragraph can be used in the identification of the organisms.

**Sinus Tracts.** For material aspirated from the maxillary or mastoid sinus, examinations should be made for bacteria and fungi. Fungal elements can be demonstrated by calcofluor white fluorescent, PAS stain, or methenamine silver stain. The latter can also be used for bacteria and some parasitic species.

## Processing of Cultures

There are a variety of organisms to recover and thus many different media are used for specimens from the ear, eye, and sinus tracts.

**Ear.** When the specimens from the ear are obtained they should be inoculated on media that will encourage growth of fastidious organisms, those microbes that may be present in small amounts, and those that may be overgrown by more aggressive bacteria. For enrichment, thioglycollate broth is suggested. Direct plating media for ear specimens includes:

- ▶ Blood agar plate (BAP)
- ▶ Chocolate agar plate
- ▶ Sabouraud dextrose agar
- ▶ CDC anaerobic blood agar
- ▶ Phenylethyl alcohol agar
- ▶ MacConkey agar
- ▶ Mycological media

The specimen should be plated at bedside when it is collected or as soon as possible in the laboratory. This is to provide an optimum sample for quick and accurate identification of the microorganisms that could cause the loss of hearing in the patient or damage to very sensitive tissue. The standard incubation time, temperature, and atmosphere for each media should be followed. When the patient is suspected of having chronic **otitis media**, careful attention should be paid to anaerobic organisms when collecting, transporting, and culturing the specimens.

**Eye.** The culture media for eye specimens is long and varied to cover a wide range of resident and pathogenic organisms that could be recovered from this delicate organ. One reference recommends tryptic soy broth, if a broth is used, to saturate the swabs prior to collection of the specimen. Other media for eye specimens includes, but is not limited, to:

▶ BAP
▶ Chocolate agar plate
▶ Thioglycollate broth
▶ Desoxycholate lactose agar
▶ Lowenstein-Jensen agar slant
▶ Sabouraud dextrose agar with antibiotics
▶ Brain-heart infusion broth with antibiotic
▶ Viral transport medium
▶ Thayer-Martin agar
▶ Pseudomonas agar
▶ Brucella blood agar
▶ Middlebrook-Cohn agar slant
▶ Nonnutrient agar plate with killed *Escherichia coli* overlay

**Sinus Tracts.** A sampling of the media for sinus specimens includes:

▶ BAP
▶ Chocolate agar plate
▶ Anaerobic blood agar plate
▶ Thioglycollate broth
▶ MacConkey agar plate

This variety will cover the resident flora and the possible pathogenic microorganisms. In cases where anaerobes predominate, such as chronic sinusitis and **mastoiditis**, careful attention must be paid by the laboratory to the effective collection, transport, and culturing of the specimen.

## OPPORTUNISTIC OR PATHOGENIC MICROORGANISMS

### Ear

Organisms that might be isolated from the external ear would be streptococci, staphylococci, *Haemophilus* species, and gram-negative rods. Bacterial pathogens frequently recovered from the middle ear are *S. pneumoniae, H. influenzae, B. catarrhalis,* group A streptococcus, and *S. aureus* in that order of prevalence. Some of the organisms are resistant to penicillin and ampicillin. From the inner ear a range of aerobes, anaerobes, fungi, and yeast is found. The usual methods for the identification of *S. pyogenes, S. pneumoniae, P. aeruginosa, H. influenzae,* and *B. catarrhalis* pertain. In children infected with human immunodeficiency virus (HIV), the common pathogens are present as in healthy children, although *S. aureus* is significantly more frequent (Marchisio, Principi, Sorella, Sala, & Tornaghi, 1996). Community-acquired *P. aeruginosa* in

nonimmunocompromised individuals tends to be associated with contaminated water. This organism has been found in infections following contact of the ear with water in swimming pools, whirlpools, or hot tubs. (High counts of this pathogenic organism can be found when the bathing water is cultured.)

Two other conditions can exist with *P. aeruginosa.* One of these has the popular name of "swimmer's ear." For people involved with aquatic sports there are reports of superficial infections of the ear canal. One study in the scientific literature (Sunstrom, Jacobson, Munck-Wikland, & Ringertz, 1996) determined that the *P. aeruginosa* in otitis externa was biochemically different from that isolated from other infections. A second more serious condition can occur in diabetic individuals and the elderly. In these patients the *P. aeruginosa* invades tissue, damaging nerve and bone. Meningitis may result. In this serious infection both antibiotics and surgery may be required for treatment. One unusual case of ear infection and contaminated water was reported in a female Greek diver with complicated suppurative otitis media. The infection was caused by a marine halophilic (salt-loving) *Vibrio alginolyticus.* Prolonged exposure to the salt water in her occupation as a diver was a major factor for this patient (Tsakris, Psifidis, & Douboyas, 1995).

### Eye

Organisms cultured from eye infections would include aerobes, facultative anaerobes, anaerobes, fungi, *Neisseria* species, *Haemophilus* species, *Mycobacterium, Nocardia* species, and gram-negative rods including *P. aeruginosa.*

Following minor trauma to the cornea, *P. aeruginosa* infections can occur. These infections are usually associated with the use of contact lenses, and more particularly, contaminated lens solution or tap water for lens care. These infections can cause corneal ulcers. If not properly treated, the corneal ulcers can progress to loss of vision. Other organisms associated with contact lens are *Bacillus* species and *Serratia* species.

### Sinus Tracts

Sinusitis is a common infection that is both polymicrobic (caused by more than one organism) and synergistic. In adults *H. influenzae* and *S. pneumoniae* are recovered in the highest numbers. Next *S. pyogenes* and *B. catarrhalis* are found in smaller amounts, and then *P. acnes.* Acute sinusitis, with a higher level of oxygen in the cells, supports the growth of aerobic organisms. Therefore anaerobes are considered pathogens in only a small number of cases of acute sinusitis. In children, *S. pneumoniae, H. influenzae,* and *B. catarrhalis* are the most likely to be found.

Chronic sinusitis may extend from the sinuses into

surrounding tissue and into intracranial spaces. The proximity of the sinuses to the central nervous system is of major importance because the infection in the sinus could result in serious complications inside the skull. Some of these complications are infection into the space around the eye, direct pressure on the major nerve of the eye, meningitis, and brain abscesses.

Anaerobes contribute to the severity and chronicity of infections that occur in the sinuses. They include species such as *Bacteroides*. *Bacteroides* species, specifically *melaninogenicus* and *oralis*, are the most important anaerobic organisms involved. These organisms possess two important virulence factors: the ability to produce β-lactamase and the ability to produce a capsule.

## MICROBIAL DISEASES OF THE EAR, EYE, AND SINUS TRACTS

### Ear

The likely diseases of the ear are mild otitis externa, severe or malignant otitis externa, and acute otitis media (AOM). The mild form is swimmer's ear, which was discussed earlier. People with type A blood have been found to have a genetic disposition to otitis externa.

The malignant form of an inflammation of the external ear is a severe infection that spreads to tissue and bone, killing the tissue it invades. The disease is associated with pain, tenderness, and pus in the canal. In the severe otitis externa there may be a pustule or cellulitis within the ear canal. Gram-positive cocci such as *S. aureus* or group A streptococcus are usually responsible for this localized infection. Small hemorrhages of the ear can be part of the picture.

Acute otitis media refers to a middle ear infection. The spread of the infection from the eustachian tube into the inner ear space occurs. Also organisms that belong to the normal flora of the mouth can find their way to the inner ear and cause infection. This condition most commonly occurs in infants and children, and in boys more than girls. AOM occurs concurrently with or subsequent to a viral respiratory infection. Children who are bottle fed while lying on their back, are teething, or have a congenital defect (such as cleft palate) have a high incidence of ear infections.

The ear infection can be present with sore throat, otalgia (earache), and fever. The physician makes the diagnosis by examining the tympanic membrane. Among the diagnostic criteria for AOM are always included the bulging eardrum and its quality of being impenetrable to light on examination. In the laboratory diagnosis, high levels of serum C-reactive protein (CRP) are found in bacterial AOM. Most microbiology specimens would involve only aerobic cultures and

show no growth in 30% to 33% of the cases. When anaerobic cultivation is performed, anaerobes are the only isolate in half and in the other 50% it would be mixed flora, anaerobic and aerobic. AOM in children and young adults, even with antibiotic treatment, can lead to mastoiditis. Several organisms have been recovered such as *S. pneumoniae, S. pyogenes, S. aureus,* coagulase-negative staphylococcus, *Klebsiella pneumoniae,* and *P. aeruginosa*. In mastoiditis there is involvement of the bony framework of the ear and some early intracranial complications (Luntz, Keren, Nusem, & Kronenberg, 1994). In a study of relapses from ear infection in adults, 100% of the isolates, including all the usual suspects, were found to be penicillin G and ampicillin resistant (Campos et al., 1995).

General otitis media has four defined stages:

1. Inflammation of the eardrum
2. Acute otitis media
3. Otitis media with secretion
4. Chronic otitis media

Several treatments are used, among them decongestants, anti-inflammatory drugs, and antibiotics. The organisms in stage three, secretory otitis media, match those in AOM very closely. It is good to establish the identity and antibiotic sensitivity of the organisms because there is increasing risk of drug failure. AOM that is persistent after initial empiric antimicrobial therapy can be caused by middle ear inflammation. There are two possible reasons for the inflammation: (1) killed bacteria, or (2) penicillin-resistant or β-lactamase-producing organisms. This usually occurs in patients who have not recently been treated (Pichichero et al., 1995). These cases can progress to the stage of chronic otitis media. A complication of chronic otitis media is mastoiditis. Medical management of stage four includes the combined treatments of surgery, drainage, and drug combinations.

Recurrent AOM is very prevalent in young children. Epidemiologic studies have suggested that prevention or reduction of the ear infections may be achieved by breast-feeding babies, eliminating tobacco smoke in the household, and using small nursery centers for preschoolers. Secondary use of antimicrobials helps somewhat. Ear tubes are no longer thought to be as effective as the antimicrobials available now. Removal of adenoids may be indicated after the ear tubes are out and AOM recurs in the child. The biggest promise of preventing otitis media lies with vaccines against the common pathogenic bacteria and viruses. Work is progressing with pneumococcal vaccines (Giebink, 1995).

Chronic otitis media results from the irritation of drainage from the middle ear (otorrhea or a "runny ear") in patients with pus in the middle ear or a perforated eardrum. The predominant organisms are *P. aeruginosa, S. aureus,* and Enterobacteriaceae. Approximately 45% of the organisms recovered in chronic otitis media are anaerobes. Although the majority of the isolates from specimens are single organisms, many are polymicrobic. Even in the latter situation *P. aeruginosa* was the most common organism and the most resistant to antimicrobials. Chronic middle ear effusions may vary by season and with the relative humidity. In rare cases, ear infections can be caused by tuberculosis, syphilis, yaws, or leprosy. A complication of chronic otitis media is mastoiditis. This condition shows predominantly anaerobic organisms.

## Eye

**Conjunctivitis.** The major types of conjunctivitis are bacterial, viral, and chlamydial. The conjunctiva can become infected by airborne bacteria-laden items, hand-to-eye contact, or spread from other parts of the eye. This condition is also called "pink eye." There is inflammation of the conjunctiva associated with markedly increased tearing and watery discharge with pus or mucus.

The likely pathogens of conjunctivitis are adenovirus, *Chlamydia trachomitis*, herpes simplex viruses (HSV), *S. aureus*, *Neisseria gonorrhoeae*, *H. influenzae*, and *S. pneumoniae*. Conjunctivitis caused by *H. influenzae* usually results in large amounts of pus. The pus should be collected on a calcium alginate swab and transported in Stuart's medium to the laboratory.

The best diagnostic tests for conjunctivitis are aerobic cultures, adenovirus cultures, Chlamydia culture, HSV culture, and Gram stain.

In neonatal conjunctivitis, infection of newborns can occur in a variety of ways. The clinical signs do not indicate the causative organism. Cultures and smear should be obtained, including viral cultures for HSV.

**Orbital Cellulitis.** The orbit of the eye can be infected in several ways: inoculation by trauma or surgery and spread of infection from the paranasal sinuses. Referring to Figure 28-3, the proximity of the sinuses to the orbit is noted, as are the many venous connections from the sinuses to the orbit. The etiologic agent is somewhat determined by the route of infection. This syndrome causes fever, an increase in WBCs, swelling of the eyelid(s), and limited movement of the eye. Orbital cellulitis is a serious condition that may produce blindness and intracranial infections. This condition may be subclassified into acute bacterial orbital cellulitis and chronic orbital cellulitis.

**Keratitis.** Predisposing factors for bacterial **keratitis** include previous eye disease, wearing contact lenses, and using topical corticosteroids. Susceptible patients are alcoholics, burn patients and other immunocompromised individuals.

Inflammation of the cornea is serious because it threatens the sight of the patient. The laboratory work-

ups should be prompt and complete. There are several types of keratitis depending on the microorganism that invades the cornea. Do note that any organism may be capable of infection if provided optimal conditions for its growth.

Bacterial keratitis can be caused by two routes: corneal injury or invasion of organisms that can penetrate intact corneas. The organisms that follow injury to the surface and cause pain, ulceration, pus, and irisitis (irritation of the iris) include *S. aureus*, *S. pneumoniae*, *P. aeruginosa*, *Citrobacter*, *Enterobacter*, *Klebsiella*, *Proteus*, and *Serratia*. *P. aeruginosa* produces the most severe infection and acts quickly. A special test for detecting the endotoxin of aerobes and facultative gram-negative bacteria is the *Limulus* lysate test. This test can be useful because gram-negative organisms are found in 60% of the cases of bacterial keratitis though they are not readily detected in Gram stains. *Mycobacterium* species can also produce chronic ulcerative keratitis. The bacteria capable of penetrating intact corneal epithelium are: *N. gonorrhoeae*, *Neisseria meningitidis*, and *Corynebacterium diphtheriae*.

Fungal keratitis may resemble bacterial keratitis with ulceration (shallow), pus ( in more than one site), and irisitis (minimal). The organisms most frequently found are *Fusarium solani*, and species of *Aspergillus*, *Acremonium*, and *Curvularia*. The cases of yeast keratitis are commonly caused by *C. albicans*.

This is a case where bilateral cultures are suggested to check for contamination. Corneal material is best obtained by scraping with the special spatula the areas where there is ulceration or pus. Try to avoid the eyelids and the eyelashes when taking the corneal scrapings. Direct inoculation is made to the appropriate media, and several slides made and fixed for routine and special stains. Use the particular design suggested ("C" shapes are popular) for inoculating media with the spatula. Do not use a cotton swab to obtain corneal specimens.

*Acanthamoeba* keratitis is the infection of the cornea by the amoeba named. Clinically it looks like other microbial infection of the cornea. The suggested media are blood agar, chocolate agar, and nonnutritive agar with an overlay of heat-killed *E. coli*. Smears should be made and stained with Gram and Giemsa stains. It will take experience for the technologist to distinguish the amoeba's trophozoites from WBCs on the smear.

This parasite has been found in eyewash stations along with other amoeba and bacteria in the water supply. An effective solution to the problem was not found. *Acanthamoeba* by themselves or mixed with other amoeba have been reported as the cause of amoebic keratitis in the last decade or so.

Viral keratitis can be caused by one of several viruses (HSV, herpes zoster, varicella, adeno- and vaccinia viruses). Epithelial debridement (the surgical removal of dead tissue) may be helpful or a cotton swab transported in viral transport media. Special stains including fluorescent antibody stains may be helpful in the laboratory diagnosis.

A summary of the microbiologic types of keratitis are listed as follows:

- ▶ Bacterial
- ▶ Mycobacterial
- ▶ Fungal
- ▶ Amoebic
- ▶ Viral

### Newborn Eye Infections

CONJUNCTIVITIS. Newborn eye infections are a specialized situation. Conjunctivitis is the most common of the eye infections of this age group. Another name for this condition is ophthalmic neonatorum. There are several etiologies of conjunctivitis so the physician should do a differential diagnosis to determine if it is infection, allergies, glaucoma, or another cause. The infections are caused by pneumococci, staphylococci, gonococci, *H. influenzae,* streptococci, adenovirus, coxsackie virus, HSV, chlamydia, rickettsia, fungi, and rarely, parasites. Many cases are self-limited.

In years past 1% silver nitrate was used routinely at birth to combat possible gonococcus in the birth canal. If there is gonococcal conjunctivitis, the neonate is treated with intravenous penicillin in the hospital and with saline washes of the eyes. Since the 1980s there has been an increasing use of 1% tetracycline ointment and erythromycin ointment. This combined treatment will hit both gonococcal and chlamydia infections in the baby's eyes.

*Chlamydia trachomatis* is found in approximately 2% to 13% of pregnant women (Freeman & Poland, 1992). It is transmitted during birth with about 30% to 50% of babies born to infected women developing conjunctivitis. Chlamydia (inclusion) conjunctivitis usually occurs at 5 to 9 days after birth or later. One symptom that is different from bacteria conjunctivitis is that it is less purulent. There is no corneal scarring with inclusion conjunctivitis. The neonate with this condition may also have pneumonia or otitis media.

Ophthalmic neonatorum can affect one or both eyes, showing lid swelling, conjunctival edema, and purulent discharge. A Gram stain should guide antimicrobial treatment to avoid blindness. A child with recurrent conjunctivitis should be checked for obstruction in the lacrimal system.

Conjunctivitis may also be caused by chemicals, specifically the silver nitrate. The inflammation is usually evident 6 to 24 hours after use of the solution. If the redness lasts for more than a day, an ophthalmologist should evaluate the case.

PERIORBITAL CELLULITIS AND ORBITAL CELLULITIS. These two conditions in newborns may coexist or one may

lead to the other. Bacterial organisms cause the cellulitis after pustules or trauma. The organisms also enter through infected paranasal sinuses, upper respiratory tract, or teeth. *S. aureus* is the most common organism. Newborns and young children are very susceptible to *H. influenzae.* These conditions are considered very serious due to medical complications, and these patients should be admitted to the hospital. Treatment with intravenous antibiotics is continued until symptoms lessen and then oral antibiotics are given for 7 to 10 days. In the rare case of mucormycosis causing cellulitis around the eye, surgery may be necessary.

DACRYOADENITIS. Many neonates are born with ductules partially open or not open. The babies experience constant tearing and a mucous discharge. The discharge should be collected and sent to the microbiology laboratory for a Gram stain and culture. The duct is usually opened by surgery or by massaging the duct.

**Congenital Infections.** Another concern with neonates are congenital infections. These occur when the pregnant woman has an infection and the fetus is affected. With toxoplasmosis the organism is passed across the placenta in the last trimester. Mothers-to-be should avoid contact with cats and uncooked meat. The mothers appear healthy but there are serious problems with the neonate including microencephaly (small brain) and with the eyes; one or both may be marked. The eye shows lesions, scars, and pigmented edges. Serologic tests can detect the antibody. Treatment varies with the severity of the lesions and inflammation.

Rubella infection in the mother can lead to cataracts in the embryo. Cataracts can also develop with the mother's infection with syphilis, and following amniocentesis. The prognosis for the baby is poor. If a well baby later contracts rubella, retinal damage may develop. Also in this case, the baby can develop glaucoma and oculomotor disorders where the eye muscles do not work properly. The baby's caretakers should be immune to rubella. Babies with birth defects due to rubella are reported to the state health department.

Though testing of parents is decreasing the incidence of congenital syphilis, problems are sometimes seen. Cataracts are a possible consequence, and some babies show pigment changes outside the iris.

Neonatal herpes simplex virus or HSV ocular infection can occur in one of two ways. One mode is the transfer of the virus from the mother to baby when it moves through the birth canal. The second way is shortly before birth if the membranes rupture. Ocular involvement occurs in about 20% of newborns with this viral infection (Oski et al., 1992).

Whether the infection attacks the embryo or the newborn eye problems and problems with other organs can affect the baby's future. Most of these situations can be prevented with good medical management of the parents-to-be. This management can prevent or alter the potential problems and minimize the subsequent transmission of infection in the nursery. If there is an infected baby, contact isolation procedures should be invoked and handwashing of health care workers increased. Special focus should be on the mother during the pregnancy and at delivery, and on the newborn postnatally.

## Sinus Tracts

**Acute Sinusitis, Community-Acquired.** Patients complain of pain in the area of the particular sinus involved (e.g., maxillary, ethmoid). This condition usually follows an upper respiratory tract viral infection and lasts 1 to 3 weeks. Other complaints include nasal congestion, rhinitis, and an abundance of exudate. Sinusitis is a common infection that is polymicrobic. Acute sinusitis, with a high oxygen level, supports aerobic organisms. In the majority of the cases, anaerobic bacteria only were isolated. In many others, they were mixed with aerobic or facultative bacteria. In a smaller number of cases aerobic or facultative organisms were isolated. In immunocompromised patients additional organisms may be involved. Laboratory tests for acute sinusitis would include aerobic cultures and Gram stain of clinical material from the appropriate sinus.

**Chronic Sinusitis, Community-Acquired.** Patients with chronic sinusitis have the same symptoms as above. In addition they often have a cough that results from postnasal drip. Extensive disease in adults was correlated with asthma, specific IgE antibodies, and eosinophilia (Newman, Platts-Mills, Phillips, Hazen, & Gross, 1994).

With a lower oxygen level, the conditions are ideal for anaerobic organisms. *Bacteroides* and anaerobic cocci are the predominant anaerobic pathogenic organisms. Streptococci and *S. aureus* are the most frequently isolated aerobic or facultative bacteria. To recover these organisms the laboratory procedures would be aerobic and anaerobic cultures plus a Gram stain of material from the sinuses.

**Hospital-Acquired Sinusitis.** This condition occurs in hospitalized patients who have prolonged contact with tubes through the nasal passages. An infection may result and the patient develops a fever with or without an increased WBC count. With aerobic cultures and Gram stain the pathogenic organisms recovered would be *S. aureus,* methicillin-resistant *S. aureus* (MRSA), and *P. aeruginosa.*

**Mucormycosis.** This condition is a potentially lethal fungal infection of the paranasal sinuses and the orbit. This infection occurs primarily in patients with complications of diabetes mellitus, but can develop in patients with altered host defense (mild diabetes, immunosuppressive therapy, alcoholic cirrhosis). The complications of mucormycosis are so serious that prompt laboratory diagnosis is absolutely necessary.

An otolaryngologist would obtain materials from the maxillary sinus by puncture. Fungal cultures of purulent matter, blood cultures, and multiple biopsies of necrotic tissue from the nose and sinuses are the primary focus of the laboratory. This condition is caused by one or more of a group of opportunistic fungal pathogens.

## SUMMARY

▶ The basic anatomy of the ear, eye, and paranasal sinus tract is unique to each organ and relates to the microbial flora found in those sites.
▶ Specimen collection from the ear, eye, and sinus tract may require a physician or special instruments.

▶ Microorganisms of all varieties, ranging from viruses to parasites, fungi to bacteria can be pathogenic for these delicate tissues.
▶ Several microbial diseases affect the ear, eye, and sinus tract, plus some less common complications.

## Review Questions

1. The majority of the sinuses around the nose naturally drain by means of:
   a. endolymph.
   b. gravity.
   c. ciliated epithelium.
   d. antibiotics.

2. Organisms routinely found in the eye include:
   a. coagulase-negative staphylococci and diphtheroids.
   b. *Branhamella catarrhalis* and *Candida albicans.*
   c. *Haemophilus influenzae* and Peptostreptococcus
   d. Diphtheroids and *Pseudomonas aeruginosa.*

3. When culturing ear infections, the pathogen most likely to be isolated is:
   a. *Staphylococcus aureus.*
   b. *Haemophilus influenzae.*
   c. *Pseudomonas aeruginosa.*
   d. *Streptococcus pneumoniae.*

4. Acute otitis media (AOM) is most likely found in which age group?
   a. Toddlers
   b. Teenagers
   c. Soccer moms
   d. Senior citizens

5. A complication of sinus infections can be:
   a. bacteriuria.
   b. bacteremia.
   c. otitis externa.
   d. brain abscesses.

6. Inflammation of the cornea can be caused by bacteria, mycobacteria, fungi, parasites, or viruses. When a yeast causes keratitis it is most likely:
   a. *Aspergillus niger.*
   b. *Candida albicans.*
   c. *Sporothrix schenkii.*
   d. *Mycobacterium leprae.*

7. The most serious ocular infection is _____. The reason for medical concern is the risk of blindness without a quick identification of the organisms and treatment.
   a. pharyngitis
   b. rhinitis
   c. endophthalmitis
   d. blepharitis

8. The doctor would make the diagnosis of AOM by examining the:
   a. results of throat cultures.
   b. titer of the *Limulus* lysate tests.
   c. condition of the tympanic membrane.
   d. report of anaerobic cultures.

9. There are noncultural detection methods for organisms from the eyes, ears, and sinus tracts. These methods can be helpful in confirming the identification when antimicrobial treatment may have started before the specimens for culture were obtained. An example of a nonculture method is:
   a. Sabouraud dextrose medium.
   b. enzyme-linked immunosorbent assay.
   c. blood cultures.
   d. chlamydial transport medium.

10. With the changes in recreation and in advances in eye care, new diseases of the ear and eye are being seen. These conditions of the 1990s include all, EXCEPT:
    a. *Pseudomonas aeruginosa* from hot tubs.
    b. *Aspergillus* following radial keratotomy.
    c. coagulase-negative staphylococci on the eye.
    d. *Acanthamoeba* in contact lens wearers.

## CASE STUDY

A 24-year-old man was found by his ophthalmologist to have keratitis. He wore soft contact lenses. The doctor obtained specimens by corneal scrapings, biopsy, and keraplasty. All specimens were sent to the laboratory and distributed to the microbiology and histopathology areas for testing. The man's contact lenses, lens storage case, and home water supply were all examined for microorganisms. From the corneal tissue samples, no pathogenic bacteria, fungi, or viruses were recovered. Organisms were observed using light and electron microscopy, but immunochemical staining was not helpful. Viable organisms were recovered from the corneal biopsy specimen. A wide range of organisms was found in the lens storage case. One of these organisms was associated with the contact lens. After prolonged culture the organism was recovered.

**Questions:**

1. What causative organism most likely caused the patient's keratitis?

2. Which stains would you suggest for the corneal scrapings?

3. This organism can cause keratitis and blindness. What steps would you suggest to contact lens wearers to avoid such serious problems?

▶ **REFERENCES &**
**RECOMMENDED READING**

Aitken, D., Hay, J., Kinnear, F. B., Kirkness, C. M., Lee, W. R., & Seal, D.V. (1996). Amebic keratitis in a wearer of disposable contact lenses due to a mixed *Vahlkampfia* and *Hartmannella* infection [Abstract]. *Ophthalmology, 103*(3), 485–494.

Alfaro, D.V., Roth, D. B., Laughlin, R. M., Goyal, M., & Ligggett, P. E. (1995). Pediatric post-traumatic endophthalmitis. [On-line]. *British Journal of Ophthalmology, 79*(10), 888–891. Abstract from: MEDLINE

Ataoglu, H., Goksu, N., Kemaloglu, Y. K., Bengisum, S., & Ozbilen, S. (1994). Preliminary report on L-forms: Possible role in the infectious origin of secretory otitis media. [On-line]. *Annals of Otol Rhinology Laryngol, 103*(6), 434–438. Abstract from: MEDLINE

Bannatyne, R. M., Clausen, C., McCarthy, L. R. (1979). Duncan, I. B. R. (Ed.). *Laboratory diagnosis of upper respiratory tract infections* (Cumulative techniques and procedures in clinical microbiology, cumitech 10). Washington, DC: American Society for Microbiology.

Bowman, E. K., Vass, A. A., Mackowski, R., Owen, B. A., & Tyndall, R. L. (1996). Quantitation of free-living amoebae and bacterial populations in eyewash stations relative to flushing frequency [Abstract]. *American Industrial Hygiene Association Journal, 57*(7), 626–633.

Brook, I. (1986). Bacterial synergy in upper respiratory infections. *Current Hospital Topics*. The Upjohn Co.

Brook, I., & Van de Heyning, P. H. (1994). Microbiology and management of otitis media [Abstract]. *Scandinavian Journal of Infectious Diseases Supplement, 93,* 20–32.

Brown, O. E., Manning, S. C., & Phillips, D. L. (1995). Lack of bacteremia in children undergoing myringotomy and tympanostomy tube placement [Abstract]. *Pediatric Infectious Disease Journal, 14*(12), 1101–1102.

Campos, J. M. (1995). *Haemophilus*. In P. R. Murray, E. J. Baron, M. A. Pfaller, F. C. Tenover, & R .H. Yoken (Eds.), *Manual of clinical microbiology* (6th ed., pp. 556–565). Washington, DC: ASM Press.

Campos, M. A., Aries, A., Rodriguez, C., Dorta, A., Betancor, L., Lopez-Aquado, D., & Sierra, A. (1995). Etiology and therapy of chronic suppurative otitis. [On-line]. *Journal of Chemotherapy, 7*(5), 427–431. Abstract from: MEDLINE

Caskey, L. J. (1995). Processing of skin and subcutaneous tissue specimens. In H. D. Isenberg, (Ed. in Chief). P. R. Murray, E. J. Baron, M. A. Pfaller, F. C. Tenover, & R. H. Yolken (Eds.), *Clinical microbiology procedures handbook* (Suppl. 1, p. 1.16.1). Washington, DC: ASM Press.

Committee on Patient Preparation and Specimen Handling. (1983). *Clinical laboratory handbook for patient preparation & specimen handling, November 1983* (Fascicle III, Microbiology). Northfield, IL: College of American Pathologists.

DeAngles, C. (1984). *Pediatric Primary Care* (3rd ed., Chap. 9). Boston: Little, Brown.

Doyle, A., Beiji, B., Early, A., Blake, A., Eustace, P., & Hone, R. (1995). Adherence of bacteria to intraocular lenses: A prospective study. [On-line]. *British Journal of Ophthalmology, 79*(4), 347–349. Abstract from: MEDLINE

Erkan, M., Aslan, T., Ozcan, M., & Koc, N. (1994). Bacteriology of antrum in adults with chronic maxillary sinusitis. [On-line]. *Laryngoscope, 104*(3 Pt1), 321–324. Abstract from: MEDLINE

Fok, T. F., Wong, W., & Cheng, A. F. (1995). Use of eye-patches in phototherapy: Effects on conjunctival bacterial pathogens and conjunctivitis. [On-line]. *Pediatric Infectious Disease Journal, 14*(12), 1091–1094. Abstract from: MEDLINE

Forbes, B. A., & Granato, P. A. (1995). Processing specimens for bacteria. In P. R. Murray, E. J. Baron, M. A. Pfaller, F. C. Tenover, & R. H. Yoken (Eds.), *Manual of clinical microbiology* (6th ed., pp. 265–281). Washington, DC: ASM Press.

Freeman, R. K., & Poland, R. L. (Eds.). (1992). *Guidelines for perinatal care* (3rd ed., Chap. 5). American Academy of Pediatrics and the American College of Obstetricians and Gynecologists.

Funke, G., Lawson, P. A., & Collins, M. D. (1995). Heterogeneity within human-derived centers for disease control and prevention (CDC) cornyform group ANF-l-like bacteria and description of *Corynebacterium auris* sp. nov [Abstract]. *International Journal of Systematic Bacteriology, 45*(4), 735–739.

Giebink, G. S. (1994). Preventing otitis media [Abstract]. *Annals of Otology Rhinology Laryngology, 163,* 20–23.

Gilligan, P. H. (1995). *Psuedomonas* and *Burkholderia*. In P. R. Murray, E. J. Baron, M. A. Pfaller, F. C. Tenover, & R. H. Yoken (Eds.), *Manual of clinical microbiology* (6th ed., pp. 509–519). Washington, DC: ASM Press.

Glasgow, B. J., Engstrom, R. E., Jr., Holland, G. N., Kneiger, A. E., & Wool, M. G. (1996). Bilateral endogenous *Fusarium* endophthalmitis associated with acquired immunodeficiency syndrome (clinical conference). [On-line]. *Archives of Ophthalmology, 114*(7), 873–877. Abstract from: MEDLINE

Hagenah, M., Bohnke, M., Engehmann, K., & Winter, R. (1995). Incidence of bacterial and fungal contamination of donor corneas preserved by organ culture [Abstract]. *Cornea, 14*(4), 423–426.

Hall, G. S., & Pezzlo, M. (1995). Ocular cultures. In H. D. Isenberg, (Ed. in Chief), P. R. Murray, E. J. Baron, M. A. Pfaller, F. C. Tenover, & R. H. Yolken (Eds.), *Clinical microbiology procedures handbook* (Suppl. 1, p. 1.13.1). Washington, DC: ASM Press.

Heaton, J. M., & Mills, R. P. (1995). Factors associated with positive bacterial cultures of chronic middle ear effusions [Abstract]. *Clinical Otolaryngology, 20*(3), 262–265.

Heidmann, D. G., Dunn, S. P., & Watts, J. C. (1995). *Aspergillus* keratitis after radial keratotomy. [On-line]. *American Journal of Ophthalmology, 120*(2), 254–256. Abstract from: MEDLINE

Infections of the head and neck. (1994). In E. J. Baron, L. R. Peterson, & S. M. Finegold (Eds.), *Bailey & Scott's diagnostic microbiology* (9th ed., Chap. 23). St. Louis: Mosby–Year Book.

Isada, C. M., Kasten, B. L., Jr., Goldman, M. P., Gray, L. D., & Aberg, J. A. (1995). *Infectious diseases handbook, including antimicrobial therapy and laboratory diagnosis*. Hudson, OH: Lexi-Comp, Inc.

Isenberg, H. D., & D'Amato, R. F. (1995). Indigenous and pathogenic microorganisms of humans. In P. R. Murray, E. J. Baron, M. A., Pfaller, F .C. Tenover, & R .H. Yoken (Eds.), *Manual of clinical microbiology* (6th ed., pp. 5–18). Washington, DC: ASM Press.

Isenberg, H. D., Schoenkhect, F. D., & vonGravenitz, A. (1979). In S. J. Rubin (Ed.), *Collection and processing of bacteriological specimens (cumulative techniques and procedures in clinical microbiology, cumitech 9)*. Washington, DC: American Society for Microbiology.

Itan, D. P., Wisnieski, S. R., Wilson, L. A., Barza, M., Vine, A. K., Doft, B. H., & Kelsey, S. F. (1996). Spectrum and susceptibilities of microbiological isolates in the endophthalmitis vitrectomy study. [On-line]. *American Journal of Ophthalmology, 122*(1), 1–17. Abstract from: MEDLINE

Jones, D. B., Liesegang, T. J., & Robinson, N. M. (1981). In J. A. Washington, II (Ed.). *Laboratory diagnosis of ocular infections (cumulative techniques and procedures in clinical microbiology, cumitech 13).* Washington, DC: American Society for Microbiology.

Jong, C. N., Olson, N. Y., Nadel, G. L., Phillips. P. S., Gill, F. F., & Neiburger, J. B. (1994). Use of nasal cytology in the diagnosis of occult chronic sinusitis in asthmatic children [Abstract]. *Annals of Allergy, 73*(6), 509–514.

Klein, J. O. (1994). Otitis media [Abstract]. *Clinical Infectious Diseases, 19*(5), 823–832.

Koneman, E. W., Allen, S. D., Janda, W. M., Schreckenberger, P. C., & Winn, W. C., Jr. (1992). *Color atlas and textbook of diagnostic microbiology* (4th ed.). Philadelphia: Lippincott.

Lawin-Brussel, C. A., Refojo, M. F., Leong, F. L., & Kenyon, K. R. (1995). Scanning electron microscopy of the early host in inflammatory response in experimental *Pseudomonas* keratitis and contact lens wear. [On-line]. *Cornea, 14*(4), 353–359. Abstract from: MEDLINE

Lee, D., Belmont, M., & Lucente, F. E. (1996). Pathologic quiz case 2. bilateral herpes zoster oticus [Abstract]. *Archives of Otolaryngology—Head and Neck Surgery, 122*(2),197–198.

Litwak, A. B. (1995). Non-CMV infectious chorioretinopathies in AIDS [Abstract]. *Optometry and Vision Science, 72*(5), 312–319.

Luntz, M., Keren, G., Nusem, S., & Kronenberg, J. (1994). Acute mastoiditis—revisited. [On-line]. *Ear Nose Throat Journal, 73*(9), 648–654. Abstract from: MEDLINE

Mandar, R., & Mikelsaar, M. (1996). Transmission of mother's microflora to the newborn at birth [Abstract]. *Biologica-Neonate, 69*(1), 30–35.

Marchisio, P., Principi, N., Sorella, S., Sala, E., & Tornaghi, R. (1996). Etiology of acute otitis media in human immunodeficiency virus-infected children [Abstract]. *Pediatric Infectious Disease Journal, 15*(1), 58–61.

Marsik, F. J. (1992, Fall). Bacteriology of infections in the pediatric population: Part 3. LabO: Microbiology News & Ideas. Cockeysville, MD: Becton Dickinson Microbiology Systems.

Merz, W. G., & Roberts, G. D. (1995). Detection and recovery of fungi from clinical specimens. In P. R. Murray, E. J. Baron, M. A. Pfaller, F. C. Tenover, & R. H. Yoken (Eds.), *Manual of clinical microbiology* (6th ed., pp. 709–721). Washington, DC: ASM Press.

Miller, J. M., & Holmes, H. T. (1995). Specimen collection, transport and storage. In P. R. Murray, E. J. Baron, M. A. Pfaller, F. C. Tenover, & R. H. Yoken (Eds.), *Manual of clinical microbiology* (6th ed., pp. 19–32). Washington, DC: ASM Press.

Newman. L. J., Platts-Mills, T. A., Phillips, C. D., Hazen, K. C., & Gross, C. W. (1994). Chronic sinusitis, relationship of computed tomographic findings to allergy, asthma, and eosinophilia [Abstract]. *Journal of the American Medical Association, 271*(5), 363–367.

Orihel, T. C., & Ash, L. R. (1995). Tissue helminths. In P. R. Murray, E. J. Baron, M.A. Pfaller, F. C. Tenover, & R. H. Yoken (Eds.), *Manual of clinical microbiology* (6th ed., pp. 1244–1256). Washington, DC: ASM Press.

Oski, F. A. (Ed. in Chief), DeAngles, C. D., Feigin, R. D., McMillan, J. A., & Warshaw, J. B. (Eds.). (1994). *Principles and practices of pediatrics* (2nd ed., pp. 884–888). Philadelphia: Lippincott.

Oyeka, C. A., Oyeka, I. C., & Okeke, G. N. (1995). Prevalence of bacterial otitis media in primary school children in Enugu Suburb, Enugu state, Nigeria. [On-line]. *West African Journal of Medicine, 14*(2), 78–81. Abstract from: MEDLINE

Pichichero, M. E., & Pichichero, C. L. (1995). Persistent acute otitis media: I. causative pathogens. [On-line]. *Pediatric Infectious Disease Journal, 14*(3), 178–183. Abstract from: MEDLINE

Post, J. C., Preston, R. A., Aul, J. J., Larkins-Pettigrew, M., Rydquist-White, J., Anderson, K. W., Wadowsky, R. M., Reagan, D. R., Walker, E. S., Kingsley, L.A., et al. (1995). Molecular analysis of bacterial pathogens in otitis media with effusion [Abstract]. *Journal of the American Medical Association, 273*(20), 1598–1604.

Power, D. A., & McCuen, P. J. (Eds.). (1988). *Manual of BBL products and laboratory procedures* (6th ed.). Cockeysville, MD: Becton Dickinson Microbiology Systems.

Ramachandran, L., Sharma, S., Sankaridurg, P. R., Vajdic, C. M., Chuck, J. A., Holden, B. A., Sweeney, D. F., & Rao, G. N. (1995). Examination of the conjunctival microbiota after 8 hours of eye closure. [On-line]. *CLAO Journal, 21*(3), 195–199. Abstract from: MEDLINE

Rodriguez, W. J., Schwartz, R. H., & Thorne, M. M. (1995). Increasing incidence of penicillin- and ampicillin-resistant middle ear pathogens. [On-line]. *Pediatric Infectious Disease Journals, 14*(12), 1075–1078. Abstract from: MEDLINE

Rothschild, M. A., Drake, W, 3rd, & Scherl, M. (1994). Cephalic zoster with laryngeal paralysis. [On-line]. *Ear Nose and Throat Journal, 73*(11), 850–852. Abstract from: MEDLINE

Samad, A., Solomon, L. D., Miller, M. A., & Mendelson, J. (1995). Anterior chamber contamination after uncomplicated phacoemulsification and intraocular lens implantation [Abstract]. *American Journal of Ophthalmology, 120*(2), 143–150.

Selection, collection, and transport of specimens for microbiological examination. (1994). In E. J. Baron, L. R. Peterson, & S. M. Finegold (Eds.), *Bailey & Scott's diagnostic microbiology* (9th ed., Chap. 7). St. Louis: Mosby–Year Book.

Shea, Y. R. (1995). Specimen collection and transport. In H. D. Isenberg, (Ed. in Chief), P. R. Murray, E. J. Baron, M. A. Pfaller, F. C. Tenover, & R. H. Yolken (Eds.), *Clinical microbiology procedures handbook* (Suppl. 1, p. 1.1.1). Washington, DC: ASM Press.

Sneed, J. O. (1995). Detection of upper respiratory tract carriers of *Staphylococcus aureus* and *Neisseria meningitidis*. In H. D. Isenberg, (Ed. in Chief), P. R. Murray, E. J. Baron, M. A. Pfaller, F. C. Tenover, & R. H. Yolken (Eds.), *Clinical microbiology procedures handbook* (Suppl. 1, p. 1.14.19). Washington, DC: ASM Press.

Sneed, J. O. (1995). Other upper respiratory tract infections. In H. D. Isenberg, (Ed. in Chief), P. R. Murray, E. J. Baron, M. A. Pfaller, F. C. Tenover, & R. H. Yolken (Eds.), *Clinical microbiology procedures handbook* (Suppl. 1, p. 1.14.18). Washington, DC: ASM Press.

Stapleton, F., Willcox, M. D., Fleming, C. M., Hickson, S., Sweeney, D. F., & Holden, E. A. (1995). Changes to the ocular biota with time in extended- and daily-wear disposable contact lens use. [Abstract]. *Infection and Immunity, 63*(11), 4501–4505.

Sundstrom, J., Jacobson, K., Munck-Wikland, E., & Ringertz, S. (1996). *Pseudomonas aeruginosa* in otitis externa: A particular variety of the bacteria? [On-line]. *Archives of Otolaryngology—Head and Neck Surgery, 122*(8), 833–836. Abstract from: MEDLINE

Steuer, M. K., Beuth, J., Hofstadter, F., Probster, L., Ko, H. L., Pulver, G., & Strutz, J. (1995). Blood group phenotype determines lectin-mediated adhesion of *Pseudomonas aeruginosa* to human outer ear canal epithelium. [On-line]. *International Journal of Microbiological, Virological, and Parasitological Infectious Diseases, 282*(3), 287–295. Abstract from: MEDLINE

Tejani, N. R., Chonmaitree, T., Rassin, T. K., Howie, V. M., Owen, M. J., & Goldman, A. S. (1995). Use of C-reactive protein in differentiation between acute bacterial and viral otitis media. [On-line]. *Pediatrics, 95*(5), 664–669. Abstract from: MEDLINE

Tsarkris, A., Psifidis, A., & Douboyas, J. (1995). Complicated suppurative otitis media in a Greek diver due to marine halophilic *Vibrio* sp. [Abstract]. *Journal of Laryngology and Otology, 109*(11), 1082–1084.

Verbraeken, H. (1995). Treatment of postoperative endophthalmitis [Abstract]. *Ophthalmologica, 209*(3), 165–171.

Wanger, A. (1995, October). *Streptococcus pneumoniae . . .* case study. *remel BACTinews 3*(4), 3.

Westergren, V., Forsum, U., & Lundgren, S. (1994). Possible errors in diagnosis of bacterial sinusitis in tracheal intubated patients. [On-line]. *Acta Anaesthesiology Scandinavica, 38*(7), 699–703. Abstract from: MEDLINE

# CHAPTER 29
# The Urinary Tract

William Nauschvetz, Ph.D.

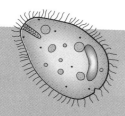

## Microbes in the News
### Vaginal Vaccine May Delay Recurrence of UTIs

An experimental vaccine may help prevent painful recurrences of urinary tract infection in millions of women prone to UTIs. In a study of 91 women susceptible to UTIs, those who received vaginal suppositories containing the vaccine showed a significant delay to reinfection compared with women who took placebo, David T. Uehling, MD, chair of the division of urology at the University of Wisconsin at Madison reported in *The Journal of Urology* (1997; 157:2049–2052). The vaccine uses whole-cell, heat-killed bacteria from ten uropathogenic isolates,

including six *Escherichia coli* strains, a strain of *Esterococcus faecalis*, and a strain of *Klebsiella pneumoniae*. While the vaccine does not promise a cure for UTIs, it seems to safely extend the interval between infections, which could help the substantial number of women who develop frequent UTIs.

La Voie, A. *Vaginal vaccine may delay recurrence of UTIs*. Medical Tribune: Obstetrician & Gynecologist Edition 04(07): 1997. Copyright 1997 Jobson Healthcare Group. Medscape.

## KEY TERMS

Acute urethral syndrome
Asymptomatic bacteriuria
Bacteriuria
Complicated urinary tract infections

Cystitis
Dysuria
Pyelonephritis
Pyuria
Significant bacteriuria

Suprapubic aspirate
Urethritis
Ureteritis
Urinary tract infection
Urine screen

# LEARNING OBJECTIVES

**Upon completion of this chapter, the student should be able to:**

1. Discuss the evolution of the term significant bacteriuria.

2. Compare and contrast the symptoms of cystitis and pyelonephritis.

3. Explain how to properly collect urine specimens from male and female patients.

4. Define the term rapid urine screen and list three examples.

5. Explain how urine is cultured and how colony counts are used to determine the concentration of bacteria in urine.

## INTRODUCTION

The urine culture is one of the most common tests ordered by physicians. In 1991, there were more than 6 million patient visits for **urinary tract infections** (UTIs). Almost 70% of the affected patients were women, and approximately one-half of all women have at least one UTI in their lives. This year, about 3% of all women will develop a UTI, and many will have more than one occurrence during the year (Kunin, 1994; Ronald & Pattullo, 1991).

The term UTI is not very specific. Patients with UTI can range from being extremely ill with bacteremia and sepsis, or they can be totally asymptomatic (see Table 29-1). To discuss the different manifestations of UTI in a more specific manner, these infections are divided into lower UTIs and upper UTIs. Lower UTI includes infection of the urethra (**urethritis**) and bladder (**cystitis**).

Upper UTI includes infection of the ureter (**ureteritis**) and kidney (**pyelonephritis**) (see Figure 29-1).

In addition, UTI can also be subdivided into "complicated" or "uncomplicated" infections. A **complicated UTI** occurs when a patient has structural, neurologic, or medical problems that interfere with normal urination. These infections are usually associated with in-dwelling catheters, stones, or congenital abnormalities. Bacteria can be difficult to eradicate from surfaces provided by the catheter or stones, and as such, these are often persistent infections. The bacteria causing complicated UTI tend to be multiresistant organisms, due to their repeated exposure to various antimicrobials. Most UTIs are uncomplicated and include those that occur primarily in young, sexually active women. Bacterial pathogens causing uncomplicated infections are generally not multiresistant to antimicrobials and generally respond well to antibiotic therapy (Kunin, 1994).

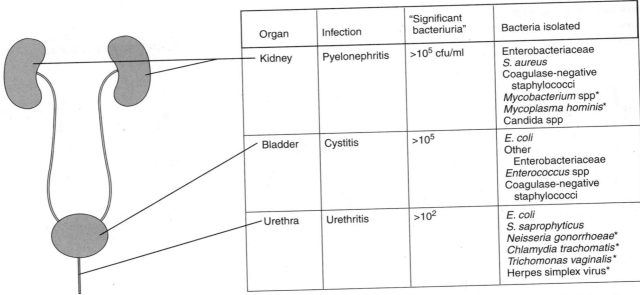

| Organ | Infection | "Significant bacteriuria" | Bacteria isolated |
|---|---|---|---|
| Kidney | Pyelonephritis | >$10^5$ cfu/ml | Enterobacteriaceae<br>S. aureus<br>Coagulase-negative<br>  staphylococci<br>Mycobacterium spp*<br>Mycoplasma hominis*<br>Candida spp |
| Bladder | Cystitis | >$10^5$ | E. coli<br>Other<br>  Enterobacteriaceae<br>Enterococcus spp<br>Coagulase-negative<br>  staphylococci |
| Urethra | Urethritis | >$10^2$ | E. coli<br>S. saprophyticus<br>Neisseria gonorrhoeae*<br>Chlamydia trachomatis*<br>Trichomonas vaginalis*<br>Herpes simplex virus* |

**FIGURE 29-1** Summary of organisms associated with major UTI, and levels of "significant bacteriuria." Agents marked with an asterisk cannot be detected with a routine urine culture.

**Table 29–1 ▶ Clinical Manifestations of Urinary Tract Infections**

| Clinical Manifestations | Symptoms |
|---|---|
| Asymptomatic bacteriuria | Bacteria, but no leukocytes in urine. The patient is asymptomatic. |
| Cystitis | Frequency, dysuria, pyuria, occasional hematuria; fever and flank pain are rare. |
| Urethritis | Frequency, dysuria, pyuria, occasional hematuria; fever is rare. |
| Pyelonephritis | Fever, chills, flank pain, frequency, dysuria, pyuria, hematuria. Patient may be bacteremic. |

## URINE

Physicians collect urine from a patient to help diagnose pyelonephritis, cystitis, and urethritis. A clean-catch midstream (CCMS) urine specimen is usually adequate for this purpose. The use of CCMS urine is relatively new. Prior to the landmark studies of Kass (1957), urine from women and children was collected by catheterization. This provided a high-quality specimen, but the procedure itself was risky because it was invasive and could start an infection. Kass found that noninvasive, clean-catch urines were able to detect pyelonephritis in asymptomatic patients, and eliminated the risks associated with catheterization. Kass also developed what could be called the "100,000 rule," which indicated that a bacterial concentration of more than 100,000 cfu/mL of a single isolate in the urine was a good predictor of pyelonephritis. On the other hand, bacterial counts of less than 100,000 cfu/mL usually indicated a contaminated urine specimen. This simplistic "100,000 rule" is how most laboratories defined **significant bacteriuria** and was used as a criterion for antimicrobial therapy.

This association of 100,000 cfu/mL and infection was determined using asymptomatic women for the diagnosis of pyelonephritis, but that concentration was also used to indicate significant bacteriuria in patients with lower UTIs, as well. Stamm and colleagues (1982) published results of a study that rocked the foundation of the "100,000 rule" by introducing the concept of low-count **bacteriuria.** They found that half the women with symptomatic cystitis and urethritis had bacterial concentrations as low as 100 cfu/mL in urine, and that by applying the 100,000 cfu/mL standard, these women may not have been correctly diagnosed or treated.

## BASIC ANATOMY OF THE URINARY TRACT SYSTEM

The urinary tract includes the kidney, ureters, bladder, and urethra. The kidney and ureters belong to the upper urinary tract, while the lower urinary tract includes the bladder and urethra.

### Upper Urinary Tract

The kidneys are bean-shaped organs, approximately 11 to 13 cm long. The renal tubules are the functional part of the kidney. One end of the renal tubule empties into one of about 500 collecting tubules, which lead urine from the tubules into a collection area called the minor calyx. Urine is then passed through the major calyx, the renal pelvis, and then into the ureter. There are two ureters, each approximately 25 cm long, each connecting a kidney to the urinary bladder.

The main functions of the kidneys are to maintain the ionic concentration and volume of body fluids and to excrete waste products that are removed from the circulatory system. The waste materials include creatinine, urea, and uric acid. The removal process sometimes results in the accumulation of crystalline compounds in the renal pelvis or calyx. These accumulated products are called renal calculi, or kidney stones (Gardner, 1975), which can cause complicated infections.

### Lower Urinary Tract

The urinary bladder is the collection site for urine that is about to be voided. The urine that accumulates in the bladder passes from the body through the urethra. The urethra leads from the urinary bladder to the exterior of the body. The male urethra is about 20 cm long and extends from the bladder to the tip of the penis. By contrast, the female urethra is only 4 cm long. It starts at the bladder and ends at the external urethral orifice, located in the vaginal vestibule. The short length of the female urethra and the location of the urethral orifice are two factors responsible for the higher rate of UTI experienced by women (Gardner, 1975).

## RESIDENT FLORA

Urine itself is normally a sterile fluid after being processed through the kidney and transported to the urinary bladder. However, the urethra is not a sterile site. Large numbers of resident bacterial flora can be present in the distal urethra, and it is necessary to consider these when trying to collect a clinically acceptable urine specimen for culture. The resident urethral flora in females changes with age. In young girls, the urethra is often colonized with gram-positive bacteria, including *Lactobacillus* species, *Corynebacterium* species, coagulase-negative *Staphylococcus*, and *Streptococcus* species. In young women, the urethra is most often colonized with lactobacilli. In elderly women, the most common types of urethral isolates are anaerobic bacteria (Kunin, 1995; Sodeman, 1995). Some bacteria, especially the Enterobacteriaceae and *Enterococcus* species, can ascend the urethra and infect the bladder. These bacteria thrive in urine and can reach concentrations greater than 1,000,000 cfu/mL.

## SPECIMEN TYPES AND COLLECTION

### Specimen Collection (Fowler, 1989; Isenberg, 1995)

Urine is used for laboratory-assisted diagnosis of UTIs. Best results are obtained when culturing the first morning void, which contains bacteria that have been incubating in the bladder overnight. Symptomatic patients can usually be diagnosed with one first-morning urine specimen. Asymptomatic patients may need to submit up to three consecutive urine specimens.

The diagnostic value of urine culture is greatly reduced when urine is contaminated with either distal urethral flora or vaginal secretions. Urine is a good growth medium for enteric bacteria, and a small number of contaminants can reproduce quickly in fresh urine left at room temperature, often resulting in false-positive urine specimens. There are urine transport systems designed to reduce the impact of contamination. Some urine collection systems include a bacteriostatic compound, such as boric acid or barium salts, to inhibit growth of bacteria in the urine during transport (see Figure 29-2) (Dorn, 1991; Lauer, Reller, & Mirrett, 1979; Nicklander, Shanhalzer, & Peterson, 1982). The effects of contamination can also be greatly reduced simply by refrigerating urine specimens if they cannot be immediately transported to the lab after collection (Lewis & Alexander, 1980).

Properly submitted urine specimens should be processed by the laboratory as soon as possible. If there is a delay in processing, the urine should again be refrigerated.

### Midstream Urine (Fowler, 1989; Isenberg, 1995; Miller & Holmes, 1995).

Women should be instructed, using diagrams if possible, on the proper methods for collecting a midstream urine specimen. The patient should:

▶ Remove undergarments to facilitate proper collection.
▶ Wash her hands with soap and water, making sure to rinse all soap from the hands.
▶ Sit facing the back of the toilet, which will naturally place the legs into a more unobstructed position.
▶ Spread her labia with one hand, while washing the exposed area around the urethral opening

with a soap solution, again ensuring that all soap is rinsed from the washed area.
▶ Begin urinating, with labia still spread.
▶ Insert a sterile collection cup into the stream *only* after urinating the first few milliliters of urine into the toilet (the flow should not be interrupted while positioning the cup).
▶ Collect up to a half-cup of urine.
▶ Carefully recap the container, being careful not to get urine on the lip of the cup.

Specimen collection for men is less complicated. The patient must use soapy water to wash his hands, cleanse the penis, and if necessary, retract the foreskin. All washed areas must be rinsed with sterile water or with gauze pads soaked with sterile water. The patient then begins urinating while keeping the foreskin pulled back. He inserts the sterile collection cup into the flow without interrupting the stream.

### Catheterized Urine (Fowler, 1989; Isenberg, 1995; Kunin, 1987; Miller & Holmes, 1995).

Physicians may have to submit a urine specimen collected by catheterization if the patient is physically unable to give a midstream urine, or if culture results from clean-catch urines are difficult to interpret. The decision to catheterize the patient is not made lightly because the procedure may actually cause a bladder infection if aseptic technique is not used.

The two general types of catheterization procedures used to collect urine are the single catheterization (also called straight catheterization and in/out catheterizations) and in-dwelling catheterization.

▶ Single catheterization: The patient must force fluids before the catheterization to extend the bladder. The urethral opening (and vaginal vestibule for women) are washed with soap and water, and the catheter is inserted into the urethra until urine begins to flow (approximately 3 inches in women, 6 inches in men). The first few milliliters are discarded, and the midstream portion is collected aseptically for culture.
▶ In-dwelling catheterization: Because in-dwelling catheters are major risk factors for nosocomial infections, they are not typically used unless patients are seriously ill or debilitated and need assistance in urinating. To collect urine from a catheter in place, the catheter port is disinfected with alcohol, and urine is aseptically aspirated from the collection port with a sterile needle and syringe. The urine is then injected into a sterile collection cup and promptly sent to the laboratory for culture. Foley catheter tips are not acceptable for culture.

### Suprapubic Aspirate.
Suprapubic aspirates (SPA) may be used to collect urine either when the patient

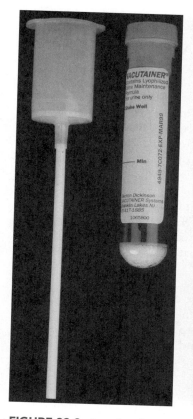
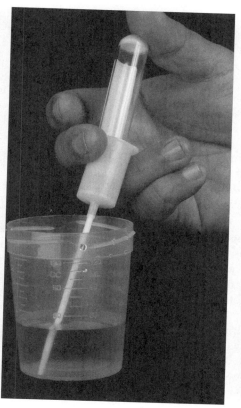
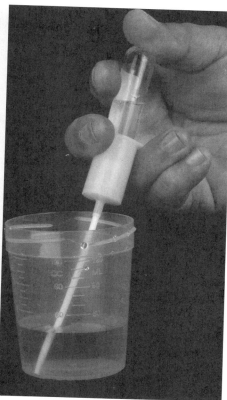

**FIGURE 29-2** A technologist fills a specialized vacutainer tube containing a bacteriostatic compound to preserve urine during transport to the laboratory.

has difficulty in giving a clean-catch urine, or when culture results from clean-catch urines seem difficult to interpret. SPA is often the preferred method for obtaining urine for culture from infants. Prior to the procedure, the patient forces fluids to inflate the bladder. The skin above the bladder is shaved and disinfected. The patient receives a local anesthetic, and the physician punctures the bladder with a needle and syringe, and withdraws approximately 20 mL of urine for culture and urinalysis.

**Bag Urine.** (Fowler, 1989; Kunin, 1987). Physicians can collect urine from children and infants using clean-catch urines, suprapubic aspirates, or by using the so-called "bag urine." The perineal area of the patient must be washed and disinfected before taping the bag over the urethral opening. The device must be removed from the patient as aseptically as possible to avoid contaminating the specimen.

## BACTERIAL DISEASES OF THE URINARY TRACT

### Lower Urinary Tract Infections

**Cystitis.** Cystitis is an infection of the urinary bladder. It occurs more often in women than in men. Cystitis in

men often indicates other problems, such as structural abnormality or immunosuppression. Risk factors in men include lack of circumcision, rectal intercourse (including practicing homosexual partners), and having a female partner who has a vaginal colonization with uropathogenic *E. coli*. Cystitis in men is usually caused by *E. coli*, *Enterococcus* species, or coagulase-negative staphylococci (Stamm & Hooten, 1993).

Cystitis can be either symptomatic or asymptomatic. Patients with asymptomatic cystitis often have bacteriuria without **pyuria**. Asymptomatic bacteriuria is common in young sexually active, elderly, or pregnant women (Gray & Malone-Lee, 1995; Nygaard & Johnson, 1996). Although **asymptomatic bacteriuria** is usually self-limiting in nonpregnant young girls, it can lead to complications in pregnant women. Up to 30% of all pregnant women with untreated bacteriuria develop pyelonephritis (Mikhail & Anyaegbunam, 1995).

In premenopausal women, cystitis is usually caused by *E. coli* or *S. saprophyticus*. In postmenopausal women, the most common causative agents are *E. coli*, other Enterobacteriaceae, and *Enterococcus* species (Nygaard & Johnson, 1996).

*Escherichia coli* causes approximately 80% of all uncomplicated UTIs. When it comes to UTIs, not all strains of *E. coli* are created equal. Uropathogenic strains of *E. coli* have certain virulence factors, such as adhesins, fimbrae, capsules, and hemolysins that facilitate infection. Bacterial fimbrae selectively bind to target tissues of the urinary tract. Bacterial capsules inhibit phagocytosis, and hemolysins may lyse phagocytic cells (Ikaheimo, Siitonen, Karkkainen, Kuosmanen, & Makela, 1993; Kunin, 1994; Miyata et al., 1994).

The second most common bacterial isolate from acute bacterial UTI is *S. saprophyticus*. It is especially common in sexually active young women (Marrie, Kwan, Noble, West, & Duffield, 1982) and may be sexually transmitted. However, *S. saprophyticus* also resides in the rectum, so nonsexual autoinfection can also occur (Rupp, Soper, & Archer, 1992).

**Urethritis.** Urethritis occurs in both men and women. In men, urethritis is often a sexually transmitted infection. The most common causative agents are *Neisseria gonorrhoeae* (causing gonococcal urethritis, or GU) and *C. trachomatis* (a major cause of nongonococcal urethritis, or NGU). Symptoms include urethral exudative discharge and **dysuria**. These bacteria cannot be detected with routine urine cultures (Fowler, 1989).

Urethritis in women can be difficult to diagnose. Women can also get GU and NGU. However, unlike their male counterparts, women often lack urethral exudates with these infections. Women with clinical urethritis can also have a condition called **acute urethral syndrome** (AUS), also referred to as pyuria/dysuria syndrome (Kunin, 1994). AUS has the clinical appearance of other lower UTI in women. However, the symptoms seem to be caused by very low concentrations (as low as 100 cfu/mL) of the pathogen. The infecting bacteria are often *E. coli* or *S. saprophyticus* (Kunin, 1994; Stamm, 1982). To diagnose urethritis in women, urine has to be screened by routine culture (to include detection of low-count bacteriuria), and a urethral swab should be submitted for the detection of *N. gonorrhoeae* and *C. trachomatis* (Fowler, 1989).

## Upper Urinary Tract Infections

**Pyelonephritis.** Pyelonephritis is an inflammation of the kidneys. Symptoms include dysuria, frequency, and urgency, and may include back pain, tenderness, and fever. The inflammation can result from a bacterial infection (usually an ascending infection) or from noninfectious causes. Ascending infections usually involve renal calculi (kidney stones) or some structural problem, such as obstruction (Kunin, 1987).

Uncomplicated pyelonephritis in young women can clinically appear as various manifestations, ranging from cystitis-like symptoms to urosepsis (growth of the UTI isolates in the bloodstream). These patients often have pyuria. *E. coli* causes approximately 80% of all uncomplicated pyelonephritis. As many as 20% of these patients may have low-count bacteriuria (Stamm & Hooten, 1993).

# SPECIMEN PROCESSING, CULTURE, AND INTERPRETATION

Many laboratories perform a quick and easy screen on urines submitted for culture. The purpose of a **urine screen** is to determine if there are high counts of bacteria or white blood cells (WBCs) in the urine. Urine with leukocytes or bacteria is processed for culture. Urine lacking bacteria or WBCs can be classified as "negative by urine screen," eliminating the need for culture.

A common screening test is the leukocyte esterase-nitrate (LE-N) dipstick. The leukocyte esterase matrix on the dipstick can detect as few as 5 WBC/hpf. The matrix for nitrate reductase equates well to the presence of 100,000 bacteria/mL. Many laboratories use a scheme in which urine specimens that are positive for either leukocyte esterase or nitrite are cultured, whereas urines negative for both reactions are listed as "negative by urine screen." Again, this test is only appropriate for CCMS urines, and should not be used to screen SPAs, catheterized urines, or urines from patients who may have AUS (Bailey, 1995; Hagay et al., 1996; Juchau & Nauschuetz, 1984; Nauschuetz, Harrison, Trevino, Becker, & Benton, 1993; Rouse, Andrews, Goldberg, & Owen, 1995; Weinberg & Gan Vanthaya, 1991).

Most laboratories use quantitative culture methods for the detection of bacterial pathogens in urine. A calibrated loop, designed to hold 0.001 mL of urine, is used to streak the specimen onto the battery of media. Typically, most laboratories use a MacConkey agar plate with either a 5% sheep blood agar (SBA) plate, or the more selective 5% SBA with CNA (colistin-nalidixic acid). The latter medium allows for more inhibition of gram-negative bacilli (refer to Color Plate 77).

The pattern of streaking urine onto the media can vary, but a "pin-wheel" streak is common (refer to Color Plate 78). The number of colonies on the plate can be used to calculate concentration of the bacteria in urine, using the formula colony-forming units/mL = number of colonies/ amount plated. For example, if 50 colonies grow on a MacConkey agar plate, then the concentration of bacteria in the urine equals 50/.001, or 50,000 cfu/mL.

The lowest bacterial concentration that can be detected using a 0.001-mL loop is 1,000 cfu/mL. However, urine specimens from patients with AUS or urines collected by catheterization or SPA may have bacterial concentrations as low as 100 cfu/mL. To detect these lower numbers, the technician must inoculate media using a 0.01-mL loop. This larger loop can detect as few as 100 cfu/mL.

There are many published guidelines and recommendations as to what constitutes a "positive" urine culture (Isenberg, 1995; Kunin, Van Arsdale, & Hua, 1993; Sodeman, 1995; Wilson, 1997). To reliably detect a "positive"

**Table 29–2** ▶ **A Scheme for Interpreting Results of Urine Cultures**

| Type of Specimen | Colony Count (cfu/mL) | Number of Isolates | Suggested Action |
|---|---|---|---|
| Catheterized urine/SPA | No growth | | Report as "no growth" |
| | > $10^2$ cfu/mL | 1 | ID/S |
| | | > 1 | Consult with MD; ID/S |
| CCMS | No growth | | Report as "no growth" |
| | $10^2$–$10^4$ | 1–2 | Descriptive ID only. Hold plates for 72 h |
| | >$10^5$ | 1–2 | Full ID/S |
| | >$10^5$ | >2 | Report as "contaminated specimen." Hold plates for 72 h. |

CCMS, clean-catch midstream; ID/S, identification/susceptibility; SPA, suprapubic aspiration

urine culture, laboratory personnel would have to know, among other things, the age and sex of the patient, the patient's symptoms, certain parts of the patient history, and the method of specimen collection. Most laboratories do not have access to most of this data. Therefore, it is up to each laboratory to define what is considered a "positive" urine culture. Table 29-2 provides guidelines when interpreting urine cultures.

▶ All growth (>$10^2$ cfu/mL) from catheterized urine or SPAs are considered significant and are worked up with full identification and susceptibility testing. Technologists call the submittors to confirm collection methods if the specimens grow multiple isolates.

▶ "Significant bacteriuria" from CCMS is considered to be greater than $10^5$ cfu/mL.

▶ If one to two isolates with concentrations less than $10^5$ cfu/mL are recovered from CCMS, the lab reports descriptive identifications and colony counts (e.g., 20,000 cfu/mL of a gram-negative bacillus) on the automated reporting system. The message also indicates these plates will be held for 72 hours. Physicians concerned about low-count bacteriuria may then request full identification and susceptibility of the isolates.

▶ Recovery of more than three isolates indicates contamination. The lab report includes a request for resubmission. These plates are also held for 72 hours to accommodate situations in which the patient may have a complicated UTI.

**Table 29–3** ▶ **Listing of Antimicrobials to Be Considered for Testing of UTI Isolates**

| Antimicrobial | Enterobacteriaceae | Pseudomonas aeruginosa and Other non-Enterobacteriaceae | Staphylococci | Enterococci |
|---|---|---|---|---|
| Carbenicillin | X | X | | |
| Cinoxacin | X | | | |
| Ciprofloxacin | | | | X |
| Ceftizoxime | | X | | |
| Lomefloxacin | X | X | X | |
| Norfloxacin | X | X | X | X |
| Ofloxacin | X | X | X | |
| Loracarbef | X | | | |
| Nitrofurantoin | X | | X | X |
| Sulfisoxazole | X | X | X | |
| Tetracycline | | X | | X |
| Trimethoprim | X | | X | |

In this medical center, representatives from the microbiology laboratory, the pharmacy, and the Infectious Disease Service negotiate which antimicrobials should be included in susceptibility reports for UTI isolates. The National Committee for Clinical Laboratory Standards (NCCLS) issues guidelines for the selection of appropriate reporting schemes. Specific antimicrobials reported by laboratories depend on hospital formulary, the specific automated or semiautomated system used in the microbiology laboratory for susceptibility determination, and cost considerations. Table 29-3 lists the suggested antimicrobials to be tested for UTI isolates (NCCLS, 1995).

## SUMMARY

▶ The term significant bacteriuria is a flexible concept, and often depends on the interpretation of physicians and microbiology laboratory at each hospital.

▶ Results from a urine culture may be meaningless if the patient does not collect the specimen properly, if the specimen is not transported properly, or if the specimen is not plated properly.

▶ Urinary tract infections can be caused by routine uropathogens, in which case they are relatively easy to detect. Symptoms can also be caused by *N. gonorrhoeae* or *C. trachomatis*, which cannot be detected with routine urine culture.

▶ Urine screening can reduce the workload on the urine culture bench by detecting urine lacking evidence of WBCs and bacteria.

▶ Rapid identification and susceptibility testing of UTI isolates is necessary to provide the physician with the best antimicrobial treatment option.

## CASE STUDY

A 30-year-old woman came to the emergency room complaining of a 2-day history of fever, chills, dysuria, and back pain. Her history indicated several similar episodes within the past 15 years. STAT urinalysis indicated increased protein, blood, and WBCs in the urine. The patient, who was also 37 weeks' pregnant, was admitted into the hospital. The patient was started on a 72-hour course of IV cefazolin.

The laboratory reported that the patient's urine had more than 100,000 cfu/mL of *E. coli*. The symptoms of her UTI resolved with treatment. She was discharged with a 10-day course of cephalexin, followed by a 30-day course of nitrofurantoin.

### Questions:

1. Based on the symptoms of the patient, what type of UTI did she have?

2. The physician put the patient on prolonged antimicrobial treatment after her symptoms resolved. Discuss why this might have been done.

3. What are the most common uropathogens associated with this type of UTI?

# Review Questions

1. Which of these cannot be submitted for culture to diagnose UTI?
   a. Bag urine
   b. Foley catheter tips
   c. Suprapubic aspirates
   d. Urine collected from an in-dwelling catheter

2. Which of the following are accepted methods for preserving bacterial counts in urine before laboratory processing?
   a. Dipslide medium
   b. Transport containing barium salts
   c. Transport containing boric acid
   d. All are acceptable.

3. Which of the following best describes pyelonephritis?
   a. Bacteriuria without pyuria and dysuria or fever.
   b. Bacteriuria, frequency, dysuria, pyuria, and occasional hematuria; patient is afebrile.
   c. Fever, flank pain, combined with lower urinary tract symptoms.
   d. Frothy vaginal discharge and pain upon urination.

4. Each of the following describes complicated urinary tract infections EXCEPT:
   a. often involve antibiotic-resistant bacteria.
   b. primarily associated with young, sexually active females.
   c. often indicates an underlying medical or anatomic problem.
   d. associated with recurrences.

5. Urinary tract infections are more common in women than in men because:
   a. the distance from the bladder to the exterior of the body is shorter in women than it is in men.
   b. the urine of men is much more acidic than that of women, and inhibits more bacteria.
   c. The distal end of the female urethra is in an area contaminated with many bacteria.
   d. a and c are true.

6. Which of the following collection methods will likely result in the best specimen from a 6-month-old child?
   a. Suprapubic aspirate
   b. Bag urine
   c. Midstream clean-catch urine
   d. Wet diaper wrung out into a sterile urine cup

7. Acute urethral syndrome:
   a. is characterized by pyuria and high-count bacteriuria.
   b. is caused by *N. gonorrhoeae* or *C. trachomatis.*
   c. may cause symptoms consistent with urethritis or cystitis.
   d. is experienced in men but never in women.

8. Many laboratories use >100,000 cfu/mL to define significant bacteriuria in:
   a. clean-catch midstream urine from asymptomatic patients.
   b. patients with acute urethral syndrome.
   c. patients with nongonococcal urethritis.
   d. in all urine collected by suprapubic aspiration.

9. Asymptomatic bacteriuria:
   a. need never be treated with antibiotics because the infection is self-limiting.
   b. is a risk to pregnant women.
   c. is seen more in men than in women.
   d. is often the result of infection with *N. gonorrhoeae*

10. Which is NOT a virulence factor for uropathogenic *E. coli*?
    a. Hemolysin
    b. Flagellum
    c. Adhesin
    d. Fimbrae

## ▶ REFERENCES & RECOMMENDED READING

Bailey, B. L., Jr. (1995). Urinalysis predictive of urine culture. *Journal of Family Practice, 40,* 45–50.

Dalet, F., & Segovia, T. (1995). Evaluation of a new agar in Uricult-Trio for rapid detection of *Escherichia coli* in urine. *Journal of Clinical Microbiology, 33,* 1395–1398.

Dorn, G. (1991). Microbial stabilization of antibiotic-containing urine samples using the FLORA-STAT urine transport system. *Journal of Clinical Microbiology, 29,* 2169–2174.

Ferguson, J., Tanner, J., & Miller, J. M. (1995). Evaluation of a new, semiquantitative screening culture device for urine specimens. *Journal of Clinical Microbiology, 33,* 1351–1353.

Fowler, J. E. (1989). Bacteriuria: General considerations. In *Urinary tract infection and inflammation* (pp. 42–43). Chicago: Year Book Medical Publishers.

Fowler, J. E. (1989). Bacteriuria in childhood. In *Urinary tract infection and inflammation* (pp. 124–129). Chicago: Year Book Medical Publishers.

Fowler, J. E. (1989). Urethral infection and inflammation. In *Urinary tract infection and inflammation* (pp. 229–252). Chicago: Year Book Medical Publishers.

Gardner, E. (1975). Kidneys, ureters, and suprarenal glands. In E. Gardner, Gray, O'Rahilley (Eds.) *Anatomy* (pp. 406–413). Philadelphia: Saunders.

Gray, R. P., & Malone-Lee, J. (1995). Review: Urinary tract infection in elderly people-time to review management? *Age and Aging, 24,* 251–353.

Hagay, Z., Levy, R., Miskin, A., Milman, D., Sharabi, H., & Insler, V. (1996). Uriscreen, a rapid enzymatic urine screening test: Useful predictor of significant bacteriuria in pregnancy. *Obstetrics and Gynecology, 87,* 410–413.

Ikaheimo, R., Siitonen, A., Karkkainen, U., Kuosmanen, P., & Makela, P. H. (1993). Characteristics of *E. coli* in acute community-acquired cystitis of adult women. *Scandinavian Journal of Infectious Disease, 25,* 705–712.

Isenberg, H. D. (1995a). Specimen collection and transport. In *Clinical microbiology procedures handbook* (pp 1.1.26–1.1.27) Washington, DC: American Society of Microbiology.

Isenberg, H. D. (1995b). Urine culture procedure. In *Clinical microbiology procedures handbook* (pp 1.17.1–1.17.15) Washington, DC: American Society of Microbiology.

Juchau, S. V., & Nauschuetz, W. F. (1984). Evaluation of a leukocyte esterase and nitrite test strip for detection of bacteriuria. *Current Microbiology, 11,* 119–122.

Kass, E. H. (1957). Bacteriuria and the diagnosis of infections of the urinary tract, with observations on the use of methionine as a urinary antiseptic. *Archives of Internal Medicine, 100,* 709–714.

Klahr, S. (1982). Structure and function of the kidneys. In J. B. Wyngaarden & L. H. Smith (Eds.), *Textbook of medicine* (pp. 443–454). Philadelphia: Saunders.

Kunin, C. (1987). The concepts of "significant bacteriuria" and asymptomatic bacteriuria, clinical syndromes and the epidemiology of urinary tract infections. In: *Detection, prevention and management of urinary tract infections,* 4th ed., pp. 57–124. Philadelphia: Lea & Febinger.

Kunin, C. (1987). Diagnostic methods. In *Detection, prevention and management of urinary tract infections,* 4th ed., pp. 195–244. Philadelphia: Lea & Febinger.

Kunin, C. M. (1994). Urinary tract infections in females. *Clinical Infectious Diseases, 18,* 1–12.

Kunin, C. M, VanArsdale, L., & Hua, T. H. (1993). A reassessment of the importance of "low-count" bacteriuria in young women with acute urinary symptoms. *Annals of Internal Medicine, 119,* 454–460.

Lauer, B. A., Reller, L. B., & Mirrett, S. (1979). Evaluation of preservative fluid for urine collected for culture. *Journal of Clinical Microbiology, 10,* 42–45.

Lewis, J. F., & Alexander, J. J. (1980). Overnight refrigeration of urine specimens for culture. *Southern Medical Journal, 73,* 351–352.

Marrie T. J., Kwan, C., Noble, M. A., West, A., & Duffield, L. (1982). *Staphylococcus saprophyticus* as a cause of urinary tract infections. *Journal of Clinical Microbiology, 16,* 427–431.

Mikhail, M. S., & Anyaegbunam, A. (1995). Lower urinary tract dysfunction in pregnancy: A review. *Obstetrical and Gynecological Survey, 50,* 675–683.

Miller, J. M., & Holmes, H. T. (1995). Specimen collection, transport and storage. In *Manual of clinical microbiology* (pp. 19–32). Washington, DC: ASM Press.

Miyata H., Kataoka, S., Moriguchi, N., Yamamoto, T., Michibata, I., Matui, K., & Maki, S. (1994). Antigenic phenotype of *Escherichia coli* in urine from patients with urinary tract infections. *Pediatric Nephrology, 8,* 267–269.

Muñoz, P., Cercenado, E., Rodriguez, C. M., Diaz, M. D., Vincente, T., & Bouza, E. (1992). The CLED agar option in urine culture routine. A prospective and comparative evaluation. *Diagnostic Microbiology and Infectious Disease, 15,* 287–290.

National Committee for Clinical Laboratory Standards. (1995). *Methods for dilution antimicrobial susceptibility tests for bacteria that grow aerobically* (3rd ed). Approved Standard M7-A3. Villanova, PA: Author.

Nauschuetz, W. F., Harrison, L. S., Trevino, S. B., Becker, G. R., & Benton, J. (1993). Two rapid urine screens for detection of bacteriuria: An evaluation. *Current Microbiology, 26,* 43–45.

Nicklander, K. K., Shanhalzer, C. J., & Peterson, L. P. (1982). Urine culture transport tubes: effect of sample volumes on bacterial toxicity of the preservative. *Journal of Clinical Microbiology, 15,* 593–595.

Nygaard, I. E., & Johnson, J. M. (1996). Urinary tract infections in older women. *American Family Physician, 53,* 175–182

Pezzlo, M. (1988). Detection of urinary tract infections by rapid methods. *Clinical Microbiology Review, 1,* 268–280.

Ronald, A. R., & Pattullo, L. S. (1991). The natural history of urinary infection in adults. *Medical Clinics of North America, 75,* 299–312

Rosenberg, M., Berger, S. A., Barki, M., Goldberg, S., & Miskin, A. (1982). Initial testing of a novel urine culture device. *Journal of Clinical Microbiology, 30,* 2686–2691.

Rouse, D. J., Andrews, W. W., Goldberg, R. L., & Owen, J. (1995). Screening and treatment of asymptomatic bacteriuria of pregnancy to prevent pyelonephritis: A cost-effectiveness and cost-benefit analysis. *Obstetrics and Gynecology, 86,* 119–123

Rupp, M. E., Soper, D. E., & Archer, G. L. (1992). Colonization of the female genital tract with *Staphylococcus saprophyticus. Journal of Clinical Microbiology, 30,* 2975–2979.

Sodeman, T. (1995). A practical strategy for diagnosis of urinary tract infections. *Clinical and Laboratory Medicine, 15,* 235–250.

Stamm, W. E., Counts, G. W., Running, K. R., Fihn, S., Turck, M., & Holmes, K. K. (1982). Diagnosis of coliform infection in acutely dysuric women. *New England Journal of Medicine, 307,* 463–467.

Stamm, W. E., & Hooten, T. M. (1993). Management of urinary tract infections in adults. *New England Journal of Medicine, 329,* 1328–1333.

Weinberg, A. G., & Vanthaya, N. G. (1991). Urine screen for bacteriuria in symptomatic pediatric patients. *Pediatric Infectious Diseases, 10,* 651–654.

Wilson, M. L. (1997). Clinically relevant, cost-effective clinical microbiology: Strategies to decrease unnecessary testing. *American Journal of Clinical Pathology, 107,* 154–167.

# CHAPTER 30
## The Genital Tract

Judith S. Heelan, Ph.D.

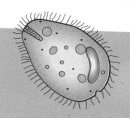

## Microbes in the News

### U.S. Requires Strep B Test in Pregnancy

Federal officials have issued guidelines to screen all pregnant women for streptococcus B infections. Although asymptomatic vaginal carriage is common, the bacteria may infect a neonate, after acquisition during passage through the birth canal. Neonatal sepsis and meningitis, with high fatality rates, may occur.

Babies at greatest risk of infection are those born to women who have already given birth to a child with a group B strep infection, infants born to mothers less than 20 years of age, premature babies, and infants born 18 hours after a woman's amniotic fluid ruptures.

Centers for Disease Control and Prevention (CDC) guidelines published in the *Morbidity and Mortality Weekly Report* were drafted with the help of repre-

sentatives from the American Academy of Pediatrics and the American College of Obstetricians and Gynecologists, and have been endorsed by both groups.

Under the guidelines, women would be tested for strep B infection between 35 and 37 weeks of pregnancy. Those having strep B infection would be informed and offered the option of receiving intravenous antibiotics during labor.

Under these recommendations, the CDC estimates that about one-fourth of all pregnant women could be treated for group B strep, and about 85% of newborn group B strep infections could be prevented.

*The Providence Journal Bulletin,* June 12, 1996.

## KEY TERMS

Bacterial vaginosis (BV)
Buboes
Clue cells
Kissing lesions

Pelvic inflammatory disease (PID)
Salpingitis
Tissue culture

Toxic shock syndrome
Nongonococcal urethritis (NGU)
Vulva

## LEARNING OBJECTIVES

**Upon completion of this chapter, the student should be able to:**

1. Describe the anatomy of the female genital tract.
2. Describe the anatomy of the male genital tract.
3. Describe the normal vaginal flora including variations at different stages of life.
4. Identify appropriate specimen types to diagnose genital tract infections.
5. List and describe opportunistic or pathogenic microorganisms associated with genital tract infections.

## INTRODUCTION

The mucosal lining of the normal human genital tract consists of stratified squamous epithelial cells. Many species of commensal microorganisms inhabit the mucosa, usually causing no harm to the host. The normal flora of the female genital tract is related to age, which affects the pH, as well as production of the female hormone, estrogen. The mucosa of the human vagina contains large amounts of glycogen, which decomposes to organic acids. The resulting acidic environment inhibits microbial growth (Tortora & Anagnostakos, 1984). In the uncircumcised man the area under the foreskin is frequently colonized by a variety of bacteria.

## BASIC ANATOMY OF THE GENITAL TRACT

Biologically, the genital tract is associated with reproduction, the mechanism by which life is sustained, and genetic material is passed from one generation to another. When the sex of an individual is determined at the moment of conception, its femaleness or maleness determines the subsequent development of genital structures (Tortora & Anagnostakos, 1984).

### Female Genital Tract

The female genital tract may be divided into the upper and lower genital tracts.

The upper genital tract includes the uterus, the ovaries, and the fallopian tubes. The uterus serves as the site of development of an implanted embryo and the site of menstruation. It is a hollow organ, shaped like an inverted pear. Tough, thick folds of parietal peritoneum, called the broad ligaments, attach the uterus to the pelvic wall. Uterine blood vessels and nerves pass through the broad ligaments. The layers of tissue that form the uterine wall, from outside to inside are called the serosa, the myometrium, and the endometrium, the mucous membrane lining the uterus.

The paired ovaries are the female gonads and are about the size and shape of almonds. They are attached to the broad ligament of the uterus by a double-layered fold of peritoneum called the mesovarium. The ovarian and the suspensory ligaments attach the ovaries to the uterus, and to the pelvic wall, respectively. The ovaries produce the female hormones estrogen and progesterone, as well as ova (see Figure 30-1).

The fallopian tubes (also called uterine tubes, or oviducts) extend laterally from the uterus and transport the ova to the uterus from the ovaries. The funnel-shaped

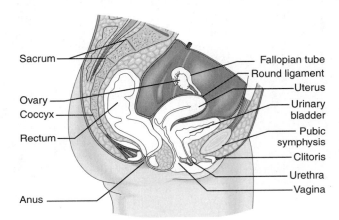

**FIGURE 30-1** Sagittal section of female genital and reproductive organs.

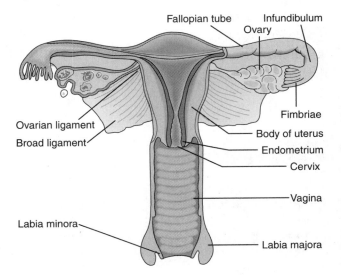

**FIGURE 30-2** Anterior view of female genital and reproductive organs.

open end of each fallopian tube (which is about 4 inches long) has long, finger-like projections, called fimbriae. It is located close to, but not directly attached to, each ovary. The fallopian tubes open into the peritoneal cavity. A potential source of infection at this site may be bacteria entering the body via the vagina.

The lower genital tract consists of the vagina, the cervix, and the external female genital structures collectively referred to as the **vulva** or pudendum. The vagina functions as a sexual organ, which receives the penis during sexual intercourse, a passageway for the menstrual flow, and the terminal portion of the birth canal. It is an elastic, muscular, tubular organ, measuring about 4 inches in length, located between the urinary bladder and the rectum. It is lined with a mucous membrane, consisting of stratified squamous epithelium and connective tissue. The cervix is the inferior narrow portion of the uterus opening into the vagina. The interior cavity is called the cervical canal (see Figure 30-2). The perineal area refers to the diamond-shaped region located between the thighs and buttocks of both men and women.

## Male Genital Tract

The male genital tract (see Figure 30-3) includes the scrotum, the testes, a duct system, and the penis. The scrotum is an outpouching of the abdominal cavity; it is covered with skin and lined with peritoneum. The testes are paired oval male reproductive glands, or gonads, measuring about 1 inch by 2 inches. These glands develop on the embryo's posterior abdominal wall, and usually enter the scrotum at about 32 weeks' gestation. Just before birth, the testes descend completely into the scrotum. They do so by passing through the inguinal canals. The arteries, veins, and nerves constitute the

spermatic cord. The male gonads produce spermatozoa and the male hormone, testosterone.

A system of ducts stores and transports sperm cells. A number of convoluted seminiferous tubules can be found in each testis (see Figure 30-4). When the sperm cells are mature, they pass from the coiled seminiferous tubules to a collection of ducts called the rete testis. The sperm are transported out of the testis through the coiled efferent ducts of the epididymis. The two epididymides are each about 1.5 inches in length; each lies along the posterior border of the testis and consists of the main duct of the epididymis.

Each duct continues as the ductus deferens (vas deferens or sperm duct). It passes from the scrotum, through the inguinal canal as part of the spermatic cord. In the pelvic cavity, it loops over the side and down the posterior surface of the urinary bladder (Solomon & Davis, 1983; Tortora & Anagnostakos, 1984). The vas deferens joins the duct from the seminal vesicles (responsible for much of the semen production) and becomes the ejaculatory duct. After passing through the prostate gland, it opens into the urethra, the single terminal duct of the system. The penis is the erectile male organ designed to deliver sperm cells into the female vagina during sexual intercourse.

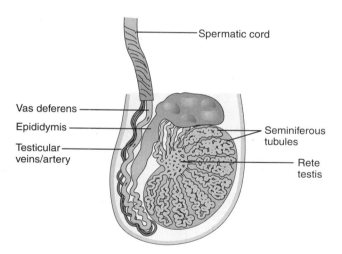

**FIGURE 30-4** Sagittal section of the male testis, showing the duct system used to store and transport sperm.

## RESIDENT FLORA

### Female

The normal flora of the female genital tract varies with age, which affects pH and hormone (estrogen) concentration. At birth, the vagina of a newborn girl is sterile, but during delivery it rapidly becomes colonized with microorganisms present in the mother's vagina, as well as with microorganisms present in the environment. Within a few days of birth, estrogen of maternal

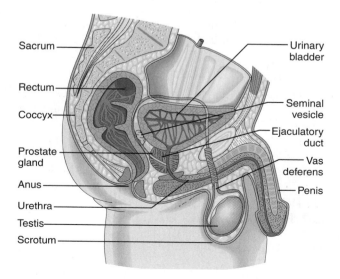

**FIGURE 30-3** Sagittal section of male genital and reproductive organs.

origin promotes glycogen deposition in the epithelium of the infant's vagina, allowing retention of the adult vaginal flora. Lactobacilli predominate in the normal host. When the estrogen level falls within a few weeks, the vaginal epithelium becomes more like surface epithelium. Staphylococci and nonspore-forming gram-positive bacilli in the *Corynebacterium* genus are commonly present in the female vagina before puberty. Micrococci and streptococci may also be present. Anaerobes and enteric bacteria (especially in girls under 2 years of age) may be present as well (Baron et al., 1993).

At puberty, when estrogen levels increase, glycogen is again deposited in the vaginal epithelium. Adult flora then colonizes the normal healthy vagina. Women of reproductive age usually are colonized with large numbers of facultative, aerobic, and anaerobic bacteria. These include lactobacilli (refer to Color Plate 79), staphylococci, streptococci, and enteric bacteria. After menopause, the vaginal flora reverts to that of prepubescence. Differences include a larger number of gram-negative bacilli, and more lactobacilli than in prepubertal girls.

## Male and Female

The vulva and penis may harbor *Mycobacterium smegmatis,* as well as other gram-positive bacteria. This is especially true beneath the foreskin of uncircumcised men. Normal urethral flora include coagulase-negative staphylococci and corynebacteria, as well as a mixture of anaerobes (Baron, Peterson, & Finegold, 1994).

## SPECIMEN TYPES AND COLLECTION

### Discharge and Secretions

**Urethral.** Both men and women may present with urethral discharge when infected with pathogens such as *Neisseria gonorrhoeae* and *Trichomonas vaginalis.* Asymptomatic infection may occur more often in women because the discharge is less pronounced and may be masked more easily. A thin urethrogenital swab is used to obtain a specimen from the urethra; the swab is inserted about 2 cm into the urethra, rotated gently, and removed. When profuse urethral discharge is present, particularly in men, the discharge may be collected without inserting the swab into the urethra. For *T. vaginalis*, material for culture and direct wet mount should be collected on rayon or Dacron-tipped swabs, and transported directly to the laboratory. Transport media, such as modified Stuart's medium, is acceptable.

**Vaginal/Cervical.** A vaginal discharge is the most common female gynecologic complaint. Such specimens are useful for the diagnosis of genital tract infections including those caused by *T. vaginalis, N. gonorrhoeae, Chlamydia trachomatis* and *Candida albicans.* **Bacterial vaginosis (BV)** is associated with production of a malodorous vaginal discharge (Koneman, Allen, Janda, Schreckenberger, & Winn, 1992). These secretions may originate in the walls of the vaginal vault, or may represent the mucopurulent discharge of cervicitis. The differentiation may be made by examination, using a speculum, of the endocervical opening. The external discharge should be wiped away, and fresh pus obtained from the cervical opening should be collected with a swab. Alternatively, a cytobrush may be used to collect infected cells, by inserting approximately ¼ inch into the endocervix. This type of specimen is particularly useful for the diagnosis of *C. trachomatis* (Baron, 1995).

## External Genital Lesion Exudates

**Vesicular.** Vesicular lesions may be found on the glans penis, vulva, perineum, buttocks, or cervix, and are usually associated with infections caused by herpes simplex virus type 2. The lesions are painful and may ulcerate. Specimens are collected by aspiration of vesicular fluid with a 27-gauge needle on a tuberculin syringe. Alternately, the vesicle may be unroofed, and the lesion base scraped with a swab or scalpel blade. The material should be transported in modified Stuart's medium, or some other suitable viral transport medium (Baron et al., 1993; Koneman et al., 1992).

**Ulcerative.** Ulcerative lesions may be present in cases of syphilis, chancroid, granuloma inguinale, and lymphogranuloma venereum. Syphilitic chancres differ from those of herpes by having indurated margins and a clean base; they are usually painless. A diagnosis of syphilis can be made by dark-field examination of lesion material for the presence of spirochetes. Chancroid ulcers are painful and do not have indurated margins (Koneman et al., 1992). Lesions of chancroid are usually ragged, necrotic, and found in pairs, where material from the first lesion autoinoculated an adjacent area (**kissing lesions**) (Baron et al., 1994).

## Miscellaneous Sites

Rectal swabs may be cultured for *N. gonorrhoeae.* Amniotic fluid infection may occur in patients in labor, with prolonged rupture of fetal membranes. Biopsies may sometimes be helpful in the diagnosis of certain genital infections. Urine specimens may provide a noninvasive method in the diagnosis of chlamydial infections.

## OPPORTUNISTIC OR PATHOGENIC BACTERIA

### True Bacteria

**Neisseria gonorrhoeae.** *N. gonorrhoeae* (the gonococcus) is a gram-negative diplococcus. The organism causes gonorrhea and may be isolated, not only from genital sites, but from rectal swabs, the conjunctiva, the oropharynx, and other body sites. The organism is extremely susceptible to temperature changes. Specimens for culture must not be refrigerated (Evangelista & Beilstein, 1993).

***Haemophilis ducreyi.*** *H. ducreyi* is a gram-negative bacillus that causes chancroid, characterized by the presence of painful ulcerative lesions.

***Calymmatobacterium granulomatis.*** *C. granulomatis* is a difficult-to-isolate bacterium that causes granuloma inguinale.

***Gardnerella vaginalis.*** *G. vaginalis* is a gram-variable bacillus that, together with other microorganisms, causes BV, characterized by the presence of a malodorous vaginal discharge.

***Mobiluncus Species.*** Species of *Mobiluncus* have been implicated, along with *G. vaginalis* in causing BV. The organisms are curved, motile, anaerobic gram-negative bacteria, which require prolonged incubation periods of 7 days to several weeks for recovery (Koneman et al., 1992).

***Streptococcus agalactiae.*** *S. agalactiae* (group B streptococcus) may reside transiently in the vagina and may act as an opportunist. Although asymptomatic carriage is common, the bacteria may infect the neonate, after acquisition during passage through the birth canal. Neonatal sepsis and meningitis, with high fatality rates, may occur (Heelan, Letourneau, & Lamarche, 1995).

***Staphylococcus aureus.*** *S. aureus* may be present in the vaginas of healthy women. Certain toxigenic strains may cause the systemic disease known as **toxic shock syndrome**. This illness, initially linked to tampon use, is a rapidly progressive illness that must be diagnosed quickly and treated with antibiotics.

## Other Microorganisms

***Mycoplasma and Ureaplasma.*** The role of *Mycoplasma hominis* and *Ureaplasma urealyticum* as causes of genital tract infection is controversial. Although often found in asymptomatic women, both organisms have been implicated as causes of **pelvic inflammatory disease (PID)**, and may also be associated with premature labor, infertility, and spontaneous abortion. Liquid specimens for culture should be promptly placed in suitable transport media because the organisms are highly susceptible to adverse environmental conditions. Swabs should also be inoculated into suitable transport media. Transport media should be frozen at −70°C, if cultures are not inoculated within a short period of time. Special culture media is required for growth of these fastidious microorganisms (Cassell, Waites, Watson, Crouse, & Harasawa, 1993).

***Chlamydia trachomatis.*** *C. trachomatis* is an obligate intracellular bacterium commonly causing sexu-

ally transmitted disease in North America and Europe. Infections and complications attributed to this organism include cervicitis, urethritis, and infertility. Infants may be infected during birth. Chlamydiae grow mainly in the columnar and squamocolumnar cells of the cervix; a cytobrush or swab is used to obtain cells for culture. Although tissue culture is the gold standard for diagnosis of *Chlamydia* infection, antigen detection and nucleic acid hybridization methods are also available. Specimens for culture must be placed in suitable transport media, and frozen at −70°C, if not cultured immediately (Baron et al., 1993).

***Treponema pallidum.*** *T. pallidum* is a slender, tightly coiled spirochete that causes syphilis. Diagnostic procedures include dark-field microscopy and a number of serologic methods (see Chapter 22).

***Trichomonas vaginalis.*** *T. vaginalis* is a flagellated protozoan frequently found in women with vaginitis. Asymptomatic carriage may occur. Diagnostic methods include wet mount preparations of vaginal discharge, urine, prostatic secretions, Pap smears, as well as culture. In a fresh wet mount, pear-shaped protozoan cells typically exhibit jerky, rapid motility. Culture considerably increases sensitivity, particularly in asymptomatic women, and in colonized men (Baron et al., 1993).

***Candida albicans.*** *C. albicans* is a yeast-like fungus normally present in small numbers as part of the normal vaginal flora. In situations where the normal flora is altered, as with antibiotic usage, overgrowth of *C. albicans* may occur, resulting in vaginitis. Diagnostic procedures include KOH prep or Gram-stained smear and culture of vaginal secretions.

## BACTERIAL DISEASES OF THE GENITAL TRACT

### Gonorrhea

Infection with *N. gonorrhoeae* may present as an asymptomatic infection or disseminated infection. In women, cervical specimens are usually the specimens of choice for culture; using a speculum, endocervical exudate is collected on a swab, and either plated directly on selective media or transported immediately to the laboratory for processing. For normally sterile body sites, a nonselective medium, such as chocolate agar, is preferred. Gram stain of exudate may show intracellular diplococci within polymorphonuclear cells (refer to Color Plate 80).

Gonorrhea in women usually presents as cervicitis; other infections include pharyngitis, anorectal infection, and cystitis. In men, urethritis is the usual presentation, although other infections listed for women, may occur. Neonatal conjunctivitis may be acquired during birth. Complications, including prostatitis and epididymitis in men, and PID in women, may occur. Disseminated gonococcal infection may occur in either sex. The most common manifestation of systemic infection is inflammation of one or more joints, known as septic arthritis. The increasing prevalence of gonococcal resistance to penicillin, as well as to other antimicrobial agents, has caused concern among public health officials (Janda, 1986).

## Syphilis

The causative agent of syphilis is the spirochete, *T. pallidum*. There has been a great increase in cases of both congenital syphilis and newly diagnosed cases of primary syphilis. Diagnostic tests for syphilis include a dark-field examination of material expressed from the syphilitic lesion for spirochetes, as well as a variety of serologic assays. The latter types of assays are more commonly used in the diagnosis of syphilis. Two types of antibodies may be detected—treponemal and nontreponemal antibodies. Nontreponemal antibodies (reagin) are produced by infected patients against tissue cells and are detected using a cardiolipin-lecithin-cholesterol antigen. These assays are usually used as screening tests for syphilis because of their ease of use and low cost. They include the rapid plasma reagin (RPR) card test, and the Venereal Disease Research Laboratory (VDRL) test. Although these assays are highly sensitive, false-positive tests may occur in patients with other conditions, such as infectious mononucleosis, autoimmune disease, and early infection with human immunodeficiency virus (HIV). Treponemal tests are used to confirm positive screening tests because they measure specific antibody to treponemes. The two treponemal assays most often used are the fluorescent treponemal antibody absorption (FTA-ABS) assay and the microhemagglutination (MHA-TP) assay; the *T. pallidum* immobilization (TPI) test is no longer widely used because it requires live *T. pallidum* spirochetes (Baron et al., 1993; Baron et al., 1994).

## Chancroid

This disease, caused by *Haemophilus ducreyi,* is characterized by the presence of painful, necrotizing ulcerative lesions at the site of inoculation. The lesions may be accompanied by inflamed, painful, swollen lymph nodes called **buboes**. Gram stain of material from the lesions may show gram-negative bacteria in a diagnostic "school of fish" formation; however, culture is the only definitive method to make a diagnosis of chancroid. The bacterium is fastidious and must be inoculated immediately onto appropriate media. *H. ducreyi* requires X factor and will grow on enriched chocolate agar. Selective media, containing vancomycin, is preferred. Incubation should be in carbon dioxide for 48 hours. At this time, pinpoint colonies may be visible. The colonies, slightly yellow, become larger with increased incubation and are easy to move around on the plate when pushed with an inoculating needle. Gram-stained colonies show the pleomorphic, gram-negative bacilli characteristic of *Haemophilus* species (Baron et al., 1993; Baron, 1995).

## Granuloma Inguinale

This slightly contagious, usually sexually transmitted, infectious disease, also called donovanosis and granuloma venereum, is caused by the encapsulated, gram-negative bacterium known as *Calymmatobacterium* (formerly *Donovania*) *granulomatis*. The primary lesion is an indurated nodule that erodes, forming a granulomatous ulcer. Diagnosis is usually made by staining ulcer scrapings, or biopsied granulation tissue, with Wright or Giemsa stains. The organisms, called "Donovan bodies," may be seen as clusters of blue- or black-staining intracellular bacteria (Baron et al., 1993).

## Bacterial Vaginosis

Formerly known as nonspecific vaginitis, the name was changed to vaginosis, because of the absence of inflammatory cells. *G. vaginalis* is the gram-variable bacillus associated with this disease, which is characterized by a foul-smelling vaginal discharge. Other microorganisms, such as the anaerobes, *Prevotella* and *Peptococcus* species, as well as *Mobiluncus* species, are thought to work synergistically with *Gardnerella* is causing this infection. The discharge consists mainly of sloughed off epithelial cells, often covered with tiny, gram-variable bacilli (**clue cells**). Diagnosis of BV can be made by culture of *G. vaginalis* on media containing human blood (human blood with Tween 80) or V agar. However, the diagnosis may be made using other criteria. In addition to the absence of abundant lactobacilli on Gram stain, which is seen in the normal vagina, clue cells and a fishy odor on the addition of a drop of 10% KOH, provide strong evidence for the clinical diagnosis of BV (Baron et al., 1994). Color Plate 81 shows the typical Gram-stained smear of vaginal secretions from a patient with BV.

## Nongonococcal Urethritis

**Nongonococcal urethritis** (**NGU**), or nonspecific urethritis, refers to an inflammation of the urethra not caused by *N. gonorrhoeae*. Although NGU affects both men and women, the term is usually reserved for men. It is usually caused by *C. trachomatis*, although *Ureaplasma urealyticum* may be associated with this usually sexually transmitted disease. Diagnosis is generally made by the absence of the gonococcus in culture of urethral specimens. *C. trachomatis* may be grown in **tissue culture**; rapid screening tests available for *Chlamydia* infections include antigen detection methods, as well as nucleic acid hybridization assays. Gen-

Probe (San Diego, California), has developed a single nucleic acid probe to detect both *C. trachomatis* and *N. gonorrhoeae*. The etiology of NGU is less clear when *C. trachomatis* is not isolated. *U. urealyticum* is strongly suspected of causing some of these cases, but asymptomatic carriage is common (Bowie & Holmes, 1980).

## Pelvic Inflammatory Disease

Pelvic inflammatory disease is a collective term given to any extensive infection of pelvic organs in women, including the uterus, fallopian tubes, or ovaries. A vaginal or uterine infection may spread into fallopian tubes, causing **salpingitis**, or to the endometrium, causing endometritis. Infection may spread into the abdominal cavity, causing peritonitis. In most cases, sexually transmitted bacteria first infect the cervix, then pass through the endometrial mucous barrier to reach the endometrium and fallopian tubes. Microorganisms most often

associated with PID include *N. gonorrhoeae* and *C. trachomatis*, although mycoplasmas and other facultative and anaerobic bacteria, often part of the normal vaginal flora, have been implicated. In the diagnosis of PID, *N. gonorrhoeae* or *C. trachomatis* may be cultured. Material for culture may include abscess or free pus, as well as a portion of abscess wall, where bacteria are more likely to be viable, rather than from the necrotic material from the center of the abscess (Baron et al., 1993). Aspirated material collected by needle and syringe is preferred to prevent contamination with vaginal flora. Aspirated material should be placed in an anaerobic transport container and sent immediately to the laboratory. Such specimens may be cultured for mycoplasmas and facultative and anaerobic bacteria, in addition to the gonococcus, and chlamydiae (Baron et al., 1994). Gram stain should always be performed. Rapid screening methods, including antigen detection methods, and nucleic acid probes are also commercially available.

## SUMMARY

► The female upper genital tract includes the uterus, ovaries, and fallopian tubes; the lower genital tract contains the vagina, cervix, and external structures referred to as the vulva.
► The male genital tract includes the scrotum, testes, a duct system, and the penis.
► The normal flora of the female genital tract varies with age, which affects pH and estrogen concentration. Normal flora may also be present beneath the foreskin of uncircumcised men.
► Specimens for culture are collected from urethral discharges, vaginal/cervical discharges, and external genital lesion exudates including vesicular and ulcerative lesions.
► Pathogenic bacteria in the genital tract include *Neisseria gonorrhoeae, Haemophilus ducreyi, Calymmatobacterium granulomatis, Gardnerella vaginalis, Mobiluncus* species, *Streptococcus agalactiae, Staphylococcus aureus, Mycoplasma hominis, Ureaplasma urealyticum, Chlamydia trachomatis, Treponema pallidum, Trichomonas vaginalis,* and *Candida albicans*.
► Among the bacterial diseases appearing in the genital tract are gonorrhea, syphilis, chancroid, granuloma inguinale, bacterial vaginosis, nongonococcal urethritis, and pelvic inflammatory disease.

## Review Questions

1. A potential source of infection in the female peritoneal cavity is:
   a. sepsis.
   b. bacteria entering the body through the vagina.
   c. bacteria in the ovaries.
   d. by aerosol contamination.

2. The vulva refers to:
   a. the male external genitalia.
   b. the female external genitalia.
   c. the uterus, ovaries, and fallopian tubes.
   d. the scrotum and testes.

3. The resident flora of the female genital tract varies with:
   a. age.
   b. estrogen.
   c. testosterone.
   d. two of the above.

4. The predominant microorganisms found in the healthy vagina of adult women are:
   a. staphylococci.
   b. streptococci.
   c. lactobacilli.
   d. gonococci.

5. The most common female gynecologic complaint is:
   a. premenstrual cramps.
   b. painful intercourse.
   c. vaginal discharge.
   d. dysmenorrhea.

6. The following microorganism may be associated with neonatal sepsis and meningitis:
   a. *Neisseria gonorrhoeae.*
   b. *Trichomonas vaginalis.*
   c. *Gardnerella vaginalis.*
   d. *Streptococcus agalactiae.*

7. The microorganism most closely associated with bacterial vaginosis is:
   a. *Neisseria gonorrhoeae.*
   b. *Trichomonas vaginalis.*
   c. *Gardnerella vaginalis.*
   d. *Streptococcus agalactiae.*

8. The microorganism that may cause neonatal conjunctivitis is:
   a. *Neisseria gonorrhoeae.*
   b. *Staphylococcus aureus.*
   c. *Treponema pallidum.*
   d. *Haemophilus ducreyi.*

9. The encapsulated, gram-negative bacterium that causes donovanosis is:
   a. *Neisseria gonorrhoeae.*
   b. *Staphylococcus aureus.*
   c. *Treponema pallidum.*
   d. *Calymmatobacterium granulomatis.*

10. An example of a serologic assay to detect "treponemal" antibodies is the:
    a. RPR card test.
    b. FTA-ABS test.
    c. VDRL assay.
    d. two of the above.

11. Microorganisms most often associated with pelvic inflammatory disease include:
    a. *Neisseria gonorrhoeae.*
    b. *Calymmatobacterium granulomatis.*
    c. *Chlamydia trachomatis.*
    d. two of the above.

12. A disease characterized by painful, necrotizing, ulcerative lesions (often called "kissing" lesions) at the site of inoculation is:
    a. granuloma inguinale.
    b. chancroid.
    c. syphilis.
    d. bacterial vaginosis.

13. A cytobrush is often used to obtain cells for culture in the diagnosis of infection with:
    a. *Chlamydia trachomatis.*
    b. *Neisseria gonorrhoeae.*
    c. *Trichomonas vaginalis.*
    d. *Treponema pallidum.*

14. Which organism has been associated with PID, but which also may cause infertility, premature labor, and spontaneous abortion?
    a. *Chlamydia trachomatis*
    b. *Neisseria gonorrhoeae*
    c. *Treponema pallidum*
    d. *Mycoplasma hominis*

15. Certain toxigenic strains of which organism, initially linked to tampon use, may cause toxic shock syndrome?
    a. *Neisseria gonorrhoeae*
    b. *Staphylococcus aureus*
    c. *Streptococcus agalactiae*
    d. *Treponema pallidum*

## CASE STUDY

A 26-year-old woman was seen in the emergency department with complaints of a painful left shoulder and left knee. She was nauseous and had vomited several times in the past 48 hours. On physical examination she had restricted motion in her shoulder and her left knee was hot and swollen. She was also noted to have a thick vaginal discharge. Her temperature was 39°C; her white blood cell count was elevated at 16,000/mm$^3$. She had a history of having several sexual partners. Cultures and Gram stains were ordered on vaginal secretions and joint fluid. Gram stains showed numerous polymorphonuclear leukocytes. Although no bacteria were seen on smear, both the vaginal and joint fluid cultures grew the causative agent. After the diagnosis was made, tests for HIV were ordered.

### Questions:

1. What is your diagnosis of this patient's infection? What is the association between the vaginal discharge and painful shoulder and knee?

2. Why was HIV testing ordered?

3. Why would there be added concern if this patient were pregnant?

## ▶ REFERENCES & RECOMMENDED READING

Baron, E. J. (1995a, May 22). Female genital tract microbiology comes out of the dark. Part I. *Advance for Medical Laboratory Professionals, 7,* 8–17.

Baron, E. J. (1995b, June 5). Vaginal discharges. Part II. *Advance for Medical Laboratory Professionals, 8,* 12–15.

Baron, E. J., Cassell, G. H., Duffy, L. B., Eschenbach, D. A., Greenwood, J. R., Harvey, S. M., Madinger, N. E., Peterson, E. M., & Waites, K. B. (1993). Laboratory diagnosis of female genital tract infections. In E. J. Baron (Ed.), *Cumitech 17A.* Washington, DC: American Society for Microbiology.

Baron, E. J., Peterson, L. R., & Finegold, S. M. (1994). Genital and sexually transmitted pathogens. In J. F. Shanahan (Ed.), *Bailey and Scott's diagnostic microbiology* (9th ed., pp. 258–273). St. Louis: Mosby.

Bowie, W. R., & Holmes, K. K. (1980). Nongonococcal urethritis. *Clinical Microbiology Newsletter, 2,* 1–3.

Cassell, G. H., Waites, K. B., Watson, H. L., Crouse, D. T., & Harasawa, R. (1993). *Ureaplasma urealyticum* intrauterine infection: Role in prematurity and disease in newborns. *Clinical Microbiology Reviews, 6,* 21–24.

Evangelista, A. T., & Beilstein, H. R. (1993). Laboratory diagnosis of gonorrhea. In C. Abramson (Ed.), *Cumitech 4A.* Washington, DC: American Society for Microbiology.

Heelan, J. S., Letourneau, C., & Lamarche, D. (1995). Detection of group B streptococci by immunoassay following enrichment in LIM-selective broth medium. *Diagnostic Microbiology and Infectious Disease, 22,* 321–324.

Janda, W. M. (1986). Neisseria update. *Clinical Microbiology Newsletter, 8,* 21–24.

Koneman, E. W., Allen, S. D., Janda, W. M., Schreckenberger, P. C., & Winn W. C., Jr. (1992). Introduction to microbiology, Part II; infections of the genital tract. In R. Winters, & A. P. Jirsa (Eds.), *Color atlas and textbook of diagnostic microbiology* (4th ed, pp. 83–88). Philadelphia: Lippincott.

Solomon, E. P., & Davis, P. W. (1983). Reproduction. In M. Brown, A. Satran, C. Field, R. Loe, and R. L. Moore (Eds.), *Human anatomy* (pp. 677–709). Philadelphia: Saunders College Publishing.

Tortora, G. J., & Anagnostakos, N. P. (1984). The reproductive system. In C. M. Wilson & R. Ginsberg (Eds.), *Principles of anatomy and physiology* (pp. 697–729). New York: Harper & Row.

# CHAPTER 31
# The Gastrointestinal Tract

Anne T. Rodgers, MT (ASCAP), Ph.D.
Geneva M. Burch, BS, MT (ASCAP, CLS, NCA), MLT (ASCAP)

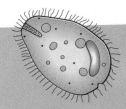

## Microbes in the News
### *Escherichia coli* Can Cause a Potentially Fatal Infection

A third-grade girl became infected with the organism and developed life-threatening complications after eating undercooked beef at a Jack in the Box restaurant. The girl's infection was one in an outbreak that affected 476 people, all of whom ate at the same restaurant in late 1995.

## KEY TERMS

Cholera
Differential media
Dysentery

Food-borne
Gastroenteritis
Normal resident flora

Selective media
Septicemia
Water-borne

## LEARNING OBJECTIVES

**Upon completion of this chapter, the student should be able to:**

1. Discuss procedures for proper collection and transport of fecal specimens.
2. Outline a protocol for direct examination and isolation of enteric pathogens from fecal specimens.
3. Discuss organisms and the diseases they cause in the gastrointestinal tract.
4. List organisms considered "enteric pathogens" and describe characteristics used for their isolation and identification.
5. Describe special problems in culturing and isolating the less common enteric pathogens, *Aeromonas, Plesiomonas, Campylobacter, Vibrio,* and *Yersinia.*

## INTRODUCTION

The gastrointestinal (GI) tract contains an enormous **normal resident flora** microorganism population that includes various bacteria, yeasts, and occasionally protozoans. Many genera are strict anaerobes but most are facultative anaerobes, being able to survive with or without oxygen. The majority of the resident flora are nonspore-forming gram-negative bacilli.

### Importance and Origin of Disease

Due to the structure and function of the digestive system, the GI tract is vulnerable to many infectious agents. Infectious agents such as bacteria, fungi, and parasites cause symptoms and disease by their invasive properties or by producing toxins.

Most infectious microorganisms that cause GI tract disease enter through the oral cavity by ingestion of food or water, by hand to mouth, or by soil contamination of food or water.

### Overview of Microorganisms

Diseases of the GI tract include **cholera, dysentery,** food poisoning, ulcers, salmonellosis, shigellosis, and **gastroenteritis**. The organisms causing these diseases can be extremely virulent. For example, the toxin produced by *Vibrio cholerae* causes extreme diarrhea and electrolyte loss, which can result in death even if small numbers of the organism are ingested. Prompt isolation and identification of the causative agent can be of the utmost importance.

Most of the organisms in the GI tract are part of the normal flora of humans and other animals. However, some are considered opportunistic pathogens and can cause disease in certain circumstances.

## BASIC ANATOMY OF THE DIGESTIVE SYSTEM

### Function

The functions of the digestive system include ingestion, digestion, absorption, and elimination. Ingestion is taking in nourishment for the body. This nourishment, in the form of food, is digested or broken down physically and chemically into small particles. These small particles are then absorbed by the GI tract and passed into the bloodstream where they are transported throughout the body and used for various body processes. During digestion chemical substances are released into the GI tract to assist the process. The leftover secretions are reabsorbed by the tract to be used again. Water, salts, and proteins are also reabsorbed. The materials not reabsorbed or used by the body are eliminated in the form of fecal waste.

### Structure

The digestive system is a long tube beginning with the mouth and ending at the anus. This tube is referred to as the GI tract or alimentary canal. The length of the tube is approximately 30 feet or 9 meters. The GI tract consists of the mouth, esophagus, stomach, small intestines, and large intestines.

The digestive system extends from the mouth through the neck and thoracic area to the abdomen and pelvic cavity. The stomach is just below the diaphragm and the intestines continue from the stomach to the anus.

The digestive system allows one-way transport of material through the GI tract. This is accomplished through the use of muscles within the system. Some muscles contract with rhythmic, wavelike contractions called peristalsis that move material forward. Elimination of fecal material is regulated by sphincter muscles in the rectum. The speed of peristalsis regulates the effectiveness of the system. For example, increased peristalsis contributes to diarrhea and decreased peristalsis results in constipation.

Four accessory organs—the liver, the gallbladder, the pancreas, and the salivary glands—secrete digestive juices at various points in the GI tract to aid in the digestive process. Figure 31-1 shows the parts of the GI tract. Table 31-1 summarizes their functions and Table 31-2 lists the secretions and functions of the accessory organs.

## RESIDENT FLORA OF THE GASTROINTESTINAL TRACT

The fetal GI tract is normally sterile. Microorganisms are first acquired from environmental contacts after birth. In adults, bacteria are present in all areas of the GI tract. The flora of the upper GI tract and the lower GI tract differ in composition.

| Table 31–1 ▶ Digestive Organs and Their Functions | |
|---|---|
| **Digestive Organs** | **Function** |
| Mouth | Chewing pulverizes food and stimulates the salivary glands. |
| Esophagus | Peristaltic muscle movement and gravity move food through the esophageal hiatus into the stomach. |
| Stomach | Hydrochloric acid, pepsin, histamine, gastrin, and intrinsic factor are secreted by the lining of the stomach. Pepsin breaks down proteins. Muscle action pulverizes food and mixes it with stomach secretions. |
| Small intestine | Carbohydrates, lipids, amino acids, and calcium are absorbed by the small intestine after digestion by various enzymes. |
| Large intestine | Absorption and secretion of water, and collection and formation of waste. |

| Table 31–2 ▶ Accessory Digestive Organs, Secretions, and Secretion Functions | | |
|---|---|---|
| **Accessory Organ** | **Secretion** | **Function** |
| Salivary glands | Ptyalin | Digests starch, forming sugars |
| Liver | Bile | Emulsifies fats |
| Gallbladder | Stores and releases bile | Emulsifies fats |
| Pancreas | Amylase, lipase, and trypsin | Breaks down starch, fats, and proteins |

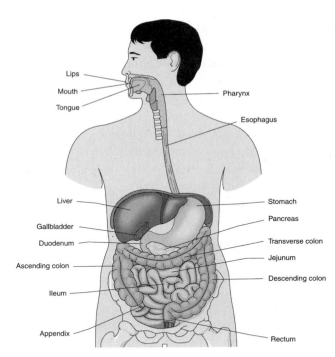

**FIGURE 31-1** Parts of the human gastrointestinal tract.

## Upper Gastrointestinal Tract Flora

Most of the flora present in the oral cavity are contained on the dorsum of the tongue, in dental plaque, and on the gums. Facultative and strict anaerobic streptococci comprise about 50% of the flora. ß-Hemolytic streptococci are not normally part of the oral resident flora. Lactobacilli, staphylococci, spirochetes, fusobacteria, bacteroides, nonpathogenic neisseria, spirillaceae, fungi, viruses, protozoa, and mycoplasmas make up approximately 25% of the oral flora. Another 25% of the flora are veillonellae and diphtheroids.

## Middle Gastrointestinal Tract Flora

The middle GI tract, the area from the throat to the small intestines, has flora derived from swallowed saliva, either mixed with food or swallowed during normal body function. Food and saliva or saliva alone pass too quickly, due to peristalsis, for flora to become established in this area in large numbers.

The acidic contents of the stomach makes this organ a hostile location for most microorganisms to survive. This environment effectively reduces the amount of flora passing into the small intestine.

## Lower Gastrointestinal Tract Flora

As in the stomach where acid produces a hostile environment, the alkalinity of the small intestine is not conducive to survival and the numbers of bacteria are low. Flora present in the small intestine may include

*Enterococcus,* diphtheroids, and lactobacilli with occasional yeast species present in some persons. Certain disease states are a result of overgrowth of the flora in the small intestine.

As food passes through the large intestine the total number of permanent resident flora increases. Resident flora compose about 8% to 25% of feces with anaerobes being the highest in numbers. The organisms present include *Escherichia coli, Klebsiella,* and other facultative gram-negative bacilli of the *Enterobacteriaceae,* anaerobes such as *Clostridium perfringens, Clostridium* species, *Bacteroides,* lactobacilli, anaerobic streptococci, staphylococci, and enterococci.

## Purpose of Resident Flora

Resident flora in the GI tract are necessary for the large intestine to function properly. Bacteria break the food down further. These products are generally used for their own metabolism, but some material is absorbed and used by the body. The large population of microorganisms also serves as a defense mechanism against disease. If small numbers of virulent organisms enter, the resident bacteria will protect their turf and basically "starve" the unwanted intruder. Without this protection, the GI tract would be more prone to disease.

# CLINICAL SPECIMENS

## Types of Specimens

The most common microbiologic specimen collected from the GI tract is feces. However, depending on the disease state, specimens can be collected by swab or directly from any individual area of the digestive system.

Oral specimens can be collected from gums, the throat, and other areas. These types of specimens are usually cultured as respiratory or wound specimens. Stomach contents can also be cultured. If the accessory organs are infected or inflamed, specimens from these areas are collected and cultured.

## Specimen Collection and Transport

For most GI diseases, the specimen of choice is feces. Specimens should be collected in clean, dry containers, not contaminated by urine, and transported to the laboratory immediately. Fecal specimens should be collected before any antimicrobial therapy is started and no preservatives should be added to specimens for bacterial culture. If plating is not done immediately, feces can be refrigerated for up to 1 hour. Fecal specimens should never be placed in an incubator because the normal flora will rapidly overgrow any pathogens present. If the specimen cannot be plated within 1 hour of collection, the specimen should be placed in a transport

media such as buffered glycerol saline or Carey-Blair transport medium. Specimens for parasite examination should be transported in the proper preservatives.

The choice of a system depends on the suspected pathogen. Table 31-3 summarizes transport methods for GI system specimens.

| Table 31–3 ▶ Transport Methods for Gastrointestinal Specimens | |
|---|---|
| **Specimen** | **Transport Method** |
| Anal swab for *N. gonorrhoeae* | *N. gonorrhoeae* transport system or inoculate immediately to Modified-Thayer-Martin media |
| Feces | Carey Blair media, buffered glycerol saline, or sterile screw-cap cup |
| Rectal swab | Swab transport system (anaerobic or other) or a gram-negative broth tube |
| Gastric lavage or washing | Sputum system or sterile screw-cap cup |
| Duodenal aspirate | Sputum system or sterile screw-cap cup |
| Sigmoidoscopy specimen | Sterile screw-cap cup or tube |
| Rectal biopsy | Sterile screw-cap cup or tube without formalin |

## Criteria for Acceptability of Specimens

Fecal specimens more than 2 hours old are unacceptable. If the transport system has an indicator, it should be checked according to the manufacturer's directions for acceptability. The specimens should not be accepted if there is urine or other extraneous material (such as toilet paper) in the container. Rectal or other swabs should not be accepted if they are dry. When an unacceptable specimen is received, the clinician ordering the specimen should be notified and a new specimen requested. The unacceptable specimen should be refrigerated until a new specimen is received, then discarded.

# SPECIMEN PROCESSING

Numerous agents of infectious disease can cause GI symptoms, some requiring special processing to ensure recovery of the agent. Therefore, it is important that the person ordering the culture request the proper type of culture. Most culture protocols are designed to detect the most common pathogens (*Salmonella, Shigella,* and *Campylobacter*). If the clinician suspects other organisms such as *Vibrio, Plesiomonas,* or *Yersinia,* the laboratory must be informed so that the proper culture protocol may be followed to ensure recovery of those pathogens. Other information that may be useful includes the travel history of the patient and information about food consumed and onset of symptoms. This information will help the medical technologist choose the most relevant culture protocol.

## Direct Examination

A Gram-stained smear of feces is not done routinely because so many bacteria are normally present in feces. For the most part, agents of GI disease cannot be presumptively identified by Gram stain. There are exceptions where examination of a direct smear in diarrheal stools may be helpful. These include Gram stain for *Staphylococcus, Vibrio,* yeast, and white blood cells (WBCs) and a methylene blue stain for WBCs. In diarrheal stools, the Gram stain may also be significant if it shows a lack of the usual gram-negative fecal flora or an overgrowth of yeast or gram-positive cocci. Examination for polymorphonuclear cells is useful in determining if an invasive pathogen is present. Liquid specimens may also be directly tested for *Clostridium difficile* toxins.

## Culture Protocol

Due to the extremely high numbers of GI resident flora present in feces, **selective media** must be used to recover GI pathogens. A clinical microbiology laboratory should routinely examine specimens for the presence of *Salmonella, Shigella, Aeromonas, Plesiomonas,* and *Campylobacter.* Isolation of *Vibrio* and *Yersinia* is usually considered a special request. However, in endemic areas such as the Gulf Coast and the lower Eastern seaboard, the protocol should include media for the recovery of *Vibrio* species. Isolates of *E. coli* are tested for enteropathogenic serotypes in certain age groups and on request.

The fecal planting protocol for isolation of *Salmonella* and *Shigella* will include primary culture media, selective **differential media**, moderately selective media, and enrichment broth. Highly selective media are not cost effective for routine use. Cultures are incubated at 35° to 37°C aerobically *NOT* in carbon dioxide. Table 31-4 shows some choices for each of these categories.

Selective differential media will separate lactose-fermenting from nonlactose-fermenting bacilli and will suppress the growth of gram-positive resident flora. MacConkey (MAC) or eosin methylene blue agar (EMB) are examples. Moderately selective media suppresses the growth of most enteric gram-negative rods in a specimen while allowing *Salmonella* and *Shigella* species to grow. Media in this category will indicate the use of sugar to produce acid and some also indicate the production of hydrogen sulfide. Hektoen enteric agar (HE), xylose-lysine-deoxycholate agar (XLD), Salmonella-Shigella agar (SS) or deoxycholate agar (DCA) are examples.

Highly selective media were developed primarily to isolate *Salmonella,* because *Salmonella* colonies are distinctive in appearance and *Shigella* and other gram-negative bacilli are inhibited. Again, these are not recommended for routine use because *Shigella* species are sometimes inhibited. Highly selective media such as brilliant green agar and bismuth sulfite agar have a fairly short shelf-life and are not used in most clinical laboratories.

An enrichment broth is used to enhance the growth of pathogens while suppressing the growth of resident flora in the early hours of culture incubation. Enrichment broths available include gram-negative broth (GN) or Hajna broth for enrichment of Salmonella and Shigella, and selenite F broth for enrichment of Salmonella.

Isolation of *Aeromonas, Campylobacter, Plesiomonas, Clostridium, Vibrio, Yersinia* and enteropathogenic *E. coli* requires the use of specific selective media. Table 31-5 summarizes these media.

*Aeromonas* should be suspected if the patient history includes drinking untreated water or any **waterborne** source of infection. Although *Aeromonas* will grow on EMB and MAC, a selective blood agar with ampicillin (BAP-AMP) is available to aid in isolation from fecal specimens.

*Campylobacter* requires a microaerophilic atmosphere for growth. Isolation media for *Campylobacter* should be incubated at 42°C in an atmosphere that contains 85% nitrogen, 10% carbon dioxide, and 5% oxygen. Several commercial kits are available that provide this microaerophilic atmosphere. Most involve a sealed plastic bag and a miniaturized gas generating system. Selective media for the isolation of *Campylobacter* has antibiotics incorporated into the media to inhibit other

## Table 31-4 ▶ Media for Culture of *Salmonella* and *Shigella* from Fecal Specimens

| Primary Culture Media | Selective Differential Media | Moderately Selective Media | Highly Selective Media | Enrichment Broth |
|---|---|---|---|---|
| Sheep blood agar | MacConkey | Salmonella-Shigella (SS) | Bismuth sulfite | Gram-negative broth |
| Phenylethyl alcohol (PEA) | Eosin methylene blue (EMB) | Hektoen | Brilliant green agar | Hajna Broth |
|  |  | Xylose-lysine-dextrose (XLD) |  | Tetrathionate broth |

| Table 31–5 ▶ Media for Culture of Less Common Fecal Pathogens | |
|---|---|
| **Organism** | **Media** |
| *Campylobacter* species | Skirrow's media |
| | Campy-BAP |
| | Campy-THIO |
| *Aeromonas hydrophilia* | BAP with ampicillin |
| | MacConkey |
| *Vibrio* species | TCBS |
| | Alkaline peptone water |
| Enteropathogenic *E. coli* | Sorbitol MacConkey agar |
| *Plesiomonas* species | Inositol brilliant green bile salts agar |
| *Yersinia enterocolitica* | CIN agar |
| *Clostridium difficile* | CCFA |
| | CDC anaerobe blood (AnBAP) |

BAP, blood agar; CCFA, cycloserine-cefoxitin-fructose agar; CDC, chenodeoxycholic; CIN, cefsulodin-irgasan-novobiocin; TCBS, thiosulfate citrate bile salts sucrose; THIO, thioglycolate

Isolation of *Yersinia* species requires selective media and incubation at 25°C. Cefsulodin-irgasan-novobiocin (CIN) agar is available for this purpose.

In recent years, attention has focused on GI disease caused by enteropathogenic *E. coli*, especially serotype O157H7. MacConkey with sorbitol rather than lactose can help to select this serotype (sorbitol negative) from nonenteropathogenic *E. coli*.

*Clostridium difficile*, the cause of pseudomembranous colitis, grows well on the selective medium CCFA (cycloserine-cefoxitin-fructose egg yolk agar) under anaerobic conditions. The toxin of *C. difficile* is detectable in fecal specimens. This is an alternate method to culture.

## Inoculation of Cultures

Media should be inoculated by use of a swab with a representative sample of the specimen. If blood, mucus, or pus is evident, these areas should be touched with the swab and inoculated to the media. Bloody areas, mucus, and pus are more likely to contain infecting organism.

## EXAMINATION OF CULTURES

Specimens are inoculated to the appropriate isolation media, incubated as appropriate for 18 to 24 hours and examined for the presence of possible pathogenic organisms. Enrichment broths for *Salmonella* and *Shigella* are subcultured to Hektoen or XLD and Salmonella-Shigella agar and incubated at 35° to 37°C for 18 to 24 hours. These plates are then examined for the presence of potential pathogens. Subculture of enrichment broths is done at the time specified by the manufacturer. If the timing is not adhered to, normal flora can overgrow and inhibit or hide the growth of pathogens.

Pathogens have characteristic growth on the selective media used for primary isolation. Table 31-6 summarizes the appearance of common pathogens on selective media.

gram-negative bacilli. Several different formulations are available. All have varying amounts of blood and antibiotics incorporated into the enriched base media. Skirrow's medium and Campy-BAP are commonly used. Skirrow's formula uses lysed horse blood with trimethoprim, vancomycin, and polymyxin B, whereas Campy-BAP uses sheep blood and adds amphotericin B and cephalothin to the above antibiotics. Some *Campylobacter* species are sensitive to cephalothin. If the numbers of *Campylobacter* are thought to be low or prolonged transport is necessary, an enrichment medium such as Campy-THIO may be used. When subculturing this medium it is important to sample the medium at least 12 cm below the surface. Microaerophilic conditions exist at this level in thioglycollate broth.

*Plesiomonas* should be suspected if the patient has a history of eating raw seafood or drinking untreated water. As with *Vibrio*, raw oysters are a common source of infection. *Plesiomonas* will grow on MAC, HE, and XLD but a selective media (inositol-brilliant green-blue salts agar) may be used to isolate the organism.

*Vibrio* species will grow on routine media, but selective media and enrichment are recommended if culture for this organism is requested. Culture for *Vibrio* is considered part of the routine protocol for fecal specimens in certain areas of the country. TCBS (thiosulfate-citrate-brom-thymol-blue-sucrose) agar is the most commonly used selective media for isolation of *Vibrio* species. Because *Vibrio* species prefer an alkaline environment for growth, alkaline peptone media is used for enrichment.

## Screening Cultures

Suspect colonies of *Salmonella* and *Shigella* may be identified by the biochemical identification system used by the laboratory or a screening protocol may be used. This protocol includes urea, triple sugar iron agar (TSI) or Kligler's iron agar (KIA) and lysine iron agar (LIA). The tubes are inoculated with the suspect colony and incubated under ambient conditions at 35° to 37°C for 18 to 24 hours. The tubes are then examined for reactions typical of *Salmonella* and *Shigella*. Motility testing by the wet mount technique is also useful. Pathogens must be definitively identified by the manual or automated method used in that laboratory.

**Table 31–6 ▶ Appearance of Common Gastrointestinal Pathogens on Differential and Selective Media**

| Media | *Salmonella* | *Shigella* | *E. coli* |
|---|---|---|---|
| MacConkey | Colorless | Colorless | Pink |
| Hektoen | Blue to blue-green with black center | Green and moist | Yellow to salmon |
| XLD | Red-yellow with black centers | Red | Large, yellow |
| SS agar | Colorless with black center | Colorless | Pink or red if grows |
| Bismuth sulfite | Dry, black colonies with brown-black precipitate | Inhibited, brown-green if grows | Brownish green if grows, usually inhibited |

Screening by the method above is only appropriate for *Salmonella* and *Shigella*. Commercial screening kits using biochemical or enzymatic reactions and latex agglutination are available to definitively identify most pathogens.

## GASTROINTESTINAL PATHOGENS AND DISEASES

### Candida albicans

*Candida albicans*, a yeast, is normal resident flora of the skin, mouth, and intestinal tract. Infections with this organism have increased in the last decade. Patients with acquired immunodeficiency syndrome (AIDS), diabetes, and those on extended antibiotic therapy or on immunosuppressive drugs are at risk for infections with *C. albicans*.

### Salmonella

Members of this genus cause salmonellosis, a gastroenteritis, enteric fever, and typhoid fever and are therefore clinically significant. Bacteremia can also occur, with or without gastroenteritis. Typhoid fever occurs at a rate of approximately 500 cases per year in the United States and gastroenteritis at a rate of about 50,000 cases. Almost half of the *Salmonella* infections (nontyphoid) occur from contaminated poultry and eggs.

### Shigella

Humans are the only host for the organism and *Shigella* is not considered part of the resident flora. Disease is transmitted by the fecal-oral route. Contaminated water and food are the usual source. *Shigella* is able to resist gastric acidity; therefore, few viable organisms are necessary to cause disease. In the United States, *Shigella sonnei* is the most common cause of infection. Infections occur most often in the summer and fall. Infections are common in sites such as nursing homes and day-care centers when handwashing is not strictly enforced.

Shigellosis or bacillary dysentery is the most common syndrome caused by *Shigella*. The symptoms range from simple gastroenteritis and diarrhea to dysentery (watery diarrhea with blood and mucus) with fever and abdominal pain. Enterotoxins produced by the organism cause fluid and electrolyte loss.

### Campylobacter

*Campylobacter jejuni* subspecies *jejuni* is the most important human pathogen in the genus. It has been recovered from up to 35% of patients with acute diarrhea. The organism is found worldwide. Most domestic animals contain the species as part of their resident flora. Human sources of infection are usually improperly cooked poultry or foods contaminated by raw poultry.

Symptoms of infection with *C. jejuni* include watery, bloody diarrhea, chills, fever, and abdominal pain. The symptoms are due to the production of a cytotoxin, enterotoxin, and cytotoxic factor. The disease is usually self-limiting and will resolve in 3 to 7 days. Only severe disease is treated.

### Vibrio

*Vibrio cholerae* is the causative agent of human cholera, which can occur as an epidemic or pandemic. The enterotoxins produced by the organism cause severe diarrheal disease resulting in life-threatening loss of fluids and electrolytes. The diarrhea is a characteristic "rice-water" stool, so called because of the flecks of mucus in the stool. Outbreaks of cholera have occurred in the United States as recently as 1991 in Texas and Louisiana. This outbreak was related to contaminated crabs, shipped in from an endemic area in South America. If a patient with diarrheal disease has consumed shellfish, had contact with seawater or traveled, the laboratory should consider *V. cholerae* as a possible cause.

*Vibrio parahaemolyticus* and *V. vulnificus* cause **food-borne** gastroenteritis from uncooked, improperly cooked, or improperly handled fish and shellfish, especially in the summer. During warm weather these bacteria can be found in salt water, including backwater, bays, and estuaries all over the world.

Symptoms of *V. parahaemolyticus* infections include abdominal cramps, nausea, vomiting, headache, chills, low-grade fever, and watery, bloody diarrhea. The illness is usually self-limiting, mild to moderate, lasting 2 to 3 days.

*Vibrio vulnificus* causes gastroenteritis, wound infections, and **septicemia**. Infections are associated with consumption of raw oysters and contact with salt or brackish water. Certain medical conditions, especially liver disease and alcoholism, predispose patients for infection by this species.

## Clostridium difficile

*Clostridium difficile*, a gram-positive anaerobic bacillus, has been implicated as the causative agent of pseudomembranous colitis and antibiotic-associated diarrhea. Many patients who are treated with antibiotics for long periods develop diarrhea. However, this is usually self-limiting and disappears when the antibiotics are discontinued. This is not the case with diarrhea due to *C. difficile*. The diarrhea is more severe and persists after antibiotics are discontinued.

*Clostridium difficile* is part of the normal intestinal flora of many animals, including humans. Confirmation of *C. difficile*-associated diarrhea and pseudomembranous colitis may be made by isolating toxin producing *C. difficile* from feces or demonstrating the toxin in fecal specimens. Because it is difficult to grow anaerobes, most laboratories identify the toxin in feces as a means of diagnosis. Many kits are available commercially for this purpose.

## Less Common Organisms

**Yersinia.** The genus *Yersinia* includes the agents of diarrheal diseases and the etiologic agent of human plague. It is the only genus in the tribe *Yersineae*, family *Enterobacteriaceae*. Three of its 11 species are considered major human pathogens: *Y. enterocolitica, Y. pseudotuberculosis,* and *Y. pestis.* Human plague is caused by *Y. pestis* and will not be discussed in detail in this chapter.

*Yersinia enterocolitica* is the most commonly isolated species in human infection and is found worldwide. Human GI infections have been linked to household pets and contaminated milk, food, and water. *Y. enterocolitica* is invasive and produces a potent enterotoxin. Symptoms are similar to acute appendicitis with diarrhea. Appendicitis does not normally cause diarrhea. *Y. enterocolitica* appears as dark red colonies with a bull's eye appearance on CIN. It is a small yellow colony on HE and small, pale, or colorless on MAC and EMB.

*Yersinia pseudotuberculosis* is a natural pathogen of rodents especially guinea pigs and part of the normal flora of domestic fowl. In humans, the toxin produced causes gastroenteritis similar to that caused by *Y. enterocolitica.*

**Aeromonas.** *Aeromonas* is presently a member of the *Vibrionaceae* family; however, a proposal has been made to place the genus into its own family to be called the *Aeromonadaceae* based on molecular genetic studies. *Aeromonas* is found in fresh and sea water and causes infections in aquatic animals, reptiles, and fish. The organisms have also been isolated from drainpipes, tap water faucets, sink traps, and distilled water supplies. These sources are the possible cause of infections in humans. Contact with and drinking these from these contaminated water sources can cause gastroenteritis in humans. Wound infections associated with contaminated water have been caused by some *Aeromonas* species.

*Aeromonas* is associated with five different clinical manifestations of gastroenteritis in humans. These include secretory with acute diarrhea and vomiting, dysenteric with blood and mucus, chronic diarrhea, cholera-like diarrhea with rice-water stool, and traveler's diarrhea. *Aeromonas* should be considered as a pathogen if the patient's infection is water-borne. Fortunately, *Aeromonas* grows well on routine media.

**Plesiomonas.** *Plesiomonas* is also a member of the *Vibrionaceae* family, and has only one species: *shigelloides*. The motile organism is ubiquitous to surface water and is also found in soil and cold-blooded animals such as frogs, snakes, turtles, and lizards. Human infections usually occur by ingestion of unwashed food or contaminated water. Infections also occur from eating raw shellfish, especially oysters, and when drinking water while traveling in foreign countries particularly Central America and Southeast Asia. However, it is less frequently isolated than *Aeromonas.*

*Plesiomonas shigelloides* causes gastroenteritis and cholecystitis in children and adults. Symptoms include mild watery diarrhea without blood or mucus. Patients with gastrointestinal cancer or immunosuppression can have severe colitis or a cholera-like disease. Infections are more prevalent in warm weather. Symptoms are the result of the organism's enterotoxin.

## SUMMARY

▶ Infections of the GI tract are common because of the structure and function of the digestive system. Many infectious agents are spread by the oral route from food and water. Diseases include gastroenteritis, food poisoning, dysentery, cholera, and salmonellosis.

▶ Resident flora of the GI tract varies with location. Most of the flora is located in the lower GI tract. About 8% to 25% of feces is composed of microorganisms. Most are nonpathogenic members of the *Enterobacteriaceae*, but some are considered opportunists. These normal microorganisms are necessary for the proper function of the digestive tract.

▶ Diagnosis of GI disease is most often made by isolation of the causative organism from feces.

Specimen collection and transport are important in ensuring the validity of the culture.

▶ Culture protocol should include differential and selective media appropriate to isolate the suspected organism. The laboratory should be informed if one of the less common pathogenic organisms is suspected.

▶ MacConkey, Hektoen, xylose-lysine-deoxycholate, and Salmonella-Shigella agars are used to isolate *Salmonella, Shigella,* and enteropathogenic *E. coli.* Enrichment broths such as gram-negative or selenite F are recommended in isolation of *Salmonella* and *Shigella.* Other selective media are used for isolation of less common organisms such as *Campylobacter, Aeromonas, Plesiomonas, Vibrio,* and *Yersinia.*

## CASE STUDY

A blood culture, wound culture, and fecal culture are requested on a 56-year-old man in the emergency department (ED). On checking his order in the computer, you notice that his liver function tests are all abnormal. The ED nurse calls the microbiology laboratory and says the man had been fishing yesterday in a salt-water estuary and was hooked in the arm by the fishhook. He came to the ED after complaining of nausea and vomiting and fever.

### Questions:

1. What organism do you suspect?

2. What culture protocol should be initiated to ensure recovery of this organism?

3. In addition to salt-water estuaries, what are other sources of infection with this organism?

4. Why did this patient have the complication of septicemia?

## Review Questions

1. Which of the following is an appropriate isolation media for the organism listed?
   a. *Vibrio cholerae*—BAP with 10% ampicillin
   b. *Aeromonas* species—TCBS
   c. *Salmonella* species—PEA
   d. Enteropathogenic *Escherichia coli*—Sorbitol-MAC

2. What medium is appropriate for isolation of *Campylobacter* species?
   a. Skirrow's medium
   b. Hektoen agar
   c. Sheep blood agar
   d. MacConkey agar

3. Of the following which would require rejection of a fecal specimen?
   a. Collection in a dry, sterile container
   b. A liquid specimen full of mucus
   c. Feces mixed with urine
   d. A specimen that has been refrigerated for an hour

4. What organism causes GI infections due to overgrowth in diabetic or immunocompromised patients?
   a. *Campylobacter* species
   b. *Candida albicans*
   c. *Aeromonas* species
   d. *Vibrio vulnificus*

5. *Shigella* infections, common in day-care centers, are transmitted from person to person most often because of:
   a. contaminated food.
   b. water that is not properly treated.
   c. poor handwashing protocols.
   d. None of the above

6. What part of the GI flora has the largest amount of normally occurring flora?
   a. Upper
   b. Middle
   c. Lower
   d. All of the above

7. What enrichment broth is recommended for isolation of *Vibrio* species?
   a. Alkaline peptone broth
   b. Carey-Blair medium
   c. GN broth
   d. Selenite F broth

8. Gram stain of a fecal sample is useful for:
   a. identification of *Salmonella*.
   b. enumeration of WBCs.
   c. assessing the degree of contamination.
   d. determining motility of *Campylobacter*.

9. Which of the following is considered highly selective media in the isolation of *Salmonella* and *Shigella*?
   a. Hektoen agar
   b. MacConkey agar
   c. Brilliant green agar
   d. CIN agar

10. Which of the following organisms must be incubated at 25°C to ensure recovery from fecal specimens?
    a. *Yersinia*
    b. *Plesiomonas*
    c. *Aeromonas*
    d. *Campylobacter*

▶ **REFERENCES & RECOMMENDED READING**

Isenberg, H. D. (Ed.). (1992). *Clinical microbiology procedures handbook* (Vol. 1 & 2). Washington, DC: American Society for Microbiology.
Koneman, E. W., Allen, S. J., Janda, W. M., Schreckenberger, P. C., & Winn, W. C., Jr. (1997). *Color atlas and textbook of diagnostic microbiology* (5th ed.). Philadelphia: Lippincott-Raven.

Mahon, C. R., & Manuselis, G., Jr. (1995). *Textbook of diagnostic microbiology*. Philadelphia: Saunders.
Rowland, Walsh, Teel, & Carnahan (1994). *Pathogenic and clinical microbiology, a laboratory manual*. Boston: Little, Brown.

# CHAPTER 32

## Skin Infections

S. Vern Juchau, Ph.D., MPH, MA

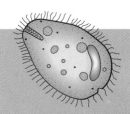

## *Microbes in the News*

### "Flesh-eating Bacteria" Cited in Four Deaths/ Fifth Victim Fighting for Her Life in Hospital

At least four Harris County deaths from the disfiguring "flesh-eating bacteria" have been reported this year, while another victim fought for her life in a local hospital Monday.

In the year's first 51 days, seven cases of the disease known as invasive group A streptococci have been treated in local hospitals. Only eight county cases were reported for all of 1994, the first year that reporting cases of the highly virulent strain of bacteria was required.

An infectious disease specialist at MacGregor Medical Association confirmed that a woman was being treated at a local hospital after surgery Saturday to remove tissue destroyed by the bacteria. She said she could provide no details because of confidentiality requirements.

The death of a man last week was revealed Friday by city Health and Human Services Department officials. His was the third 1995 death reported in the city. The Harris County Health Department has reported two cases this year, including one fatality. The city has had four cases reported this year, while the report on a fifth case is now being prepared and is not yet part of official figures.

A city epidemiologist said Monday that Houston hospitals reported four cases of the disease last year, but she could not say how many, if any, were fatal. Epidemiologists are investigating the city cases to see if there is any link.

Dubbed "flesh-eating bacteria" by tabloids after an outbreak killed at least 12 people in Great Britain last year, the bacteria has been around a long, long time. A researcher with the Baylor College of Medicine has said there are two subtypes of strep A that differ genetically from others that do not attack human flesh with such drastic consequences. Extremely rare, the invasive form of the bacteria struck 10,000 to 15,000 Americans in 1993, the federal Centers for Disease Control and Prevention has said.

The invasive form produces toxins that kill the affected flesh, exacerbating the effects of the infection. Though victims usually have cuts or bruises in the infected area because of trauma, such trauma is not necessary before an infection erupts. Other researchers have postulated that tissue damaged by bruising or cuts provides an ideal breeding ground for the bacteria.

Treatment includes intravenous antibiotics and, if necessary, surgery to remove the disfigured, necrotic flesh often destroyed by the bacteria. Experts differ in their estimates but say death occurs in 50% to 80% of all cases of invasive strep infections. The initial symptoms are similar to that of a flulike illness, including high fever and joint aches that occur before the visible effects on the skin appear. Once that sets in, it (the infection) can progress in a matter of hours.

Source: *Houston Chronicle*, February 1995

## KEY TERMS

Cutaneous
Dermis
Epidermis
Macule

Necrosis
Necrotizing fasciitis
Papule

Subcutaneous
Ulcer
Vesicle

## LEARNING OBJECTIVES

**Upon completion of this chapter, the student should be able to:**

1. Describe the common bacterial causes of skin and wound infections.
2. Have an understanding of specimens that may yield positive results in the diagnosis of skin infections.
3. Understand that culture is usually necessary for the correct diagnosis and proper treatment of skin infections.
4. Describe characteristic features of skin infections.
5. Describe the vast variety of bacteria responsible for skin infections.

## INTRODUCTION

The skin is the natural habitat of millions of bacteria. It is no wonder then that skin infections are common. The fact that they are not more common is because the skin is a natural barrier to infection, containing its own defense mechanisms, and because the majority of bacteria present on the skin do not normally invade the skin, but live there as commensals. Infection normally occurs when the skin is broken through trauma and even then by only a small fraction of the bacterial population of the skin. That is the reason we add antiseptic to wounds and bandage them: to kill or inhibit the organisms already present and to keep out others that may come into contact with the wound.

A variety of well defined skin infections can occur, such as impetigo, folliculitis, furunculosis, erysipelas, cellulitis, **necrotizing fasciitis**, and others. The result-

ing morphologic characteristics manifest can provide a clue to the diagnostician as to the possible etiologic agent(s) involved.

### Types of Lesions

**Macules.** A **macule** is a flat lesion of any size or shape that only differs from the surrounding tissue on the surface in color.

**Papules.** A **papule** is a solid, elevated skin lesion that can be felt (i.e., palpable). They may be any color. Maculopapular refers to any skin eruption that contains both macules and papules.

**Plaques.** A plaque is a large, solid lesion that is palpable. It is essentially a large papule or a coalition of papules.

**Nodules.** A nodule is essentially a papule that extends beneath as well as above the surface. It may extend into the dermis as well as into subcutaneous tissue. The clinician will wish to determine if the nodule is hard or soft, fixed or movable, painful or painless and if it is warm to the touch.

**Vesicles and Bullae.** These are elevated lesions that contain fluid. **Vesicles** are smaller than 0.5 cm in diameter and bullae are greater than 0.5 cm in diameter.

**Pustules.** Pustules are raised lesions containing pus and varying in size, shape, and color.

**Ulcers.** An **ulcer** is a depression in the skin in which the epidermidis and at least the upper layer of the dermis has been destroyed. They have various shapes, borders, and exudates, which provide diagnostic clues. They are more common on pressure areas of the body and over bony prominences and in body folds.

**Cysts.** A cyst is a closed sac with a semisolid or fluid material inside.

## Types of Bacterial Invasion

Epidermal manifestations of bacterial involvement can be categorized into three types:

1. Pathogens that invade the skin and cause moderate to severe damage because of virulent properties that they possess.
2. Opportunists that gain entry through breaks in the skin and cause damage mostly because they are foreign and the body responds to their presence.
3. Organisms that initially invade some other system and develop skin manifestations after becoming systemic. These organisms often spread through the bloodstream. Their skin damage may be only secondary to the original problem, but the skin damage may be the manifestation that the patient recognizes first and for which treatment is sought.

## BASIC ANATOMY OF THE SKIN

The skin is a large organ system that has the primary function of protecting the body. It resists punctures, cuts, and tearing, is flexible, and heals quickly. It is one of the few organs that replaces lost or damaged cells so quickly and easily. It forms callouses to help protect areas of great wear or friction, equivalent to making its own padding. It creates an environment that is unfriendly to bacteria due to high salt or oil concentrations.

The skin is divided into two main layers, the **epidermis** and the **dermis** (see Figure 32-1). The epidermis is the outer layer of skin, approximately 0.4 to 0.6 mm thick, on the average, but ranges from .05 mm on the eyelids to 1.5 mm on the palms and soles. The epidermis is made up of stratified epithelium, the tough outer layer of skin that forms a physical barrier to the outside.

Underneath the epidermis lies the dermis, which ranges from 0.3 mm on the eyelid to 3.0 mm on the back. It is composed of connective tissue and contains the hair follicles, nerves, and blood vessels. The epider-

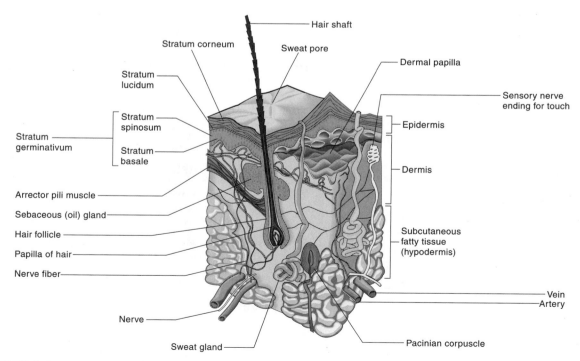

**FIGURE 32-1** Basic anatomy of the skin.

mis and the dermis make up the **cutaneous** tissue of the body. That layer of tissue below the cutaneous layer is called **subcutaneous** tissue.

## RESIDENT FLORA

Microorganisms of many types literally cover the human body. The composition of the resident flora of the skin is constantly changing, depending on the habitat, work environment, state of cleanliness, activity of skin glands, and the close contact of the host with different sources of bacteria. There may be significant differences between individuals.

Certain species such as *Staphylococcus epidermidis* and *Propionibacterium* species may be found anywhere on the skin. Others tend to be more localized. For example, the corynebacteria are more likely to be found in moist areas. The skin flora is resistant to the lipids and fatty acids of the skin, which tend to kill other bacteria.

The normal flora of the human skin includes:

A. Gram-positive organisms
1. Bacillus
2. Diphtheroids
3. Micrococcus
4. Mycobacterium
5. Peptococcus
6. *Propionibacterium acnes*
7. *Staphylococcus aureus*
8. *Staphylococcus epidermidis*
9. Streptococci
10. Yeast

B. Gram-negative organisms
1. Acinetobacter
2. Other gram-negative bacilli

Those most commonly found include *Staphylococcus* species, *Corynebacterium* species (see Figure 32-2 and refer to Color Plate 82), *Propionibacterium* species, *Mycobacterium* species (see Figure 32-3), and various yeasts. Areas adjacent to body orifices often have a population reflecting the population of the orifice. For example, gram-negative enteric bacilli may be readily isolated from the skin surrounding the anus.

## SPECIMEN TYPES AND COLLECTION

Although a swab may be the easiest way to collect a specimen for microbiologic testing, it is usually not the best way. Whenever possible, it is advisable to get an aspirate of at least a few milliliters from a closed abscess using a needle and syringe. Before obtaining this specimen, the overlying skin should be carefully disinfected to avoid contaminating the specimen with normal skin flora. The specimen thus obtained will serve as its own transport medium and provide plenty of material with which to work.

From an open wound, it is preferable to clean out the purulent material, which will contain large numbers of contaminating skin flora, and swab the posterior wall of the wound or abscess. This, then, should be placed in a transport medium for transfer to the laboratory to avoid drying out of the specimen. Excised tissue specimens are also good diagnostic specimens, especially if contaminated areas can be avoided. For deep wounds,

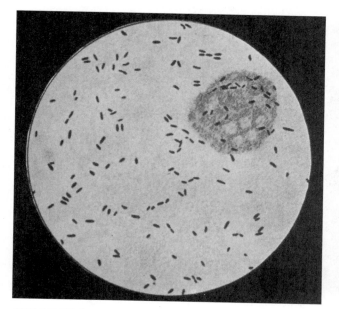

**FIGURE 32-2** *Corynebacterium acnes* from pustule on the face. (Courtesy of Centers for Disease Control and Prevention, Atlanta, GA)

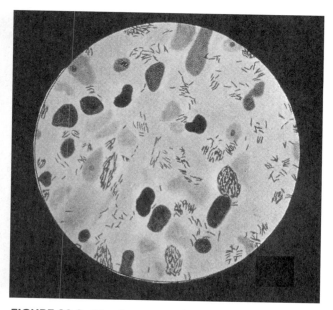

**FIGURE 32-3** *Mycobacterium leprae* from leprosy skin lesion. (Courtesy of Centers for Disease Control and Prevention, Atlanta, GA)

culture should include attempts to grow anaerobic organisms. For these, it is necessary to transport specimens under anaerobic conditions, either by using an anaerobic transport medium or by placing the specimen in an anaerobic atmosphere during transport. Skin scrapings may also serve as suitable specimens from dry lesions.

Whenever possible, specimens should be taken before therapy is initiated. Because specimens from the skin are often contaminated with skin flora, it is important to culture the specimens as soon as possible to avoid overgrowth of nonsignificant bacteria that will make it difficult to recover slow-growing organisms such as mycobacteria. If transport is to be delayed, specimens should be refrigerated. All specimens should be submitted in sterile containers.

Tissue should be submitted in sterile normal saline. If culture for *Mycobacteria* species is desired, the tissue should be submitted in sterile Middlebrook 7H9 or 7H11 broth. Tissue is the preferred specimen for suspected mycobacterial skin infections. The yield from swabs of open lesions is very poor.

For determination of bacterial load, as in cases of leprosy, skin smears and nasal scrapings are often used. Slitting and scraping skin lesions, or the earlobe if no lesions are present, will provide a specimen suitable for this determination. Ideally, skin-slit smears should be collected from several areas showing the most active skin eruptions.

## OPPORTUNISTIC OR PATHOGENIC BACTERIA

It is often a dilemma for the clinical microbiologist to determine which isolates from a superficial site are etiologic agents of the disease process and which are merely there because they normally reside on the skin. Under certain conditions or in an immunocompromised host, normal flora can become opportunistic or even invasive pathogens. Wound flora depends on the site of the wound, how the wound was inflicted, what degree of environmental contamination occurred, and the immunocompetence of the host.

### Opportunists

Opportunistic bacteria most likely to be isolated from wound infections are listed in Table 32-1.

## BACTERIAL DISEASES OF WOUNDS AND OTHER SUPERFICIAL SITES

### Staphylococcal Infections

Staphylococci are the most common cause of skin diseases and superficial wound infections. Staphylococcal infections are suppurative, cause **necrosis** of

### Table 32–1 ▶ Opportunistic Skin Pathogens

| Gram-Negative Organisms | Gram-Positive Organisms |
|---|---|
| *Acinetobacter* species | *Bacillus anthracis* (rare) |
| *Bacterioides* | *Candida albicans* |
| *Eikenella corrodens* (rare) | *Clostridium* |
| *Escherichia coli* | Enterococci |
| *Flavobacteria* | *Erysipelothrix rhusiopathiae* |
| *Fusobacterium* | *Mycobacteria* species |
| Enterobacteriaceae | *Nocardia asteroides* |
| *Pasteurella multocida* | *Peptostreptococcus* |
| *Prevotella* species | *Staphylococcus aureus* |
| *Propionibacterium acnes* | *Staphylococcus epidermidis* |
| *Proteus* species | Streptococci (groups A, B, D and microaerophilic) |
| *Pseudomonas pseudomallei* | |
| *Xanthomonas maltophilia* | |

local tissues, and tend to form pus-filled abscesses. They may cause boils, furuncles, pustules in the newborn, and superficial folliculitis. Staphylococci are the major cause of suppurative parotitis and frequently cause cellulitis. They are the most common cause of mastitis in women and wound infections in all humans. They produce powerful exotoxins that may have severe effects on the skin. Staphylococcal enterotoxin B is even capable of causing dermatitis when applied to intact skin. There is evidence that *S. aureus* may play a role in the pathogenesis of atopic dermatitis.

### Streptococcal Infections

*Streptococcus pyogenes* is known by several names, among them, group A ß-hemolytic streptococcus is the most accurate and descriptive. This is often shortened to group A strep. These are gram-positive cocci that occur in chains (see Figure 32-4).

*Streptococcus pyogenes* is associated with or the cause of several conditions affecting the skin. Among these are toxic shock syndrome, erysipelas, necrotizing fasciitis (caused by the so-called "flesh-eating bacteria"), and streptococcal pharyngitis ("strep throat"). Invasive group A streptococcus infections appear to have been increasing in recent years. These infections are more common in infants and the elderly. In a study performed in Canada, it was found that 56% of patients with invasive streptococcal infections had underlying chronic diseases. Risk factors included infection with human immunodeficiency virus (HIV), cancer, diabetes, alcohol abuse, and chickenpox. Fourteen percent of the cases were nosocomial and were often

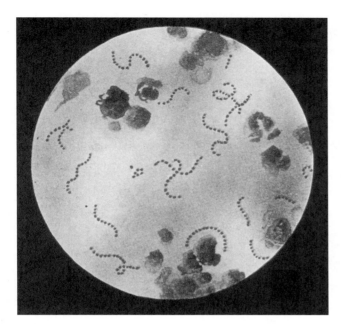

**FIGURE 32-4** *Streptococcus pyogenes* in short chains, from pus. (Courtesy of Centers for Disease Control and Prevention, Atlanta, GA)

associated with outbreaks, indicating the contagious nature of these infections.

These organisms have thus far been susceptible to penicillin, but some infections have been resistant to erythromycin, a penicillin alternative used for patients allergic to penicillin. Treatment with antibiotics alone is most inadequate, partly because the circulation to the gangrenous area is damaged, and the organisms are isolated from the penicillin. Aggressive surgical debridement must be used to treat these infections successfully.

*Streptococcus pyogenes* is a skillful opponent with many tools at its disposal. Streptolysins O and S, hyaluronidase, pyrogens, toxins, all contribute. If it eventually adds penicillin resistance, or resistance to other drugs, it will become an even more formidable opponent.

## Necrotizing Fasciitis

Necrotizing fasciitis is a soft tissue infection of the layer of tissue between the skin and muscle, which progresses rapidly and is life-threatening. It is usually caused by toxin-producing, virulent bacteria. It is accompanied by fever, toxicity, and perhaps local pain. It occurs more commonly in patients who are immunosuppressed or have underlying vascular disease. There is some evidence that pregnancy may predispose a woman to necrotizing fasciitis. The abdominal wall, perineum, and extremities are the most common sites of infection. Necrotizing fasciitis may begin as an innocuous break in the skin—a cut or scratch or a chickenpox lesion that is scratched. Surgical wounds may also serve as entry points for organisms. Once the organisms enter, they produce toxins and erode the fas-

cia (layer just beneath the skin). The nerve endings are also damaged, so the patient may not complain of any pain until after much damage is done.

The majority of cases yield a mixture of organisms on culture of the wound. When multiple organisms are involved, necrotizing fasciitis is usually caused by enteric pathogens. When only a single organism is involved, it is usually a member of the skin flora. Aerobic or facultative bacteria only are recovered in about 10% of cases, anaerobic bacteria are the only isolates in about 22% of cases, and mixed aerobic-anaerobic flora are recovered in about 68% of cases. An average of four to five isolates per specimen are recovered. Organisms recovered tend to reflect the flora of the anatomic location of the infected site. Anaerobic bacteria outnumber aerobic bacteria at all sites, but are most commonly isolated from the buttocks, trunk, neck, external genitalia, and inguinal areas. *S. pyogenes, S. aureus,* and *E. coli* are the most common aerobic causes of this affliction. Predominating anaerobic isolates are *Peptostreptococcus* species, *Prevotella* species, *Porphyromonas* species, *Bacteroides fragilis* group, and *Clostridium* species. Isolates tend to correspond to certain clinical findings or predisposing conditions: *B. fragilis* group, *Clostridium* species, *S. aureus, Prevotella* species, and group A streptococci are associated with edema; *Enterobacteriaceae* and *Clostridium* species with gas formation; *Bacteroides* species are associated with a foul odor; *Clostridium* species with trauma; *Bacteroides* species, *Enterobacteriaceae,* and *S. aureus* with diabetes; group A streptococci with varicella; *Pseudomonas aeruginosa* with burn infections; and *Pseudomonas* species and *Enterobacteriaceae* with cancer and immunosuppression. The damage to tissue and the systemic toxicity that occurs are thought to be due to the release of endogenous cytokines and toxins of the bacteria. If debridement is not initiated fairly early in the course of the disease, the mortality rate is high.

*Streptococcus pyogenes* infections are not uncommon, but necrotizing fasciitis is a relatively rare complication of these infections. A cluster of necrotizing fasciitis infections in England was highly publicized in 1994. These infections were *not* an outbreak of a rapidly spreading, easily communicated organism. The cases were caused by several different M-types, indicating that these cases were caused by different organisms. In past years, the incidence of necrotizing fasciitis has remained steady. Studies in Scandinavia, England, and the United States indicate these rates are not changing. Drug resistance to penicillin, which is already found in staphylococci and other organisms, emerging in *S. pyogenes* would be of even more serious consequence.

Diagnosis of necrotizing fasciitis is a clinical judgment. Laboratory testing may supplement, but rapid treatment, including surgical debridement, should begin before the laboratory results are complete in most cases. This creates a dilemma for the clinician who must distinguish among necrotizing fasciitis and other infections that present similar symptoms.

## Mycobacterial Infections

Mycobacteria are a diverse group of microorganisms that stain with acid-fast stains. They are gram-positive bacilli, fastidious in nature and have a tendency to be slow growers.

**Leprosy.** Leprosy is not as prevalent as it used to be. This can be attributed in large part to the initiation of multidrug therapy introduced in 1981. In fact, in the last 10 years the prevalence of leprosy has decreased from 10 to 12 million cases to about 2.5 million cases worldwide. This disease occurs only in humans and animals. To date no other source has been found, but it has been speculated that some environmental sources may occur. Leprosy has become rare in the United States, but it is still prevalent in developing countries. The disease affects more men than women, and the average age at onset is between 10 and 20 years. The portal of entry of the organism is thought to be primarily through breaks in the skin, but some evidence suggests that entrance through the respiratory tract may have some importance. Subclinical infections do occur as evidenced by high antibody titer to *Mycobacterium leprae* in the blood of contacts of leprosy patients. Only a small percentage of contacts develop the disease.

*Mycobacterium leprae* is an obligately intracellular parasite and may be found in a variety of cells in infected individuals including macrophages, Schwann cells, muscle cells, and endothelial cells. However, it affects primarily skin and peripheral nervous tissue. It is easier to detect than it used to be because of the advent of techniques such as the polymerase chain reaction (PCR), and it is now considered to be a curable disease. Eradication is a future possibility.

Several animals are susceptible to infection with this organism, including the nine-banded armadillo, which is quite commonly infected in Louisiana (about 20%). The most common source of infections appears to be family members or children.

Patients with leprosy exhibit a variety of different manifestations that seem to correlate with the host's susceptibility to *M. leprae*. The spectrum of disease ranges between the lepromatous form and the tuberculoid form with five classification groups being used worldwide. The tuberculoid form is characterized by the formation of lesions, usually single, which are erythematous or hypopigmented macules having a slightly elevated border. Patients sometimes lose their hair and find their sense of touch to be impaired. Acid-fast bacilli are not usually seen in the tissues, but granulomas with giant cells surrounded by lymphocytes are seen in the dermis and sometimes in the epidermis. Lepromatous leprosy is characterized by the forma-

tion of diffuse macules, papules, and nodules. Acid-fast bacilli may be found in skin smears or biopsies of macules or papules.

It is important to determine the bacterial load in cases of leprosy because it is an indication of the patient's susceptibility to *M. leprae*. Skin smears and nasal scrapings are commonly examined. The morphologic index, which is a measure of viable cells, is used to monitor the effectiveness of treatment.

Serologic tests may also be done to aid in diagnosis of leprosy, but the sensitivity of available tests is poor. PCR has recently been shown to be very sensitive and may become the method of choice for detecting *M. leprae* infections.

**Nontuberculosis Mycobacteria Infections.** The source of these infections is mainly environmental. When these organisms are isolated in association with an infection, it is important to verify that they indeed are the causative agent and not just an environmental contaminant. Contamination of laboratory equipment or reagents can often be determined when the same organism is isolated from several specimens processed over a short time. The nontuberculous mycobacteria can be found in many places in the environment in all areas of the world. They may be found in the soil or water or on the skin and in the stools of healthy individuals. Some of them, however, such as *M. haemophilum, M. ulcerans, M. genavense,* and *M. szulgai* have never been isolated from the environment, even though the epidemiology of infections caused by them often suggests environmental sources. In a study done in Africa, 67 strains of mycobacteria were isolated from skin scrapings of forearms and thighs. The predominant isolate was strains belonging to the *Mycobacterium avium complex* (MAC). Other isolates from the skin, which may represent only colonization, include *M. intracellulare, M. scrofulaceum, M. chelonae, M. fortuitum, M. malmoense,* and *M. flavescens. M. gordonae, M. fortuitum, M. terrae, M. simiae, M. flavescens, M. scrofulaceum* and MAC may also be isolated from the stools of healthy individuals. Skin and intestinal tract colonizations probably originate from environmental sources.

Nontuberculous mycobacteria may be isolated from postinfection abscesses. These are most commonly due to contamination of the injection solution. *M. fortuitum* and *M. chelonae* are well known to be implicated in these infections. It is important to ensure that the solutions used for injection are sterile.

*Mycobacterium ulcerans* causes skin ulcers known as Buruli ulcers. This ulcer is characterized by necrosis of the dermis and underlying layers of skin, often causing massive destruction of those tissues. They are most commonly found on the limbs, but may be present on other areas of the body. After healing, the victim may be left with gross deformities. To date it has only been reported from tropical countries in Africa and central and southeast Asia. Its source appears to be environmental although it has not yet been isolated from the environment.

Among the rapid growing mycobacteria, *M. fortuitum* and *M. chelonae* are the most likely to be involved in skin infections. They are common in the environment, grow in 3 to 7 days, and may grow on routine media as well as specific mycobacterial media. Infection may be acquired after a minor wound has occurred in the outside environment or through surgical intervention. The vast majority of cutaneous mycobacterial infections are caused by members of this group. Two-thirds of cutaneous infections caused by this group are caused by *M. fortuitum* and one-third are caused by *M. chelonae*. Infections with this group manifest in the skin more than half the time. Most cases occur after surgery with the rest resulting from trauma or secondary infections of primary skin infections caused by other organisms. Lesions may present in a variety of forms, but in most cases they eventually become ulcers. Patients with sarcoidosis are especially subject to infections with these organisms and may present with nasal and oral lesions that are erosive.

*Mycobacterium marinum* is a common cause of skin infections associated with water and fish. It is a cause of fish infections and aquarium owners are at risk for infection with this organism. Cutaneous infections with this organism used to be called "swimming pool granuloma," but proper chlorination of swimming pools has caused this source of infection to disappear. However, virtually any water-related activity has the potential of exposing the participant to infection, and infection is most common in those who have water-related hobbies or activities.

## Boils, Furuncles, Pustules, Superficial Abscesses

Boils, or furuncles, are skin infections of hair follicles, sebaceous glands, or sweat glands. They often follow acne conditions. If the infection occurs at the base of an eyelash, a stye is formed. Often, the patient is infected with his own carried strain of staphylococci, which is usually carried in the nose.

If the infection of a furuncle spreads to the subcutaneous tissue, one or more abscesses may develop, which are known as carbuncles. These are more common on the back of the neck, but may be found elsewhere. This infection may spread further into the bloodstream and become quite serious.

Bullous impetigo is a very communicable skin infection of the superficial layers of the skin characterized by large blisters that are teeming with staphylococci. This infection is most common in children and is spread from person to person via contaminated fomites. Staphy-

lococcal strains involved produce exfoliatin and so this is a localized form of scalded skin syndrome.

*Staphylococcus epidermidis* is associated with pimples and is often accompanied by *P. acnes*. *P. acnes* probably plays an important role in the pathogenesis of acne vulgaris, but it is not clear that it ever acts alone. It appears to contribute to the duration and severity of inflammation. This gram-positive bacillus constitutes a large portion of the normal flora of skin. It makes its appearance when the host reaches puberty and reaches a population of about $10^5$ colony-forming units per hair follicle. *P. acnes* produces a number of extracellular enzymes and other proteins that probably play a role in the course of acne. Although not strict anaerobes, they are more likely to be isolated from anaerobic than from aerobic cultures.

## Impetigo

The etiologic agents of impetigo are *S. aureus* and *S. pyogenes*. They often are both isolated from patients with impetigo. Impetigo may be spread through skin-to-skin contact.

The early lesion is a vesicle or pustule surrounded by erythema. It progresses rapidly to develop a yellow-brown crust. It may then penetrate deeper into the dermis creating a crater-like ulcer called ecthyma (see Figure 32-5).

About 75% of cases are in people less than 25 years of age, and 35% are in those less than 10 years of age. In Europe, most cases are caused by *S. aureus;* in the United States, the majority of infections are caused by *S. pyogenes*.

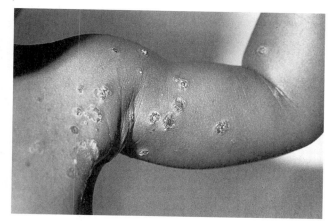

**FIGURE 32-5** Impetigo. (Courtesy of Robert A. Silverman, M.D. Clinical Associate Professor, Department of Pediatrics, Georgetown University)

## Cellulitis

Cellulitis is often caused by streptococci and staphylococci. Streptococci involved may be aerobic or anaerobic. However, the most common anaerobic cause of cellulitis is the clostridia. It is not unusual for mixtures of bacteria to be involved with cellulitis. In children less than 3 years of age, *Haemophilus influenzae*, a fastidious gram-negative bacillus, is often the etiologic agent. It may sometimes be caused by other organisms such as nongroup A streptococci, *P. aeruginosa,* or *Campylobacter fetus.*

Cellulitis is a rapidly advancing deep inflammation of the skin characterized by swelling and erythema. It involves the dermis and subcutaneous tissue. Often spread to the lymphatic tissue is involved, which may progress to septicemia. It typically occurs near surgical wounds or cutaneous ulcers, but may develop in normal skin (see Figure 32-6).

A subcutaneous form of cellulitis, caused by streptococci, is called erysipelas. It differs from other forms of cellulitis by prominently involving the lymphatic tissue, creating a streaking effect. It is superficial and has sharper margins than ordinary cellulitis. It commonly affects the legs, ears, and face.

Identification of the infectious agent is best done by culture. Culture of the area with the greatest inflammation, using an aspirate of the area, is the most productive.

## Anthrax

Anthrax is a rare disease in the United States and Europe. However, it is still common in parts of Africa, Asia, and Eastern Europe. It is caused by *Bacillus anthracis,* a spore-forming gram-positive bacillus that is encapsulated. It primarily occurs in herbivorous animals and humans become infected when they come in contact with animals or animal products. In developed areas, it is usually acquired through occupational exposure to animal products such as leather. Cutaneous anthrax accounts for more than 95% of anthrax cases, and lesions are normally found on exposed surfaces that have received a minor trauma such as an abrasion. The organisms grow rapidly, releasing toxins that produce marked inflammatory edema and necrosis. The incubation period is 1 to 3 days after which the initial lesion is a small itching papule that may be mistaken for an insect bite. This develops into a vesicle surrounded by a broad area of edema. The lesion evolves into a hemorrhagic necrotic area often covered by an eschar. The bacilli can be demonstrated in a Gram-stained smear from the lesion. From the cutaneous lesion, the bacilli may become bacteremic and cause systemic symptoms, including fever, hypotension, and septic shock. The infection may be confused with several other types of infections, but diagnosticians should be alerted to anthrax when a painless ulcer surrounded by a zone of edema is present. Recovery of the organism from infected tissue or blood culture is confirmatory. If cutaneous anthrax is untreated, death occurs in 5% to 20% of cases.

## Wound Infections

**Traumatic.** Traumatic wounds are often infected by members of the normal skin flora, including *S. aureus, S. pyogenes, P. aeruginosa, E. coli, Acinetobacter* species, *Proteus* species, enterococci, and flavobacteria. Environmentally contaminated wounds may be infected with the anaerobic clostridia. These include the agents of gas gangrene including *Clostridium perfringens* (see Figure 32-7), *Clostridium septicum,* and *Clostridium novyii.* If the wound is not deep, these

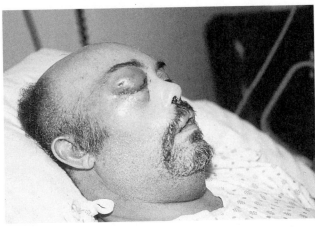

**FIGURE 32-6** Cellulitis. (Courtesy of Dr. Mark Dougherty, Lexington, KY)

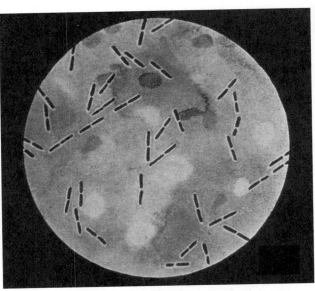

**FIGURE 32-7** *Clostridium perfringens.* Gas bacillus from gas gangrene. (Courtesy of Centers for Disease Control and Prevention, Atlanta, GA)

organisms may be present but not cause any problems. *Clostridium tetani* may be a problem in nonimmunized individuals if the wound is deep.

**ANIMAL BITE WOUNDS.** Bite wounds by dogs and cats, when infected, usually become infected with the normal flora of the biting animal. Bite wounds by dogs are often infected with *Pasteurella multocida,* and bite wounds by both dogs and cats may become infected with *Bacteroides* and *Prevotella* species. The latter two are anaerobic gram-negative rods that are difficult for the average clinical laboratory to identify because the species involved do not appear in the data bases of anaerobic identification kits.

**HUMAN BITE WOUNDS.** Human bite wounds are generally more serious than animal bite wounds. Humans carry more pathogens in their oral cavity than do animals, and human bites are more likely to result in a serious infection. *S. aureus, Eikenella corrodens, Haemophilus* species, and anaerobic bacteria are likely causes. Anaerobic bacteria are involved more than 50% of the time.

## Scalded Skin Syndrome

This is a condition in which superficial layers of the skin peel off just as they would if large areas of the body had been scalded. It is caused by certain strains of *S. aureus* that carry a phage that produces exfoliatin, an exotoxin responsible for separation of layers of the skin. Two distinct toxins may be produced, one chromosomally mediated and one mediated by a phage. A single strain of *S. aureus* may contain either or both. The skin peeling may occur at sites remote from the location of the infected site. The toxins are absorbed into the bloodstream and may cause peeling at sites remote from the primary site of infection. This disease is found more commonly in children less than 5 years of age, although it may occur in adults. It tends to occur on the face, axilla, and groin first, later spreading to other parts of the body. It generally results from a localized infection that may or may not be easy to locate.

## Actinomycosis

Several members of the genus *Actinomyces* may cause skin infections, but *Actinomyces israelii* is most common in humans. These are gram-positive, branching, nonspore-forming anaerobic bacilli that live as commensals in the oral cavity and respiratory and digestive tracts. Infections are rare in modern day. Around half of all infections are on the head or neck. These organisms are thought to be transmitted by flies and can be isolated from healthy animals. Not surprisingly, infections from it are most common in rural settings. Infections tend to be deep abscesses or ulcers developing after a mucosal injury. The formation of sulfur granules at the infection site is characteristic of this organism. The organisms are difficult to isolate in culture because of their fastidious nature. Thus, they are only cultured from active infections about 30% of the time. A microscopic examination of lesion material characteristically reveals sulfur granules that contain branching, pleomorphic, gram-positive rods. One must be aware that *Nocardia* can also form sulfur granules so it is not an absolute sign of actinomycosis.

Actinomycosis usually presents as a palpable mass, which may be reddish purple, on the head or neck, sometimes painful. The most common sites are the lower jaw and the cheek. In 40% to 60% of the patients, a draining sinus may be present, but it is often not present when the patient is first seen. Tissue surrounding the mass is usually quite firm. Isolates are universally sensitive to penicillin and therapy is usually successful.

## Nocardia Infections

Six species of *Nocardia* cause infections in humans. Of these, *N. otitidiscaviarum, N. brasiliensis,* and *N. asteroides* are the most common. *N. asteroides* is responsible for about 90% of human infections, and the other two species account for most of the rest. *N. asteroides* is more commonly seen as opportunistic infections in immunocompromised hosts, whereas *N. brasiliensis* causes disease in immunocompetent individuals. They are gram-positive filamentous bacteria commonly found in soil. They are aerobic and stain with acid-fast stains.

Primary skin infections are usually caused by *N. brasiliensis* and only occasionally by the other two species. Cutaneous manifestations present in many different ways from lymphoid tissue involvement to superficial ulcers, abscesses, pustules, and cellulitis. Subcutaneous infections can include actinomycotic mycetoma, a chronic granulomatous mass with multiple draining sinuses. Subcutaneous infections usually are a result of trauma involving soil contact.

## SYSTEMIC INFECTIONS WITH SKIN INVOLVEMENT

Almost any infection that is bacteremic may lead to skin lesions. This is particularly true if the patient is immunocompromised. For example, *Mycoplasma hominis*, which is not usually found in skin infections, has been reported to cause sternal wound infections after cardiac surgery.

In effect, any organism that is present in the bloodstream may find a home in a wound where it may be filtered out due to poor circulation in the area or the presence of scar tissue that impedes blood flow. Once there, if conditions are right, the organism will multiply. Its growth, toxic and invasive properties, and metabolic substances thrown off during metabolism and death may cause tissue damage.

## Organisms That May Be Involved

Bacteria that may be involved in systemic infections with skin involvement are shown in Table 32-2.

## Lyme Disease

Lyme disease is a global disease with major geographic foci. The etiologic agent is *Borrelia burgdorferi*. It is transmitted to mammalian host by ticks of the genus *Ixodes* and by the lone star tick (*Amblyomma americanum*). Each stage of the tick life cycle must have a blood meal giving them three opportunities to transmit an infection. A history of contact with a tick, along with typical symptoms, should alert clinicians and laboratorians to the possibility of this diagnosis. Although this is primarily a systemic infection, one of its hallmarks is a skin inflammation known as erythema migrans, which occurs in 70% of infected humans. Erythema migrans consists of expanding circular skin lesions surrounding the area of the tick bite with central clearing and a bright red outer border. About half the patients have more than one lesion resulting from hematogenous spread of the spirochetes near the skin surface. The spirochetes may be isolated from biopsies taken at the border of the lesions. However, diagnosis is usually made through serologic testing and observation of clinical symptoms.

## Cat Scratch Disease

Cat scratch disease is caused primarily by *Bartonella henselae,* but some cases may be caused by *Afipia felis.* These organisms are difficult to cultivate, and diagnosis is usually made serologically. An interesting observation of *B. henselae* is that if a drop of broth from a blood culture infected with this organism contains some red blood cells, the bacteria may be seen entering and leaving the blood cells. Blood culture has been the most effective method for culturing these organisms.

As the name implies, this infection is strongly associated with a cat scratch or bite. *B. henselae* has been isolated from the blood of cats indicating that cats serve as a reservoir of infection for humans. However, one-third of patients have had no association with cats and probably pick up the organism from the soil where it is indigenous. Soil is probably also the source of infection for the cat.

Cat scratch disease is usually a self-limited disease, but will usually respond to ciprofloxacin if treatment is deemed necessary.

## Tuberculosis of the Skin

As with leprosy, the source of this infection is human or animal with no environmental reservoir being known. Cutaneous infections with *M. tuberculosis* are not very common, but they are likely to increase as the population becomes more and more immunocompromised. It is important to be able to diagnose these infections so that adequate therapy can be carried out.

Cutaneous manifestations of tuberculosis usually occur after pulmonary infection has occurred. From the primary site of infection, the bacteria migrate via the lymph and bloodstream to set up a secondary site of infection wherever fixed macrophages phagocytize them. The cell-mediated immune response that results leads to an intense inflammatory reaction at the site of deposition. This generally appears as a small brownish red papule, which, after several weeks, evolves into an ulcer, usually less than 1 cm in diameter, but occasionally as large as 5 cm. The lesions may present as abscesses or chronic draining sinuses. They occur mainly on the face and extremities in children, but other sites, particularly those recently involved in trauma of some kind may be affected. Both initial and mature lesions may be mistaken for

| Table 32–2 ▶ Bacteria Involved in Systemic Infections with Skin Involvement | | |
|---|---|---|
| **Gram-Negative** | **Gram-Positive** | **Other** |
| *Afipia felis* | *Candida albicans* (rare) | *Borrelia burgdorferi* |
| *Bartonella* | *Mycobacterium tuberculosis* | *Treponema* species |
| *Francisella tularensis* | *Staphylococcus aureus* | |
| *Haemophilus influenzae* | *Streptococcus pyogenes* | |
| *Neisseria gonorrhoeae* | | |
| *Neisseria meningitidis* | | |
| *Pasteurella pestis* | | |
| *Salmonella typhi* | | |
| *Streptobacillus moniliformis* | | |
| Many others, particularly in the immunocompromised | | |

other infections so culture is necessary. It is wise to do a direct smear of the lesion and stain it by acid-fast staining if tuberculosis is considered in the differential diagnosis. A problem with this is that many forms of cutaneous tuberculosis do not typically have many mycobacteria present in the skin so that acid-fast smears are usually negative. Culture may be positive, but it takes weeks for the organism to grow in culture. Fortunately, more rapid techniques, such as DNA detection, are becoming available but at present are available only in specialized laboratories.

Persons who have already developed an immune response to *M. tuberculosis*, as demonstrated by a positive tuberculin reaction, develop granulomatous lesions that are warty in appearance. Because most people who develop extrapulmonary tuberculosis are already immune, this is the most common type of tuberculous skin infection. In endemic areas, it is most commonly seen in children who inoculate their extremities or buttocks while playing. In other areas, it may be seen as the result of occupational exposure among butchers, farmers, or morticians. Over time, the warty lesions may develop fissures that can become secondarily infected with other bacteria.

Patients with active deep tissue tuberculosis may be inoculated at other body sites by organisms shed from the deeper tissues. These lesions are often found around body openings, such as the anus or mouth, which lead to the site of infection. This type of infection is rare, but when it does occur, it develops necrotic ulcers with acid-fast bacilli easily demonstrated.

## Toxic Shock Syndrome

Toxic shock syndrome is not really a systemic infection with skin manifestations, but rather a localized infection with systemic manifestations, some of which are dramatic skin effects. It became well known in the late 1970s and early 1980s when cases were associated with superabsorbent tampons that were left in long enough for staphylococci to use them as a focus of infection. It is characterized by rash and desquamation of the skin, along with fever and severe shock. It was caused by strains of *S. aureus* that produce toxin TSST-1. It may be associated with localized staphylococcal infections in both sexes.

Group A streptococci cause a toxic shock-like syndrome that is a disease that is invasive and bacteremic. Although toxin plays a major part in this syndrome, other factors are involved, such as M proteins, capsular polysaccharides, and other enzymes excreted by the organism. More than half the patients have severe soft tissue infections, such as necrotizing fasciitis. Patients are usually young, normally healthy individuals. It usually starts with localized pain and influenza-like symptoms. The mortality rate approaches 30%. The dominant virulence factor appears to be extracellular proteins called streptococcal pyrogenic exotoxins. Overall, cases of this syndrome are relatively rare because most people are immune to one or more of the virulence factors or lack the required antigen receptors. Rapid diagnosis of these infections is important because they tend to quickly progress to hypotension, organ failure, and death. Penicillin is the treatment of choice for most streptococcal infections, but an inhibitor of protein synthesis, such as clindamycin, may be more effective for treatment of toxic shock-like syndrome.

## Scarlet Fever

Scarlet fever is caused by *S. pyogenes* strains that produce a toxin responsible for a diffuse rash on the body. Because the first infection results in an immunity to the toxin, subsequent infections with toxin producing *S. pyogenes* will not produce the rash.

A scarlet fever-like syndrome can occur with pharyngeal infection by *Arcanobacterium haemolyticum*. This manifests as an extensive exanthematous eruption of the skin on the trunk and proximal areas of the extremities. This, like scarlet fever, may be diagnosed by isolating the organism from a throat culture.

## SUMMARY

► Skin infections may be caused by essentially any species of bacteria that have the potential to cause disease in humans, particularly in immunocompromised humans. The most common skin invaders are *Staphylococcus aureus, Streptococcus pyogenes,* and various anaerobic bacteria.
► Skin infections may range from a small papule or vesicle to extensive deep necrosis of tissue. Serious systemic manifestations, such as toxic shock syndrome or scalded skin syndrome, may also occur.

► The etiologic agents of most skin infections may be readily determined through culture and microscopy. However, a few are difficult to diagnose and may require other techniques such as serology or polymerase chain reaction.
► Many skin and wound infections are polymicrobial, and all organisms recovered should be identified.
► A patient history is important in determining the most likely source and etiologic agent of infection.

## CASE STUDY

A 40-year-old Hispanic woman was seen for a chronic draining wound and an abnormal chest film. The patient was in excellent health until 4 to 5 months previous to being seen, when she was struck by her right scapula by a refrigerator door. One to 2 months later she noted a raised pustule over the area in question. The patient was seen by her primary care physician who opened the lesion and prescribed ciprofloxacin. Over the next month she noticed what she felt were some bone fragments coming from this site as well as clear fluid. An x-ray done of the chest and scapula revealed possible osteomyelitis of the right scapula and an abnormal left chest. The patient was referred to both an orthopedic surgeon and a pulmonologist.

The orthopedic surgeon did initial debridement and culture. *P. acnes* was initially grown and the patient was placed on high-dose penicillin. The wound did not heal and presented to the infectious disease specialist as a fistula with surrounding discoloration. Specimens were obtained for culture.

**Questions:**

1. Imagine you are the microbiologist tasked with the responsibility of culturing these specimens. What organisms would you suspect might be responsible for this infection?

2. What is the significance of *P. acnes* in this case?

## Review Questions

1. Which of the following are part of the normal flora of the skin?
   a. *Salmonella* and *Shigella*
   b. Corynebacteria and *Staphylococcus epidermidis*
   c. *Mycobacterium leprae* and *Erysipelothrix rhusiopathiae*
   d. *Haemophilus influenzae* and *Nocardia brasiliensis*

2. What are the best specimens to obtain for culture of skin lesions?
   a. Dry swabs
   b. Pus from the surface of the wound
   c. Blood and hair
   d. Aspirate from a closed abscess or tissue

3. Opportunists generally invade the skin through:
   a. the mouth.
   b. breaks in the skin.
   c. the respiratory tract.
   d. by directly penetrating the skin.

4. What are the most common bacterial agents of skin and wound infections?
   a. Viruses and fungi
   b. *Staphylococcus epidermidis* and viridans streptococci

   c. *Staphylococcus aureus, Streptococcus pyogenes,* and anaerobic bacteria
   d. Mycobacteria

5. Which bacteria commonly cause impetigo?
   a. *Streptococcus pyogenes* and *Staphylococcus aureus*
   b. *Erysipelothrix rhusiopathiae*
   c. *Mycobacterium marinum*
   d. *Corynebacterium minutissimum*

6. What is the skin infection caused by *Erysipelothrix rhusiopathiae* called?
   a. Impetigo
   b. Erythrasma
   c. Leprosy
   d. Erysipeloid

7. Which description fits *Bacillus anthracis?*
   a. Gram-negative coccobacillus
   b. Gram-positive, spore-forming bacillus
   c. Gram-positive coccus occurring in chains
   d. Filamentous bacillus that is anaerobic

8. What is the most common cause of actinomycosis in humans?
   a. Anaerobic streptococci
   b. *Actinomyces israelii*
   c. *Actinomyces brasiliensis*
   d. *Actinomyces otitivariscarium*

9. Skin infections with severe systemic manifestations that include desquamation (peeling) of the skin include which of the following?
   a. Toxic shock syndrome and scalded skin syndrome
   b. Necrotizing fasciitis
   c. Leprosy
   d. Cat scratch fever

10. Material from an infected dog bite wound was Gram stained. Microscopic examination of the stained smear showed gram-negative coccobacilli. What is the most likely organism that will be isolated?
    a. *Escherichia coli*
    b. *Pasteurella multocida*
    c. *Franciscella tularensis*
    d. A *Clostridium* species

## ▶ REFERENCES & RECOMMENDED READING

Agger, W. A., & Mardan, A. (1995). *Pseudomonas aeruginosa* infections of intact skin. *Clinical Infectious Diseases, 20*(2), 302–308.

Alexander, C. J., Citron, D. M., Gerardo, S. H., Claros, M. C., Talan, D., & Goldstein, E. J. C. (1977). Characterization of saccharolytic *Bacteroides* and *Prevotella* isolates from infected dog and cat bite wounds in humans. *Journal of Clinical Microbiology, 35*(2), 406–411.

Brogan, T. V., Nizet, V., Waldhausen, J. H., Rubens, C. E., & Clarke, W. R. (1995). Group A streptococcal necrotizing fasciitis complicating primary varicella: A series of fourteen patients. *Pediatric Infectious Disease Journal, 14*(7), 588–594.

Brook, I., & Frazier, E. H. (1995). Clinical and microbiological features of necrotizing fasciitis. *Journal of Clinical Microbiology, 33*(9), 2382–2387.

Cockerell, C. J., & Bottone, E. J. (1995). *Bartonella* infections. Evolution from the esoteric. *American Journal of Clinical Pathology, 104*(5), 487–490.

Davies, H. D., McGeer, A., Schwartz, B., Green, K., Cann, D., Simor, A. E., & Low, D. E. (1966). Invasive group A streptococcal infections in Ontario, Canada. *New England Journal of Medicine, 335*(8), 547–554.

Degitz, K. (1996). Detection of mycobacterial DNA in the skin. *Archives of Dermatology 132*, 71–75.

Eisenstadt, D. O., & Hall, G. S. (1995). Microbiology and classification of Mycobacteria. *Clinics in Dermatology, 13*(3), 197–206.

Feingold, D. S. (1996). Group A streptococcal infections. *Archives of Dermatology, 132*, 67–70.

Freland, C., Fur, J. L., Nemirovsky-Trebucq, B., Lelong, P., & Boiron, P. (1995). Primary cutaneous nocardiosis caused by *Nocardia otitidiscaviarum*: Two cases and a review of the literature. *Journal of Tropical Medicine and Hygiene, 98*, 395–403.

Funke, G., Von Graevenitz, A., Clarridge, J. E., & Bernard, K. A. (1997). Clinical microbiology of coryneform bacteria. *Clinical Microbiology Reviews, 10*(1), 125–169.

Gaston, D. A., & Zurowski, S. M. (1996). *Arcanobacterium haemolyticum* pharyngitis and exanthem. *Archives of Dermatology, 132*, 61–64.

Gluckman, S. J. (1995). Mycobacterium marinum. *Clinics in Dermatology, 13*(3), 273–276.

Green, R. J., Defoe, D. C., & Raffin, T. A. (1996). Necrotizing fasciitis. *Chest, 110*(1), 219–229.

Groves, R. (1995). Unusual cutaneous mycobacterial diseases. *Clinics in Dermatology, 13*(3), 257–263.

Habif, T. P. (1996). *Clinical dermatology*. St. Louis: Mosby.

Hechemy, K. (1994). Lyme disease: Issues and perspectives. *The Loop, 21*(6), 1–7.

Kodama, B. F., Fitzpatrick, J. E., & Gentry, R. H. (1994). *Cutis, 54*(4), 279–280.

Macgregor, R. R. (1995). Cutaneous tuberculosis. *Clinics in Dermatology, 13*(3), 245–255.

Mallon, E., & McKee, P. H. (1997). Extraordinary case report: Cutaneous anthrax. *The American Journal of Dermatopathology, 19*(1), 79–82.

McHenry, C. R., Azar, T., Ramahi, A. J., & Collins, P. L. (1996). Monomicrobial necrotizing fasciitis complicating pregnancy and puerperium. *Obstetrics and Gynecology, 87* (5 Pt 2), 823–826.

Murray, P. R., Baron, E. J., Pfaller, M. A., Tenover, F. C., & Yolken, R. H. (Eds.). (1995). *Manual of clinical microbiology*. Washington, DC: ASM Press.

Noble, W. C. (Ed.). (1992). *The skin microflora and microbial skin disease*. Cambridge: Cambridge University Press.

Pollack, S. (1996). Staphylococcal scalded skin syndrome. *Pediatrics in Review, 17*(1), 18.

Portaels, F. (1995). Epidemiology of mycobacterial diseases. *Clinics in Dermatology, 13*(3), 207–222.

Sanders, C. V., & Nesbitt, L. T., Jr. (Eds.) (1995). *The skin and infection*. Baltimore: Williams & Wilkins.

Sastry, V., & Brennan, P. J. (1995). Cutaneous infections with rapidly growing mycobacteria. *Clinics in Dermatology, 13*(3), 265–271.

Saubolle, M. A., Kiehn, T. E., White, M. H., Rudinsky, M. F., & Armstrong, D. (1996). *Mycobacterium haemophilum*: Microbiology and expanding clinical and geographic spectra of disease in humans. *Clinical Microbiological Reviews, 9*(4), 435–447.

Seddon, M., Parr, D., & Ellis-Pegler, R. B. (1995). Lymphocutaneous *Nocardia brasiliensis* infection: A case report and review. *New Zealand Medical Journal, 108*, 384–385.

Sherris, J. C. (Ed.). (1990). *Medical microbiology: An introduction to infectious diseases*. Norwalk, CT: Appleton & Lange.

Smyth, E. G., & Weinbren, M. J. (1993). *Mycoplasma hominis* sternal wound infection and bacteremia. *Journal of Infection, 26*, 315–319.

Sriskandan, S., Moyes, D., Buttery, L. K., Krausz, T., Evans, T. J., Polak, J., & Cohen, J. (1996). *Journal of Infectious Diseases, 173*(6), 1399–1407.

Stewart, M. G., & Sulek, M. (1993). Pediatric actinomycosis of the head and neck. *ENT Journal, 72*(9), 615–619.

Strange, P., Skov, L., Lisby, S., Nielsen, P. L., & Baadsgaard, O. (1996). Staphylococcal enterotoxin B applied on intact normal and intact atopic skin induces dermatitis. *Archives of Dermatology, 132*, 27–33.

Sugita, Y. (1995). Leprosy. *Clinics in Dermatology, 13*(3), 235–243.

Tierno, P. M., & Hanna, B. A. (1993). Toxic shock syndrome: An epilogue. *Clinical Microbiology Updates, 6*(1), 1–6.

Vartivarian, S. E., Papadakis, K. A., Palacios, J. A., Manning, J. T., Jr., & Anaissie, E. J. (1994). Mucocutaneous and soft tissue infections caused by *Xanthomonas maltophilia*. *Annals of Internal Medicine, 121*(12), 969–973.

Yamada, H., Yudate, T., Orita, T., & Tezuka, T. (1996). Serum levels of anti-*Staphylococcus aureus*-specific IgE in patients with atopic dermatitis. *Journal of Clinical and Laboratory Immunology, 48*, 167–175.

# CHAPTER 33
## Deep Tissues and Internal Organ Sites

Susan Fraser, MD

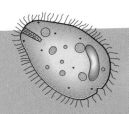

### Microbes in the News

Tuberculosis, caused by *Mycobacterium tuberculosis,* is the major infectious cause of death in the world today. In the United States, approximately 80% of infections are isolated to the lung, but *M. tuberculosis* can infect almost any deep tissue, including the lymph nodes, pleura, genitourinary system, bones, joints, meninges around the brain, peritoneum, and so on. The epidemic of infection with human immunodeficiency virus (HIV) has led to an alarming rise in the number of reported cases of tuberculosis, and especially of multidrug resistant tuberculosis (MDR-TB.) Risk factors for MDR-TB include living in or immigrating from a country where tuberculosis is endemic, poverty, alcoholism, intravenous drug abuse, and infection with HIV. Health care providers and laboratory workers must always consider tuberculosis as a potential cause of infection in nearly any human tissue or organ.

---

**INTRODUCTION**

**BASIC ANATOMY**
Deep Tissues (Fascia, Muscle, and Tendons, the Breast)
Bone and Bone Marrow
Lymph Nodes
The Abdominal Cavity and Its Organs
Heart Valves and Blood Vessels
Brain

**RESIDENT FLORA**
Skin Overlying Tissues and Organs
Gastrointestinal System

**SPECIMEN TYPES AND COLLECTION**
Tissue Biopsies
Aspirates
Swabs

**OPPORTUNISTIC OR PATHOGENIC ORGANISMS**
Pathogenic Bacteria
Anaerobic Bacteria
Fungi
Mycobacteria
Viruses
Atypical and Unusual Organisms

**DISEASES OF THESE SYSTEMS AND ORGANS**
Deep Tissues
Lymph Nodes
The Abdominal Cavity and Its Organs
Bone
Bone Marrow
Heart Valves and Blood Vessels

---

## KEY TERMS

Abscess
Bacteremia
Empyema
Fasciitis
Infective endocarditis (IE)

Lymphadenitis
Mastitis
Mediastinitis
Mycotic aneurysm
Myositis

Osteomyelitis
Peritonitis
Pyogenic
Suppurate
Tendinitis

## LEARNING OBJECTIVES

**Upon completion of this chapter, the student should be able to:**

1. Understand the basic anatomy of the human deep tissues and internal organ systems as well as how these sites may become infected.
2. Describe the proper handling of specimens obtained from deep tissues and internal organs when submitted to the microbiology laboratory.
3. List the organisms that can be isolated from infections in various deep tissues.
4. Discuss the infectious diseases that may occur in these systems.
5. Suggest additional tests that may be helpful in identifying the specific cause of an infection in one of these systems if standard procedures are not diagnostic.

## INTRODUCTION

This chapter introduces you to the key elements in processing specimens obtained from deep tissues and internal organs. First, the basic anatomy of the systems is covered, followed by a discussion of the resident flora that can invade these sites, either directly from adjacent tissues or from blood. Specimen types and their collection, and how they should be handled once received in the microbiology laboratory, are reviewed.

The common opportunistic and pathogenic organisms that may infect deep tissues are discussed, with a few comments on more unusual pathogens. Finally, we review the infectious diseases of the internal organs and systems, including comments on how to assist health care providers regarding proper submission procedures, as well as suggesting additional tests that can be performed when standard testing is nondiagnostic.

## BASIC ANATOMY

The deep tissues and internal organs of the human body are protected from the environment by skin and mucous membranes, as well as tissue planes specific to the individual organ. The deep tissue and organ sites discussed include fascia, muscles, tendons, joints, bones, bone marrow, and lymph nodes; the cardiovascular system including the heart, heart valves, veins and arteries; the abdominal cavity and its organs including the liver, pancreas, spleen, kidneys and peritoneum; the breast; and the brain.

The fascia is a fibrous band of tissue that lies deep to the skin and separates muscle groups and other organs from each other. Individual muscles are enclosed in sheaths that merge with tendons to attach muscle to bone, whereas other organs have membranes such as the pericardial sac, which surrounds the heart, or the pleura, which surrounds the lungs. The meninges surround the spinal cord and brain, whereas the peritoneum is a membrane that lines abdominopelvic walls and surrounds most of the abdominal organs. Some organs have cap-sules, including those surrounding the liver, spleen, kidneys, and thyroid gland.

Infections can occur not only in these tissues, but also in those spaces between the protective membranes, capsules, or sheaths and their associated organs. Examples of tissue infections include **fasciitis**, which is an infection of the fascia, or **osteomyelitis**, infection in bone. Examples of space infections include an abscess in the subcapsular space of the kidney (commonly associated with pyelonephritis), **peritonitis** that may develop in the abdominal cavity with or without a specific organ infection, or **empyema**, which is an infection within the pleural cavity between the lung and the thoracic cage.

## Deep Tissues (Fascia, Muscles, and Tendons, the Breast)

The fascia is a special fibrous layer of tissue present in multiple regions of the body. In general, it acts as a protective layer between the fat, which lies underneath the skin, and the deeper tissues. Usually muscles lie just beneath the fascia. Because of the proximity of fascia to both skin and muscle, it is easy to visualize how a skin infection can spread deeper to involve fascia (fasciitis) and muscle (**myositis**) (see Figure 33-1).

Tendons are specialized tissues that connect muscles to bone at the joints. You can easily see the tendons in your hands, wrists, feet, and ankles. Tendons lie very near the skin in many areas of the body and are at risk for infection (**tendinitis**) whenever the skin in that area is damaged.

Embryologically considered to be a modified sweat gland, the breast is comprised of a complex array of specialized glands and ducts that can produce and transport milk. Most infections of the breast (**mastitis**) occur in women, but men can also be affected.

## Bone and Bone Marrow

Bones are usually well protected by skin, layers of fat, fascia, and muscle. Any bone in the body can develop an infection (osteomyelitis), but the long bones of the

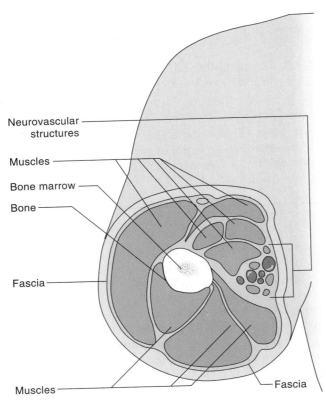

Neurovascular structures

Muscles

Bone marrow

Bone

Fascia

Muscles

Fascia

**FIGURE 33-1** The anatomic relationship between the skin, muscles, fascia, and bone.

arms and legs, as well as the vertebrae, or spinal column, are at particular risk of becoming infected when **bacteremia** occurs. Although bones are made of extremely hard and resilient material, when infected they produce enzymes and create cellular reactions in the host, which contributes to further destruction of the local tissue.

Bone marrow is the soft organic material that fills the central cavities of bone. Red blood cells, white blood cells, platelets, and other cells are produced in the bone marrow. When the bone marrow is infected, the cell production may be reduced or increased depending on the specific infecting agent.

## Lymph Nodes

Lymph nodes are small organs of the lymphatic system where white cells congregate. They are grouped in certain regions of the body, with channels connecting the entire lymph system of the body. Eventually lymph is returned to the blood. When an infection occurs (**lymphadenitis**), the activated white cells, which have phagocytized bacteria, travel to lymph nodes and cause them to swell. They can sometimes become quite tender, with local erythema and warmth, and will even **suppurate** (develop an **abscess**). The most easily palpated lymph nodes are in the neck, the axillae (armpits), and the groin.

## The Abdominal Cavity and Its Organs

The abdomen contains multiple solid organs plus the stomach and intestines. The peritoneum is a strong serous membrane that lines the abdominopelvic walls and covers the intestines. Infection of this membrane is called peritonitis. There is always a very small amount of fluid in the peritoneal cavity. When fluid accumulates (usually due to severe liver or kidney disease) ascites develops, and this fluid can also become infected, causing peritonitis.

Each organ in the abdominal cavity has its own blood supply. The spleen is part of the lymphatic system and receives a large arterial blood supply, as do the kidneys. These organs are more at risk for bacteremic infections than the liver, through which almost all venous blood from the abdomen drains. The liver, therefore, is more at risk for infections spreading from other abdominal or pelvic organs (see Figure 33-2).

## Heart Valves and Blood Vessels

The heart is located just behind the sternum in the thoracic cavity. The aorta is the large artery that leaves the heart to distribute blood to the rest of the body, and the vena cavae (inferior and superior) bring blood back from the body to the right atrium of the heart. The four valves in the heart, any of which can be infected, include the tricuspid, pulmonary, mitral, and aortic.

## Brain

The brain is a sensitive organ that lies well protected inside the skull. It receives its blood supply from four different arteries. Its proximal position to the ears, mastoids, sinuses, and mouth place it at some risk for becoming infected, and yet brain abscesses are uncommon.

## RESIDENT FLORA

Any tissue or organ that lies underneath the skin or mucous membranes can become infected when there is a break in the integrity of the barrier. A break can be caused by diseases of the skin, accidental abrasions, lacerations or other traumatic injuries, or by surgical incisions and manipulations. Examples include necrotizing fasciitis or myositis after skin trauma, and brain abscesses following sinus or neurosurgical procedures. Sometimes microorganisms introduced through skin, airways, or the gastrointestinal tract can travel through the blood (bacteremia, fungemia, parasitemia) and lodge in distant organs, causing infection. Examples include **infective endocarditis (IE)** in an intravenous drug user and splenic abscess from an infected intravenous catheter. Deep tissues or organs can also be infected by local extension of bacteria or fungi, usually due to inflammation of nearby tissues following natural disease, surgical injury, or trauma.

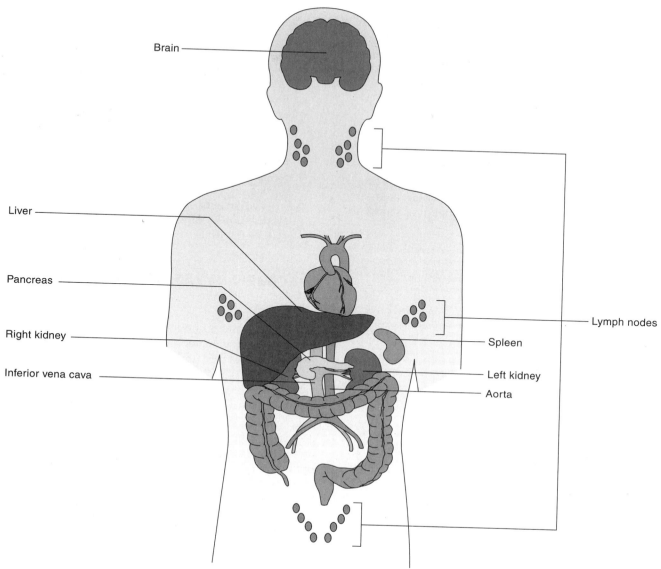

**FIGURE 33-2** The location of the major organs and deep tissue sites.

In all of the above situations, the infecting microorganisms are frequently a part of the patient's normal flora and will vary depending on the actual site(s) involved. The microbiologic flora of the head and neck, which could cause a brain abscess after head trauma, differ from the skin flora of the leg, which might cause osteomyelitis after a gunshot wound. The lower gastrointestinal tract organisms implicated in liver abscesses following appendectomy are different from the oral flora that may cause endocarditis after dental procedures.

## Skin Overlying Tissues and Organs

The microbiologic flora of the skin is not quite uniform over the entire body. Some organisms, such as *Staphylococcus aureus,* the coagulase-negative staphylococci, and *Proprionibacterium acnes* are found on skin throughout the body, but *S. aureus* may be found in higher numbers in the anterior nares (nose), groin, and armpits. *P. acnes,* however, is more commonly found on skin of the head, neck, and upper torso than anywhere else on the body. Enterococci are not usually cultured from areas above the waist, but because of their presence in the gastrointestinal tract, can be found on the skin of the buttocks, perineum, and groin. The Enterobacteriaceae are more commonly found in the genital and perineal skin, similar to the enterococci.

Generally, the following organisms can be considered to be part of the normal skin flora, and they play important roles in causing deep tissue and organ infections when skin integrity is compromised.

**Facultative Gram-Positive Cocci.** *Staphylococcus aureus,* the coagulase-negative staphylococci including *S. epidermidis, Streptococcus pyogenes* (group A strep),

*Streptococcus agalactiae* (group B strep), group G streptococci, viridans streptococci, and other streptococcal species, including the microaerobic or nutritionally deficient streptococci, *Micrococcus* species, and *Enterococcus* species, are commonly cultured from skin surfaces. Any one of these may act as an opportunist in causing deep tissue infection, either alone or in combination with other organisms.

**Gram-Negative Bacteria.** *Escherichia coli, Proteus vulgaris, Morganella* species, *Providencia* species, *Klebsiella pneumoniae* and other bacteria from the Enterobacteriaceae, *Pseudomonas* species, and *Neisseria* species are found on skin less commonly than the gram-positive cocci and are less frequently isolated in serious deep tissue and organ infections.

**Gram-Positive Bacilli.** *Bacillus* species and *Corynebacterium* species, as well as other diphtheroids, can commonly be isolated from skin, and occasionally cultured from deep infections.

**Anaerobic Bacteria.** Although rarely isolated as sole pathogens, anaerobic bacteria are routinely isolated from mixed deep tissue infections in nearly any body site. *P. acnes, Peptostreptococcus* species, *Clostridium* species, and *Eubacterium* species are commonly found on human skin; less frequently seen are *Lactobacillus, Bacteroides, Prevotella, Fusobacterium,* and other anaerobic species.

**Fungi.** *Candida albicans,* other *Candida* species, *Malassezia furfur (Pityrosporum orbiculare), Trichosporon beigelii,* and the dermatophytes are commonly found on skin. *C. albicans* and the other *Candida* species are the most significant fungal causes of deep tissue and organ infections.

## Gastrointestinal System

The gastrointestinal (GI) tract harbors numerous organisms, varying from region to region. The Enterobacteriaceae and enterococci are found more commonly in the lower intestine, whereas *Streptococcus pneumoniae* and *Haemophilus influenzae* may colonize the upper GI tract, but are not as commonly found in the intestines. Anaerobes, which make up over 99% of normal enteric flora, can be found throughout the GI tract, although some are much more common oral than lower tract isolates and vice versa. Therefore, infections associated with the GI tract may have markedly different etiologies according to the specific site of involvement.

Because deep tissue and solid organ infections are not as commonly associated with oral flora, and the oral flora is fairly similar to that found in the nasopharynx (see next section), specific organisms of the upper GI tract will not be listed. The following organisms are commonly found in the intestines and can be significantly involved in deep tissue and organ infections

within the abdominal cavity, and in some cases may be involved with infectious processes above the diaphragm.

▶ Gram-positive anaerobes: *Peptostreptococcus, Clostridium, Bifidobacterium eubacterium, Lactobacillus, Peptococcus, Actinomyces* species, and less commonly, *Propionibacterium* species
▶ Gram-negative anaerobes: *Bacteroides fragilis* group, other *Bacteroides,* pigmented and other *Prevotella, Fusobacterium, Veillonella* species, and other gram-negative bacilli and cocci
▶ Aerobes and facultative bacteria: Enterobacteriaceae, especially *E. coli,* the enterococci, and streptococci; less common are *S. aureus, Pseudomonas,* other gram-negative bacilli, and *Candida* species

## SPECIMEN TYPES AND COLLECTION

Ideally, specimens obtained from deep tissue and internal organ sites should be either tissue biopsies or frankly purulent material obtained directly from the infected area before antimicrobial therapy is started. A Gram stain should be performed on any submitted fluid or pus. Most deep tissue and organ specimens should automatically be cultured for both aerobes and anaerobes, with cultures for fungi, mycobacteria, and less common pathogens at the discretion of the submitting clinician in consultation with the microbiology laboratory personnel. If the specimen is obtained through infected skin or normally nonsterile body sites (e.g., the oral cavity), then there is a significant chance that the culture will be contaminated, particularly with anaerobes, and the results compromised.

Specimens may be submitted on swabs, in syringes, or in sterile containers. They should be brought directly to the microbiology laboratory and processed quickly to prevent death of sensitive organisms. In general, the faster the appropriate plating procedures are performed, the more complete and accurate the results will be. The biggest concern with specimens from deep tissues and organs is the potential loss of anaerobic organisms if the specimen is not submitted in proper anaerobic transport conditions or plated and placed in the anaerobic incubation chamber expeditiously. Although refrigeration of specimens may lead to the loss of temperature- or oxygen-sensitive organisms, sometimes it is necessary to refrigerate specimens for a short period, and most pathogens will remain viable.

## Tissue Biopsies

A biopsy of deep tissue is usually performed by a surgeon who, after sterilizing the overlying skin, obtains a sample of tissue under direct visualization. Examples include open biopsies of muscle, lymph nodes, abdominal organs, peritoneum, heart valves at open heart surgery, and brain. Sometimes, a needle biopsy is performed, whereby a large hollow-bore, tapered needle is inserted into solid tissue (e.g., liver or bone marrow) and then withdrawn. The tissue remains in the needle and is then ejected into sterile containers for processing in the microbiology and pathology labs.

An appropriate clinical history should accompany the specimen and can sometimes lead the microbiologist to perform pertinent additional testing. For instance, if a chronic granulomatous process is suspected, but the clinician only requests routine bacteriology studies of a lymph node or other tissue, the microbiologist can intercept the specimen and suggest to the clinician that fungal and mycobacterial testing may also be useful. Usually the health care providers are appreciative of such efforts, and the additional information provided on behalf of the patient may save a significant amount of time and expense in additional hospital costs and repeat procedures if the first samples were nondiagnostic.

A good tissue biopsy specimen should be divided, with one part to go to the microbiology lab and the other part submitted to pathology. The tissue may be placed into sterile saline for transport, but should never be placed into a fixative, such as formalin, before submission to the microbiology laboratory. When the sample arrives in the microbiology lab, the tissue should be processed in a laminar flow cabinet by a technician wearing gloves. In some cases, the tissue should be processed in the anaerobic chamber to optimize recovery of these organisms. The tissue should be sterilely ground or minced with forceps and scissors, and then appropriate smears and plating of culture media performed.

**Direct Smears.** A Gram stain should be performed on all tissue specimens and then other smears depending on the request from the submitting clinician and the history provided. If fungal and mycobacterial smears are ordered, the majority of the tissue submitted to the microbiology lab should be submitted to these areas for appropriate processing, and then acid-fast, modified acid-fast, fluorochrome, acridine orange, calcofluor white, and other stains performed as indicated.

**Culture Media.** After mincing or grinding the tissue specimen, and adding a small amount of sterile nutritive broth to the specimen to keep it moist, samples should be plated onto standard media: blood agar, MacConkey agar, Columbia agar with colistin and nalidixic acid (CNA), thioglycolate broth, and anaerobic blood agar. By inoculating thioglycolate broth, both aerobes and anaerobes can grow, so that if the standard solid media fails to yield an organism, then growth in the broth can be Gram stained and replated.

When unusual pathogens are suspected (e.g., *Brucella, Bartonella, Mycoplasma,* etc.), then additional special media can be inoculated in an attempt to isolate these organisms. Buffered charcoal yeast agar can be used to isolate *Nocardia,* brain-heart infusion agar for *Bartonella,* and specific agars for isolating *Brucella, Mycoplasma,* and many other less commonly encountered organisms. If culturing for fungi, an appropriate battery of mycologic agars should be inoculated, and if culturing for mycobacteria, appropriate solid and liquid media should be inoculated following decontamination procedures of the submitted specimen.

## Aspirates

Deep body fluids that may be aspirated, usually with needle and syringe, include pleural fluid, peritoneal fluid, and joint fluids. A collection of pus anywhere in the human body can be aspirated and submitted to the laboratory for smears and cultures. Sometimes the pus comes from within an organ (e.g., brain, liver, splenic abscesses) or from an infection in a space around or near other organs (e.g., retroperitoneal space abscess). Aspirated pus should be left in a sterile, capped syringe with the needle removed, or injected into a sterile container for transport to the lab. Aspirates are handled in a similar fashion to tissue samples, except that mincing the specimen is usually unnecessary.

**Direct Smears.** Aspirates of pus from normally sterile sites require immediate attention in the laboratory, with at least a Gram stain performed expeditiously. In most cases, a general quantification of the numbers of white and red blood cells (few, moderate, or many) should be noted, and then the specific bacteria or other organisms described. Most bacteria Gram stain easily, and many yeasts can also be seen on Gram stain. In certain situations when fungal or mycobacterial diseases are suspected, then special stains should also be performed.

**Culture Media.** Pus should be inoculated onto blood, MacConkey, and anaerobic agars, and into thioglycolate broth. If the smear shows many gram-negative bacilli and a few gram-positive cocci, then Columbia CNA agar should also be inoculated to enhance recovery of the gram-positive organisms. When anaerobes are highly suspected, cooked meat broth may increase the chances of their recovery over thioglycolate broth. When fungi or mycobacteria are suspected, then appropriate fungal and mycobacterial media should also be inoculated after the usual decontamination and concentration procedures are performed.

## Swabs

Cotton-tipped or calcium alginate-tipped swabs with plastic shafts are commonly used to obtain samples from deep tissue infections. Swabs for this purpose are manufactured for both aerobic transport as well as for anaerobic transport of specimens. Those for aerobic transport usually have a small glass ampule of transport media at the end of the tube. After the material is obtained on the swab, and the swab reinserted into its container, then the ampule of glass is broken, allowing the media to moisten the specimen and protect it during transport and refrigeration if necessary. Several different companies manufacture anaerobic transport devices for aspirated as well as swabbed specimens. Any swab submitted for anaerobic culture in an appropriate transport container should be processed in an anaerobic chamber.

When swabs are received in the laboratory, ideally the clinician will provide three separate specimens: one swab for smear, one for inoculating culture media, and one in an anaerobic transport container. If only one swab is submitted, the results may be compromised by lack of sufficient material. The swab should be used to inoculate all sterile media and can then be smeared onto a glass slide for Gram stain. Swabs are not recommended when submitting specimens for fungal or mycobacterial smears and cultures.

## OPPORTUNISTIC OR PATHOGENIC ORGANISMS

### Pathogenic Bacteria

Bacteria that are not considered to be normal flora can act primarily as pathogens when they are introduced into the susceptible human. The following examples include many organisms that may be found in animals or the environment, or in rare instances may be repeatedly isolated from a human chronic carrier. In parentheses are the most common or significant human diseases or deep tissue infections that may be caused by the named microbe.

**Gram-Positive Cocci.** Almost all of the gram-positive cocci (*Staphylococcus, Streptococcus,* and *Enterococcus* species) can be considered members of the human normal flora.

**Gram-Positive Bacilli.** *Corynebacterium diphtheriae* (diptheria), *Listeria monocytogenes* (meningitis), *Bacillus anthracis* (anthrax), and *Rhodococcus equi* (lung abscess) are examples of pathogenic gram-positive rods that can cause deep tissue infections.

**Gram-Negative Cocci.** *Neisseria gonorrhoeae* (pelvic inflammatory disease), *Neisseria meningitidis* (bacteremia and occasional deep tissue infections), and *Kingella* species (bone and joint infections) are pathogenic gram-negative cocci that cause deep tissue and organ infections.

**Gram-Negative Bacilli.** *Salmonella* species (spleen abscess, osteomyelitis), *Shigella* species (pericardial infections), *Francisella tularensis* (lymphadenitis), *Haemophilus ducreii* (adenopathy and lymph node abscesses), and *Yersinia pestis* (plague and lymph node abscess) are a few of the gram-negative bacilli that are not considered part of the normal flora and can cause significant human disease.

## Anaerobic Bacteria

The mucous membranes, GI tract, and skin are colonized with many species of anaerobic bacteria that have been associated with human illness and deep tissue infections. When associated with deep tissue infections, these organisms are commonly seen as part of mixed flora in abscesses, but have also been isolated from bone, joint, and other types of infections as sole infecting agents.

**Opportunists.** *Bacteroides, Prevotella,* and *Fusobacterium* are gram-negative bacilli that can act as opportunists. *Peptostreptococcus, Clostridium, Eubacterium, Propionibacterium, Lactobacillus,* and *Actinomyces* species are anaerobic gram-positive cocci and bacilli that can be isolated from deep tissue infections.

**Pathogens.** *Clostridium perfringens* is the best known anaerobic gram-positive bacillus that can cause deep tissue infections (gas gangrene) but is not considered to be a part of the human normal flora.

## Fungi

*Candida* species are well known yeasts that are considered normal human flora and are fully capable of causing opportunistic infections in the susceptible host. They can cause deep tissue abscesses, endocarditis, osteomyelitis, and many other infections. Molds, such as *Aspergillus* species, and the zygomycetes can occasionally be cultured from human skin or mucous membranes, and have also been opportunistic causes of deep tissue infections (brain abscess), usually in an immunocompromised human.

Some of the more common fungi that act as pathogens (not part of the normal flora) in causing deep tissue or organ infections include *Histoplasma capsulatum* (**mediastinitis**), *Coccidioides immitis* (muscle and bone infections), and *Blastomyces dermatitidis* (bone and joint infections).

## Mycobacteria

Several species of *Mycobacterium* can be found in the mouth and upper respiratory and gastrointestinal tracts and do not cause illness in most people. However, in certain predisposed individuals, the mycobacteria can act as opportunists and cause lung abscesses, lymph node and bone marrow infections, and other deep infections.

*Mycobacterium tuberculosis* is the most common mycobacterial cause of deep tissue infections. It is not a part of the normal human flora and is therefore considered to be pathogenic whenever it is isolated. Examples of deep tissue sites that may be infected by *M. tuberculosis* include the lymph nodes, pleural space, kidneys, genitourinary system, bones, joints, meninges around the brain and spinal cord, abdominal peritoneum, bone marrow, liver, spleen, pancreas, bowel, and others.

## Viruses

Many viruses cause systemic or disseminated disease in humans. Except for HIV and the herpesviruses (herpes simplex viruses, and Epstein-Barr virus), most viruses are not known to survive for an extended period in the human. They usually are killed by the host, or the host is killed by the virus infection. A variety of culture, antigen, and antibody assays and molecular techniques have been developed to diagnose human viral infections with greater accuracy. These are discussed in the virology section of this book.

## Atypical and Unusual Organisms

Many parasites and worms can cause infection of deep tissues in humans. A brief list includes the filaria (*Wuchereria bancrofti, Dirofilaria, Loa loa*), *Taenia, Echinococcus, Entamoeba histolytica, Trypanosoma cruzi,* and *Leishmania* species. Spirochetal organisms that can cause deep organ and tissue infections include the etiologic agents of Lyme disease (*Borrelia burgdorferi*), Rocky Mountain spotted fever (*Rickettsia rickettsiae*), and syphilis (*Treponema pallidum*). Other organisms that cause deep infections include *Nocardia* (lymphadenitis, brain abscess, pneumonia), *Coxiella burnetii,* which is the etiologic agent of Q fever, and the *Chlamydia* and *Mycoplasma* species.

The microbiology laboratory can assist in culturing a few of the above organisms with the use of special media or techniques (e.g., *Nocardia, Mycoplasma, Leishmania*), but in many cases either a pathologist makes the diagnosis with special stains, or more advanced techniques must be used. These may include immunofluorescence, polymerase chain reaction (PCR), or other molecular techniques.

## DISEASES OF THESE SYSTEMS AND ORGANS

Infectious diseases (see Table 33-1) continue to be a major cause of death in populations around the world. Just as different geographic areas in the world may differ in terms of frequency of certain reported diseases, various pathogenic organisms will cause infections in different organs and body systems. Although many syndromes of infectious diseases are predictable, numerous opportunistic and pathogenic organisms have unique interactions with the human host. In addition, although many bacteria, fungi, and viruses are capable of infecting several different organ systems, a few pathogens infect certain organ systems in characteristic ways. For instance, the viridans streptococci can cause valvular endocarditis, but rarely cause disease elsewhere in the body. A number of bacteria and fungi can cause nodular lymphadenitis (*Nocardia* species and *Sporothrix schenkii* are two examples), and a knowledge of these organisms coupled with an understanding of how tissues should be processed for optimal yield of infecting microorganisms, will make the competent diagnostic microbiologist an invaluable asset in the health care arena.

The infectious diseases in deep organs and tissues of the body can present themselves in a myriad of ways, and yet the final diagnosis in most cases is found when appropriate samples of tissue and body fluids are submitted to the microbiology laboratory. With the advent of advanced diagnostic techniques, including PCR, immunofluorescence, and many others, the diagnostic capabilities of laboratories have expanded dramatically. However, the basic microbiologic techniques that have been used for decades to process and examine human specimens remain the foundation on which clinicians place their initial trust, primarily because most infections are caused by known bacteria. The Gram stain, standard fungal and mycobacterologic stains, in addition to appropriate culture techniques are still used to diagnose the majority of infections in humans.

## Deep Tissues

The tissues deep to the skin include fascia, muscles, and tendons, as well as vascular and nerve structures that can be affected by local infections. In general, these deep tissues are infected by local extension from an infection on the skin (cellulitis) or occasionally by transport of microbes through the bloodstream, which are then, usually by chance, deposited in the affected site. Infections in these tissues are usually characterized by inflammation ("itis" means inflammation), which clinically presents as pain, redness, and swelling in or over the affected area.

Collections of pus develop when local inflammatory effects draw white blood cells to the infected area. The white blood cells plus offending microbes plus the cellular by-products and debris formed by the interactions of all these cells describe the composition of pus. If pus is not formed, then actual samples of tissue may contain significant numbers of infectious organisms, so that they can be seen in smears or cultured.

**Fasciitis (Inflammation of Fascia).** Fasciitis, or more traditionally, necrotizing fasciitis, is a severe bacterial infection that involves the subcutaneous soft tissues, particularly the fascia. It is preceded by some sort of skin injury, which sometimes may go unnoticed. This infection can occur at any age, including infancy. Pre-

## Table 33–1 ▶ Summary of Deep Tissue and Organ Sites and Their Infectious Organisms

| | Fascia | Muscle | Tendons | Breast | Lymph Nodes | Liver | Spleen | Pancreas | Peritoneum | Brain | Heart Valves | Bone |
|---|---|---|---|---|---|---|---|---|---|---|---|---|
| Aerobic gram-positive cocci | S. pyogenes, S. aureus, streptococci, staphylococci, enterococci | S. aureus, S. pyogenes, S. pneumoniae, streptococci | S. aureus, S. pyogenes, coagulase negative staphylococci, streptococci | S. aureus, staphylococci, streptococci | S. aureus, S. pyogenes, S. pneumoniae, staphylococci, streptococci | S. aureus, streptococci, enterococci, staphylococci | S. aureus, streptococcus, staphylococci | S. aureus, staphylococci, streptococci, enterococci | S. pyogenes, S. pneumoniae, S. aureus, staphylococci, enterococci, streptococci | S. aureus, S. pneumoniae, staphylococci, streptococci | S. aureus, staphylococci, viridans streptococci, other streptococci, enterococci | S. aureus, S. pyogenes, S. agalactiae |
| Aerobic gram-negative bacilli | E. coli, Enterobacteriaceae, Pseudomonas | E. coli, Salmonella, Klebsiella, Enterobacter, Enterobacteriaceae, Pseudomonas, Aeromonas, Vibrio vulnificus, S. typhi, Legionella | | | Enterobacteriaceae, Pseudomonas, Bartonella, Yersinia, Haemophilus, Salmonella, Y. pestis, F. tularensis, P. pseudomallei | E. coli, Enterobacteriaceae, Yersinia enterocolitica, Pseudomonas | Salmonella species, Enterobacteriaceae | E. coli, Enterobacteriaceae, Pseudomonas | E. coli, K. pneumoniae, other Enterobacteriaceae, Pseudomonas, Acinetobacter, Haemophilus | H. influenzae, P. aeruginosa | (rare) | E. coli, P. aeruginosa, Enterobacteriaceae, Salmonella, H. influenzae, Brucella, Pasteurella, Eikenella |
| Aerobic gram-positive bacilli | Corynebacterium | | Corynebacterium, Nocardia | | C. diphtheriae, L. monocytogenes, B. anthracis | Corynebacterium | | Corynebacterium | Corynebacterium, Nocardia | | | |
| Aerobic gram-negative cocci | | | N. gonorrhoeae, Moraxella | | | | | | N. gonorrhoeae | | | |
| Anaerobic gram-positive cocci | Peptostreptococcus | Peptostreptococcus | | Peptostreptococcus | Peptostreptococcus | Peptostreptococcus | Peptostreptococcus | Peptostreptococcus | Peptostreptococcus | | | Peptostreptococcus |
| Anaerobic gram-negative bacilli | Bacteroides, Fusobacterium | Bacteroides | | Bacteroides species | | B. fragilis, Bacteroides species, Fusobacterium, Actinomyces | | B. fragilis, Bacteroides species | B. fragilis, Bacteroides species, Bilophila | Bacteroides, Prevotella | | Fusobacterium, Prevotella, Porphyromonas, Bacteroides |
| Anaerobic gram-positive bacilli | Clostridium | C. perfringens, Clostridium species, Bacillus | | | | | | | Clostridium species | | | P. acnes, Actinomyces |
| Fungi | | Coccidioides, Candida species, Cryptococcus, Aspergillus, other molds | Sporothrix schenkii | | H. capsulatum, C. immitis, C. neoformans, Aspergillus | C. albicans, Candida species | Candida species, H. capsulatum, C. neoformans | C. albicans, Candida species | C. albicans, Candida species, C. immitis | Candida species, Aspergillus, Rhizopus, other molds | (rare) | Coccidioides, Blastomyces, Cryptococcus, Sporothrix |
| Mycobacteria | | M. tuberculosis, Mycobacterium species | M. marinum, Mycobacterium species | | M. tuberculosis, Mycobacterium species | | M. tuberculosis, Mycobacterium species | | M. tuberculosis | | | M. tuberculosis |
| Viruses | | HIV, influenza, dengue, Coxsackievirus s, echoviruses, EBV, CMV | rubella | | EBV, CMV, measles, rubella, HIV, HSV, adenoviruses | | | | | | | |
| Other organisms | | Trichinella, Taenia solium, Toxoplasma, Sarcocystis, Rickettsia | | | T. pallidum, C. trachomatis | E. histolytica, Echinococcus | Pneumocystis | | C. trachomatis, E. histolytica, S. stercoralis | Taenia solium, Toxoplasma gondii | | |

CMV, cytomegalovirus; EBV, Epstein-Barr virus; HIV, human immunodeficiency virus; HSV, herpes simplex virus disposing illnesses that may place a patient at higher risk of acquiring a necrotizing fasciitis include diabetes, alcoholism, cirrhosis, corticosteroid use, and intravenous drug abuse.

**Myositis.** Myositis (inflammation of muscle) is an infection of muscle that can be caused by bacteria, mycobacteria, viruses, fungi, or parasites. Pyomyositis specifically is caused by an acute bacterial infection of skeletal muscle. Myositis may be present without evidence of any other infection elsewhere in the body, or it can be associated with either local infection (e.g., gas gangrene that spreads from skin through fascia to muscle) or some systemic process, such as a viral illness.

**CLINICAL FEATURES.** The presentation of a patient with myositis can be very distinctive, with localized muscle pain, swelling, and tenderness, or rather nonspecific, such as in the case of a viral illness, where diffuse myalgias are present. Depending on the underlying illness, the patient can be extremely toxic (gas gangrene) or only mildly ill appearing. Usually some elevation of the temperature is present, as is a leukocytosis. In the case of a parasitic muscle infection, peripheral eosinophilia may be present.

**ORGANISMS INVOLVED.** Bacterial causes of myositis are varied. If due to local extension from a skin wound, then the usual skin organisms including anaerobes are implicated. When an isolated pyogenic myositis is present, then almost any bacteria that could have seeded the muscle through hematogenous spread may be suspected. Consider *S. aureus,* group A streptococcus, *S. pneumoniae,* other aerobic and anaerobic streptococci, any of the species of Enterobacteriaceae including *E. coli, Salmonella, Klebsiella,* and *Enterobacter,* anaerobes including *Peptostreptococcus, C. perfringens* and other *Clostridium* species, *Bacteroides,* other gram-negative anaerobic bacilli, and *Aeromonas hydrophila* in the differential diagnosis.

*Mycobacterium tuberculosis* is a well known cause of psoas muscle abscess, although *S. aureus* is seen in this entity more commonly. Mycobacteria other than *M. tuberculosis,* fungi such as *C. immitis, Candida* species, *Cryptococcus* and the molds (e.g., *Aspergillus*) can rarely cause myositis. Parasites that can be implicated include *Trichinella spiralis, Toxoplasma, Taenia solium,* and *Sarcocystis.* Viral causes of myositis include HIV, influenza, dengue, coxsackievirus B, echovirus, Epstein-Barr virus and cytomegalovirus. Infections with *Legionella,* spirochetes or rickettsiae may cause myositis.

**LABORATORY DIAGNOSIS.** The laboratory can assist in the diagnosis of myositis whenever tissue or pus is submitted. When a patient is systemically ill, blood cultures can be helpful in identifying bacteremia (*N. meningitidis,* causes of infectious endocarditis) or mycobacteremia or fungemia. Special Isolator® blood cultures can assist in identifying these last organisms.

When processing pus from muscles, or the tissue itself, standard bacteriologic procedures are used: a Gram stain is performed, and the clinical material is inoculated onto media for incubation under aerobic as well as anaerobic conditions. When indicated by the clinical history or smear, fungal and mycobacterial smears and cultures can also be obtained.

**Tendons.** Tenosynovitis is an infection/inflammation of a tendon and its associated sheath.

**CLINICAL FEATURES.** Clinically, a patient with tenosynovitis will present with pain, swelling, and sometimes warmth and erythema over a tendon or group of tendons. There is usually limited range of motion of the nearby joints. This infection may be associated with a local wound or skin infection, such as cellulitis, or can appear on its own. The classic case of tenosynovitis is that of a young sexually active patient who has disseminated gonococcal infection, where the symptoms usually involve the tendons of the hands and wrists.

**ORGANISMS INVOLVED.** Implicated organisms include all of those bacteria that may cause cellulitis (see Chapter 32). In addition, consider *N. gonorrhoeae, Moraxella, Nocardia, Sporothrix schenkii, Mycobacterium marinum* and other nontuberculous mycobacteria, and rubella.

**LABORATORY DIAGNOSIS.** Sometimes the etiology of tenosynovitis must be deduced by the clinical picture of the patient and cultures from associated skin infections, or, as in the case of disseminated gonorrhea, from genital, throat, or rectal cultures. The surgeon may be able to obtain swabs or tissue from infected tendons. As with any other tissue, smears should be made, and tissue placed onto appropriate media for isolating both aerobic and anaerobic bacteria. In many cases, fungal and mycobacterial smears and cultures should also be performed, and this can be dictated by the specific history with guidance from the clinician.

**Mastitis and Breast Abscess.** Infections of the breast occur almost always in women, frequently associated with pregnancy and breast-feeding. Several organisms, both common and uncommon, have been documented to cause mastitis or abscesses of the breast.

**CLINICAL FEATURES.** Breast infections manifest with breast tenderness, redness that may be wedge-shaped corresponding to the affected lobe, fevers, chills, and malaise. Sometimes fluid or pus can be discharged from the nipple. When an abscess is present, a mass, which may be fluctuant, can often be documented.

**ORGANISMS INVOLVED.** Mastitis associated with breast-feeding has occurred in epidemics and is most commonly caused by *S. aureus.* Other organisms that have caused puerperal mastitis include the coagulase-negative staphylococci, ß-hemolytic streptococci, *Enterococcus faecalis, Haemophilus parainfluenzae, E. coli,* and *Klebsiella* species.

Mastitis that occurs later in life, is not associated with breast-feeding, and is frequently chronic is called periductal mastitis. Anaerobic bacteria play a significant role in the pathogenesis of this illness, with most cultures showing mixed flora of from two to five organisms on average. *S. aureus,* coagulase-negative staphylococci, and the α-hemolytic streptococci are the predominant facultative bacteria, with *Bacteroides* species (not *B. fragilis*) and *Peptostreptococcus* species the most common anaerobic organisms isolated.

When breast abscess occurs, the most commonly isolated bacteria is *S. aureus,* but cultures are frequently mixed, with anaerobes present in the majority of mixed cultures. As with mastitis, staphylococci and streptococci are the most common facultative organisms isolated, and peptostreptococci and *Bacteroides* species are the most common anaerobic isolates. Unusual causes of breast abscesses or infections include the gram-negative bacilli, parasites, *Taenia* species, fungi to include *H. capsulatum, Cryptococcus neoformans* and *Candida* species, *Actinomyces israelii* and *M. tuberculosis.*

**LABORATORY DIAGNOSIS.** Fluid or pus expressed from the nipple, needle-aspirated fluid or pus, or breast tissue obtained at surgery may be submitted to the laboratory for processing. Unless a nonbacterial infection is suspected, the clinician will usually only request Gram stain and culture. Because anaerobic bacteria play an important role in the etiology of breast infections, any material should be routinely inoculated into media appropriate for isolating both aerobic and anaerobic organisms, and incubated appropriately. When unusual infections, such as fungal or mycobacterial are clinically suspected or suggested by the smear, then other special stains and inoculation of appropriate media should be performed as indicated.

## Lymph Nodes

Lymphadenitis, or infection in the lymph nodes, can be acute or chronic in nature and has a multitude of potential causes. Sometimes, only one lymph node or group of nodes is involved, and sometimes there is a more diffuse or disseminated process with several lymph nodes or groups of nodes infected. A bacterial, fungal, or mycobacterial infection distal to the involved lymph node(s) may be present and could suggest the etiology of the lymphadenitis. In many cases, however, no obvious local clues are present. The evaluation of the patient then must include obtaining a complete history to include episodes of injury, exposures to animals, foods, environments or other persons with infections, and any other accompanying complaints.

**Clinical Features.** When acute, the patient usually has typical signs of infection to include fever with swelling and pain at the site and may have leukocytosis. The lymph node or nodes may be draining pus or other material or could be erythematous, enlarged, and fluctuant. In the more chronic situation, the lymph nodes are usually swollen, may or may not be tender, or draining, but there is usually no significant warmth to the nodes. Occasionally the lymph channels leading to the nodes are also swollen and tender. This is called lymphangitis.

**Organisms Involved.** Bacterial causes of acute infections in the lymph nodes include *S. aureus, S. pyogenes,* gram-negative bacilli to include the Enterobacteriaceae, and *Pseudomonas* and *Yersinia* species. Other causes include anaerobic organisms such as *Peptostreptococcus,* the etiologic agent of cat scratch disease (*Bartonella henselae*), *H. ducreyi, M. tuberculosis,* the atypical mycobacteria, and *Salmonella typhi.* Rare bacterial causes of lymphadenitis include *C. diphtheriae, Brucella abortus, Leptospira, Y. pestis, L. monocytogenes, B. anthracis, F. tularensis, T. pallidum, Streptobacillus moniliformis, Spirillum minus,* and *Pseudomonas pseudomallei.*

Fungal species that can cause lymphadenitis include *H. capsulatum, C. immitis, C. neoformans, Aspergillus* and other molds, and *Paracoccidioides brasiliensis.* Multiple viruses are capable of causing lymphadenitis, the most famous of which is probably Epstein-Barr virus, which causes infectious mononucleosis. Other viruses to consider include cytomegalovirus, measles, rubella, dengue, the herpesviruses, adenoviruses, and HIV.

*Chlamydia trachomatis* can cause lymphadenitis. The rickettsial organisms, protozoa, and helminths are all capable of causing lymphadenitis, but they are rare.

**Laboratory Diagnosis.** When evaluating lymphadenitis, the clinician may be able to submit aspirated pus or an entire lymph node for processing. Occasionally a swab of pus or discharge from a group of nodes is submitted. This may be adequate for diagnosing a **pyogenic** abscess with *S. aureus* or *S. pyogenes,* but will be less helpful if a less common organism is the cause. Once the specimen is received in the lab, tissue is minced, and then either pus or tissue is Gram stained and plated on the usual aerobic and anaerobic media. Depending on the clinical situation, it may be necessary to perform fungal smears and cultures, mycobacterial smears and cultures, or culture the material on other specialized media (e.g., for *Bartonella*). Cultures should be held for several days to weeks to allow for the growth of unusual organisms.

Some of the sample may be inoculated into viral culture media if a viral etiology is suspected. Newer identification techniques, including DNA probes, PCR, and immunostaining may be used by the pathologists or microbiologists to identify the very rare causes of lymphadenitis, depending on the clinical suspicion.

## The Abdominal Cavity and Its Organs

The abdominal cavity contains the stomach, intestines, and pelvic organs, all of which are discussed in other chapters. The liver, spleen, kidney, pancreas, and peritoneal fluid space are discussed in this chapter. These organs may become involved with infections due to local spread of enteric organisms or because of bloodborne pathogens that happen to "land" in the organ of interest. Infections within the abdominal cavity can be divided into peritonitis, which is a general inflammation of the peritoneal space and adjacent tissues, and frank abscess. An intra-abdominal abscess can occur in the peritoneal space, or in specific organs, such as the liver, pancreas, and spleen.

**Peritonitis.** Peritonitis (inflammation of the peritoneum) may occur spontaneously, in the setting of ascites (collection of fluid in the abdomen) and alcoholic cirrhosis, or secondarily, as a result of another primary intra-abdominal infectious process. Occasionally, patients who are receiving dialysis through a peritoneal dialysis catheter can develop peritonitis, almost always associated with a catheter infection, or sometimes due to a break in sterile technique. Any peritonitis is capable of progressing to a localized abscess. The microbes involved in abscesses are generally similar to those that account for cases of secondary peritonitis.

**CLINICAL FEATURES.** Most patients with peritonitis are ill, with fever, abdominal pain, and other symptoms localized to the GI tract, such as nausea, vomiting, or diarrhea. If associated with ascites or cirrhosis, the clinical signs can be quite subtle, and include mild mental status changes in the patient with low-grade fevers and no abdominal tenderness. If peritonitis is due to a general infection after a ruptured bowel, then the signs are more obvious, with decreased bowel sounds, abdominal tenderness, sometimes severe, and higher fevers. The clinical scenario can vary, but any injury to or disease of the bowel can lead to perforation and leaking of enteric flora into the peritoneum, where it can cause peritonitis.

**ORGANISMS INVOLVED.** With primary peritonitis associated with ascites, the infectious etiologies are almost uniformly bacterial, and not necessarily associated with the bowel, especially in children with nephrotic syndrome. Bacterial agents include *S. pyogenes* and other streptococci, gram-negative bacilli, especially *E. coli* and *K. pneumoniae*, *S. pneumoniae*, staphylococci, enterococci and anaerobes, especially *Bacteroides* species. Rare causes of primary peritonitis include the sexually transmitted pathogens *N. gonorrhoeae* and *C. trachomatis*, and occasionally *M. tuberculosis* or *C. immitis* can be isolated.

When a peritoneal dialysis catheter is in place, the organisms involved are more likely to be common skin commensals (*S. epidermidis*, *S. aureus*, diphtheroids), gram-negative bacilli, especially *E. coli*, the other Enterobacteriaceae, and *Pseudomonas*. Less common causes of catheter-associated peritonitis include *C. albicans*, *Acinetobacter* species, the molds, *Nocardia*, and *M. tuberculosis*.

With secondary peritonitis, the most commonly isolated pathogens are anaerobic enteric bacteria, followed by the Enterobacteriaceae, *P. aeruginosa*, *S.*

*aureus*, and the enterococci. Because *Candida* can be a commensal of the GI tract, it can occasionally be isolated. Infrequent causes of secondary peritonitis are *N. gonorrhoeae*, *M. tuberculosis*, *Entamoeba histolytica*, or *Strongyloides stercoralis*.

**LABORATORY DIAGNOSIS.** In primary peritonitis, a sample of the ascitic fluid is aspirated and sent to the lab for studies. Usually a cell count and differential are ordered, as well as routine chemistry tests. Undiluted samples should be submitted in sterile containers, and Gram stain performed. Inoculation of culture media for aerobes and anaerobes is indicated in all cases. Placement of larger amounts of the fluid into blood culture bottles (both aerobic and anaerobic) will increase the yield of positive cultures.

For some cases of secondary peritonitis, when there is enough peritoneal fluid, the lab may receive an aspirate in much the same manner as above. In the vast majority of cases of secondary peritonitis, a surgical procedure must be performed, and material for culture is obtained intraoperatively. Swabs for both aerobic and anaerobic transport should be submitted to the lab. They should be appropriately plated, and smears made. Yeasts will stain on Gram stain and *Candida* species grow on blood agar, so unless strongly clinically suspected, additional smears and cultures for fungi and mycobacteria are not usually necessary.

**Hepatic Abscess.** Liver abscesses can occur as a complication of peritonitis, appendicitis, diverticulitis, or cholecystitis. They are also seen following surgical procedures in the abdomen, such as tumor resection or liver transplantation. Most abscesses are comprised of bacteria, but amebic, mycobacterial, and fungal liver abscesses can also be seen.

**CLINICAL FEATURES.** Most patients with liver abscess will have fever and chills with right upper abdominal pain, and sometimes cough or pleuritic chest pain. The liver is usually tender.

**ORGANISMS INVOLVED.** Pyogenic (bacterial) liver abscesses are usually polymicrobial in nature, which is a reflection of their enteric origin. At least half contain anaerobic bacteria, including the gram-positive cocci (*Peptostreptococcus*, *Peptococcus*), *Bacteroides* species, *Fusobacterium* species and *Actinomyces* species. *S. aureus*, the enterobacteriaceae, *Yersinia enterocolitica*, *Candida* species and streptococci, including group A strep, are the more common facultative and aerobic organisms recovered. The mycobacteria and molds are cultured infrequently. *E. histolytica* and *Echinococcus* can also cause hepatic abscess, but are rare in the United States.

**LABORATORY DIAGNOSIS.** Pus obtained at surgery or by needle aspiration is processed in the same manner as those for peritonitis. If an amoebic or echinococcal abscess is suspected, the diagnosis is usually made by the pathologist. Depending on the clinical scenario, stains and cultures for mycobacteria may be performed.

**Pancreatic Abscess.** Pancreatic abscesses usually develop after an episode of acute pancreatitis, although surgical procedures that invade the retroperitoneal space, perforated stomach ulcers, and prior episodes of pancreatitis with presence of a pseudocyst predispose patients to acquiring these infections.

CLINICAL FEATURES. Patients frequently complain of abdominal pain radiating to the back, similar to complaints of pancreatitis without infection. Usually fever, nausea, vomiting, and poor response to therapies directed at treating simple pancreatitis suggest the diagnosis of an abscess or infected pseudocyst. The white blood cell count is high, and the patient appears ill.

ORGANISMS INVOLVED. The bacteria that cause pancreatic abscess are those that cause any peritoneal abscess, namely the enteric organisms. Approximately half of pancreatic abscesses are polymicrobic in nature, which is not surprising when considering the underlying predispositions of these patients. *M. tuberculosis* is an unusual cause of pancreatitis.

LABORATORY DIAGNOSIS. After identifying a fluid-filled space in the pancreas, needle aspiration or direct surgical exploration can be used to obtain pus. Rarely is true tissue obtained because the pancreas is not easily biopsied. The microbiology laboratory should process these specimens in the same manner as with any other intra-abdominal abscess (see procedures and discussion above).

## Bone

Osteomyelitis, or infection of the bone, can occur from direct extension of infection from adjacent soft tissues or by hematogenous spread. The hematogenous route is the most common route for children and infants to acquire osteomyelitis, and in these cases the infection is almost always due to a single pathogen. The long bones are most commonly affected when the infection is acquired hematogenously, due to the anatomy of the blood vessels in bone. The vertebral bodies can also acquire infection, usually also from hematogenous spread. Sometimes the vertebral bodies are infected in association with past surgery or trauma in the local area.

Osteomyelitis can also occur in the setting of infection in nearby tissues, which nearly always lack an adequate blood supply as in the patient with peripheral vascular disease or diabetes, or by surgical or accidental trauma and chronic nonhealing wounds. This kind of osteomyelitis is termed "contiguous focus." In these cases, infection may be caused by a single organism, but in many cases, especially those associated with diabetic foot ulcers, the bone infection is polymicrobic.

Both hematogenously acquired bone infections, as well as contiguous focus osteomyelitis can progress to a chronic condition that requires long-term antibiotics for control. These patients are rarely cured without amputation or wide debridement.

**Clinical Features.** Symptoms may range from vague and nonspecific, especially in the infant or young child, to severe bone pain, fever, immobility, swelling, and erythema over the involved area.

**Organisms Involved.** Any organism that can cause a blood-borne infection is capable of causing osteomyelitis. However, some organisms are seen much more frequently than others, and in certain situations the etiologic agent may be predicted. *S. aureus* is the most common organism isolated from bone infections in all age groups. In infants, *E. coli* and *S. agalactiae* can also be isolated with some frequency. In children, *S. pyogenes* remains, and, until the use of the HiB vaccine, *H. influenzae* was a common cause of osteomyelitis. In patients with sickle cell disease, infection with *Salmonella* species is well documented in bone as well as spleen. Unusual organisms including the molds, yeasts, atypical mycobacteria, and others have been documented to cause osteomyelitis.

The vertebral bodies are often infected by hematogenous spread with *S. aureus*. *P. aeruginosa* (especially in intravenous drug users) is another common isolate. Infection can result from organisms normally found in the genitourinary tract, on the skin, the respiratory tract and oral mucosa, or from unknown sources. Obviously, it is not easy to predict the infectious agent in osteomyelitis. *Brucella* species and *M. tuberculosis* are important causes of vertebral osteomyelitis.

In cases where the bone has become infected by a contiguous focus of infection, the implicated organism is usually involved in the local process. For example, a sacral decubitus ulcer that invades bone is likely to have *S. aureus,* enterobacteriaceae, enterococci, or enteric anaerobes as the etiology. Diabetic foot ulcers that invade into bone can have similar organisms, as well as *P. aeruginosa.*

**Laboratory Diagnosis.** Bone biopsy must be performed to accurately diagnose the exact infectious cause of osteomyelitis, especially in those infections where more than one bacteria is found in adjacently infected tissues. Occasionally, the blood culture will be positive with the same organism as that invading bone. Once the surgeon obtains a bone biopsy, it should be placed in a sterile container and immediately carried to the microbiology laboratory. Ideally, if anaerobes are to be recovered, the work on the specimen should be performed in an anaerobic chamber.

The bone is ground up, sometimes with the addition of a small amount of sterile broth. Bacterial and mycobacterial smears can be made from the solution, and then pieces of bone and solution are inoculated onto appropriate aerobic and anaerobic media. Intact bone pieces must be inoculated onto fungal media for adequate recovery of some fungi.

## Bone Marrow

Bone marrow biopsies are performed in certain situations when an infectious disease is strongly suspected, but other diagnostic modalities have failed to make the diagnosis. The classic situation is that of fever of unknown origin. Because certain organisms have reputations for being found only in the bone marrow, despite aggressive attempts to isolate them from blood and other sources, a bone marrow aspirate and biopsy are a part of the work-up of difficult-to-diagnose diseases.

**Clinical Features.** In general, patients who have bone marrow biopsies or aspirates submitted to the microbiology laboratory for diagnosis are febrile, with unexplained constitutional symptoms or cytopenias that are not otherwise explained. Usually, blood cultures have been drawn and other body fluids submitted for evaluation, without diagnostic results.

**Organisms Involved.** Although any organism that can cause blood-borne infection can be isolated from the bone marrow, this invasive test is not usually meant to diagnose the more common bacteria or yeast infections. Usually, the clinician is looking for *M. tuberculosis, Brucella* species, *H. capsulatum, B. dermatitidis,* atypical mycobacteria such as *Mycobacterium avium-intracellulare complex,* fungi, or *Leishmania* species.

**Laboratory Diagnosis.** Bone marrow aspirates and cultures are not always routinely cultured for the common bacteria because these organisms usually do not escape detection when other methods (e.g., blood culture) have been used, and frequently bone marrow cultures are contaminated by coagulase-negative staphylococci or other common skin organisms. However, the aspirate can be placed directly into an Isolator® tube in which lytic agents will lyse the cells, releasing potential pathogens so the microbiologist can more easily culture them.

In general, the microbiology laboratory will receive a specimen of the bone marrow biopsy tissue, which should be expeditiously processed. For recovery of anaerobes, processing is ideally performed in an anaerobic chamber. The tissue can be moistened with a small amount of broth to assist in making the correct consistency for smears (Gram stain, fungal, mycobacterial), and is then plated onto appropriate fungal and mycobacterial media. Under certain circumstances, special media for the isolation of *Brucella* should also be inoculated, and special media for growing *Leishmania* organisms can also be prepared and inoculated.

## Heart Valves and Blood Vessels

Endocarditis, or infection of the endocardium or heart valves, has been attributed to almost all aerobic as well as several anaerobic bacteria, as well as yeasts and fungi. Microscopic breaks in the skin and mucous membranes can lead to bacteremia with organisms that commonly colonize the skin. Although in the majority of these cases the bacteremia is cleared quickly, in certain circumstances the microbes will lodge on a valve, in the endomyocardium, or in a blood vessel. There, the organism will multiply and continually release daughter organisms into the bloodstream or cause local tissue destruction.

Clinical situations leading to bacteremia include dental procedures, needle punctures, surgical procedures, and endoscopic procedures. Doing something as simple as brushing teeth can lead to transient bacteremias. The tissues that may become infected include all four heart valves, both native and prosthetic, the endocardium of the heart, and the endothelium of both veins and arteries. An infected artery that becomes dilated is usually called a **mycotic aneurysm**, and an infected vein is termed suppurative phlebitis.

**Clinical Features.** The patient with an endovascular infection is usually febrile, with chills, and often many constitutional complaints such as fatigue, muscle pain, joint aches, and headaches. In arterial or heart valve infections, small emboli can escape and lodge in the blood vessels of the distal extremities or in other organs. These are called septic emboli and can be sought on physical examination. When a vein or superficial artery is infected, there is usually significant pain, erythema, swelling, and sometimes pus at the area.

**Organisms Involved.** Infection of heart valves can be caused by nearly any bacteria or fungus, although several common bacteria make up the majority of cases. The staphylococci, including both *S. aureus* and the coagulase-negative staphylococci, enterococci, viridans streptococci, and other streptococci cause the vast majority of cases of endocarditis. Less commonly isolated are the gram-negative bacilli, fungi, and anaerobic and unusual bacteria.

Suppurative phlebitis is almost always associated with an infected intravenous catheter and may be caused by *S. aureus,* the Enterobacteriaceae, coagulase-negative staphylococci, and other bacteria. *Candida* species, *M. furfur,* and anaerobes are uncommonly isolated from these infections.

Mycotic aneurysm does not only refer to arterial infections caused by fungi. Those microbes that can cause these infections include staphylococci, *Salmonella* species, streptococci including *S. pyogenes* and *S. pneumoniae, H. influenzae,* gram-negative bacilli from the family Enterobacteriaceae, *P. aeruginosa,* enterococci, *Brucella* species, *Campylobacter fetus,* anaerobic bacteria, especially *Clostridium septicum,* and fungi to include *Candida, Histoplasma, Aspergillus,* and *Blastomyces* species.

**Laboratory Diagnosis.** The laboratory may already be aware of the specific agent of one of the above intravascular infections because of positive blood cultures. Frequently in these cases the infected valve, artery, or vein must be surgically excised, and the microbiology section will have the opportunity to process the tissue for smears and culture. As with any deep tissue culture, the specimen should be processed for both anaerobes and aerobes, and when requested or suggested by the clinical scenario, fungal and other studies should also be performed. Tissue should be ground up, and then Gram stained, stained for fungi if appropriate, and plated onto anaerobic, aerobic, and fungal media.

Swabs of pus may also be submitted. These can be plated according to the request (for aerobic culture, anaerobic, or both), and Gram stained.

## SUMMARY

▶ Human deep tissues and internal organs can become infected by normal human flora that colonize any nonsterile part of the body or by outside pathogens, either from direct spread of the organisms into a traumatized wound, or by blood carrying the organisms to the deep tissue site.

▶ Specimens obtained from deep tissues and organs submitted to the microbiology laboratory should be processed expeditiously; at least a Gram stain along with aerobic and anaerobic cultures are done on every routine specimen, with fungal and mycobacterial stains and cultures performed on other samples as dictated by the body site or other clinical history or at the request of the clinician.

▶ As a group, the anaerobic bacteria that are usually considered normal flora are the most common isolates from abscesses in normally sterile human body sites.

▶ The single most commonly isolated organism from deep tissue infections is *Staphylococcus aureus.*

▶ An understanding of the diversity of potentially infectious microorganisms that can be involved in deep tissue and organ infections will enhance the microbiologists' ability to recover these isolates using thorough standard and recently developed techniques.

## CASE STUDY

A 53-year-old man with leukemia who has recently undergone bone marrow transplantation (BMT) presents with abdominal pain and fevers. His post-BMT course had been complicated by fevers, neutropenia, an upper gastrointestinal bleed, and a central venous catheter infection. He had received antibiotics, and with a return of his leukocytes, improved. It is now 1 month later. He has noticed fevers to 101°F and vague abdominal discomfort. A liver ultrasound shows a collection of fluid in the left lobe of the liver.

**Questions:**

1. What is the diagnosis?

2. List the possible pathogenic organisms that might be involved.

3. What recommendations will you give the clinicians when they ask you how to submit the aspirated material?

# Review Questions

**1.** What would be the most likely Gram stain finding in a specimen obtained from a patient with a pancreatic abscess following cholecystitis (infection in the bile ducts)?
   a. Many white blood cells, no organisms seen
   b. Few white blood cells, few gram-negative coccobacilli
   c. Many white blood cells, moderate gram-negative bacilli, moderate gram-positive cocci
   d. Few white blood cells, many gram-positive cocci in chains

**2.** The most common cause of osteomyelitis is:
   a. *Streptococcus pyogenes.*
   b. *Staphylococcus aureus.*
   c. *Pseudomonas aeruginosa.*
   d. *Enterococcus faecium.*

**3.** You receive a specimen from the neurosurgical operating room labeled "brain abscess." No other clinical information is given. What is the minimum processing that this specimen requires?
   a. Gram stain, culture for aerobic and anaerobic bacteria
   b. Gram stain, fungal stain, culture for aerobic and anaerobic bacteria, and fungi
   c. Gram stain, fungal stain, mycobacterial stain, culture for aerobic and anaerobic bacteria, fungi and mycobacteria
   d. Gram stain, culture for aerobic bacteria

**4.** The medical student from the HIV ward brings a specimen labeled "lymph node aspirate" to your lab for processing. The patient has fevers, weight loss, a cough with bloody sputum, and two other enlarged cervical lymph nodes. What is the minimum processing that this specimen requires?
   a. Gram stain, culture for aerobic and anaerobic bacteria
   b. Gram stain, fungal stain, culture for aerobic and anaerobic bacteria and fungi
   c. Gram stain, fungal stain, mycobacterial stain, culture for aerobic and anaerobic bacteria, fungi and mycobacteria
   d. Mycobacterial stain and culture

**5.** When a deep tissue infection in the abdomen is cultured, what group of organisms is most commonly found in polymicrobic infections?
   a. Facultative gram-positive cocci
   b. Facultative gram-negative bacilli
   c. Aerobic gram-negative bacilli
   d. Anaerobes

**6.** The single most common organism isolated from deep tissue infections is:
   a. *S. aureus.*
   b. *M. tuberculosis.*
   c. *E. coli.*
   d. *B. fragilis.*

**7.** Which tissue is *M. tuberculosis* least likely to infect?
   a. Lung
   b. Bone
   c. Lymph node
   d. Brain

**8.** Which of the following is considered to be a common pathogenic (not opportunistic) cause of human deep tissue infections?
   a. *S. aureus*
   b. *S. epidermidis*
   c. *Candida albicans*
   d. *Clostridium perfringens*

**9.** Which of the following is considered to be an opportunistic cause of human deep tissue infections?
   a. *M. tuberculosis*
   b. *E. coli*
   c. *N. gonorrhoeae*
   d. *H. capsulatum*

**10.** You perform a Gram stain on a tissue sample submitted for routine bacterial studies and labeled "peritoneum." You document many white blood cells and no bacteria, but see many budding yeastlike cells. What is your next course of action?
   a. In addition to inoculating standard aerobic and anaerobic media, inform the clinician of your findings and bring any remaining specimen to the fungal lab for special stains and plating.
   b. Inoculate the specimen only onto standard aerobic and anaerobic bacterial culture media because that was what was requested on the lab slip, and if the yeast is a *Candida* species, it should grow on this media anyway.
   c. Discard any standard bacterial media already inoculated, and bring any remaining specimen directly to the fungal lab for special stains and plating.
   d. Call your supervisor for advice.

▶ **REFERENCES &
RECOMMENDED READING**

Anderson, C. B., Butcher, H. R., & Ballinger, W. F. (1974). Mycotic aneurysms. *Archives of Surgery, 109,* 712–717.

Barnes, P. F., DeCock, K. M., Reynolds, T. N., & Ralls, P. W. (1987). A comparison of amebic and pyogenic abscess of the liver. *Medicine, 66*(6), 472–483.

Baron, E. J., Peterson, L. R., & Finegold, S. M. (Eds.). (1994). *Bailey and Scott's diagnostic microbiology.* St. Louis: Mosby.

Carithers, H. A. (1985). Cat-scratch disease. An overview based on a study of 1200 patients. *American Journal of Diseases in Children, 139*(11), 1124–1133.

Christin, L., & Sarosi, G. A. (1992). Pyomyositis in North America: Case reports and review. *Clinical Infectious Diseases, 15*(4), 668–677.

Demers, B., Simor, E. E., Vellend, H., Schlievert, P. M., Byrne, S., Jamieson, F., Walmsley, S., & Low, D. E. (1993). Severe invasive group A streptococcal infections in Ontario, Canada: 1987–1991. *Clinical Infectious Diseases, 16*(6), 792–800.

Finegold, S. M. (1977). Abdominal and perineal infections. In S. M. Finegold (Ed.)., *Anaerobic bacteria in human disease* (pp. 257–313). New York: Academic Press.

Freidig, E. E., McClure, S. P., Wilson, W. R., Banks, P. M., & Washington, J. A., II. (1986). Clinical-histologic-microbiologic analysis of 419 lymph node biopsy specimens. *Reviews of Infectious Diseases, 8*(3), 322–328.

Fry, D. E. (Ed.). (1995). *Surgical infections.* Boston: Little, Brown.

Giuliano, A., Lewis, F., Jr., Hadley, K., & Blaisdell, F. W. (1977). Bacteriology of necrotizing fasciitis. *American Journal of Surgery, 134*(1), 52–57.

Johnson, R. A., Zajac, R. A., & Evans, M. E. (1986). Suppurative thrombophlebitis: Correlation between pathogen and underlying disease. *Infection Control, 7,* 582–585.

Kaplan, K. (1985). Brain abscess. *Medical Clinics of North America, 69,* 345–360.

Lorber, B., & Swenson, R. M. (1975). The bacteriology of intra-abdominal infections. *Surgery Clinics of North America, 55,* 1349–1354.

Mandell, G. L., Bennett, J. E., & Dolin, R. (Eds.). (1995). *Principles and practice of infectious diseases.* New York: Churchill Livingstone.

Nelken, N., Isnatius, J., Skinner, M., & Christensen, N. (1987). Changing clinical spectrum of splenic abscess. A multicenter study and review of the literature. *American Journal of Surgery, 154*(1), 27–34.

Nichols, R. L. (1985). Intra-abdominal infections: An overview. *Reviews of Infectious Diseases, 7*(Suppl. 4), S709–1715.

Perry, C. R., Pearson, R. L., & Miller, G. A. (1991). Accuracy of cultures of material from swabbing of the superficial aspect of the wound and needle biopsy in the preoperative assessment of osteomyelitis. *Journal of Bone and Joint Surgery, 73(A),* 745–749.

Rea, W. J., & Wyrick W. J., Jr. (1970). Necrotizing fasciitis. *Annals of Surgery, 172,* 957–964.

Surani, S., Chandna, H., & Weinstein, R. A. (1993). Breast abscess: Coagulase-negative *Staphylococcus* as a sole pathogen. *Clinical Infectious Diseases, 17,* 701–704.

Washington, J. A., II. (1982). The role of the microbiology laboratory in the diagnosis and antimicrobial treatment of infective endocarditis. *Mayo Clinic Proceedings, 57*(1), 22–32.

Wilcox, C. M., & Dismukes, W. E. (1987). Spontaneous bacterial peritonitis: A review of pathogenesis, diagnosis and treatment. *Medicine, 66,* 447–456.

# Mycology

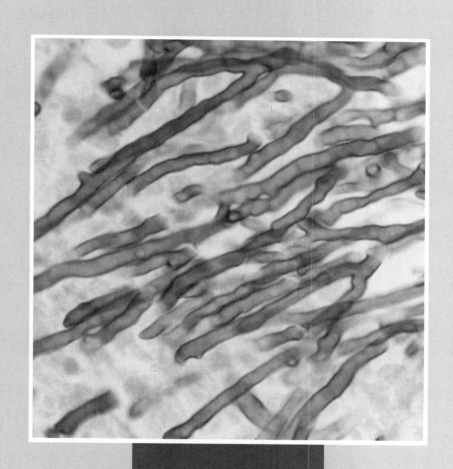

# CHAPTER 34
# Basic Concepts and Techniques in Mycology

Anne T. Rodgers, MT (ASCP) PhD, James A. Miller, MD

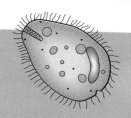

## Microbes in the News

### The terminator: (mucormycosis)

A case study in the January 1995 issue of *Discover* described a patient who appeared to have sinusitis but eventually dies of mucormycosis. Mucormycosis is a rare, potentially fatal fungal infection with the fungus *Mucor*, which infects persons with diabetes in ketoacidosis.

Source: Abigail Zuger, The terminator, *Discover*, *16*(1), 23–24.

INTRODUCTION

GENERAL CHARACTERISTICS OF FUNGI

REPRODUCTION OF FUNGI
Sexual Spores
Asexual Spores

CLASSIFICATION OF FUNGI

GENERAL APPROACH TO THE IDENTIFICATION OF FUNGI
Characteristics of Fungi in Direct Examination of Clinical Specimens
Cultures of Fungi

ANTIFUNGAL AGENTS AND SUSCEPTIBILITY TESTING

## KEY TERMS

Ascospore
Aseptate
Basidiospore
Budding
Chitin
Conidium (pl. conidia)
Conidiophore
Dematiaceous
Dimorphic

Ergosterol
Hyphae
Melanin
Mold
Mushroom
Mycelium
Mycology
Mycosis(es)

Pseudohyphae
Saprophyte
Septate
Sporangiophore
Sporangiospore
Sporangium (pl. sporangia)
Yeast
Zygospore

## LEARNING OBJECTIVES

Upon successful completion of this chapter, the student should be able to:

1. Name the divisions, subdivisions, and classes of fungi that contain species of medical relevance to man.

2. Describe general nutritional, growth, and isolation requirements of fungi.

3. List and discuss media used to isolate and identify fungi.

4. Identify and describe types of colonial morphology, hyphae, and sexual and asexual spores used to identify the filamentous fungi.

5. List and discuss steps in a general approach for identification of fungi in the mycology laboratory.

6. Name and discuss antifungal drugs used to treat fungal infections.

## INTRODUCTION

**Mycology** is the branch of microbiology that involves the study of fungi. Fungi are microorganisms that include **molds**, **yeasts**, and **mushrooms**. The clinical microbiologist is interested in those fungi that cause disease. Although there are more than 50,000 species of fungi, relatively few of these are true pathogens in humans. Some species are plant pathogens. Most fungi are **saprophytes** in nature. However, any of these can potentially cause infections in humans, given the right circumstances. Many fungi are readily recognized to have an important role in the ecologic balance of the earth. The molds are especially important decomposers of organic matter. Symbiotic fungi have mutualistic relationships with the roots of plants. Mushrooms are important as food sources, although some of the mushrooms may produce deadly toxins. Yeasts are used in fermentation of wine and beer as well as in bread making. Some wonderfully tasting cheeses are the result of the action of molds. Molds may also produce antimicrobial substances such as penicillin and cephalosporin antibiotics, which have revolutionized the treatment of infectious diseases.

This section concerns itself with the fungi that cause disease in humans. These fungal diseases are called **mycoses**. They may be classified by the tissue or body site infected. Table 34-1 summarizes the mycoses.

Of those fungi causing mycoses, fewer than 100

species are true pathogens and have the capacity to cause infection in a normal host. Most of these cause superficial skin or subcutaneous infections. A very few cause the classic systemic or deep fungal infections. The vast majority of fungi are of low virulence and do not cause disease in humans under normal circumstances. However, a host with altered resistance is susceptible to infection by a wide variety of fungi usually considered nonpathogenic. Such patients may be immunosuppressed as a result of disease or immunosuppressive drug therapy. Included among these patients are those who have certain cancers and those who are infected by the human immunodeficiency virus (HIV). The incidence of opportunistic fungal infections has been steadily increasing so that they are now the most common fungal infections encountered in hospitalized patients.

Reservoirs of potentially pathogenic fungi are everywhere. Two common reservoirs are animals and soil. Susceptible hosts come into contact with them in the environment, where these fungi are often transmitted by inhalation of spores or introduction through some trauma such as a puncture wound. Another source includes yeasts, which are a part of the normal flora in humans or animals. This chapter introduces the concepts and techniques basic to an understanding of medical mycology. The remaining chapters in this section deal with collection and processing of fungal specimens and the identification and characteristics of the most common causative agents of fungal infections.

## GENERAL CHARACTERISTICS OF FUNGI

The fungi are a diverse group of organisms that includes the yeasts, molds, mushrooms, rusts, and smuts. The fungi are eukaryotic, meaning their cells have a membrane-bound nucleus and cell organelles. The cell membranes are rich in lipid compounds called sterols. The most important of these is **ergosterol**. Like plants, they possess cell walls composed of complex polysaccharides, but unlike plants they lack chlorophyll.

| Table 34–1 ▶ Classification of Mycoses | |
|---|---|
| **Mycosis** | **Affected Tissue** |
| Superficial | Outermost layers of skin and hair |
| Cutaneous | Keratin in skin, hair, and nails and causes inflammation in the skin |
| Subcutaneous | Soft tissue, muscles, and bones immediately below the skin |
| Systemic | Involve the deep tissues and organs of the body |

The fungi may be unicellular such as the yeasts or multicellular such as the molds. Molds are filamentous, which means that they are composed of elongated tube-like filaments called **hyphae**. The hyphae may be **septate** or **aseptate**. Septate hyphae contain crosswalls called septa (sing. septum) that divide the hyphae into separate cells. Hyphae lacking these structures are aseptate, and there is no distinct separation of the cytoplasm of individual cells. These differences are illustrated in Figure 34-1. Molds grow by elongation and branching of the hyphae to form a mass of hyphae called a **mycelium**.

Yeasts are oval to round cells. When yeasts grow in culture, they produce moist, creamy colonies, resembling bacterial colonies. Yeasts often reproduce by a process called **budding** in which a small outgrowth called a blastoconidium is produced from the parent cells. Budding of yeast is shown in Figure 34-2. In some species the buds elongate and resemble the hyphae of molds. These **pseudohyphae** (false hyphae) can be distinguished from true hyphae by the constriction between cells. Figure 34-3 shows the difference between true hyphae and pseudohyphae.

## REPRODUCTION OF FUNGI

Reproduction of fungi may be sexual or asexual, through the production of spores or other structures resembling spores. A true spore is a reproductive structure formed either by meiosis (sexual) or cleavage (asexual). Although many species are able to produce more than one type of asexual spore, any given fungus can produce only one kind of sexual spore.

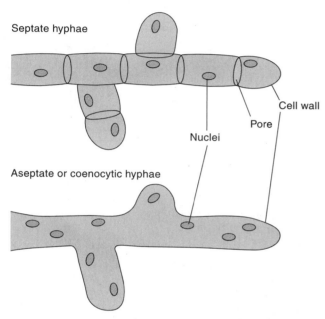

**FIGURE 34-1** Microscopic appearance of hyphae. Septate hyphae with crosswalls are compared to aseptate hyphae that lack these.

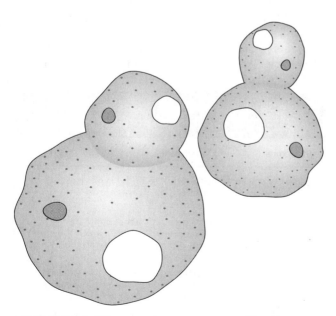

**FIGURE 34-2** Microscopic appearance of budding yeast cells.

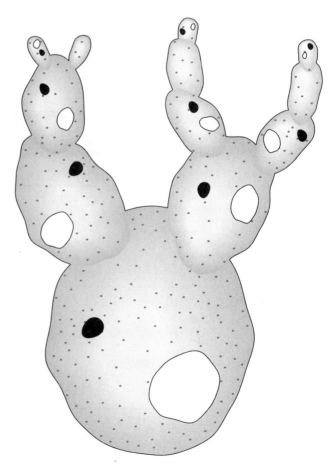

**FIGURE 34-3** Microscopic appearance of yeast with pseudohyphae.

## Sexual Spores

Under most circumstances fungi reproduce by forming asexual spores. However, sexual spores may be produced under certain environmental conditions, resulting in individuals with new genetic combinations. Production of sexual spores usually requires mating of two separate strains of the fungus. Because these conditions are not often met in the clinical laboratory, sexual spores are rarely seen in clinical specimens. Some fungi are homothallic and may produce sexual spores in culture. Sexual spores are of three types: (1) **ascospores**, (2) **zygospores**, and (3) **basidiospores** as illustrated in Table 34-2. Ascospores are contained in an ascus, which is a sac that gives rise to the ascospores. In some cases the asci may be contained in a fruiting body called an ascocarp. Examples are shown in Table 34-3.

## Asexual Spores

There are two major types of asexual spores, **sporangiospores** and **conidia**. These spores may be produced by a variety of supporting structures, which often are characteristic of a particular species. These and other reproductive bodies are commonly used as a basis for identification and classification of medically important fungi in the clinical laboratory.

**Sporangiospores.** Sporangiospores are true spores formed by cleavage following nuclear fusion and mitosis from a **sporangium** (pl. sporangia). A sporangium may be supported by a specialized hyphal structure

### Table 34–3 ▶ Ascocarp Morphology

| Ascocarp | Definition | Diagram |
|---|---|---|
| Cleistothecium | A saclike fruiting body that contains randomly distributed asci. The asci are released when the cleistothecium ruptures. | |
| Perithecium | A fruiting body having asci in layers. It contains a small opening through which asci or ascospores escape. | |

called a **sporangiophore**, much like a tree trunk supports the branches of a tree. These features are summarized in Table 34-4 and diagrammed in Figure 34-4. Sporangiospores are produced by a single class of fungi, the *Zygomycetes.*

**Conidia.** Conidia (sing. conidium) are produced by most of the medically important fungi, except for the *Zygomycetes.* Technically, conidia are not true spores, but are asexual sporelike structures not formed by cleavage or conjugation. However, for practical purposes they are often referred to as spores. Conidia are most often produced either directly from the hyphae or yeast cells or from specialized supporting cells called **conidiophores.** The conidiophores act like stalks supporting the conidia. In other cases there are other specialized supporting cells, such as annellides or phialides. An annellide is a cell that gives rise to conidia by successive elongation resulting in a tapered tip. A phialide

### Table 34–2 ▶ Sexual Spores Produced by Fungi

| Type of Spore | How Formed | Diagram |
|---|---|---|
| Ascospores | Haploid cells formed after meiosis from the fusion of a male and female nucleus inside an ascus (sac) | |
| Basidiospores | Spores on the end of a club-shaped cell containing the haploid nuclei resulting from the fusion of two compatible hyphae or yeast cells | |
| Zygospore | The fusion of two compatible hyphae to form a thick-walled protective structure | |

### Table 34–4 ▶ Structures Associated with Sporangiospore Production

| Structure | Description |
|---|---|
| Sporangiospore | Asexual spore of the zygomycetes produced by cleavage from a sporangium |
| Sporangium (pl. sporangia) | Saclike structure that contains sporangiospores, from which they are produced by cleavage from the membrane |
| Sporangiophore | A stalklike structure that rises from the hyphae and from which the sporangium arises by swelling at the tip |
| Columella | A swollen portion of the sporangiophore that extends into the sporangium |

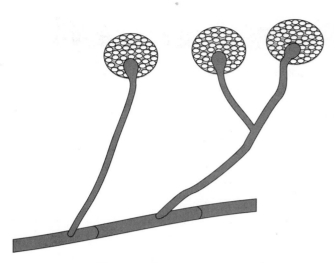

**FIGURE 34-4** Diagram of microscopic appearance of sporangiospore production.

| Table 34–5 ▶ Commonly Observed Conidia | | |
|---|---|---|
| **Type of Spore** | **How Formed** | **Diagram** |
| Arthroconidium | Modification of hyphal cell | |
| Blastoconidium | A bud coming off a parent cell | |
| Chlamydoconidium | Round, thick-walled, structures formed at the end, sides, or within the strand of a hypha or pseudohypha | |
| Macroconidium | The larger of two conidia, formed by the same fungus, generally multicellular | |
| Microconidium | Smaller of two conidia formed by the same fungus, generally unicellular | |

also gives rise to conidia but remains fixed and does not increase in length as the conidia are formed and released. Conidia, which are relatively large, sometimes multicelled, are referred to as macroconidia. Smaller conidia in species that produce two types of conidia are called microconidia. Occasionally conidia may be contained in saclike structures called pycnidia, which must be distinguished from saclike ascocarps. Figure 34-5 illustrates examples of aerial conidia production.

Conidia are also formed directly from the hyphae. Chlamydoconidia are round, enlarged conidia within or at the end of hyphae. Arthroconidia are boxcar-like conidia formed by modification of a hyphal cell. Table 34-5 defines and illustrates commonly observed conidia and supporting structures.

## CLASSIFICATION OF FUNGI

Even though asexual spores are most often observed in clinical specimens, the type of sexual spore produced,

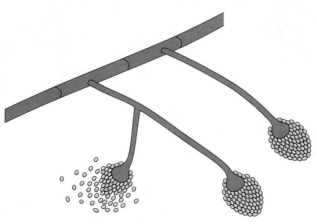

**FIGURE 34-5** Examples of aerial conidia production.

or lack thereof, is the primary criterion used to separate fungi into classes. There are four basic phyla of fungi: (1) *Zygomycota,* (2) *Ascomycota,* (3) *Basidiomycota,* and (4) *Deuteromycota.* No sexual spores have been identified for the *Deuteromycota,* which are sometimes referred to as imperfect fungi (Fungi Imperfecti). Table 34-6 lists the four phyla and some of their major characteristics. The *Zygomycota, Ascomycota,* and *Basidiomycota,* each contain only one class, *Zygomycetes, Ascomycetes,* and *Basidiomycetes,* respectively.

Although the *Zygomycetes* are defined by their ability to form sexual zygospores, these are almost never seen in clinical specimens. However, the medically important *Zygomycetes* also have two distinctive characteristics that are observed in the clinical laboratory: (1) They produce aseptate hyphae, and (2) they produce asexual sporangiospores. None of the other medically important fungi has these characteristics. One exception is *Coccidioides immitis,* which produces spherules and endospores resembling sporangia and sporangiospores (see Chapter 38).

Most of the clinically important fungi for which a sexual state has been defined are *Ascomycetes.* On occasion ascospores are produced in cultures observed in the clinical laboratory. When a sexual state for one of the imperfect fungi is discovered, it most commonly has been proven to be an ascomycete.

| | | | | Predominant Cell Wall |
|---|---|---|---|---|
| **Table 34–6 ▶ Characteristics of the Four Fungal Phyla** | | | | |
| **Phylum** | **Sexual Spore** | **Asexual Spore** | **Hyphae** | **Polysaccharide** |
| Zygomycota | Zygospore | Sporangiospore | Aseptate | Chitin |
| Ascomycota | Ascospore | Conidium | Septate | Glucan and mannan |
| Basidiomycota | Basidiospore | Conidium | Septate | Chitin and mannan |
| Deuteromycota | None | Conidium | Septate | Chitin and glucan |

## GENERAL APPROACH TO THE IDENTIFICATION OF FUNGI

Although there are a number of techniques and procedures to be learned and mastered in the clinical mycology laboratory, a much greater emphasis is placed on morphologic assessment than in the bacteriology laboratory. Biochemical testing of the fungi, particularly the molds, is of limited value. Microscopic morphology in culture and direct preparations of clinical specimens is of paramount importance in fungal identification.

### Characteristics of Fungi in Direct Examination of Clinical Specimens

Whenever possible a clinical specimen or tissue section should be examined directly in the evaluation of a fungal infection. The initial examination using direct microscopic evaluation is especially important because it provides the physician with a rapid source of information that can assist in diagnosis and treatment. This information may also help the microbiologist decide how to more effectively isolate and culture the etiologic agent.

Some fungi have characteristic morphology and can be identified conclusively from their microscopic appearance in tissues and other specimens. Other fungi can be visualized in these specimens, but cannot be further characterized until cultures are performed and evaluated. Table 34-7 lists the various forms that may be observed in direct examination of clinical specimens. The parasitic yeast forms of the **dimorphic** pathogenic fungi are quite distinctive. The presence of pseudohyphae suggests *Candida* or *Trichosporon* organisms; the demonstration of a capsule is indicative of *Cryptococcus neoformans.* The presence of spherules and endospores suggests *C. immitis,* but must be distinguished from the sporangia of the *Zygomycetes,* which are occasionally seen in sinus or nasal specimens.

If nonseptate hyphae are observed, this indicates that the organism is a zygomycete. Septate hyphae are much less specific. However, one group of organisms produces hyphae that contain a brown **melanin** pigment. These are the **dematiaceous** (dark) fungi. The hyphae appear brown in unstained preparations. The other septate hyphae are hyaline or clear and may be difficult to see in unstained preparations. Some organisms grow in small colonies in tissues. These may be recognized as granules or grains. If the organisms are dematiaceous, these grains will be black or dark brown. Some dematiaceous organisms produce round sclerotic bodies that resemble yeast.

Visualization of fungi in direct preparations may be aided by digesting cells or mucous with 10% potassium hydroxide (KOH) preparation. There are also a number of special stains that can be used to enhance visualization or in some cases even provide definitive identification of certain fungi. Table 34-8 lists some of the more useful methods and stains for direct microscopic detection of fungi. Special stains such as methenamine silver, periodic acid-Schiff (PAS) and alcian blue/mucicarmine are most commonly performed by histology departments for the clinical mycology laboratory. Methods for KOH preparation and the India ink preparation are given in Chapter 35.

### Cultures of Fungi

When processing and evaluating specimens for fungal cultures it is important to have a clear understanding of the clinical situation so that appropriate specimens are taken and appropriate procedures are performed.

**Table 34–7 ▶ Characteristics of Fungi in Direct Examination of Clinical Specimens**

| Structures Observed in Clinical Specimens |
|---|
| 1. yeasts |
| 2. yeasts and pseudohyphae |
| 3. spherules |
| 4. nonseptate hyphae |
| 5. hyaline septate hyphae |
| 6. dematiaceous septate hyphae |
| 7. sclerotic bodies |
| 8. granules/colonies |

## Table 34–8 ▶ Methods Used for Microscopic Examination of Fungi

| Method | Application |
|---|---|
| Potassium hydroxide (KOH) prep | Detection of fungal elements in skin and mouth scrapings, sputum, and secretions |
| Calcofluor white | Enhance detection of fungal elements by fluorescence |
| India ink preparation | Demonstrate capsule of *Cryptococcus neoformans* in cerebrospinal fluid and other fluids |
| Alcian blue/mucicarmine stains | Demonstrate capsule of *C. neoformans* in tissue and smears |
| Periodic acid-Schiff (PAS) stain | Stain fungal elements in smears and tissue for best detail |
| Methenamine silver stain | Stain fungal elements in smears and tissue. Most sensitive |
| Giemsa stain | Demonstrate yeast in bone marrow smears |
| Papanicolaou stain | Used on body fluids and sputum samples to visualize dimorphic fungi |

The subsequent chapters in this section about clinical mycology provide the kind of clinical information necessary to make these decisions.

As a general rule specimens for fungal cultures should be placed on several different media to enhance recovery. Because some fungi grow quite slowly, media containing inhibitory substances may be needed to prevent overgrowth of contaminating bacteria. Moreover, certain pathogenic fungi will grow on inhibitory media while saprophytes often do not. In general, media for fungal cultures contain fewer nutrients than those used for bacterial cultures. Nutritionally poor media also may enhance the production of reproductive structures in fungi. Because molds are identified by these characteristics, it is important to maximize spore production.

The choice of incubation conditions also depends on the clinical situation and type of specimen. In general, molds grow best in ambient (room air) conditions. Incubators can be set at 30°C to standardize these conditions. Some fungi can grow at higher temperatures and the ability to grow at elevated temperatures may be of diagnostic importance. Some yeasts may exhibit enhanced growth at body temperature. Demonstration of thermal dimorphism is necessary for identification of certain pathogenic fungi (see Chapter 38).

When dealing with fungal cultures, attention to laboratory safety cannot be overstressed. Cultures should always be evaluated under a biologic safety hood. Tubed media are preferred over plate media because the chance of transmission of aerosolized spores is much lower. In addition, tubed media will not dry out over prolonged incubation.

**Yeasts.** The approach to yeast cultures is somewhat different from the molds, in that carbohydrate utilization is much more important. However, microscopic studies are still important, because it is necessary to ensure that the assimilation and fermentation tests are appropriate for the kind of organism cultured (see Chapter 41).

**Nonculture Methods of Identification.** Because fungi generally grow more slowly than bacteria, identification can be a slow process. In some cases a rapid diagnosis is extremely important, particularly in the immunocompromised patient. Several more rapid methods of diagnosis have come on the market in recent years, which are helpful in making at least a presumptive diagnosis of a mycotic infection. There are DNA probes now available for some of the dimorphic pathogens and *C. neoformans*. Cryptococcal antigen can also be detected in fluids where the number of organisms is too low to be detected in direct examination. Fluorescent antibody stains were once felt to be a promising method for specific identification of certain fungi. However, specificity is very limited because of cross-reactions, and these stains are no longer used.

Serologic testing of patients for serum antibodies to the systemic fungi and certain saprophytes can be helpful in diagnosis and management of some patients. Cross-reactivity is also a problem with these tests. Moreover, some of these tests are not very sensitive in detecting infection. Additionally, it may be difficult to separate previous infection or exposure from current active disease.

## ANTIFUNGAL AGENTS AND SUSCEPTIBILITY TESTING

Until recently there have been few drugs that could be used effectively to treat serious systemic fungal infections. With the increase in deep fungal infections as a serious health problem in immunocompromised patients, research in this area has increased, and new drugs are being developed. One problem with antifungal drug therapy is the toxicity of many of the agents. Because of the similarities between mammalian cells and fungal cells, drugs that affect fungi can cause toxic reactions in humans. Research has been directed toward the production of less toxic but effective agents.

Three basic kinds of drugs are used to treat systemic fungal infections. Amphotericin B is the principal polyene antibiotic. It binds to ergosterol, which is the major lipid compound in the cell membrane of fungi. This causes membrane damage and changes the permeability of the cell membrane. It is the most established systemic agent but is very toxic. 5-Fluorocytosine inhibits pyrimidine synthesis and thus interferes with nucleic acid synthesis. It is principally a second-line drug used to treat some yeast infections, often in combination with amphotericin B. Most of the newer drugs are azoles, which affect

## Table 34–9 ▶ Antifungal Drugs and Their Uses

| Antifungal Agents | Activity | Examples | Use |
|---|---|---|---|
| Polyene macrolides | Bind to ergosterol, alter membrane function | amphotericin B | Systemic, topical, oral |
| | | nystatin | |
| 5-Fluorocytosine | Inhibits nucleic acid synthesis | 5-FC | Systemic |
| Azols | Impair ergosterol synthesis of membranes | miconazole | Topical and systemic |
| | | ketoconazole | Topical and systemic |
| | | fluconazole | Systemic |
| | | itraconazole | Systemic |
| | | clotrimazole | Topical |
| Griseofulvin | Antibiotic, fungistatic, binds to lipid | griseofulvin | Systemic for refractory dermatophyte infections |
| Allylamine | Inhibits membrane sterol production | naftifine | Topical for dermatophytes |
| | | terbinafine | Topical, systemic for dermatophytes |

lipid membrane synthesis. Some of these can be taken orally, in contrast to amphotericin B, which must be given intravenously. The azoles vary in toxicity. Drugs include miconazole, ketoconazol, fluconazole, and itraconazole. Table 34-9 summarizes antifungal drugs and their uses.

Unlike antibiotic sensitivity testing in bacteria, antifungal susceptibility in the laboratory is in its infancy. Although methods are being developed. it is much more difficult to test the agents because of their chemi-cal properties and poor solubility. Moreover, the fungal organisms themselves grow slowly when compared to bacteria and it is difficult to standardize testing conditions. Only a few studies have compared in vitro sensitivity results with clinical effectiveness of the drug in patients. Further controlled studies need to be done before routine testing of antifungal drug susceptibility will be applicable to the community hospital clinical laboratory.

## SUMMARY

▶ Mycology is the branch of microbiology that involves the study of fungi. These include molds, yeasts, and mushrooms. Medical mycology concerns fungi that cause disease in humans.

▶ Fungi are eukaryotic and have true membrane-bound nuclei. The cell membranes are rich in sterol lipids, especially ergosterol. They have rigid polysaccharide cell walls but lack chlorophyll.

▶ Molds are comprised of filamentous cells called hyphae. Septate hyphae have crosswalls (septa) dividing the cells, whereas aseptate hyphae do not.

▶ Yeasts are round cells and reproduce by budding.

▶ Fungi are classified by the type of sexual spores which, may be produced. These include zygospores (*Zygomycota*), ascospores (*Ascomycota*), and basidiospores (*Basidiomycota*). Deuteromycetes are imperfect fungi, which do not produce sexual spores.

▶ Identification of fungi in the clinical laboratory involves direct microscopic examination of specimens and cultures. Molds are most commonly identified morphologically by the kinds of reproductive structures produced. Biochemical tests are more important in yeast identification.

▶ Antifungal drugs tend to be quite toxic to humans. Therefore, serious, deep fungal infections are more difficult to treat than bacterial infections. Antifungal susceptibility testing in the laboratory needs more development before it can be routinely applied in the clinical laboratory.

# Review Questions

1. The drug amphotericin B interferes with permeability of the fungus cell wall because of its affinity for which substance in the cell wall?
   a. Glycogen
   b. Chitin
   c. Ergosterol
   d. Melanin

2. All except which of the following are characteristic of fungi?
   a. Cell wall
   b. Chlorophyll
   c. Membrane-bound nucleus
   d. Ergosterol

3. Which of the following criteria are used to classify fungi into phyla?
   a. Asexual spore type and hyphae type
   b. Asexual spore type and the major component of the cell wall
   c. Sexual spore type
   d. Hyphae type and the major component of the cell wall

4. Which of the following is a sexual spore?
   a. Arthroconidium
   b. Chlamydoconidium
   c. Sporangiospore
   d. Zygospore

5. Which of the following best stains fungal elements in smears for detail?
   a. Papanicolaou
   b. Giesma stain
   c. India ink
   d. Periodic acid-Schiff

6. The hypha pictured in Figure 34-6 is:
   a. septate.
   b. nonseptate.

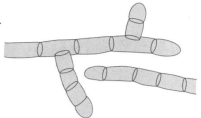

**FIGURE 34-6**

7. Sporangiospores are typical of which group of fungi?
   a. Zygomycetes
   b. Ascomycetes
   c. Basidiomycetes
   d. Yeasts

8. No sexual spores have been identified for members of the class:
   a. *Ascomycota.*
   b. *Basidiomycota.*
   c. *Zygomycota.*
   d. *Deuteromycota.*

9. Which of the following is associated with conidia production?
   a. Sporangiospore
   b. Ascocarp
   c. Phialide
   d. All of the above

10. A bud coming off a parent cell is called a:
    a. conidiophore.
    b. blastoconidium.
    c. arthroconidium.
    d. macroconidium.

## ▶ REFERENCES & RECOMMENDED READING

Baron, E. J., Peterson, L. R., & Finegold, S. M. (Eds.). (1994). *Bailey and Scott's diagnostic microbiology* (9th ed.). St. Louis: Mosby.

Campbell, M. C., & Stewart, J. L. (1980). *The medical mycology handbook.* New York: Wiley.

Espinal-Ingroff, A., & Fuller, M. A. C. (1992). Antifungal agents and susceptibility testing. In P. Murray (Ed.). *Manual of clinical microbiology* (6th ed., pp. 1405–1414). Washington, DC: ASM Press.

Georgopapadakou, G., & Walsh, T. J. (1994, April 15). Human mycoses: Drugs and targets for emerging pathogens. *Science, 264,* 371–373.

Howard, B. J., et al. (1994). *Clinical and pathogenic microbiology.* St. Louis: Mosby.

Koneman, E. W., & Roberts, G. D. (1985). *Practical laboratory mycology* (3rd. ed.). Baltimore: Williams & Wilkins.

Kwon-Chung, K. J., & Bennett, J. E. (1992). *Medical mycology.* Philadelphia: Lea & Febiger.

Larone, D. H. (1993). *Medically important fungi: A guide to identification* (2nd ed.). Washington, DC: American Society for Microbiology.

National Committee for Clinical Laboratory Standards. (1992, December). *Reference method for broth dilution antifungal susceptibility testing of yeasts: Proposed standard M-27-P.*

Reese, R. E., & Betts, R. F. (Eds.). (1991). *A practical approach to infectious diseases* (3rd ed.). Boston: Little, Brown.

Sarosi, G. A., & Davies, S. F. (1994). Therapy for fungal infections. *Mayo Clinic Proceedings, 69,* 1111–1117.

Sherris, J. C. (Ed.). (1990). *Medical microbiology: An introduction to infectious diseases* (2nd ed.). New York: Elsevier.

Sternberg, S. (1994). The emerging fungal threat. *Science, 266,* 5191 (p.1632).

Zuger, A. (1995). The terminator. *Discover, 16*(1), 23–24.

# CHAPTER 35

# Collection and Processing of Fungal Specimens

Anne T. Rodgers, MT (ASCP), PhD, James A. Miller, MD

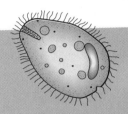

## Microbes in the News

### "The Heart of the Sixties"

It was reported in *Newsweek,* that Bob Dylan, rock star of the sixties was hospitalized with an illness called histoplasmosis, a usually mild illness that occurs when a fungus is inhaled. In Dylan's case, the lining of the sac surrounding the heart was also involved, usually a life-threatening complication. Because his tour scheduled for August was not canceled, *Newsweek* reported that he probably will be all right. *Newsweek,* June 9, 1997.

## KEY TERMS

| | | |
|---|---|---|
| Ambient | Texture | Umbonate |
| Histopathologic stains | Topography | Verrucose |
| Rugose | | |

## LEARNING OBJECTIVES

**Upon successful completion of this chapter, the student should be able to:**

1. Describe appropriate methods for fungus specimen collection.

2. List media appropriate for isolation and identification of fungi.

3. Describe the various procedures used in direct examination of fungus cultures. Name structures that are shown by the method.

4. List and discuss procedures used to identify and report fungus isolates including yeasts.

5. List the macroscopic and microscopic observations that should be made when reading a fungus culture.

# INTRODUCTION

As with bacteria, the ability to isolate and identify fungi begins with appropriate specimens and collection of those specimens. Some of the same considerations discussed in specimen collection for bacterial cultures apply to fungal cultures. These include knowledge of the resident flora of a particular site and proper procedures for collection, processing, and planting of the specimen. An understanding of the types of media available and their use will increase the chances of isolating a causative agent. Knowledge of the clinical aspects of various infections is also extremely valuable in ensuring that proper specimens are obtained and appropriate laboratory procedures are instituted.

In this chapter, specimens, media, and procedures for isolation will be discussed. In addition, general guidelines for identification of fungal groups will be covered. Specific characteristics of genera and species will be discussed in the chapters covering those groups.

| Table 35–1 ▶ Collections of Specimens for Fungal Culture | |
|---|---|
| **Specimen Type** | **Recommendations for Collection** |
| Respiratory specimens | Sputum should be a fresh morning specimen. Collect in a sterile screw-top container and transport immediately. |
| Pus, drainage, and exudates | Aspirate with sterile syringe and place in sterile container. |
| Vaginal material | Collect with sterile swabs and place in sterile container. |
| Tissue | Collect aseptically from the center and edge of lesion. Keep moist with sterile water and transport in sterile container. |
| Bone marrow | Aspirate aseptically and place in sterile container. SPS or heparin may be added as an anticoagulant. |
| Cerebrospinal fluid (CSF) | Collect in a sterile container and transport immediately. |
| Urine | A catheterized specimen is preferred, but a fresh early morning clean-catch specimen may be used. |
| Nails | Clean with 70% alcohol, collect whole nail or scrapings, and transport in a clean envelope. |
| Skin scrapings | Clean with 70% alcohol, collect scrapings, and transport in a clean envelope. |
| Hair | Collect at least 10 affected hairs with shaft. Place hairs between two clean glass slides and transport in envelope. |
| Body fluids | Collect aseptically in a sterile container. |

# COLLECTION AND TRANSPORT OF SPECIMENS FOR FUNGUS CULTURE

## Collection and Transport

Quality of specimens for fungal culture is an important consideration in successful isolation of the etiologic agents of mycoses. To ensure recovery of the etiologic agent, collection should be appropriate to the specimen. Transportation to the laboratory must be rapid, and the specimen should be processed promptly. Table 35-1 summarizes the main specimen types and their recommended method of collection.

## Processing of Specimens

The method used for processing of clinical specimens for fungal culture depends on the type of specimen and the quality of the specimen. If specimens are not acceptable, even proper processing will not ensure recovery of the causative agent. Table 35-2 lists common specimen types, processing technique, and unacceptable specimens. Specimens that come from normally sterile sites or that have scant resident bacterial flora need little additional processing and may be inoculated directly on culture media. Table 35-3 lists specimens that may be inoculated directly and describes the method for inoculation of culture media.

# CULTURE MEDIA AND INCUBATION REQUIREMENTS

## Culture Media

A variety of media are available for isolation of fungi and yeasts from clinical specimens. As with bacteriologic

| Table 35–2 ▶ Direct Inoculation of Specimens | |
|---|---|
| **Type of Specimen** | **Processing and Inoculation** |
| Aspirates and exudates | Inoculate culture tubes with 2–3 drops and streak. |
| Bone marrow aspirates | Inoculate culture tubes with 2–3 drops and streak. |
| CSF and body fluids | Centrifuge and inoculate media directly with sediment. If clotted, mince clot and divide among culture tubes. |
| Vaginal swabs | Directly swab the media surface. |
| Urine | Centrifuge and inoculate media directly with sediment. |
| Hairs and skin scrapings | Press specimen onto surface of medium. |
| Nail | Mince or grind, divide evenly and press onto medium surface. |
| Bronchial washings | Inoculate with up to 0.5 mL fluid for each tube. May also be concentrated as for CSF. |

## Table 35–3 ▶ Common Specimen Types

| Specimen | Method for Processing | Criteria for Rejection |
|---|---|---|
| Urine | Concentrate by centrifugation | Specimens > 50 mL or 24-h specimens |
| Sputum | Inoculate bloody or puslike material | 24-h collections |
| Corneal scrapings | Collected by physician and inoculated at bedside | Dried specimens and swabs not acceptable |
| Body fluids (including CSF) | Concentrate if > 2 mL; inoculate sediment directly | Swabs not acceptable |
| Stool | Freshly passed feces; inoculate directly | Swabs not acceptable |

media, the choice depends on several factors including availability, laboratory preference, and cost. The media listed here are only suggestions, based on current references. Actual practice in individual laboratories may vary. Media available for culture of molds and yeasts generally falls into three groups, primary plating media, media for observation of microscopic morphology, and special purpose media. Primary plating media include media with and without antibacterial agents and enriched media for the isolation of the dimorphic fungi. Antibacterial agents such as chloramphenicol and gentamicin are added to media to inhibit the growth of bacteria, allowing any fungi present to grow. The addition of cycloheximide to a medium will inhibit some of the saprophytic fungi and allow the growth of slow-growing fungi such as the dermatophytes. If a medium containing cycloheximide is used an additional medium should be planted with it so that other fungi, when present, may be isolated. Enriched media are used when dimorphic fungi are suspected. Some common primary isolation media are Sabouraud's dextrose media, inhibitory mold agar, brain-heart infusion agar (with or without blood and antibiotics) and Mycosel.

Media for the observation of microscopic morphology are used when observation of reproductive structures is desired. Fungi are stimulated to produce reproductive structures and resting structures on nutritionally poor media. Media such as potato dextrose agar and cornmeal agar contain only basic ingredients to allow the fungus to survive. Potato dextrose agar is used in slide cultures and cornmeal agar is used to observe the pseudohyphae and blastoconidia of yeasts. Special purpose media include media for testing biochemical reactions and pigment production. Examples of special purpose media would be dermatophyte test medium, Birdseed (Niger seed) agar, and V-8 juice agar. The reader is referred to specific manufacturers for specifications regarding the makeup of these media. Table 35-4 lists the more common fungal and yeast isolation media and their use.

## Incubation Requirements

Most molds grow best at room temperature in a range from 26° to 30°C. Yeasts and the yeast phase of the dimorphic fungi grow best at 35° to 37°C. A source of moisture must be provided as even tubed media will dry out before some of the slower growing fungi appear. For the most part, fungi will grow under **ambient** (room air) conditions and need no enrichment of the atmosphere.

## Table 35–4 ▶ Primary Culture Media for Fungus Cultures

| Medium | Purpose | Manufacturer |
|---|---|---|
| Sabouraud dextrose | Saprophytes and pathogens | Difco, BBL |
| Inhibitory mold agar (IMA) | Pathogens except for dermatophytes | BBL |
| Mycosel | Dermatophytes | BBL |
| Dermatophyte test medium (DTM) | Dermatophytes (screening) | Difco, BBL |
| Brain-heart infusion (BHI) | Saprophytes and pathogens | Difco, BBL |
| Brain-heart infusion with antibiotics | Systemic pathogens (dimorphic), except dermatophytes | Difco, BBL |
| Mycobiotic | Pathogens, especially dermatophytes | Difco |
| SABHI | Saprophytes and pathogens | Difco, BBL |

List of Media Manufacturers:
Difco Laboratories Incorporated, Detroit, Michigan; BBL, Becton Dickinson Microbiology Systems, Cockeysville, MD; Remel (Distributor), Lenexa, Kansas

## DIRECT EXAMINATION OF SPECIMENS

Several techniques are used in addition to culture to examine specimens for fungal organisms. These include the potassium hydroxide (KOH) prep, India ink prep, various histopathology (tissue) stains, and calcofluor white and fluorescent Antibody stains. The Gram stain is usually not useful in direct examination of specimens for fungi. Two exceptions are Gram stain for yeasts, *Actinomyces* and *Nocardia*. Gram reactions for these organisms will be covered in those specific chapters.

### KOH Preparation

The KOH preparation is used to examine material from specimens directly. The KOH will clear cellular debris and make fungal elements such as hyphae, pseudohyphae, and spores more apparent. This method works well for skin scrapings, pus material, sputum, hair, and nails.

### India Ink Preparation

The India ink preparation is used as a "negative stain" to demonstrate the capsules of *Cryptococcus neoformans*. India ink does not actually stain cellular material but provides a black background against which capsules appear as large refractile clear spaces. When a sample containing *C. neoformans* is added to India ink,

the organism appears as a wide, clear refractile area (the capsule) with a yeast form inside. The yeast cell may or may not have a bud. This direct stain is especially useful for CSF specimens and may be used for urine sediments. In specimens with numerous white blood cells, red blood cells, or other fluids, care must be taken in interpreting the smear. Leukocytes, especially polymorphonuclear leukocytes, may be mistaken for cryptococci because of their clear cytoplasm and nuclear lobes.

### Calcofluor White Stain

The calcofluor white stain may be used to stain fungal elements found in clinical specimens. Calcofluor white will fluoresce when a fluorescent microscope is used. Calcofluor white binds to fungal cell wall polysaccharide and fluoresces as it is exposed to ultraviolet light (Kwon-Chung & Bennett, 1992).

### Fluorescent Antibody Stains

Specific reagents for fluorescent antibody stains are available for some of the fungi. However, specificity is very poor and cross-reactions are common.

### DNA Probes

DNA probes are now available for some of the dimorphic pathogens and *C. neoformans*. The probe

---

# PROCEDURE 35-1
## KOH Preparation

### Principle:

Clinical specimens mixed with 15% potassium hydroxide (KOH) will clear rapidly, while fungal elements that contain chitin will clear more slowly. Thus hyphae, pseudohyphae, spherules, and granules will be visible, even in material that is originally cloudy because of pus, cellular material, or mucus.

### Method:

1. Place the material on a clean glass slide. Add a drop of 15% KOH solution and mix. Coverslip.
2. Pass the slide through a flame to warm it and speed up the clearing process. Do not allow to overheat.
3. Examine the preparation microscopically using low power. Make sure that the light is adjusted so that hyaline structures are visible (use re-

duced light). Phase microscopy may aid in making fungal elements visible.
4. Although permanent preparations may not be made using this method, allowing the slide to sit overnight may allow additional clearing to occur. Slides initially negative for fungi should be reexamined in this way.

### Quality Control:

A portion of a viscous specimen such as sputum should be treated with the KOH solution prior to use to ensure sufficient clearing occurs.

### Expected Results:

Fungal structures such as spherules, yeast cells, pseudohyphae, and hyphae that were obliterated by cellular material or mucus will be visible after clearing occurs.

## PROCEDURE 35-2
## India Ink Preparation

### Principle:

India ink does not stain cellular material. When added to a preparation it provides a black background against which the capsules of *C. neoformans* in clinical specimens may be visualized.

### Method:

1. Dilute India ink (Stanford or Pelikan) 1 drop to 9 drops water.
2. Place 1 drop diluted India ink on slide.
3. Add 1 drop of CSF sediment and mix gently.
4. Coverslip. Examine with high dry objective of microscope for capsules.

### Quality Control:

It is important that the India ink be diluted and that the sediment used is not too thick. White cells, especially polymorphonuclear cells, present in infected CSF or urine may also show a refractile appearance and the cytoplasm with the lobes inside may give the appearance of a "yeast" surrounded by an unstained capsule. In this case care should be taken to look for true budding. Note that the capsule of *C. neoformans* is generally larger in diameter than the cytoplasm of the normal polymorphonuclear leukocyte.

### Expected Results:

*Cryptococcus neoformans* will appear as a budding, yeast organism that may be spherical or oval. The budding yeast will be surrounded by a wide capsule. The capsule may be generally twice the diameter of the yeast cell. The capsule gives a halo effect due to the unstained material surrounding the yeast cell.

---

for each organism consists of strands of DNA, which can hybridize with RNA material from an unknown fungus. The combination can be detected by luminescence. Commercially available systems have reached the market and promise to be the most accurate and rapid method for identification of these pathogens.

## Tissue Stains

In many cases, causative fungal agents are difficult to grow in the laboratory. **Histopathologic stains** then become the primary means of diagnosis of those mycoses. Stains for tissue sections include the periodic acid-Schiff (PAS) stain, Gomori methenamine silver (GMS), Giemsa stain, modified acid-fast stain, and the hematoxylin and eosin stain (H&E). These are the most commonly used stains for diagnosis of mycoses in tissue sections. Since the histopathology laboratory is separate from the mycology laboratory, and the stains are performed there, this text will not cover specific procedures. Applications for these stains will be covered in later chapters.

## IDENTIFICATION PROCEDURES

### Tease Preparation

Once the culture has grown and reproductive structures have formed, a direct microscopic examination of the culture may be done using the tease prep technique. A small amount of the fungus culture, taken midway between the center and edge of the culture is placed in a drop of lactophenol cotton blue and gently teased apart using two dissecting needles. A coverslip is then placed on the slide. The prep is examined microscopically under low power for hyphal structures, conidia, and spores. Patience is necessary in performing this technique because the first attempts may yield only free spores. Several preps may have to be made before intact reproductive structures are seen. However, even with the obvious disadvantages to this technique, valuable information about the fungal group may be obtained.

### Scotch Tape Technique

Some mycologists prefer the scotch tape technique to the tease prep for the microscopic examination of cultures. The sticky side of a piece of clear cellophane tape is first applied to the surface of a mold colony. The tape is then placed sticky side down on a glass slide and examined under the microscope. Spores and hyphae that have adhered to the tape can be evaluated through the tape, which acts as a coverslip. The advantage of this technique is that it is rapid and does not require manual manipulation of the mycelium as in the tease prep. The disadvantage is that often the spores adhere to the tape but the fruiting heads and supporting structures are left behind. Moreover, the tape is not as optically clear as a glass coverslip and it may be difficult to discern fine structure.

## PROCEDURE 35-3
## Fungal Tease Mount

### Principle:

A small portion of a growing fungal culture is "teased" apart on a slide, a stain such as lactophenol cotton blue (LPCB) is added and the slide is examined under the microscope (see Figure 35-1).

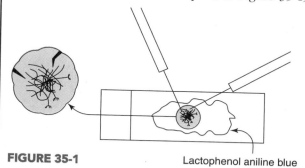

**FIGURE 35-1**          Lactophenol aniline blue

### Method:

1. Put one drop of LPCB on a slide.
2. Using a flamed and cooled inoculating probe, pick up a small portion of a fungal colony and place in the drop of LPCB on the slide.
3. Using a second probe, *gently!!* tease apart the hyphae so that there is a thin layer.

4. Place a coverslip on the slide. Avoid pressing hard on the coverslip so that structures are not unduly disturbed.
5. Allow the slide to sit for a few minutes if desired to let the dye penetrate the structures and examine under the microscope.

### Quality Control:

Preparations will be better if samples are taken between the center and the edge of the colony. Mycelia in the center may be sterile, whereas mycelia near the edge may not have produced reproductive structures. Only a small amount is necessary. The final preparation should be relatively thin.

### Expected Results:

Tease preparations are useful to examine the colony immediately after it matures. However, teasing apart the hyphae will often disturb the reproductive structures. The slide culture method is recommended to observe reproductive structures in a more natural state. The tease prep can give valuable preliminary information such as hyphal septa, color, and shape of spores.

## Slide Culture

A major disadvantage of the tease preparation of a fungus culture is that the spores may be removed from the aerial mycelium and may not maintain a typical appearance. Also, matted hyphae may be difficult to separate, obscuring detail of the reproductive structures. However, a slide culture will provide a monolayer and enable the fungus to be observed without disturbing the aerial mycelium and other characteristic structures. A slide culture is made by using spores from an unknown culture, and provides a valuable aid in the identification process. The procedure is given in Procedure 35-4.

## Yeast Identification Procedures

Several methods are used to identify yeasts that are not used for filamentous molds. These include the wet mount, germ tube test, cornmeal agar, urea agar, and biochemical tests including carbohydrate assimilation. The germ tube test is used to presumptively identify *Candida albicans*. A positive urea will eliminate *Candida* species and suggest *Cryptococcus* species or *Trichosporon* or *Rhodotorula* species. Morphology on

cornmeal agar is used to confirm biochemical identification of various yeasts. A wet mount, emulsifying a portion of suspected yeast in saline will rapidly differentiate yeast cells from bacteria. These tests will be covered in more detail in Chapter 41.

## Reading Cultures

After a fungus is isolated both macroscopic and microscopic observations should be made to gather data for final identification of the fungus or yeast.

**Macroscopic Observations.** Macroscopic observations include the medium used, the rate of growth, temperature requirements, and colony morphology. Rate of growth can be helpful because the Zygomycetes such as *Mucor* and *Rhizopus* tend to be rather rapid growers, sometimes appearing in 1 to 2 days. Pathogens such as the dermatophytes tend to take a week or more to appear. It is important to keep fungus cultures several weeks before reporting them as "no growth."

The first observation regarding colony morphology is whether the colony is a yeast or a mold. If the colony is creamy, a yeast should be suspected. Other observa-

# PROCEDURE 35-4
## Slide Culture

### Principle:

A portion of a fungal colony is inoculated onto a medium such as potato dextrose agar, a coverslip is added, and the culture is then allowed to grow undisturbed until reproductive structures appear. The coverslip is removed and mounted on a glass slide with lactophenol cotton blue (LCPB) and examined microscopically. When properly done, this procedure enables the medical technologist to examine reproductive structures of fungi in an undisturbed state (see Figure 35-2).

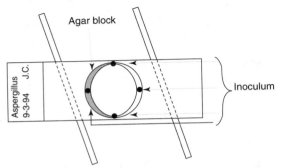

**FIGURE 35-2**

### Method:

1. Prepare slide culture "sets" by autoclaving glass slides, a coverslip (larger than the agar plug to be used), wedge of filter paper, and pieces of applicator sticks in glass 10 × 100 Petri dishes. The slide should be placed on the sticks to raise it off of the bottom of the dish. Glass rods may be used in place of the sticks. Autoclave at 15 lb, 121°C for 15 minutes, and dry in a hot air oven.
2. Prepare plugs of potato dextrose agar from a plate by cutting with the end of a sterilized 16 × 75 glass test tube.
3. Using a sterile scalpel or spatula, transfer a plug of agar, aseptically to the sterile slide in the glass Petri dish prepared in #1.
4. Using a sterile inoculating probe, inoculate four areas on the edge of the plug and the middle of the plug with a small amount of the mold colony.
5. Flame the coverslip in alcohol, cool, and place on the top of the agar plug. Add sterile distilled water to the dish (enough to wet the filter paper), and replace the cover of the dish.
6. Incubate the dish at room temperature or 30°C for a week or longer or until mature growth is apparent. (Some saprophytes may grow more rapidly.) A dissecting microscope may be used to check the progress of the culture. *DO NOT* remove the top of the dish when checking the culture in this manner.
7. Add sterile distilled water aseptically at regular intervals so the culture does not dry out.
8. After growth has matured, carefully remove the coverslip with flamed and cooled forceps and place fungi side down in a drop or two of LCPB on a second slide. The second slide need not be sterile. If the coverslip "sticks," it may be gently pried loose using a sterile inoculating probe.
9. Allow the preparation to sit for at least 20 minutes to allow staining with the LPCB. Overnight is preferred.
10. Examine under low power to observe the hyphae and types of spores and their arrangement on the mycelium. Confirm detail with high dry power.
11. Autoclave, wash and "recycle" the glass culture sets.

### Quality Control:

It is imperative that the culture be kept in a moist environment during the incubation time. Some fungi may take up to 2 weeks to produce visible fruiting bodies and other reproductive structures. Asepsis is important because of the ease with which fungal cultures may be contaminated. Care should be taken when removing the coverslip from the culture so that the fungal elements are not disturbed.

### Expected Results:

Look for fungal elements; hyphae, fruiting bodies and other structures, on the outer edge of the circle formed by the plug. Examine the whole coverslip before discarding. Use 10× magnification to scan and go to 100× to examine individual structures.

# PROCEDURE 35-5
## Germ Tube Test

### Principle:

*Candida albicans* will produce germ tubes (lateral hyphal filaments) when incubated in serum (human or bovine). This method affords a rapid easy method for the presumptive identification of *C. albicans*.

### Method:

1. Place 0.5 mL of human or bovine serum into a small glass test tube.
2. Inoculate a loopful of yeast culture into the serum. Include controls. (*C. albicans*, positive; *Candida tropicalis*, negative). To inoculate touch the tip of a sterile Pasteur pipe to the yeast colony. Place the pipe in the tube with the serum.
3. Incubate in a waterbath at 37°C for 2 hours.
4. Place a drop of the yeast-serum mixture on a clean glass slide with the Pasteur pipe.
5. Coverslip and examine under the low-power objective of the microscope.

### Quality Control:

Controls must be included because arthrospores of *Geotrichum* may be mistaken for germ tubes.

### Expected Results:

The formation of lateral hyphal filaments off of the yeast cell is a positive test. Germ tubes have two parallel sides and are not constricted at the point of origin.

### Reference:

Eisenberg, H. D. (1992). *Clinical microbiology procedures handbook*. Washington, DC: American Society for Microbiology.

---

tions must be made in the case of the molds. Each colony should be evaluated on the basis of pigment produced, the surface **topography**, and the surface **texture**. Fungi produce a variety of pigments. Pigment may appear in three places: the top of the colony (surface pigment), the underside of the colony (reverse pigment), and diffused into the medium (diffusible pigment). Careful observation of the pigment will help to classify fungi into groups.

The topography of the colony refers to the surface features of the colony, that is, "hills and valleys" formed as the colony grows. Because growth of the aerial mycelia may obscure this characteristic, topography may be best observed by looking at the underside of the colony. Colonies may be **rugose**, **umbonate**, **verrucose**, or flat. Rugose colonies have furrows radiating from the center to the edge of the colony. Umbonate colonies have a raised center but may also exhibit furrows around the central "button." Verrucose colonies have a wrinkled surface. Figure 35-3 illustrates these characteristics. Topography is difficult to determine when tube media are used and is less important than texture when making a final identification of a mold.

Texture is described using terms such as woolly, cottony, granular, powdery, velvety, or glabrous. Texture is derived from the height of the aerial mycelium and the type of spores produced by the mold. Woolly or cottony colonies have a dense, high aerial mycelium. Granular or

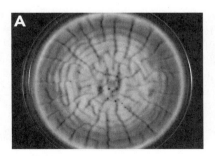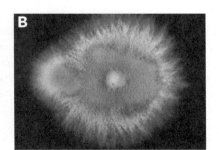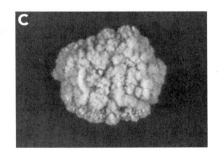

**FIGURE 35-3** Fungus culture topography. **A.** Verrucose. **B.** Rugose. **C.** Umbonate

---

# PROCEDURE 35-6
## Cornmeal Tween 80

### Principle:

Pseudohyphae, blastospores, and chlamydospores are produced on a nutritionally poor media such as cornmeal Tween 80 agar. These characteristics can be used to differentiate *C. albicans* from other species of *Candida* as well as other yeasts such as *Saccharomyces* and *Torulopsis*.

### Method:

1. Divide a Petri dish containing cornmeal agar with or without Tween 80 into two halves with a marking pen. Label with the culture number.
2. Make two separate streaks approximately 1.5 cm long and 1 cm apart using a sterile inoculating needle with a fresh yeast isolate. DO NOT dig into the agar.
3. Flame the needle, allow it to cool and make an "S"-shaped streak across the two lines.

4. Flame coverslip and place directly over the inoculation.
5. Incubate at room temperature for 72 hours.
6. Remove the Petri dish lid and observe each section with the low-power objective through the coverslip:

### Quality Control:

Include an isolate of *C. albicans* as a control.

### Expected Results:

Along the streak *C. albicans* produces characteristic thick-walled round terminal chlamydospores and pseudomycelia bearing clusters of blastospores.

---

powdery colonies have very flat aerial mycelia but produce large numbers of conidia, giving the powdery/granular appearance. Velvety colonies resemble velvet fabric because they produce low, very dense aerial mycelia. Fungi that produce no aerial mycelium and yeasts will show a waxy or glabrous morphology.

**Microscopic Observations.** Microscopic morphology of the fungus is observed using the tease preparation or the slide culture. The slide culture is preferred because reproductive structures may be observed in an undisturbed state. Microscopic observations that should be made include the type of hyphae, type of spores, and the manner in which the spores are produced.

### Final Identification

Identification of fungi is not difficult if the student uses all of the information derived from macroscopic and microscopic observations. As you are making macroscopic and microscopic observations it is important to avoid letting one characteristic cause you to jump to conclusions. Identification of fungi is rather like putting together bits and pieces of a puzzle. Be sure and check to see that all the pieces of the puzzle fit together before reporting a final identification. Occasionally, confirmatory

tests are necessary. These are most often used in the case of yeasts. A variety of rapid biochemical kits are available for this purpose and will be discussed later. Specific confirmatory tests for fungi will be discussed in those chapters.

## REPORTING CULTURE RESULTS

Direct examination should be done on all specimens submitted and the results reported. Although final reports for cultures may not be available for several weeks, preliminary results should be issued any time there is new information.

### Critical Values

Certain direct examination results and culture reports are considered significant findings and should be reported immediately to the physician. In this way clinicians are alerted to potentially life-threatening infections. The following are considered critical values and reported immediately; true hyphae in a clinical specimen, fungi seen in a normally sterile specimen, and yeast resembling *Cryptococcus* (McGinnis, 1992).

# SUMMARY

► Proper specimen collection for fungal specimens requires knowledge of clinical aspects of the patient's infection, resident normal flora, proper collection techniques, and an understanding of types of media and other tests available.

► Fungal cultures should be inoculated on to a variety of media for optimal recovery of organisms. These include general purpose media, enriched media, and inhibitory media. Nutritionally poor media are used to enhance production of reproductive structures for microscopic morphology.

► Direct examination of specimens for fungi should be performed in all cases if possible. KOH preparation clears all debris that can

obscure fungi in skin scrapings, pus, and sputum. India ink preparation reveals capsules of *Cryptococcus neoformans* in fluids. Calcofluor white enhances detection by fluorescence. Histopathologic tissue stains enhance detection by selectively staining fungal elements.

► Identification of molds in culture uses observations of growth rate, temperature requirements, colony morphology, and microscopic morphology of hyphae and reproductive structures. The microscopic examination can be performed using the tease preparation, scotch tape technique, and slide culture.

► Identification of yeasts uses wet mounts, the germ tube test, morphology on cornmeal agar, and biochemical tests including carbohydrate utilization.

## CASE STUDY

A 15-year-old boy injured his eye when a friend struck him in the face with a twig. Over the next few days he developed an ulcer and cloudiness in his cornea associated with some decrease in vision. His ophthalmologist suspected a fungal infection, and submitted corneal scrapings to the laboratory.

**Questions:**

1. What is the first thing you should do with the specimen after receiving it in the mycology laboratory?

2. What media should be planted?

3. Under what conditions should it be incubated?

4. What would you expect to see on the direct examination with KOH?

## Review Questions

1. The function of 15% KOH in the direct examination of skin, hair, and nail scrapings is to:
   a. preserve fungal elements.
   b. kill contaminating bacteria.
   c. clear and dissolve debris.
   d. fix preparation for subsequent staining.

2. All of the following are commonly used methods for the microscopic examination of filamentous molds, EXCEPT:
   a. tease mount.
   b. Gram stain.
   c. scotch tape technique.
   d. microslide culture.

3. A medium appropriate for use in making a slide culture preparation is:
   a. brain-heart infusion.
   b. potato dextrose agar.
   c. blood agar.
   d. V-8 juice agar.

4. India ink is useful for the microscopic demonstration of:
   a. hyphae.
   b. chlamydospores.
   c. capsules.
   d. sporangia.

5. One of the better media for routine isolation of fungi is:
   a. Sabouraud's dextrose agar.
   b. SIM medium.
   c. chocolate agar.
   d. corn meal agar.

6. Which of the following is most often used to prepare a slide from a tease prep of a plate culture for microscopic observation of a dermatophyte?
   a. Lactophenol cotton blue
   b. Potassium hydroxide
   c. Iodine solution
   d. Gram stain

7. In which of the following specimens is it important to perform a direct examination for fungi in addition to setting up a fungal culture?
   a. Skin scrapings
   b. Bronchial washings
   c. Cerebrospinal fluid
   d. All of the above

8. Which of the following would be expected to have moist, creamy or glabrous colonies?
   a. Saprophytic molds
   b. Dermatophytes
   c. Zygomycetes
   d. Yeasts

9. A slide culture is useful to demonstrate which of the following?
   a. Conidia production
   b. Germ tube production
   c. Capsule formation
   d. All of the above

10. Tease preparation reveals a mold with septate hyphae. Which of the following might be seen in a slide culture of this organism?
    a. Sporangia
    b. Capsules
    c. Macroconidia
    d. All of the above

## ▶ REFERENCES & RECOMMENDED READING

Baron, E. J., Peterson, L. R., & Finegold, S. M. (1994). *Bailey and Scott's diagnostic microbiology* (9th ed.). St. Louis: Mosby.

Difco Laboratories. (1984). *Difco manual* (10th ed.). Detroit, MI: Author.

Eisenberg, H. D. (Ed.). (1992). *Clinical microbiology procedures handbook*. Washington, DC: American Society for Microbiology.

Howard, B. J., et al. (1994). *Clinical and pathogenic microbiology*. St. Louis: Mosby.

Kern, M. E. (1985). *Medical mycology, a self instructional text*. Philadelphia: Davis.

Koneman, E. W., & Roberts, G. D. (1985). *Practical laboratory mycology* (3rd ed.). Baltimore: Williams & Wilkins.

Kwon-Chung, K. J., & Bennett, J. E. (1992). *Medical mycology*. Philadelphia: Lea & Febiger.

Larone, D. H. (1993). *Medically important fungi: A guide to identification* (2nd ed.). Washington, DC: American Society for Microbiology.

Murray, P. R. (Ed.). (1995). *Manual of clinical microbiology* (6th ed.). Washington, DC: ASM Press.

Power, D. A., (Ed.). (1988). *Manual of BBL products and laboratory procedures* (6th ed.). Cockeysville, MD: Becton Dickinson Microbiology Systems.

Sherris, J. C. (Ed.). (1990). *Medical microbiology: An introduction to infectious diseases* (2nd ed.). New York: Elsevier.

# CHAPTER 36
# Dermatophytes and Other Agents of Superficial Mycoses

James A. Miller, MD, Anne T. Rodgers, MT (ASCP), PhD

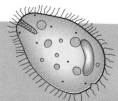

## Microbes in the News
### Ringworm and Club Lamb Fungus

Sheep exhibitors should take special care when examining their sheep for the show ring. Washing and shearing removes the natural lanolin and suint that protects sheep from getting some diseases. Exhibitors should be aware of ringworm and a ringworm-like disease that can be transmitted from infected sheep to humans. One ringworm type disease, caused by fungus, is currently being called "club lamb" fungus.

Ringworm of animals is caused by two genera of fungi—Microsporum and Trichophyton. In most cases, these fungi are obligate parasites of the skin and hair (wool). They are highly contagious from animal to animal, particularly in dense population conditions. The infections not only transmit readily to other animals, but they often transmit to human attendants of the animals and cause severe skin lesions. Infection results from direct contact with infected animals as well as by indirect contact through clippers, brushes, combs, blankets and contaminated pens. Although the disease is not life-threatening, it has reached epidemic proportions in some western states.

Wolverton, D., & Doane, T. *Ringworm and Club Lamb Fungus.*
http://www.ianr.unl.edu/pubs/nebfacts/nf91-29.htm

## KEY TERMS

Arthroconidia
Chlamydoconidia
Cutaneous
Dematiaceous
Dermatophyte
Ectothrix
Endothrix

Favic chandelier
Id reaction
Intertriginous
Keratin
KOH preparation
Lipophilic
Macroconidia

Microconidia
Pectinate body
Racquet hyphae
Ringworm
Spiral hyphae
Tinea

# LEARNING OBJECTIVES

**Upon successful completion of this chapter, the student should be able to:**

1. Identify the etiologic agents of the superficial mycoses: tinea versicolor, tinea nigra, black piedra, white piedra.

2. Identify and describe the clinical disease for each of the superficial mycoses discussed.

3. Discuss laboratory procedures for direct examination and cultural characteristics for the identification of these organisms.

4. Identify the etiologic agents of the dermatomycoses.

5. Identify and describe colonial and microscopic morphology of the dermatophytes.

6. List laboratory procedures and culture media used for the isolation and identification of these organisms.

7. Identify and discuss the clinical diseases caused by the dermatophytes including anatomic site of infection.

## INTRODUCTION

The cutaneous mycoses are among the most common fungal infections of humans and animals. In this group of infections the fungi are confined to the outer keratin layer of the skin. **Keratin** is the protective surface of the skin produced by cells of the epidermis as they mature and die. Because hair and nails are made of modified keratin, they are often involved in these infections as well. The fungal organisms do not invade the deeper layers of the skin and thus do not cause destruction or life-threatening infections.

Several of the **cutaneous** fungi produce a pattern of infection called **tinea**, which means wormlike. This refers to the irregular undulating pattern of the advancing edge of the lesions. Hence many of these infections are referred to as **"ringworm"** infections.

These diseases include a group of unrelated superficial infections and infections caused by a homogeneous group of fungi known as **dermatophytes**.

## SUPERFICIAL MYCOSES

In this group of infections the fungi are confined to the keratin layer of the skin or hair. Because the organisms are relatively innocuous and do not extend into the living cells of the epidermis, the body produces no tissue reaction to the fungi. Table 36-1 lists the superficial mycoses and their causative agents.

### Tinea Versicolor (Pityriasis Versicolor)

**Clinical Disease.** Tinea versicolor is caused by *Malassezia furfur,* a yeastlike organism commonly found on the skin. Relatively few individuals actually develop the lesions of tinea versicolor. The organism lives only in the keratin layer of the skin. Overgrowth of the organism results in the characteristic depigmented or discolored lesions typical of tinea versi-

| Table 36–1 ▶ Superficial Mycoses | |
|---|---|
| **Disease** | **Agent** |
| Tinea versicolor (Pityriasis versicolor) | *Malassezia furfur* |
| Tinea nigra | *Pheoanellomyces werneckii (Exophiala werneckii)* |
| Black piedra | *Piedraia hortae* |
| White piedra | *Trichosporon beigelii* |

color. The lesions are usually found on the chest or trunk. Adults are more commonly affected than children. Early infections most commonly involve loss of normal pigment in the skin, which may be easier to detect following sun exposure. The lesions may be slightly scaly. Chronic infections often produce darker, discolored lesions. There usually are no symptoms of irritation, and the disease is primarily a cosmetic problem. Topical agents can clear the lesions, but susceptible individuals are prone to recurrences.

**Direct Examination.** Examination of skin scrapings in **KOH preparations** is the most important laboratory test in the evaluation of patients with tinea versicolor. The organism appears as clusters of small yeast forms mixed with branched hyphae, giving the appearance of "spaghetti and meatballs." Figure 36-1 depicts a typical KOH preparation from a patient with tinea versicolor.

**Cultural Characteristics.** Because the appearance of the organism in a KOH preparation is diagnostic, culture is not usually necessary. Although the organism can grow well on a variety of fungal media, it is **lipophilic**. This means that the culture must be covered by a layer of sterile olive oil for the organism to grow. *M. furfur* has been increasingly recovered from blood cultures from patients on total parenteral nutrition therapy. As normal flora in the skin, the organism gains access to the bloodstream by way of the in-dwelling deep venous

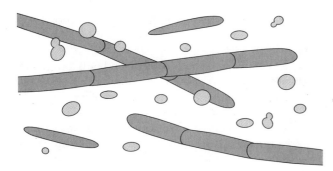

**FIGURE 36-1** *Malassezia furfur* KOH preparation of skin scrapings, with "spaghetti and meatballs" appearance.

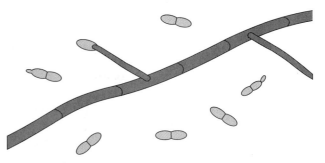

**FIGURE 36-2** Microscopic appearance of *Phaeoannellomyces werneckii* young culture.

catheter. Subculture to solid media from the primary blood culture liquid medium must be overlaid with olive oil for the organism to grow.

## Tinea Nigra

Tinea nigra, also known as tinea nigra palmaris, is caused by *Phaeoannellomyces werneckii* (*Exophiala werneckii*), which is a **dematiaceous** fungus. Dematiaceous means dark or pigmented and refers to fungi whose hyphae contain a brown pigment in the cell wall.

**Clinical Disease.** Tinea nigra most commonly occurs in the tropics, but has been seen worldwide. The lesions are most common on the palms of the hands. The fungus is confined to the keratin layer, and there is no reaction by the body to it. Because the fungus is pigmented, the lesions appear as brown or black spreading, round, flat plaques. The lesions may be confused with moles or melanoma. The organism is found on decaying vegetation and soil and is introduced into the surface of the skin from natural sources. The lesions are readily treated with topical agents that dissolve keratin.

**Direct Examination.** KOH preparation of skin scrapings from the lesions of tinea nigra will reveal the pigmented hyphae.

**Cultural Characteristics.** Because the lesions are characteristic, culture is usually not necessary. *P. werneckii* grows slowly on fungal media, often requiring several weeks before growth is observed. Early cultures are moist and consist of yeastlike cells present in pairs resembling safety pins. Later the organism becomes mycelial with dark mold colonies. Conidia are produced from annellides. Figure 36-2 depicts the microscopic features of *P. werneckii*.

## Black Piedra

Piedra is a fungal infection of the hair, without any involvement of the hair follicle. Two forms exist: (1) black piedra caused by *Piedraia hortae* and (2) white piedra caused by *Trichosporon beigelii*.

**Clinical Disease.** Black piedra is a disease primarily found in the tropics. The fungus attaches to the hair shaft producing small nodules that are black and very hard. The nodule may be too small to be detected visually, but produces a "clicking" sound when a comb is passed through the hair. The affected hair may become brittle and break, but otherwise there are no adverse effects.

**Direct Examination.** KOH preparation of affected hair will reveal packed hyphae. Ascii with ascospores may be present.

**Cultural Characteristics.** Culture is not necessary for diagnosis. *P. hortae* is dematiaceous (dark), producing brown to black slow-growing colonies. The hyphae may produce **chlamydoconidia**. Sometimes ascii and ascospores are present.

## White Piedra

**Clinical Disease.** White piedra is found in warm temperate areas of the world. It is associated with poor hygiene. Hair of the beard, axilla (armpit), and groin are frequently involved. The infection consists of a loose soft mass of fungal hyphae around the hair shaft. The granule is characteristically white. Cutting of the hair below the infection is curative, although topical antifungal agents may be used. The causative agent *T. beigelii* has also been increasingly associated with opportunistic infections in compromised hosts (see Chapter 39).

**Direct Examination.** KOH preparation of infected hair reveals the loosely packed hyphae, often with **arthroconidia** (arthrospores). Blastoconidia may also be present.

**Cultural Characteristics.** *Trichosporon beigelii* grows well on routine fungal media producing creamy yeastlike colonies within a few days. Later the colonies become moldlike. Blastoconidia and arthroconidia are produced. The organism is usually urease positive. Commercial yeast identification systems may be used for identification (see Chapter 41).

## DERMATOPHYTES

The dermatophytes are a relatively homogeneous group of fungi that cause a variety of infections of the skin, hair, and nails. The organisms probably originated as soil-inhabiting fungi, but have adapted to keratin. Some species are still found in the soil, but many now are principally associated with humans and animals. There are approximately 40 species of dermatophytes comprising three genera in the anamorph or imperfect state: *Trichophyton, Epidermophyton,* and *Microsporum.* All of the organisms for which a perfect or teleomorphic state has been found are ascomycetes, belonging to the genus *Arthroderma.* It is interesting that in some cases more than one anamorph species derive from a single teleomorph species.

### Clinical Diseases

The dermatophytes cause ringworm infections. The organisms are confined to the superficial epidermis or hair shaft. Although the deeper tissues are not involved, the body often produces a prominent inflammatory reaction to metabolic products of the fungus or as a result of allergy to the fungus. A classification of disease based on the particular organism causing the infection is unsatisfactory because a single species of a dermatophyte can cause a variety of clinical manifestations in different parts of the body, and the same clinical picture can be caused by dermatophytes of different species. Therefore most dermatologists use a classification based on the part of the body affected (see Table 36-2). The term tinea refers to the ringworm infection. Not all persons are equally susceptible. Some persons are plagued by persistent or recurrent infections, whereas others seem completely resistant to many of the dermatophyte infections.

**Tinea Pedis (Athlete's Foot).** Athlete's foot is the most common of the dermatophyte infections. The moist, warm environment of the spaces between the toes

provides the ideal setting for this fungal infection. Maceration of the tissues encourages the infection. Most commonly the disease is manifested by cracks or fissures in the skin between the third, fourth, and fifth toes (**intertriginous** infection). However, some very susceptible individuals develop more extensive involvement of the foot, sometimes associated with allergic manifestations. These patients may have crusted, scaly lesions or even blisters or ulcers. Although the intertriginous infections usually respond quickly to therapy with topical antifungal agents, the more extensive forms are often very difficult to eradicate. The most common organisms causing tinea pedis are *Trichophyton mentagrophytes, Trichophyton rubrum,* and *Epidermophyton floccosum.*

**Tinea Unguium (Ringworm of the Nails).** Tinea unguium is infection of the nail by a dermatophyte. The yeast *Candida albicans* can produce a very similar infection. Therefore, examination of scrapings of the nail by KOH preparation is vital in distinguishing these infections. The dermatophyte infection may be associated with production of soft, cheesy keratin debris within and under the nail or may result in pitted, grooved nails with loss of nail substance. The most common dermatophytes involved are *T. mentagrophytes, T. rubrum,* and *E. floccosum.* Of these, *T. rubrum* results in persistent infections that are very resistant to treatment. Topical antifungal agents have little effect. Systemic griseofulvin therapy can inhibit growth of the fungus. This therapy must be continued until the area of involvement grows out and can be cut away.

**Tinea Cruris (Jock Itch).** Tinea cruris is a dermatophyte infection of the groin area. Warm, moist macerated skin predisposes to the infection. The lesions spread away from the site of initial infection in a ring-like pattern. The edges are red; the center portions usually become scaly and brown. *E. floccosum* has traditionally been the most common causative organism, but recently *T. rubrum* has become more common. The infection is easily treated with topical antifungal agents.

**Tinea Corporis (Ringworm of the Body).** Ringworm of the body is associated with spreading scaly lesions. The margins are usually red while the central portion becomes scaly. Sometimes the central portions heal spontaneously. Highly susceptible individuals may have more inflammatory lesions and blisters. Almost any of the dermatophytes may be involved. Most cases respond to topical antifungal agents.

**Tinea Barbae (Ringworm of the Beard Area).** Infections of the hair of the beard area (see Figure 36-3) used to be more common when men obtained shaves at barber shops, and razors were not cleaned carefully between customers. The infection may be mild, resembling those of tinea corporis or may be extremely inflammatory associated with pustular infections of the hair follicles. The most commonly involved organisms are *Trichophyton verrucosum* and *T. mentagrophytes.*

| Table 36-2 ► Clinical Classification of Ringworm Infections | |
|---|---|
| **Clinical Disease** | **Common Name** |
| Tinea pedis | Athlete's foot |
| Tinea unguium | Ringworm of the nails |
| Tinea cruris | Jock itch, ringworm of the groin |
| Tinea corporis | Ringworm of the body |
| Tinea barbae | Ringworm of the beard |
| Tinea capitis | Ringworm of the scalp |
| Tinea favosa | Favus hair infection |
| Tinea imbricata | Asian ringworm |

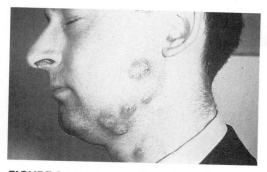

**FIGURE 36-3** Tinea barbae. (Courtesy of the Centers for Disease Control and Prevention, Atlanta, GA)

Many of the cases resolve spontaneously after a few weeks. Griseofulvin therapy will speed recovery.

**Tinea Capitis (Ringworm of the Scalp).** Tinea capitis is a dermatophyte infection of the hair of the scalp. It is common in children, but tends to disappear after puberty and is uncommon in adults. The infection may produce white patches on the hair or may become very inflammatory, associated with hair follicle involvement. **Ectothrix** infections involve the outer surface of the hair, whereas in **endothrix** infections, hyphae and arthroconidia are present within the hair shaft. Use of ultraviolet light (Wood's lamp) can demonstrate areas of infection that do not have scaly patches. These infected hairs exhibit bright green fluorescence. Until about 20 years ago, most of the infections in the United States were caused by *Microsporum audouinii,* which was contagious and rapidly spread among siblings and playmates. However, today the organism is rarely found and most infections are caused by *Trichophyton tonsurans* and *Microsporum canis.* Tinea capitis infections of all types are much less common today than they were 20 to 30 years ago.

Some tinea capitis infections resolve spontaneously. Topical antifungal agents cannot cure the infection but may help in local control. Griseofulvin therapy can cure the infections, but the treatment must be continued until the infected hair has grown out and the organisms can be eliminated by scrubs or cutting of the hair.

**Tinea Favosa and Tinea Imbriata.** Tinea favosa is a dermatophyte infection of the hair on which thick crusts are produced, associated with raw weeping wounds. *Trichophyton schoenleinii* causes most cases. Griseofulvin therapy is necessary to cure the infection.

Tinea imbricata is caused by *Trichophyton concentricum.* It produces concentric rings over the body in a mosaic pattern. The infection occurs principally in the islands of the Southwest Pacific and in South Asia among Indonesians and Polynesians. Susceptibility to infection is genetically determined as an autosomal recessive trait. Only homozygous individuals get the infection.

**The Id Reaction.** Occasionally patients with a dermatophyte infection on one part of the body will pre-

sent with skin lesions elsewhere, which look like additional areas of infection. Skin scrapings and cultures of the lesions will reveal no fungi. These lesions are an allergic reaction to the infection elsewhere on the body. The **id reaction** can occur anywhere on the body and be associated with any type of ringworm infection. However, the most common lesions involve the hands in association with tinea pedis. Treatment of the primary site of infection will result in clearing of the id reaction.

## Laboratory Identification of Dermatophytes

**Direct Examination.** Direct microscopic examination of skin or nail scrapings and infected hair using KOH preparation is the most useful approach to the patient with a dermatophyte infection. (See Chapter 35 for procedure.) The KOH digests the keratin and skin cells leaving the hyphae of the dermatophyte visible. Several minutes should be allowed for the KOH to clear the debris before the slide is examined, otherwise the hyphae may be missed. Nail scrapings are the most difficult because of the longer digestion time required and the low number of hyphae usually present. Examination of infected hair will reveal either ectothrix or endothrix infection, providing some clue to the causative agent. *T. tonsurans* and *Trichophyton violaceum* are most likely to cause endothrix infection. In addition to hyphae, arthroconidia will be visible on or within the hair.

The KOH preparation is also useful to help distinguish infections due to *Candida. Candida* is a genus of several species of yeast that may produce skin and nail infections very similar to dermatophyte infections (see Chapter 41). In *Candida* infections, yeast cells and pseudohyphae will be observed.

**Culture.** Dermatophytes grow slowly in culture. Sabouraud's agar provides an ideal medium, but because of the slow growth of the dermatophytes, may become contaminated by bacteria or saprophytic fungi. Therefore, media with inhibitory substances such as cyclohexamide and antibiotics should also be used.

Colonial morphology is helpful in identifying the dermatophytes, but considerable overlap exists among the species. Most have white, cream, tan, or gray surfaces. The reverse side of the colonies may show pigment production characteristic of a particular species. For example, *M. canis* often has a bright yellow reverse pigment, and *T. rubrum* will produce a deep red reverse pigment. Pigment production may be enhanced by using cornmeal agar.

**Microscopic Morphology.** Some of the dermatophytes produce very characteristic **macroconidia** and are readily identified in tease preparations and slide cultures. This is particularly true for *E. floccosum* and many of the *Microsporum* species, except for *M.*

*audouinii*. The *Trichophyton species* produce few macroconidia but arrangement of **microconidia** may be diagnostic in some cases. Other species may have characteristic chlamydoconidia. Some of the dermatophytes produce unusual hyphae which also may be characteristic of certain species. Figure 36-4 illustrates some of these unusual hyphal forms. Often the dermatophytes produce no single diagnostic feature. In these cases, final identification depends on careful observation of all of these morphologic features.

**Additional Diagnostic Tests.** There are other tests that may be helpful in identification of some of the dermatophytes, particularly those without diagnostic conidia (see Table 36-3). Urease production will help distinguish *T. mentagrophytes* (positive) from *T. rubrum* (negative). Other organisms will also produce urease so that the test is best done only when the choices have been narrowed to *T. mentagrophytes* and *T. rubrum*. These two organisms can also be distinguished by the hair penetration test. When placed on clipped hair in a moist environment *T. mentagrophytes* will penetrate into the hair shaft but *T. rubrum* will not. This is detected by examining the hair under the microscope. This test is not used much any longer because it requires hair that has not been subjected to harsh chemicals in shampoo or other grooming items.

Special media may aid in identification of some of the *Trichophyton* species. There are seven of these Trichophyton agars numbered 1 through 7, although use of Trichophyton agar numbers 1 and 4 will be all that are required in most cases. Trichophyton agar number 1 is base medium with casein; the other agars contain certain added vitamins. Trichophyton agar number 4 contains thiamine, which is required for growth of most strains of *T. violaceum, T. verrucosum,* and *T. tonsurans*.

Unlike the other *Microsporum* species, *M. audouinii* rarely produces conidia. Despite this it can be identified by a failure to grow on rice grain medium or pol-

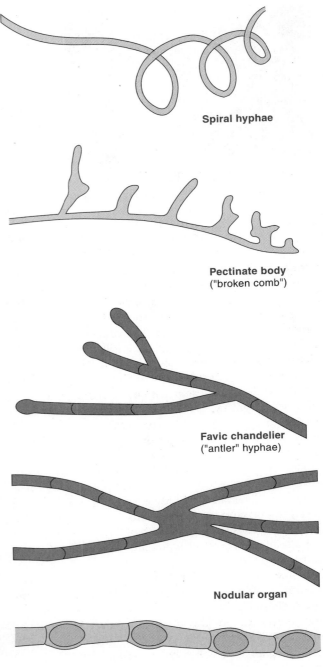

**Spiral hyphae**

**Pectinate body** ("broken comb")

**Favic chandelier** ("antler" hyphae)

**Nodular organ**

**Racquet hyphae**

**FIGURE 36-4** Unusual hyphae associated with dermatophytes.

ished rice grains, which readily support growth of other *Microsporum* species. Use of polished white rice eliminates the need to keep special media on hand.

## Mycology of Specific Organisms

Although there are at least 40 species of dermatophytes, only those organisms that commonly cause human infections are described here. The key to the

| Table 36-3 ▶ Selected Diagnostic Tests in Dermatophyte Identification | |
|---|---|
| **Diagnostic Test** | **Expected Result** |
| Urease | T. mentagrophytes—positive within 7 d T. rubrum—negative |
| In vitro hair penetration | T. mentagrophytes—positive T. rubrum—negative |
| Growth on polished rice grains | M. audouinii—no growth Other Microsporum species—growth |
| Growth on Trichophyton agars | T. violaceum—enhanced with thiamine (agar no. 4) T. verrucosum—enhanced with thiamine (agar no. 4) T. tonsurans—enhanced with thiamine (agar no. 4) |

**Table 36–4 ▶ General Differential Characteristics of the Dermatophytes**

| Organism | Source | Macroconidia | Microconidia |
|---|---|---|---|
| Epidermophyton | Skin and nails | Club-shaped, multiseptate, borne in clusters | None |
| Microsporum | Skin and hair | Cylindrical to spindle-shaped, multiseptate, borne singly. Exception: *M. audouinii* rarely produces conidia | Uncommon |
| Trichophyton | Skin, hair, and nails | Pencil to cigar shaped, scant to absent | Often predominant, arrangement may be diagnostic |

identification of these fungi lies in the accumulation of a variety of observations about the unknown culture. Table 36-4 lists characteristics of the three genera of dermatophytes. Particular attention should be paid to the following:

1. Source of specimen
2. Color of colony surface
3. Color of colony reverse
4. Presence and type of macroconidia
5. Presence and type of microconidia
6. Unusual hyphal morphology
7. Additional diagnostic tests where appropriate

**Epidermophyton floccosum (see Figure 36-5).** This is the only pathogenic species of the genus. *Epidermophyton* colonies are brown and not distinctive. Macroconidia are club shaped with smooth walls and borne in clusters. Microconidia are not produced.

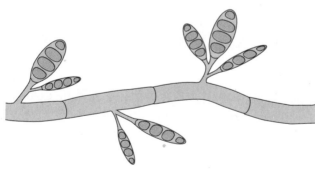

**FIGURE 36-5** Microscopic appearance of *Epidermophyton floccosum*.

**Microsporum canis (see Figure 36-6).** The organism is most often transmitted from cats or dogs. Colonies are white to pale yellow with a very characteristic deep yellow reverse. Macroconidia are spindle shaped with pointed tips, rough surface, and cross septa. *Microsporum canis* var. *distortum* produces macroconidia that are distinctively bent and distorted, but is rarely associated with human infections.

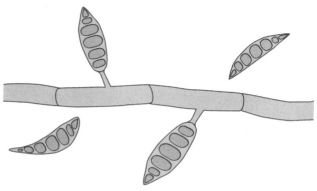

**FIGURE 36-6** Microscopic appearance of *Microsporum canis*.

**Microsporum gypseum (see Figure 36-7).** Colonies tend to be tan to brown with a powdery surface. The reverse appearance is variable. Macroconidia are spindle shaped with blunt rounded ends (cf. *M. canis*, which has pointed ends).

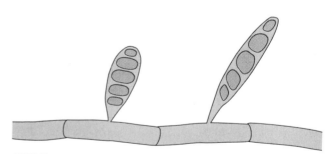

**FIGURE 36-7** Microscopic appearance of *Microsporum gypseum*.

**Microsporum audouinii (see Figure 36-8).** The colonies of *M. audouinii* are usually white. The reverse may have orange pigment. *M. audouinii* rarely produces conidia but terminal chlamydoconidia are sometimes produced. Abnormal hyphal forms such as racquet hyphae and especially pectinate hyphae may be seen. The pectinate hyphae resemble a broken comb.

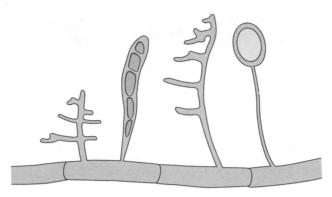

**FIGURE 36-8** Microscopic appearance of *Microsporum audouinii.*

### Trichophyton mentagrophytes (see Figure 36-9).

This fungus is one of the most common agents of a number of different dermatophyte infections in humans. Colonies are cream colored to white with variable pigment visible on the reverse. Microconidia are few, thin walled and smooth. Macroconidia are numerous and borne in grapelike clusters. Spiral hyphae and nodular organs are common. The fungus is differentiated from *T. rubrum* by positive urea agar, positive hair penetration test, and lack of pigment production on cornmeal agar.

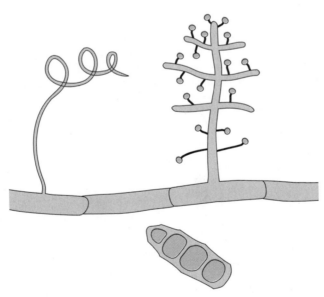

**FIGURE 36-9** Microscopic appearance of *Trichophyton.*

### Trichophyton rubrum (see Figure 36-10).

This organism is a common cause of ringworm infections and causes the most severe cases of tinea pedis and tinea unguium. Colonies are white with a distinctive red pigment produced on the reverse side. Pigment production is enhanced on cornmeal agar. Macroconidia are very rare; when present they have a broad attachment to the

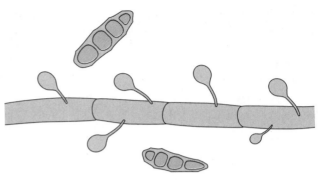

**FIGURE 36-10** Microscopic appearance of *Trichophyton rubrum.*

hyphae. Microconidia are borne singly along the hyphae. Urease is not produced and hair is not penetrated.

### Trichophyton tonsurans (see Figure 36-11).

*T. tonsurans* is now the most common cause of tinea capitis. Colonies are highly variable. Macroconidia are irregular but are usually not produced. Microconidia are tear drop or balloon shaped. Chlamydoconidia and arthroconidia may be produced. The organism requires thiamine for growth and thus shows increased growth on Trichophyton agar number 4 compared to the base medium Trichophyton agar number 1.

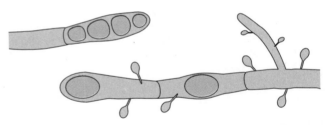

**FIGURE 36-11** Microscopic appearance of *Trichophyton tonsurans.*

### Trichophyton violaceum (see Figure 36-12).

Colonies are folded and waxy with a purple color both on the surface and reverse of the colony. Aerial conidia are usually not produced, but chlamydoconidia may be formed on thiamine enriched agar (Trichophyton agar number 4).

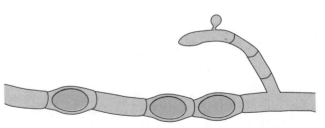

**FIGURE 36-12** Microscopic appearance of *Trichophyton violaceum.*

*Trichophyton schoenleinii* (see Figure 36-13). Colonies are white and waxy. Aerial conidia are not formed, but chlamydoconidia may be numerous. This organism produces characteristic antler-like hyphae called favic chandeliers. It is the organism responsible for the severe favic hair infection.

*Trichophyton verrucosum* (see Figure 36-14). The organism is most often contracted from cattle. Colonies are gray to white and may have a central knoblike projection. On the usual isolation media only chains of chlamydoconidia are produced. The organism requires thiamine and will produce "rat tail" macroconidia as well as microconidia on Trichophyton agar number 4.

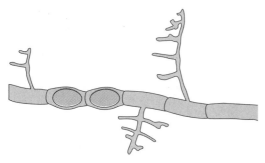

**FIGURE 36-13** Microscopic appearance of *Trichophyton schoenleinii.*

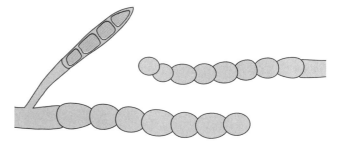

**FIGURE 36-14** Microscopic appearance of *Trichophyton verrucosum.*

## SUMMARY

▶ Superficial and cutaneous infections are confined to the outer layer of the skin. Hair and nails may be affected because they are modified keratin.

▶ The superficial infections include tinea versicolor, tinea nigra, black piedra, and white piedra. These are generally innocuous and more of a nuisance.

▶ The dermatophyte infections are known as ringworm infections (also called tinea). Classification is based on the part of the body involved.

▶ The dermatophytes include various species of the genus *Epidermophyton, Microsporum,* or *Trichophyton.*

▶ *Epidermophyton* produces club-shaped macroconidia and microconidia in culture.

▶ *Trichophyton* species produce scant or no macroconidia. Microconidia may be predominant in some species. Identification may require additional diagnostic tests.

## CASE STUDY

A 16-year-old man presented to his physician with an itchy, scaly, red rash on his hands. He had been spending his summer vacation participating on a swimming team at the YMCA. Physical examination revealed some cracks and fissures in the skin between the fourth and fifth toes of both feet. There was some inflammation and scaling of the skin adjacent to the fifth toe on the left foot. Except for the hands, no additional skin rash was detected. KOH preparation of the lesions on the foot revealed fungal hyphae. However, repeated KOH preparation of the rash from the hands revealed no hyphae at all.

### Questions:

1. What is your diagnosis?
2. Why was the KOH preparation from the hands negative?
3. What are some of the organisms likely to be involved?

# Review Questions

1. A patient presents with a chronic infection of the fingernails. Which of the following organisms is the most likely cause?
   a. *Microsporum canis*
   b. *Trichophyton rubrum*
   c. *Microsporum audouinii*
   d. *Microsporum gypseum*

2. A culture of skin scrapings reveals a fungus that produces club-shaped macroconidia and no microconidia. Which of the following organisms is most likely?
   a. *Epidermophyton floccosum*
   b. *Microsporum canis*
   c. *Trichophyton tonsurans*
   d. *Microsporum gypseum*

3. *Trichophyton mentagrophytes* can be distinguished from *Trichophyton rubrum* by which of the following?
   a. Hair penetration by *Trichophyton mentagrophytes*
   b. Urease production by *Trichophyton mentagrophytes*
   c. Red pigment production by *Trichophyton rubrum*
   d. All of the above

4. The most common cause of tinea capitis in the United States today is:
   a. *Malassezia furfur.*
   b. *Trichosporon beigelii.*
   c. *Piedraia hortae.*
   d. *Trichophyton tonsurans.*

5. Which of the following are characteristic of dermatophytes?
   a. Dematiaceous hyphae
   b. "Spaghetti and meatballs"
   c. Spiral hyphae
   d. Clusters of yeast

6. Addition of which of the following to the culture media will aid in the identification of the species of *Trichophyton?*
   a. Olive oil
   b. Blood
   c. Vitamin C
   d. Thiamine

7. *Epidermophyton floccosum* is associated with which of the following?
   a. Ectothrix hair infection
   b. Endothrix hair infection
   c. Favus hair infection
   d. None of the above

8. Which of the following causes tinea cruris (jock itch)?
   a. *Malassezia furfur*
   b. *Epidermophyton floccosum*
   c. *Phaeoannellomyces werneckii*
   d. *Piedraia hortae*

9. Which of the following organisms is most likely to be transmitted by contact with animals?
   a. *Trichosporon beigelii*
   b. *Microsporum gypseum*
   c. *Malassezia furfur*
   d. *Microsporum canis*

10. Use of polished rice grains or rice grain medium will aid in the identification of which of the following?
    a. *Trichophyton rubrum*
    b. *Trichophyton mentagrophytes*
    c. *Microsporum audouinii*
    d. *Epidermophyton floccosum*

## ▶ REFERENCES & RECOMMENDED READING

Larone, D. H. (1995). *Medically important fungi, a guide to identification* (3rd ed.). Washington, DC: ASM Press.

Marcon, M. J., & Powell, D. A. (1992). Human infections due to *Malassezia* spp. *Clinical Microbiology Reviews, 5,* 101–119.

Rippon, J. W. (1988). *Medical mycology: The pathogenic fungi and the pathogenic actinomycetes.* (3rd ed.). Philadelphia: Saunders.

Shadomy, H. J., & Philpot, C. M. (1980). Utilization of standard laboratory methods in the laboratory diagnosis of problem dermatophytes. *American Journal of Clinical Pathology, 74,* 197–201.

Weitzman, I., & Summerbell, R. C. (1995). The dermatophytes. *Clinical Microbiology Reviews, 8,* 240–259.

# CHAPTER 37
## Agents of Subcutaneous Mycoses

James A. Miller, MD, Anne T. Rodgers, MT (ASCP), PhD

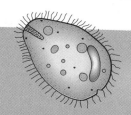

## Microbes in the News
### Madura Foot in New Jersey

A 56-year old Indian woman presented at a hospital in New Jersey with a painful and swollen left foot. The woman had previously lived in Western India where she frequently walked barefoot through marshy, wet fields. Excision of the lesion on her foot revealed chronic inflammation, granulation of tissue and focal abscess formation. Microscopic examination revealed small colonies of gram-positive, filamentous organisms suggestive of Actinomyces. A diagnosis of Madura Foot was made, based on the woman's past residence in an endemic area and the characteristic localized abscesses containing a granule or clusters of granules. The woman was treated and released; follow-up five months later revealed slow, gradual improvement.

Source: Grigoriu et al. (1995), Tropical Diseases in Urban New Jersey. *Infect Med* 12(9):460–469.

**INTRODUCTION**

**CLINICAL DISEASES**
Chromoblastomycosis
Cystic Chromomycosis
Mycetoma
Sporotrichosis

**LABORATORY EVALUATION AND DIAGNOSIS OF SUBCUTANEOUS MYCOSES**
Characteristics of Dematiaceous Fungi
Agents of Chromoblastomycosis

Agents of Cystic Chromomycosis and Mycetoma
*Sporothrix schenckii*

## KEY TERMS

Abscess
Annellide
Chromoblastomycosis
Chromomycosis
Cleistothecium

Dematiaceous
Dimorphic
Madura foot
Mycetoma

Neurotropic
Phaeohyphomycosis
Phialide
Sclerotic bodies

## LEARNING OBJECTIVES

**Upon successful completion of this chapter, the student should be able to:**

1. Name the etiologic agents of the subcutaneous mycoses and mycetomas.
2. Identify and describe the colonial and microscopic morphology for agents of the subcutaneous mycoses and mycetomas.
3. List laboratory procedures used for the isolation and identification of these organisms.
4. Describe the clinical diseases chromoblastomycosis, cystic chromomycosis, and mycetoma.
5. Identify and describe the causative agent of and disease sporotrichosis.

# INTRODUCTION

The subcutaneous mycoses include a variety of clinical infections originating when fungi have been introduced by trauma into the deep tissues of the skin. Many of the fungi causing these subcutaneous infections are **dematiaceous** or pigmented fungi. The hyphae themselves contain brown or black melanin pigment in the cell walls. The infections caused by these organisms are called **chromomycoses**, referring to the pigmented nature of the fungi. Some of the infections are also referred to as **phaeohyphomycoses** where the prefix *phaeo* refers to dark pigmentation.

# CLINICAL DISEASES

## Chromoblastomycosis

**Chromoblastomycosis** is a specific kind of chromomycosis, manifested as a verrucous dermatitis caused by various dematiaceous fungi. There are four important organisms causing the disease:

- ▶ *Fonsecaea pedrosi*
- ▶ *Fonsecaea compacta*
- ▶ *Phialophora verrucosa*
- ▶ *Cladosporium carrionii*

The term verrucous dermatitis refers to wartlike nodules on the skin produced in response to the fungi. The infection is almost exclusively a disease of the tropics even though it can also be found in temperate climates. It occurs on exposed areas of the skin where the fungi are introduced by trauma from their natural habitat as saprophytes in soil and decaying wood. The fungi appear as round, thick-walled brown bodies called **sclerotic bodies**. A photomicrograph of sclerotic bodies is shown in Color Plate 83. Even though several different organisms that may cause chromoblastomycosis, all of them have the same appearance in the infected tissues. These sclerotic bodies resemble yeasts, but they reproduce by splitting. Because they are dematiaceous they are readily identified in unstained potassium hydroxide (KOH) preparations, aspirates, and biopsies. In their natural habitat the organisms are molds.

The lesions of chromoblastomycosis may remain localized or may spread in the adjacent subcutaneous tissues. Although the lesions can be quite disfiguring, there is usually little disability, and some patients may go for many years without treatment. Localized lesions can be cured by surgical excision. More extensive lesions can be treated by antifungal drugs, especially 5-fluorocytosine.

## Cystic Chromomycosis

Cystic chromomycosis, also known as phaeomycotic cyst, is a localized subcutaneous **abscess** caused by dematiaceous fungi. Most cases in the United States are caused by *Exophiala jeanselmeii,* with a smaller number caused by *Wangiella dermatitidis*. Injury to the skin introduces the organism. Because the organisms can be found on decaying wood, splinters may carry the organism into the skin (refer to Color Plate 84). The lesion becomes an isolated subcutaneous nodule or abscess, which remains cystlike. Complete surgical excision will usually cure the infection. The organisms are generally resistant to antifungal drugs.

## Mycetoma

A **mycetoma** is a destructive abscess within which the fungi grow as compact colonies. These colonies form small grains or granules that are visible to the naked eye. Most of these infections occur on the extremities, particularly the foot, where the organisms have most likely been inoculated by trauma. The abscesses do not remain localized, but cause extensive destruction of the tissues, including muscle and bone. The affected extremity is swollen and exhibits multiple nodules with draining sinuses over the surface. Pus exuding from the sinuses contains the granules of fungal colonies, composed of matted hyphae. When the infection is caused by dematiaceous fungi, the granules are dark brown or black. Other fungi produce white to pale yellow grains.

Mycetoma was first described in India, where it was called **Madura foot**. The causative agent of Madura foot is *Madurella mycetomatis,* a dematiaceous fungus found in India, but not in the United States. In the United States most cases of mycetoma are caused by *Pseudoallescheria boydii,* which is not dematiaceous. Occasional cases of mycetoma can be caused by common saprophytic fungi, especially *Acremonium* species and the dematiaceous *Curvularia* species.

Mycetomas of the extremities are difficult to treat because the organisms are highly resistant to antifungal drugs. Localized infection may be cured by surgical excision but more advanced lesions require extensive surgical debridement and drainage. In some cases amputation may be the only effective treatment.

Certain filamentous bacteria can cause infections that are clinically identical to mycotic mycetoma. These infections are called actinomycotic mycetoma and are caused by various species of *Nocardia, Streptomyces,* and *Actinomadura* (see Chapter 12). In these cases the discharged granules are composed of matted filamentous bacteria, which are gram-positive. The distinction between these infections is important because actinomycotic mycetoma can be cured by antibiotics directed against bacteria and does not usually require extensive surgical intervention.

## Sporotrichosis

Sporotrichosis is caused by the **dimorphic** pathogenic fungus, *Sporothrix schenckii*. The clinical manifestations of a typical case of sporotrichosis are so characteristic that often a diagnosis can be made just from the patient's description of the infection. The primary lesions are usually located on the extremities, especially the hands and fingers. They present as a nonhealing sore, either nodules or an ulcer. This is followed by inflammation spreading away from the primary lesion following the distribution of the lymphatic drainage. The secondary lesions are nodular and may ulcerate at the skin surface. Regional lymph nodes then become enlarged and inflamed. The typical case is easily cured by antifungal drugs. Disseminated infections are rare.

*Sporothrix schenkii* is commonly found in decaying vegetation, particularly sphagnum moss (Powell et al., 1978). The organism is introduced by trauma into the skin and subcutaneous tissues. Rose gardeners and nursery workers are particularly susceptible. In nature *S. schenkii* is a dematiaceous mold. However, when introduced into tissue, it converts to a parasitic yeast form. It is the yeast form that will be observed in tissue sections and smears. Color Plate 85 depicts the yeast of *S. schenkii* in tissue. Culture of infected exudate from the lesions will yield the mold phase at room temperature.

## LABORATORY EVALUATION AND DIAGNOSIS OF SUBCUTANEOUS MYCOSES

Some of the agents of subcutaneous mycoses are among the most difficult medically important fungi to identify. This is particularly true of the agents of chromomycosis. As with the other molds, identification is primarily based on the appearance of spores and hyphae in culture. Biochemical tests are of limited usefulness. Many of the organisms grow slowly in culture. Moreover, they may not produce unique conidia, and identification will depend on the accumulation of data from careful observation of microscopic structures.

## Characteristics of Dematiaceous Fungi

Although the dematiaceous fungi are not necessarily closely related, it is useful to consider them as a group because they can be distinguished easily in cultures and smears due to the presence of melanin pigment in their cell walls. In smears and wet mounts the hyphae are brown when compared to the clear hyphae of other molds. The mycelia formed of these hyphae will result in colonies that are dark brown or black, occasionally olive. More importantly, the reverse side of the colonies will be black, indicating that the dark color on the surface is not due only to pigmentation of conidia but also to the hyphae themselves.

Young colonies of some dematiaceous fungi produce yeastlike cells. This results in growth that is moist, soft, pasty and shiny, showing yeastlike characteristics. As the colonies mature, they become velvety, fuzzy, or wooly due to development of aerial hyphae.

Conidia are produced from annellides or phialides or directly from the hyphae. An **annellide** is a supporting structure that gives rise to conidia by successive elongation leading to a tapered end. A **phialide** is a supporting structure that stays fixed in length as conidia are produced. Among the dematiaceous fungi, phialides are often vase or cup-shaped with a small collar.

The agents of chromoblastomycosis, particularly, exhibit four types of conidia production, which may be present in a variety of combinations These are illustrated in Figure 37-1.

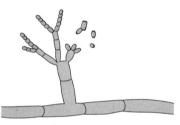

Cladosporium type

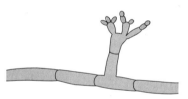

Fonsecaea type

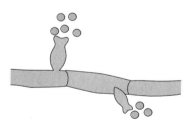

Phialophora type

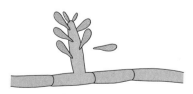

Rhinocladiella type

**FIGURE 37-1** Types of conidia production of agents of chromomycosis.

1. Cladosporium type: Conidia arise in chains from the conidiophore and leave thick scars as they detach.
2. Fonsecaea type: Several conidia arise from narrow projections at the end of a conidiophore. Long chains are not produced.
3. Phialophora type: Conidia arise from the end of vase-shaped phialides, resembling flowers in a vase.
4. Rhinocladiella type: Conidia arise from the end and sides of erect conidiophores.

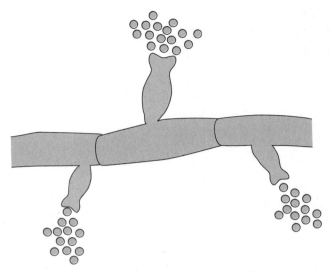

FIGURE 37-3 Microscopic morphology of *Phialophora verrucosa*, conidia production.

## Agents of Chromoblastomycosis

***Fonsecaea pedrosi.*** This is the most common agent of chromoblastomycosis. Growth is slow, 2 to 3 weeks. The surface of the colony is black, gray, or olive, the reverse is black. Hyphae are brown and septate. All four types of conidia production may be observed. Fonsecae and Rhinocladiella types usually predominate, but diagnosis is enhanced by finding all four types of conidiation.

***Fonsecaea compacta* (see Figure 37-2).** Growth is very slow, up to 1 month. Colonies are black or dark green; reverse is black. Hyphae are brown and septate. Sporulation is predominately Fonsecaea type with fruiting heads short and compact, hence the species name. Other spore types may also occur.

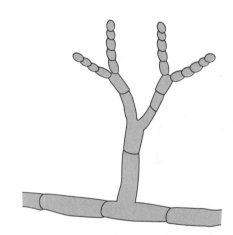

FIGURE 37-4 Microscopic morphology of *Cladosporium carrionii*, conidia production.

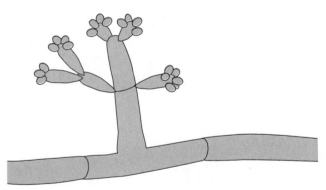

FIGURE 37-2 Microscopic morphology of *Fonsecaea compacta*, conidia production.

***Phialophora verrucosa* (see Figure 37-3).** This is a common cause of chromoblastomycosis. Growth is slow, up to 2 weeks. Colonies are brown to olive gray, reverse is black. Hyphae are brown and septate. Only Phialophora sporulation takes place. The phialides resemble a vase and produce conidia resembling flowers in the vase.

***Cladosporium carrionii* (see Figure 37-4).** This organism is uncommon in the United States and is usually found in Venezuela, South Africa, and Australia. Growth is slow, 3 weeks. Colonies are gray, dark green, or brown, reverse is black. Only Cladosporium sporula-

tion is produced, resulting in long chains of conidia. It is distinguished from *Xylohypha bantiana* by inability to grow at 42°C.

## Agents of Cystic Chromomycosis and Mycetoma

***Exophiala jeanselmei* (see Figure 37-5).** This is the most common etiologic agent of cystic chromomycosis and a common cause of mycetoma. The organism is dematiaceous. It grows slowly at room temperature and not at all at 37° to 40°C. Colonies are black, moist and yeastlike at first. Later they become velvety and gray. The reverse is black. Young cultures contain yeastlike cells. Later brown hyphae develop, producing annellides. Oval conidia collect at the tip of the annellides, and then fall in clusters along the conidiophores.

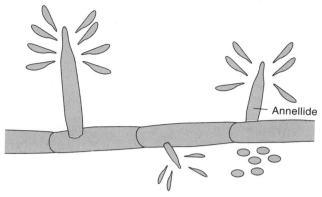

**FIGURE 37-5** Microscopic morphology of *Exophiala jeanselmei*, conidia production.

### Wangiella dermatitidis (see Figure 37-6).

This organism causes cystic chromomycosis, but also has been implicated in deeper infections, including some in the central nervous system. It is found worldwide, but most commonly in Japan. The organism is dematiaceous. Growth is yeastlike at first. Aerial hyphae develop only after several weeks and may require subcultures. Colonies are black to olive; reverse is black. When hyphae form, they are brown and produce phialides that do not have the usual cuplike or vaselike configuration of other dematiaceous fungi. The phialides are cylindrical, resembling annellides. Conidia accumulate along the phialides, similar to the way conidia are distributed over the annellides of *E. jeanselmei*.

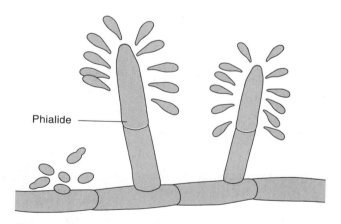

**FIGURE 37-6** Microscopic morphology of *Wangiella dermatitidis*, conidia production and yeastlike cells.

### Xylohypha bantiana (see Figure 37-7).

This organism is **neurotrophic** and causes brain abscesses. Extreme care is recommended when handling the organism; all procedures should be carried out in a biologic safety hood. The organism grows slowly, producing black or gray colonies. Reverse is black. The organism will grow at 42°C distinguishing it from *C. carrionii,* which it resembles. Hyphae are brown and septate. Conidia are

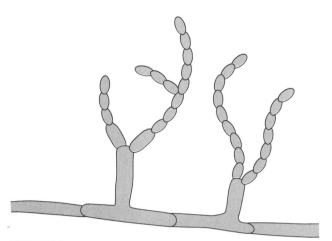

**FIGURE 37-7** Microscopic morphology of *Xylohypha bantiana*, conidia production.

borne in long chains from branching conidiophores. The chains of conidia are generally longer than those of *C. carrionii*. Although they resemble *Cladosporium,* the conidia do not have thick detachment scars.

### Madurella species.

*Madurella mycetomatis* causes madura foot in India. *Madurella grisea* causes similar infection in the Western hemisphere. Both organisms are difficult to identify because conidia production is poor, especially with *M. grisea*. Both organisms are dematiaceous. Pigment production varies but the colony reverse is dark brown. *M. mycetomatis* grows best at 37°C, whereas *M. grisea* grows slowly at room temperature and not at all at 37°C. They are often sterile in the laboratory. *M. mycetomatis* may produce chlamydospores. *M. grisea* rarely produces conidia.

### Pseudallescheria boydii (Scedosporium apiospermum).

This organism is the most common cause of mycotic mycetoma. It also may cause opportunistic infections in other organs. The organism is not dematiaceous in tissues and the grains in infected material are white to yellow. *P. boydii* is the name of the sexual or teleomorphic state. Teleomorphic names are not commonly used in clinical medical mycology but because ascospores may be seen in cultures, the teleomorphic name is traditionally used for this organism. The asexual or anamorph state is *S. apiospermum,* although other teleomorphic organisms may also assume this anamorphic state. *S. apiospermum* was previously called *Monosporium apiospermum,* a name that is incorrect but descriptively appropriate. The organism grows moderately rapidly, producing white cottony colonies that become gray or brown with age. The reverse also turns dark with age, the organism becoming dematiaceous only in mature colonies. Single oval conidia are produced on top of conidiophores (annellides) resulting in structures resembling sperm (see Figure 37-8). The conidia are occasionally larger and round. The conidiophores may be long or short. Often they will be

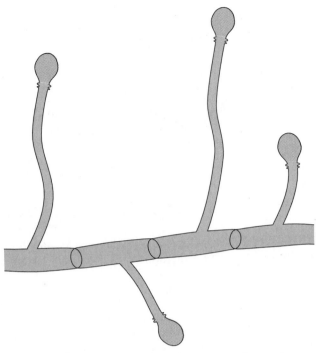

**FIGURE 37-8** Microscopic morphology of *Pseudo-allescheria boydii, Scedosporium apiospermum.* Anamorph phase, conidia production.

found in clusters, resembling sheaves of grain (Graphium anamorph form). Because the organism is homothallic, sexual spores are frequently seen in cultures grown on cornmeal agar (Padhye, 1995). The sexual spores are ascospores that are contained in large sacs called **cleistothecia** (see Figure 37-9). The sac ruptures at maturity releasing the ascospores.

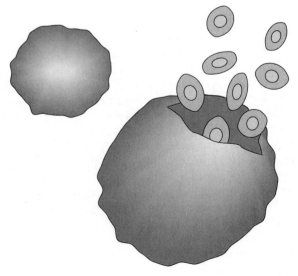

**FIGURE 37-9** Microscopic morphology of *Pseudo-allescheria,* Cleistothecia with ascospores.

## Sporothrix schenkii

The agent of sporotrichosis is dimorphic, existing as a mold in its natural habitat, but converting to a yeast when it infects tissue. This transformation most likely represents an adaptation by the organism to a hostile environment, particularly elevated temperature. Other organisms exhibiting thermal dimorphism are discussed in detail in Chapter 38.

**Direct Examination.** In infected tissues the organism is a small yeast (see Figure 37-10) that often is elongated or cigar shaped. The organism is nearly impossible to recognize in unstained smears or KOH preparations. Special stains, particularly periodic acid-Schiff or methenamine silver are usually required to identify the yeasts. It may be necessary to pretreat the pus or tissue with diastase to digest away carbohydrate debris, which may be confused with the organism.

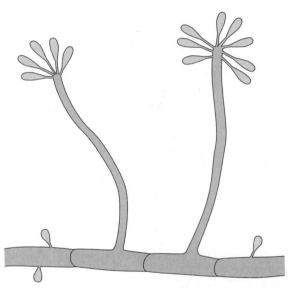

**FIGURE 37-10** Microscopic morphology of *Sporothrix schenkii,* mold phase with conidia production.

**Culture Characteristics.** At room temperature the organism grows rapidly within a few days. Initially the colonies are white, but subsequently become brown or black, considered dematiaceous. When the mold is subcultured and incubated at 35° to 37°C, the organism converts to the yeast form. Brain-heart infusion agar with blood enhances the yeast conversion. Colonies are white to tan, smooth and creamy. Demonstration of thermal dimorphism is more easily demonstrated for *S. schenkii* than for the systemic dimorphic pathogens discussed in Chapter 38.

**Microscopic Characteristics.** The mold phase produces thin septate hyphae that give rise to slender, tapering conidiophores. Oval to round conidia are produced on top of the conidiophores in clusters like delicate petals on the head of a flower (see Figure 37-10). Sometimes single conidia are produced along the hyphae.

Identification is confirmed by yeast conversion. Smears of the yeast colonies reveal very small yeast varying from round to oval to cigar shaped (see Figure 37-11). They are approximately 3 μm in diameter. The elongated cells may grow up to 10 μm in length.

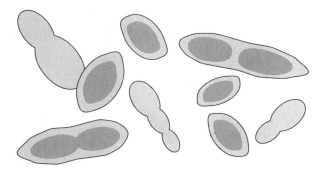

**FIGURE 37-11** Microscopic morphology of *Sporothrix schenkii*, yeast phase from culture at 37°C.

## SUMMARY

▶ Many of the subcutaneous infections are caused by dematiaceous (pigmented) fungi.

▶ Organisms are introduced into the subcutaneous tissues from their natural habitat by trauma.

▶ Chromoblastomycosis is a verrucous (wartlike) skin infection caused by several dematiaceous fungi. In the tissues they all appear as sclerotic bodies. In culture they are all molds.

▶ Cystic chromomycosis is a localized abscess most often caused by either *Exophiala jeanselmei* or *Wangiella dermatitidis*.

▶ Mycotic mycetoma is a destructive abscess caused by fungi in which the organisms form colonies of matted hyphae in the infected tissues

and pus. Mycetoma can be caused by dematiaceous fungi, *Pseudoallescheria boydii*, or a variety of hyaline saprophytic fungi.

▶ *Xylohypha bantiana* is a neurotropic dematiaceous fungus that causes brain abscesses.

▶ Sporotrichosis is a lymphocutaneous infection with very characteristic clinical features. It is caused by *Sporothrix schenckii*, a dimorphic fungus. It is a dematiaceous mold found in decaying vegetation, but changes to a small pleomorphic yeast when introduced into tissues. Thermal dimorphism can be demonstrated in the laboratory.

## CASE STUDY

A 54-year-old woman presented to her physician because of a nonhealing wound on her finger. The patient stated that she had developed a painful swollen index finger several weeks before. Eventually the wound broke down and formed an ulcer that would not heal. Recently she had developed some red, painful streaks along her forearm and a swollen nodule over her elbow. The patient was an executive with a major computer software corporation. In her leisure time she was an avid rose gardener and had won several prizes for her roses.

### Questions:

1. What disease does the patient have? What is the causative organism?

2. If you wish to demonstrate the organism in a direct preparation from the finger wound, how would you process the specimen? What would you expect to see?

3. How would you confirm the identity of the organism in culture?

# Review Questions

1. A patient presents with chromoblastomycosis. A sample of the infected material is sent to the laboratory for direct examination by KOH prep. Which of the following would you expect to see?
   a. Pigmented hyphae
   b. Pigmented sclerotic bodies
   c. Pigmented conidia
   d. All of the above

2. Which of the following organisms causes chromo-blastomycosis?
   a. *Fonsecaea pedrosi*
   b. *Cladosporium carrionii*
   c. *Phialophora verrucosa*
   d. All of the above

3. A patient presents with mycotic mycetoma of the foot. Small granules are recovered from pus draining from the infection. What are these granules composed of?
   a. Masses of hyphae
   b. Masses of white blood cells
   c. Sclerotic bodies
   d. Ascospores

4. Which of the following organisms is dimorphic?
   a. *Pseudoallescheria boydii*
   b. *Exophiala jeanselmei*
   c. *Sporothrix schenkii*
   d. *Fonsecaea pedrosi*

5. Growth in culture at 42°C will help distinguish which of the following organisms?
   a. *Sporothrix schenkii* from *Pseudoallescheria boydii*
   b. *Phialophora verrucosa* from *Cladosporium carrionii*
   c. *Fonsecaea pedrosi* from *Fonsecaea compacta*
   d. *Wangiella dermatitidis* from *Exophiala jeanselmei*

6. *Pseudoallescheria boydii* produces which of the following type(s) of conidia production?
   a. Cladosporium type
   b. Rhinocladiella type
   c. Phialophora type
   d. None of the above

7. *Exophiala jeanselmei* may cause mycotic mycetoma of the extremities. What color granules will it produce?
   a. White
   b. Yellow
   c. Black
   d. Red

8. Which of the following organisms is most likely to produce sexual spores in culture?
   a. *Sporothrix schenkii*
   b. *Pseudoallescheria boydii*
   c. *Phialophora verrucosa*
   d. *Wangiella dermatitidis*

9. Which of the following organisms is dematiaceous?
   a. *Fonsecaea pedrosi*
   b. *Phialophora verrucosa*
   c. *Xylohypha bantiana*
   d. All of the above

10. Which of the following organisms produces vase-shaped phialides?
    a. *Phialophora verrucosa*
    b. *Sporothrix schenkii*
    c. *Pseudoallescheria boydii*
    d. *Xylohypha bantiana*

## ▶ REFERENCES & RECOMMENDED READING

Borges, M. G. Jr., Warren, S., White, W., & Pellettiere, E. V. (1991). Pulmonary phaeohyphomycosis due to *Xylohypha bantiana*. *Archives of Pathology and Laboratory Medicine, 115*, 627–629.

Larone, D. H. (1995). *Medically important fungi: A guide to identification* (3rd ed.) Washington, DC: ASM Press.

Padhye, A. (1995), Fungi causing eumycotic mycetoma. In P. Murray, (Ed.). *Manual of clinical microbiology* (6th ed. pp. 847–854). Washington, DC: ASM Press.

Padhye, A. A., McGinnis M. R., & Ajello, L. (1978). Thermotolerance of *Wangiella dermatitidis*. *Journal of Clinical Microbiology, 8*, 424–426.

Powell, K. E., Taylor, A., Phillips, B. J., Blackey, D. L., Campbell, D. L., Kaufman, L., & Kaplan, W. (1978). Cutaneous sporotrichosis in forestry workers. Epidemic due to contaminated sphagnum moss. *Journal of the American Medical Association, 240*, 232–235.

Rippon, J. W. (1988). *Medical mycology. The pathogenic fungi and the pathogenic actinomycetes* (3rd ed.). Philadelphia: Saunders.

Schell, W. A., Pasarelli, L., Salkin, I. F., & McGinnis, M. R. *Bipolaris, Exophiala, Scedosporium, Sporothrix,* and other dematiaceous fungi. In P. Murray (Ed.). *Manual of clinical microbiology* (6th ed., pp. 825–846). Washington, DC: ASM Press.

# CHAPTER 38
# Systemic Dimorphic Fungi

James A. Miller, MD, Anne T. Rodgers, MT (ASCP) PhD

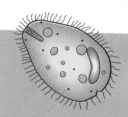

## Microbes in the News
### Rotavirus-associated Diarrhea: A Global Problem

Severe diarrhea is a major cause of morbidity and mortality, most commonly affecting children aged under 5 years and the elderly. A recent estimate suggested 1.1–1.7 billion episodes of acute diarrhea occur yearly among the world's 500 million young children. Surveys conducted since the identification of rotaviruses in 1973 have shown they are a major cause of infection, accounting for about 900,000 deaths per year. Rotaviruses are transmitted via the fecal-oral route, and the infectious dose is about 10-100 particles per ml. All diagnostic techniques (electron microscopy, enzyme-linked immunosorbent assays, latex agglutination tests and polyacrylamide gel electrophoresis) have a sensitivity of $10^{5-7}$ particles per gram of specimen. Polymerase chain reaction (PCR) is capable of detecting less than 10 virions per ml.

(*The International Journal of Clinical Chemistry,* 15:11-13, 1996).

## KEY TERMS

Arthroconidia
Conidia
Dimorphic
Disseminated
Endemic
Endospore
Exoantigen immunodiffusion

Fulminant infection
Inhibitory media
Opportunistic fungi
Parasitic phase
Primary infection
Saprophytic phase

Spherule
Systemic
Teleomorphic
True pathogen
Tuberculate macroconidia
Valley fever

## LEARNING OBJECTIVES

**Upon successful completion of this chapter, the student should be able to:**

1. Identify the etiologic agents of the systemic mycoses.
2. List the areas and organs of the body that are affected by the systemic mycoses.
3. Identify and describe the colonial and microscopic morphologies of these organisms.

4. Differentiate colonial and microscopic morphology at 37°C and at room temperature.
5. List procedures and culture media used for the isolation and identification of these organisms. Select confirmatory methods of identification.
6. Associate the fungus with its source of infection and discuss necessary safety precautions for the handling of cultures.

## INTRODUCTION

The systemic mycoses fall into two general categories: (1) infections caused by true pathogenic fungi, and (2) those caused by **opportunistic fungi**. The **true pathogens** have the capacity to produce disease in the normal host when the inoculum is of sufficient size. The opportunistic organisms on the other hand only cause disease when the host's resistance is altered.

### CHARACTERISTICS OF TRUE PATHOGENIC FUNGI

1. Capacity to cause infection in normal host
2. Most commonly skin or subcutaneous pathogens
3. Systemic pathogenic fungi
   a. Dimorphic
   b. Restricted geographic distribution
   c. Primary lung infection
   d. Infections often asymptomatic
   e. Most infections resolve spontaneously
   f. Resistance to reinfection
   g. Parasitic phase not infectious

The true **systemic** pathogens include *Histoplasma capsulatum, Coccidioides immitis, Blastomyces dermatitidis,* and *Paracoccidioides brasiliensis.* These organisms are characteristically **dimorphic** and exhibit transformation from a mycelial form in their natural habitat, called the **saprophytic phase** to another form found in infected tissues, called the **parasitic phase**. Generally

the parasitic form is a yeast except for *C. immitis,* which becomes a large **spherule** containing **endospores**. The appearances of the dimorphic pathogenic fungi are summarized in Table 38-1. The transformation probably represents an adaptation of the organism to an unfavorable environment, including elevated temperature and altered nutrients. The parasitic forms are quite characteristic and can be identified in specially stained tissue sections and smears of infected material.

### Infections Caused by Systemic Dimorphic Fungi

In most instances the organisms are introduced as a **primary infection** in the lungs by inhalation of **conidia** from the mycelial form. Transmission of the parasitic phase is extremely rare and patients with these diseases are not considered contagious. Most of the primary lung infections are asymptomatic or of short duration and resolve completely. Resolution often is accompanied by resistance to reinfection. Only a small percentage of patients develop more serious disease following the initial lung infection. This may be manifested by progressive infection in the lungs or by spread to other organs throughout the body. Dissemination can occur even in the absence of any clinical signs of pulmonary infection, and patients may present months or years later with infections at distant sites.

### Table 38–1 ► Dimorphic Pathogenic Fungi

| Disease | Organism | Saprophytic Phase | Parasitic Phase |
|---|---|---|---|
| Histoplasmosis | *Histoplasma capsulatum* | Septate hyphae, **tuberculate macroconidia**, microconidia | Small, oval yeast, 2–5 µm |
| Coccidiodomycosis | *Coccidioides immitis* | Septate hyphae, alternating arthroconidia | Large spherule, 10–80 µm with endospores |
| Blastomycosis | *Blastomyces dermatitidis* | Septate hyphae, single round or pyriform conidia attached to conidiophores or hyphae | Yeast, 8–15 µm with thick refractile cell wall and single broad-based bud |
| Paracoccidiomycosis (South American blastomycosis) | *Paracoccidioides brasiliensis* | Septate hyphae, chlamydoconidia, arthroconidia, pyriform conidia | Yeast, 30 µm with multiple radial buds, "ship's wheel" |

**Geographic Distribution.** The systemic pathogenic fungi have a very restricted geographic distribution. In the **endemic** areas infections are very common. Therefore, health care workers may encounter patients with advanced or **disseminated** infections frequently even though they represent only a small fraction of the total number of cases.

**Infections in Immunocompromised Hosts.** Immunocompromised patients may also acquire infections caused by true systemic pathogenic fungi. Infections in these patients are often atypical and more severe than in patients with normal immune function. This is especially true for patients with acquired immunodeficiency syndrome (AIDS) in whom these infections can be devastating.

## Evaluation of Clinical Specimens

In many respects the dimorphic pathogens are evaluated in the laboratory using techniques common to all fungi (see Chapters 34 and 35). However, because these organisms have characteristic forms, microscopic evaluation of clinical specimens and tissue samples assumes an even greater importance. Moreover, these organisms may be slow growing, and a diagnosis based on culture results may be delayed several weeks.

**Demonstration of Thermal Dimorphism.** Conversion of the mold form to the parasitic phase should be demonstrated if possible, because the mold form may not exhibit unique morphology. Yeast conversion requires transferring the isolate to a richer medium such as brain-heart infusion agar with blood and incubating it at 37°C. Conversion may require multiple subcultures and several weeks of incubation.

**Exoantigen Immunodiffusion Test.** The exoantigen test (see Figure 38-1) allows for identification of an unknown isolate more rapidly from the mold state. In this test soluble antigens are extracted from the mold cultures and concentrated. The concentrate is then placed in immunodiffusion agar and diffused for 24 hours against antisera of a known control organism. Antigen extract from the same known organism is used as a positive control. A precipitin line identical with the control is considered positive.

## HISTOPLASMA CAPSULATUM

*Histoplasma capsulatum* is an ascomycete (perfect state: *Ajellomyces capsulatus*). It grows as a mold in nature, producing both microconidia and macroconidia. The parasitic phase is a small oval yeast 2 to 5 μm in diameter, somewhat smaller than a red blood cell.

## Geographic Distribution and Natural Habitat

*Histoplasma capsulatum* is found worldwide, but abundant growth is restricted. In the United States it is

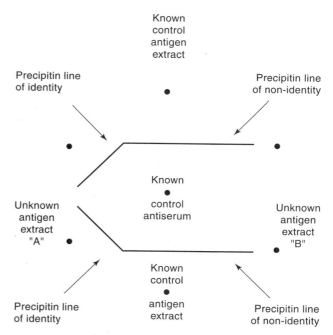

EXOANTIGEN IMMUNODIFFUSION TEST

**FIGURE 38-1** Exoantigen immundiffusion test.

most heavily endemic in the Midwest along the drainage pattern of the Ohio, Tennessee, and Mississippi rivers. There are other isolated endemic pockets in the United States, South America, Europe, and Indonesia. *H. capsulatum* thrives best in soil with high nitrogen content. It is frequently found where there are bird or bat droppings (guano). In the United States it is especially prevalent where there is a high concentration of starlings. Outside the endemic area *H. capsulatum* may be found in large numbers in closed environments such as bird roosts, chicken coops, or bat caves.

## Clinical Disease

Histoplasmosis may manifest itself in a perplexing variety of clinical forms. Of all the fungal diseases it most closely resembles tuberculosis. Patients acquire the infection by inhaling conidia from the mold phase into the lungs. In the lungs the organism converts to the parasitic yeast form. Hyphae do not develop in tissue under ordinary circumstances. The initial lung infection may or may not produce clinical symptoms. However, even those patients who have asymptomatic lung infection may develop infections in other organs at a later time.

**Infection in the Normal Host.** Most patients with pulmonary histoplasmosis are asymptomatic or have mild flulike symptoms. Some patients have more intense and prolonged respiratory symptoms, including cough, shortness of breath, and fever. Nodular infiltrates in the lungs and enlarged lymph nodes will be visible in chest radiographs. Some patients will have other allergic symptoms.

Patients who have a very heavy exposure to *Histoplasma* conidia develop acute pulmonary histoplasmosis. The disease usually appears 2 to 3 weeks after exposure with flulike symptoms. Often the lung infiltrates in chest x-rays appear far more extensive than the patient's clinical illness would suggest. If the patient has had histoplasmosis previously, then symptoms of acute pulmonary histoplasmosis occur within a few days, reflecting prior immunologic stimulation. Most patients with primary pulmonary histoplasmosis recover completely without requiring antifungal drug therapy. Healing of the lung lesions often results in calcifications, visible in chest x-rays years later. Some patients have progressive infections, requiring antifungal drug therapy. These progressive infections may stay confined to the lungs, often resembling tuberculosis, or may occur in other organs as a result of dissemination of the organisms.

**Infection in the Abnormal Host.** Opportunistic histoplasmosis occurs when there is an underlying abnormality in the patient. One form is called chronic pulmonary histoplasmosis, associated with pulmonary emphysema in cigarette smokers. Patients with emphysema have enlarged air sacs caused by destruction of lung tissue. These structural abnormalities are more susceptible to infection than normal lung tissue. In most patients the disease is self-limiting and resolves spontaneously. However, some patients have more progressive disease, requiring therapy.

The second form of opportunistic histoplasmosis is disseminated histoplasmosis in which organisms have spread from the lungs to other parts of the body. In some patients a defect in the immune system is obvious. In other cases an immune defect is suspected but not proven. Severe **fulminant infections** occur most commonly in infants and in patients with AIDS. The disease is rapidly fatal if not treated. Amphotericin may cure some patients but the mortality rate is still high. Organisms can be demonstrated in smears and cultures of bone marrow, blood, and sputum.

## Laboratory Evaluation and Diagnosis

Confirmation of the diagnosis of histoplasmosis requires identifying the organism recovered from infected tissue. Serologic testing for various antibodies in serum can be helpful but usually is not definitive. Appropriate specimens for smears and cultures are determined by the clinical characteristics of the patient. Direct examination of smears and tissues will reveal the parasitic yeast form, whereas cultures will yield the mold form.

**Direct Examination.** In infected tissues, *H. capsulatum* is a small oval yeast, approximately 4 μm in diameter. The yeast is nearly impossible to detect in unstained specimens. The organism is phagocytized by macrophages or histiocytes (from which the name histoplasmosis is derived). The organisms will be seen in the cytoplasm of these cells unless the tissue has undergone cell death and breakdown (necrosis) as a result of the infection. *H. capsulatum* parasitizing a macrophage is shown in Figure 38-2.

Parasitized histiocytes are most commonly seen in disseminated histoplasmosis. The organism can be visualized in the cells by a variety of stains including Wright-Giemsa, periodic acid-Schiff (PAS), and methenamine silver (see Figure 38-3).

Free organisms within dead cell debris are characteristic of chronic respiratory infections with histoplasmosis. In these cases and in cases where the organisms are not numerous, the methenamine silver stain is preferred because of its much greater sensitivity. In the silver

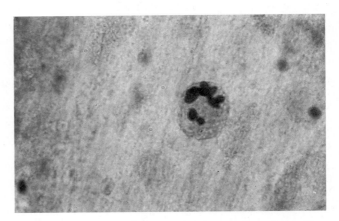

**FIGURE 38-2** *Histoplasma capsulatum* yeast parasitizing histiocytes (macrophages). Methenamine silver stain.

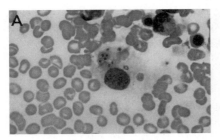 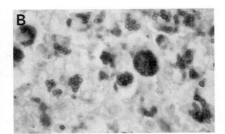 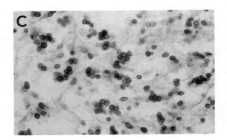

**FIGURE 38-3** *Histoplasma capsulatum* yeast. **A.** Disseminated histoplasmosis, bone marrow histiocyte parasitized by *H. capsulatum* yeast; Wright-Giemsa stain. **B.** Disseminated histoplasmosis; histiocytes of spleen parasitized by *H. capsulatum* yeast. PAS stain. **C.** Pulmonary histoplasmosis; yeast in cell debris. Methenamine silver stain.

stain the organism will appear somewhat larger than in the other stains because metallic silver is precipitated on the surface of the organisms. The organisms tend to be uniform; budding is uncommonly observed. With careful observation the organism can be identified with a high degree of accuracy. However, in necrotic debris there may be small calcified bodies similar in size and shape to *Histoplasma* organisms (see Figure 38-4). Care must be taken not to confuse these with *Histoplasma* yeasts.

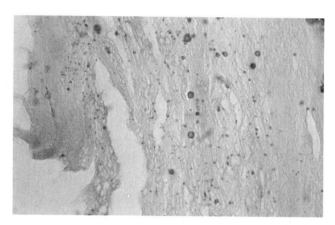

**FIGURE 38-4** Calcified bodies resembling *H. capsulatum*.

**Culture.** *Histoplasma capsulatum* grows slowly in culture, sometimes requiring up to 6 weeks for visible growth. Specimens should be cultured on several media including blood agar and Sabouraud's agar and incubated at room temperature (25°C). Specimens such as sputum can easily become overgrown by contaminating bacteria or yeast unless precautions are taken. **Inhibitory media** containing antibiotics or yeast extract must be used for those specimens (see Chapter 35). Blood cultures in patients with disseminated histoplasmosis yield best results when lysis centrifugation (Isolator) or biphasic techniques are used (Paya, Roberts, & Cockerill, 1987). *H. capsulatum* grows as a relatively nondescript mold in culture. The colonies are generally white to tan and cannot be distinguished from many other fungi including *Blastomyces*. The mold produces two types of conidia (see Figures 38-5 and 38-6). The small microconidia (2–5 μm), generally appear first. The large macroconidia measure 10 to 15 μm and are tuberculate, that is, they have a rough knobby or bumpy surface.

Confirmation that the organism is *H. capsulatum* requires conversion to the parasitic yeast phase or characteristic **exoantigen immunodiffusion**. Demonstration of yeast conversion may be difficult and require several attempts. The organism is transferred to a rich agar containing blood, cysteine, or glutamine. It is then incubated at 37°C. The conversion may require 1 to 2 weeks to achieve. Often the cultures contain a mixture of yeast and hyphae.

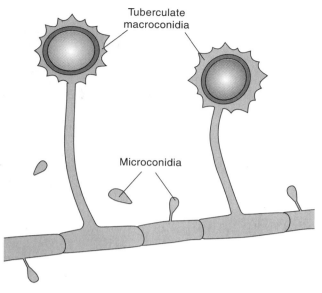

**FIGURE 38-5** *Histoplasma capsulatum*, mold phase tuberculate macroconidia and microconidia.

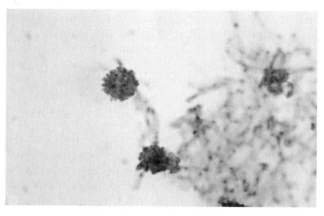

**FIGURE 38-6** *Histoplasma capsulatum*, mold phase, tuberculate macroconidia.

## COCCIDIOIDES IMMITIS

Coccidioidomycosis is among the most fascinating of all fungal infections. It is caused by *C. immitis,* a dimorphic fungus that inhabits a very specialized environment. The saprophytic phase is a mold that produces highly infectious **arthroconidia** (arthrospores) (see Figure 38-7). The parasitic phase is a large spherule that develops endospores (see Figure 38-8*A*). When the spherule becomes too large, it ruptures releasing endospores into the surrounding tissue (see Figure 38-8*B*). These endospores are then capable of developing into spherules, thus perpetuating the infection. Should the spherules become exposed to the outside environment, they convert back to the mold phase producing septate hyphae.

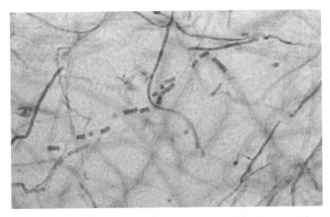

**FIGURE 38-7** *Coccidioides immitis*, mold phase with arthroconidia.

## Geographic Distribution and Natural Habitat

*Coccidioides immitis* has a very restricted geographic distribution. The most highly endemic areas are in the desert southwest of the United States and adjacent Mexico. There are other endemic foci in Central and South America. This habitat is called the Lower Sonoran Life Zone, which is semi-arid, rainfall occurring in one short season of the year. The organism lives in the soil. The organisms are disseminated by the winds that stir up the dusty soil.

## Clinical Disease

*Coccidioides immitis* is the most virulent of all the fungi. Inhalation of only a few arthroconidia will cause infection. Therefore, in the endemic areas infection is nearly universal. Fortunately, the vast majority of patients recover completely, most without treatment. Primary infection is in the lungs, resulting from inhalation of arthroconidia. More than half the infected patients have no symptoms. Only positive skin tests later provide evidence of the previous infection. Patients who do have symptomatic primary pulmonary infections generally have a flulike illness that can vary considerably in severity. Inhalation of large numbers of arthroconidia in dusty environments is more likely to produce severe symptoms. The clinical illness is called **valley fever**, named after the San Joaquin Valley in California. Many patients have allergic manifestations in the skin and joints ("desert rheumatism" and "desert bumps"). The vast majority of patients get well without any antifungal drug therapy. Fewer than 10% of patients have persistent disease, and most of those patients have benign, non–life-threatening complications. These may include the persistence of mild pneumonia or cavities in the lungs. Some patients develop a nodule in the lung called a coccidioma, which is identical to the histoplasmoma previously described. The coccidioma is of no clinical significance except that it may mimic lung cancer in a chest x-ray.

## Laboratory Evaluation and Diagnosis

Extreme care must be taken in the mycology laboratory when dealing with *C. immitis* because the arthroconidia are highly infectious. Because the spherules themselves are not infectious, direct microscopic examination of specimens and tissues is very important. For patients with pulmonary infections, sputum and other lower respiratory specimens will contain the spherules. In patients with disseminated disease the site of infection will determine the most appropriate specimen.

**Direct Examination.** The spherules of *C. immitis* are among the most easily identifiable structures in the microbiology laboratory. They may be identified in direct wet mounts of specimens or may be stained by a variety of stains. Among the fungal stains, methenamine silver is the most sensitive but PAS or Gridley stains provide much better detail.

When mature, the spherules measure up to 80 μm in diameter and are filled with round endospores measuring 2 to 5 μm in diameter (see Figures 38-8*A* & *B*).

Problems in recognition may occur in a variety of

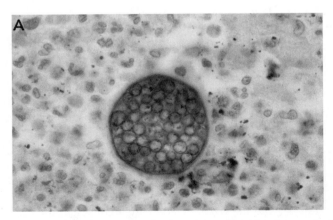

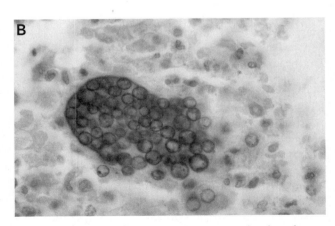

**FIGURE 38-8** *Coccidioides immitis*, parasitic phase. **A.** Spherule containing endospores. **B.** Ruptured spherule releasing endospores.

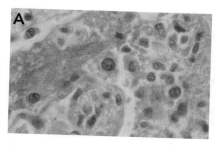
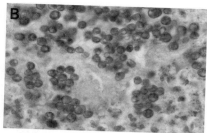
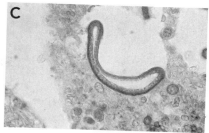

**FIGURE 38-9** *Coccidioides immitis,* parasitic phase. **A.** Immature spherule, which can be confused with yeast of *Blastomyces.* **B.** Released endospores, which can be confused with small yeast. **C.** Collapsed spherule following release of endospores.

circumstances, however. When the spherules are not mature they may resemble other large yeasts, particularly *Blastomyces* (see Figure 38-9*A*). Released endospores may be confused with a variety of smaller yeasts including *Cryptococcus* (see Figure 38-9*B*). Careful examination, however, will reveal the typical internal structure of *Coccidioides*. Moreover, *Coccidioides* spherules do not have buds or pseudohyphae as do true yeasts.

In some specimens only collapsed spherules may be present. The endospores have been released and only the cell wall remains (see Figure 38-9*C*). These structures are easily overlooked if the specimens are not carefully examined.

**Culture.** *Coccidioides immitis* grows rapidly on a wide variety of media. The colonies develop rapidly, within a few days. They are nondescript, usually white and cottony. Arthroconidia develop readily. Because these conidia are so highly infectious, Petri dishes should never be used. Only a few conidia released into the air can cause infection in technologists throughout the laboratory room. All cultures should be handled in a biologic safety hood. Once growth is sufficient, the cultures can be sterilized by pouring formaldehyde or phenol over the agar slants. Then tease preps can be

made for microscopic examination to identify the arthroconidia. A diagrammatic representation of *C. immitis* with arthroconidia is depicted in Figure 38-10. These are boxcar-like and are found in the septate hyphae in a pattern alternating with empty hyphal cells. Exoantigen immunodiffusion is the preferred method to confirm the culture diagnosis of *C. immitis* and has the advantage of being able to be performed on cultures that have been sterilized by phenol.

## BLASTOMYCES DERMATITIDIS

*Blastomyces dermatitidis* is a dimorphic ascomycete (**teleomorphic** state: *Ajellomyces dermatitidis*). Thus the perfect state is closely related to *H. capsulatum* (*Ajellomyces capsulatus*). The organism is a mold in nature but converts to a yeast when it infects tissues. The yeast is fairly uniform in size varying from 8 to 15 µm in diameter. It produces a characteristic single broad-based bud (see Figure 38-11).

### Geographic Distribution and Natural Habitat

The distribution and ecology of *B. dermatitidis* is much more difficult to define than for *Histoplasma* or *Coccidioides*. The infections are most commonly found in the Midwest along the drainage of the Mississippi River, as well as along the St. Lawrence River, Great

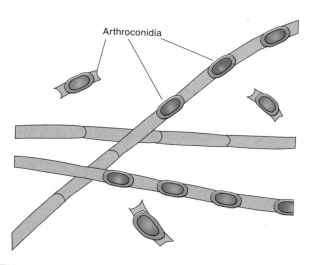

**FIGURE 38-10** Diagram of *C. immitis,* mold phase with alternating arthroconidia.

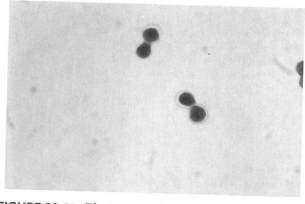

**FIGURE 38-11** *Blastomyces dermatitidis,* yeast phase.

Lakes, and in the southeastern states. There have also been cases in Africa and sporadic infections in Europe. Thus the old name of North American blastomycosis is no longer appropriate.

The fungus is felt to inhabit the soil, but it has only rarely been recovered from its natural habitat. Soil moisture and animal excreta may be important because the organism has been isolated from the soil associated with beaver ponds (Klein et al., 1986). The fungus may be dormant much of the year and only active at certain times (Rippon, 1988).

## Clinical Disease

Although blastomycosis was originally recognized as a skin infection, all evidence now indicates that the cutaneous infections are secondary, following current or previous lung infections. The pulmonary infections are caused by inhalation of conidia from the mold phase. The initial lung infection may or may not be symptomatic. The primary infection may resolve spontaneously or may cause progressive lung infection.

Whether or not the primary lung infections heal, the organisms may disseminate throughout the body. The most common site of extrapulmonary infection is in the skin. The skin infections are verrucous (wartlike) and ulcerating. They may be quite extensive and destructive, leaving deforming scars.

The second most common site of dissemination is to bones. These lesions may clinically resemble bacterial osteomyelitis or malignant tumors. Blastomycosis can also be septicemic involving almost any organ system in the body. Immunocompromised patients, including patients with AIDS, are increasingly susceptible to severe disseminated disease.

## Laboratory Evaluation and Diagnosis

**Direct Examination.** Because the yeast of *B. dermatitidis* is so characteristic, direct microscopic examination of clinical specimens and tissues is the most useful method for the rapid detection of the organisms. The yeast may be found in sputum and lower respiratory specimens in patients with active pneumonia in a high percentage of cases. It may also be found in infected tissue and pus from skin and other involved organs. Because there may be relatively few organisms compared to the extensive tissue reaction, it is important to examine all specimens thoroughly and carefully. The organism can be identified with a wide variety of stains, but also is visible in KOH preparations of sputum and pus.

The yeast of *B. dermatitidis* varies from 8 to 15 μm in diameter. It has a thick, refractile cell wall. In alcohol- or formalin-fixed specimens the cell body retracts away from the cell wall, producing an artifactual clear space around the cell body, which is very characteristic of the organism (see Figure 38-12). This artifact may not be

seen in wet preparations. The yeast produces a single broad-based bud, which helps distinguish it from cryptococci and other yeasts that have narrow pinched-off buds. The yeasts also typically are uniform distinguishing them from the more varied cryptococci.

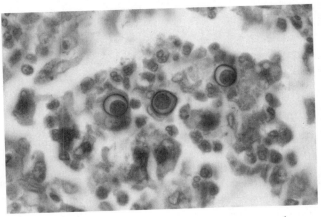

**FIGURE 38-12** *Blastomyces dermatitidis*, yeast phase in tissue. Note retraction artifact of cell body from cell wall. PAS stain.

**Culture.** *Blastomyces dermatitidis* generally grows well in culture, although there is considerable variability. Usually growth is evident within a few days to a week on a variety of media. The colonies of *B. dermatitidis* are not distinctive and can resemble a number of saprophytes. They vary from white to brown and from waxy to cotton-like. Some strains have concentric rings. Single round to pyriform conidia are produced on the hyphae, closely resembling the saprophyte *Chrysosporium* species (see Figure 38-13).

Confirmation that the fungus is *B. dermatitidis* requires demonstration of dimorphism. Yeast conversion is relatively simple and is accomplished by transferring the mold form to a rich nutrient agar containing blood and incubating this at 37°C. Yeastlike colonies will appear within a few days to weeks. The yeast cells will exhibit the typical microscopic morphology of *B. dermatitidis*

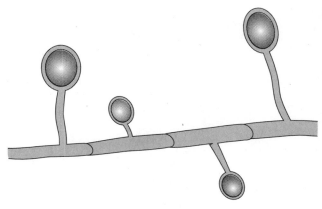

**FIGURE 38-13** *Blastomyces dermatitidis*, microscopic appearance of mold phase.

in most cases. However, some strains will be composed of smaller yeast resembling *H. capsulatum*. The exoantigen immunodiffusion test (see above) can also be used to identify the organism from the mycelial phase.

## PARACOCCIDIOIDES BRASILIENSIS

Paracoccidioidomycosis is generally confined to Central and South America and is not commonly found in other parts of the world. In fact, it is often referred to as South American blastomycosis. However, cases have been seen outside endemic areas, including the United States. All of these have occurred in patients who have visited or lived in an endemic area. With increasing world travel and immigration it is reasonable to suspect that the infection will be seen more frequently in the United States.

*Paracoccidioides brasiliensis* is dimorphic. The saprophytic form is a mold producing a variety of spores none of which are characteristic. On the other hand, the parasitic form is among the most distinctive of all organisms. This parasitic form is a relatively large yeast that produces multiple radial buds resembling a ship's wheel (see Figure 38-14).

### Geographic Distribution and Natural Habitat

*Paracoccidioides brasiliensis* is found from Mexico to Argentina. Clinical infections are most commonly found in Brazil (80%), Columbia, and Venezuela. The organism appears concentrated in humid forests where there is abundant summer rainfall and short winters. It may be associated with excreta of water fowl, but the organism has rarely been isolated from the natural habitat (Brummer, Castaneda, & Restrepo, 1993).

### Clinical Disease

In the usual case primary infection occurs in the lungs, but it is almost always subclinical and inappar-

ent. Most patients with clinical disease present with chronic adult paracoccidioidomycosis. Men are 13 times more likely than women to have this infection, even though skin test reactivity in the endemic areas has an equal male to female ratio (Brummer et al., 1993). Thus, women appear to be more resistant to clinical disease, possibly because estrogen hormones can inhibit yeast transformation (Restrepo et al., 1984).

Chronic adult infection may be limited to the lungs, but more commonly is disseminated to other organs. By far the most common form is the mucocutaneous infection that occurs in the area of the mouth, lips, and nose. The infection presents as ulcers that are initially painless but may become very painful when advanced. Regional lymph nodes are often enlarged due to the infection. Some patients present with infections localized to a single organ, most commonly the adrenal gland. Multifocal infections can be widespread throughout the body. The infections respond well to the newer antifungal drugs.

### Laboratory Evaluation and Diagnosis

**Direct Examination.** Because the parasitic form of *P. brasiliensis* is so characteristic, direct examination of clinical specimens provides the best and most rapid diagnosis. Specimens may include respiratory secretions, exudate from ulcers, or tissue biopsies. KOH preparation of sputum may reveal the organisms, but special stains may be necessary when examining infected tissue.

Microscopic examination reveals the characteristic large yeasts. When mature these measure up to 30 µm, sometimes larger. Radial, narrow-based buds surround the yeast (see Figure 38-15), resembling a ship's wheel. When there are fewer buds, the organism resembles a "Mickey Mouse cap."

**Culture.** *Paracoccidioides brasiliensis* grows as a mold on a variety of media at room temperature. The growth

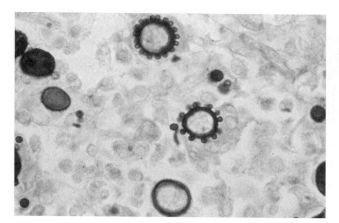

**FIGURE 38-14** *Paracoccidioides brasiliensis*, yeast phase with radial buds.

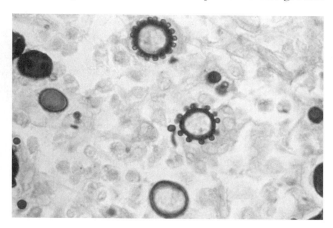

**FIGURE 38-15** *Paracoccidioides brasiliensis*, yeast phase, tissue section. Methenamine silver stain.

rate is slow so that media containing antibiotics should be used to suppress bacterial contamination. The mold produces a variety of spores including conidia, which resemble those of *B. dermatitidis,* arthroconidia, and chlamydospores. None of these are distinctive enough to be diagnostic. A diagram of the mold phase of *P. brasiliensis* is depicted in Figure 38-16.

On blood-containing agar at 37°C the organism converts to the yeast form. This growth is more rapid than the mold phase. Examination of smears from the yeast colonies reveals the diagnostic yeast morphology. The exoantigen immunodiffusion test can be used for identification but generally is not necessary because the yeast conversion is usually successful and timely.

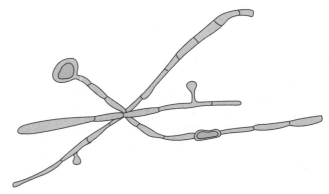

**FIGURE 38-16** *Paracoccidioides brasiliensis,* diagram of microscopic appearance of mold phase.

## SUMMARY

▶ The systemic true pathogenic fungi are dimorphic and transform from a mold form in their natural habitat to a parasitic form when they cause infections. The parasitic form is a yeast except for *Coccidioides immitis,* which is a spherule with endospores.

▶ Primary infections of the systemic dimorphic pathogens are in the lungs. Infections in other parts of the body are the result of dissemination.

▶ The systemic dimorphic pathogens have a restricted geographic distribution. In the endemic areas these infections are very common.

## CASE STUDY

A 45-year-old male patient developed a flulike respiratory infection. He worked in a cotton textile mill in eastern North Carolina, and had never been outside of the state of North Carolina in his life. His job in the mill was to receive and open the bales of cotton that had been shipped in from other parts of the United States including Arizona.

The flulike illness became progressively severe, and the patient developed signs of high fever and pneumonia. He was admitted to the hospital, but died within a few days, before a definitive diagnosis could be made.

An autopsy was performed, which revealed infection involving many organs of the body, including lungs, liver, lymph nodes, spleen, kidneys, and adrenal glands. Sections of the involved tissues revealed large spherules as shown in Figure 38-17. Within a week culture grew a white mold that produced arthroconidia.

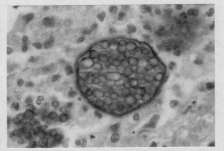

**FIGURE 38-17** Photomicrograph of structures found in tissue of patient.

**Questions:**

1. What is the name of the organism that caused the infection? What is the disease called?

2. What is the relationship of the white mold grown in culture to the spherule seen in tissue sections?

3. Because the patient had never traveled outside the state of North Carolina, how did he contract the infection?

4. Is the type of clinical infection this patient had typical of most infections caused by this organism?

► *Histoplasma capsulatum* is found most frequently in the Midwest, but there are other endemic foci in the United States, South America, and Europe. *H. capsulatum* is a mold producing tuberculate macroconidia and microconidia. The parasitic form is a small oval yeast, difficult to visualize without special stains. Lung disease often resembles tuberculosis. Disseminated disease may be mild, moderate, or fulminant.

► *Coccidioides immitis* is found in the deserts of the southwestern United States, Mexico, and similar areas in South America. The organism lives in the soil as a mold and produces highly infectious arthroconidia. When it infects tissues, it transforms into a large spherule containing endospores. The primary infection is flulike and called "valley fever." Most cases resolve spontaneously. Progressive lung infections and disseminated infections are uncommon, but serious.

► *Blastomyces dermatitidis* is the least characterized epidemiologically of the systemic dimorphic fungi. It is a nondescript mold producing conidia that are not distinctive. The parasitic phase is a very characteristic large yeast that produces a single broad-based bud. Primary infections are more likely to be symptomatic and require treatment than the other systemic infections. The most common sites of dissemination are to skin and bones.

► *Paracoccidioides brasiliensis* causes South American blastomycosis. The mold form is nondescript. The parasitic yeast is distinctive with multiple radial buds resembling a ship's wheel. Primary infection is usually inapparent with most patients presenting with disseminated mucocutaneous infections of the mouth and face.

## Review Questions

1. Which of the following characteristics is NOT generally associated with the systemic true pathogenic fungi?
   a. Dimorphic
   b. Restricted geographic distribution
   c. Infections often asymptomatic
   d. Normal flora in humans
   e. Parasitic phase not contagious

2. Which of the following is (are) characteristic of *Histoplasma capsulatum?*
   a. Tuberculate macroconidia
   b. Microconidia
   c. Small oval yeast
   d. All of the above

3. Which of the following organisms produces arthroconidia?
   a. *Coccidioides immitis*
   b. *Histoplasma capsulatum*
   c. *Blastomyces dermatitidis*
   d. *Paracoccidioides brasiliensis*

4. Which of the following is characteristic of the yeast phase of *Histoplasma capsulatum?*
   a. Has a mucoid capsule
   b. Has multiple radial buds
   c. Yeast with a single broad-based bud
   e. None of the above

5. A sample of infected skin from a patient with cutaneous blastomycosis is submitted to the laboratory and examined directly under the microscope. Which of the following is likely to be seen?
   a. Large yeast with single broad-based bud
   b. Tuberculate macroconidia
   c. Septate hyphae
   d. Arthroconidia

6. Which of the following tests are useful in identifying *Histoplasma capsulatum* in culture?
   a. Exoantigen immunodiffusion
   b. Nucleic acid probes
   c. Thermal dimorphism
   d. All of the above

7. Which of the following cities is found in an area endemic for histoplasmosis?
   a. Boston, Massachusetts
   b. Bakersfield, California
   c. Nashville, Tennessee
   d. El Paso, Texas

8. Which of the following is considered to be the most infectious agent?
   a. Yeast of *Histoplasma capsulatum*
   b. Arthroconidia of *Coccidioides immitis*
   c. Spherule of *Coccidioides immitis*
   d. Endospore of *Coccidioides immitis*

9. KOH preparation from an ulcer in the mouth reveals a large yeast surrounded by small radial buds. What is the identity of the organism?
   a. *Paracoccidioides brasiliensis*
   b. *Coccidioides immitis*
   c. *Histoplasma capsulatum*
   d. *Blastomyces dermatitidis*

**10.** Biopsy of an ulcer in the mouth reveals yeast forms characteristic of *Histoplasma capsulatum.* Which of the following statements concerning this patient's infection is true?

    a. The organism was introduced into the ulcer by an injury from a chicken bone.

    b. The organism spread to the mouth from the lungs.

    c. The organism was transmitted from the hands of the patient's dentist.

    d. The patient drank water from a contaminated pond.

▶ **REFERENCES & RECOMMENDED READING**

Brummer, E., Castaneda, E., & Restropo, A. (1993). Paracoccidioidomycosis, an update. *Clinical Microbiology Reviews, 6,* 89–117.

Darling, S. T. (1906). A protozoan general infection producing pseudotubercules in the lungs and focal necrosis in the liver, spleen and lymph nodes. *Journal of the American Medical Association, 46,* 1283–1285.

Drutz, D. J., & Catanzaro, A. (1978). Coccidioidomycosis. *American Review of Respiratory Disease, 117,* 559–585.

Goodwin, R. A. Jr., & Des Perez, R. M. (1978). Histoplasmosis. *American Review of Respiratory Disease, 117,* 929–956.

Klein, B. S., (1986). Isolation of *Blastomyces dermatitidis* in soil associated with outbreaks of blastomycosis in Wisconsin. *New England Journal of Medicine, 314,* 529–534.

Larson, D. M., Eckman, M. R., Alber, R. L., & Goldschmidt, V. G. (1983). Primary cutaneous (inoculation) blastomycosis: An occupational hazard to pathologists. *American Journal of Clinical Pathology, 79,* 253–255.

Pya, C. V., Roberts, G. D., & Cockerill, F. R. (1987). Laboratory methods for the diagnosis of disseminated histoplasmosis: Clinical implication of the lysis-centrifugation blood culture technique. *Mayo Clinic Proceedings, 62,* 480–485.

Restrepo, A., Salazar, M. E., Cano, L. E., Stover, E. P., Feldman, D., & Stevens, D. A. (1984). Estrogens inhibit mycelium to yeast transformation in the fungus *Paracoccidioides brasiliensis:* Implication for resistance of females to paracoccidioidomycosis. *Infection and Immunity, 46,* 346–353.

Rippon, J. W. (1988). *Medical mycology: The pathogenic fungi and the pathogenic actinomycetes* (3rd ed.). Philadelphia: Saunders.

Sarosi, G. A., & Davies, S. F. (1979). Blastomycosis. *American Review of Respiratory Disease, 120,* 911–938.

Wheat, J. (1995). Endemic mycoses in AIDS: A clinical review. *Clinical Microbiology Reviews, 8,* 146–159.

Wheat, L. J., Kohler, R. B., & Tewari, R. P. (1986). Diagnosis of disseminated histoplasmosis by detection of *Histoplasma capsulatum* antigen in serum and urine specimens. *New England Journal of Medicine, 314,* 83–88.

# CHAPTER 39
# Opportunistic Fungi

James A. Miller, MD, Anne T. Rodgers, MT (ASCP) PhD

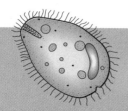

## Microbes in the News

### Over-the-Counter Drugs and Drug Resistance

The widespread use of over-the-counter azole-based agents to treat common fungal infections, such as vulvovaginal candidiasis, may be accelerating the development of azole-resistant strains of fungal infections. According to Dr. John E. Bennett at a grand rounds lecture on investigational systemic antifungal agents sponsored by the National Institute of Allergy and Infectious Diseases, the emergence of these new strains of *Candida* underscore the need for newer, more effective antifungal agents. "Because the use of azoles has so recently exploded, we don't know yet what the full impact on drug resistance is going to be," Dr. Bennett said. Hospitals would be especially at risk for the transmission of azole-resistant *Candida*.

Drug manufacturers are currently performing trials on a new category of antifungal drugs called lipopeptides to determine their effectiveness against *Aspergillus* and *Candida*. Potential resistance against these drugs is still unknown.

Source: Bykowski, M. *Skin & Allergy News* 29(2): 14, 1998.

## KEY TERMS

| | | |
|---|---|---|
| Aseptate hyphae | India ink preparation | Opportunistic |
| Conidia | Ketoacidosis | Pseudohyphae |
| Fungus ball | KOH preparation | Saprophytes |
| Hyaline hyphomycetes | Mucopolysaccharide capsule | Septate hyphae |
| Immunosuppressed | Normal flora | Sporangium |

Upon successful completion of this chapter, the student should be able to:

1. Identify etiologic agents causing opportunistic fungal infections and their clinical manifestations.
2. Identify and describe colonial and microscopic morphologies of the agents that cause opportunistic fungal infections.
3. Discuss the value of direct examination of the specimens and describe laboratory findings by this method.
4. Explain how a common contaminant can be determined to be etiologically significant.

## INTRODUCTION

Only a very small percentage of fungi are true pathogens and have the capacity to cause disease in the normal host. The vast majority of fungi are **opportunistic**, that is, they only cause disease when the host's resistance is altered. The most common factors predisposing to opportunistic fungal infections are:

▶ Immune deficiencies
▶ Immunosuppressive drugs
▶ Corticosteroids
▶ Malignancies (especially lymphoid)
▶ Organ transplantation
▶ Antibiotics
▶ Diabetes mellitus
▶ Trauma

Common to many of these is an alteration in the immune response, especially of the T-cell lymphocyte system. Whereas primary T-cell immunodeficiencies are uncommon, acquired T-cell deficiencies are becoming increasingly common now that acquired immunodeficiency syndrome (AIDS) is reaching epidemic proportions. Opportunistic fungal infections are extremely common in patients with AIDS and are often a cause of death. Immunosuppressive and corticosteroid drugs primarily depress the T-cell immune system. Lymphoid malignancies such as lymphoma and leukemia produce cells that do not have normal immune function and that destroy the lymph nodes and bone marrow where these cells are normally produced.

Antibiotics deserve special mention as promoters of opportunistic fungal infections. These are often associated with infections caused by yeasts that can be considered part of the **normal flora** of the body. They are usually present in quite low numbers, often held in check by the bacteria that are also normal flora in the same site. Antibiotics used to treat a bacterial infection may have the unintended consequence of depressing these normal bacteria as well. When that happens, fungi that are not susceptible to antibiotics overgrow in the area, leading to infection.

The opportunistic fungi are ubiquitous and do not have a restricted geographic distribution. Some of these organisms are normal flora in humans and animals; others are **saprophytes** in nature. Unlike the systemic dimorphic pathogenic fungi, the opportunistic fungi exhibit no change in morphology from the saprophytic to the parasitic phase. Fungi, which are molds in nature, exist in the hyphal form when they cause infections; yeast also remain yeast in infections.

As steroid and immunosuppressive therapy, organ transplantation, and AIDS infections have increased, the incidence of these fungal infections has risen, and they are now the most common fungal infections encountered in hospitalized patients. Theoretically any fungal species is capable of causing infection given the opportunity. However, most of the opportunistic fungal infections are caused by species of *Candida, Cryptococcus, Aspergillus,* and the *Zygomycetes.*

There are some pitfalls to beware of in evaluating clinical specimens from patients suspected of having opportunistic fungal infections. Because the organisms involved are common saprophytes or normal flora, it may be difficult to distinguish organisms that are causing infection from those that have contaminated the clinical specimen. Whereas in the past saprophytic fungi were often discarded as airborne contaminants, that practice should no longer be continued, and the recovered organisms should be evaluated as fully as possible. Physicians caring for these patients will ultimately need to decide whether an organism is responsible for the patient's illness.

## CRYPTOCOCCOSIS

Cryptococcosis is an infection caused by one of a number of species of the yeast organism *Cryptococcus. Cryptococcus neoformans* is the principal pathogen in this group, and this section deals with infections caused by this organism. For a discussion of the characteristics of other species of *Cryptococcus* see Chapter 41.

## Mycology

*Cryptococcus neoformans* is a pleomorphic yeast, that is, the cells vary considerably in size. The organism produces single or multiple narrow base buds (blastoconidia), which when mature detach to become new organisms (see Figure 39-1).

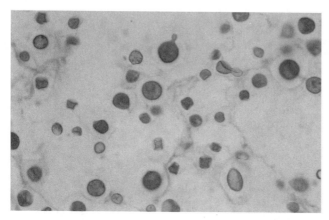

**FIGURE 39-1** *Cryptococcus neoformans* demonstrating pleomorphic budding yeast. Periodic acid-Schiff stain.

The most characteristic feature is the presence of an acid **mucopolysaccharide capsule** around the yeast cells. The capsule is exhibited in the electron micrograph shown in Figure 39-2.

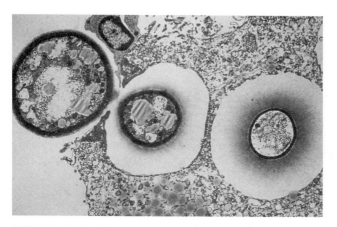

**FIGURE 39-2** *Cryptococcus neoformans* demonstrating capsule.

The capsule can be detected in **India ink preparations** (see Chapter 35) and by special stains specific for acid mucopolysaccharide, such as alcian blue and mucicarmine. No other yeasts, including other species of *Cryptococcus,* produce such a capsule. Thus its recognition in clinical specimens provides conclusive evidence that the yeast is *C. neoformans*. Rare variants of *C. neoformans* do not possess a capsule and thus are capsular deficient. These variants do not appear to be as virulent as the capsule-producing organism.

Cryptococcus is a saprophyte in the intestine of various species of birds, particularly the pigeon. It probably does not cause infection in the birds because the body temperature of birds averages 42°C, and the organism does not grow well at that temperature. The organism is transmitted via the excreta of these birds in which it remains viable for long periods of time (Mitchell & Perfect, 1995).

## Clinical Disease

The portal of entry for *C. neoformans* is the respiratory tract. Therefore, primary infections are in the lung. The pulmonary infections may be asymptomatic or may produce a variety of signs and symptoms that mimic other lung infections or lung cancer. It is not possible to make a clinical diagnosis of pulmonary cryptococcus without identifying the organism in infected clinical specimens.

Whether or not *C. neoformans* produces symptoms of the lung infection, it can spread to other organs in the body. The central nervous system (CNS) is by far the most common site of dissemination. Meningitis is most frequent but actual infections of brain tissue can also occur. Cryptococcal meningitis is a chronic infection and does not often present with devastating symptoms of acute bacterial meningitis. Headache is the most common symptom, with neck rigidity and alteration of consciousness seen in many patients as well. The diagnosis is made by lumbar puncture (spinal tap). Cell counts of cerebrospinal fluid (CSF) vary, but usually exhibit increased lymphocytes. Protein is usually elevated and glucose is low. The diagnosis is confirmed by identifying organisms in India ink preparation or culture or by demonstrating cryptococcal antigen.

About 10% of patients with disseminated cryptococcus will develop cutaneous or bone infections. Disseminated cryptococcosis can affect any organ of the body and in some cases there are multiple sites of infection. The organism can even be recovered in blood and bone marrow cultures.

Treatment of cryptococcosis requires use of antifungal drugs. A variety of drugs may be effective, and the choice will depend on the clinical setting. To a great extent, prognosis for recovery will depend on the patient's underlying clinical status. In AIDS patients, for example, silent persistent infection is common even after apparently successful treatment (Bozzett et al., 1991).

## Direct Evaluation of Clinical Specimens

The capsule is the key to the pathogenicity of *C. neoformans*. It is also the key to its diagnosis. The capsule offers some protection of the organism from host defenses. Thus there may be large numbers of cryptococcal organisms in infected tissue with very little host inflammatory response. Yeast may be demonstrated in a number of ways in clinical specimens, but identification of the mucopolysaccharide capsule confirms that the organism is *C. neoformans.*

The India ink preparation is the most rapid way to diagnose *C. neoformans* in fluid specimens (see Figure 39-3). The procedure is detailed in Chapter 35 (Procedure 35-3). Unfortunately a positive India ink preparation is only demonstrated in approximately one-half the patients with subsequently proven cryptococcal meningitis due to low numbers of organisms in the CSF. In these cases demonstration of cryptococcal antigen is more sensitive, but takes somewhat longer to perform.

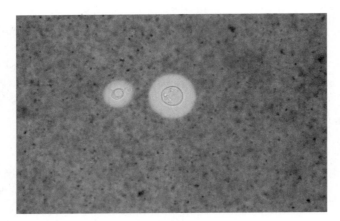

**FIGURE 39-3** *Cryptococcus neoformans,* India ink preparation.

*Cryptococcus neoformans* is a yeast that under ordinary circumstances does not produce **pseudohyphae**. For practical purposes observation of pseudohyphae will indicate that the organism is not *C. neoformans,* but represents some other yeast, particularly *Candida* species. However, on rare occasions pseudohyphae will be produced by *C. neoformans* (see Figure 39-4).

## CANDIDIASIS

Candidiasis, also known as candidosis, is caused by one of several species of *Candida* organisms (see

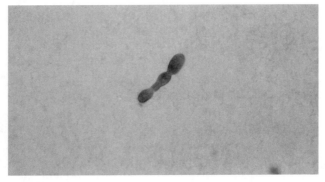

**FIGURE 39-4** *Cryptococcus neoformans* demonstrating rare example of pseudohyphae in CSF specimen.

Chapter 41). These are commonly encountered yeasts that produce pseudohyphae. All of the *Candida* species are capable of producing disease in the compromised host, but the principal pathogen is *Candida albicans.*

## Mycology

*Candida albicans* exists in low numbers as normal flora in the mouth and intestinal tract of humans and animals. This is one organism with which it may be difficult to distinguish contamination of culture material by normal flora from true disease-causing organisms. The organisms readily produce pseudohyphae and do not have capsules, distinguishing them from *C. neoformans.* Microscopic features of *C. albicans* with pseudohyphae are shown in Figure 39-5.

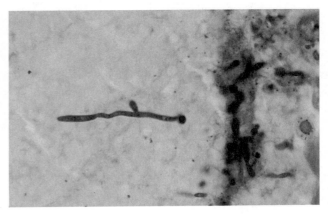

**FIGURE 39-5** *Candida albicans* with pseudohyphae. Periodic acid-Schiff stain.

## Clinical Disease

*Candida albicans* causes a wide variety of opportunistic infections some of which are trivial and others of which have a high mortality rate. Factors predisposing to *Candida* infections are similar to those usually associated with opportunistic fungal infections. However, because *C. albicans* is part of the normal flora of humans, there is increased emphasis on those factors that cause an imbalance in the normal flora. Thus there is particular emphasis on use of antibiotics, presence of deep venous catheters, and prolonged hospitalization.

Factors predisposing to disseminated candida infections include:

▶ Malignancy (hematologic)
▶ Long-term antibiotics
▶ Prolonged hospitalization
▶ Antineoplastic drugs
▶ Deep venous catheters
▶ AIDS

Cutaneous infections may mimic ringworm infections caused by dermatophytes (see Chapter 36). The organisms most commonly infect tissues that are warm, moist, and easily macerated. Nails may also be infected.

The most common mucocutaneous infections are vaginal candidiasis, usually referred to as vaginal yeast infections. Symptoms may be quite unpleasant but are not life-threatening. Candidiasis in the mouth is commonly referred to as thrush. The organisms produce a white coating of the tongue and mucous membranes. It is commonly seen in infants who do not have a well developed immune system and in adults on antibiotic therapy. It may also be the first sign that AIDS is developing in patients infected with human immunodeficiency virus (HIV). Organisms may extend to the esophagus and gastrointestinal tract or bronchial tree. Chronic mucocutaneous candidiasis occurs in children with certain congenital immune deficiencies.

Systemic candidal infections are always very serious infections that may have a high rate of mortality. This is particularly true for infections of the heart valves, brain, and meninges. When septicemia occurs, abscess can develop in almost any organ of the body.

## Direct Evaluation of Clinical Specimens

*Candida* organisms are readily visualized in a wide variety of clinical specimens. Cutaneous and mucocutaneous infections are best evaluated by examining scrapings of the lesions by **KOH preparation**. The organisms will appear as budding yeast with pseudohyphae. Because other yeasts may also produce pseudohyphae, identification of the organism as *Candida* is only presumptive in direct preparations, and definitive identification requires culture of the organism. Even though *C. albicans* is the principal pathogen, other *Candida* species will appear similar microscopically.

Vaginal infections can be detected by direct wet prep of vaginal swab material, but also can be identified in Pap smears (see Figure 39-6). The Pap stain is useful for evaluating cells as well as microbiologic organisms and can detect *Candida* infections in esophageal brush-

ings, bronchoscopic specimens, and fluids. Gram stain of sputum specimens will often reveal *Candida* organisms, but it is impossible to distinguish normal flora from organisms causing infection. In specimens where these are a low number of organisms, detection can be enhanced by using special stains for fungi, including methenamine silver or periodic acid-Schiff (PAS). Figure 39-7 demonstrates the enhanced detection of *Candida* by methenamine silver stain.

## ASPERGILLOSIS

Aspergillosis refers to a variety of infections and allergic disorders caused by any of a number of species of the genus *Aspergillus*. *Aspergillus* is a very common saprophytic fungus, and opportunistic infections are likewise very common. Whereas it was a common practice in past decades to discard cultures containing *Aspergillus* as contaminated, this is no longer acceptable practice.

## Mycology

The genus has several hundred species, but only a few are commonly associated with human infections. *Aspergillus fumigatus, Aspergillus flavus,* and *Aspergillus niger* are most often encountered in disease. *Aspergillus* is a mold organism, producing only **septate hyphae**. It is often encountered as a bread mold or as a contaminant in air-conditioning units. In fact, there has been increased recovery of aspergillus from respiratory specimens and even pulmonary infections in compromised patients during periods of hospital renovation, particularly involving air filtration and ventilation systems (Arnow, Anderson, Mainous, & Smith, 1978; Sarubbi, Kopf, Wilson, McGinnis, & Rutala, 1982). *Aspergillus* is not a part of the normal flora of humans.

In culture, the organism produces conidiophores from the hyphae. The reproductive structures are demon-

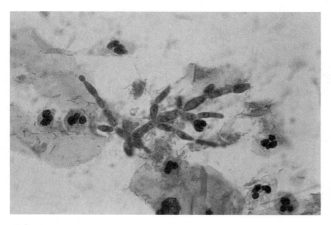

**FIGURE 39-6** *Candida* species in Pap smear.

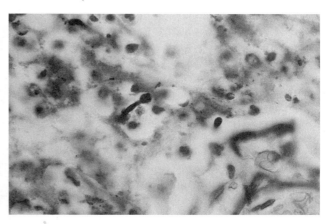

**FIGURE 39-7** Photograph of *Candida albicans* shows enhanced detection in methenamine silver stain.

strated in Figure 39-8. These conidiophores develop a swelling on the end called a vesicle. Phialides are produced from the vesicle and **conidia** are produced from the phialides. The arrangement of phialides on the vesicle is used in the identification of the various species of aspergillus (see Chapter 37).

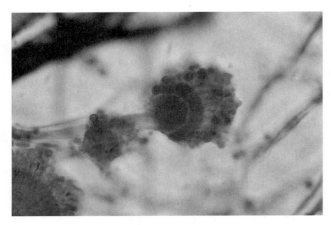

**FIGURE 39-8** Fruiting head of *Aspergillus* species from culture.

## Clinical Disease

Aspergillus is capable of causing a wide variety of infections in compromised hosts. It is also associated with serious allergies of the respiratory system. Most infections involve the respiratory tract because the organisms most commonly gain entrance to the body when airborne conidia are inhaled through the nose into the lungs.

When aspergillus infects the lungs it can cause a severe bronchial infection producing a membrane of organisms and inflammation covering the surface of the airways. More commonly it causes pneumonia in the compromised patient. The pneumonia is often associated with death and breakdown of lung tissue, and there may be large numbers of hyphae growing in the dead tissue. These are shown in Figure 39-9. Aspergillus preferentially seeks out blood vessels, which leads to two serious complications. When the organisms invade the vessels, this interrupts blood flow and results in obstruction of the vessel. The loss of blood flow leads to death of tissue. Access to the blood vessels also allows the organisms to spread to other parts of the body, resulting in disseminated infections.

Sinonasal infections develop when the conidia lodge in the nose. In the most severe cases the organism can destroy the bones of the sinuses and base of the skull, and from there gain access to the brain. CNS aspergillosis can also arise from dissemination of organisms from lung infections. They can lead to abscesses in the brain or to meningitis. Disseminated aspergillus can involve almost any organ, with kidney, liver, and heart valves among the most common. Inva-

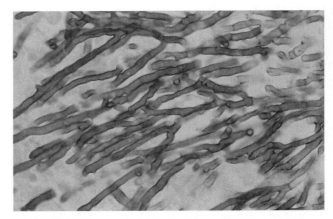

**FIGURE 39-9** Septate hyphae of *Aspergillus* species in lung tissue. Methenamine silver stain.

sive aspergillus infections are difficult to treat and carry a high mortality rate.

An aspergilloma is the result of colonization of a pre-existing cavity by *Aspergillus,* and as such is not an invasive infection. The lung is the most common site, but nasal cavity and sinuses can also develop aspergillomas. In the lung, aspergillus spores are inhaled into old healed cavities of tuberculosis or lung cysts. The spores develop into hyphae that grow in a large mass producing a **fungus ball** (see Figure 39-10). The aspergilloma is this mass of hyphae. It usually does not result in invasion of tissue but may lead to bleeding into the cavity.

*Aspergillus* also causes serious allergic disorders in susceptible people. It can produce symptoms very much like asthma. The bronchi can contain plugs of mucus within which the hyphae are found. Paradoxically, despite the presence of fungal hyphae, the patients are treated with corticosteroids because the reaction is one of hypersensitivity, not invasive infection. Similar allergic manifestations can be found in nasal and sinus tissue.

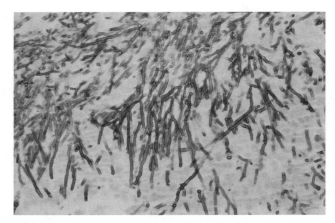

**FIGURE 39-10** Mass of hyphae of aspergilloma. Methenamine silver stain.

## Direct Evaluation of Clinical Specimens

Direct examination of clinical specimens is important in evaluating patients with suspected aspergillosis. Because *Aspergillus* is a common contaminant in cultures, recovery of hyphae in the clinical specimens confirms that the organism recovered in the culture is associated with aspergillosis. Figure 39-11 shows hyphae of *Aspergillus* in a sputum specimen.

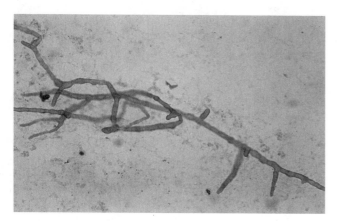

**FIGURE 39-11** *Aspergillus* species hyphae in sputum.

Specimens can be examined by wet preparations but visualization of the hyphae is enhanced following digestion of tissue or mucus by KOH. The final diagnosis requires recovery of the organism in culture.

In certain circumstances a definitive diagnosis of aspergillosis can be made from direct examination or stained specimens. This is possible when the characteristic conidiophores and reproductive structures are observed. These structures may be present when there is sufficient oxygen to which large numbers of organisms are exposed, as in the case of aspergilloma (fungus ball) of the lung or sinonasal tissues. The fruiting heads of *Aspergillus* from an aspergilloma of the lung are shown in Figure 39-12.

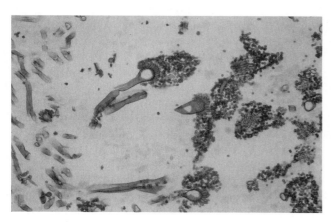

**FIGURE 39-12** Fruiting heads (reproductive structures) from *aspergilloma*. Methenamine silver stain.

## ZYGOMYCOSIS

Zygomycosis is an infection caused by a member of the class of fungi called Zygomycetes. The organisms are common environmental saprophytes. They are frequently found in soil and on plants and fruit. Like *Aspergillus* they are common bread molds. Although *Rhizopus* species are most often associated with infection, the disease is known also as mucormycosis, named for another genus of Zygomycetes, *Mucor*.

### Mycology

The Zygomycetes are molds that form broad **aseptate hyphae**. Occasional septa will be produced in older growth, but never to the extent seen with *Aspergillus* or the other hyaline Hyphomycetes. The organisms derive their class name from their production of zygospores, which are sexual spores produced by the teleomorphic or perfect state. However, these are of no practical importance in identification or classification.

Unlike the **hyaline hyphomycetes**, which produce a variety of conidia, the Zygomycetes produce asexual sporangiospores. These spores are contained within a saclike structure called a **sporangium**. The appearance of the sporangia and supporting structures are used to identify the most common genera of the Zygomycetes (see Chapter 37). Species identification is more difficult and usually is unnecessary in the clinical setting.

*Rhizopus* is the most common of the organisms encountered, both as an environmental contaminant and in disease. Other organisms likely to be found in infections include *Mucor* species, *Rhizomucor* species, and *Absidia* species. The organisms all have similar cultural characteristics. They grow rapidly producing wooly colonies that can fill a Petri dish within 2 or 3 days. The rapid growth can also occur in tissues, leading to a medical emergency in patients with rhinocerebral zygomycosis (see below).

### Clinical Disease

The Zygomycetes are opportunistic, producing infection in the compromised host. As such, zygomycosis is increasing in incidence in conjunction with the increase in organ transplantation and use of chemotherapeutic agents and corticosteroids. In addition however, zygomycosis is particularly associated with diabetes mellitus. It is not high blood sugar levels, but rather **ketoacidosis** that predisposes to infection by the Zygomycetes.

Common to all of the invasive infections is the tendency for the infections to progress rapidly. This is the result of rapid growth rate of the organisms and the propensity for the organisms to invade blood vessels. The tendency toward vascular invasion is more striking for the Zygomycetes than for *Aspergillus*. It results in death of tissue supplied by these blood vessels as well as spread to other areas of the body.

Rhinocerebral zygomycosis can be a very rapidly progressive infection that can lead to extensive destruction of tissues and death of the patient within a few days. It is similar to but even more rapidly destructive than sinonasal aspergillosis. The nasal passages and sinuses develop a progressive destructive infection sometimes eroding through the bones of the sinuses and skull. This can result in breakdown of tissues of the face and even loss of an eye. When the organisms invade blood vessels and bones of the skull they gain access to the brain. Treatment requires a combination of antifungal drugs and surgical debridement of the infected tissues. If the patient is diabetic, acidosis must be corrected. Mortality rate is high, up to 65%.

Thoracic infections usually involve the lung and result from inhalation of airborne spores. There may be extensive tissue destruction associated with vascular invasion by the fungi. Dissemination can occur throughout the body. The mortality rate is even higher than with rhinocerebral zygomycosis. Abdominal infections are rare and usually involve the intestinal tract.

Colonization of cavitary spaces is uncommon compared to *Aspergillus,* but can occur with species of *Mucor.* This is especially true in the nasal passages. In such infections various spore structures can be seen.

## Direct Evaluation of Clinical Specimens

Because of the rapidly progressive nature and high mortality rate of zygomycete infections, direct examination of clinical specimens is of paramount importance. Waiting a matter of only a few days for culture results may turn a potentially treatable infection into a fatal one. Because the organisms produce broad, ribbon-like aseptate hyphae, they can be identified as Zygomycetes in unstained and stained clinical specimens. Although identification of the particular genus of Zygomycete requires recovery in culture, the physician only needs to know that the organism is a Zygomycete to initiate appropriate therapy.

The organisms have very characteristic hyphae (see Figure 39-13). They are broad often with irregular swellings. The lack of septa confirms that the organisms are Zygomycetes. However, the finding of an occasional septum does not exclude the diagnosis of zygomycosis because older organisms do develop a few septa. The hyphae are often folded over themselves, which may give the appearance of septa. In tissue sections, cross-sections of the organisms may appear round and should not be confused with spherules or sporangia.

In ordinary circumstances sporangia and sporangiospores are not observed in clinical specimens. However, in the rare occurrence of the development of a "fungus ball" in a lung cavity or in the nose or sinuses, sporangia may develop (see Figure 39-14).

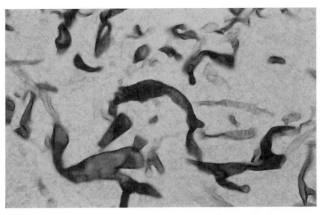

**FIGURE 39-13** *Zygomycete* demonstrating broad, aseptate hyphae. Methenamine silver stain.

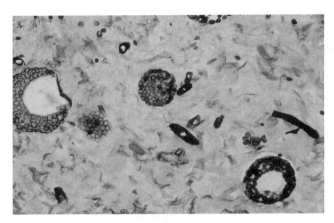

**FIGURE 39-14** Sporangia of zygomycete in nasal tissue. Methenamine silver stain.

## LESS COMMON OPPORTUNISTIC FUNGI

Among the less common opportunistic fungi there are a few organisms worthy of mention because of special clinical situations associated with them. Cultural characteristics of these organisms are covered in Chapters 37 and 38.

### Fusarium Species

*Fusarium* is among the most common of the saprophytic molds and thus is a common contaminant in cultures. However, it is increasingly becoming associated with a variety of infections. Traditionally it has been proven to cause infections of the eye following injury to the cornea or contact lens wear. Cutaneous infections are also relatively common in traumatized skin and in **immunosuppressed** patients. However, *Fusarium* skin infections are most characteristically associated with burns. Disseminated infections can occur in patients with severe burns or more commonly in patients who are immunosuppressed or undergoing cancer chemotherapy. The organisms gain access to the bloodstream either from a skin or burn infection or through the respiratory tract by inhalation of airborne conidia. Of all the mold organisms, *Fusarium* is the most readily recovered from blood cultures (Nelson, Digneni, & Anaissie, 1994).

Treatment of patients with serious *Fusarium* infections can be successful if there is correction of the underlying host defect. Low white blood cell counts associated with chemotherapy are directly related to progression of the infections. Treatment will only be successful when bone marrow function and white blood cell counts are returned to normal. Even then less than 30% of disseminated infections can be successfully treated by antifungal drugs (Nelson et al., 1994).

In the laboratory, the fungal nature of the infections can be recognized through direct examination of clinical specimens and tissues sections. Septate fungal hyphae will be observed (see Figure 39-15). It is not possible to distinguish these hyphae from other hyaline hyphomycetes such as *Aspergillus*. Positive identification requires culture of the organisms. However, in the clinical setting of a patient with serious burns, observation of septate fungal hyphae in tissue or blood cultures should be presumed to be *Fusarium* species until proven otherwise.

## Penicillium marneffei

*Penicillium* species are very common saprophytic molds. Infections caused by these organisms are extremely rare, even in compromised hosts. However, one species of *Penicillium* can cause serious disseminated infections in immunocompromised hosts. That organism is *Penicillium marneffei*.

*Penicillium marneffei* is not native to North America, but is found most commonly in southeast Asia and China. However, it is seen with increasing frequency in the United States among AIDS patients who have lived

or traveled in southeast Asia. It is unclear whether immunocompetent patients are also at risk of infection.

Unlike other species of *Penicillium*, *P. marneffei* is dimorphic and converts to a yeast in the parasite phase. Thus, in infected tissues the organisms will be observed as small oval yeastlike bodies 3 to 8 µm long. They have a central cross septum. The organisms can also be recovered as "yeasts" in blood cultures incubated at 35°C. In ordinary fungal cultures at room temperature the organism is a mold, producing septate hyaline hyphae and the typical conidiophores and conidia of other *Penicillium* species (see Chapter 37). The organism characteristically develops a red pigment after a few days in culture.

## Trichosporon Species

*Trichosporon beigelii* has been discussed in Chapter 36 as the cause of white piedra. However, on rare occasions it and *Trichosporon capitatum* (*Blastoschizomyces capitatus*) can cause invasive infections in compromised patients, particularly those with acute leukemia. The patients often have septicemia and the organisms can be recovered in blood culture. In biopsy material and blood cultures the organisms are pleomorphic yeasts that produce blastoconidia (budding yeast), anthroconidia, and pseudohyphae. These are shown in Figure 39-16.

## Torulopsis glabrata (Candida glabrata)

*Torulopsis glabrata* is considered to be a species of *Candida* by some mycologists. It is a common organism, part of the normal flora of the skin of humans. It has been seen in invasive infections, particularly in the bloodstream, urinary tract, and lungs in immunosuppressed patients. The organism is a small yeast that does not produce pseudohyphae. It can be confused morphologically with *Histoplasma capsulatum*. However, it is not dimorphic and can readily be distinguished from *H. capsulatum* in culture.

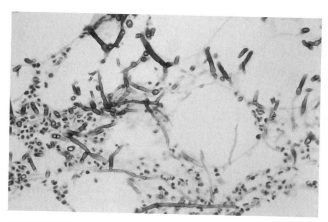

**FIGURE 39-15** Hyphae of *Fusarium* species in tissue, which cannot be distinguished from *Aspergillus* and other hyphomycetes. Methenamine silver stain.

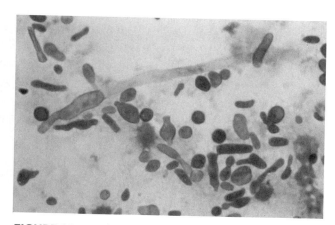

**FIGURE 39-16** Photograph of *Trichosporon beigelii* demonstrating yeast, pseudohyphae, and arthrospores. Periodic acid-Schiff stain.

## SUMMARY

▶ Opportunistic fungi only cause disease when the host's resistance is altered. Factors predisposing to opportunistic infections include primary or secondary immune deficiencies, antibiotic therapy, or other disease states.

▶ Any fungal species is capable of causing an infection, given the opportunity. However, the vast majority of such infections are caused by species of *Candida, Cryptococcus, Aspergillus,* or the Zygomycetes.

▶ *Cryptococcus neoformans* is a pleomorphic yeast with a mucoid capsule, which is the key to identification in direct examination of clinical specimens. India ink preparation reveals the capsule in fluid specimens. The respiratory tract is the portal of entry in most cases, but dissemination to other organs frequently occurs. Cryptococcal meningitis is the most common form of disseminated infection.

▶ *Candida albicans* is part of the normal flora in the mouth and intestine. It can cause a wide variety of opportunistic infections from trivial to very serious with high mortality rates. *Candida* is a yeast that produces pseudohyphae that are easily recognized in direct examination of clinical specimens. It may be difficult to distinguish infection from colonization.

▶ *Aspergillus* is a common saprophytic mold that can cause a variety of infections, especially of the respiratory tract. These may be invasive infections or colonization of preexisting cavities. Septate hyphae are observed in direct examination of clinical specimens. These cannot be distinguished from hyphae of other molds, unless reproductive structures are also present.

▶ The Zygomycetes are also common environmental saprophytes, but can be recognized in direct examination because they form aseptate hyphae. They also produce sporangiospores, which are only rarely observed in clinical specimens. Opportunistic zygomycosis may affect the nasal and sinus tissues, respiratory tract or other organs. There is a propensity for the organisms to invade blood vessels. In addition to immunosuppressed states, the infections are also associated with diabetic ketoacidosis.

▶ *Fusarium* species may cause eye infections or may infect patients with serious burns. *Penicillium marneffei* is dimorphic and converts from a mold to a yeast. It is most commonly associated with AIDS.

▶ *Trichosporon* species and *Torulopsis (Candida) glabrata* are yeasts that can cause bloodstream infections in immunosuppressed patients and patients with leukemia.

## CASE STUDY

A 62-year-old male patient had a 15-year history of autoimmune hemolytic anemia. He had been treated with corticosteroid drugs and had responded well. However, when the steroids were stopped, the anemia recurred. Steroids were reinstituted and he was also treated with immunosuppressive and cytotoxic drugs. Approximately 1 month later he presented with a swollen abdomen, fever, and severe headache. He was noted to have an unstable gait. Some fluid was removed from the abdominal cavity by needle and syringe. This fluid was thick, viscous, and very mucoid. A spinal tap revealed elevated cerebrospinal fluid pressure. The fluid had a low glucose value and elevated protein. Lymphocytes were moderately increased, but there were no neutrophils.

### Questions

1. What diagnosis do you suspect? Why?

2. What is the most rapid test you could perform to confirm this diagnosis? What other tests might be helpful?

3. Do you expect other organ systems to be involved in this case? Why?

## Review Questions

1. Which of the following provides definitive evidence that the patient has an opportunistic infection of the lung?
   a. Presence of yeast and pseudohyphae in direct examination of sputum
   b. Presence of *Candida albicans* in culture of sputum
   c. Presence of *Aspergillus* species in sputum culture
   d. None of the above

2. KOH prep of sinus tissue reveals broad, non-septate fungal hyphae. Which of the following organisms is most likely present?
   a. *Candida albicans*
   b. *Aspergillus* species
   c. *Fusarium* species
   d. *Rhizopus* species

3. Which of the following provides the most definitive evidence that a patient has pulmonary aspergillosis?
   a. Presence of fungal hyphae in sputum smears
   b. Presence of *Aspergillus niger* in sputum culture
   c. Presence of pseudohyphae in sputum smear
   d. Presence of fungal hyphae in sputum smear and *Aspergillus fumigatus* in sputum culture

4. A yeast is recovered from a sputum culture. Which of the following would provide definitive evidence that the yeast is *Cryptococcus neoformans?*
   a. Positive Gram stain
   b. Positive alcian blue stain
   c. Positive methenamine silver stain
   d. Positive PAS stain

5. Which of the following organisms is dimorphic?
   a. *Penicillium marneffei*
   b. *Candida albicans*
   c. *Aspergillus niger*
   d. *Trichosporon beigelii*

6. Which of the following organisms is part of the normal flora of the mouth and intestinal tract of humans?
   a. *Aspergillus flavus*
   b. *Rhizopus* species
   c. *Candida albicans*
   d. *Fusarium* species

7. Observation of yeast with pseudohyphae is presumptive evidence of which of the following?
   a. *Candida albicans*
   b. *Penicillium marneffei*
   c. *Aspergillus niger*
   d. All of the above

8. Which of the following predispose to an opportunistic infection?
   a. Anticancer chemotherapy
   b. Antibiotic therapy
   c. Diabetes mellitus
   d. All of the above

9. Which of the following is presumptive evidence that an observed organism is *Aspergillus* species?
   a. Yeast with pseudohyphae
   b. Calcium oxalate crystals
   c. Aseptate hyphae
   d. Positive India ink preparation

10. Which of the following tests can distinguish meningitis caused by *Cryptococcus neoformans* from meningitis caused by *Candida albicans?*
    a. India ink prep of spinal fluid
    b. Demonstration of thermal dimorphism
    c. KOH prep of spinal fluid
    d. All of the above

▶ **REFERENCES & RECOMMENDED READING**

Arnow, P. M., Anderson, R. L., Mainous, P. D., & Smith, E. J. (1978). Pulmonary aspergillosis during hospital renovation. *American Review of Respiratory Disease, 118,* 49–53.

Bozzette, S. A., Larsen, R. A., Chiu, J., Leal, M. A., Jacobsen, J., and The California Collaborative Treatment Group. (1991). A placebo-controlled trial of maintenance therapy with fluconazole after treatment of cryptococcal meningitis in the acquired immunodeficiency syndrome. *New England Journal of Medicine, 324,* 580–584.

Erke, K. H., (1976). Light microscopy of basidia, basidiospores and nuclei in spores and hyphae of *Filobasidiella neoformans* (*Cryptococcus neoformans*). *Journal of Bacteriology, 128,* 445–455.

Gordon, M. A., & Devine, J. (1970). Filamentous and endogenous sporulation in *Cryptococcus neoformans. Sabouraudia, 8,* 227–234.

Hazen, K. (1995). New and emerging yeast pathogens. *Clinical Microbiology Reviews, 8,* 462–478.

Lee, S. H., Barns, W. G., & Schaetzel, W. P. (1986). Pulmonary aspergillosis and the importance of oxalate crystal recognition in cytology specimens. *Archives of Pathology and Laboratory Medicine, 110,* 1176–1179.

Mead, J. H., Lupton, G. P., Dillavou, C. L., & Odom, R. B. (1979). Cutaneous rhizopus infection. Occurrence as a postoperative complication associated with an elasticized adhesive dressing. *Journal of the American Medical Association, 242,* 272–274.

Mitchell, T. G., & Perfect, J. R. (1995). Cryptococcosis in the era of AIDS—100 years after discovery of *Cryptococcus neoformans. Clinical Microbiology Reviews, 8,* 515–548.

Musial, C. E., Cockerill, F. R., & Roberts, G. D. (1988). Fungal infections of the immunocompromised host: Clinical and laboratory aspects. *Clinical Microbiology Reviews, 1,* 349–364.

Nelson, P. E., Digneni, M. C., & Anaissie, E. J. (1994). Taxonomy, biology, and clinical aspects of *Fusarium* sp. *Clinical Microbiology Reviews, 7,* 49–504.

Rippon, J. W. (1988). *Medical mycology: The pathogenic fungi and the pathogenic actinomycetes.* Philadelphia: Saunders.

Sarubbi, F. A., Kopf, H. B., Wilson, M. B., McGinnis, M. R., & Rutala, W. A. (1982). Increased recovery of *Aspergillus flavus* from respiratory specimens during hospital construction. *American Review of Respiratory Disease, 125,* 33–38.

Wheeler, M. S., McGinnis, M. R., Schell, M. S., & Walker, D. H. (1981). Fusarium infections in burned patients. *American Journal of Clinical Pathology, 75,* 304–311.

# CHAPTER 40

# Saprobic Fungi Encountered in Clinical Specimens

James A. Miller, MD., Anne T. Rodgers, MT (ASCP), PhD

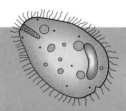

## Microbes in the News

### Fungal Infections a Risk for Liver Transplant Patients

Fungal infections remain a risk for orthotopic liver transplant recipients, despite recent improvements in antifungal therapy. Most infections occur within the first month after the transplant and are caused by *Candida albicans*. However, other *Candida* species and *Aspergillus* species are also responsible for infections. According to Dr. Susan Hadley of the Beth Israel Deaconess Medical Center in Massachusetts, *Aspergillus* species are the most common mycelial fungi causing infection and are responsible for almost 100% mortality rates.

Early detection of these organisms is ideal, but difficult because of a lack of signs and symptoms in the patient. While assays to detect organism-specific antibodies exist, sensitivity for *Candida* species has been low. Researchers have had more luck with the *Aspergillus*-antigen detection test. Other methods of detection are routine fungal surveillance cultures of the oral cavity, the rectum, and stool, wounds, and urine, but experts are mixed on their usefulness.

Source: Hadley, S. (1997) Fungal Infections in Liver Transplant Recipients, *Infect Med* 14(4):311–318.

## KEY TERMS

Annellide
Apophysis
Cleistothecium
Conidiophore
Dematiaceous

Hyaline
Macroconidia
Merosporangium
Metula

Phialide
Rhizoid
Sporangium
Sporangiophore

**Upon successful completion of this chapter, the student should be able to:**

1. Describe the colonial and microsopic (slide culture) morphology of the commonly isolated saprophytic fungi.
2. Compare and contrast the microscopic morphology of the zygomycetes.
3. Compare the microscopic morphology of *Aspergillus fumigatus, Aspergillus flavus,* and *Aspergillus niger.*
4. Compare and contrast the microscopic morphology of the dematiaceous hyphomycetes.

## INTRODUCTION

The fungi discussed here are not true pathogens because they do not ordinarily cause disease in the normal human host. However, as shown in Chapter 39, any fungus is capable of causing infection given the right circumstances, when the host is compromised. Therefore, although these fungi are often referred to as saprobic fungi or saprophytes, they are fully capable of causing disease in such patients. In hospitalized patients, infections due to these organisms are more common than those due to the true pathogens, systemic and cutaneous.

The saprophytic molds are most commonly identified by careful observation of morphologic features in the culture. Cultural characteristics of importance in identification of saprophytic molds include:

▶ Growth rate
▶ Temperature requirements
▶ Colony morphology
 — Surface
 — Reverse
 — Pigmentation
▶ Microscopic morphology
 — Types of hyphae
 — Reproductive structures

Gross colony features are important but can be highly variable among different strains of the same species. Microscopic features are more important and include types of hyphae and reproductive structures. In some cases, the reproductive structures are highly characteristic and provide definitive identification. In other cases a variety of spores may be produced. Some organisms produce reproductive structures reluctantly. In these cases sporulation may be stimulated by using different media, such as cornmeal or potato dextrose agar.

Biochemical tests used to identify bacteria and yeast organisms are not generally of any importance in identifying saprobic molds. Molecular methods including DNA probes are being developed to identify some pathogenic fungi but are not available for the saprophytes.

Although there are thousands of species of fungi, only a few of the most common saprophytes are included in this chapter. Nevertheless, this will account for most of the fungi encountered in the clinical laboratory. For more unusual organisms the student is referred to definitive texts of laboratory mycology (Larone, 1995; Murray, 1995; Rippon, 1988).

## ZYGOMYCETES

The zygomycetes are common environmental contaminants and important causes of opportunistlc fungal infection (see Chapter 39). The organisms characteristically produce aseptate hyphae, although occasional septa can be produced in older colonies and derive their name from the sexual spores they produce, called zygospores. These spores are rarely encountered in clinical specimens. More importantly, for purposes of identification, the organisms produce sporangiospores, which are asexual spores contained within sacs called sporangia. The organisms typically grow very rapidly and can fill a Petri dish or agar slant within only a few days. Genus identification is based on characteristics of the following microscopic structures (see Figure 40-1*A*).

1. **Rhizoids**: rootlike structures along the hyphae
2. **Sporangium** (pl. sporangia): saclike structures containing the sporangiospores
3. **Sporangiophore**: stalk from the hyphae supporting the sporangium
4. Columella: swelling at the top of the sporangiophore.
5. **Apophysis**: a collar-like structure just below the columella

Species identification is difficult and is usually unnecessary in clinical situations.

### *Rhizopus* Species

**Colonies.** Growth is rapid; the organism can fill a Petri dish within a few days. The colonies are like wool or cotton candy. Small black dots appear on the surface as sporangia develop. The organism grows well at room temperature and also at temperatures up to 45°C.

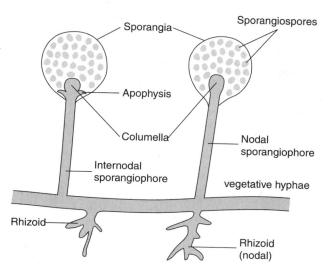

**FIGURE 40-1A** Microscopic morphology of the zygomycetes.

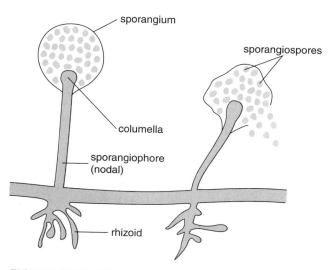

**FIGURE 40-1B** Microscopic morphology of *Rhizopus* species.

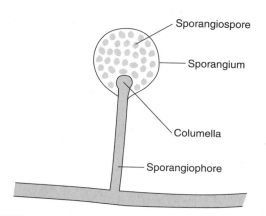

**FIGURE 40-1C** Microscopic morphology of *Mucor* species.

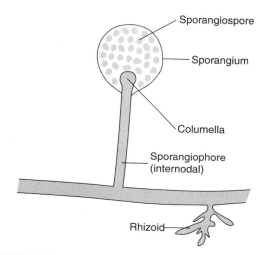

**FIGURE 40-1D** Microscopic morphology of *Rhizomucor* species.

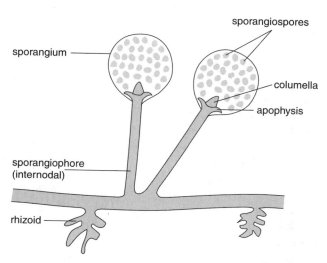

**FIGURE 40-1E** Microscopic morphology of *Absidia* species.

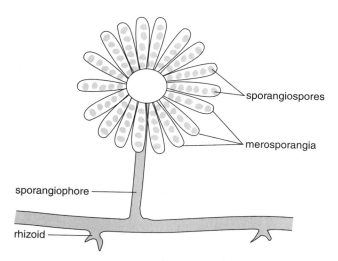

**FIGURE 40-1F** Microscopic morphology of *Syncephalastrum* species.

**Microscopic (see Figure 40-1B).** Hyphae are broad and aseptate. The organisms characteristically produce rhizoids. Sporangiophores have a nodal arrangement, which means they arise from the hyphae at the point where the rhizoids are produced, much like a tree trunk arising from its roots. Columella is round and the apophysis is inconspicuous.

## Mucor Species

**Colonies.** Colonies are like wool or cotton candy and growth is rapid, similar to *Rhizopus*. However, the organism does *not* grow well at 37°C or above.

**Microscopic (see Figure 40-1C).** Hyphae are aseptate. No rhizoids are produced, a key feature in distinguishing *Mucor* from *Rhizopus* and the other common Zygomycetes. Columella can vary in shape. No apophysis is produced.

## Rhizomucor Species

**Colonies.** Colonies are like cotton candy similar to the other Zygomycetes. Growth can occur at temperatures up to 50°C.

**Microscopic (see Figure 40-1D).** Rhizoids are produced but may be inconspicuous. The sporangiophores arise from hyphae between the rhizoids, not directly from them (internodal). Columella is round and apophysis is absent. Hyphae are aseptate.

## Absidia Species

**Colonies.** Growth is rapid and colonies are similar to other Zygomycetes. Growth may occur at temperatures up to 45°C.

**Microscopic (see Figure 40-1E).** Hyphae are aseptate. Rhizoids are produced, but usually are sparse, and must be carefully searched for. Internodal sporangiophores are produced from hyphae between the rhizoids. Columella may be pointed and there is a prominent apophysis, helping to distinguish *Absidia* from *Rhizomucor* and *Rhizopus*.

## Syncephalastrum Species

**Colonies.** Growth is rapid. Colonies are white at first and then turn dark gray.

**Microscopic (see Figure 40-1F).** The key characteristic of *Syncephalastrum* is the production of a **merosporangium**, which is tube like. Mesosporangia may be confused with the fruiting heads of *Aspergillus* species. However, careful examination will reveal that chains of sporangiospores are contained inside the thin-walled merosporangia and there are no **phialides** or conidia. Rhizoids are formed but are primitive.

# DEMATIACEOUS HYPHOMYCETES

As we learned in Chapter 36, **dematiaceous** fungi are characterized by the presence of dark brown melanin pigment in their cell walls. Colonies produced by these fungi are dark brown or black. Because the pigmented hyphae, not the spores, are responsible for the dark color, the reverse of the colonies is also black.

The dematiaceous fungi produce conidia. The size, shape, and arrangement of the conidia form the basis for identification of these organisms.

## Curvularia Species

*Curvularia* is a very common environmental contaminant, but also may cause infections of the cornea of the eye, nasal sinuses, and subcutaneous tissues.

**Colonies.** Growth is rapid with mature colonies within a few days. Colonies are dark brown or black and fuzzy.

**Microscopic (see Figure 40-2A).** Hyphae are septate and brown (dematiaceous). **Macroconidia** are produced from **conidiophores**. The macroconidia are curved (hence the name) and have transverse septa.

## Alternaria Species

*Alternaria* is one of the most common environmental contaminants encountered in the clinical laboratory. The highly characteristic macroconidia are often observed contaminating sputum, other respiratory specimens, and even Pap smears.

**Colonies.** Growth is rapid. The colonies are white to dirty gray at first, later becoming dark gray. Reverse is dark. Surface tends to be wooly.

**Microscopic (see Figure 40-2B).** Hyphae are septate and brown. Conidiophores are also septate. The macroconidia are club-shaped and produced in chains. There are alternating longitudinal and transverse septa, a characteristic from which the organism draws its name.

## Cladosporium Species

The pathogenic *Cladosporium carrionii* and the morphologically similar *Xylohypha bantiana* have been discussed in Chapter 37. Many other species of *Cladosporium* are common environmental contaminants. In past years some of these were referred to as *Hormodendrum* species.

**Colonies.** Growth is moderate with best growth at room temperature and poor or no growth at 37°C. Colonies are velvety and vary from olive to black. Reverse is black.

**Microscopic (see Figure 40-2C).** The hyphae are septate and brown. Conidiophores are branched like tree limbs. Oval microconidia are produced in chains.

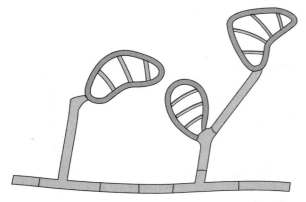

**FIGURE 40-2A** Microscopic morphology of *Curvularia* species.

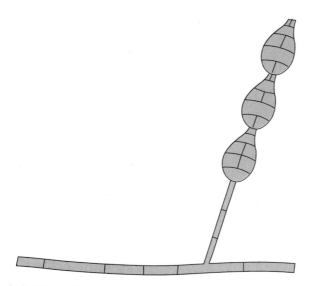

**FIGURE 40-2B** Microscopic morphology of *Alternaria* species.

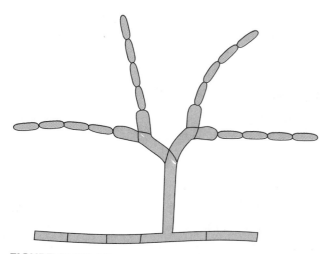

**FIGURE 40-2C** Microscopic morphology of *Cladosporium* species.

# HYALINE HYPHOMYCETES

**Hyaline** hyphomycetes are very common environmental contaminants, although several of them are also among the most common causes of opportunistic fungal infections (see Chapter 39). All of these organisms produce clear septate hyphae that cannot be distinguished from one another. Identification in the clinical laboratory depends on recognition of characteristic conidia production.

## Aspergillus Species

There are many species of *Aspergillus,* but only three of the most important are described here: *Aspergillus fumigatus, Aspergillus flavus,* and *Aspergillus niger.* In most clinical situations it is not necessary to further speciate the other *Aspergillus* organisms. *Aspergillus* species are extremely common environmental contaminants. However, as discussed in Chapter 39, *Aspergillus* is among the most common causes of fungal infection in the compromised host. *A. fumigatus* is responsible for most of these infections.

*Aspergillus* produces conidia from phialides that develop from a swollen vesicle at the tip of the conidiopore (see Figure 40-3A). The phialides were formerly referred to as sterigmata. *Aspergillus* also has a teleomorphic or perfect state and may produce ascospores in **cleistothecia**. However, these are rarely observed in clinical specimens, and even more rarely with the clinically important species.

**Colonies.** Growth of most species is rapid, within a few days. *A. fumigatus* typically exhibits a gray-green powdery or velvety surface as conidia are produced. However, there is marked variation among strains, including some that have a brown surface. Different appearances can result when other culture media are used.

*Aspergillus niger* often is yellow at first but turns black as the conidia are produced. *A. flavus* most commonly has an olive surface.

**Microscopic.** General appearance of *Aspergillus* species is shown in Figure 40-3A. Speciation depends on the arrangement of phialides over the vesicle. The vesicle may be completely or only partially covered. Some species possess only a single row of phialides (*A. fumigatus*), whereas other species develop a second supporting structure between the phialide and the vesicle called a **metula**. Differentiation of *A. fumigatus, A. niger,* and *A. flavus* is shown in Figure 40-3B.

## Penicillium Species

Various species of *Penicillium* are directly beneficial, providing the antibiotic penicillin as well as various blue

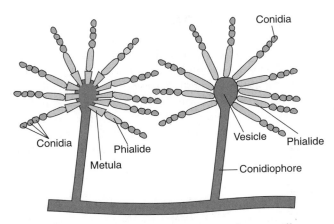

**FIGURE 40-3A** General morphology of *Aspergillus* species.

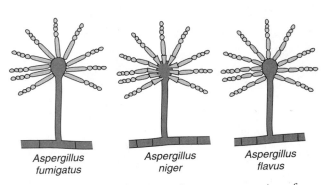

**FIGURE 40-3B** Comparison of common species of *Aspergillus*.

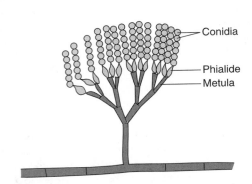

**FIGURE 40-3C** Microscopic morphology of *Penicillium*.

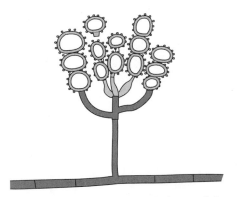

**FIGURE 40-3D** Microscopic morphology of *Scopulariopsis* species.

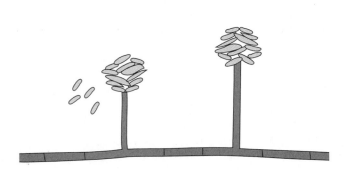

**FIGURE 40-3E** Microscopic morphology of *Acremonium* species.

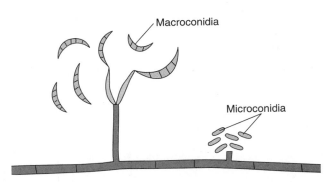

**FIGURE 40-3F** Microscopic morphology of *Fusarium* species.

cheeses. They are known as common environmental contaminants but may also cause a variety of opportunistic infections in compromised hosts. *Penicillium marneffei* is a dimorphic fungus, discussed in Chapter 39. It is found in east Asia and is not native to the United States. It is most commonly found in patients with acquired immunodeficiency syndrome (AIDS) who have lived or traveled in Asia.

**Colonies.** Growth is rapid, within a few days. Most species develop a powdery blue-green surface. *P. marneffei* characteristically produces a red pigment but other *Penicillium* species may also be red.

**Microscopic (see Figure 40-3C).** Conidia are produced from phialides, which have a brush-like arrangement. Metulae connected to the conidiophores support the phialides. The conidia are round.

## Scopulariopsis Species

**Colonies.** Growth is rapid, within a few days. Colonies are white at first, becoming tan.

**Microscopic (see Figure 40-3D).** Although there is a brush-like arrangement of the conidia-bearing cells, these are **annellides** rather than phialides. Therefore, these structures elongate as the conidia are produced. When the conidia are released, a short piece is left at the site of attachment. The conidia are rough and knobby. Although not macroconidia, they are somewhat larger than those of *Penicillium*.

## Acremonium Species

*Acremonium* species are common contaminants, but also are agents of eye and subcutaneous fungal infections.

**Colonies.** Growth is rapid, within a few days. Colonies are white at first, becoming pale pink or salmon colored.

**Microscopic (see Figure 40-3E).** Conidia occur in tight clusters on top of tapered phialides that form directly from the hyphae. The conidia are elongated and their tight arrangement resembles the surface of a brain. It is for this reason that the organism was formerly called *Cephalosporium* species. The conidia resemble the microconidia of *Fusarium*.

## Fusarium Species

*Fusarium* species are frequent contaminants in culture, but also are relatively common causes of opportunistic infections (see Chapter 39). It is most commonly associated with infections of the eye and with burns.

**Colonies.** Growth is rapid, within a few days. Colonies are often purple in the center and pale at the periphery.

**Microscopic (see Figure 40-3F).** *Fusarium* species produce two kinds of conidia. The most characteristic are sickle-shaped macroconidia that are produced from phialides on conidiophores. Oval microconidia, very similar to those of *Acremonium* species are also produced from conidiophores. Usually the microconidia are not as tightly clustered as those of *Acremonium* species.

## SUMMARY

▶ Saprophytic molds may be encountered in the clinical laboratory either as contaminants in culture or as causes of opportunistic infections. Although there are thousands of species of saprophytic molds only the most commonly encountered organisms have been described in this chapter.

▶ The identification of saprophytic molds is almost exclusively based on morphologic features in culture, especially reproductive structures. In this chapter key characteristics have been chosen to provide a logical scheme for identification of these molds.

▶ The Zygomycetes possess aseptate hyphae and produce sporangiospores from sporangia.

▶ Dematiaceous hyphomycetes are dark because the hyphae contain melanin pigment. These organisms produce conidia, which provide the basis for identification.

▶ Hyaline hyphomycetes possess clear nonpigmented hyphae. The colonies may exhibit a variety of colors, due to conidia production. Identification of the organisms depends on recognition of characteristic conidia microscopically.

## Review Questions

1. Which of the following is (are) not characteristic of Zygomycetes?
   a. Aseptate hyphae
   b. Columella
   c. Vesicle
   d. Rhizoids

2. Which of the following organisms is dimorphic?
   a. *Penicillium marneffei*
   b. *Aspergillus flavus*
   c. *Aureobasidium pullulans*
   d. *Sepedonium* species

3. Which of the following organisms produce macroconidia?
   a. *Sepedonium* species
   b. *Fusarium* species
   c. *Curvularia* species
   d. All of the above

4. Which of the following organisms possess dematiaceous, septate hyphae?
   a. *Bipolaris* species
   b. *Aspergillus niger*
   c. *Rhizopus* species
   d. *Acremonium* species

## CASE STUDY

A 25-year-old male patient underwent endoscopic sinus surgery for chronic, recurrent episodes of sinusitis. He also had a history of food allergies in childhood and seasonal allergic rhinitis (hay fever). Microscopic examination of the sinus tissue revealed numerous eosinophils and impacted mucus. Culture of the sinus tissue revealed well developed fuzzy dark brown mold colonies in 4 days. Colony reverse was black. Curved macroconidia with transverse septa were produced from conidiophores.

**Questions:**

1. What is the name of the organism cultured?

2. What is the significance of the organism in this case?

3. What other organisms might also have been expected in this culture?

---

5. Which of the following is NOT characteristic of *Penicillium* species?
   a. Phialides
   b. Conidiophore
   c. Tuberculate macroconidia
   d. Metula

6. Which of the saprophytic fungi may be confused with a dimorphic pathogen?
   a. *Aspergillus fumigatus*
   b. *Chrysosporium* species
   c. *Paecilomyces* species
   d. *Cladosporium* species

7. Which of the following organisms produce rhizoids?
   a. *Mucor* species
   b. *Absidia* species
   c. *Alternaria* species
   d. All of the above

8. Which of the following organisms produces a vesicle?
   a. *Aspergillus fumigatus*
   b. *Aspergillus flavus*
   c. *Aspergillus niger*
   d. All of the above

9. Blue-green colonies are commonly observed with which of the following organisms?
   a. *Rhizopus* species
   b. *Curvularia* species
   c. *Alternaria* species
   d. None of the above

10. Which of the following are most likely to be confused with *Aspergillus* species microscopically?
    a. *Syncephalastrum* species
    b. *Alternaria* species
    c. *Mucor* species
    d. *Sepedonium* species

---

▶ **REFERENCES & RECOMMENDED READING**

Larone, D. H. (1995). *Medically important fungi: A guide to identification* (3rd ed.). Washington DC: ASM Press.

McGinnis, M. R. (1980). *Laboratory handbook of medical mycology.* New York: Academic Press.

Murray, P. (Ed.). (1995). *Manual of clinical microbiology* (6th ed.). Washington, DC: ASM Press.

Rippon, J. W. (1988). *Medical mycology: The pathogenic fungi and the pathogenic actinomycetes* (3rd ed.). Philadelphia: Saunders.

Torres, C. et al. (1996). Allergic fungal sinusitis: A clinico-pathologic study of 16 cases. *Human Pathology, 27,* 793–799.

# CHAPTER 41

## Yeasts

Anne T. Rodgers MT (ASCP), PhD., James A. Miller, MD

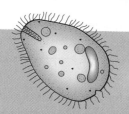

## Microbes in the News

### *Candida* Intestinal Yeast Infections

People can experience an overgrowth of yeast in the intestines when they inadvertently kill good bacteria by using antibiotics, eating too much sugar (which feeds the yeast), eating almost no vegetables (which are essential for proper pH), or generally abuse their bodies so that their immunity is lowered. When *Candida* thrives inside the intestines long enough, it can root through the intestinal wall and enter into the bloodstream. Then it spreads through-out the body and is labeled "systemic *Candida*." Chronic *Candida* infections often cause liver toxemia which allows multiple allergies to food, pollen, and chemicals. What is observed as being a "beer gut" is often just the bloatedness that accompanies a strong yeast infection.

Forrest, M. *Candida Intestinal Yeast Infections Treatment by Electro-Medicine.* http://www.ioa.com/~drangonfly/candida.html

## KEY TERMS

Assimilation
Blastoconidium (blastospore)
Chlamydospore (chlamydoconidium)
Germ tube
Pseudohyphae
Yeast

## LEARNING OBJECTIVES

**Upon successful completion of this chapter, the student should be able to:**

1. Describe the following identification procedures and discuss their use in identification of yeasts:
   a. India ink
   b. germ tube
   c. Assimilation tests and fermentation tests
2. Describe the characteristic microscopic appearance, colony morphology, and key biochemical reactions or tests for the identification of the yeasts described in this chapter.
3. Describe the appearance of yeast organisms on Sabouraud's's dextrose agar and Chlamydospore agar.
4. Discuss the clinical relevance of yeasts and list specimens where they are most often isolated.
5. List and describe rapid methods for the identification of yeast isolates.

## INTRODUCTION

With the increase in immunocompromised patients and patients with acquired immunodeficiency syndrome (AIDS), **yeast** infections have become more important. In the past, only two species of yeasts, *Candida albicans* and *Cryptococcus neoformans,* were considered to be pathogens and cause disease. Presumptive identification of these two organisms was relatively straightforward. Cultures that were **germ tube** negative and capsule negative were signed out as *Candida* species, not *albicans*. Cultures producing germ tubes were identified as *Candida albicans,* and yeasts positive for capsules by the India ink examination were reported as *Cryptococcus neoformans*. Today, however, the technologist must, in most cases, identify yeasts to species. This is necessary because species formerly considered opportunists or normal flora may cause life-threatening infections in the immunocompromised host. Thus, knowledge of the cultural, morphologic, and biochemical characteristics of yeasts is important to the medical technologist.

## CLINICAL SIGNIFICANCE OF YEASTS

Yeasts are ubiquitous in nature and found as normal flora in many parts of the body, especially the genital tract, upper respiratory tract, and the gastrointestinal tract. Yeasts are found widely in nature and involved in the breakdown of organic matter. Fermentation products of yeasts are necessary in the production of many foods and beverages, including bread, doughnuts, beer, and wine. However, yeasts are also the causative agents of several disease states including meningitis, thrush, and systemic infections in the immunocompromised host. Yeast infections are transmitted in several ways including direct contact and aerosols. The most common entry site is the respiratory tract. Other infections result from the overgrowth of yeasts normally resident in a particular body site. Yeasts are not generally considered strict pathogens but will cause infection in hosts whose immune system or other defenses have been altered or compromised in some way. Yeasts are increasingly isolated in the clinical microbiology laboratory from specimens from patients who are being treated with chemotherapy or antibiotics and in patients with AIDS. In cultures, the most commonly isolated genera are *Candida* and *Cryptococcus*. A more complete discussion of infections with *Candida* and *Cryptococcus* may be found in Chapter 39.

## IDENTIFICATION PROCEDURES FOR YEASTS

Several methods are used to identify yeasts that are not used for filamentous molds. These include the wet or direct mount, India ink test, germ tube test, microscopic characteristics on cornmeal agar, and biochemical tests including carbohydrate **assimilation**.

### Identification of Yeasts from Clinical Specimens

Unlike the filamentous molds, identification of yeasts must include tests other than microscopic morphology. A variety of tests are used for direct examination to confirm the presence of a yeast and to determine germ tube and capsule production. A positive germ tube or presence of a capsule can presumptively identify a yeast as *Candida* or *Cryptococcus,* respectively. Then the isolate may be inoculated on cornmeal agar to determine the production of **blastoconidia**, **pseudohyphae**, and **chlamydospores (chlamydoconidia)**. Biochemical tests are also performed to determine the species of yeast present.

### Direct Examination

Most yeasts will grow well on standard bacteriologic media. Yeast colonies are often mistaken for staphylococci because yeast colonies are white to off-white in color on the standard sheep blood agar used in bacteriology cultures. A wet or direct mount, performed by emulsifying a portion of suspected yeast in saline or lactophenol, will rapidly differentiate yeast cells from bacteria. Figure 41-1 shows budding yeast cells.

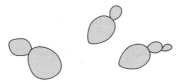

**FIGURE 41-1** Budding yeast as seen in wet preparation.

Capsules may be detected by the India ink test. It is performed by adding a drop of India ink to a portion of a yeast colony that has been emulsified in a drop of saline or water. The India ink will not stain capsules, and the capsule will appear as a large halo surrounding the yeast cell. Figure 41-2 shows the appearance of a yeast surrounded by a capsule in the India ink stain.

Some yeasts, especially *C. albicans,* will form germ tubes rapidly in serum-based media. The germ tube test

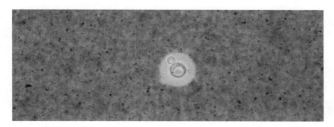

**FIGURE 41-2** India ink stain, encapsulated yeast. (Courtesy of James A. Miller, MD)

is performed by suspending yeast cells in bovine or human serum, incubating at 35°C to 2 to 3 hours, and examining for the presence of germ tubes, which are shown in Figure 41-3. These tests are discussed in detail in Chapter 35.

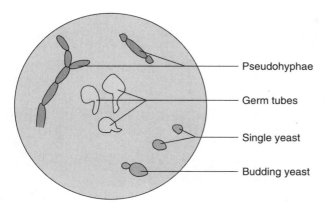

**FIGURE 41-3** Germ tubes and other structures seen in the germ tube test.

## Microscopic Examination

Cornmeal agar (CMA) with Tween 80 is used to demonstrate production of pseudohyphae, blastoconidia, and chlamydospores. This media, like potato dextrose agar, encourages the production of blastoconidia, pseudohyphae, true hyphae, and chlamydospores. These structures, illustrated in Figure 41-4, can be used to differentiate the various genera and species of yeasts. Table 41-1 summarizes the microscopic characteristics of commonly encountered yeasts.

## Biochemical Characteristics

Unlike the filamentous molds, biochemical characteristics of the yeasts are important in identification. Many of the tests are the same as those for bacteria. One of the more important biochemical characteristics is the ability of yeast organisms to utilize carbohydrates. Tests for carbohydrate utilization by yeasts include fermentation and assimilation tests. Fermentation tests detect whether or not the yeast can produce acid from the carbohydrate under anaerobic conditions. Assimilation tests simply detect whether the yeast can utilize the carbohydrate as a sole carbon source without regard to whether acid or gas is produced. Most of the methods used today for determining carbohydrate use are based on assimilation rather than fermentation.

Other biochemical tests useful in differentiating yeasts are the urease test and nitrate assimilation test. In the urease test, organisms that produce urease split urea, producing ammonia. The ammonia causes a rise in pH and a color change in the indicator system. The urease test is useful in identification of *Cryptococcus* species and *Rhodotorula* species. The nitrate assimilation test is similar to the carbohydrate assimilation tests in that in the latter, nitrate is provided as the sole source of nitrogen and in the former carbohydrates are the sole source of carbon. This test can be helpful in identification of *Cryptococcus, Hansenula, Rhodotorula,* and *Trichosporon.* Today, biochemical characteristics of the yeasts are most often determined by rapid methods that incorporate panels of biochemical tests. These commercial systems enable the laboratory to identify most yeast isolates within 24 to 72 hours.

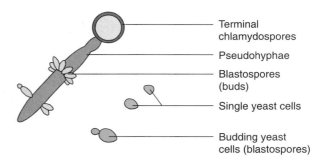

**FIGURE 41-4** Morphologic characteristics seen in yeast isolates.

**Table 41–1 ▶ Microscopic Characteristics of Commonly Isolated Yeasts**

| Organism | Pseudohyphae | Germ Tube Production | Morphology on CMA with Tween 80 |
|---|---|---|---|
| *Candida albicans* | yes | yes | Pseudohyphae, clusters of blastoconidia and terminal chlamydospores |
| *Candida tropicalis* | yes | no | Long branching pseudohyphae; blastoconidia produced along the pseudohyphae singly, or in small groups |
| *Candida keyfur* | yes | no | Long branching pseudohyphae and blastoconidia of varying lengths clustering in parallel lines with the pseudohyphae ("logs in a stream") |
| *Candida parapsilosis* | yes | no | Branched pseudohyphae with a few blastoconidia borne singly or in small groups along pseudohyphae. Pseudohyphae may be short and crooked. Occasional large hyphal elements ("giant cells") |
| *Candida krusei* | yes | no | Branched pseudohyphae with long blastoconidia borne at the ends of a pseudohyphal branch. "Crossed matchsticks" or "treelike" appearance |
| *Candida guillermondi* | yes | no | Short, slightly curved pseudohyphae with few blastoconidia clustered at constrictions of the pseudohyphae |
| *Cryptococcus neoformans* | no | no | Single or budding yeast cells |
| *Geotrichum candidum* | no | no | Hyphae with arthroconidia |

Table 41-2 summarizes the biochemical characteristics of the more common yeast isolates.

## Commercial Yeast Identification Systems

Several commercial systems are available for identification of yeasts. These systems include sugar assimilation and other biochemical tests to determine the identity of a particular yeast isolate. It is important to remember, however, that biochemical characteristics determined by these systems must be supplemented with morphologic studies and the germ tube test before a final identification may be made. All require a pure culture isolate on nonselective media such as Sabouraud's dextrose agar. Table 41-2 summarizes the biochemical and morphologic characteristics for each of the yeasts discussed in this chapter.

Two commonly used manual systems are the API 20C AUX (BioMerieux Vitek Inc.) and the Uni-Yeast Tek system (Remel, Lenexa, KS). These panels of biochemical tests use growth and assimilation methods and require 24 to 72 hours for a final result. There are an increasing number of more rapid tests coming on the market including the IDS Rapid ID Yeast Plus System (Innovative Diagnostics Systems & Remel, Lenexa, KS). These rely on enzymatic reactions and have a much shorter turn-around time (as little as 4 hours in some cases).

In addition to manual systems, automated systems are available for identification of yeasts. Presently these are available as supplements to the more established automated bacterial identification systems such as the Automicrobic (BioMerieux-Vitek) and the Microscan Rapid Yeast Identification Panel (Dade/Microscan, West Sacramento, CA).

**API 20C AUX System.** This system uses a modification of the auxanographic sugar assimilation test developed by Wickerham. It consists of a plastic strip with cupules containing dehydrated carbohydrate substrates. The API 20C strip is pictured in Figure 41-5. A standardized suspension of yeast in basal medium is added and the strip is incubated at 30°C for 24 to 72 hours. The cupules are examined for growth at 24, 48, and 72 hours. Turbidity greater than the control cupule indicates a positive result. Identification is made by comparing the pattern of reactions with the manufacturer's differential charts. A portion of an API 20C strip showing growth in the cupules is seen in Figure 41-6.

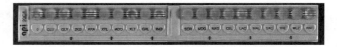

**FIGURE 41-5** API 20C AUX strip. (Courtesy of James A. Miller, MD)

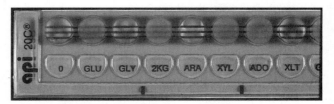

**FIGURE 41-6** API 20C AUX strip showing growth. (Courtesy of James A. Miller, MD)

## Table 41-2 ▶ Biochemical Characteristics of Common Yeast Isolates

| Organism | Assimilations | | | | | | | | | | | | Fermentations | | | | | | Other Tests | |
|---|---|---|---|---|---|---|---|---|---|---|---|---|---|---|---|---|---|---|---|---|
|  | DEXTROSE | MALTOSE | SUCROSE | LACTOSE | GALACTOSE | MELLIBIOSE | CELLOBIOSE | INOSITOL | XYLOSE | RAFFINOSE | TREHALOSE | DULCITOL | DEXTROSE | MALTOSE | SUCROSE | LACTOSE | GALACTOSE | TREHALOSE | NITRATE | UREASE |
| *Candida albicans* | + | + | + | 0 | + | 0 | 0 | 0 | + | 0 | + | 0 | + | + | 0 | 0 | w | V | 0 | 0 |
| *Candida tropicalis* | + | + | V | 0 | + | 0 | V | 0 | + | 0 | + | 0 | + | + | V | 0 | V | V | 0 | 0 |
| *Candida keyfur* | + | 0 | + | + | + | 0 | + | 0 | V | + | 0 | 0 | + | 0 | + | + | + | 0 | 0 | 0 |
| *C. parapsilosis* | + | + | + | 0 | + | 0 | 0 | 0 | + | 0 | + | 0 | + | 0 | 0 | 0 | V | 0 | 0 | 0 |
| *Candida krusei* | + | 0 | 0 | 0 | 0 | 0 | 0 | 0 | 0 | 0 | 0 | 0 | + | 0 | 0 | 0 | 0 | 0 | 0 | V |
| *C. guillermondi* | + | + | + | 0 | + | + | + | 0 | + | + | + | + | + | 0 | w | 0 | w | w | 0 | 0 |
| *Geotrichum candidum* | + | 0 | 0 | 0 | + | 0 | 0 | 0 | + | 0 | 0 | 0 | 0 | 0 | 0 | 0 | 0 | 0 | 0 | 0 |
| *Cryptococcus neoformans* | + | + | + | 0 | + | 0 | V | + | + | V | + | + | 0 | 0 | 0 | 0 | 0 | 0 | 0 | 0 |

w, weak reactions; V, strain variation.

**Uni Tek Yeast System.** The Uni Tek Yeast system consists of a germ tube test (GBE), a sucrose assimilation test (SAM), and a wheel containing carbohydrate and biochemical substrates (see Color Plate 86). In the center of the wheel is a well with cornmeal agar that is used to assess the microscopic morphology of the yeast isolate.

**Microscan Rapid Yeast Identification Panel.** The Microscan Rapid Yeast Identification system consists of a microtiter plate containing dehydrated biochemical substrates as shown in Figure 41-7. A standardized suspension of the test organism is added to the wells and incubated. After 4 hours, the panel is read using a Microscan instrument and the yeast is identified based on the pattern of reactions. In this particular panel, more than 25 substrates are used.

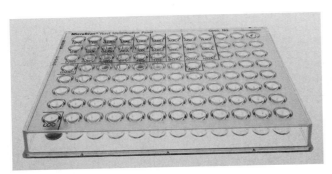

**FIGURE 41-7** Microscan microtiter plate. (Courtesy Dade Microscan Inc.)

## CANDIDA

Candidiasis, caused by *C. albicans,* is the most common of the yeast infections. (See Chapter 39 for a discussion of the disease.) Infections due to other *Candida* species are increasing in frequency in immunocompromised patients. Thus, isolation of these organisms is more frequent than in the past and species other than *C. albicans* must be recognized and identified.

### Candida albicans

**Colonies.** Growth on Sabouraud's dextrose agar at 25°C is rapid, 48 to 72 hours. Colonies are smooth, shiny, and white to cream in color. As the colonies mature, pseudohyphae and hyphae (a mycelial fringe) appear at the edge of the colony, which has the appearance of pseudopods or "feet."

**Microscopic and Biochemical Characteristics.** On cornmeal agar with Tween 80, *C. albicans* forms pseudohyphae, clusters of blastoconidia at the constrictions of the pseudohyphae, and terminal chlamydospores as shown in Figure 41-8. Pseudohyphae may be distinguished from true hyphae by the presence of a constriction at each septum. *C. albicans* is sucrose

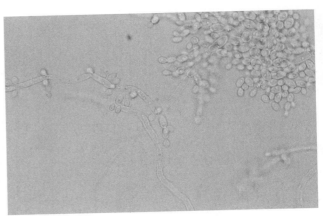

**FIGURE 41-8** Microscopic morphology of *Candida albicans* on cornmeal agar. CMA with Tween 80, ×100. (Courtesy Remel Inc., Lenexa, KS)

positive. The characteristic microscopic morphology on cornmeal agar, production of germ tubes, and positive sucrose is sufficient in most laboratories to identify the organism.

### Candida tropicalis

**Colonies.** Growth on Sabouraud's dextrose agar at 25°C is rapid, 48 to 72 hours. Colonies are smooth, shiny, and white to cream in color. As the colonies mature, pseudohyphae and true hyphae (a mycelial fringe) appear.

**Microscopic and Biochemical Characteristics.** On cornmeal agar with Tween 80, *C. tropicalis* forms long branching pseudohyphae. Blastoconidia are produced along the pseudohyphae singly or in small groups. If chlamydospores are produced they tend to be pear- or tear-shaped rather than round as in *C. albicans*. Figure 41-9 shows the appearance of *C. tropicalis* on cornmeal agar. Microscopic morphology and characteristic biochemical reactions are necessary to definitively identify the organism (see Table 41-2).

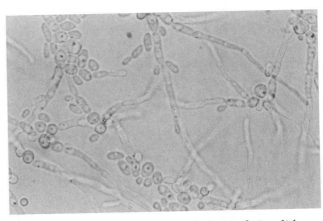

**FIGURE 41-9** Microscopic morphology of *Candida tropicalis* on cornmeal agar. CMA with Tween 80, ×100. (Courtesy Remel Inc., Lenexa, KS)

## Candida keyfur (pseudotropicalis)

**Colonies.** Growth on Sabouraud's dextrose agar at 25°C is rapid, 48 to 72 hours. Colonies are smooth, shiny, and white to cream in color.

**Microscopic and Biochemical Characteristics.** On cornmeal agar with Tween 80, *C. keyfur* forms long branching pseudohyphae and blastoconidia of varying lengths, which tend to cluster in parallel lines with the pseudohyphae giving the classical "logs in a stream" appearance. To most observers, the blastoconidia look like logs that have jammed together while trying to move through a small space. Figure 41-10 shows the typical morphology on cornmeal agar. The microscopic morphology on cornmeal agar and characteristic biochemical reactions are necessary to definitively identify the organism (see Table 41-2).

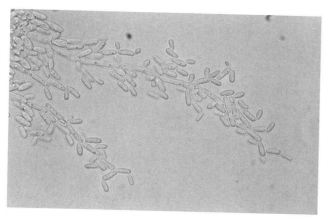

**FIGURE 41-10** Microscopic morphology of *Candida keyfur* on cornmeal agar. CMA with Tween 80, ×100. (Courtesy Remel Inc., Lenexa, KS)

## Candida parapsilosis

**Colonies.** Growth on Sabouraud's dextrose agar at 25°C is rapid, 48 to 72 hours. Colonies are smooth, shiny, and white to cream in color. Some strains produce a lacy or wrinkled topography as the colony ages. On cornmeal, the colonies may give a "spider-like" appearance, which is distinctive under low power.

**Microscopic and Biochemical Characteristics.** On cornmeal agar with Tween 80, *C. parapsilosis* forms branched pseudohyphae with a few blastoconidia borne singly or in small groups along the pseudohyphae. Often the pseudohyphae are short and may appear crooked. Occasionally the organism will produce large hyphal elements ("giant cells"). Figure 41-11 shows the typical morphology on cornmeal agar. Although the microscopic morphology on cornmeal agar is fairly distinct, both morphology and biochemical reactions are necessary to definitively identify the organism (see Table 41-2).

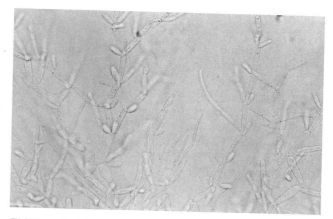

**FIGURE 41-11** Microscopic morphology of *Candida parapsilosis* on cornmeal agar. CMA with Tween 80, ×100. (Courtesy Remel Inc., Lenexa, KS)

## Candida krusei

**Colonies.** Growth on Sabouraud's dextrose agar at 25°C is rapid, 48 to 72 hours. Colonies are dry, flat, and white to cream in color. As the colonies mature, pseudohyphae and hyphae (a mycelial fringe) may appear.

**Microscopic and Biochemical Characteristics.** On cornmeal agar with Tween 80, *C. krusei* forms branched pseudohyphae with long blastoconidia borne at the ends of a pseudohyphae branch. This gives the appearance of "crossed matchsticks" or a "treelike" configuration as seen in Figure 41-12. Another opportunistic yeast, *Blastoschizomyces capitatus* has very long blastoconidia and may be confused with *C. krusei*. Therefore, biochemical reactions are necessary to definitively identify the organism (See Table 41-2).

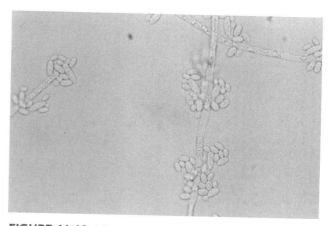

**FIGURE 41-12** Microscopic morphology of *Candida krusei* on cornmeal agar. CMA with Tween 80, ×100. (Courtesy Remel Inc., Lenexa, KS)

## Candida guillermondi

**Colonies.** Growth on Sabouraud's dextrose agar at 25°C is rapid, 48 to 72 hours. Colonies are white to cream colored, flat, with a lacy or wrinkled topography becoming pinkish in color with age.

**Microscopic and Biochemical Characteristics.** On cornmeal agar with Tween 80, *C. guillermondi* forms short pseudohyphae that may be slightly curved. Few blastoconidia are produced, but when present are clustered at the constrictions (septa) of the pseudohyphae. Small yeast cells may also be seen. Figure 41-13 shows the typical appearance of *C. guillermondi* on cornmeal agar. The microscopic morphology on cornmeal agar and characteristic biochemical reactions are necessary to definitively identify the organism (see Table 41-2).

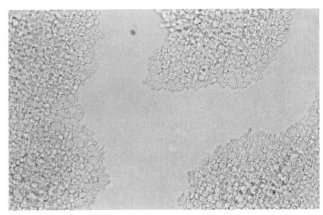

**FIGURE 41-13** Microscopic morphology of *Candida guillermondi* on cornmeal agar. CMA with Tween 80, ×100. (Courtesy Remel Inc., Lenexa, KS)

### Candida glabrata (Torulopsis glabrata)

**Colonies.** Growth on Sabouraud's dextrose agar at 25°C is rapid, 48 to 72 hours. Colonies are cream colored, soft, smooth, and glossy. No pseudohyphae or mycelial fringes are present.

**Microscopic and Biochemical Characteristics.** On cornmeal agar with Tween 80, *C. glabrata* does not form pseudohyphae, blastoconidia, or chlamydospores. Masses of yeast forms are seen. Therefore, biochemical reactions are necessary to definitively identify the organism (see Table 41-2).

## CRYPTOCOCCUS

### Cryptococcus neoformans

*Cryptococcus neoformans* is the causative agent of cryptococcosis, a systemic infection often seen in patients with AIDS or immunocompromised patients. The organism may be recovered from cerebrospinal fluid, urine, and blood specimens in these patients. For additional information on the clinical disease see Chapter 39. A rapid presumptive means of identification is the India ink test, which detects the distinctive capsule of *C. neoformans*. Another presumptive identification test is the detection of cryptococcal antigen in specimens. Final identification must be made by isolating the organism and inoculating biochemical test media.

**Colonies.** Growth on Sabouraud's dextrose agar at 25°C is rapid, 48 to 72 hours. Colonies are white to cream, smooth, and mucoid. Yeast cells with thick capsules will form very mucoid colonies, which may tend to run together.

**Microscopic and Biochemical Characteristics.** Morphology on cornmeal agar is not useful in identification because no pseudohyphae are formed and only masses of yeast cells will be seen. Niger seed agar may be used to differentiate *C. neoformans* from other *Cryptococcus* species. *C. neoformans* forms dark brown colonies on this medium, whereas other species of *Cryptococcus* form white or greenish colonies. Generally, the presence of a positive India ink test and a positive cryptococcal antigen test are sufficient to identify this organism.

### Other Cryptococcus Species

Other *Cryptococcus* species are isolated more frequently today in specimens from immunocompromised hosts. Two of these include *Cryptococcus albidus* and *Cryptococcus laurentii*.

Colony morphology is similar to *C. neoformans*. The Niger seed agar test is useful in differentiating *C. neoformans* from the other *Cryptococcus* species, but biochemical tests must be done to definitively identify the organisms.

## OTHER OPPORTUNISTIC YEASTS

### Rhodotorula rubra

*Rhodotorula rubra* may occasionally be isolated from clinical specimens as a contaminant. It does not usually cause infection. The organism grows readily on most bacteriologic media and on Sabouraud's agar within 24 to 48 hours and can be identified by its distinctive red to coral-red pigment. On cornmeal agar, masses of yeast cells will be seen. The organism does not produce pseudohyphae, blastoconidia, or chlamydospores.

### Geotrichum candidum

This organism is the causative agent of geotrichosis. Growth on Sabouraud's dextrose agar at 25°C is rapid, 48 to 72 hours. The colonies appear moist at first, but older colonies have a wrinkled appearance. The organism is a mold that forms yeastlike colonies, which mature to become moldlike. A distinctive morphologic characteristic of this organism is the formation of arthroconidia rather than pseudohyphae on cornmeal agar. These arthroconidia are continuous along the hyphae. It is important to distinguish *Geotrichum* from *Coccidioides immitis,* because *C. immitis* also forms arthroconidia. The arthroconidia of *C. immitis* have an alternating pattern (see Chapter 38). On cornmeal agar the arthroconidia of *Geotrichum* germinate at the corners producing structures resembling a hockey stick (see Figure 41-14).

### Hansenula anomala

Another yeast isolated with increasing frequency in catheter-related infections is *Hansenula anomala*. Its colony morphology varies and thus it may appear at first to be *Candida* or *Cryptococcus*. However, micro-

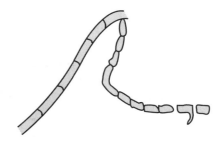

**FIGURE 41-14** Microscopic morphology of *Geotrichum candidum* on cornmeal agar. Hockey stick-shaped arthroconidia.

scopic morphology on cornmeal agar will be variable and, therefore, biochemical testing must be done to make a final identification of *Hansenula*.

## SUMMARY

▶ Yeasts are of increasing importance as causative agents of infections in the immunocompromised host. Patients receiving chemotherapy, on extensive antibiotic therapy, with AIDS, or with other conditions that weaken the immune system or destroy normal flora are at increased risk of opportunistic yeast infections that may be life-threatening.

▶ Yeasts cannot be identified on the basis of microscopic morphology alone. Additional tests such as germ tube or capsule formation, carbohydrate utilization, and other biochemical reactions must be used to definitively identify genera and species.

▶ *Candida* species are identified by their colony morphology, the germ tube test, microscopic morphology on cornmeal agar, and biochemical tests. *Candida albicans* produces germ tubes

## CASE STUDY

A culture is requested on a portion of a heart valve allograft that has been replaced in surgery. The tissue is minced and placed on blood agar and chocolate agar and in thioglycollate broth. After 24 hours incubation at 37°C, the thioglycollate appears cloudy and both the blood agar and chocolate agar show moderate growth of white, glossy colonies that are catalase positive. The direct Gram stain reveals a few large oval cells with a single bud.

### Questions:

1. What test should be done on this isolate to confirm that a yeast is present?

2. What test should be done on this isolate to rule out *Candida albicans*? *Cryptococcus neoformans*?

3. If the isolate is *Candida albicans,* what would you expect to see microscopically on cornmeal agar?

and is sucrose positive. On cornmeal agar, it produces clusters of blastoconidia and terminal thick-walled chlamydospores. Other *Candida* species have fairly distinct morphology on cornmeal agar, but must be identified by biochemical reaction patterns.

## Review Questions

1. A yeast isolate is germ tube positive and sucrose positive. On cornmeal agar pseudohyphae, clusters of blastoconidia and terminal chlamydospores are seen. The organism may be identified as:
   a. *Geotrichum candidum*.
   b. *Candida albicans*.
   c. *Candida keyfur*.
   d. *Candida tropicalis*.

2. Speciation of *Candida* (other than *albicans*) requires results of which tests?
   a. Antibiotic sensitivity
   b. Serologic tests
   c. Special stains
   d. Sugar assimilations

3. A presumptive identification of *Cryptococcus* in a case of meningitis can be reported if the following is/are seen:
   a. small yeast forms in CSF macrophages.
   b. creamy colonies with pseudohyphae.
   c. encapsulated yeast cells in India ink prep of CSF.
   d. hyphal fragments in KOH prep of sputum.

4. Which of the following species produce germ tubes?
   a. *Geotrichum candidum*
   b. *Candida albicans*
   c. *Candida glabrata*
   d. *Rhodotorula rubra*

5. Which of the following tests can differentiate *Candida albicans* from *Candida krusei*?
   a. Sucrose assimilation
   b. Dextrose assimilation
   c. Growth at 37°Candida
   d. Urease

6. A yeast forms long blastoconidia that tend to form parallel lines with the pseudohyphae, giving the appearance of "logs in a steam." It does not assimilate maltose or melibiose. What is the identity of this organism?
   a. *Candida albicans*
   b. *Candida tropicalis*
   c. *Candida keyfur*
   d. *Candida parapsilosis*

7. A yeast colony with a red pigment is isolated. What is the most likely identity of this isolate?
   a. *Geotrichum candidum*
   b. *Candida albicans*
   c. *Candida glabrata*
   d. *Rhodotorula rubra*

8. Which of the following forms arthroconidia on cornmeal agar?
   a. *Geotrichum candidum*
   b. *Candida albicans*
   c. *Candida glabrata*
   d. *Candida tropicalis*

9. A test that will differentiate *Cryptococcus neoformans* from other *Cryptococcus* species is:
   a. sucrose assimilation.
   b. urease test.
   c. capsule formation.
   d. Niger seed agar.

10. Which of the following conditions or treatments predisposes patients to yeast infections?
    a. Antibiotic therapy
    b. AIDS
    c. Cancer chemotherapy
    d. All of the above

## ▶ REFERENCES & RECOMMENDED READING

Baron, E. J., Peterson, L. R., & Finegold, S. M. (1994). *Bailey & Scott's diagnostic microbiology* (9th ed.) St. Louis: Mosby.

Difco Laboratories. (1984). *Difco manual* (10th ed.). Detroit, MI: Author.

Kern, M. E., & Blevins, K. S. (1997). *Medical mycology, a self instructional text* (2nd ed.). Philadelphia: Davis.

Kwon-Chung, K. J., & Bennett, J. E. (1992). *Medical mycology*. Philadelphia: Lea & Febiger.

Larone, D. H. (1995). *Medically important fungi: A guide to identification* (3rd ed.). Washington, DC: ASM Press.

McGinnis, M. R. (1992). Mycology. In H. D. Eisenberg (Ed.). *Clinical microbiology procedures handbook*. Washington, DC: American Society for Microbiology.

Murray, P. R., Baron, E. J., Pfaller, M. A., Tenover, F. C., & Volken, R. H. (1995). *Manual of clinical microbiology* (6th ed.). Washington, DC: ASM Press.

Power, D. A. (Ed.) (1988). *Manual of BBL products and laboratory procedures* (6th ed.). Cockeysville, MD: Becton Dickinson Microbiology Systems.

Rippon, J. W. (1988). *Medical mycology: The pathogenic fungi and the pathogenic actinomycetes* (3rd ed.). Philadelphia: Saunders.

Sherris, J. C. (Ed.). (1990). *Medical microbiology: An introduction to infectious diseases* (2nd ed.). New York: Elsevier.

# SECTION IV

# Parasitology

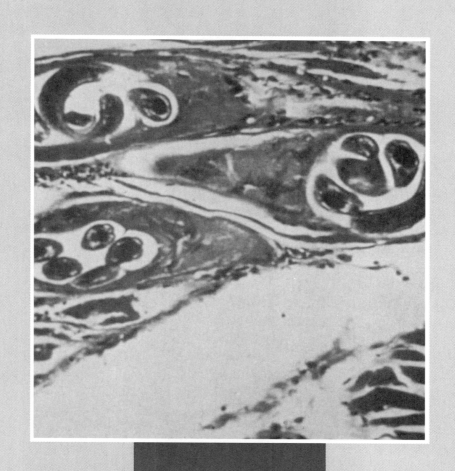

# CHAPTER 42
# Basic Concepts and Techniques in Parasitology

Lisa Shimeld, MS

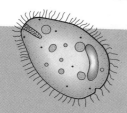

## Microbes in the News
### Outbreak of *Cryptosporidium* in Las Vegas a Mystery

*Cryptosporidium*, a protozoan parasite that is usually transmitted by contaminated water, caused illness in over 100 persons in the Las Vegas area during the Spring of 1994 and contributed to the death of 19 AIDS patients. Prior to this there were 23 cryptosporidiosis-related AIDS deaths in all of 1993 and only 8 cases of *Cryptosporidium* infection in 1992 in Nevada. The number of new cases dropped off after March of 1994 but this appears to be the largest cluster of cases in the United States since the parasite was detected in Milwaukee's water in 1993. Over 400,000 were sickened and over 100 died in Milwaukee at that time.

Source: *The Press-Enterprise*, May 25, 1994, Page B1.

## KEY TERMS

Accidental parasite
Carrier
Cercariae
Cilia
Ciliate
Commensal
Commensalism
Complex life cycle

Conjugation
Cyst
Cysticercus
Dead-end host
Definitive host
Dioecious
Direct life cycle
Direct wet film

Duodenal
Ectoparasite
Endoparasite
Enteric capsule
Eosinophilia
Facultative parasite
Fomite
Gametocyte

## KEY TERMS (cont.)

| | | |
|---|---|---|
| Gastric juice | Microfilaria | SAF |
| Granulocyte | Micronucleus | Schizogony |
| Helminth | Monecious | Scolex |
| Hermaphroditic | Mutualism | sIgA |
| Host | Night soil | Simple life cycle |
| IgE | Obligate parasite | Sporozoan |
| IgM | Oocyst | String test |
| Incidental parasite | Parasite | Symbionts |
| Indirect life cycle | Parasitism | Symbiosis |
| Intermediate host | Phoresis | Temporary parasite |
| Lymphokines | Proglottid | Trophozoite |
| Macronucleus | PVA | Vector |
| Metazoan | Reservoir host | Zoonosis |

## LEARNING OBJECTIVES

**Upon successful completion of this chapter, the student should be able to:**

1. Define key terms.
2. Discuss parasitic adaptations and the transmission of parasites.
3. List and briefly describe the methods used to diagnose parasitic infections.
4. Distinguish between and give examples of simple and complex parasitic life cycles.
5. Describe the host's immune response to parasitic infection.
6. List the major taxonomic categories of parasitic protozoans and helminths.

## INTRODUCTION

Parasitology is the study of invertebrates that are human pathogens and is an area of importance to the clinical microbiologist. The basic principles discussed in earlier chapters apply as well to parasitology. The conditions influencing the development of parasitic disease are similar, if not the same, as in other microbial infections. Parasitic infections are detected by microscopic examination, cultivation, or immunodiagnostic (serologic) methods. These techniques, sample collection, and specific organisms are discussed in the other chapters in this section. There are two catagories of human parasites: the unicellular protozoans and the multicellular metazoans.

Protozoans are members of the kingdom Protista and are classified into phyla according to their mode of motility and reproduction. Four protozoan phyla are parasitic in humans: Sarcomastigophora, Apicomplexa, Ciliophora, and Microspora. Phylum Sarcomastigophora includes the amebas (motile by means of pseudopods) and the flagellates; both reproduce asexually by binary fission. *Entamoeba histolytica* is an ameba that often causes dysentery in persons who consume cysts in feces-contaminated food or water. *Trichomonas vaginalis* is a flagellate that causes a common sexually transmitted infection. Phylum Apicomplexa, or the **sporozoans**, are protozoans that are nonmotile when mature and have alternating sexual and asexual generations in their life cycle. *Cryptosporidium* is a sporozoan that is transmitted in contaminated water and has contributed to the deaths of 19 patients with acquired immunodeficiency syndrome (AIDS) in the Las Vegas area in 1994. (See Microbes in the News.) Members of phylum Ciliophora are motile by means of cilia and they reproduce by binary fission or sexual conjugation followed by binary fission. *Balandidium coli* is a ciliate that is an occasional intestinal parasite of humans. Finally, phylum Microspora includes tiny, intracellular parasites that may be transmitted by direct contact or by some intermediate host. *Enterocytozoan bieneusi* is a member that causes enteritis in patients with AIDS.

The **metazoans** are divided into two groups: **helminths** and arthropods. Only the helminths are discussed in this text. Helminths are sometimes referred to as the worms and those that are parasitic in humans are members of two phyla: Aschelminthes and Platyhelminthes. Parasitic members of Aschelminthes, or the roundworms, are in class Nematoda. *Necator americanus* is the common hookworm. Phylum Platyhelminthes, or the flatworms, has parasitic members in two classes: the Cestodes, or the tapeworms, and the Trematodes, also referred to as the flukes. Species of the tapeworm *Taenia* are transmitted to humans through the consumption of undercooked, contaminated beef or pork. *Schistosoma mansoni* is a blood fluke that has a complex life cycle including a snail intermediate host.

## SYMBIOTIC RELATIONSHIPS

Many different relationships exist between organisms. When two dissimilar species live in close association with each other it is referred to as **symbiosis**. Usually, one partner lives on or in the body of the other. Both partners are referred to as **symbionts**.

When organisms are merely traveling together and neither symbiont is metabolically dependent on the other, the relationship is termed **phoresis**. Barnacles living on crustaceans or on other mollusks are examples of phoresis.

When both partners benefit from the relationship then it is called **mutualism**. Lichens are an example of a mutualistic relationship. Lichens are slow-growing organisms that live on rocks and consist of a fungus and an algae or a cyanobacterium. The fungal component of the lichen anchors the organism to the rock and provides protection against desiccation. The algae or cyanobacterium provides nutrients in the form of carbohydrates that it produces by photosynthesis. Neither partner would be able to survive in this harsh environment without the other.

The word **commensalism** is derived from Latin and means "eating at the same table." In this type of relationship one partner, the **commensal**, benefits while the other partner, the **host**, neither benefits nor is harmed. This often involves the commensal feeding on scraps of food captured by the host. An example of a commensal is the remora, a slender fish that attaches to a host, such as a larger fish, by means of a modified dorsal fin. The remora feeds on scraps of food that are unwanted or unusable by its host.

**Parasitism** is the result when one symbiont causes some harm to or lives at the expense of the other partner. The **parasite** is the smaller of the two organisms. It lives on or inside of the host and is metabolically dependent on the host. Metabolic dependence may be for nutrients or for cofactors and vitamins, or for some developmental stimulus. The host may provide the parasite with a hormone that stimulates the parasite to develop into the next stage of its life cycle.

**Ectoparasites** live on the host or in cavities that open to the surface, such as the ears. Examples of ectoparasites include ticks, lice, and mites. **Endoparasites** live in the body of the host. They may reside in cells, in blood or other tissues, in organs, the alimentary canal, or in the body cavity. Parasitic protozoans and helminths are examples of endoparasites.

Some organisms are **facultative parasites**, meaning that they are not usually parasitic but can be if an opportunity presents itself. **Obligate parasites** spend at least part of and maybe all of their life cycle as parasites. When a parasite infects some species other than its usual host it is referred to as an **accidental** or **incidental parasite**. This is the case with *Dipylidium caninum*, a tapeworm that usually infects dogs and cats but is sometimes seen in humans, especially children (see Figure 42-1). Human infection with *Dipylidium* is an example of a **zoonosis**, which is a disease of animals that is transmitted to humans. Because it is unlikely that the life cycle of *Dipylidium* will have an opportunity to continue under these circumstances the human is a **dead-end host**. **Temporary parasites**, such as ticks, only visit the parasite to feed.

## HOSTS

Parasitic life cycles involve one or most hosts (see Figure 45-1). In most cases each type of host is limited to one or maybe two species of organism making the parasitic relationship very specific. The host in which the parasite reaches sexual maturity and reproduces sexually is referred to as the **definitive** or final **host**. Dogs and humans are definitive hosts in the life cycle of *D. caninum*. In parasites that only reproduce asexually, such as many parasitic protozoans, the host in which the parasites spends the majority of its life cycle is called the definitive host. Humans or other mammals serve as definitive hosts for the protozoan, *Giardia*.

**Intermediate hosts** harbor an immature stage of the parasite. A parasitic life cycle may include one or more intermediate hosts. Asexual reproduction of the parasite may occur in one or more intermediate hosts. Arthropods such as ticks and mites and mollusks, especially snails, are common intermediate hosts.

A **reservoir host** serves as a source of the parasite that can be transmitted to humans or domestic animals. For example, many wild mammals such as beavers and muskrats serve as reservoirs of the protozoan parasite, *Giardia lamblia*. Cysts are introduced into mountain streams when infected animals defecate in the water. *Giardia* is transmitted to humans when they drink untreated, contaminated water.

## PARASITIC ADAPTATIONS

Parasitic organisms are highly evolved for a specialized kind of existence. Parasitic life styles probably arose in organisms that adapted to selective pressures in their current environment in ways that allowed them

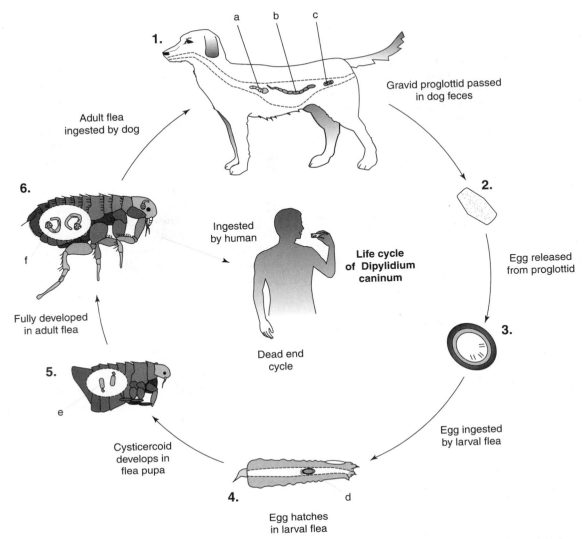

**FIGURE 42-1** Life cycle of *Dipylidium caninum*. *1*. Dog ingests *6*, mature flea containing *f*, fully developed cysticercoid. *A*. cysticercoid develops into adult tapeworm that resides in the small intestine of the dog. *C*. Gravid proglottids are passed in the dog's feces and *3*, eggs are relased from the proglottid. Eggs are ingested by larval fleas and hatched (*d*) in the gastrointestinal tract. The *e*, cysticercoid develops in the flea and pupa and the cysticercoid is fully developed (*f*) in the adult flea. When an adult flea containing a cysticercoid is ingested by a human, it develops into an adult tapeworm. The cycle dead ends in the human host because it is unlikely that larval fleas will have an opportunity to ingest the eggs.

to participate in facultatively parasitic relationships. This concept is called preadaptation and may have involved morphologic and physiologic changes in the parasite. Such changes might have included modifications that allowed the parasite to attach to a host and to resist the enzymatic activity of the host.

Ectoparasites may have evolved from predators of the blood or secretions of the host. Endoparasites may have been introduced to the alimentary canal of the host by accidental ingestion. Within the protected environment provided by the host, parasites continued to adapt, eliminating enzymatic pathways that could be provided by their host and "streamlining" body systems

they no longer needed. For example, tapeworms lack a digestive system, relying instead on predigested food obtained from the host's intestines. Many helminths lack a nervous system and some parasitic protozoans are nonmotile. Eventually, as these changes accumulated they led to an obligate relationship.

An exception to this concept of "streamlining" is the reproductive ability of most helminths as compared to similar free-living organisms. It is unlikely that any given parasitic egg or infective larvae will find its way to a suitable host, so it is necessary for helminths to produce large numbers of eggs or larvae. This increases the likelihood that the next generation of the parasitic organism will survive. Asexual reproduction of larval stages of parasites within intermediate hosts also increases the chances of contacting the next intermediate host or the definitive host.

Living inside of the host creates some unique obstacles for endoparasites. These include surviving in an environment with a high osmotic pressure, low oxygen, and, in many cases, exposure to the strongly acidic secretions of the gastrointestinal system. Successful parasites of the digestive system include protozoans that form cysts and helminths with resilient cuticles and eggs. Endoparasites must also be able to evade the host's immune response and may do so by residing in protected areas or by changing antigenic determinants on their surface.

## TRANSMISSION OF PARASITIC DISEASES

Three elements are necessary for the transmission of parasitic diseases. They are: (1) a source of infection, (2) a mode of transmission, and (3) a susceptible host. The source of infection may be the cyst or, less often, the **trophozoite** form of a protozoan. Eggs or infective

larvae are the source of infection for parasitic helminths. Several routes of transmission exist including ingestion of contaminated food or water, direct contact with the same or another host, injection of the parasite by an arthropod vector, penetration of the skin by an infective stage of the parasite, transplacental infection, and respiratory transmission.

Food and water are the routes of transmission for some protozoan parasites such as *E. hystolytica* (see Figure 45-2). Food may be contaminated with *Entamoeba* cysts by symptomatic or asymptomatic **carriers** due to poor hygiene of food handlers. In many areas, feces-contaminated water is the primary means of transmission. The use of **night soil** (human feces) to fertilize agricultural crops is common in third world nations and is also associated with transmission of *E. histolytica*. Night soil also transmits many bacterial, viral, and other parasitic diseases.

Person-to-person transmission is observed in people who live in close contact with many other people. This often occurs in prisons, orphanages, and mental hospitals. Transmission by direct contact may involve the oral-fecal route with the same or another host as occurs with eggs of the pinworm, *Enterobius vermicularis*. Respiratory infection with *Enterobius* is also possible

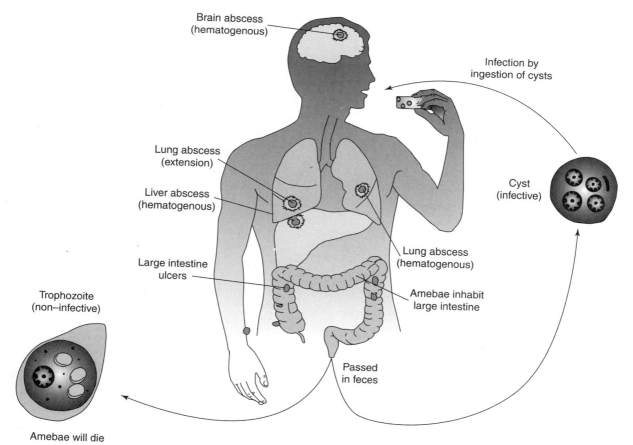

**FIGURE 42-2** Life cycle of *Entamoeba histolytica*.

because the light eggs are easily airborne. Infection is established when the eggs are inhaled and swallowed. Sexual contact is another type of direct contact that allows the transmission of protozoans lacking a cyst stage. *T. vaginalis* trophozoites are often transmitted in this manner. The trophozoites are also transmitted by **fomites** such as soiled clothing.

Arthropods that transmit parasites serve as mechanical or biologic **vectors**. Arthropods act as mechanical vectors when they passively transmit the parasite, as for example on the leg of a fly. *E. histolytica* cysts are sometimes transmitted from human feces to food in this manner. When a portion of the parasitic life cycle occurs in an arthropod it is a biologic vector and an intermediate host. The parasite is transmitted to a human host by the bite of the arthropod vector. Many parasitic protozoans such as *Plasmodium* and *Trypanosoma* are transmitted to humans by arthropod vectors. Four species of *Plasmodium* cause malaria in humans and are vectored by the *Anopheles* mosquito. Diseases caused by *Trypanosoma* include African sleeping sickness and Chagas disease. Arthropod vectors that transmit these diseases are the tsetse fly (*Glossina*) and the reduviid bug.

The infective larvae of *S. mansoni* are referred to as **cercariae** and are released into water by infected snails serving as intermediate hosts. Cercariae have forked tails and anterior penetrating glands. The glands aid the schistosome in the infection of humans or some other host. Humans are infected by penetration of unbroken skin when they enter water containing cercariae.

When maternal infection with *Toxoplasma gondii* occurs it results in congenital infection of the central nervous system of the fetus. Infection of the mother occurs on accidental ingestion of **oocysts** from cat feces or by ingestion of undercooked, cyst-containing meat such as beef, pork, or lamb.

## REPRODUCTION OF PARASITES

Because of the difficulties faced in finding suitable hosts, most parasitic organisms have evolved mechanisms to increase their reproductive potential. This is important to help ensure success of the species because the odds against finding an appropriate host are enormous. Both sexual and asexual reproduction are observed in many protozoans and helminths.

### Asexual Reproduction of Parasites

Asexual reproduction of parasitic organisms can be accomplished by several mechanisms including mitotic fission, **schizogony**, and budding. Many protozoans reproduce asexually by the first two methods, whereas budding is seen primarily in some larval helminths.

Simple mitotic fission is common among protozoan parasites and is the only means of reproduction in some groups, such as most members of the phylum Sarcomastigophora. Mitotic fission produces two daughter cells. *E. histolytica* and *T. vaginalis* are examples of protozoans that reproduce by mitotic fission.

Many protozoan parasites have increased their reproductive potential with a method known as schizogony, or multiple fission. In this process the nucleus undergoes several mitotic divisions after which the cytoplasm is divided among the daughter cells. *Plasmodium* is a protozoan parasite that reproduces asexually by schizogony.

Some juvenile helminths are able to increase their numbers by budding. This greatly increases the numbers of worms that develop in a host that consumes a single egg. The **cysticercus** or larval form of some tapeworms in the genus *Taenia* bud to increase their numbers. The cysticercus is sometimes referred to as a bladderworm.

### Sexual Reproduction of Parasites

Sexual reproduction in parasitic organisms is accomplished in several ways. Protozoans reproduce by **conjugation** and the production of **gametocytes**. Helminths reproduce by cross-fertilization and self-fertilization. With the exception of self-fertilization, sexual reproduction leads to greater genetic diversity and an increased chance for survival.

*Balantidium coli* is a **ciliate** that is sometimes parasitic in humans, causing a disease called balantidium dysentery. This organism can reproduce asexually by fission or sexually by conjugation. During conjugation two of the organisms fuse and exchange genetic material. After separation the organisms continue to reproduce by fission.

Sexual reproduction of *Plasmodium* begins with the production and fusion of gametocytes. The gametocytes are produced and fuse in a human or other vertebrate host and are then ingested by a feeding *Anopheles* mosquito. The sexual portion of the malarial life cycle is completed within the gut of the mosquito.

Many cestodes and trematodes are **hermaphroditic** or **monecious**, meaning that one individual contains both male and female reproductive organs. Most of these parasites can self-fertilize, a process that is also referred to as "selfing," whereas others can cross-fertilize with another individual. Some are only capable of cross-fertilization.

## PARASITIC LIFE CYCLES

Parasitic life cycles are complex and have exacting physical and biologic requirements. Parasitic organisms must overcome many adverse conditions to ensure continuation of the species. In addition, the odds against the successful transfer of the parasite to another suitable host are enormous. In part these obstacles are overcome through greatly increased reproductive potential and by mechanisms that protect the parasite from the host and the harsh environment outside of the host.

There are two basic types of parasitic life cycles: **direct** or **simple life cycles** involving only a definitive host and **indirect** or **complex life cycles** with a definitive host and one or more intermediate hosts. Both types of life cycles are seen in the protozoans and the helminths.

## Direct Life Cycles

Many parasitic organisms have a single host and are transmitted from one host to another by direct contact or by ingestion of a resistant form such as a **cyst**. *T. vaginalis* is a protozoan parasite that does not produce a resistant cyst. It can survive for a short time outside of the host and is usually transmitted by direct contact or by fomites. *G. lamblia* does form resistant cysts. Transmission of *Giardia* is achieved when these cysts are ingested by a host.

In many organisms with direct life cycles eggs, cysts or oocysts are passed in the feces of the host. Because of limited resources, such as nutrients, the parasite must be transmitted to a suitable host within a finite time. During this time the parasite may need to develop into the infective stage. Successful transmission of the parasite depends on several factors including where the infective stage is deposited and the frequency of host contact with the infective stage. An example of a direct life cycle is illustrated by *E. histolytica* in Figure 42-2.

## Indirect Life Cycles

Many parasitic protozoans and helminths have complex life cycles. These life cycles are even more restrictive than are direct life cycles. This is due to the complications introduced by the need for one or more intermediate hosts and in many cases further development of the parasite will only occur in a specific environment. For example, eggs of the lung fluke, *Paragonimus westermani* will only develop into infective metacercariae in an aquatic environment with the appropriate species of snail and crustacean available to serve as intermediate hosts (Figure 42-3).

## HOST-PARASITE RELATIONS

Parasitism exerts evolutionary pressure on both the parasite and the host. It is a type of selective pressure that results in the development of individuals better able to participate in parasitic relationships. Parasitic infection does not always result in disease. Often a state of equilibrium exists between the parasite and the

host. Some organisms such as *E. histolytica* are commensals in one individual but are invasive in others or in the same individual under different circumstances causing significant damage in the host. Many parasitic infections are chronic and asymptomatic. These asymptomatic infections are important to the epidemiology of parasitic disease with carriers contributing to transmission of the parasitic organism.

Parasitic infection can produce a variety of detrimental effects on the host due to mechanical and chemical damage and the impairment of vital functions. Parasites also compete with the host for vital nutrients and some feed on host tissue. Injury to the host varies in severity.

Mechanical damage can be caused by the hooks and suckers of helminths. For example, the hooks that tapeworms use to attach to the intestinal mucosa can cause significant damage, especially when the host is heavily infected. Tapeworms also absorb vitamin $B_{12}$ from the host leading to anemia. *G. lamblia* is a protozoan that attaches to the intestinal mucosa of its host by means of a ventrally located sucker. Hosts heavily infected with *Giardia* experience difficulty absorbing nutrients. This phenomena is referred to as giardial malabsorption syndrome. Parasitic eggs can also cause mechanical damage to the host. Sharp spines on the eggs of schistosomes damage blood vessels of the host. Large numbers of nematodes such as *Ascaris* cause intestinal obstruction in the host. Other kinds of mechanical damage include chewing, perforation of the skin and other organs, cell destruction, and pressure caused by the formation of a cyst.

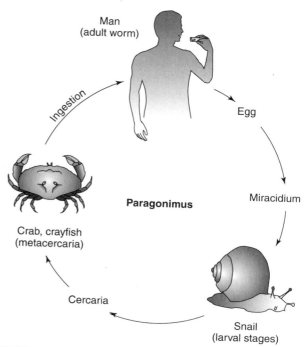

**FIGURE 42-3** Life cycle of *Paragonimus westermani*.

Chemical damage to the host may be due to secretion or excretions produced by the parasite. Excretions of the parasite can act as toxins, decreasing host vitality. Examples of secretions that cause host damage include the proteolytic enzymes of *Entamoeba,* the penetrating enzymes of *Schistosoma,* and the anticoagulating factors produced by many hookworms.

## THE IMMUNOLOGY OF PARASITIC INFECTION

Through the process of evolution, host organisms have developed a variety of defenses against parasitic infection while parasitic organisms have developed mechanisms to overcome them. If a host's specific and nonspecific defenses are able to prevent the establishment and survival of a parasite, then the host is resistant, or immune, to that parasite. The host is susceptible if the parasite is able to overcome these defenses to establish an infection or cause disease. Specific defenses to parasitism involve the host's immune system and the production of protein molecules called antibodies and sensitized T cells. Nonspecific mechanisms of defense include the physical barrier created by the skin and mucous membranes, phagocytic cells such as macrophages and **granulocytes**, and chemical factors such as lymphokines, sebum, and **gastric juice**.

### Host Response to Parasitic Infection

Host responses to parasitic infection are varied and include inflammation, the production of chemical substances such as **lymphokines**, the formation of specific antibodies and T cells and **eosinophilia**. Inflammation may be a reaction to the parasite or products of the parasite. It mobilizes the body's defenses against infection and aids in the repair of damaged tissues. Sensitized T cells are produced in response to parasitic infection. When stimulated by parasitic antigens, T cells known as delayed hypersensitivity T cells, or $T_d$ cells, secrete lymphokines. These small, protein molecules initiate other aspects of the immune response such as attraction of macrophages to the site of infection. Eosinophilia refers to the presence of large numbers of eosinophils in the blood and is associated with many helminth infections. Evidence suggests that eosinophils have a cytotoxic effect on helminths.

Parasitic organisms are antigenically complex and have evolved mechanisms that help them to resist the host's immune response. Although elevated levels of **IgM** and **IgE** are seen in some parasitic infections, these antibodies are often less effective against the organisms due to their large size. **sIgA** and IgM antibodies are formed against the flagella and attachment disk of *Giardia;* however, they are ineffective against the protozoan. This is due at least in part to the ability of *Giardia,* as well as many other parasitic organisms, to rapidly change their surface antigens, rendering the antibodies ineffective and evading the host's immune response. Other parasites that are able to change their surface antigens include *S. mansoni* and the trypanosomes. These organisms may be able to produce hundreds or even thousands of different surface antigens making the prospect for the development of effective vaccines difficult at best.

### Parasitic Infection and the Immunocompromised Host

Many parasitic organisms only cause disease in immunocompromised persons. This is usually the case with *T. gondii, Pneumocystis carinii* and the microsporidia. There are numerous ways in which the host can become immunocompromised, including but not limited to, hospitalization, surgery, chemotherapy (especially corticosteroids), and immunosuppressive diseases such as AIDS. Parasitic disease itself compromises the immune system by making the host more susceptible to other pathogenic organisms. Secondary infections with another agent, such as the host's normal flora, are commonly associated with many parasitic infections.

## AN OVERVIEW OF SOME IMPORTANT PARASITES

What follows is a partial list of important groups of human parasites and some animal parasites that are occasional parasites of humans. This list includes protozoans and helminths.

### Protozoan Parasites

*Phylum Sarcomastigophora.* Members of this phylum are motile by means of pseudopods, flagella, or both. Trophozoites are often the active, feeding, and reproducing form of these organisms and many species can form resistant cysts. Reproduction is primarily by mitotic fission with sexual reproduction occurring in some flagellate species. Transmission varies and includes direct contact, ingestion of cysts in food or water, or by an arthropod vector. Both direct and indirect life cycles occur. These organisms may parasitize the alimentary canal, the blood, or other tissues. Some species are commensals of the alimentary canal. Included in this phylum are the two subphyla: Sarcodina, the amebas and Mastigophora, the flagellates. Both subphyla have free-living as well as parasitic forms. *E. histolytica* is a member of subphylum Sarcodina; *G. lamblia* is a member of Mastigophora. Both of these organisms cause disease in humans.

*Phylum Apicomplexa.* This phylum was formally referred to as Sporozoa. All members are obligate parasites of tissues and are nonmotile when mature. They have complex life cycles alternating between sexual and asexual generations. Transmission is by direct contact, ingestion of feces-contaminated water, as zoonoses by domestic animals, or by an arthropod vector. *Plasmodium* and *Cryptosporidium* are representative genera of the phylum Apicomplexa.

*Phylum Ciliophora.* These organisms are motile by means of **cilia**. Their life cycle consists of a trophozoite and a cyst. Reproduction is by mitotic fission or by conjugation. Many species are multinucleate, having one or more **macronuclei** and **micronuclei**. The only member of Ciliophora that is parasitic in humans is *B. coli* and it is often a commensal of the alimentary canal. When *Balantidium* is invasive it causes a condition known as balantidium dysentery.

*Phylum Microspora.* Members of this phylum were formally classified with the Sporozoa. These organisms are tiny, intracellular parasites that infect many vertebrates and invertebrates. Transmission is by direct contact or by an intermediate host. They lack mitochondria but have a coiled organelle referred to as the polar filament. The polar filament is extruded from a spore to inject infectious material into the host. After completion of a complex life cycle, additional spores are produced. Due to their small size (1–4 μm) electron microscopy is required to recognize and identify microsporidia (Neva & Brown, 1994). Although they are most often associated with disease in immunocompromised persons, they also cause disease in immunocompetent individuals. A representative member causing enteritis in AIDS patients is *E. bieneusi* (Neva & Brown, 1994). Treatment is not available at this time and serologic tests for diagnosis are under development.

## The Helminths

*Phylum Aschelminthes.* Members of this phylum that parasitize humans are in the class Nematoda and are referred to as roundworms. They are multicellular and have a complete digestive system, meaning that they have both a mouth and an anus. Nematodes are covered by a tough cuticle and have separate sexes (**dioecious**). Reproduction is sexual. Some nematodes are free-living in soil, whereas others parasitize a variety of plants and animals. In some cases the entire life cycle is spent in a single host, or part of the cycle is completed in the soil. Some nematodes require an intermediate host. Human infection with nematodes is transmitted by ingestion of eggs or infective larvae, or by penetration of the skin by larvae. In humans, nematodes are parasites of the intestines or other tissues. *Ascaris lumbricoides* is a large nematode (averages 30 cm in length) having infective eggs. The larvae of the hookworm, *N. americanus* inhabits the soil and penetrates the skin of humans on contact.

*Phylum Platyhelminthes.* The Platyhelminthes are multicellular flatworms having long, bilaterally symmetrical bodies and incomplete digestive systems. This means that food enters and waste exits through one opening. Some species absorb nutrients through their cuticle. Species that infect humans are members of the classes Trematoda (the flukes) and Cestoda (the tapeworms).

*Class Trematoda.* The flukes have leaf-shaped or elongated bodies and suckers or hooks attach the organism to the host. The suckers also draw fluids from host tissue. Trematodes are hermaphroditic and can cross-fertilize with another individual or in many cases self-fertilize. Flukes have complex life cycles with one or more intermediate hosts. Human infection occurs by ingestion or penetration of an infective larvae. Flukes are named according to the tissue they inhabit in the definitive host. Examples of trematodes are the blood fluke, *S. mansoni,* and the lung fluke, *P. westermani.*

*Class Cestoda.* The cestodes or the tapeworms have long ribbon-like, segmented bodies. Adult tapeworms inhabit the small intestine and lack a digestive system. Nutrients are absorbed through the cuticle. Most species have complex life cycles. A specialized attachment organ called the **scolex** is located at the anterior end and has hooks, suckers, or both. The segments of the tapeworm are called **proglottids** and contain male and female sex organs. Tapeworms cross-fertilize or self-fertilize and eggs are produced in the proglottids. As the tapeworm grows, proglottids are pushed to the posterior end where they eventually break free to be passed in the host's feces. The eggs must be ingested by the intermediate host for the life cycle to be completed. Humans may serve as the definitive host or as the intermediate host. *Taenia saginata* is a tapeworm in which humans are the definitive host; humans are the intermediate host for *Echinococcus granulosus.*

## TECHNIQUES FOR PARASITIC EXAMINATION

A variety of techniques are used to detect and identify parasitic infections. Some are used routinely and others have limited applications. The methods mentioned here are discussed in detail in the other chapters in this section.

## Examination of Fecal Specimens

The examination of fecal samples for parasitic organisms begins with the determination of its physical characteristics such as consistency. Examination of unpreserved fecal samples will yield some clues as to what kinds of parasites it might contain (Markell et al., 1992). For example, protozoan trophozoites are usually found in soft or liquid stools, whereas cysts are seen in fully formed stools. Unpreserved specimens are examined for helminths on the surface and in the interior of the fecal sample. Whole worms or proglottids may be evident in stool specimens. Microscopic examination may reveal protozoan trophozoites or cysts, or helminth eggs. The presence of blood and mucus suggests intestinal ulceration as seen in infections with *E. histolytica* and *B. coli*.

If unpreserved, the age of the fecal sample is critical. Specimens that cannot be promptly examined within the appropriate time must be preserved in a fixative solution such as **PVA** or **SAF**.

Several techniques are available for more detailed examination of fecal samples. Because no one technique is completely reliable it is advisable to use at least two methods. A **direct wet film** is used to detect cysts and helminth eggs. Direct wet films are made by mixing a small portion of the fecal sample with a drop of normal saline on a clean slide. After adding a coverslip the unstained preparation is examined. Wet films allow for determination of trophozoite motility that may provide clues as to the identity of the parasite. Other slides may be stained with iodine for easier viewing of protozoan cysts. Permanent preparations are recommended for the protozoans and may be stained with iron hematoxylin or Gomori's trichrome stain.

Protozoan trophozoites and cysts and helminth eggs may be more easily viewed after treating the fecal sample with a concentration technique. A variety of methods are available to separate cysts and eggs from the bulk of the fecal sample based on differences in specific gravity using flotation or sedimentation. The ethyl acetate concentration method is useful to detect both cysts and eggs. Other concentration methods have more limited applications.

A commercial kit is available to collect eggs of the pinworm, *Enterobius*, or cellophane tape can be used. After the tape is pressed against the perianal area of the infected person, it is applied to a slide and microscopically examined for the presence of eggs.

In some cases it is necessary to sample the **duodenal** contents. It is helpful to do so when examining for the larvae of *Strongyloides*, the eggs of *Fasciola* and the protozoans, *Giardia* and *Cryptosporidium*. One method used to obtain these samples is the **enteric capsule** or the **string test** (see Figure 42-4). A gelatin capsule containing a weighted line is swallowed by the patient. One end of the line protrudes from a hole in the capsule and is taped to the patient's cheek. After 4 hours, the line is pulled up and is examined microscopically for the presence of parasites. A biopsy of the intestinal mucosa may also reveal intestinal parasites.

## Examination of Blood Specimens

A number of parasites may be detected in blood preparations such as *Plasmodium, Trypanosoma, Leishmania,* and **microfilariae**. Although trypanosomes and microfilariae may exhibit motility in fresh, whole blood it is more common that a permanent preparation be examined. Always use clean, grease-free, unscratched slides that have been washed in detergent followed by 70% ethyl alcohol (Garcia & Bruckner, 1993). Whole blood, buffy coat preparations, or concentrated blood may be used. Thick or thin blood films are stained with Giemsa's or Wright's stain.

Thick and thin blood smears are used to detect *Plasmodium, Trypanosoma,* and microfilariae. When making these smears the preparation must be thin enough to avoid obscuring the parasites with blood cells; ideally it should be one layer of cells thick. Thick preparations will contain more organisms per field; however, the technique causes some distortion. Buffy coat preparations concentrate the white blood cells and are especially useful for detecting *Leishmania* as well as trypanosomes.

## Examination of Cerebrospinal Fluid

Cerebrospinal fluid (CSF) is examined for *Toxoplasma,* trypanosomes, and eosinophilia, an indicator of some other parasitic infections. CSF is best examined promptly—within 20 minutes of collection is recommended. CSF is often centrifuged before examination to concentrate parasitic organisms and aid in their identification. *Naegleria* is an ameba that is detected by the presence of motile trophozoites in CSF.

## Examination of Tissues and Organs

Tissues and organs may be sampled for parasitic infection by biopsy or aspiration. Biopsies involve the removal and microscopic examination of a tissue sample. Spleen, liver, and bone marrow biopsies are used to diagnose

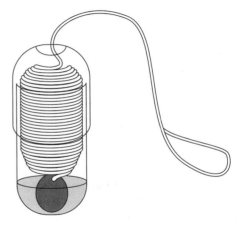

**FIGURE 42-4** Enteric capsule used to sample duodenal contents.

visceral leishmaniasis; *Schistosoma* eggs are sometimes demonstrated in rectal mucosa or in mucosa of the bladder wall. *Trichinella* larvae may be found in biopsies of voluntary muscle or the diaphragm. Aspiration to obtain samples usually involves the removal of fluid from an abscess to examine for evidence of parasites. Involved lymph nodes are aspirated to detect trypanosomes. They may also be cultured or inoculated into an animal to recover trypanosomes, *Toxoplasma* and *Leishmania* (Neva & Brown, 1994). Skin scrapings or snips are useful for the identification of some infections such as leishmania and trypanosomiasis. Giemsa's and Wright's stain are commonly used to stain tissue samples.

## Examination of Sputum

Pulmonary infection with *Paragonimus* or *Entamoeba* may be detected by examination of sputum. *Paragonimus* eggs are often swallowed and evident in feces. Other organisms such as *Ascaris* or *Cryptosporidium* are sometimes evident in sputum. The best sample for examination is induced, free of saliva, and collected early in the morning (Markell et al., 1992). Fresh sputum is examined by wet mount or is fixed with PVA.

## Examination of Urine and Vaginal Secretions

*Trichomonas vaginalis* is detected in wet mounts of urine, vaginal secretions, or prostate exudate by the presence of motile trophozoites possessing an undulating membrane. *Schistosoma* eggs or occasionally the eggs of other helminths are sometimes found in urine.

## Culture Methods

A variety of culture media have been developed to support the growth of parasitic organisms. *E. histolytica* grows well on nutrient media containing rice flour and bacteria under partially anaerobic conditions (Neva & Brown, 1994). *Leishmania* and trypanosomes are often cultured in *Novy*, MacNeal, Nicolle (NNN) liquid media with added fetal calf serum or insect hemolymph. Other parasites are recovered by tissue culture or by inoculation into an animal such as mice or rats.

## Immunodiagnostic Techniques

Immunodiagnostic (serologic) tests are used when conventional methods such as identification of the parasite in the patient's tissues, body fluids, or excretions fail to yield results. Many test kits and reagents are commercially available; however, cross-reaction with other antigens is possible, seriously limiting the usefulness of these tests.

Immunodiagnostic tests are not performed routinely in the diagnostic microbiology laboratory because they are not economically practical and in many cases a specific test does not exist. Table 42-1 lists several serologic tests used to diagnose parasitic disease.

### Table 42–1 ▶ Serologic Tests Used to Diagnose Parasitic Disease

| Test Method | Major Features | Application |
|---|---|---|
| Complement fixation (CF) | Sensitized sheep red blood cells (RBC) added to test serum and antigen after incubation. | Chagas' disease |
| | Unfixed complement hemolyzes sheep RBCs | *Leishmania* |
| | Degree of hemolysis inversely proportional to amount of antibody in original sample | *Paragonimus* |
| Agglutination | Latex beads or formalin-fixed parasite is exposed to test serum. | Chagas' disease |
| | Agglutination indicates specific antibody to parasite is present. | |
| Radio-immunoassay primarily (RIA) | Tracer isotope-tagged antibody is mixed with test sample. | |
| | If the parasite is present the parasite antigen-tagged antibody binds to it and can be measured. | |
| Western blot | Antigen separated by electrophoresis, blotted onto a membrane, cut into strips, and exposed to test serum | Schistosomiasis |
| | After exposing to test serum the sample is incubated and examined. | |
| | Sensitive to small amounts of antibody | |
| | Difficult to interpret | |
| | Always use controls | |
| Ouchterlony gel diffusion | Wells in a gel-filled Petri plate are filled with antigen or antibody | Amoebiasis |
| | The antigen and antibody diffuse toward each other. | Various helminths |
| | A spur-shaped band of precipitate between the wells indicates a positive reaction. | |

## SUMMARY

▶ Parasitology is the study of unicellular and multicellular organisms that parasitize humans. These organisms include the protozoans, the helminths, and some arthropods.

▶ When two organisms live together the relationship is referred to as symbiosis. Symbionts that cause harm to, or that live at the expense of their partner, are known as parasites.

▶ The host in which a parasite reaches sexual maturity is called a definitive host. An intermediate host is one in which the immature stage of the parasite resides. A reservoir host harbors the same stage of the parasite that is found in humans.

▶ Parasites are highly evolved for a specialized type of life. Many of the systems of parasitic organisms (primarily in the helminths) are streamlined for life in the protected environment provided by the host.

▶ Most parasitic organisms reproduce in large numbers to increase the likelihood that their next generation will survive.

▶ The three elements necessary for the transmission of parasitic disease are a source of infection, a mode of transmission, and a susceptible host.

▶ Asexual and sexual reproduction are observed in many protozoa and helminths. Asexual reproduction includes mitotic fission, schizogony, and budding. Sexual reproduction includes conjugation and the production of gametocytes.

▶ Parasitic life cycles include direct and indirect life cycles.

▶ A host is susceptible to a parasite if the parasite is able to overcome the immune system of the host. Host responses to parasitic infection include lymphokines, the formation of antibodies and T cells, and eosinophilia.

▶ A variety of techniques are used for parasitic examination. Specimens include fecal material, blood, tissue biopsy, sputum, urine, and vaginal smears.

## Review Questions

1. Which of the following are metazoans?
   a. Ticks
   b. Helminths
   c. Protozoans
   d. Both a and b are metazoans.

2. Which of the following best defines "reservoir host"?
   a. A reservoir host is the host in which asexual reproduction of the parasite occurs.
   b. All hosts in the parasitic life cycle are reservoir hosts.
   c. An organism that harbors the same stage of the parasite that is found in humans.
   d. A reservoir host is an organism that accidentally infected with a parasite that normally infects another species.

3. How do parasitic organisms overcome the difficulties they face in transmitting the next generation to a suitable host?
   a. They do so by producing resistant eggs or cysts.
   b. Parasitic organisms have a greater reproductive potential than do most free-living species thus increasing the chances of transfer to a suitable host.

   c. Some parasitic organisms increase their numbers by reproducing asexually in the intermediate host making it more likely that they will make their way to a suitable host.
   d. Most parasitic organisms produce toxins that discourage unsuitable hosts.

4. Which of the following are necessary for the transmission of parasitic disease to occur?
   a. A susceptible host
   b. A mode of transmission
   c. A source of infection
   d. All of the above are necessary for the transmission of parasitic disease.

5. A stool sample is collected from a patient suspected of infection with *Entamoeba histolytica*. The stool sample is liquid. What stage of the life cycle of *Entamoeba* is most likely to be observed in the specimen?
   a. The resistant cyst
   b. The trophozoite
   c. An immature cyst
   d. The tryptomastigote

6. Individuals infected with *Taenia* species may undergo an increased parasitic burden by which of the following?
    a. Schizogony of the *Taenia* egg that was originally ingested
    b. Fission of the adult worm in the host's intestine
    c. Budding of the cysticercus
    d. Conjugation between adult worms

7. Monecious helminths are able to:
    a. self-fertilize.
    b. mate with another worm.
    c. reproduce by the production of eggs only.
    d. Only a and b are true.

8. Eggs of *Paragonimus westermani* are only able to develop into metacercariae if they:
    a. are ingested by a susceptible human within 2 months of their release from the adult worm.

    b. incubate in warm soil for a summer before they are ingested.
    c. are deposited into an aquatic environment with the appropriate species of snail.
    d. are transmitted to humans by the bite of an infected arthropod.

9. *Giardia lamblia* is able to resist the host's defenses by:
    a. changing surface antigens.
    b. residing inside of host cells.
    c. encysting.
    d. killing T cells.

10. Direct wet films of fecal samples are examined to detect:
    a. protozoan cysts and helminth eggs.
    b. *Plasmodium* and other sporozoans.
    c. many species of arthropods.
    d. microsporidians.

▶ **REFERENCES & RECOMMENDED READING**

Baron, E. J., Peterson, L. R., & Finegold, S. M. (1990). *Bailey and Scott's diagnostic microbiology* (8th ed.). St. Louis: Mosby.

Coleman, R. M., Lombard, M. F., Sicard, R. E. (1989). *Fundamental immunology*. Dubuque, IA: Wm. C. Brown.

Garcia, L. S., & Bruckner, D. A. (1993). *Diagnostic medical parasitology* (2nd ed.). Washington, DC: American Society for Microbiology.

Goodgame, R. M., et al. (1993). Intensity of infection in AIDS-associated cryptosporidiosis. *Journal of Infectious Diseases, 167*, 704–709.

Kuby, J. (1994). *Immunology* (2nd ed.). New York: Freeman.

Lee, C. H., et al. (1993). Nucleotide sequence variation in *Pneumocystis carinii* strains that infect humans. *Journal of Clinical Microbiology, 31*, 754–757.

Markell, E. K., Voge, M., & John, D. T. (1992). *Medical parasitology* (7th ed.). Philadelphia: Saunders.

Miller, B. F., & Keane, C. B. (1987). *Encyclopedia and dictionary of medicine, nursing and allied health* (4th ed.). Philadelphia: Saunders.

Neva, F. A., & Brown, H. W. (1994). *Basic clinical parasitology* (6th ed.). East Norwalk, CT: Appleton & Lange.

Olsen, O. W. (1986). *Animal parasites: Their life cycles and ecology*. New York: Dover.

Perry, N. (1990). *Symbiosis: Nature in partnership*. London: Blandford.

Schmidt, G. D., & Roberts, L. S. (1989). *Foundations of parasitology* (4th ed.). St. Louis: Times Mirror/Mosby.

*Scientific American: A Special Issue*. (1994). Life, death and the immune system. New York: Freeman.

Thomas, C. L. (Ed.). (1997). *Taber's cyclopedic medical dictionary* (18th ed.). Philadelphia: Davis.

Tortora, G. J., Funke, B. R., & Case, C. C. (1992). *Microbiology: An introduction* (4th ed.). Redwood City, CA: Benjamin/Cummings.

Waterborne Bug May Have Killed 19 in Las Vegas. *The Press-Enterprise*, 25 May 1994.

Wyler, D. J. (Ed.). (1990). *Modern parasite biology: Cellular, immunological and molecular aspects*. New York: Freeman.

# CHAPTER 43

# Specimen Collection and Processing for Parasite Examinations

Bardwell J. Eberly, MT (ASCAP), SM

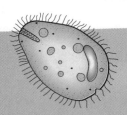

## Microbes in the News

### State Issues Drinking Water Warning for People With Immune Deficiencies

The State of Hawaii Department of Health has followed the lead of two federal agencies in issuing a water warning for people with immune deficiencies. Individuals who take immunosuppressive drugs for cancer or after transplant surgery and who have tested positive for HIV/AIDS should be careful in their consumption of tap water.

Bruce Anderson of the Health Department has stated that most of Hawaii's drinking water is from ground water sources and is not vulnerable to conta-

mination. However, areas that tap river, lake, and stream sources are susceptible to the parasite cryptosporidium. These areas include Makawao, Kula, parts of Lahaina on the island of Maui, and Waimea on the island of Hawaii.

For those individuals who may be at risk, the Department of Health recommends boiling tap water for a least 1 minute or using a home filtration device.

Source: *Honolulu Advertiser*, July 1995.

## KEY TERMS

Amastigote
Diurnal periodicity
Endemic
Hematuria
Immunosuppressed / immunodeficiencies / immuno-

competent / immunocompromised
Intraerythrocytic
Minced
Nocturnal periodicity
Nonperiodic periodicity

Oocyst
Perianal
Promastigote
Thick smear
Thin smear

## LEARNING OBJECTIVES

**Upon successful completion of this chapter, the student should be able to:**

1. List the general requirements for specimen collection for parasite examination.

2. List the specimen of choice to detect pinworm, *Naegleria, Acanthamoeba, Cryptosporidium, Babesia,* and intestinal parasites.

3. Describe the direct microscopic examination procedures for fecal, duodenal, perianal, and sigmoidoscopic specimens.

4. Describe the general concentrated techniques for performing formalin-ethyl acetate procedure, modified acid-fast stain, and peripheral blood smears.

5. List the stains used for routine parasitic examination and describe the purpose of each stain.

6. List the serodiagnostic techniques used for detection of parasite-specific antibody or antigen from clinical specimens and describe the principle for each technique.

## INTRODUCTION

To provide accurate and relevant information to a physician, it is most important to collect and handle the sample properly. Adequate instructions and proper containers for collection of specimens should be provided to the physician, nursing staff, or patient to ensure that a satisfactory specimen will be received for examination. Inadequate and poorly preserved specimens are of little or no value in establishing a diagnosis and can often lead to poor management of care.

## SPECIMEN COLLECTION AND PROCESSING

### Fecal

To rule out intestinal parasites, a fecal specimen should be collected before the administration of barium, bismuth, antidiarrheal medication, oily laxatives, or any antacids. Antibiotics cause temporary decrease or absence of organisms. Reliable diagnosis may not be possible until 2 or more weeks, *after* the last dose is taken. Barium, bismuth, and nonabsorbable antacids render the stool unsatisfactory for examination. These substances reduce the visibility of detecting intestinal parasite in wet mounts and permanent preparations (Howard, Keiser, Smith, Weissfeld, & Tilton, 1994). Specimens should be collected 7 to 10 days *after* the compounds are given.

The fecal specimen should be collected in a clean, dry, wide-mouthed container. Contamination of fecal material with water or urine should be avoided. Water may contain free-living saprophytes that may be mistaken for parasites. Urine may destroy protozoan trophozoites (Howard et al., 1994). A minimum of two specimens collected on alternating days is recommended for routine examination. Deliver each collection to the laboratory within 30 minutes.

The fecal material may be refrigerated for 2 to 3 days if there is a delay in the transportation of the sample to the laboratory. An alternate method would be to place the fecal material in a commercial two-vial preservative system kit (ParaPak). The kit consists of 10% formalin and polyvinyl alcohol (PVA). The 10% formalin preserves helminth eggs, larvae, and protozoan cysts. PVA preserves all stages of protozoan for an indeterminate time.

If fresh stool is submitted to the laboratory within 30 minutes, a direct wet mount and macroscopic examination for stool consistency, color, and gross and occult blood should be performed. The direct wet mount examination will detect motile protozoan trophozoites and other intestinal parasites. Adding iodine solution to the preparation will enhance the morphologic characteristics of the cysts and kill the trophozoite stages of the parasite (Murray, Baron, Pfaller, Tenover, & Yolken, 1995).

Profuse and watery stools, with or without mucus, collected from **immunocompetent** or **immunosuppressed** patients should be submitted in the commercial two-vial preservative system kit. Permanent mounts should be prepared from formalin and PVA vials. The prepared smear from the 10% formalin should be stained with the modified Kinyoun stain and examined for *Cryptosporidium, Isospora,* and *Cyclospora* **oocysts**. Smear prepared from the PVA preserved vial should be stained with trichrome stain and examined for protozoan cysts and trophozoites.

### Pinworm Examination

Pinworm infection is highly prevalent throughout the world and is suspected in children with **perianal** itching, insomnia, or restlessness (Brown, 1975). The causative agent is *Enterobius vermicularis.* The adult female does not hatch her eggs in the intestine but migrates to the outer portion of the anus to deposit her eggs. The specimen of choice is the cellulose acetate (Scotch tape) test or the pinworm paddle (Howard et al., 1994; Koneman, Allen, Janda, Schreckenberger, & Winn, 1992). Ideally, the sample should be collected at home by the parents. The sticky side of the paddle is pressed onto the perianal area of the child, preferably in the morning before a bowel movement. Paddle or tape is delivered to the lab and directly observed under the microscope for *E. vermicularis* eggs.

## Urine

If schistosomal **hematuria** is suspected, a midday voided urine is collected. A 10-mL aliquot of urine is centrifuged and wet mounts are prepared from the sediment. A saline preparation is examined under low-power magnification for the diagnostic egg stage of *S. haematobium* and confirmed under high dry. If unable to examine urine immediately, the specimen should be preserved with 10% formalin.

## Sputum

On rare occasions, expectorated sputa are examined for larval migrations of hookworms, *Ascaris lumbricoides* or *S. stercoralis* and eggs of *Paragonimus westermani*. If the sputum is unusually thick and mucoid, an equal volume of 3% *N*-acetyl-L-cysteine or 3% sodium hydroxide is added to liquefy the specimen. The sample is mixed for 2 to 3 minutes, strained through a funnel/filter device into a 15-mL conical tube and centrifuged. From the sediment, saline and iodine wet mounts are set up for examination. If for any reason the examination of the sputum sediment is delayed, 10% formalin should be added to preserve helminth eggs and larvae (refer to Color Plates 87 and 88).

## Duodenal

When multiple fecal examinations are negative for ova and parasites, duodenal contents are collected via a nasogastric intubation. The contents are examined for the rhaditiform larva of *S. stercoralis*, trophozoite/cyst stage of *Giardia lamblia*, or oocysts of *Cryptosporidium* and/or *Isospora* (refer to Color Plates 89 and 90). In addition to the contents, duodenal material could be collected with the string test (Entero-Test) (Isenberg, 1992.) On receipt in the laboratory, the specimen should be processed as soon as possible. The bile-stained mucus is squeezed or scraped off the line onto a Petri dish or microscope slide. Direct wet mounts are prepared and examined for *S. stercoralis* larva, *G. lamblia* trophozoites, or cysts. In addition to the wet mounts, permanent smears should be prepared and stained with trichrome or modified Kinyoun stain. If there is a delay in processing the sample, 10% formalin and PVA should be used as preservatives (Aldeen, Hale,

Robison, & Carroll, 1995; Garcia & Shimizu, 1993; Melvin & Brooke, 1980).

Aspirated material with a volume greater than 1 ml should be centrifuged at 500*g* (1,600–1,800 rpm) for 10 minutes. Wet mounts are prepared and examined as soon as possible. Permanent smears should be included and stained with trichrome and modified Kinyoun stain. If there is a delay in the examination process, the sample should be preserved in 10% formalin and PVA.

## Cerebrospinal Fluid

Members of the genera *Toxoplasma, Naegleria, Trypanosoma,* and *Acanthamoeba* exhibit a predilection for the central nervous system (Dalton & Nottebart, 1986). In patients with suspected meningitis, a lumbar puncture is performed and cerebrospinal fluid (CSF) is submitted for examination. The specimen is centrifuged at 250*g* (1,200–1,300 rpm) for 10 minutes and processed in a biologic safety cabinet. With the technologist wearing gloves, the supernatant except for 0.5 mL of fluid is carefully removed and transferred to a sterile tube. The remaining fluid (0.5 mL) is mixed with the sediment. Using a sterile pipet, 2 to 3 drops of sediment is inoculated to the center of a nonnutrient agar seeded with *Escherichia coli*. The plate is sealed with parafilm, incubated upright at 37°C, and examined daily for a period of 10 days for cysts.

In addition to culture, smears are prepared from the CSF sediment and stained with Giemsa and trichrome stains. Wet mounts are also prepared and examined under phase microscopy for motile trophozoites (Koneman et al., 1992).

## Vaginal Swab

*Trichomonas vaginalis* is considered to be one of the most common of the sexually transmitted disease organisms. Scrapings or vaginal swabs are collected and placed in normal saline for examination. On receipt, a wet mount is prepared and examined for the jerky motility that is characteristic of *T. vaginalis*.

## Corneal Scraping/Keratitis

Eye infections caused by the free-living protozoan *Acanthamoeba* has been associated with contaminated lens solution that was prepared by the user. Early symptoms include red, irritated eyes, pain, and no discharge. Later in the course of infection, the pain can become severe, the cornea can develop opaque areas (ring infiltrates), and blindness can occur (Garcia & Shimizu, 1993).

If *Acanthamoeba* keratitis is suspected, corneal scrapings should be directly inoculated to a nonnutrient agar plate seeded with *E. coli*. The plate is sealed with parafilm, incubated upright at 37°C without carbon dioxide, and examined daily for a period of 10 days for cysts of *Acanthamoeba.* A calcofluor white preparation is prepared from the scrap fragments and examined under a fluorescent microscope for *Acanthamoeba* cysts (Gorbach, Bartlett, & Blacklow, 1992).

If the homemade contact lens solution is submitted for examination, gloves should be worn and the processing of samples should be done in a biologic safety cabinet. Centrifuge solutions greater than 2 mL at 250$g$ (gravity) forces for 10 minutes. If less than 2 mL of solution is received, inoculate directly onto a nonnutrient agar plate seeded with *E. coli.* Seal plate with parafilm to avoid dehydration, incubate upright at 37°C without carbon dioxide, and examine daily for cysts (refer to Color Plates 91, 92, and 93).

## Aspirates/Sigmoidoscopic Specimens

When multiple fecal examinations are negative for parasites, specimens such as aspirates from deep, seeded liver abscess or scraping from ulcerated areas of the intestinal mucosa are collected and submitted for parasitic examination. Such specimens are usually submitted for the diagnosis of extraintestinal amebiasis. One drop of the specimen is mixed directly on a microscope slide with 3 drops of PVA. The emulsion is then spread over one-third of the slide. The slide is placed in drying oven for 30 to 45 minutes, stained with trichrome stain and examined for protozoan trophozoites and cysts (Gorbach et al., 1992; Howard et al., 1994).

If *Cryptosporidium, Isospora,* or *Cyclospora* is suspected, a permanent prep should be stained with modified Kinyoun acid-fast stain and examined for oocysts.

For bone marrow or lymph node aspirates, smears should be prepared, stained by Giemsa stain, and examined for *Leishmania* or *Trypanosoma* species, if these parasites are suspected. The remaining portion of the aspirate should be processed by the histopathology section and smear preparations evaluated by a pathologist.

## Biopsies

For suspected cases of cutaneous parasitic infection, biopsies should be submitted in a sterile container with adequate amount of saline to prevent dehydration of the tissue. For skin snips (punch biopsy) suspicious for leishmaniasis, a portion of the skin snip should be **minced** and inoculated to Nicolle-Novy-McNeal (NNN) media with guinea pig or sheep blood. The culture is incubated at 25°C in the dark and examined weekly for a period of 4 weeks. If the culture is suspicious for growth, thin smears are prepared, stained by Giemsa stain, and evaluated for **promastigotes** of *Leishmania donovani* (refer to Color Plates 94 and 95).

In addition to culture, touch preps of the skin snip (punch biopsy) should be stained with Giemsa stain and examined for **amastigote** stages of *Leishmania* within the macrophages.

The remaining portion of the tissue biopsies, skin snips suspected for *Onchocerca volvulus* or *Mansonella streptocerca,* and lymph nodes should be processed by the histopathology section and smear preparations evaluated by a pathologist.

## Blood

For the diagnosis of *Plasmodium* and *Babesia* species and filarial nematodes, whole blood with or without anticoagulant is the specimen of choice. For a patient who has lived and traveled in an area **endemic** for malaria, the blood is collected on the first visit and at 6-hour intervals thereafter (Brown, 1975). Thin and thick smears are prepared from the peripheral blood and stained with Giemsa stain. Blood should be examined 3 to 4 successive days until the diagnostic characteristics for malarial parasites is confirmed.

To rule out babesiosis, thin and thick smears are prepared from the peripheral blood, stained with Giemsa stain and examined for **intraerythrocytic** parasites. Travel history of the patient should be provided to assist in the laboratory diagnosis of differentiating *Babesia* species from *Plasmodium* species.

Time of collection, clinical symptoms, and travel history of a patient could assist in the recovery of filarial nematodes from blood. Blood should be collected after 10 PM to recover and identify microfilariae (**nocturnal periodicity**) of *Wuchereria bancrofti and Brugia malayi.* For Pacific Islanders who reside in the South Pacific (Brown, 1975), the microfilariae of *W. bancrofti* is **nonperiodic** and blood samples can be collected randomly. If blood is collected between 11 AM and 1 PM, the microfilariae (**diurnal periodicity**) of *Loa loa* can be recovered on the peripheral smear. Thin smears are prepared and stained with Giemsa stain.

Summary of body sites, specimen source, collection methods, and recommended stains are shown in Table 43-1.

## DIRECT EXAMINATION

## Fecal

If fresh stool is submitted, the specimen should be examined macroscopically for barium, oily laxatives, or any antacids that may render the specimen unacceptable for ova and parasite examination. Consistency of the stool may indicate the type of protozoan present. Trophozoites may be recovered from diarrhetic (loose and watery) stool, both trophozoites and cysts from soft stool, and cysts from formed stool (Murray et al., 1995). If gross blood and mucus are present, it may indicate ulcers or purulent abscesses where amebae may be concentrated (Koneman et al., 1992).

For the detection of motility of amoebae trophozoites and flagellates from fresh stool, the direct examination (wet mount) is performed. Place a drop of saline

## Table 43–1 ▶ Specimen Collection and Processing for Parasites

| Site | Specimen Source | Collection Method | Recommended Stain |
|---|---|---|---|
| Blood | Smear or whole blood | Fresh thick and thin preps | Giemsa stain |
| | Anticoagulated blood | EDTA (1st choice) | Giemsa stain |
| | | Heparin (2nd choice) | Giemsa stain |
| Bone marrow | Aspirate | Sterile test tube | Giemsa stain |
| Central nervous system | Spinal fluid | Sterile test tube | Trichrome stain |
| | | | Giemsa stain |
| Eye | Contact lens | Sterile container with saline | Calcofluor white (cyst only) |
| | Lens solution | Sterile test tube | Giemsa (trophozoite and cysts) |
| | Scrapings | Sterile container with saline | |
| Intestinal tract | Fresh stool | Clean, dry container | Dobell and O'Connor iodine solution |
| | Preserved stool | PVA and 10% formalin | Trichrome stain |
| | Anal impression smear | Pinworm paddle/Scotch tape | |
| | Duodenal contents | Entero-Test or aspirate | Dobell and O'Connor iodine solution |
| | | | Trichrome stain (trophozoite and cysts) |
| | | | Modified Kinyoun stain (oocyst) |
| | Sigmoidoscopic | PVA | Trichrome |
| | | 10% Formalin | Modified Kinyoun stain (oocyst) |
| Lymph node | Aspirate | Sterile test tube | Giemsa stain |
| Muscle | Biopsy | Sterile container | Hematoxylin and eosin (routine histology) |
| Respiratory | Sputum | Sterile container | Saline and Dobell and O'Connor iodine solution |
| | Bronchial washing | Sterile container | Hematoxylin and eosin, Silver methenamine stain (routine histology) |
| | Adult worms | Sterile container | Modified Kinyoun stain (oocyst) |
| Skin snips | Punch biopsy | Sterile container | Giemsa stain |
| Urogenital | Vaginal discharge | Saline swab | Saline and Dobell and O'Connor iodine solution |
| | Urine | Sterile container | Saline and Dobell and O'Connor iodine solution |

and a drop of iodine on opposite ends of a slide. With an applicator stick or disposable pipet, pick up a very small portion of the specimen or mucus and add to each solution. Make a suspension dense enough to read a newspaper print in each solution. If the suspension is too thick, the diagnostic characteristics of the parasite may be obscure; too thin, parasitic forms in low numbers may be diluted out and missed (Koneman et al., 1992). Avoid large particles on the slide. Cover each preparation with a coverglass and seal with melted vaspar to prevent dehydration of mounted specimen. Systematically scan the entire saline prep under low power magnification and iodine prep under high dry. Quantitate organisms observed.

## String Test (Entero-Test)

This test consists of a coiled nylon string in a weighted gelatin capsule with the free end to be attached to the mouth of the patient. The capsule is swallowed, dissolves in the stomach, and travels to the duodenum and jejunum. After 4 hours the line is retrieved, placed in a container, and delivered to the laboratory. Using gloved two fingers or a glass slide, the bile-stained mucus is squeezed or scraped into a plastic container or Petri dish. Several drops of mucus are obtained for a wet mount and permanent prep. Examine saline preparation under low-power magnification for helminth eggs, larvae, trophozoites, and motility. The diagnostic characteristics of trophozoites should be confirmed with iodine under high-power magnification (see Figures 43-1, 43-2 and 43-3).

For the permanent prep, place one drop of mucus on a 1 × 3 inch slide with 2 to 3 drops of PVA. Mix the mucus and PVA with an applicator stick. Spread the suspension over one-third of the surface of the slide, preferably in the middle of the slide. Air dry overnight at room temperature or at 40° to 43°C for 30 to 45 min-

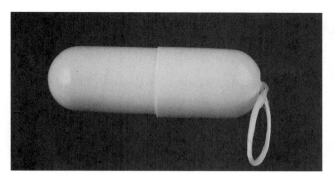

**FIGURE 43-1** Entero-Test capsule used to sample duodenal contents.

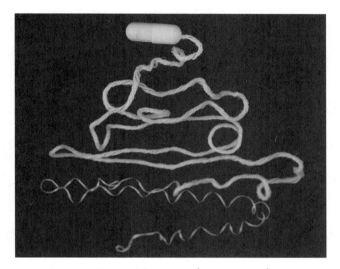

**FIGURE 43-2** Entero-Test capsule, unwound.

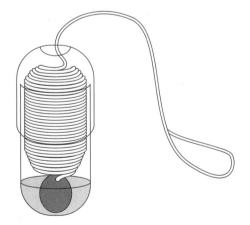

**FIGURE 43-3** Entero-Test.

utes. Stain prep with trichrome stain and examine under oil immersion for protozoan trophozoites and cysts. Quantitate if parasites observed.

## Pinworm Examination

Tape pinworm paddle onto a 3 × 2 inch slide and examine the entire paddle under low-power magnifica-

tion for *E. vermicularis* ova or larvae. Refer to Chapter 46 for diagram on a positive pinworm examination.

## Aspirates/Sigmoidoscopic Specimen

The specimen should be processed immediately on receipt. Aspirates greater than 1 mL should be centrifuged for 10 minutes at 500*g*. Wet mounts and permanent smears should be prepared, stained with trichrome and modified Kinyoun stains, and examined for protozoan and oocysts, respectively.

## CONCENTRATION TECHNIQUES FOR DETECTION OF PARASITES

### Formalin-Ethyl Acetate Concentration

The sedimentation method of fecal concentration has become part of the routine procedure for ova and parasite examination. The most popular method is the formalin-ethyl acetate concentration. It is the easiest to perform and the least subject to technical error. The specimen can be fresh or stool preserved in 10% formalin or PVA (refer to Color Plates 96 through 100).

The procedure for the microscopic examination of fecal specimens by formalin-ethyl acetate concentration follows.

For the preparation of the permanent stain smear, 2 to 3 mL of PVA suspension is poured into a test tube and centrifuged at 500*g* for 10 minutes. Decant the supernatant. Mix sediment with an applicator stick and roll the applicator stick across one-third of the surface of a microscope slide, forming a thin film. Place smear in a drying incubator for 30 to 45 minutes. Stain with trichrome stain, coverslip and examine for protozoan trophozoite and cyst stages.

### Modified Kinyoun (Acid-Fast) Stain

Profuse and watery stools, with or without mucus, collected from immunocompetent or immunosuppressed patients should be submitted in 10% formalin if *Cryptosporidium, Isospora,* and *Cyclospora* are suspected. Oocysts, the infective stage for these organisms, vary in size for each genus, cannot be detected on formalin-ethyl acetate wet mounts or trichrome stain. Permanent smear preparations are prepared from formalin-fixed material or sediment from formalin-ethyl acetate concentration if the centrifugation was at 500*g* for 10 minutes (Garcia & Bruchkner, 1993). Mix 1 drop of the fecal sediment with a dab of rabbit serum onto a 2 × 3 inch microscope slide. Make smear approximately the size of a nickel and place in a drying incubator for 30 to 45 minutes to be dry. Remove slide and place on staining rack.

Procedural guideline for the modified Kinyoun follows.

# PROCEDURE 43-1
## Formalin-Ethyl Acetate Concentration

### Principle:

Because the number of parasitic forms on a wet mount or stained smear may be too low, concentrating the sample would increase the probability of detecting and identifying any diagnostic parasitic stage. The procedure is efficient for the recovery of helminth eggs, larvae, and protozoan cysts that have been preserved with 10% formalin.

### Method:

1. Large amount of preserved fecal material (4–6 mL) is poured through a funnel/filter device to give a sediment of 0.5 to 0.75 mL in a 15-mL conical centrifuge tube.
2. Add tap water to the 15-mL mark and centrifuge at 650$g$ (1,500–1,600 rpm) for 1 minute.
3. Decant supernatant into a discard container.
4. Add 8 to 9 mL of 10% formalin to the conical tube and resuspend sediment.
5. Add approximately 3 to 4 mL of ethyl acetate. Stopper the tube, and shake it vigorously for 30 seconds. Hold tube so the stopper is directed away from your face. After 15 to 30 seconds wait, carefully remove the stopper.
6. Centrifuge for 1 minute at 500$g$. Four layers should result: (1) ethyl acetate layer, (2) debris plug, (3) formalin layer, and (4) sediment.

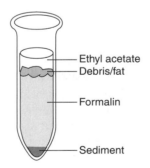

Ethyl acetate
Debris/fat

Formalin

Sediment

**FIGURE 43-4** Sedimentation tube after centrifugation.

With an applicator stick, free the debris plug from the sides of the tube. Carefully decant the top three layers. Wipe the sides of the tube with a cotton-tipped swab. Mix the sediment with the small amount of fluid that drains back from the sides of the tube.

7. Add a few drops of 10% formalin to the sediment if necessary.
8. Prepare a saline and iodine wet mounts from the sediment. The suspension should be dense enough to read a newspaper print in each solution.
9. Cover each preparation with a coverglass and seal with melted vaspar to prevent dehydration.
10. Systematically, scan the entire saline prep under low-power magnification and iodine prep under high dry. Examine for helminth eggs, larvae, or protozoan cysts.

### Quality Control:

1. Check formalin and saline each time they are used. Reagents should appear clear, without any visible contamination.
2. Concentrate known positive specimens and verify organism recovery at least quarterly and after the centrifuge has been recalibrated.

### Expected Results:

1. Protozoan cysts, helminth eggs and larvae may be seen and identified. Protozoan trophozoites are less likely to be seen.
2. Results obtained should be confirmed by a permanent stain (trichrome) smear. Some protozoa are very small and difficult to be identified by the direct wet smears alone.

### References:

Garcia & Bruckner, 1993; Isenberg, 1992; Koneman et al., 1992; Melvin & Brooke, 1980.

## Blood

For the detection of intraerythrocytic parasites and filarial nematodes, thin and thick blood smears are prepared, separately or combination of both (Garcia & Bruchkner, 1993), from whole or anticoagulated blood.

A **thin smear** (for species identification) (Howard et al., 1994) is prepared in the same manner as a differential smear for white blood cell count on an alcohol-cleaned microscopic slide. The **thick smear** (to detect light parasitic infection or when thin film is negative)

# PROCEDURE 43-2
## Modified Kinyoun Acid-Fast Stain

### Principles:

*Cryptosporidium, Isospora* and *Cyclospora* species have now been recognized as a cause of severe diarrhea in immunodeficient patients, and can cause transient diarrhea in immunocompetent individuals. Because the oocysts cannot be detected on a trichrome-stained smear, modified Kinyoun acid-fast stain is recommended. The following procedure may be used on formalin-fixed material or sediments from formalin-ethyl acetate concentration.

### Method:

1. Flood smear(s) with carbol fuchsin stain. Let stand at room temperature for 5 minutes. DO NOT HEAT.
2. Rinse with tap water and drain.
3. Decolorize with 3% HCl (acid-alcohol) for 2 minutes, or until no more color runs off the slide.
4. Rinse with tap water and drain.
5. Counterstain with brilliant green K stain for 2 minutes.
6. Rinse with tap water and drain.
7. Thoroughly air dry smear(s).
8. Place a drop of permount onto the smear and cover with a coverglass.
9. Examine smear microscopically with 40X objective. Examine at least 200 to 300 high-power fields.

### Quality Control:

1. A positive control slide of *Cryptosporidium parvum* and negative control slide without *C. parvum* from 10% formalin preserved specimen will be stained and processed with each staining batch run and with each new reagent prepared.
2. Check preparation of sample (macroscopically) for adherence to the slide.

### Expected Results:

1. Oocysts of *Cryptosporidium, Isospora,* and *Cyclospora* species will be readily seen.
2. *Cyclospora* oocysts (8–9 μm in diameter) are twice the size of *Cryptosporidium* oocysts (4–5 μm in diameter) and tend to be acid-fast variable.
3. There is usually a range of color intensity of the oocyst from pink to red to deep purple.
4. Oocysts will stain pink to red to deep purple and the background would be green due to the counterstain, brilliant green K.

### References:

Isenberg, 1992; Murray et al., 1995)

---

(Howard et al., 1994) is prepared at the opposite end by placing 1 drop of blood onto the slide. Using the pointed edge of a glass slide, the blood is spread over an area about the size of a dime. The thickness of the smear should be 50 μm or less (Brown, 1975) or dense enough to read a newspaper print through it. Allow the thick smear to air dry for 6 to 8 hours or overnight. The thin smear is fixed in methanol and air dried in a vertical position with the thick film up. When the slide is completely dry, the slide is stained with 1 part Giemsa stock solution with 50 parts of phosphate buffer for 50 minutes. The slide is then rinsed with buffered or tap water. Drain and allow the slide to air dry in a vertical position with the thin film up. Add a coverslip to the slide and examine for the presence of blood or tissue parasites (*Plasmodium* species, *Babesia* species, filarial nematodes, etc.).

## STAINS

### Dobell and O'Connor's Iodine Solution

In the direct and formalin-ethyl acetate examination, Dobell and O'Connor's iodine solution (Melvin & Brooke, 1980) is used in the iodine mount to stain the cyst's cytoplasm and nuclear material. It is a weak solution and is stable for a period of 3 weeks. If it appears faded or control organisms are not properly stained, a pinch of iodine crystals can be added and the solution is shaken until the color is a "strong tea" appearance. The remaining solution should be stored in a brown bottle.

If the cyst of a protozoan is stained properly, the cytoplasm is yellow and the chromatin material stains brown to black. The glycogen mass, if present within the cytoplasm, would stain reddish brown. Chromotoidal bars (bodies) would be less visible in the iodine solution than the saline prep.

# PROCEDURE 43-3
## Wheatley's Modification of Gomori's Trichrome Stain

### Principle:

A rapid, simple procedure that produces uniformly well stained smears of intestinal protozoa, human cells, yeast cells, and artifact material. It facilitates the identification of trophozoites and cysts, confirmation of species, and as a permanent record of organisms recovered.

### Method:

Technique for PVA-fixed specimens
1. Place prepared slide(s) in staining rack into the first coplin jar. Stain smears according to the staining time given:

| COPLIN JAR | REAGENT | STAINING TIME: |
|---|---|---|
| # 1 | 70% ethanol plus iodine | 10–20 minutes |
| # 2 | 70% ethanol | 5 minutes |
| # 3 | 70% ethanol | 5 minutes |
| # 4 | Trichrome stain | 8 minutes |
| # 5 | 90% glacial acetic acid alcohol | 3–5 seconds (briefly dip in and out) |
| # 6 | 95% ethanol | rinse briefly |
| # 7 | 95% ethanol | rinse briefly |
| # 8 | absolute alcohol | 5 minutes |
| # 9 | carbo-xylene | 5 minutes |
| #10 | xylene | 10 minutes |

2. Remove slide from #10 coplin jar and add several drops of permount onto smear. Carefully place a 22 × 40 mm coverslip on the smear. Avoid bubble formation.
3. Allow smear to dry overnight or 1 hour at 37°C.
4. Examine smear microscopically with 100X objective. Examine at least 200 to 300 oil immersion fields.

### Quality Control:

1. Prepare and stain a smear of PVA fixed fecal specimen containing protozoa or PVA-preserved negative stool specimen to which buffy coat cells have been added weekly.
2. Include a quality control smear when the decolorizing reagent has been changed, new lot of reagents have been added, or new reagents have been added to the dish.
3. Cover all staining dishes to prevent evaporation.
4. If xylene becomes cloudy, replace before staining.

### Expected Results:

1. Protozoan trophozoites and cysts will be readily seen.
2. Cytoplasm of trophozoites or cysts stain blue-green, and chromatin material, chromotoidal bodies, red blood cells (ingested), and bacteria stain red or purplish red.
3. Background material appears green and larvae or eggs stain red.

### References:

Isenberg, 1992; Melvin & Brooke, 1980

## Wheatley's Modification of Gomori's Trichrome Stain

Permanent stains are recommended for routine ova and parasite examination. They are used to identify trophozoite and cyst forms, for confirmation of species, and as a permanent record of the organisms recovered from concentrated techniques (Isenberg, 1992). A permanent stain that is stable, rapid, and used to stain fecal smears prepared from fresh, sediment (formalin-ethyl acetate) or preservative (PVA) specimen is Wheatley's modification of Gomori's trichrome stain. Intestinal protozoan, human cells (polymorphonucleated cells, red blood cells, macrophages, etc.), yeast or mold, and artifact materials are stained uniformly. The cytoplasm of trophozoites or cysts is stained blue-green, and chromatin material, chromotoidal bodies, red blood cells (ingested), and bacteria stained red or purplish red. Background material appears green and larvae or eggs would stain red.

## Giemsa Stain

For the detection of blood and tissue parasites, the most dependable stain is Giemsa stain with azure B. It will stain and differentiate cellular elements from intraerythrocytic parasites. Red blood cells stain pale red, the nuclei of polymorphonucleated white blood cells stain purple with pale purple cytoplasm, and neutrophilic and eosinophilic granules stain deep pink to purple and bright purple to red, respectively. Nuclear material of intraerythrocytic and blood parasites (*Plasmodium* species, *Babesia* species, etc.) would stain red to purple red with a blue cytoplasm and Schuffner's granules within the red blood cell would stain red. The

sheath of microfilariae (*W. bancrofti* or *B. malayi*) may or may not stain with Giemsa but the nuclei would stain blue to purple (Isenberg, 1992).

A summary of stains, applications, and purposes is shown in Table 43-2.

## Table 43–2 ▶ Stains Used for Parasites

| Stain | Application | Purpose |
|---|---|---|
| Dobell and O'Connor's iodine solution | Fresh and preserved stool, duodenal contents, sputum, vaginal discharge, urine | Stain cyst's cytoplasm (yellow) and nuclear material (brown to black) |
| Wheatley's modification of Gomori's trichrome stain | Preserved stool, duodenal contents, sigmoidoscopic, spinal fluid | Used to identify trophozoites and cysts, for confirmation of species, and as a permanent record of organisms recovered. |
| | | Cytoplasm of trophozoites or cysts stain blue-green, and chromatin material, chromotoidal bodies, and blood cells (ingested), and bacteria stain red or purplish red. Background material appears green and larvae or eggs stain red. |
| Modified Kinyoun acid-fast stain | Stool, bronchial washing and sigmoidoscopic in 10% formalin | Stains the oocyst of *Cryptosporidium*, *Isospora*, and *Cyclospora* pink to red to deep purple. Background material appears green or blue depending on the counterstain used. |
| Giemsa stain | Blood with or without anticoagulant, punch biopsy, bone marrow or lymph node aspirate, contact lens solution | Stains the nuclear material of intraerythrocytic parasite red to purple red with a blue cytoplasm. Schuffner's granules within the erytrocyte would stain red. Microfilariae sheath may or may not stain but the nuclei would stain blue to purple. |

## SUMMARY

▶ For accurate and reliable identification, specimens must be collected and handled properly.

▶ The type of material to be examined depends on the parasite and its location within the host.

▶ Fecal specimens should be submitted in a two-vial preservative system kit, whereas urine, aspirates, or biopsy samples should be delivered to the laboratory immediately after collection.

▶ Collection of cerebrospinal fluid (CSF), tissue, or corneal scrapings from the affected site must be obtained aseptically and kept at room tempera-

ture. Personnel must take added precautions by wearing gloves and processing the sample in a biologic safety cabinet.

▶ Types of procedures used to recover and identify parasites are direct wet mounts, concentration techniques, permanent stain preparations, and cultivation.

▶ When the direct and concentrated techniques are negative for parasites, serodiagnostic tests for antibody or antigen detection are requested when the suspected parasite is not generally found in stool examination, aspirates, or tissue samples.

## Review Questions

1. Parasites that may be found in sputum specimens include:
   a. *Paragonimus westermani* and *Entamoeba coli*.
   b. *Iodamoeba butschlii* and *Ascaris lumbricoides*.
   c. *Strongyloides stercoralis* and *Entamoeba hartmanii*.
   d. *Paragonimus westermani* and hookworm.

2. The trophozoite stage of a parasite can be recovered from a soft fecal specimen submitted for parasitic examination if the specimen:
   a. is incubated at 37°C for 24 hours.
   b. is placed in 10% formalin 15 minutes after defecation.
   c. is stored at refrigerator temperature.
   d. is placed into PVA solution 30 minutes after defecation.

## CASE STUDY

A 3-year-old girl was referred for evaluation of diarrhea. One month prior, the patient had been having chronic abdominal pain and gas to frank diarrhea for the preceding 1 to 2 weeks. On the morning of her evaluation, the patient's diarrhea was yellow, foul-smelling, and frothy. Specimen was collected for culture and ova and parasite examination. After 48 hours, the stool culture was reported as negative for enteric pathogens and the ova and parasite examination was positive for pear-shaped trophozoites 12 to 15 μm long with two bilateral nuclei.

**Questions:**

1. Which parasite was found in the stool specimen?

2. How is this parasite transmitted?

3. How can infection with this organism be prevented?

---

3. In cases of suspected infection with *Enterobius vermicularis*, the preferred specimen is:
   a. fresh stool.
   b. formalin-preserved stool.
   c. cellulose acetate.
   d. string test.

4. *Schistosoma haematobium* is best detected by examination of:
   a. urine sediment.
   b. rectal biopsy.
   c. fecal specimen.
   d. culture material.

5. When stool examination is negative, the preferred specimen for the diagnosis of paragonimiasis is:
   a. bile drainage.
   b. duodenal contents.
   c. expectorated sputum.
   d. rectal biopsy.

6. *Enterobius vermicularis* infection is usually diagnosed by:
   a. finding adult worms in feces.
   b. finding larvae in feces.
   c. finding larvae in perianal specimens.
   d. finding eggs in perianal specimens.

7. In which specimen is the eggs of *Schistosoma haematobium* most likely to be found?
   a. Sputum
   b. Feces

   c. Urine
   d. Perianal

8. Immunocompromised hosts have been found to have an increased susceptibility to:
   a. *Babesia*.
   b. *Cryptosporidium*.
   c. *Strongyloides*.
   d. *Cyclospora*.
   e. all of the above
   f. none of the above

9. Knowledge of its nocturnal periodicity is especially important in the diagnosis of:
   a. *Loa loa*.
   b. *Dracunculus* species.
   c. *Wuchereria bancrofti*.
   d. *Plasmodium* species.

10. Hematuria is a typical sign of human infection caused by:
    a. *Trichinella spiralis*.
    b. *Trichomonas vaginalis*.
    c. *Schistosoma haematobium*.
    d. *Trichomonas hominis*.

## ▶ REFERENCES & RECOMMENDED READING

Aldeen, W. E., Hale, D., Robison, A. J., & Carroll, K. (1995). Evaluation of a commercially available ELISA assay for detection of *Giardia lamblia* in fecal specimens. *Diagnostic Microbiology and Infectious Disease, 21,* 77–79.

Brown, H. W. (1975). *Basic clinical parasitology* (4th ed.). New York: Appleton-Century-Crofts.

Dalton, H. P. & Nottebart, H. C., Jr. (1986). *Interpretative medical microbiology.* New York: Churchill Livingstone.

Garcia, L. S., & Shimizu, R. Y. (1993). Medical parasitology: Update on diagnostic techniques and laboratory safety. *Laboratory Medicine, 24,* 81–87.

Garcia, L. S., & Bruckner, D. A. (1993). *Diagnostic medical parasitology* (2nd ed.). Washington, DC: ASM Press.

Gorbach, S. L., Bartlett, J. G., & Blacklow, N. R. (1992). *Infectious disease.* Philadelphia: Saunders.

Hiatt, R. A., Markell, E. K., & Ng, E. (1995). How many stool examinations are necessary to detect pathogenic intestinal protozoa? *American Journal of Tropical Medicine, 53,* 36–39.

Howard, B. J., Keiser, J. F., Smith, T. F., Weissfield, A. S., & Tilton, R. C. (1994). *Clinical and pathogenic microbiology* (2nd ed.). St. Louis: Mosby–Year Book.

Isenberg, H. D. (1992). *Clinical microbiology procedures handbook.* Washington, DC: ASM Press.

Koneman, E. W., Allen, S. D., Janda, W. M., Schreckenberger, P. C., & Winn, W. C., Jr. (1992). *Diagnostic microbiology* (4th ed.). Philadelphia: Lippincott.

Melvin, D., & Brooke, M. (1980). *Laboratory procedures for the diagnosis of intestinal parasites.* Atlanta, GA: Centers for Disease Control.

Morris, A. J., Smith, L. K., Mirrett, S., & Reller, L. B. (1996). Cost and time savings following introduction of rejection criteria for clinical specimens. *Journal of Clinical Microbiology, 34,* 355–357.

Murray, P. R., Baron, E. J., Pfaller, M. A., Tenover, F. C., & Yolken, R. H. (1995). *Manual of clinical microbiology* (6th ed.). Washington, DC: ASM Press.

Scheffler, E. H., & Van Etta, L. L. (1994). Evaluation of rapid commercial enzyme immunoassay for detection of *Giardia lamblia* in formalin-preserved stool specimens. *Journal of Clinical Microbiology, 32,* 1807–1808.

# CHAPTER 44
# Intestinal and Atrial Protozoans

Lisa Shimeld, MS

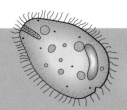

## Microbes in the News

### *Cryptosporidium* Infections Associated with Swimming Pools—Dane County, Wisconsin, 1993

An estimated 403,000 people with cryptosporidiosis were reported in March and April of 1993 in the Milwaukee area. In late August 1993, two clusters of persons with laboratory-confirmed cryptosporidiosis were identified in Dane County (approximately 80 miles west of Milwaukee). Cryptosporidiosis is a diarrheal disease that is caused by the protozoan pathogen *Cryptosporidium parvum*. The disease is most often transmitted by ingestion of the oocyst stage of *Cryptosporidium* in water contaminated with sewage.

The outbreak investigation determined that several members of a girls' swim team had reported experiencing severe diarrhea to their physicians. One of the girls had a laboratory-confirmed case of cryptosporidiosis. The swimming pool where the team practiced was inspected by public health officials, and 31 of the other patrons using the pool were interviewed. Seventeen of the 31 patrons (55%) reported having watery diarrhea for 2 or more days with onset during July or August. Eight of the 17 (47%) experienced the diarrhea for more than 5 days. Four persons who reported seeking medical care tested positive for cryptosporidiosis.

Public health nurses identified a second cluster of nine individuals with laboratory-confirmed cryptosporidiosis in Dane County by following up case reports submitted by physicians. Seven of these people reported swimming at a large outdoor pool. A phone survey of Dane County residents coupled with laboratory confirmation of cryptosporidiosis helped public health officials estimate the scope of the outbreak.

As a result of the investigation, Dane County, state, and local public health officials implemented five recommendations. The recommendations were (1) closing pools linked to infection and hyperchlorinating the pools to achieve disinfection; (2) advising all area pool managers of the increased potential for waterborne transmission of *Cryptosporidium;* (3) posting signs at area pools stating that persons with diarrhea or those who have had diarrhea in the last 14 days should not enter the pool; (4) notifying area physicians of the increased potential for cryptosporidiosis in the community and requesting that patients with watery diarrhea be tested for *Cryptosporidium;* and (5) maintaining laboratory-based surveillance in the community to determine whether transmission was occurring at other sites.

Source: Bongard, J., et al. (1994, August). *Cryptosporidium* infections associated with swimming pools—Dane County, Wisconsin, 1993. *MedNews.* Online: America Online. 12 January, 1997. This article can be found at http://ch.nus.sg/MEDLINE/aug94/7381_html

## KEY TERMS

Ameboma
Amebiasis
Amebic dysentery
Axostyle
Balantidiasis
Chromatodial body
Cryptosporidiosis
Extraintestinal amebiasis
Formalin-ethyl acetate sedimentation

Giardial malabsorption syndrome
Giardiasis
Gingival pockets
Isosporiasis
Linin
Macrogametes
Microgametes
Oocyst
Parabasal bodies

Pellicle
Peripheral chromatin
Polar tube
Proteolytic enzymes
Sheather's sugar concentration flocculation
Sigmoidoscopic aspirates
Spontaneous recovery
Trichomoniasis
Undulating membrane

## LEARNING OBJECTIVES

Upon successful completion of this chapter, the student should be able to:

1. Define the key terms.
2. Give examples of intestinal and atrial protozoans that cause disease in humans.
3. Describe the characteristics of intestinal and atrial protozoans that cause disease in humans.
4. Discuss the life cycles of the protozoans covered in this chapter.

5. Indicate how human infections with intestinal and atrial protozoans are diagnosed.
6. Give an example of drugs that are used to treat these infections.
7. Explain how intestinal and atrial protozoans are transmitted to humans.
8. Differentiate intestinal and atrial protozoans of humans from the artifacts that may be found in clinical samples.

## INTRODUCTION

As mentioned in Chapter 42, the protozoans are unicellular eucaryotes and are classified into four groups. These groups are the ameba, the flagellates, the ciliates, and the coccidia and microsporidians. This chapter considers the intestinal protozoa of humans and those that inhabit the mouth, the upper respiratory tract, and the urogenital tract. Although several species of lumen-dwelling protozoa are parasitic, many are commensals and others are of questionable pathogenicity. Protozoan parasites of the blood and tissues are discussed in Chapter 45.

## AMEBA

The ameba are primitive protozoans and are the least evolved members of kingdom Protista. They are members of the phylum Sarcomastigopora, which also includes the flagellates. Ameba are motile by cytoplasmic extensions called pseudopods and most species have cyst and trophozoite stages in their life cycle. The cyst stage is the infective stage and humans acquire the

organism by ingesting it in feces-contaminated water or food. The active (or vegetative) stage that feeds and moves is called the trophozoite. In most species of ameba the trophozoite is not infectious because it is unable to survive the harsh conditions of the stomach. Ingestion of trophozoites does not result in infection.

*Entamoeba histolytica* is the most important intestinal pathogenic ameba in humans. Estimates of the prevalence of infection with *E. histolytica* are 10% worldwide. Another potential pathogenic ameba is *Blastocystis hominis,* an unusual organism that is commonly found in human feces. Although it was once considered a fungus it is now believed to be a protozoan. The classification of *Blastocystis* is still the subject of debate. Some authors include *Blastocystis* with the coccidians, whereas others consider the organism an ameba. *B. hominis* moves and feeds with pseudopodia and for that reason is included in this section (see Table 44-1).

Most ameba that occur in humans are commensals and a few are of questionable pathogenicity. Ameba species found in humans that are nonpathogenic include *Entamoeba gingivalis, Entamoeba coli, Endolimax nana,* and *Iodamoeba butschlii. Entamoeba hartmanni* is of questionable pathogenicity and was once considered a

## Table 44–1 ► Characteristics to Identify Intestinal Ameba: Trophozoite Form

| Characteristic | Entamoeba histolytica | Entamoeba hartmanni | Entamoeba coli | Endolimax nana | Iodamoeba butschlii |
|---|---|---|---|---|---|
| Comments | Ingested RBCs may be seen in vacuoles | Bacteria may be seen in vacuoles; no RBCs are seen | Bacteria may be seen in vacuoles, no RBCs are seen | Bacteria may be seen in vacuoles, no RBCs seen | Bacteria may be seen in vacuoles, no RBCs are seen |
| Cytoplasm | Granular endoplasm; wide, clear ectoplasm | Finely granular, no clear distinction between ectoplasm and endoplasm | Granular, no clear distinction between ectoplasm and endoplasm | Granular, multiple vacuoles | Coarsely granular with multiple vacuoles |
| Diameter (μm) | 10–60 | 5–12 | 15–50 | 6–12 | 10–20 |
| Karyosome | Single, small, centrally located | Small, centrally located; rarely eccentric | Large, irregular, usually eccentric | Large, irregular shapes | Large, central, surrounded by refractile granules |
| Motility | Rapid amoeboid with blunt or long, thin pseudopods | Slow by a single pseudopod | Sluggish with multiple blunt, broad pseudopods | Sluggish | Sluggish |
| Nucleus | Single—difficult to see in unstained preparations | Single—difficult to see in unstained preparations | Single—easy to see in unstained preparations | Single, lobulated | Single and large—difficult to see in unstained preparations |
| Size Usual range (μm) | 15–20 | 8–10 | 20–25 | 8–10 | 12–15 |

RBC, red blood cell

smaller variant of *E. histolytica*. Most clinicians believe that *E. hartmanni* is nonpathogenic. All of these species inhabit the large intestine with the exception of *E. gingivalis*, which is found in the mouth. The five species of ameba that are usually commensals (or questionable) in humans are described here so that they can be distinguished from the pathogenic *E. histolytica*. Another species, *Entamoeba polecki*, is an intestinal parasite in pigs and monkeys and is morphologically similar to *E. histolytica*. It is also a rare incidental parasite of humans and may cause diarrhea. (See Figure 44-1 for geographic distribution of various infectious diseases.)

## Entamoeba histolytica

*Entamoeba histolytica* is a relatively common intestinal parasite with cosmopolitan distribution. Infection with *E. histolytica* occurs from pole to pole but is most common in underdeveloped tropical countries. The disease caused by *E. histolytica* is called **amebiasis** or **amebic dysentery**. The ameba was first described in 1875 by Losch, who discovered the ameba in the feces of a young Russian man with severe dysentery. He also experimentally produced intestinal lesions in a dog, providing further evidence of the pathogenic nature of the ameba. The pathogenicity of *E. histolytica* was definitely established in 1913 when Walker and Sellards fed cysts to volunteers. The experiment led to the development of intestinal lesions in many of the volunteers.

*Entamoeba histolytica* is distinguished from other intestinal ameba primarily on the basis of morphology. Trophozoites are round or oval, and vary in size from 10 to 60 μm. They average slightly more than 20 μm (see Figure 44-2). One or more blunt or thin pseudopods may be observed. Trophozoites are usually actively motile in freshly passed feces. Motility can often be enhanced by warming a wet mount of the feces on a slide warmer. This is only helpful with viable cells and will not revive ameba that have been kept for too long at room temperature (Markell, Voge, & John, 1992).

A clear, wide, refractive ectoplasm surrounds a highly granulated endoplasm in *E. histolytica*. There are usually no bacteria seen in the endoplasm of trophozoites but red blood cells in various stages of digestion may be observed in invasive cases. Freshly ingested red blood cells appear as pale greenish, refractive bodies in the cytoplasm. A clearly defined nucleus is observed on staining with hematoxylin or trichrome and is one of the most characteristic features of *E. histolytica*. The inside of the nuclear envelope is uniformly lined with fine granules of chromatin (referred to as **peripheral chromatin**) and a small but well defined karyosome is centrally located. Thin fibrils made of **linin** radiate from around the karyosome to the periphery of the nucleus. Variations in nuclear structure do occur and some examples are shown in Figure 44-3.

The cysts of *E. histolytica* are round, oval, or irregular in shape and have a hyaline wall (see Figure 44-4). The average diameter of the cysts is 10 to 20 μm and when observed in unstained preparations they are

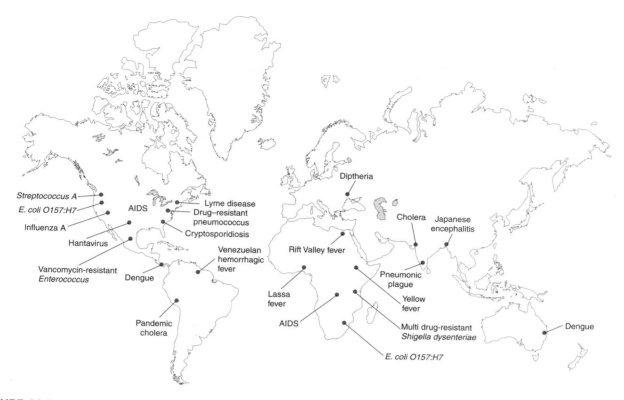

**FIGURE 44-1** Geographic distribution of various infectious diseases.

highly refractive. Cysts contain one, two, or four nuclei (or rarely more) that are usually not visible in unstained preparations. Cysts may also contain one or more **chromatodial bodies** that are composed primarily of crystalline RNA. In unstained preparations these elongated bar-shaped bodies appear as clear spaces in the cytoplasm. They may be short, or only slightly shorter than the diameter of the cyst, and have rounded or square ends. Occasionally, chromatodial bodies are cigar-shaped or ovoid. One or more chromatodial bodies are often seen flanking a glycogen vacuole in cysts having one or two nuclei but are usually not present in (mature) cysts with four nuclei. Glycogen vacuoles and

chromatodial bodies may represent stores of food. Chromatodial bodies are named for their similar appearance to the chromatin of the nucleus when stained with hematoxylin. In trichrome preparations chromatodial bodies stain bright red.

An estimated 10% of the world's population is infected with *E. histolytica* with the highest prevalence rates occurring in areas of crowding and poor sanitation, especially in the tropics. Africa, India, Latin America, and Southeast Asia have significant health problems associated with the ameba. Prevalence rates as high as 50% to 80% have been reported from some tropical areas. In all areas where *E. histolytica* occurs 85% to 95% of infections are asymptomatic. There are an esti-

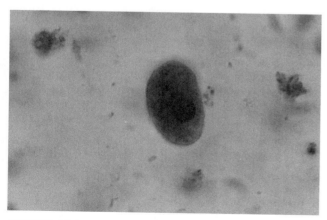

**FIGURE 44-2** Trophozoites of *E. histolytica*.

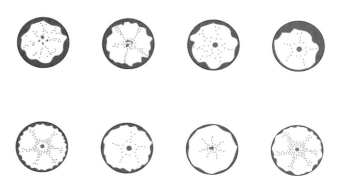

**FIGURE 44-3** Nuclear variations in *E. histolytica*.

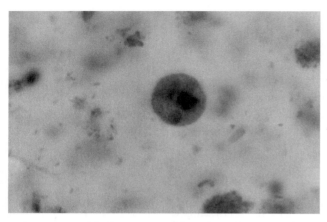

**FIGURE 44-4** Trichrome- and hematoxylin-stained *E. histolytica* cysts with chromatodial bodies.

mated 50 million cases worldwide of amebiasis with 40,000 to 50,000 deaths annually (KnowledgeBase: Amebiasis).

Infection with *E. histolytica* occurs when the cyst stage is ingested in food or water contaminated with feces. Person-to-person transmission of amebiasis is also possible. This usually occurs through anal intercourse and amebiasis is seen with increasing frequency in homosexual men in the United States. The use of night soil (human feces as fertilizer) also contributes to the transmission of *E. histolytica*. Asymptomatic carriers of *E. histolytica* are more important in the epidemiology of amebiasis than are symptomatic individuals. The feces of asymptomatic carriers contain the infective cyst stage of the parasite, whereas individuals with diarrhea or dysentery pass the noninfective trophozoite.

On ingestion, each cyst produces eight trophozoites, which are released in the small intestine. In most cases *E. histolytica* resides in the large intestine of the host as a harmless commensal feeding on resident bacteria and yeasts. In other individuals the ameba becomes invasive, producing **proteolytic enzymes** that allow the organism to penetrate the intestinal mucosa and invade other parts of the body.

The primary infection may be subclinical, or the patient may experience symptoms that include anorexia, weight loss, abdominal pain and cramps, and chronic diarrhea or dysentery. Once the barrier provided by the intestinal mucosa is penetrated, the proteolytic enzymes released by the ameba produce flask-shaped lesions called **amebomas**. The ameba feeds on host red blood cells and other tissues. Secondary infection of the lesion by the normal flora of the gastrointestinal tract, especially *Escherichia coli,* is common and results in a fever. The trophozoites may "hitch a ride" to other parts of the body through the circulatory or lymphatic system resulting in **extraintestinal amebiasis**. This secondary infection with *E. histolytica* may occur in the liver, lungs, brain, and occasionally other sites (see Figure 44-5). Uncomplicated attacks last up to 2 weeks and recur-

rences are common unless diagnosis is made and the individual is successfully treated. An adapted version of the clinical classification developed by the World Health Organization (WHO) in their report on amebiasis in 1969 is shown as follows:

**I.** Asymptomatic infections (85–95% of cases)
**II.** Symptomatic infections (5–15% of cases)
    **A.** Intestinal amebiasis
        **1.** Dysentery
        **2.** Chronic diarrhea
    **B.** Extraintestinal amebiasis (about 5% of symptomatic cases)
        **1.** Hepatic
        **2.** Pulmonary
        **3.** Other sites are very rare

All percentages given are approximate.

Diagnosis of amebiasis is based primary on the presence of *E. histolytica* trophozoites or cysts in the feces, or by examination of **sigmoidoscopic aspirates** (Figure 44-6). Three or more fecal samples may be required for successful diagnosis because trophozoites may be passed intermittently in active cases. Fecal samples may be concentrated to detect cysts. Some serologic tests have been developed for *E. histolytica* but are not yet routinely used. They include enzyme immunoassays that can detect *E. histolytica* with a sensitivity that is probably superior to traditional microscopic examinations (Ryan, 1994). The potential value of these tests for routine use remains to be established. Extraintestinal amebiasis is more difficult to diagnose than intestinal amebiasis. Serologic tests that detect antibodies in the blood in response to *E. histolytica* can be helpful, but are often negative in asymptomatic individuals. Several instant tests, such as a latex agglutination test, are commercially available.

Several drugs are used to treat amebiasis. The choice depends primarily on the clinical stage of the infection. Metronidazole (Flagyl) and iodoquinol are antiparasitic drugs that are often used to treat amebiasis. Nausea is a possible side effect of these drugs and may necessitate intravenous therapy until the medication can be tolerated by mouth. Investigational drugs including dehydroemetine (Mebadin) and diloxanide furoate (Furamide) are also available. Early treatment is usually effective in elimination of amebiasis but the death rate is high in untreated individuals. Commensal ameba are usually not treated.

Prevention of amebiasis is largely dependent on the availability of pure water. Implementation of water treatment and adequate facilities for sewage processing helps to break the chain of transmission. When necessary, water is easily disinfected by boiling or treating with iodine. When traveling to countries where amebiasis is endemic, avoid drinking unbottled water (it is preferable to drink water bottled in the United States) or using ice cubes that could be made from contami-

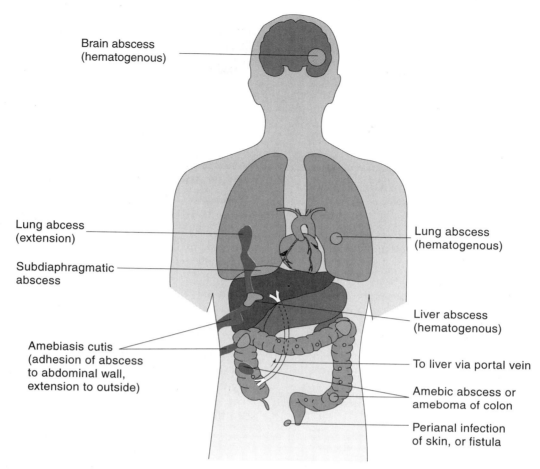

Brain abscess
(hematogenous)

Lung abcess
(extension)

Subdiaphragmatic
abscess

Amebiasis cutis
(adhesion of abscess
to abdominal wall,
extension to outside)

Lung abscess
(hematogenous)

Liver abscess
(hematogenous)

To liver via portal vein

Amebic abscess or
ameboma of colon

Perianal infection
of skin, or fistula

**FIGURE 44-5** Common sites of lesions in amebiasis.

nated water. Also avoid eating fresh fruits and vegetables (that are unpeeled) that may have been watered or washed with contaminated water.

## Blastocystis hominis

*Blastocystis hominis* is an interesting and somewhat controversial organism. It is a common resident of the

gastrointestinal tract and is frequently found in fecal specimens. Once classified as a fungus, *Blastocystis* is now considered a protozoan. This reclassification is primarily due to the inability of *B. hominis* to grow on artificial media used in mycology, and the fact that it reproduces by binary fission and sporulation rather than budding. There is also some controversy over whether *B. hominis* is always a commensal or if it can

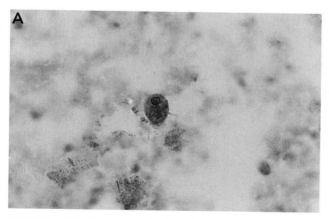
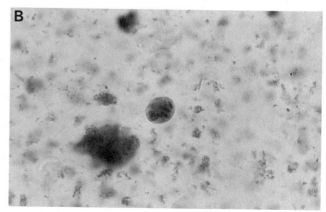

**FIGURE 44-6** *Entoamoeba histolytica*. **A.** trophozoite; **B.** cyst.

be pathogenic causing diarrhea and other symptoms. Although the protozoan is frequently found in the feces of people who are free of symptoms, it is also observed in symptomatic individuals in the absence of other pathogenic microorganisms. Evidence linking *B. hominis* to disease is incomplete; however, it has never been demonstrated to be invasive and no toxins have been identified.

*Blastocystis hominis* is usually round but several morphologic forms have been identified (see Figure 44-7). The organism varies in size from 5 to 30 μm and is a strict anaerobe. A membrane-bound central body takes up to 90% of the cell and functions in sexual and asexual reproduction. *B. hominis* feeds on bacteria and debris in the intestine. The protozoan moves and feeds with pseudopodia (Figure 44-8).

Although the primary means of transmission of *B. hominis* is not yet well defined, it is assumed to be acquired through the oral-fecal route in contaminated food or water. Symptoms are most frequently exhibited in immunocompromised patients, especially in those with acquired immunodeficiency syndrome (AIDS), and with individuals who have traveled abroad. Sympto-

matic patients experience diarrhea, abdominal cramps, nausea, vomiting, and fever.

Diagnosis is based on identification of *B. hominis* in the fecal specimens of patients who lack any other organisms that might cause similar symptoms. Wet mounts may not reveal the protozoan and it is easiest to observe in trichrome stains. Metronidazole and other drugs are used to treat symptomatic infections.

## Ameba That Are Usually Commensals in Humans

*Entamoeba gingivalis* is a nonpathogenic resident of the mouth that resides in the tartar of the teeth and **gingival pockets**. The prevalence of *E. gingivalis* ranges from 10% in persons with healthy mouths to 95% in individuals with diseased teeth and gums (Neva & Brown, 1994). Although the presence of the ameba is common in individuals with pyorrhea, no link has been established between the two. A large number of vacuoles containing bacteria and host cells in various stages of digestion can be observed.

*Entamoeba hartmanni* (see Figure 44-9) is considered by most clinicians to be nonpathogenic and was long considered a small variant of *E. histolytica*. Prevalence of 10% to 20% infection with *E. hartmanni* is seen throughout the world. Because the morphologic

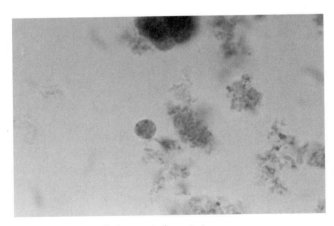

**FIGURE 44-7** *Blastocystis hominis.*

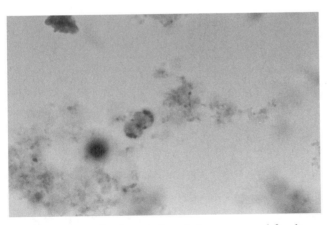

**FIGURE 44-8** *Blastocystis hominis* moves and feeds with pseudopodia.

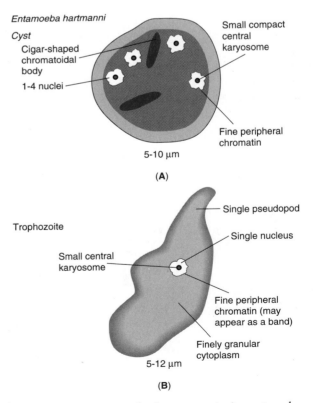

**FIGURE 44-9** *Entamoeba hartmanni.* **A.** cyst and **B.** trophozoite.

similarities between the two are confusing, they are separated primarily on the basis of size. Their characteristic nuclei also aid in identification of the amoeba. The round trophozoites of *E. hartmanni* range from 5 to 12 µm in diameter and are usually well below the 20 µm average of *E. histolytica*. Mature cysts have four nuclei and are often irregularly shaped. Cysts range in size from 5 to 10 µm. Nuclear variations are seen in *E. hartmanni* and are the same as those seen in *E. histolytica*. There are significant serologic differences between the two ameba.

*Entamoeba coli* is another nonpathogenic ameba that may inhabit the large intestine and is occasionally observed in human feces (see Figure 44-10). The trophozoites of *E. coli* range from 15 to 50 µm and often are slightly larger than the trophozoites of *E. histolytica*. Although bacteria are often present in vacuoles, red blood cells are rarely ingested by *Entamoeba coli*. *E. coli* cysts range in size from 10 to 35 µm and are definitely larger than those of *E. histolytica*. *E. coli* cysts contain from one to eight nuclei.

The similarities in their morphologies makes it somewhat difficult to distinguish between the two ameba. This confusion can lead to unnecessary treatment of a nonpathogenic ameba or omission of appropriate therapy for a pathogen (Markell et al., 1992).

*Endolimax nana* is a small ameba that resides in the large intestine as a commensal when the cyst is ingested in feces-contaminated food or water. The prevalence of infection with *E. nana* reflects the level of sanitation. Trophozoites of *E. nana* range in size from 6 to 12 µm. The nucleus lacks peripheral chromatin and contains a large, irregular karyosome that is attached to the nuclear envelope. *E. nana* cysts are 5 to 10 µm and lack chromatodial bodies. Mature cysts have four nuclei. The trophozoite and cyst stage of *E. nana* are shown in Figure 44-11.

*Iodamoeba butschlii* is another ameba that is an intestinal commensal in humans and other primates and pigs. It is the most common intestinal ameba in swine. The rate of prevalence of human infection with *I. butschlii* is 4% to 8% worldwide. Trophozoites range from 10 to 20 µm in diameter or length (see Figure 44-12). The entire cytoplasm of the trophozoite is granulated and there is no clear demarcation between the ectoplasm and endoplasm. A large, eccentric karyosome is present in the nucleus. The nuclear envelope lacks peripheral chromatin. Cysts of *I. butschlii* are usually oval and vary in size from 8 to 20 µm. The cyst of this ameba often has a large glycogen mass that appears reddish brown when stained with iodine.

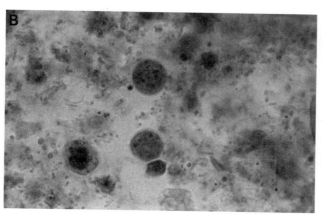

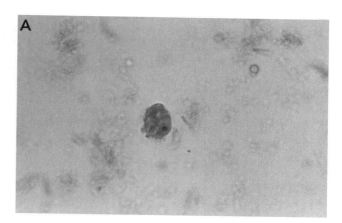

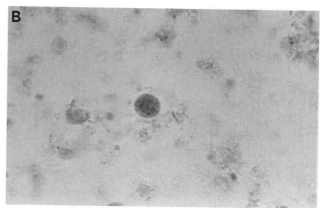

**FIGURE 44-10** *Entamoeba coli.* **A.** cyst and **B.** trophozoite.

**FIGURE 44-11** *Endolimax nana.* **A.** cyst and **B.** trophozoite.

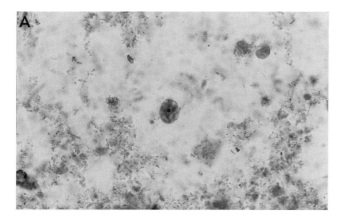

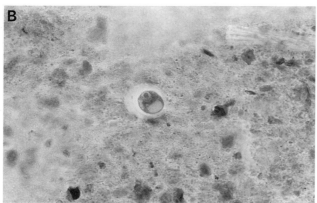

**FIGURE 44-12** *Iodamoeba butschlii.* **A.** cyst and **B.** trophozoite.

## FLAGELLATES

The flagellates are also members of the phylum Sarcomastigopora, but unlike the ameba they are motile by one or more long, thin cytoplasmic extensions called flagella. Flagellates are surrounded by a semi-rigid **pellicle** giving them a more definite shape than the ameba. A number of flagellates are parasites of humans and infect the intestinal tract, blood, and other tissues. The lumen-dwelling flagellates are the topic of this chapter. Flagellates that infect the blood and other tissues are discussed in Chapter 45.

Three species of flagellates are clinically significant. The two most important are *Giardia lamblia,* the cause of giardiasis, and *Trichomonas vaginalis,* the cause of **trichomoniasis**. *Dientamoeba fragilis* is the third and was once considered an ameba. It has been reclassified as a flagellate for several reasons that are discussed later in this section. No cyst stage is observed in the life cycle and the organism causes a variety of symptoms in some infected individuals. Transmission of *Dientamoeba fragilis* may be by way of the egg of an intestinal nematode. Infection with *G. lamblia* most often occurs when the cyst stage is ingested in feces-contaminated water. Two *G. lamblia* trophozoites are released in the intes-

tine from each cyst. Trophozoites of the organism can be transmitted through anal intercourse. *G. lamblia* resides in the lumen of the intestine and relies on the intestinal contents and the occasional ingestion of host epithelial cells for nutrition. *T. vaginalis* lacks a cyst stage in its life cycle and is transmitted by direct contact with an infected individual (usually by sexual contact) or by fomites, such as soiled clothing.

Several species of flagellates are commensals in humans and include *Trichomonas hominis, Chilomastix masnili,* and *Dientamoeba fragilis.* These organisms are described in this section so that they may be distinguished from *G. lamblia* and *T. vaginalis* in clinical specimens.

### Intestinal Flagellates

*Giardia lamblia.* *Giardia lamblia* is a cosmopolitan intestinal parasite of humans and is the most common intestinal parasite of humans in the United States. Prevalence rates of *Giardia* infected individuals range from 1.5% to 20% in the United States. The bilaterally symmetrical, teardrop-shaped trophozoite of *Giardia* ranges in length from 12 to 15 μm. The trophozoite contains two nuclei each having a large, centrally located karyosome (see Figure 44-13). In addition to

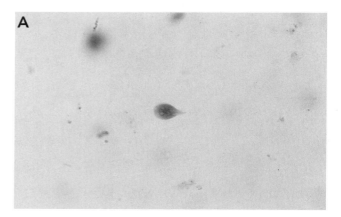

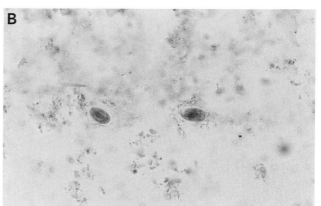

**FIGURE 44-13** *Giardia lamblia.* **A.** trophozoite and **B.** cyst.

the nuclei, two dark-staining **parabasal bodies** can be observed in each trophozoite. The organism has four pair of flagella that propel it with a characteristic rapid, jerky, twisting motion that has been compared to a falling leaf. The anterior end of the cell is broad and round; the posterior end tapers into a point. The dorsal side of the cell is convex and smooth, and the anterior portion of the flat ventral side is modified into a large sucking disk. The oval cysts of *G. lamblia* vary from 9 to 12 μm in diameter and have two or four nuclei.

Infection with *G. lamblia* most often occurs when the cyst stage of the organism is ingested and may result in development of **giardiasis**. The cysts are found in water contaminated with sewage or in water from mountain streams or rivers contaminated by the feces of infected wild animals. *G. lamblia* infects many species of warm-blooded animals and they play an important role in the epidemiology of giardiasis. Infected food handlers who practice poor hygiene can also transmit the parasite to other individuals. Infection with *G. lamblia* is more often observed in children (especially in the 6–10-year age group) than in adults and outbreaks have been reported in day care centers and nurseries.

After passing through the hostile environment of the stomach, each cyst releases two trophozoites. *G. lamblia* trophozoites reside in the upper part of the small intestine. They attach to the mucosal lining by means of the ventral sucking disk and reproduce by binary fission. The sucking disks allow the trophozoites to withstand the peristalsic action of the intestine. For this reason, the trophozoites are not frequently passed, except in fluid feces. The nutritional needs of the trophozoite are met by absorbing the contents of the intestine and by the occasional ingestion of host epithelial cells through the sucking disk. The trophozoite may penetrate the intestinal mucosa and is sometimes found in the gallbladder and in biliary drainage.

After the infection is established, symptomatic individuals may present with mild to severe symptoms. They include abdominal discomfort, abdominal gas and distention, and severe, chronic, foul-smelling diarrhea. These symptoms lead to eventual weight loss. Severe damage to the intestinal mucosa caused by the sucking disks of *Giardia* is common in heavily infected people. This, coupled with the uptake of bile salts by *Giardia*, inhibits the absorption of lipids and a variety of other bowel function abnormalities. They are known collectively as **giardial malabsorption syndrome**.

Diagnosis of infection with *G. lamblia* is based on serologic tests and the detection of cysts in formed feces and trophozoites and cysts in diarrheic feces. It is important to examine fecal samples immediately after collection for the easy to recognize trophozoites because they disintegrate rapidly. A portion of the sample may be preserved for later examination for the presence of cysts. Samples should be collected at inter-

vals that are several days apart because the cysts are often passed sporadically. Trophozoites may sometimes be collected by biopsy.

Even if untreated most cases of giardiasis end in **spontaneous recovery** over a period of time and is probably due to T-cell activity. Quinacrine hydrochloride (Atabrine) is commonly used to treat giardiasis.

***Dientamoeba fragilis.*** Although many clinicians consider *D. fragilis* to be a harmless commensal when it occurs in the gastrointestinal tract of humans, some infected individuals do experience symptoms. Diarrhea and abdominal pain are most common, but some patients also experience bloody stools, abdominal gas, and fatigue or weakness. Estimates of symptomatic infections vary from 15% to 27% (Markell et al., 1992). *D. fragilis* was formally classified as an ameba but was reclassified as a flagellate in recent years. Although this unusual protozoan has some ameba-like characteristics it is now considered a flagellate. This is due primarily to the lack of a cyst stage in its life cycle, and its binucleate condition.

*Dientamoeba fragilis* trophozoites range in size from 3 to 18 μm but average from 7 to 12 μm (see Figure 44-14). Most trophozoites are binucleate (up to 80%) but occasionally cells with three or four nuclei are observed. No cyst stage has been identified. *D. fragilis* resides in the mucosal crypts of the large intestine and rarely ingests red blood cells. Broad pseudopodia with leaflike serrated margins are characteristic of the parasite. The nuclei are not easily observed in unstained preparations but are prominent when stained with iron hematoxylin. The nuclear envelope is thin and lacks peripheral chromatin. A large mass made of four to eight chromatin granules is located near the center of the nucleus. *D. fragilis* is actively motile in freshly passed feces but quickly round up on cooling.

Some questions remain to be answered concerning the transmission of *D. fragilis*, but it is unlikely to be acquired through the oral-fecal route. Some researchers think that the protozoan is transmitted by ingestion of

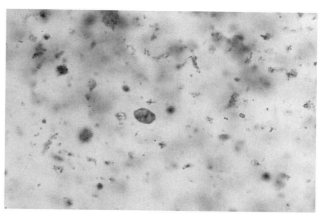

**FIGURE 44-14** *Dientamoeba fragilis* trophozoites.

the eggs of the nematode parasite, *Enterobius vermicularis*. Structures resembling *D. fragilis* have been observed in the nematode eggs and a significant number of persons infected with the nematode are coinfected with *Dientamoeba*. This evidence suggests that the connection between *D. fragilis* and the nematode is more than casual. Infected individuals are treated with iodoquinol. Tetracycline is an alternate treatment.

***Chilomastix mesnili.*** *Chilomastix mesnili* is a commensal that resides in the cecum of some chimpanzees and other monkeys, pigs and other mammals, including humans. Human infection most often occurs by ingestion of cysts in sewage-contaminated water. Prevalence of human infection with the flagellate is about 3.5% in the United States and 6% of the world population. *C. mesnili* must be differentiated from *G. lamblia*, *D. fragilis*, and other flagellates that may be in human feces.

Both the trophozoite and cyst of *C. mesnili* have a single nucleus that can be seen in stained preparations (see Figure 44-15). The nucleus is located at the anterior end of the cell and the nuclear chromatin is in the form of granules. The trophozoites vary in length from 10 to 20 μm and have a teardrop shape that is similar to *G. lamblia*. Oval trophozoites are sometimes observed. Three flagella originating from kinetophores are located at the anterior end and a groove runs in a spiral along the length of the cell. A cytosome (oral depression) is located at the anterior end of the cell. This structure is surrounded by fibrils and accompanied by a short flagellum that is characteristic of *C. mesnili*. The short flagellum is curved making it look somewhat like a shepherd's crook.

Cysts of *C. mesnili* are usually seen in formed stools. They vary in length from 6 to 10 μm and are thick walled. A nipple-like protuberance at the anterior end of the cell gives the cyst a unique and characteristic lemon shape. When stained a single large nucleus and the curved cytosomal flagellum is apparent.

## Other Flagellates That Occur in Humans

Trichomonads are flagellates that possess an **axostyle** and an **undulating membrane**. An axostyle is a tube-like organelle that runs along the length of some flagellated protozoans. The axostyle protrudes and raises a segment of the pellicle into a long fold called the undulating membrane. The undulating membrane assists in motility giving the protozoan a characteristic rotary motion. Many species have an anterior tuft of flagella. Their distinctive morphology and motility makes the flagellates easy to recognize in clinical specimens.

Flagellates occur in the mouth, intestine, or vagina of most vertebrates and at least three species are commonly found in humans. They are *Trichomonas tenax*, *Trichomonas hominis*, and *Trichomonas vaginalis*. Like most members of the genus *Trichomonas*, these three species do not form cysts. *T. vaginalis* is the only flagellate that is a pathogen in the vagina of humans. Flagellates that are parasites of the blood and tissues are discussed in Chapter 45.

*Trichomonas tenax* is a commensal in the mouth of some humans and has cosmopolitan distribution. This small flagellate ranges in size from 6 to 10 μm in length (see Figure 44-16). It was first discovered in the tartar of human teeth. It is most often observed in the mouths of individuals with pyorrhea.

*Trichomonas hominis* is an intestinal commensal in some humans. Although it is not pathogenic it is an indication of direct fecal contamination because it does not form cysts. Cells range from 7 to 15 μm in length and possess four flagella and an undulating membrane (see Figure 44-17). A single anterior nucleus and a costa are also characteristic of *T. hominis*. A costa is a thin, curved rod that is about the same length as the undulating membrane. This unique feature is an important diagnostic feature of *T. hominis*.

It is easier to identify the living organism than it is in stained preparations. The rotary motion typical of some flagellates is observed in living trophozoites. Iron

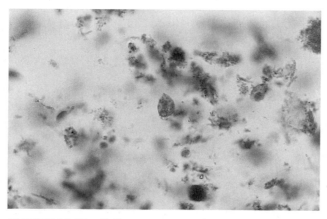

**FIGURE 44-15** *Chilomastix mesnili.* **A.** trophozoite and **B.** cyst.

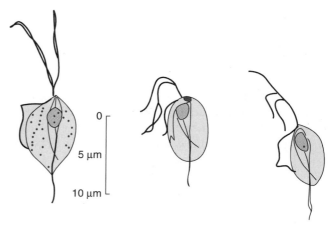

**FIGURE 44-16** *Trichomonas tenax.*

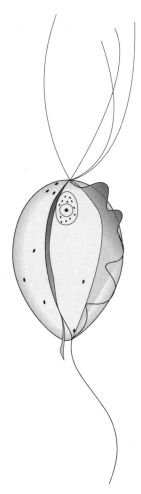

**FIGURE 44-17** *Trichomonas hominis.*

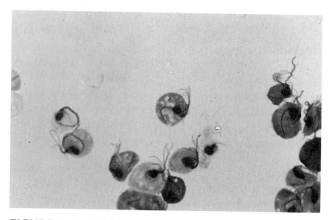

**FIGURE 44-18** *Trichomonas vaginalis.*

hematoxylin does not stain the flagella and the undulating membrane well but the nucleus and costa are easily observed.

**Trichomonas vaginalis.** *Trichomonas vaginalis* is the only flagellate that is a parasite of the human urogenital system. The disease caused by *T. vaginalis* is trichomoniasis. Because this protozoan does not form cysts, it is transmitted by direct contact with an infected individual (usually sexual contact) or by fomites. *T. vaginalis* usually ranges from 5 to 15 μm long, but can reach a length of 30 μm (see Figure 44-18). Although *T. vaginalis* is closely related to *T. hominis,* the two flagellates can be distinguished based on differences in their morphologies. This usually is not a practical necessity because the organisms are site specific.

The anterior end of *T. vaginalis* is rounded; the posterior end tapers to a point. Its undulating membrane is shorter than that in *T. hominis.* The undulating membrane of *T. vaginalis* originates at the anterior end and extends about half the length of the cell. In living preparations *T. vaginalis* displays a jerky motion that is similar to *T. hominis.*

The prevalence of infection with *T. vaginalis* is about 10% to 25% in women and is much lower in men. Women with symptomatic infections most often experience a frequent and sometimes profuse creamy or yellowish discharge. Other possible symptoms include burning, itching and bright red spots on the vaginal mucosa. Infected men are often symptomatic but possibly serious symptoms occur when the prostate, seminal vesicles, and upper urinary system are infected. A thin discharge and an enlarged and tender prostate are indicative of this type of involvement.

Diagnosis of *T. vaginalis* is based on demonstration of trichomonads in wet film preparations. Phase contrast microscopy is best for viewing flagella and undulating membranes. The undulating membrane can be seen "rippling" for several hours after the protozoan stops moving. In infected women, *T. vaginalis* can usually be identified in vaginal secretions or in urethral discharge. In men, the flagellate may be found in the urethral discharge, prostatic secretions, or centrifuged urine. Culture methods using artificial media are sometimes used in identification of *T. vaginalis.* Some serologic tests are available including indirect hemagglutination (IHA). The drug of choice for trichomoniasis is metronidazole (Flagyl).

## CILIATES

The ciliates are the most highly evolved protozoans and most species have trophozoite and cyst stages in their life cycle. *Balantidium coli* is the only ciliate that is a pathogen in humans.

### Balantidium coli

Human infection with *B. coli* is seen primarily in the tropics. This protozoan occurs primarily in pigs and is an occasional parasite in humans. The incidence of *Balantidium* in humans is very low. When infection with *Balantidium* occurs the protozoan usually resides as a commensal in the intestine. Heavy infections can result in lesions and dysentery, which is referred to as **balantidiasis**. This ciliate is the largest protozoan infecting humans, with oval trophozoites ranging from 50 to 100 μm long and 40 to 70 μm wide (see Figure 44-19). The cyst of *B. coli* is also oval and varies from 50 to 70 μm. Oval trophozoites are completely covered with cilia. They contain a large, kidney-shaped nucleus and one or more small micronuclei. A cytosome is located at the posterior end of the cell.

Infection with *B. coli* occurs when cysts are ingested in contaminated water or food. Trophozoites reproduce by conjugation (micronuclei are exchanged) followed by binary fission in the lumen or wall of the colon where lesions form. Balantidiasis is diagnosed by identification of trophozoites in diarrheic feces and occasionally cysts in formed stools. Symptomatic infections are treated with tetracycline or metronidazole. Hogs should be considered the primary source of potential infection.

## COCCIDIA AND MICROSPORIDIA

The clinically significant intestinal coccidia of humans include *Cryptosporidium parvum, Isospora belli,* and the microsporidians. These intracellular parasites have

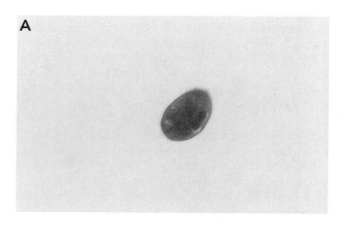

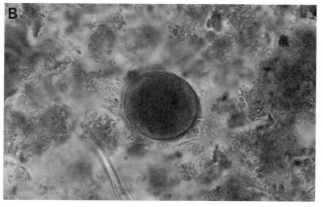

**FIGURE 44-19** *Balantidium coli.* **A.** trophozoite and **B.** cyst.

alternating sexual and asexual phases in their life cycles. *C. parvum* is the agent of **cryptosporidiosis**, a disease that is asymptomatic or mild in healthy individuals, but can be fatal in the immunocompromised. **Isosporiasis** is caused by *I. belli* and like cryptosporidiosis is most serious in immunocompromised patients. The microsporidia are a group of coccidians that are widely distributed in nature. They are considered primitive eucaryotes due to their lack of some organelles. Several genera including *Enterocytozoan* and *Microsporidium* are representative of the microsporidians.

### Cryptosporidium parvum

*Cryptosporidium parvum* infects numerous species of birds and animals, including humans. *C. parvum* does not appear to be host specific and sometimes causes a mild, self-limiting disease called cryptosporidiosis in the immunocompetent. A more serious, even life-threatening disease develops in immunocompromised individuals. Cryptosporidiosis has become one of the more important opportunistic infections in patients with AIDS. Although much remains to be learned about the epidemiology of cryptosporidiosis, estimates suggest the prevalence in AIDS patients may be as high as 15%.

*Cryptosporidium parvum* is transmitted through ingestion of the infectious **oocyst** in fecal-contaminated food or water, oral-anal sexual contact, or by direct contact with an infected individual or animal. *C. parvum* is also a zoonosis and cattle are considered a potential reservoir of the organism. Cryptosporidiosis is sometimes seen in children and outbreaks have been reported in day care centers.

Oocysts release the sporozoite stage about 1 to 2 weeks after infection occurs. The sporozoites penetrate host cells and reside between the cytoplasm and the plasma membrane, where they undergo two asexual generations. **Microgametes** and **macrogametes** are also produced in the epithelial cells. These male and female gametes mate and form zygotes. Thick-walled, infectious oocysts develop from the zygotes and are released in the feces of the infected individual.

On infection with *C. parvum,* individuals having a healthy immune system are asymptomatic or may develop mild, self-limiting disease. Symptoms include watery diarrhea with mucus, nausea, vomiting, malabsorption, and a slight fever. Immunocompromised patients, especially those with AIDS, can develop severe, chronic and potentially fatal diarrhea. The disease is not always confined to the gastrointestinal tract in the immunocompromised individual. Cases of severe respiratory tract infection have been reported in AIDS patients. Because there is no totally effective treatment available at this time, the prognosis is poor for immunocompromised patients diagnosed with cryptosporidiosis. Diagnosis is based on the identification of the small (4–5 μm) oval or round oocysts in fecal specimens. The oocysts are often difficult to see without special staining by methods that include modified acid-fast (cells stain pink to red, Giemsa and the direct, fluorescent antibody technique. Four sporozoites are apparent in some oocysts. Any oocysts that float to the surface of wet preparations may be detected by focusing directly under the cover glass (Garcia & Bruckner, 1993). Oocysts are more likely to be detected by concentration of the fecal specimen using the **formalin-ethyl acetate sedimentation** or **Sheather's sugar concentration flocculation** methods. A test using monoclonal antibodies is commercially available.

### Isospora belli

Although the epidemiology of *I. belli* is not completely understood it is known to be transmitted by ingestion of mature oocysts in contaminated food and water and by some sexual practices. Once in the intestine *Isospora* penetrates epithelial cells where it repeatedly undergoes asexual reproduction. Large portions of the intestinal surface are destroyed in this process. The sexual phase of its life cycle results in oocysts that are released in the feces. Maturation of the oocyst occurs in the intestine. Immature oocysts contain a single mass that develops into two sporozoites in the mature oocyst (see Figure 44-20).

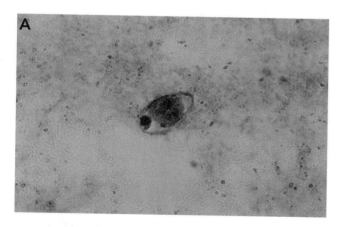

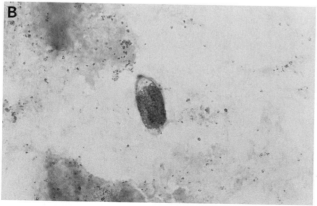

**FIGURE 44-20** *Isospora bellia.* **A.** immature and **B.** mature cyst; modified acid-fast stain.

Isosporiasis is diagnosed by the detection of immature or mature oocysts in fecal specimens. Mature cysts are elongated and oval. They vary from 20 to 30 μm in length to 10 to 20 μm in width. Oocysts are easily detected in wet preparations. Examination of fresh or concentrated material in a direct smear is preferable to a stained smear. Oocysts collected in concentration sediment from polyvinyl alcohol (PVA) may be difficult to detect.

Infection with *I. belli* is often asymptomatic and self-limited, but some individuals experience mild to severe symptoms ranging from mild gastrointestinal discomfort to severe and sometimes fatal dysentery. A combination of trimethoprim and sulfamethoxazole and other drugs are fairly effective in the treatment of isosporiasis in the immunocompromised and others.

## Microsporidia

The microsporidians are widely distributed in nature where they are obligate intracellular parasites of a variety of animals, especially invertebrates. As a group, the microsporidians range in size from 1.5 to 5.0 μm. Unfortunately, those microsporidians that infect humans tend to be small (1.5–2.0 μm), making them difficult to detect using traditional microscopic techniques. Newer diagnostic methods, including serologic tests, have made it easier to diagnose the microsporidians. Until recently not much was known about these tiny eucaryotic microorganisms. Our increased understanding of opportunistic infections in immunocompromised individuals has shed some light on a number of pathogenic agents including the microsporidians.

Five genera of microsporidians have been reported in humans. They are *Encephalitozoon*, *Pleistophora*, *Nosema*, *Microsporidium*, and *Enterocytozoon*. Of these *Encephalitozoon*, *Pleistophora*, and *Nosema* have been reported in patients with AIDS. *Microsporidium* and *Nosema* have caused corneal infections in humans. *Enterocytozoon bieneusi* is the only microsporidian that is reported to cause intestinal infections in AIDS patients.

The microsporidians are characterized by having spores that contain a **polar tube**. Reproduction is by production of these spores. The microsporidians infect humans by using the polar tube as an extrusion mechanism for injecting the contents of the spore into host cells. Microsporidian infections can also be acquired by inhalation of the spores. Classification of the microsporidians is based on spore size, configuration of the nuclei in the spores, and the number of tubule coils in the spore.

Diagnosis of infection with microsporidia is by the observation of spores in biopsy material. The spores stain poorly by most techniques but are most easily detected in Giemsa-stained preparations. Species identification can only be made by electron microscopy. Serologic tests for microsporidians are becoming increasingly available.

A review of the lumen-dwelling protozoans that cause disease in humans is shown in Table 44-2.

## Table 44–2 ▶ Lumen-Dwelling Protozoan Infections of Humans

| Disease | Parasite | Means of Human Infection | Location of Parasite in Humans | Other Sites of Infection | Clinical Features | Laboratory Diagnosis |
|---|---|---|---|---|---|---|
| Amebiasis | *Entamoeba histolytica* | Ingestion of cysts | Large intestine | Liver, lungs, brain, etc. | Diarrhea, dysentery, etc. | Trophozoites or cysts in feces or tissue aspirate, serologic tests |
| Giardiasis | *Giardia lamblia* | Ingestion of cysts | Attached to small intestine | Bile duct, gallbladder | Diarrhea, cramps, gas, malabsorption | Trophozoites or cysts in feces, duodenal aspirate, string test |
| Trichomoniasis | *Trichomonas vaginalis* | Sexual intercourse, fomites | Vagina, urethra | Prostate, seminal vesicles | Vaginal or urethral dishcarge, itching, burning | Trophozoites in vaginal or urethral discharge |
| Balantidiasis | *Balantidium coli* | Ingestion of cysts | Large intestine | None | Diarrhea | Trophozoites or cysts in feces |
| Intestinal infection with coccidia and microsporidia | A variety of coccidians and microsporidians | Ingestion of oocysts, spores of microsporidia | Intestinal epithelium | Respiratory tract | Diarrhea, abdominal pain, etc. | Oocysts in stools, intestinal biopsy, electron microscopy |

## ARTIFACTS THAT RESEMBLE PROTOZOANS FOUND IN FECES

Of all the specimens in which protozoan parasites must be differentiated from artifacts, fecal samples are the most difficult. Feces are made of several components including undigested food, digestive by-products, epithelial cells and mucus from the digestive tract, and a variety of microbes such as bacteria and yeasts. Many artifacts are incorrectly identified as protozoan trophozoites and cysts. Incorrect identifications can be minimized by training, adherence to protocols, quality control measures, reference materials, and the use of consultants.

Free-living ameba that are found in fecal specimens, or as water contaminants, can be differentiated from parasitic ameba based on morphology and sometimes on the basis of cultivation. It is extremely important that care is taken to avoid the contamination of specimens during collection. Fecal specimens should be examined as soon as possible after passage.

Intestinal yeasts and other fungi provide the clinician with perhaps the greatest source of confusion. Plant cells are commonly found in fecal specimens and can be differentiated from parasitic organisms by their thick cellulose walls and striations. Air bubbles, fat globules, mucus, and starch granules have been mistaken for protozoan cysts (see Table 44-3). Figure 44-21 illustrates some of the artifacts that may be found in fecal specimens.

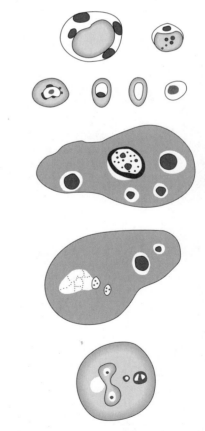

**FIGURE 44-21** Various structures that may be found in fecal preparations.

## Table 44–3 ▶ Artifacts That Resemble Lumen-Dwelling Protozoan Parasites

| Artifacts | Resemblance |
| --- | --- |
| Free-living ameba, flagellates, ciliates | Parasitic ameba, flagellates, ciliates |
| Yeast cells | *Cryptosporidium parvum*, microsporidia, protozoan cysts |
| Bacteria | Microsporidia |
| Plant cells | Protozoan cysts |
| Human cells | |
|   Old (disintegrating) PMNs | *Entamoeba histolytica* cyst |
|   Red blood cells | *Cryptosporidium* species |
|   Epithelial cells | Amebic trophozoites |
|   Macrophages | *E. histolytica* trophozoites |
| Air bubbles | |

PMN, polymorphonuclear leukocyte

## SUMMARY

Numerous species of protozoa may reside in the gastrointestinal and urogenital tracts of humans. Although most of these microbes are harmless commensals some cause mild to severe, and even life-threatening disease. These protozoans are discussed in Chapter 46. Several tables and illustrations in this chapter will assist in the diagnosis of diseases caused by lumen-dwelling protozoa. The protozoa that infect blood and other tissues are discussed in the next chapter.

## CASE STUDY

A 46-year-old male patient is admitted to the hospital with severe dysentery, fever, and hepatomegaly. Trophozoites with thin pseudopodia and a single nucleus having a distinct, central endosome are recovered from a liver biopsy. Although no cysts are detected in a fecal specimen collected from the patient, some trophozoites are identified. The genus and species of the infecting protozoan is most likely:

**Questions:**

1.
   a. *Endolimax nana*
   b. *Chilomastix mesnili*
   c. *Isospora belli*
   d. *Entamoeba histolytica*
   e. *Blastocystis hominis*

2. Cysts of the protozoan in question number 1 could have which of the following characteristics?
   a. Chromatodial bodies
   b. Two nuclei
   c. Four nuclei
   d. All of the above

3. What staining technique would be most appropriate to identify the trophozoites and cysts of the protozoan in question number 1?
   a. Giemsa staining
   b. Trichrome staining
   c. Modified acid-fast staining
   d. Gram staining

## Review Questions

1. One possible result of giardiasis is malabsorption syndrome. It is most likely due to which of the following?
   a. Multiplication of *Giardia* trophozoites in the intestinal lining
   b. The effects of a toxin produced by *Giardia*
   c. The production of bile salts by *Giardia*
   d. Damage to the intestinal lining caused by *Giardia*'s sucking disk

2. While residing in the human intestine *Giardia lamblia* relies on _____ for nutrition.
   a. the contents of the intestine and occasional ingestion of host epithelial cells
   b. host red blood cells
   c. ingestion of other protozoans residing there
   d. All of the above

3. Which of the following protozoans have a cytosome and a short flagellum that resembles a shepherd's crook?
   a. *Chilomastix mesnili*
   b. *Trichomonas vaginalis*
   c. *Giardia lamblia*
   d. *Blastocystis hominis*

4. What role to micronuclei play in the life cycle of *Balantidium coli?*
   a. They are the infectious stage of the protozoan.
   b. They are exchanged during conjugation.
   c. They allow *Balantidium* to resist antiparasitic drugs.
   d. They regulate the rate of binary fission.

5. Persons with which of the following occupations would be most likely to become infected with *Balantidium coli?*
   a. Turkey ranchers
   b. Pork ranchers
   c. Sewage workers
   d. Nurses

6. Which of the following is least likely to be found in a fecal specimen?
   a. *Entamoeba coli*
   b. *Entamoeba hartmanni*
   c. *Entamoeba histolytica*
   d. *Entamoeba gingivalis*

7. Why are asymptomatic individuals who are infected with *Giardia lamblia* more important in the epidemiology of giardiasis than are symptomatic individuals who are experiencing severe diarrhea?
   a. Because asymptomatic individuals pass large numbers of the trophozoite in their feces which are noninfectious
   b. Because symptomatic individuals only pass the noninfectious trophozoite stage in their feces
   c. Because asymptomatic individuals pass the infectious cyst stage in their feces
   d. Because symptomatic individuals pass the infectious cyst stage in their feces

8. *Trichomonas hominis* can be distinguished from *Trichomonas vaginalis* based on:
   a. *T. hominis* is usually found in fecal specimens and not in vaginal smears.
   b. *T. hominis* possesses a costa, which is not present in *T. vaginalis*.
   c. *T. vaginalis* trophozoites are usually much larger than the trophozoites of *T. hominis*.
   d. Only a and b are true.

9. A 24-year-old woman seeks medical attention for what she believes is a severe yeast infection after an over-the-counter yeast medication fails to work. The symptoms that she is experiencing include a profuse, foul-smelling, whitish, vaginal discharge and bright red spots on the vaginal mucosa. She also reported severe itching of the vaginal mucosa and burning on urination. Which of the following is identified in a vaginal smear of the patient?
   a. Oval cysts with four nuclei and chromatodial bodies
   b. A teardrop-shaped trophozoite with an undulating membrane that begins at the anterior end of the cell and extends about half the length of the cell
   c. An oval trophozoite with cilia and a cytosome
   d. Tiny bacteria-like cells that cannot be adequately observed with light microscopy

10. The physician might prescribe which of the following to treat the young woman in question #9?
    a. Metronidazole
    b. Penicillin
    c. Monostat
    d. Amoxycillin

## ▶ REFERENCES & RECOMMENDED READING

Baron, E. J., Peterson, L. R., & Finegold, S. M. (1994). *Bailey and Scott's diagnostic microbiology* (9th ed.) St. Louis: Mosby.

Bongard, J., et al. (1994, August). *Cryptosporidium* infections associated with swimming pools—Dane County, Wisconsin, 1993. *MedNews.* Online. America Online. 12 January, 1997.

Centers for Disease Control and Prevention. (1995, September 25) *Cryptosporidiosis: A guide for persons with HIV/AIDS, Document # 578001.* Atlanta: Author.

Centers for Disease Control and Prevention. (1995, September 28). *Cryptosporidiosis: Fact sheet Document #578000.* Atlanta: Author.

Coleman, R. M., et al. (1989). *Fundamental immunology.* Dubuque, IA: Wm. C. Brown.

Delost, M. D. (1997). *Introduction to diagnostic microbiology: A text and workbook.* St. Louis: Mosby.

Elford, B. C., & Ferguson, D. (1993, March). Secretory processes in *Plasmodium. Parasitology Today, 9,* 80–81.

Garcia, L. S., Bruckner, D. A. (1993). *Diagnostic medical parasitology* (2nd ed.). Washington, DC: American Society for Microbiology.

Goodgame, R. M., et al. (1993). Intensity of infection in AIDS-associated cryptosporidiosis. *Journal of Infectious Diseases, 167,* 704–709.

Greenberg, P. D. (1997, January 13). Diagnosing *Cryptosporidium parvum* in AIDS patients with severe diarrhea. *Pharmaceutical Information Network ACG95 Highlights Bulletin #3.5.* Online. America Online.

Kuby, J. (1994). *Immunology* (2nd ed.). New York: Freeman.

Lee, C. H., et al. (1993). Nucleotide sequence variation in *Pneumocystis carinii* strains that infect humans. *Journal of Clinical Microbiology, 31,* 754–757.

Markell, E. K., Voge, M., & John, D. T. (1992). *Medical parasitology* (7th ed.). Philadelphia: Saunders.

Miller, B. F., & Keane, C. B. (1987). *Encyclopedia and dictionary of medicine, nursing and allied health* (4th ed.). Philadelphia: Saunders.

Neva, F. A., & Brown, H. W. (1994). *Basic clinical parasitology* (6th ed.). East Norwalk, CT: Appleton & Lange.

Olsen, O. W. (1986). *Animal parasites: Their life cycles and ecology.* New York: Dover.

Petersen, C. (1995). *Cryptosporidium* and the food supply. *The Lancet, 345,* 1128–1129.

Ryan, K. J. (Ed.). (1994). *Sherris: Medical microbiology: An introduction to infectious diseases* (3rd ed.). Stamford, CT: Appleton & Lange.

Schmidt, G. D., & Roberts, L. S. (1989). *Foundations of parasitology* (4th ed.). St. Louis: Times Mirror/Mosby.

*Scientific American: A Special Issue.* (1994). Life, death and the immune system. New York: Freeman.

Thomas, C. L. (Ed.). (1997). *Taber's cyclopedic medical dictionary* (18th ed.). Philadelphia: Davis.

Tortora, G. J., Funke, B. R., & Case, C. C. (1992). *Microbiology: An introduction* (4th ed.). Redwood City, CA: Benjamin/Cummings.

"Waterborne Bug May Have Killed 19 in Las Vegas." *The Press-Enterprise,* 25 May 1994.

Wyler, D. J. (Ed.). (1990). *Modern parasite biology: Cellular, immunological and molecular aspects.* New York: Freeman.

# CHAPTER 45

# Plasmodia and Other Blood and Tissue Protozoans

Lisa Shimeld, MS

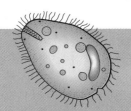

## Microbes in the News

### An Amazon Adventure—Malaria

There are few malaria cases in the United States because the mosquito that transmits malaria does not live in the states. According to the CDC (Centers for Disease Control), there were 1,014 cases in the United States. Most of these were tourists, foreign diplomats, or military personnel who returned to the United States after a long trip or deployment. Only five cases were actually transmitted and received in the United States. Most cases were diagnosed in the big cities (New York, Los Angeles, and Chicago). One of the largest rises of the cases of malaria was when the soldiers from the Vietnam War came back to America. Another large rise was when the US peacekeepers came back from Somalia. Of the people who enter the United States, most malaria cases come from India and Niger. Travelers to malaria-infected areas should take proper safety measures. These include using mosquito nets while sleeping and applying bug repellant every one to two hours.

Burns, J. (1997). *An Amazon Adventure—Malaria*. http://168.216.238.53/amazon/malaria.htm

## KEY TERMS

Babesiosis
Black water fever
Chagoma
Granulomatous amebic
  encephalitis (GAE)
Hemoflagellates
Hemozoin
Kissing bug

Leishmaniasis
Malarial paroxysm
Malignant jaundice
Primary ameba meningoen-
  cephalitis (PAM)
Quartan
Reduviid bug

Sandfly
Tachyzoite
Tertian
Texas cattle fever
Tsetse fly
Ulcerative acanthameba
  keratitis

## LEARNING OBJECTIVES

**Upon successful completion of this chapter, the student should be able to:**

1. Define the key terms.
2. List and describe the characteristics of the protozoans discussed in this chapter.
3. Discuss the life cycles of the protozoans covered in this chapter.

4. Indicate diseases caused by plasmodia and other blood and tissue protozoans are diagnosed.
5. Give an example of drug used to treat these infections.
6. Describe how the protozoans discussed in this chapter are transmitted to humans.

## INTRODUCTION

Numerous protozoans parasitize the blood and tissues of humans and other animals. Some cause diseases of great economic importance, such as malaria and African sleeping sickness, whereas others are rather uncommon. Infection with these protozoans occurs in a variety of ways. Ameba, like *Acanthamoeba* and *Naegleria,* may infect humans by invasion of the mucous membranes when they swim in contaminated water, or by improper disinfection of contact lenses. Others, are vectored by a blood-sucking arthropod that might also serve as an intermediate or definitive host. This is the case with *Plasmodium* species, the cause of malaria, the trypanosomes, that cause African sleeping sickness and Chagas' disease, and *Babesia* species, the cause of **babesiosis**, a disease that is somewhat similar to malaria.

## AMEBA

Only two genera of ameba are occasional parasites of human tissues originating in sites other than the gastrointestinal tract. They are *Acanthamoeba* and *Naegleria*. Although clinical reports of both ameba have increased in recent years, they are still not commonly encountered in the clinical laboratory. Both are discussed briefly in this chapter.

### Acanthamoeba Species and Naegleria fowleri

*Acanthamoeba* species and *Naegleria fowleri* are small, free-living ameba that are abundant in nature, but are not commonly recognized clinically. These protozoans are found living in fresh water, soil, hot tubs, air-conditioning systems, dust, air, and compost. *Naegleria* has a flagellated stage in its life cycle, and thus is sometimes referred to as an ameboflagellate (see Figure 45-1). It can temporarily transform to the flagellated stage when introduced into water. The amebic form of *Acanthamoeba* species and *N. fowleri* can pass through, and infect, the mucous membranes of the nasal sinuses

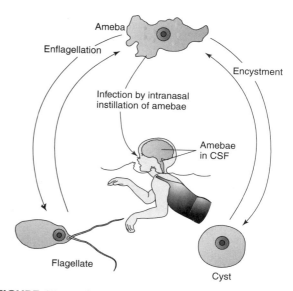

**FIGURE 45-1** Life cycle of *Naegleria.*

and spread along nerves to the brain and central nervous system (CNS).

Prior to 1989, very few cases of infection with *Acanthamoeba* species or *N. fowleri* were reported. Since then, over 140 cases of **primary ameba meningoencephalitis (PAM)** caused by *N. fowleri,* and in excess of 40 cases of **granulomatous amebic encephalitis (GAE)** caused by *Acanthamoeba* species, have been documented. Additionally, there have been over 250 cases of **ulcerative acanthameba keratitis** in contact lens wearers, most of which were related to poor lens hygiene. The tests used to diagnose *Acanthamoeba* and *Naegleria* are not commonly performed in the diagnostic microbiology laboratory and so these organisms are mentioned only briefly here.

Only a few cases of PAM (caused by *N. fowleri*) are reported in the United States each year. Most are acquired by children when they swim in contaminated ponds or streams. After infecting the nasal mucosa, the organism spreads to the brain. The trophozoite of *Naegleria* has broad, lobed pseudopodia and exhibits active motility when examined in a wet mount preparation (see Figure 45-2). The thin-walled cyst is sometimes found encysted in tissue. Although infection with *N. fowleri* is uncommon, it is almost always 100% fatal. Diagnosis is usually made at autopsy.

Acanthameba keratitis is acquired by swimming in fresh water in which cysts are present, using contaminated hot tubs, inadequate disinfection of contact lenses, contamination of homemade saline solution, and wearing

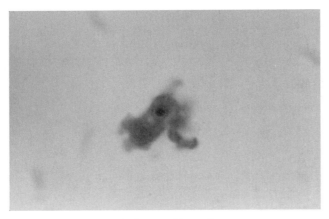

**FIGURE 45-2** Morphology of *Naegleria*.

contact lenses while swimming (see Figure 45-3). The early stages of the infection are characterized by mild inflammation, which progresses to severe pain. If undiagnosed and untreated, the damage caused in acanthameba keratitis is often so severe that corneal transplant or even removal of the eye may be required. The trophozoites of *Acanthamoeba* species are larger and more sluggish than those of *Naegleria* and have spiny pseudopods (see Figure 45-4). There is no flagellated stage in the life cycle. The cysts of *Acanthamoeba* may also be found encysted in tissue. Infection with *Acanthamoeba* is diagnosed by the presence of trophozoites and cysts in stained scrapings of the cornea.

## MASTIGOPHORA, OR THE HEMOFLAGELLATES

Several species of flagellates infect the blood and tissues, causing significant diseases in humans. These flagellates are also known as the **hemoflagellates** and include species of the genera *Trypanosoma* and *Leishmania*. They are all transmitted to humans by the bite of a blood-sucking arthropod. The hemoflagellates that cause disease in humans are the trypanosomes and leishmania.

### Trypanosomes

The trypanosomes that most often cause disease in humans include three species: *Trypanosoma brucei* subspecies *gambiense*, *Trypanosoma brucei* subspecies *rhodiense*, and *Trypanosoma cruzi*. These pleomor-

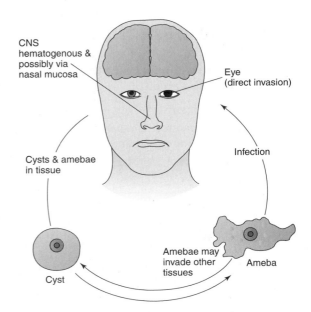

**FIGURE 45-3** Life cycle of *Acanthamoeba*.

phic protozoans have several stages in their life cycles as shown in Table 45-1. Some of their general features are included in Table 45-2.

Two subspecies of *T. brucei*, *T. brucei gambiense* and *T. brucei rhodiense*, cause African sleeping sick-

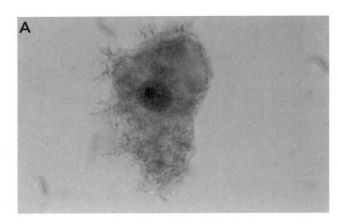

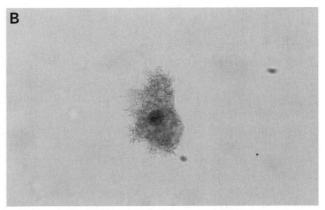

**FIGURE 45-4** Morphology of *Acanthamoeba*. **A.** Trophozoite; **B.** Cyst.

ness. Both are vectored to humans by the bite of infected arthropods of the genus *Glossina,* which is commonly called the **tsetse fly** (see Figure 45-5). The tryptomastigote stage is introduced into the blood of the human host and a hard nodule forms where the bite occurred (refer to Color Plates 102 and 103).

The Gambian form of African sleeping sickness is more common than the sporadic Rhodiesian type. The acute stage of both varieties of the disease begin with an invasion of the blood and lymph nodes by the protozoan. Symptoms often include night sweats, high fever, and joint and muscle pain. If the patient is untreated,

the chronic form develops in 6 months to a year in the Gambian form, and in as little as 1 month in the Rhodiesian form. As the chronic stage continues, the patient eventually becomes comatose and death occurs in 2 to 3 years.

Diagnosis of African sleeping sickness is made by observation of tryptomastigotes in lymph node aspirates early in the disease. Giemsa- or Wright-stained peripheral blood smears contain the tryptomastigotes as the infection progresses. Wet mounts reveal motile tryptomastigotes that vary from 12 to 40 μm in length. The two species of *T. brucei* are usually not differentiated.

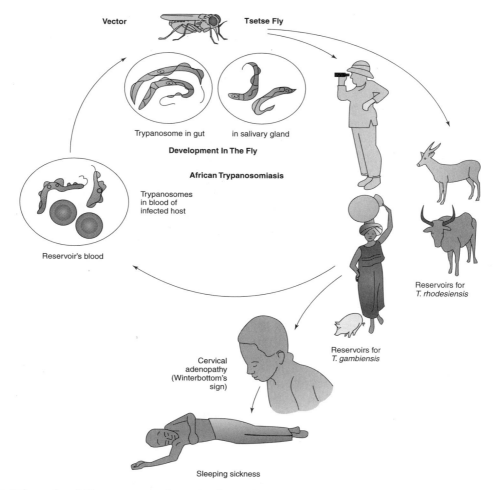

**FIGURE 45-5** Life cycle of *Trypanosoma brucei* subspecies.

## Table 45–1 ▶ Life Cycle Stages of Trypanosomes

| Name of Life Cycle Stage | Alternate Name | Host in Which Stage is Found | Intracellular/Extracellular |
|---|---|---|---|
| Amastigote | Leishmanial form | Humans—in various tissues | Intracellular |
| Promastigote | Leptomonal form | Arthropod | Extracellular |
| Epimastigote | Crithidial form | Arthropod | Extracellular |
| Tryptomastigote | Trypanosomal form | Arthropod and humans | Extracellular |

## Table 45–2 ▶ General Features of Trypanosomes That Cause Disease in Humans

| Organism | Disease | Arthropod Vector | Geographic Distribution | Reservoirs |
|---|---|---|---|---|
| T. brucei gambiense | African sleeping sickness | Glossina—tsetse fly | Central and Western Africa | Wild animals |
| T. cruzi | American trypanosomiasis or Chagas' disease | Panstrongylus—reduviid or kissing bug | South America | Humans and animals |
| T. brucei rhodiense | Eastern African sleeping sickness | Glossina—tsetse fly | Eastern Africa | Humans |

*Trypanosoma cruzi* is the cause of American trypanosomiasis, or Chagas' disease and begins with the bite of an infected fly of the genus *Panstrongylus*. Common names for the arthropod include the **reduviid** or **kissing bug**. The bite most often takes place at night and on the face of the victim. The metacyclic tryptomastigote of *T. cruzi* is deposited on the skin of the human by the fly and enters the body when the bite is scratched. A hard, red **chagoma** develops at the site of the bite. The tryptomastigote enters various host cells, especially phagocytes, where it transforms into the amastigote phase. Asexual reproduction of the amastigote occurs and results in lysis of the infected cell. The infection spreads as the newly produced amastigotes enter and reproduce in other host cells. The acute stage lasts from 1 to 4 months, and symptoms experienced include fever, headache, muscle ache, cardiac abnormalities, and others (refer to Color Plates 104 and 105).

### Leishmania Species

Several species of *Leishmania* cause cutaneous, mucocutaneous, or visceral **leishmaniasis** in humans (see Table 45-3). The leishmania are vectored to humans by the bite of the female **sandfly** (genus *Lutzomyia* or *Plebotomus*), or, occasionally, the stable or dog fly, *Stomoxys*. Several animals serve as reservoirs of *Leishmania* including a variety of rodents and dogs. After biting a human, the sandfly regurgitates the promastigote stage of *Leishmania,* which enters the bloodstream through the bite (see Figure 45-6). The promastigote develops into the amastigote, which then multiplies in macrophages located in the host's skin. Cutaneous leishmaniasis is confined to the skin and lymphophatics where it causes chronic ulcerations; the ulcers occur in the oral or nasal cavities in mucocutaneous leishmaniasis. The primary infection in visceral leishmaniasis occurs in the skin and progresses to invade the visceral organs. In visceral leishmaniasis, the host experiences symptoms that include chills and shaking, sweating, weight loss, and hepatosplenomegaly as the protozoan disseminates through the body. Additional sandflies acquire the parasite when they ingest infected macrophages during a blood meal from a human or animal reservoir.

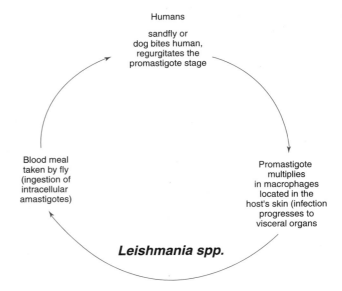

Humans

sandfly or dog bites human, regurgitates the promastigote stage

Blood meal taken by fly (ingestion of intracellular amastigotes)

Promastigote multiplies in macrophages located in the host's skin (infection progresses to visceral organs

*Leishmania spp.*

**FIGURE 45-6** Life cycle of *Leishmania*.

Identification of the amastigote form of *Leishmania* is diagnostic of infection in humans. It is found in macrophages of the skin lesion with *L. tropica* and *L. mexicana*. The amastigote is isolated at the edge of the skin lesion in *L. braziliensis* infections. Tissue samples from the spleen, lymph nodes, liver, and bone marrow are required to locate the amastigote in infections with *L. donovan*. Pentavalent antimony and amphotericin B are two drugs used to treat leishmaniasis.

## SPOROZOA

The sporozoans are intracellular parasites that are vectored by a blood-sucking arthropod. Sporozoans that cause disease in humans include species in the genera *Plasmodium* and *Babesia*. Four species of *Plasmodium* cause malaria in humans, a disease of great economic importance that occurs in more than 100 countries worldwide. Two species of *Babesia* cause babesiosis, a disease that is somewhat similar to malaria, but is much less common. Neither malaria or babesiosis is commonly encountered by clinicians in

| Table 45–3 ► Species of *Leishmania* Causing Disease in Humans and Their Geographic Distribution | | |
|---|---|---|
| **Species of Leishmania** | **Disease Caused by This Species** | **Geographic Distribution** |
| *L. braziliensis* | Mucocutaneous leishmaniasis (New World mucocutaneous leishmaniasis) | Rural and forested Central and South America |
| *L. donovani* | Visceral leishmaniasis (Kalazar) | Central and South America, India, China, E. Africa, Mediterranean |
| *L. mexicana* | Cutaneous leishmaniasis (New World leishmaniasis) | Rural Central and South America |
| *L. tropica* | Cutaneous leishmaniasis (Old World cutaneous leishmaniasis) | Near East, Middle East, Mediterranean, India, Africa |

the United States. When they are, most cases have been imported from other countries.

## Plasmodium Species

Four species of *Plasmodium* including *P. falciparum, P. ovale, P. vivax,* and *P. malariae,* cause malaria in humans. These intracellular parasites have complex life cycles that involve an intermediate and definitive host. *Plasmodium*'s sexual phase is called sporogeny and takes place in its definitive host, the *Anopheles* mosquito. Asexual reproduction, or schizogony, occurs in the human intermediate host. *Plasmodium*'s life cycle is outlined in Figure 45-7. The major characteristics of each of the four species are compared in Table 45-4.

Human infection with *Plasmodium* begins with the bite of an infected *Anopheles* mosquito. A few cases of transmission of malaria from the sharing of needles between drug addicts and by blood transfusions have been documented. The sporozoite stage of *Plasmodium* resides in the salivary glands of the mosquito. It is introduced to a human when the arthropod takes a

blood meal. The sporozoites enter the bloodstream, then host liver cells, enlarge, and undergo multiple fission (schizogony). Eventually, the infected cells lyse, releasing merozoites into the blood, which invade erythrocytes (RBCs). Ring-stage trophozoites develop in the RBCs utilizing hemoglobin to produce the malarial pigment, **hemozoin**. This pigment is of diagnostic importance because it stains as black granules in Giemsa- or Wright-stained blood smears.

After further development of the protozoan, the RBCs lyse releasing the parasite and its metabolic by-products into the bloodstream. The malarial waste products are toxic to the human host. Their release into the blood causes **malarial paroxysm**, which is characterized by shaking chills followed by fever. Periodicity of the paroxysms varies with the infecting species of *Plasmodium* and is either **tertian** (beginning 3 days after the first paroxysm) or **quartan** (beginning 4 days after the first paroxysm). Eventually, some of the merozoites develop into male and female gametocytes. Sporogony (sexual reproduction of *Plasmodium*) is initiated when gametocytes are ingested by an *Anopheles* mosquito taking a blood meal from an infected human.

Malarial symptoms begin with a low-grade fever, headache, and anorexia. As RBCs burst and patients undergo paroxysms, they experience chills, followed by fever, flushed skin, and pain in the back and limbs. As the fever subsides, the patient sweats profusely and sleeps until the next paroxysm. The destruction of RBCs can be significant enough to cause anemia. The hemozoin pigment that is released with the parasite during the lysis of RBCs is sometimes passed in the patient's urine resulting in what is known as **black water fever**.

Malaria occurs anywhere in the world where the *Anopheles* mosquito is found. A few hundred cases of malaria are reported in the United States each year, most of which are imported. A handful of cases are thought to be acquired locally from infected *Anopheles* mosquitoes (see Case Studies 1 and 2). Malaria was a serious problem in the United States until the introduction of DDT and the eradication of most *Anopheles* mosquitoes.

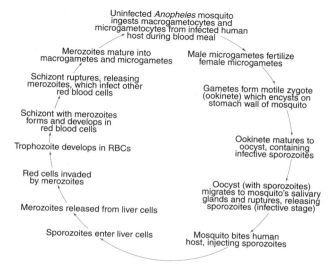

**FIGURE 45-7** Life cycle of *Plasmodium.*

### Table 45–4 ▶ Major Differentiating Characteristics of the Four Species of *Plasmodium*

| Characteristic | P. falciparum | P. malariae | P. ovale | P. vivax |
|---|---|---|---|---|
| Periodicity | Tertian | Quartan | Tertian | Tertian |
| Dots (hemozoin)/clefts | Rare Mauer's clefts | None | Schuffner's dots at all stages. Darker than P. vivax | Schuffner's dots except in early ring stage |
| Early ring stage | Small, multiple rings. Double-nuclei and signet-ring forms seen | Usually only one per host cell | Usually only one per host cell | Usually only one per host cell, double nuclei possible |
| Mature ring stage | Small, round, rare | Ribbon, band or amoeboid forms | Larger but otherwise similar to P. malariae | Large, amoeboid with cytoplasms filling host cell |
| Schizonts | 8–16 merozoites per schizont. Rare in peripheral blood | 6–12 merozoites per schizont. Coarse, granular hemozoin | 8 merozoites | 12–24 merozoites per schizont |
| Gametocytes | Crescent shaped | Round with coarse, unevenly distributed pigment | Similar to P. malariae | Large, round, almost fill host cell. Coarse hemozoin |
| Size of RBCs | Normal | Normal | 1.5 times normal, oval with irregular margin | 1.5–2 times normal |
| Other | Usually see only early ring and gametocytes | All stages observed but few rings and gametocytes | Difficult to differentiate because similar to all but P. falciparum | Usually infect young RBCs, all stages found in peripheral blood |

RBCs, red blood cells

The four species of *Plasmodium* can and should be differentiated. It is important to determine if the infecting species is *P. falciparum* because it causes the most severe and fatal form of the disease. Chloroquine is commonly used to treat malaria, but *P. falciparum* is becoming increasingly resistant to the drug (refer to Color Plates 106 and 107).

## *Babesia* Species

Five species of the tick-vectored sporozoan *Babesia* infect domestic and wild animals:

▶ *Babesia bovis*     cattle
▶ *Babesia divergens*  cattle
▶ *Babesia equi*      horses
▶ *Babesia microti*    rodents
▶ *Babesia canis*     dogs

Sometimes these infections are undetectable, but at other times they are of economic importance and include **Texas cattle fever** and **malignant jaundice** in dogs. Two species of *Babesia*, *B. microti* and *B. equi*, are incidental parasites of humans causing babesiosis. *B. microti* is endemic in the southern New England States, Texas, and in other parts of the United States, and causes most of the human infections there. *B. equi* is also seen in the United States and in other parts of the

world including South America, Europe, Africa, Asia, India and Russia (refer to Color Plate 108).

Several species of *Ixodes* ticks vector *Babesia*. The ticks become infected with the sporozoan when it is transmitted to them by their infected mother, or when they take a blood meal from a *Babesia*-infected mammal (Figure 45-8). The protozoan enters RBCs of the host and produces ringlike structures resembling *Plas-*

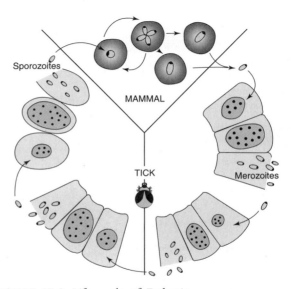

**FIGURE 45-8** Life cycle of *Babesia*.

*modium* (Figure 45-9). Several protozoans may infect a single RBC.

Babesiosis is usually self-limiting in humans. After a 1- to 4-week incubation period, symptoms develop gradually and begin with a fever. Headache, chills, sweating, fatigue, and weakness are also experienced. This disease lacks the periodic recurrence that is characteristic of malaria. People who have had splenectomies are at a higher risk of babesiosis than are other individuals. This is probably because the splenectomy affects their susceptibility to infection and the severity of the resulting illness.

Human infections most often occur in late summer and early fall, and not suprisingly, in tick-infested areas. Diagnosis of babesiosis in humans is by the detection of the parasite in Giemsa-stained blood films. It is best to use a thick blood smear because few organisms are seen in early stages of the disease. *Babesia* can be differentiated from *Plasmodium* because it does not produce the pigment, hemozoin, that is typical of malarial infections. Also, the other stages of *Plasmodium* that are seen in the blood of malaria patients are lacking in babesiosis. A few serologic tests for babesiosis are also available. A combination of quinine-clindamycin is effective in eliminating babesiosis when treatment is indicated.

## COCCIDIA

*Toxoplasma gondii* is the only coccidian that infects human tissues and is not an atrial or intestinal parasite. Like other coccidians, *Toxoplasma* has a complex life cycle and is an obligate, intracellular parasite. Most infections with *Toxoplasma* are clinically insignificant, but the organism has become an important, often fatal parasite, in seriously immunocompromised patients.

### *Toxoplasma gondii*

Although considered a coccidian by many microbiologists, the classification of *Toxoplasma gondii* is still somewhat questionable. Some include *Toxoplasma* with the sporozoans because it is an obligate intracellular parasite with a complex life cycle, but it is included with the coccidians even more often, and will be here as well. The entire life cycle of *T. gondii,* including sexual and asexual reproduction, occurs in the gastrointestinal tract of its definitive host, the cat (see Figure 45-10). This cosmopolitan, protozoan parasite can infect most mammals, including humans, causing toxoplasmosis. Maternal infection with *T. gondii* results in infection of the fetus and causes the tragic disease, congenital toxoplasmosis.

Three stages occur in the life cycle of *T. gondii* including an oocyst, trophozoite (also called **tachyzoite**),

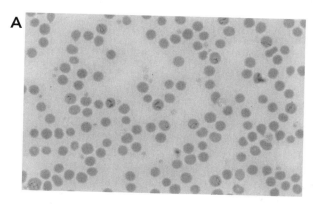
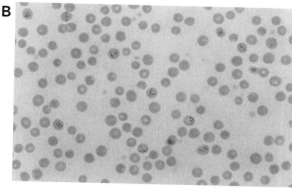
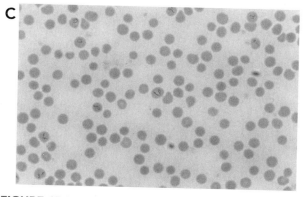

**FIGURE 45-9** Morphology of *Babesia.*

**Natural Cycle**                    **Accidental Cycle**

Cat or other feline—definitive host

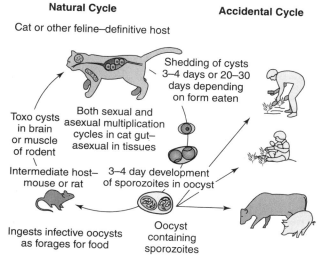

**FIGURE 45-10** Transmission cycle of *Toxoplasma gondii.*

and tissue cyst (see Figure 45-11). Infection occurs on ingestion of the oocyst stage that is passed in cat feces or ingestion of the tissue cyst in undercooked meat such as beef, pork, and bear. Although approximately one-half of all Americans are infected with *Toxoplasma,* the majority of these infections are asymptomatic and self-limiting. Clinical disease caused by *T. gondii* exhibits three major forms: (1) asymptomatic and self-limiting, or symptomatic and mild; (2) highly lethal infection of the severely immunocompromised; and (3) congenital infection of the fetus.

Infections with *T. gondii* in immunocompetent individuals usually does not produce symptoms, but if they do occur they are mild and may include fever and fatigue. Toxoplasmosis in the immunocompromised individual is quite serious. The protozoan often disseminates throughout the patient's body and is often fatal. Toxoplasmosis has become a common cause of death in patients with acquired immunodeficiency syndrome (AIDS). Congenital toxoplasmosis only occurs if a woman is infected with *Toxoplasma* during pregnancy. The protozoan invades the CNS of the fetus and the severity of damage depends on the trimester of pregnancy in which the infection occurred.

Three morphologic forms of *T. gondii* exist. The oocyst is oval and varies from 10 to 12 μm in diameter, and its thick resistant wall is destroyed by chemicals such as formalin and iodine and heat in excess of 66°C. Although the center of immature oocysts lack internal structure, mature ones contain two sporocysts. Even later in the development of the oocyst, four sporozoites may be observed in each sporocyst. It is this form of the parasite that spreads the organism from cats to other mammals by the fecal-oral route.

Trophozoites, or tachyzoites, are crescent-shaped and vary from 3 to 7 μm in length. This asexual form of *Toxoplasma* is responsible for cell invasion of the host organism. It is unable to resist digestive enzymes and cannot cause infection if ingested.

The tissue cyst is similar in appearance to the oocyst but ranges from 10 to 200 μm in diameter. Although its thick wall is able to resist digestive enzymes, the tissue cyst is destroyed by freezing and thawing and normal cooking temperatures. This stage causes infection when it is consumed in undercooked meat.

Diagnosis of toxoplasmosis is through demonstration of trophozoite in tissue sections stained with hematoxylin-eosin, Wright-Giemsa or periodic acid-Schiff (PAS). Serologic tests including the enzyme-linked immunosorbent assay (ELISA) are also available (refer to Color Plates 109 and 110).

## UNCONVENTIONAL PROTOZOANS FOUND IN BLOOD AND TISSUE SPECIMENS

Because the classification of *Pneumocystis carinii* is questionable, it is included here as an unconventional protozoan found in blood and tissue specimens. Although virtually unheard of prior to 1981, this unusual pathogen is now a significant cause of death in the severely immunocompromised, including patients with AIDS and cancer.

### Pneumocystis carinii

*Pneumocystis carinii* is an unusual organism whose classification is questionable. Long considered a protozoan by many, evidence provided by RNA sequencing, including cell wall structure, and reproduction suggest that it may actually be a fungus. Until a consensus is reached we will consider *P. carinii* as an unconventional protozoan found in blood and tissue specimens (refer to Color Plates 111 and 112).

*Pneumocystis carinii* is widespread in nature and has been found in a number of mammals including dogs, cats, rodents, sheep, and others. Human infection is usually asymptomatic, except in immunocompromised patients such as premature infants and patients with AIDS and leukemia. The life cycle of *Pneumocystis* has two stages, neither of which is intracellular (see Figure 45-12). The trophozoite stage ranges from 1 to 4 μm in diameter and is covered with tiny projections that attach the organism to host epithelial cells. The

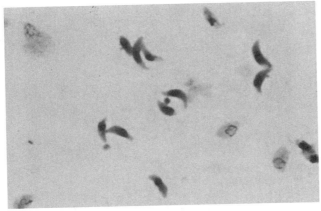

**FIGURE 45-11** Morphology of *Toxoplasma gondii.*

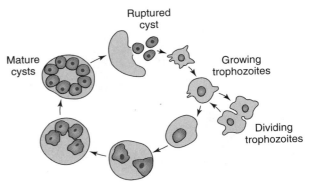

Ruptured cyst

Mature cysts

Growing trophozoites

Dividing trophozoites

**FIGURE 45-12** Life cycle of *Pneumocysti carinii.*

resistant cyst stage varies in diameter from 5 to 8 μm and when inhaled is the infectious stage.

The lungs are the typical site of infection, but the organism may disseminate to the eye, bone marrow, liver, and spleen in AIDS patients. Introcystic bodies are released in the lungs from the cyst and develop into trophozoites. Asexual reproduction occurs on the surface of epithelial cells and once again produces the cyst stage. Infection with *P. carinii* is serious and potentially fatal in immunocompromised patients and can result in symptomatic pneumonitis in premature infants. A rapidly progressive pneumonia often occurs in infected AIDS and leukemia patients and is a leading cause of death.

Diagnosis of *P. carinii* infection is through observation of the trophozoite or cyst in lung secretions or tissue sections. Specimens are stained with modified Gomori methenamine silver nitrate, Giemsa, or toluidine blue O.

## SUMMARY

▶ *Acanthamoeba* and *Naegleria* are the only two parasites of humans that originate in sites other than the gastrointestinal tract.

▶ Neither *Acanthamoeba* or *Naegleria* is commonly recognized clinically. *Naegleria fowleri* occasionally causes primary ameba meningoencephalitis (PAM). *Acanthamoeba* species occasionally cause granulomatous amoebic encephalitis (GAE) and ulcerative acanthamoeba keratitis.

▶ The Hemoflagellates include *Trypanosoma* and *Leishmania*. Both are vectored by the bite of a blood-sucking arthropod.

▶ *Trypanosoma brucei* subspecies *gambiense, T. brucei* subspecies *rhodiense,* and *T. cruzi* are the three trypanosomes that most often cause disease in humans.

▶ Several species of *Leishmania* cause cutaneous, mucocutaneous, and visceral leishmaniasis in humans and are vectored by the sandfly.

▶ Sporozoans are intracellular parasites vectored to humans by the bite of a blood-sucking arthropod. They have complex life cycles with an intermediate and definitive host.

▶ Four species of *Plasmodium* cause malaria in humans and are vectored by the *Anopheles* mosquito. Two species of *Babesia* cause babesiosis (a malaria-like disease) in humans.

▶ *Toxoplasma gondii* is the only coccidian included in this chapter.

▶ *Toxoplasma* has a complex life cycle and infects most mammals, including humans.

▶ Because of the questions related to the classification of *Pneumocystis carinii* it is included in this section.

▶ Although *P. carinii* is common in nature, human infection is usually asymptomatic. The infection can be serious and fatal in premature infants and patients with AIDS and leukemia.

## CASE STUDY 1

On June 22, 1996, a 53-year-old man residing in Tift County, Georgia, was admitted to a hospital due to a 12-day history of fever, chills, fatigue, and myalgias. His temperature on admission was 105.6°F and laboratory examinations demonstrated moderate anemia. On June 26, a peripheral blood smear demonstrated intracellular parasites that were identified as *Plasmodium vivax*. This diagnosis was confirmed by the Centers for Disease Control and Prevention by examination of a blood smear and serologic testing. After treatment with chloroquine phosphate and primaquine phosphate, all symptoms were resolved and examination of peripheral blood smears were clear of infection.

### Questions:

1. What staining technique(s) would be appropriate for the peripheral blood smear taken from the patient?

2. How is malaria transmitted to humans?

3. List the four species of *Plasmodium* that cause malaria in humans.

## CASE STUDY 2

On August 2, 1988, a migrant worker who lived in a canyon near the Lake Hodges reservoir (25 miles north of San Diego) was diagnosed with *P. vivax* infection. Twelve other workers who lived in the same area had symptoms suggestive of the infection and were subsequently diagnosed with malaria. Further investigation resulted in identification of an additional 30 infected persons in the same area. All denied previous infection with malaria, intravenous drug use, and blood transfusions in the past 3 years.

The majority of the infected individuals lived in a canyon area and either slept in the open or in shelters made of cardboard or plastic tarpaulins, and were located within 5 feet of open water. Traps placed in the canyon caught *Anopheles hermsi* mosquitoes, a competent malaria vector. All infected persons were treated with chloroquine by the San Diego County Department of Health Services.

**Questions:**

1. What gender of *Anopheles* mosquito transmits *Plasmodium* to humans?

2. During what time(s) of day are mosquito bites most common?

3. What actions could be taken to help prevent the transmission of malaria?

4. Why is proximity to water significant to the transmission of malaria?

## CASE STUDY 3

A 30-year-old homosexual man was well until January 1981 when he developed esophageal and oral candidiasis. He was treated with amphotericin B, which resolved the infection. The man was hospitalized in February 1981 for *Pneumocystis* pneumonia and was successfully treated with trimethoprim-sulfamethoxazole (TMP/SMX). The esophageal candidiasis recurred after the pneumonia was diagnosed and an esophageal biopsy revealed that he also had cytomegalovirus (CMV).

(Note: This case study was one of the first cases of pneumocystis pneumonia that led to the identification of HIV. It was reprinted by CDC as a part of their 50th year anniversary.)

**Questions:**

1. What can you conclude about the overall health of the patient?

2. What is the most probable source of the candidiasis?

## Review Questions

Use the following case study for questions 1–3.

An optometrist sees a 17-year-old contact lens wearing male patient who complains of chronic irritation of his left eye. On examination, the optometrist does not see anything unusual, and recommends that the patient not wear his contacts for 1 week. She reschedules a return visit for the patient in 1 week.

Four days later the patient calls to tell the doctor that the eye has not improved and is now extremely painful. The optometrist refers the patient to an ophthalmologist. After questioning the patient, the optometrist learned that the patient prepares his own saline solution and uses a cold disinfection method.

1. Based on the information that is provided what would be your tentative diagnosis?
   a. Infection with *Staphylococcus aureus*
   b. Mucocutaneous leishmaniasis
   c. A corneal abrasion
   d. *Acanthamoeba* keratitis

2. If your tentative diagnosis is correct, what test(s) would you order to confirm your suspicions?
   a. An ELISA to detect antibodies.
   b. Place a few drops of a fluorescent dye in the eye and examine under a fluorescent light to check for the abrasion.
   c. Take a corneal scraping to stain and examine for the presence of trophozoites and cysts.
   d. Culture a sample of the patient's tears on mannitol salt agar and examine for yellow colonies.

3. Assuming that a corneal abrasion is not the cause of the problem, what life style stages are possible in the infectious agent?
   a. A trophozoite only
   b. A trophozoite and a cyst
   c. A trophozoite, a cyst, and a flagellated stage in water
   d. Grapelike clusters of round bacterial cells

Questions 4–8. Choose the correct response for each of the possible pathogens.

4. *Toxoplasma gondii:*
   a. Black water fever, *Anopheles* mosquito
   b. Crithidial form of the disease, epimastigote stage of the parasite
   c. An individual who has had a splenectomy, *Ixoides* ticks
   d. Oocysts, a congenital infection of the CNS of a fetus

5. *Plasmodium:*
   a. Black water fever, *Anopheles* mosquito
   b. Crithidial form of the disease, epimastigote stage of the parasite
   c. An individual who has had a splenectomy, *Ixoides* ticks
   d. Oocysts, a congenital infection of the CNS of a fetus

6. *Naegleria fowleri:*
   a. Black water fever, *Anopheles* mosquito
   b. Crithidial form of the disease, epimastigote stage of the parasite
   c. An individual who has had a splenectomy, *Ixoides* ticks
   d. A hot tub, a disease that is usually diagnosed at autopsy

7. *Trypanosoma* species:
   a. Black water fever, *Anopheles* mosquito
   b. Crithidial form of the disease, epimastigote stage of the parasite
   c. An individual who has had a splenectomy, *Ixoides* ticks
   d. Oocysts, a congenital infection of the CNS of a fetus

8. *Babesia* species:
   a. Black water fever, *Anopheles* mosquito
   b. Crithidial form of the disease, epimastigote stage of the parasite
   c. An individual who has had a splenectomy, *Ixoides* ticks
   d. Oocysts, a congenital infection of the CNS of a fetus

Use the following information for questions 9 and 10.

After being bitten by an infected arthropod, the patient experiences a high fever, night sweats, and joint and muscle pain. The chronic form of the disease develops in about 9 months.

9. The causative agent is:
   a. *Acanthamoeba.*
   b. *Plasmodium.*
   c. *Leishmania.*
   d. *Trypanosoma.*

10. What life cycle stages of the parasite could be observed in the patient's blood?
    a. Tryptomastigote
    b. Ring-stage trophozoite
    c. Amastigote
    d. Both a and c

## ▶ REFERENCES & RECOMMENDED READING

Centers for Disease Control and Prevention. (1996). *Pneumocystis* pneumonia—Los Angeles. *Morbidity and Mortality Weekly Report, 45*(34), 729–733.

Centers for Disease Control and Prevention. (1995). 1995 Revised guidelines for prophylaxis against *Pneumocystis carinii* pneumonia for children infected with or perinatally exposed to human immunodeficiency virus. *Morbidity and Mortality Weekly Report, 44* (RR-4).

Centers for Disease Control and Prevention. (1997). Probable locally acquired mosquito-transmitted *Plasmodium vivax* infection—Georgia, 1996. *Morbidity and Mortality Weekly Report, 46,* 264–267.

Centers for Disease Control and Prevention. (1996). Imported malaria and use of malaria chemoprophylaxis by travelers—Kentucky, Maryland, and United States, 1993–1994. *Morbidity and Mortality Weekly Report, 45*(43), 944–947.

Centers for Disease Control and Prevention. (1991). Treatment of severe *Plasmodium falciparum* malaria with quinidine gluconate. *Morbidity and Mortality Weekly Report, 40*(14), 240.

Centers for Disease Control and Prevention. (1991). Mosquito-transmitted malaria—California and Florida, 1990. *Morbidity and Mortality Weekly Report, 40*(6), 106–108.

Centers for Disease Control and Prevention. (1990). Transmission of *Plasmodium vivax* malaria—San Diego County, California, 1988 and 1989. *Morbidity and Mortality Weekly Report, 39*(6), 91–94.

Centers for Disease Control and Prevention. (1995). Malaria surveillance—United States, 1992. *Morbidity and Mortality Weekly Report, 44*(SS-5).

Centers for Disease Control and Prevention. (1991). Guidelines for prophylaxis against *Pneumocystis carinii* pneumonia for children infected with human immunodeficiency virus. *Morbidity and Mortality Weekly Report, 40*(RR-2).

Centers for Disease Control and Prevention. (1997). AIDS rates. *Morbidity and Mortality Weekly Report, 46*(15), 333–334.

Coleman, R. M., et al. (1989). *Fundamental immunology.* Dubuque, IA: Wm. C. Brown.

Delost, M. D. (1997). *Introduction to diagnostic microbiology: A text and workbook.* St. Louis: Mosby.

Elford, B. C., Ferguson, D. (1993, March). Secretory processes in *Plasmodium. Parasitology Today, 9,* 80–81.

Garcia, L. S., & Bruckner, D. A. (1993). *Diagnostic medical parasitology* (2nd ed.). Washington, DC: American Society for Microbiology.

Kuby, J. (1994). *Immunology* (2nd ed.). New York: Freeman.

Lee, C. H., et al. (1993). Nucleotide sequence variation in *Pneumocystis carinii* strains that infect humans. *Journal of Clinical Microbiology, 31,* 754–757.

Markell, E. K., Voge, M., & John, D. T. (1992). *Medical Parasitology* (7th ed.). Philadelphia: Saunders.

Miller, B. F., & Keane, Brackman, C. (1987). *Encyclopedia and dictionary of medicine, nursing and allied health* (4th ed.). Philadelphia: Saunders.

Neva, F. A., & Brown, H. W. (1994). *Basic clinical parasitology* (6th ed.). East Norwalk, CT: Appleton & Lange.

Olsen, O. W. (1986). *Animal parasites: Their life cycles and ecology.* New York: Dover.

Ryan, K. J. (Ed.). (1994). *Sherris: Medical microbiology: An introduction to infectious diseases.* (3rd ed.). Stamford, CT: Appleton & Lange.

Schmidt, G. D., & Roberts, L. S. (1989). *Foundations of parasitology* (4th ed.). St. Louis: Times Mirror/Mosby.

*Scientific American: A Special Issue.* (1994). Life, death and the immune system. New York: Freeman.

Simonds, R. J., Lindegren, M. L., Thomas, P., et al. (1995). Prophylaxis against *Pneumocystis carinii* pneumonia among children with perinatally acquired HIV infection in the United States. *New England Journal of Medicine, 332,* 786–790.

Thomas, C. L. (Ed.). (1997). *Taber's cyclopedic medical dictionary* (18th ed.). Philadelphia: Davis.

# CHAPTER 46
# Intestinal Helminths

Lisa Shimeld, MS

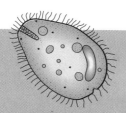

## Microbes in the News
### Pork Tapeworm Found in New Jersey

Over the last few years medical professionals in the United States have been encountering more patients with diseases that are typically found in tropical countries. This rise is due in part to increased immigration and global travel. For example, a 41-year-old woman, formerly a native of Mexico, presented at an emergency room in New Jersey with a progressively worsening headache, an unsteady gait, and vomiting. MRI of the brain revealed dilatation of the lateral and third ventricles and a cystic mass in the fourth ventricle, causing obstructive hydrocephalus and associated ton- silar herniation. After surgical intervention, the patient underwent another MRI that revealed a small, mural nodule within a cyst that suggested the presence of a scolex and a diagnosis of neurocysticercosis (NCC). The CDC performed an immunoelectrotransfer blot assay on serum; this was positive for *Taenia solium,* or the pork tapeworm. Later pathological examination of the tissue upon surgical removal revealed the par- tially destroyed scolex and larval form of *T. solium.*

Source: Grigoriu et al., Tropical Diseases in Urban New Jersey, *Infect Med 12*(9): 460–469, 1995

## INTRODUCTION

## NEMATODES

*Enterobius vermicularis*

*Trichuris trichiura*

*Ascaris lumbricoides*

*Necator americanus* and
  *Ancylostoma duodenale*

*Strongyloides stercoralis*

## CESTODES

*Taenia saginata* and *Taenia
  solium*

*Diphyllobothrium latum*

## TREMATODES

*Clonorchis sinesis*

*Paragonimus westermani*

## KEY TERMS

Ascariasis
Cercariae
Copulatory bursa
Coracidia
Cysticerci
Enterobiasis

Internal autoinfection
Mebendazole
Metacercariae
Miracidium
Oncosphere

Piperazine
Plerocercoid
Procercoid
Redia
Thiabendazole

## LEARNING OBJECTIVES

Upon successful completion of this chapter, the student should be able to:

1. Define the key terms.
2. List and describe the characteristics of the intestinal helminths discussed in this chapter.
3. Discuss the life cycles of the intestinal helminths covered in this chapter.

4. Indicate how the diseases caused by intestinal helminths are diagnosed.
5. Give an example of drugs that are used to treat these infections.
6. Describe how the intestinal helminths discussed in this chapter are transmitted to humans.

## INTRODUCTION

This chapter discusses helminths that reside in the human intestinal tract and those that are diagnosed by the presence of their eggs in the feces. Some of these parasites are flatworms and members of the phylum Platyhelminthes. The two classes of human parasites in this phylum include class Trematoda, or the flukes, and Cestoda, the tapeworms. The roundworms that are intestinal parasites are members of phylum Aschelminthes, class Nematoda. Life cycles of more common intestinal helminths are discussed. Brief mention of some helminths that are uncommon in humans is included so that they can be differentiated from the others in clinical specimens.

## NEMATODES

The nematodes, or roundworms, are members of the phylum Aschelminthes. Although most roundworms are free-living (primarily in soil or in water), numerous species are parasites of plants, humans, and other animals. Some parasitic species spend a portion of their life cycle free-living in soil where they feed on bacteria. Six nematodes are intestinal parasites of humans. They lack the succession of larval stages seen in the flatworms. Nematodes that cause human intestinal infections include *Enterobius vermicularis* (pinworm), *Trichuris trichiura* (whipworm), *Ascaris lumbricoides* (large intestinal roundworm), *Necator americanus* (New World hookworm), *Ancylostoma duodenale* (Old World hookworm), and *Strongyloides stercoralis* (threadworm). Some species that normally infect other animals are incidental parasites of humans and are described later in this chapter. Blood and tissue helminths are discussed in Chapter 47.

Nematodes are long, cylindrical worms whose bodies are covered by a tough cuticle and tapered at both ends. The nematodes have a complete digestive system with both a mouth and an anus. Longitudinal muscle fibers allow the roundworms to move with a side-to-side whipping motion. The nematodes are dioecious, meaning that the sexes are separate. Males are typically

smaller than females. The females are extremely prolific, producing hundreds, or thousands of eggs that must incubate or embryonate outside of the host, after which they are infectious to another individual. Some intestinal nematodes infect humans on ingestion of the egg passed in contaminated food or hands. Others have eggs that hatch outside of the host, often in soil, and the larva is the infectious stage in those organisms.

### Enterobius vermicularis

*Enterobius vermicularis*, the pinworm, has cosmopolitan distribution but is more common in temperate parts of the world. **Enterobiasis** (pinworm infection) is caused by ingestion of the embryonated egg in infected food, contaminated hands, or by soiled clothing or bedding. Pinworm infection is most common in children. The entire life cycle is spent in a human host and is shown in Figure 46-1. Adult worms and an embryonated egg are shown in Figure 46-2.

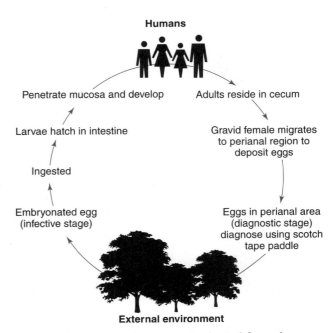

**Humans**

Penetrate mucosa and develop

Adults reside in cecum

Larvae hatch in intestine

Gravid female migrates to perianal region to deposit eggs

Ingested

Embryonated egg (infective stage)

Eggs in perianal area (diagnostic stage) diagnose using scotch tape paddle

**External environment**

**FIGURE 46-1** *Enterobius vermicularis*, life cycle.

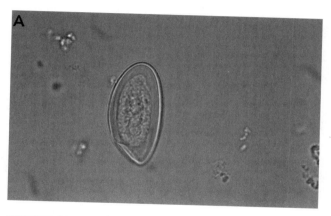
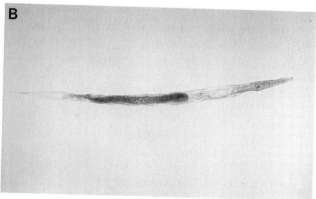

**FIGURE 46-2** Embryonated eggs (**A**) and adult worm (**B**) of *E. vermicularis*.

The pinworm is named for its shape. A bulge is present at the anterior end and tapers into a long posterior end, making the worm resemble a pin. Adult worms vary from 5 to 10 mm in length and reside in the large intestine. Female worms migrate to the anus at night and lay their eggs in the perianal folds of the infected individual. The eggs may not be detected in the feces. Specimens are best obtained in the morning by the "Scotch tape" method (see Figure 46-3) and should be collected before bathing or defecation. A small paddle with a piece of cellophane tape (sticky side facing outward) is pressed against the perianal area and examined microscopically for the presence of eggs. Occasionally, female worms are observed protruding from, or near, the anus.

Severe local itching of the perianal skin is common in pinworm infection and so is bleeding due to scratching by the infected individual. **Mebendazole**, a broad-spectrum antihelminth drug, and **piperazine** are commonly used to treat enterobiasis.

## Trichuris trichiura

*Trichuris trichiura* has cosmopolitan distribution with approximately 1 billion people infected world-

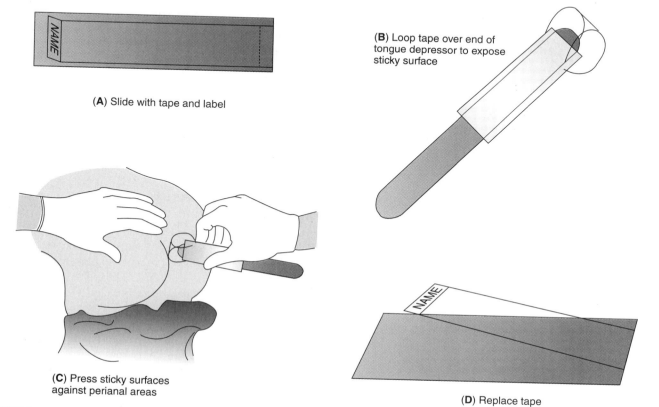

(A) Slide with tape and label

(B) Loop tape over end of tongue depressor to expose sticky surface

(C) Press sticky surfaces against perianal areas

(D) Replace tape

**FIGURE 46-3** The "Scotch tape" method for detection of pinworms.

wide. Whipworm infections occur primarily in under-developed tropical countries but about 2 million individuals in the southeastern United States are infected as well. The infection is most often seen in children and is associated with poor hygiene, especially hand-washing. It is also common in parts of the world where night soil (human feces used as fertilizer) is used in agriculture.

*Trichuris trichiura* is referred to as the whipworm due to the morphology of the adult worms. The anterior two-thirds of the worm is long and threadlike; the posterior end is thick and resembles a tiny handle. The thin portion of the male worm is coiled, but the female's is straight. Adult worms vary from 30 to 55 mm in length (see Figure 46-4). Infection occurs on ingestion of embryonated eggs containing the first stage larva in contaminated food or water.

After ingestion, the eggs hatch in the duodenum where they take 1 month to mature. The adult worms migrate and reside in the cecum. After copulation, the female worm produces between 3,000 and 10,000 eggs a day, which are passed from the host in their feces. When deposited in soil, the eggs must incubate for at least 10 days to become fully embryonated and infectious. The embryonated eggs are ingested in contaminated food or water, or if individuals have contact with

contaminated soil (without washing their hands) infection occurs.

Light infections with whipworms are usually asymptomatic or subclinical. Symptoms in heavy infections include nausea, abdominal pain, diarrhea, dysentery, and sometimes malabsorption. The growth of infected children may be stunted. Severe mucosal damage is common in heavy infections and can result in blood loss and anemia. Colonic or rectal prolapse is sometimes observed in individuals with heavy worm loads.

Diagnosis is based on the fecal presence of oval or football-shaped eggs having polar plugs at both ends. Stool concentration methods may be necessary to recover the eggs in light infections but are not necessary in heavy infections. Mebendazole is the drug of choice but the cure rate is only 60% to 70%.

## Ascaris lumbricoides

*Ascaris lumbricoides* is the largest nematode that causes intestinal infection in humans. The infection is called **ascariasis** and is common worldwide. Ascariasis is often seen in the United States. The adult worms can reach an alarming 30 cm (about 1 foot) in length (see Figure 46-5*A*). Eggs of *Ascaris* are passed in the feces of the infected individual and hatch in soil where they feed on bacteria (Figure 46-5*B* and *C*).

Human infection occurs when individuals walk barefooted on contaminated soil. The tiny larvae penetrate the skin of the foot, enter a blood or lymph vessel, and are carried to the lungs. The larvae cause irritation of the lungs and can result in pneumonia. Larvae are coughed up in sputum, swallowed, and are carried to the small intestine where they mature into adult worms that feed on partially digested food. Except in heavy infections the nematodes usually cause few symptoms (see Figure 46-6).

Diagnosis is based on detection of eggs in the feces of the patient or by emergence of adult worms from the anus. Mebendazole is commonly used to treat ascariasis.

## Necator americanus and Ancylostoma duodenale

*Necator americanus* and *Ancylostoma duodenale* are discussed here together because their life cycles are virtually identical and their morphologies are very similar. *N. americanus* is often referred to as the New World hookworm, and *A. duodenale* is called the Old World hookworm. Human infection with hookworms has cosmopolitan distribution between the latitudes of 45° north and 30° south. *Necator* occurs primarily in the tropical areas of Africa and Asia and in the southeastern United States. The worm was introduced to the United States with the African slave trade. *Ancylostoma* is seen most often in the Mediterranean basin, the Middle East, northern India, China, and Japan. Approximately 700

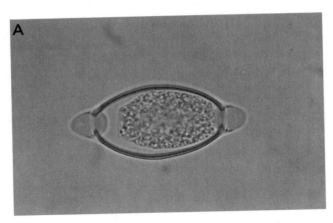

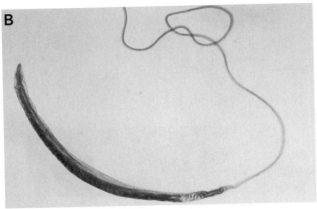

**FIGURE 46-4** Embryonated egg **(A)** and adult worm **(B)** of *T. trichiura.*

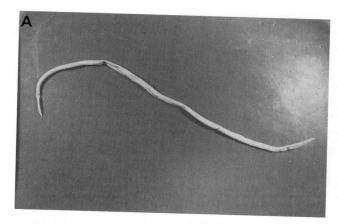

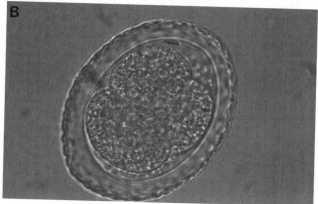

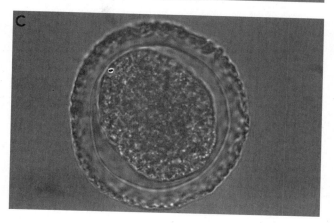

**FIGURE 46-5** Adult worm **(A)**, fertilized, unembryonated egg **(B)**, and unfertilized egg **(C)**, of *A. lumbricoides.*

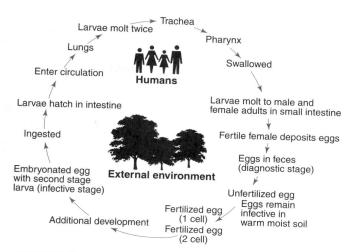

**FIGURE 46-6** *Ascaris lumbricoides,* life cycle.

After copulation, the female worm produces 10,000 to 20,000 eggs a day, which are passed from the host in their feces. The eggs are usually in the four- to eight-cell stage when they are passed from the host (see Figure 46-7*B*). They have a thin shell and vary from 40 to 60 µm in length. The eggs must be passed onto shady, well drained soil to hatch (in 48 hours) into the rhabdi-

million people worldwide are infected with hookworms and 50,000 to 60,000 deaths occur annually.

The adult worms are about 10 mm in length and the head is often observed curving in a direction opposite of the body (see Figure 46-7*A*). Hooks surrounding the mouth of the worm are used for attachment to the intestinal mucosa and to obtain blood from the host's tissues. Male hookworms have a unique fan-shaped **copulatory bursa**. Although differentiation of the worms is not usually attempted it can be accomplished by comparison of the morphology of the oral cavities.

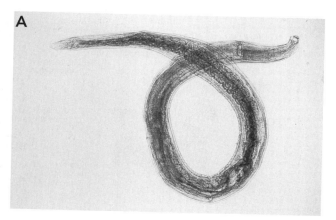

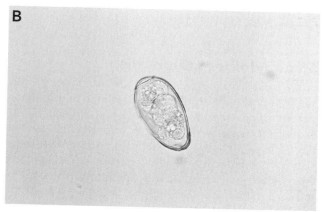

**FIGURE 47-7** *Necator americanus* and *Ancylostoma duodenale.* **A.** Adult worm; **B.** Egg.

tiform larva (Ryan, 1994). The larvae are free-living in soil where they feed on bacteria. Human infection occurs when the larvae penetrate the skin of barefooted individuals who walk on contaminated soil. After penetrating the skin of the host, the larvae enter a blood or lymph vessel and pass through the right side of the heart and into the lungs. They are coughed up in sputum and swallowed, and take up residence on the small intestine (see Figure 46-8).

As seen in many of the intestinal helminths, light infections are usually asymptomatic. The initial skin infection often causes a rash and swelling, usually between the toes of the victim. Pulmonary symptoms may occur and are similar to ascariasis, but are less frequent and less severe. Both hookworms extract blood from their host and other bleeding occurs due to the migration of the worms. Anemia is common in heavy infections and heart failure occurs in some children.

Diagnosis is based on the detection of eggs in the feces. Usually no attempt is made to differentiate between *Necator* and *Ancylostoma*. Treatment involves correction of the anemia (often by iron replacement) and pyrantel pamoate or mebendazole. Both drugs are extremely effective.

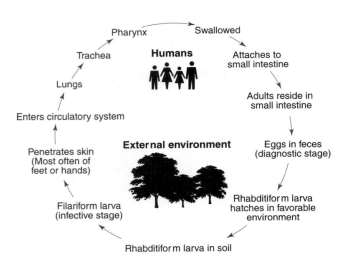

**FIGURE 46-8** Hookworm life cycle.

## *Strongyloides stercoralis*

*Strongyloides stercoralis,* or the threadworm, is the smallest of the intestinal nematodes infecting humans. Adult worms reach only 2 mm in length. Infection with *Strongyloides* occurs primarily in tropical climates. The life cycle of *Strongyloides* includes an egg, two larval stages (rhabditiform and filariform), and the adult worm (see Figure 46-9). The males are rarely observed in infected individuals because they are passed from the gut shortly after copulation with the female worm.

The pregnant female penetrates the mucosa of the duodenum where she deposits her eggs, which hatch

into rhabditiform larvae. The larvae vary from 16 to 200 μm in length and resemble hookworms, but have a shorter buccal cavity (see Figure 46-10). The rhabditiform larvae reenter the lumen of the gut and are passed from the host in their feces.

Rhabditiform larvae hatch in the soil into filariform larvae. Human infection occurs when the larvae penetrate the skin. As in ascariasis, the larvae are transported to the lungs by the circulatory system. They are coughed up and swallowed, and mature in the small intestine. The rhabditiform larvae can mature in the soil and pass through several generations before the infectious rhabditiform is again produced.

Pulmonary symptoms, again similar to ascariasis, occur in some hosts, but intestinal infections are usually asymptomatic. In heavy intestinal infections, abdominal symptoms including pain and tenderness, vomiting, diarrhea, and malabsorption may be observed. The parasitic burden of the host is increased by **internal autoinfection** of the nematode without the usual soil

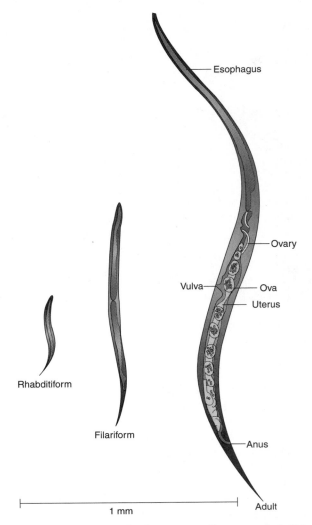

**FIGURE 46-9** *Strongyloides stercoralis*—egg, rhabditiform and filariform larvae, and adult worm.

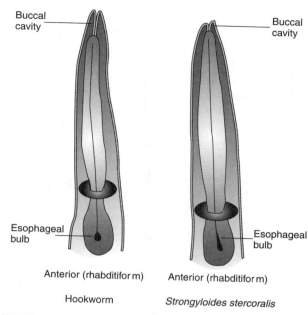

Buccal cavity

Esophageal bulb

Anterior (rhabditiform)

Hookworm

Buccal cavity

Esophageal bulb

Anterior (rhabditiform)

*Strongyloides stercoralis*

**FIGURE 46-10** *S. stercoralis* and *N. americanus*, comparison of buccal cavities.

phase. This ability is unique (among the intestinal nematodes) to *Strongyloides*.

Diagnosis is based on identification of rhabditiform larvae in the feces. It is important to examine freshly voided specimens so as not to confuse the larvae with

hatching hookworm eggs. All health care personnel should wear gloves and a gown when handling specimens to avoid infection with rhabditiform larvae. Infected individuals are usually treated with **thiabendazole**, but this treatment is not 100% effective. For this reason the feces must be rechecked to see if retreatment is necessary.

## CESTODES

The tapeworms, or cestodes, are members of the phylum Platyhelminthes, class Cestoda. All cestodes have segmented bodies and are parasitic. Species that infect humans have complex life cycles that involve a definitive and an intermediate host. Humans serve as the definitive host in some tapeworm life cycles, or as an acceptable alternate definitive host, as in *Taenia solium*. In other tapeworm species, humans serve as an intermediate host to a larval form of the worm. Tapeworms have flat, ribbon-like bodies that vary from a few millimeters to over 20 meters in length (see Figure 46-11). They lack a digestive system and absorb predigested food through their cuticle. The body consists of a scolex, or head, a neck, and hundreds to thousands of body segments called proglottids. The scolex has suckers and sometimes small hooks that attach the worm to the mucosa of the host's small intestine. The neck is attached to the scolex and is the site of proglottid production.

Tapeworms are monecious, meaning that both male

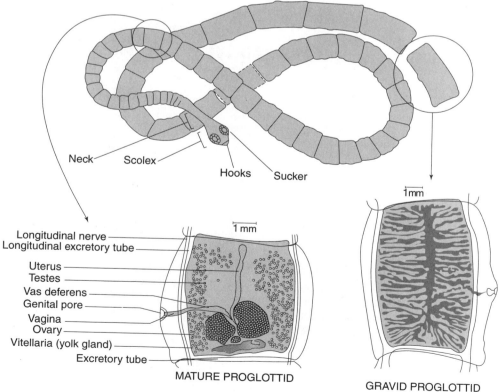

Neck  Scolex  Hooks  Sucker

1 mm

Longitudinal nerve
Longitudinal excretory tube

Uterus
Testes
Vas deferens
Genital pore
Vagina
Ovary
Vitellaria (yolk gland)
Excretory tube

MATURE PROGLOTTID

1 mm

GRAVID PROGLOTTID

**FIGURE 46-11** Generalized tapeworm anatomy.

and female reproductive organs are contained in one individual. Each proglottid is a complete reproductive unit that produces hundreds of eggs. As new, immature proglottids are formed the existing ones are pushed toward the posterior end of the worm where they mature. Once the proglottid produces eggs it is referred to as gravid, which means pregnant (see Figure 46-12). Eventually, the gravid proglottids break off of the posterior end and are passed from the host in their feces. The proglottids of some tapeworm species are large enough to be observed with the naked eye, whereas others are only visible microscopically.

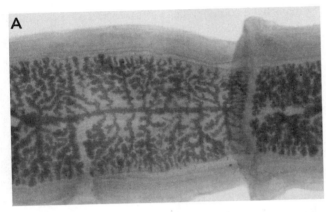

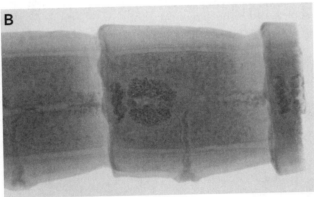

**FIGURE 46-12** Immature, mature, and gravid proglottids.

## *Taenia saginata* and *Taenia solium*

Many similarities exist between the life cycles and human infection with *Taenia saginata* (the beef tapeworm) and *Taenia solium* (the pork tapeworm) and so they are discussed together. Both organisms have cosmopolitan distribution, but occur primarily in Latin America, Asia, and Africa. Human infection is associated with the ingestion of larvae in contaminated, undercooked beef or pork, and occasionally by other infected herbivores. *T. solium* is also transmitted to humans by the ingestion of eggs through the use of night soil and by poor hygiene. The eggs of *T. saginata* are not believed to be infectious to humans.

Humans are the definitive host for both *T. saginata* and *T. solium;* humans and pigs can serve as the intermediate host for *T. solium.* Bovines (cattle), and occasionally other herbivores, are the intermediate hosts for *T. saginata.* The life cycle of *T. saginata* is shown in Figure 46-13 and that of *T. solium* in Figure 46-14. The two organisms are compared in Figure 46-15.

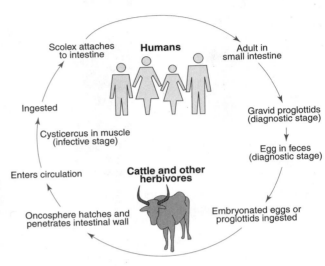

**FIGURE 46-13** Life cycle of *T. saginata.*

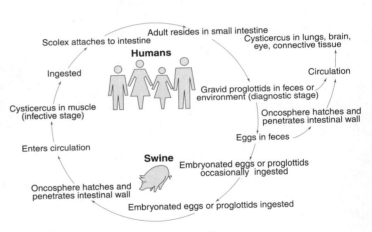

**FIGURE 46-14** Life cycle of *T. solium.*

Gravid proglottids containing thousands of eggs are passed in the feces of humans that are infected with *T. saginata.* When the contaminated feces are used to fertilize pastures that cattle graze on, the eggs are ingested. The eggs hatch into larva that penetrate the intestinal wall, migrate to muscle tissue, and encyst as **cysticerci.** New human infections occur on the consumption of raw or undercooked (rare) beef containing the cysticerci. When humans ingest contaminated beef, everything but the tapeworm's scolex is digested. The life cycle of *T. saginata* continues when the scolex attaches to the human's small intestine and begins the

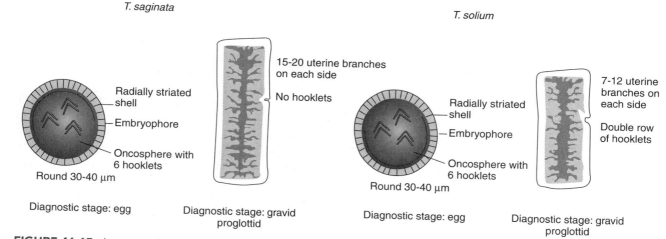

**FIGURE 46-15** A comparison of *T. saginata* and *T. solium*, showing eggs and proglottids.

production of new proglottids. The adult tapeworm can reach a length of 4 to 10 meters.

Human infection with *T. saginata* is diagnosed based on the presence of proglottids or eggs (or both) in the feces. Infection can be prevented by avoiding the use of night soil as fertilizer and by the inspection of beef. Infected, or "measly," beef can be detected by examination for cysticerci, which are visible to the naked eye. Most infected individuals harbor only one tapeworm and are asymptomatic. Some individuals experience nausea, diarrhea, and weight loss. Praziquantel or niclosamide are used to treat infected humans and are highly effective in a single-dose oral preparation.

Adult *T. solium* also reside in the small intestine of infected humans, who pass the proglottids and eggs in their feces. When the proglottids or eggs are ingested by pigs, they hatch into a larval form called the **oncosphere**, which penetrates the intestinal wall and enters the circulatory system. The oncospheres migrate to and encyst in muscle tissue as a cysticercus. Humans become infected when they consume undercooked pork containing cysticerci. A difference between *T. solium* and the beef tapeworm is that autoinfection of humans with *T. solium* can occur when they ingest the eggs due to poor hygiene practices. When *T. solium* cysticerci are ingested by humans, the infection is similar to what occurs with *T. saginata*. Ingestion of *T. solium* eggs by humans follows the same course as is seen in pigs. An oncosphere hatches from the egg, penetrates the intestinal wall, enters the circulatory system, and encysts as the cysticercus in muscles, the heart, the liver, the lungs, the brain, and the eyes. Brain infections usually result in central nervous system symptoms including fever and headache and the mortality rate approaches 50%. Prolonged treatment with praziquantel or albendazole are fairly effective.

## Diphyllobothrium latum

*Diphyllobothrium latum* is known as the fish tapeworm or the broad tapeworm. Humans become infected when they eat raw (sushi or sashimi) or undercooked contaminated fish including salmon, trout, perch, and pike. It is referred to as the broad tapeworm due to the width of its proglottids. *D. latum* is the largest tapeworm that infects humans. It can reach a length of 10 meters and may have as many as 3,000 to 4,000 proglottids. Humans, dogs, and cats serve as the definitive hosts of *D. latum;* crustaceans (such as the genus *Cyclops*) and fish serve as intermediate hosts.

Two sucking grooves attach the worm to the intestinal mucosa of infected humans (or dogs or cats) (see Figures 46-16 and 46-17). Over 1 million eggs a day are released in the feces of the infected individual. The eggs are released from the uterine pore of the tapeworm, rather than in proglottids that break off of the end of other tapeworm species. Another difference between it and other tapeworms is that the eggs of *D. latum* are operculated.

When the eggs are released into freshwater they hatch and release a ciliated, free-swimming larva called the **coracidia**. The coracidia must be ingested by a suitable crustacean within a few days for the life cycle to proceed where it develops into the second larval form know as the **procercoid**. The life cycle continues when the infected crustacean is consumed by one of the fish mentioned earlier. In the fish, larvae migrate to muscle tissue and develop into the infectious **plerocercoid**. Humans are infected when they consume the plerocercoid in raw, undercooked or pickled contaminated fish.

Infection with the fish tapeworm is seen most often in countries with cool climates such as Russia, Switzerland, and the Scandinavian countries. It also occurs in

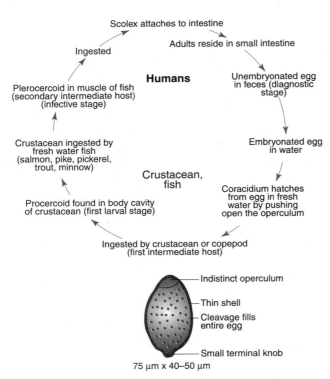

FIGURE 46-16 Life cycle and egg of *D. latum*.

Italy, Japan, Chile, and in North America. Most infections are asymptomatic, but in persons with heavy worm loads a variety of symptoms may be experienced. These include abdominal distention, abdominal cramps, flatulence, belching, and diarrhea. Intestinal or biliary blockage is also possible. Diagnosis is based on the presence of eggs in the feces. Praziquantel or niclosimide is used successfully to treat fish tapeworm infections. Human infection can be avoided by cooking fish or freezing it at −10°C for 48 hours before consumption. Prevention of untreated sewage into streams and lakes is also important in breaking *D. latum*'s life cycle.

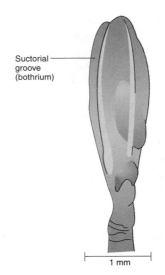

FIGURE 46-17 The scolex of *D. latum*.

# TREMATODES

The flukes are flat, leaf-shaped helminths whose bodies lack the segmentation that is seen in the tapeworms. They are members of the phylum Platyhelminthes, class Trematoda, and are also known as the trematodes. The flukes have complex life cycles with several stages of sexual and asexual reproduction. The life cycle includes a definitive host and at least two intermediate hosts. Trematodes that are intestinal parasites of humans (at least during some portion of their life cycle) are monecious.

A generalized adult fluke is seen in Figure 46-18. The adult worm has an oral sucker that opens into its digestive system. Nutrients are drawn from the host's tissue through the oral sucker and are also absorbed through the worm's body surface. Trematodes lack an anus so waste is excreted through the oral sucker. A ventral sucker attaches the fluke to the host.

Although some variations occur from species to species in the life cycles of trematodes, the general course of events occur as follows. The adult worm lays eggs that are passed from the human host in their feces. In order for the life cycle to continue the eggs must be deposited in freshwater. A ciliated, free-swimming larva called the **miracidium** emerges from the egg and enters a snail, which is the first intermediate host. Several stages of asexual reproduction occur in the snail and include production of larval **redia** and free-swimming larval **cercariae**. The cercariae exit the snail by boring through its tissues and encyst on a plant (such as water chestnuts) or enter a second intermediate host as a **metacercariae**. Freshwater fish or crustaceans such as crabs commonly serve as the second intermediate host. Humans become infected when they consume a contaminated plant or crustacean. The metacercariae encyst in the human's intestinal tract then migrate to various parts of the body. The site of maturation into the adult worm varies with the species of trematode and could be the lungs or liver. Specific life cycles are included in the discussions of each fluke.

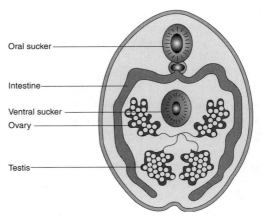

FIGURE 46-18 Generalized fluke anatomy.

## Clonorchis sinesis

*Clonorchis sinesis* is known as the oriental liver fluke and is seen almost exclusively in populations that routinely consume raw fish. Humans, pigs, and cattle serve as definitive hosts of *Clonorchis,* snails and fish are the first and second intermediate hosts (see Figure 46-19 and refer to Color Plate 112).

The use of human and animal feces as fertilizer that contaminates ponds where fish are caught propagates the life cycle. Individuals with light infections usually experience mild symptoms, primarily indigestion. Heavily infected individuals may experience obstruction of the bile duct and jaundice. Praziquantel is most often used to treat *Clonorchis* infections.

## Paragonimus westermani

*Paragonimus westermani,* or the lung fluke, has cosmopolitan distribution, but is most often seen in Eastern Asia. Although several species of *Paragonimus* infect humans, *P. westermani* is most often seen. About 5 million individuals are infected. The adult worm resides in the bronchioles of humans and other mammals and reaches a length of 12 mm. Eggs are released into the sputum of the infected individual and many of them are swallowed to be released in the host's feces. The egg varies from 50 to 90 μm in length. The life cycle of *Paragonimus* is shown in Figure 46-20 and the adult worm and operculated egg are seen in Color Plate 113.

Most individuals with lung fluke infection are asymptomatic, but some ectopic infections of the brain do occur. Lung infections sometimes result in the formation of fibrous capsules that surround and enclose the parasite. Eggs in the feces are diagnostic of *Paragonimus,* but may not be detected for the first 3 months of the infection. Bithionol and praziquantel are commonly used to treat lung fluke infections and complete cooking of shellfish can prevent the disease from occurring.

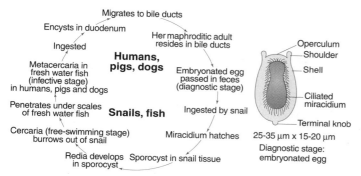

**FIGURE 46-19** Eggs **(A)** and life cycle **(B)** of *C. sinesis.*

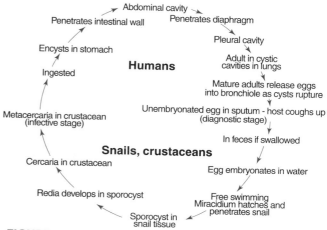

**FIGURE 46-20** Life cycle of *P. westermani.*

## SUMMARY

▶ Nematodes (roundworms) are members of the phylum Aschelminthes and have long, cylindrical bodies, a complete digestive system and are dioecious.

▶ *Enterobius vermicularis,* the pinworm, causes enterobiasis on ingestion of the embryonated egg. *Trichuris trichiura,* the whipworm, is seen most often in underdeveloped countries. *Ascaris lumbricoides* is the largest nematode infecting humans.

▶ *Necator americanus* and *Ancylostoma duodenale* are called hookworms and have nearly identical life cycles and morphologies. *Strongyloides stercoralis,* the threadworm, is the smallest nematode to infect humans.

▶ The tapeworms are members of the phylum Platyhelminthes, class Cestoda. All are parasitic, have flattened, segmented bodies, complex life cycles, and are monecious.

▶ *Taenia saginata* and *Taenia solium* are tapeworms that share many similarities. Both occur primarily in Latin America, Asia, and Africa. *Diphyllobothrium latum* is the fish tapeworm, or the broad tapeworm.

▶ The flukes are flat and leaf-shaped and lack segmentation. They are members of phylum Platyhelminthes, class Trematoda. Flukes have complex life cycles and are monecious.

▶ *Clonorchis sinesis* is the oriental liver fluke and is seen in populations that eat raw fish. *Paragonimus westermani,* the lung fluke, is most often seen in Eastern Asia.

## CASE STUDY

A 49-year-old man, a recent Russian immigrant, is admitted to the hospital for a possible intestinal blockage. When taking the patient's history, the physician learned that the patient has been experiencing chronic diarrhea, flatulence, and abdominal cramps. Further questioning revealed that the consumption of pickled fish, usually pike, was common in the patient's home village. Cestode eggs but no proglottids were recovered from the patient's feces. Based on this information answer the following questions.

**Questions:**

1. What genus and species of cestode is the most likely culprit?

2. Why were no proglottids recovered from the patient's fecal sample?

3. How could the infection have been avoided?

4. What treatment is recommended for treatment of infections with this cestode?

## Review Questions

1. Nematodes that parasitize humans spend:
   a. their entire life cycle in the human host.
   b. a portion of their life cycle in the human host and a portion in soil.
   c. a portion of their life cycle in an arthropod vector.
   d. Both b and c are true.

2. A 3-year-old boy is examined in an outpatient clinic for itching and bleeding of the perianal skin. His mother observed a small, round worm protruding from his anus but did not have the presence of mind to bring the worm to the doctor. Which of the following did the doctor most likely give the mother for use on the child to aid in diagnosis? Which drug is likely to have been prescribed?
   a. Nothing, metronidazole
   b. A small jar of formalin, Flagyl
   c. Nothing, but she ordered a lung biopsy, an iron supplement
   d. A small paddle covered with sticky tape, mebendazole

3. A 47-year-old female Korean immigrant presents with chronic indigestion and mild jaundice. The physician determines that sushi dishes are a favorite of the patient. While in Korea, the patient worked as a fisherwoman. What is the likely diagnosis and treatment?
   a. *Clonorchis sinesis,* praziquantel
   b. *Necator americanus,* mebendazole
   c. *Paragonimus westermani,* bithionol
   d. *Hymenolepsis diminuta,* no treatment is necessary unless the symptoms worsen

4. A patient is infected with *Necator americanus.* How did the infection probably occur?
   a. By ingesting contaminated water chestnuts
   b. By ingesting contaminated bamboo
   c. By ingesting undercooked beef
   d. By walking barefooted on contaminated soil

5. Infection with which of the following parasites is most likely to result in the development of serious symptoms?
   a. *Ascaris lumbricoides*
   b. *Taenia saginata*
   c. *Taenia solium* eggs
   d. *Taenia solium* cysticerci

6. Human infection with _____ may occur on ingestion of infected grain or grain products.
   a. *Clonorchis sinesis*
   b. *Hymenolepsis diminuta*
   c. *Fasciolopsis buski*
   d. *Necator americanus*

7. A resident specializing in tropical medicine examines a 7-year-old girl. She is obviously small for her age and is anemic. The child has experienced alternating bouts of diarrhea and dysentery for at least 6 months. A fecal examination reveals football-shaped eggs with polar plugs at both ends. How was the child most likely infected?
   a. By eating raw fish
   b. By eating contaminated water chestnuts
   c. Oral-fecal route
   d. By playing in contaminated soil

8. What drug is prescribed to the child in question 7?
   a. Flagyl
   b. Ampicillin and tetracycline
   c. Mebendazole
   d. Pyrantel pamoate

9. A difference between *Diphyllobothrium latum* and many other tapeworms is:
   a. *D. latum* is vectored to humans by beetles.
   b. that it is the only tapeworm in which the patient requires no chemotherapy.
   c. that is the only tapeworm that lacks an intermediate host.
   d. that its eggs are released through a uterine pore rather than in proglottids.

10. How are infections with *Necator americanus* and *Ancylostoma duodenale* differentiated?
   a. On the basis of the morphology of the adult worms
   b. On the basis of egg morphology
   c. Based on patient symptoms
   d. None of the above

## ▶ REFERENCES & RECOMMENDED READING

Baron, E. J., Peterson, L. R., & Finegold, S. M. (1994). *Bailey and Scott's diagnostic microbiology* (9th ed.). St. Louis: Mosby.

Coleman, R. M., et al. (1989). *Fundamental immunology*. Dubuque, IA: Wm. C. Brown.

Delost, M. D. (1997). *Introduction to diagnostic microbiology: A text and workbook*. St. Louis: Mosby.

Garcia, L. S., & Bruckner, D. A. (1993). *Diagnostic medical parasitology* (2nd ed.). Washington, DC: American Society for Microbiology.

Kuby, J. (1994). *Immunology* (2nd ed.). New York: Freeman.

Markell, E. K., Voge, M., & John, D. T. (1992). *Medical parasitology* (7th ed.). Philadelphia: Saunders.

Miller, B. F., & Keane, C. B. (1987). *Encyclopedia and dictionary of medicine, nursing and allied health* (4th ed.). Philadelphia: Saunders.

Neva, F. A., & Brown, H. W. (1994). *Basic clinical parasitology* (6th ed.). East Norwalk, CT: Appleton & Lange.

Olsen, O. W. (1986). *Animal parasites: Their life cycles and ecology*. New York: Dover.

Ryan, K. J. (Ed.). (1994). *Sherris: Medical microbiology: An introduction to infectious diseases* (3rd ed.). Stamford, CT: Appleton & Lange.

Schmidt, G. D., & Roberts, L. S. (1989). *Foundations of parasitology* (4th ed.). St. Louis: Times Mirror/Mosby.

*Scientific American: A Special Issue*. (1994). Life, death and the immune system. New York: Freeman.

Thomas, C. L. (Ed.). (1997). *Taber's cyclopedic medical dictionary* (17th ed.). Philadelphia: Davis.

Tortora, G. J., Funke, B. R., & Case, C. C. (1992). *Microbiology: An introduction* (4th ed.). Redwood City, CA: Benjamin/Cummings.

Wyler, D. J. (Ed.). (1990). *Modern parasite biology: Cellular, immunological and molecular aspects*. New York: Freeman.

# CHAPTER 47

# Blood and Tissue Helminths

Jeffrey J. Adamovicz, PhD

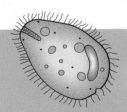

## *Microbes in the News*

### Dracunculiasis Prevalent in 18 Developing Countries

Pakistan is the first country to have completely eliminated dracunculiasis during the global program for dracunculiasis eradication, having reported zero cases every month since October 1993. Globally, the achieved reduction in cases has been about 97% during the past decade, from an estimated 3.5 million cases in 1986 to about 100,000 cases worldwide during 1995. As of December 1995, five countries reported fewer than 100 cases for the entire year, in addition to Pakistan with its zero cases. If the more than 80% reduction in cases seen in recent months is sustained, dracunculiasis will indeed soon become the first parasitic disease ever to be eradicated (World Health Organization, Division of Control of Tropical Diseases).

**INTRODUCTION**

**NEMATODES**
*Trichinella spiralis*
Filarial Nematodes

**CESTODES**
*Echinococcus granulosus*

**TREMATODES**
*Schistosoma mansoni,*
*Schistosoma japonicum,* and
*Schistosoma haematobium*

**UNCOMMON HELMINTHS**
*Dracunculus medinensis*

## KEY TERMS

Bancroftian
Brugian
Calabar swelling
Cystic hydatid disease
Dracunculiasis
Elephantitis
Filarial

Filariasis
Kampala eye worm
Knott's technique
Loiasis
Mansonelliasis
Microfilariae

Onchocerciasis
Oncosphere
River blindness
Robles disease
Sowda
Stroblia

## LEARNING OBJECTIVES

**Upon successful completion of this chapter, the student should be able to:**

1. Identify the current and future laboratory tests used to diagnose helminth infections.
2. Understand the importance of insect vectors in the transmission of helminth disease.
3. Relate periodicity to the collection of clinical samples for diagnosis of filarial disease.
4. Identify the role that dogs play as reservoirs of helminth disease for humans.
5. Understand the role that geography and weather play in spreading/restricting helminth infections.

## INTRODUCTION

A major group of human parasites are the blood and tissue helminths. These multicellular organisms are important agents of disease throughout the world. Taxonomically the helminths are composed of the phylum Aschelminthes, containing the class Nematoda (roundworms), and the phylum Platyhelminthes which includes the trematodes or flukes, and the cestodes or tapeworms. The increased mobility of today's human population has allowed travel to or from areas of endemic helminth disease to areas where the medical/laboratory staff are unfamiliar with the disease or its diagnosis. This has created an expanded need for the clinical laboratory to identify disease-causing helminths and to confirm helminthic infection in people. During the last 5 years, many new laboratory methods have been created to facilitate accurate and rapid diagnosis of parasitic infection. Many of these methods are available only in specialty or reference laboratories; therefore, most laboratories still perform the traditional identification tests.

## NEMATODES

### Trichinella spiralis

**Epidemiology.** *Trichinella spiralis,* the causative agent of trichinosis, is transmitted from animal to humans by ingestion of undercooked meat containing cysts. The most common reservoir of the disease for humans is the domestic pig, but any carnivorous or omnivorous animal can be infected and carry cysts. Because the parasite lacks host specificity it has a worldwide distribution, but the number of infected people is unknown. The disease is most common in areas of the world where the chain of transmission between infected animals is unbroken and meat for human consumption is undercooked. This disease occurs in about 200,000 people per year in the United States and is under public health surveillance (Case definitions, 1997).

**Etiology and Pathology.** Most cases of trichinosis, especially in healthy adults, are asymptomatic, but severe symptoms may manifest with heavy parasite burdens or poor health. A common transmission cycle includes the consumption of cyst-carrying rats by domestic pigs and subsequent consumption of the pigs by people. Symptoms of *T. spiralis* infection can be divided into three clinical stages: intestinal, disseminated, and convalescent. The intestinal stage occurs 2 to 7 days after infection and produces nonspecific physical findings to include diarrhea and abdominal pain. These symptoms occur after the ingested cyst is digested and the larva embeds itself in the upper small intestine. The larva matures in the small intestine to the adult form through four molts over the course of 3 days. The adults mate in the gut lumen; the female then embeds itself in the mucosa and produces up to 1,500 larvae over the course of her life. After mating, the male may remain in the lumen for several weeks but is usually rapidly expelled. The female may continue to produce larvae over the next few weeks to months depending on the immune state and health of the host but is also eventually expelled.

During the second week of infection and for up to 12 weeks the larvae penetrate the gut mucosa and enter the bloodstream and lymphatics and quickly invade the striated skeletal muscle. Many of these larvae are destroyed by the body during the invasion of the muscle tissue, but many are able to invade individual muscle cells and encyst. The larvae seem to prefer the most active muscle tissue cells and are able to subvert the muscle cell for its own purposes. The larvae will grow to a length of about 1,100 µm but this is difficult to measure because the larvae are coiled within the cyst. The cysts are arranged as elongated lemon shapes parallel to the muscle fiber and are visible to the naked eye. The disease manifestations include fever, weakness, muscle soreness, and periorbital edema. The fever may be intermittent as seen in protozoan infections. The majority of people eventually develop splinter hemorrhages under the nail beds. Although generally asymptomatic, invasion of the heart muscle occurs in the majority of patients. This facet of the infection can be associated with heart palpitations, difficult breathing, arrhythmias, and sometimes death. Less common symptoms include headaches and a fine macular rash.

The third stage of the disease occurs when the adults

are expelled from the gut and the migrating larvae have encysted or been destroyed. The clinical symptoms begin to diminish and eventually disappear with the exception of the eosinophilia, which may remain elevated for months. During this phase the encysted larvae are slowly destroyed by the body's granulomatous response and eventually calcify. This response is usually incomplete as viable larvae have been recovered from cysts that are up to 15 years old. It is during this stage that measurement of serum antibodies becomes useful.

This disease can be prevented by the proper handling and preparation of meat and meat products. Cooking meat (> 58.3°C, 20 min/lb) or freezing meat (−15°C for 20 days) will kill the cysts. All utensils that come in contact with meat or meat by-products should be thoroughly cleaned. If the disease is contracted it can be treated with mebendazole. The use of steroids is recommended for patients with heart and or central nervous system (CNS) involvement.

**Identification.** It is extremely rare to identify the disease during the intestinal stage because adults or larvae are rarely identified in the feces. The disease is frequently misidentified as gastroenteritis during the first week. Examination of the peripheral blood usually reveals increased numbers of leukocytes and eosinophils. Eosinophilia is frequently noted throughout the course of the disease and is a hallmark of many helminth infections. During the disseminated stage of the disease the first diagnostic "window of opportunity" opens. The opportunity to diagnose the disease increases with time and the basis of these tests are described below.

**TRADITIONAL.** Examination of peripheral blood sediment treated with 3% acetic acid should reveal the presence of larvae during the dissemination stage of the disease. The size of the migrating larvae averages from 100 to 150 μm long by 6 to 8 μm wide. The larvae may also be recovered from cerebrospinal fluid (CSF) of patients with CNS symptoms. During the end of the disseminated and convalescent stage, the identification of fresh noncalcified cysts is considered diagnostic. This is generally accomplished by microscopic examination of a muscle biopsy for cysts (refer to Color Plate 114). This is followed by pepsin digestion of the muscle tissue and sedimentation to recover viable larvae.

**IMMUNOLOGIC.** Several approaches have been taken with these techniques. Delayed hypersensitivity following intradermal injection of larvae extracts indicates exposure (but not active infection) to *Trichinella*. This test is rapid and produces a result within 20 minutes but cannot be given until 3 weeks after infection. The test will remain positive for up to 7 years after exposure. The second type of test detects parasite antigens in tissue or fluids. This assay is an enzyme-linked immunosorbent assay (ELISA) test but is insensitive because it can only detect antigen in less than half of infected patients. The advantage of this test is that it is 100% specific for *Trichinella* with no cross-reactivity to other nematode antigens (Lewis & Maizels, 1993).

## Filarial Nematodes

Human infections by **filarial** nematodes are mediated by arthropod vectors. These vectors are primarily biting insects such as mosquitoes and flies. Disease distribution is therefore associated with the range of the insect vector. There are seven known filarial helminths that infect primarily humans; five of these are discussed below. It is important to differentiate the parasites that require humans to complete their life cycle from zoonotic infections in which humans are not the primary or definitive host. Zoonotic **filariasis** occurs when humans are infected with larva that cannot complete their life cycle in humans. The filaria that normally infect animals other than humans include *Dirofilaria* species. The human filarial infections can be subclassified as lymphatic (e.g., **bancroftian** and **brugian**) and nonlymphatic (e.g., **loiasis, onchocerciasis** and **mansonelliasis**). In lymphatic infections, the larval stage of the parasite enters the wound caused by an insect bite. The larva becomes an adult in the lymph vessels then the adults mate and produce **microfilariae**. The microfilariae eventually enter the bloodstream and are subsequently acquired by the vector (e.g., biting insect). An interesting adaptation of the parasite to its host and vector is the phenomenon of periodicity. Periodicity is the association of the appearance of microfilariae in the peripheral blood with the feeding habits of the mosquito. The microfilariae are either nocturnal (circulate in the blood at night), diurnal (appear during the day), or neither (microfilariae are present in the blood continuously). It is important to note that these definitions are not absolute, that is, it is possible to detect nocturnal microfilariae from daytime blood samples with a sufficiently sensitive technique. The pathology of bancroftian and brugian filariasis is caused by damage to the lymphatic vessels by adult worms. The tissue damage caused by agents of nonlymphatic filariasis is a result of migration of either adult worms or microfilaria. The epidemiology, etiology, pathology, and identification of human filiarial nematodes are discussed below.

### *Wuchereria bancrofti* and *Brugia malayi.*

**EPIDEMIOLOGY.** In 1977, lymphatic filariasis was targeted by the World Health Organization (WHO) for eradication but today there are still an estimated 119 million infected humans (Michael, Bundy, & Grenfell, 1996). The majority of infections are caused by *W. bancrofti,* which has a worldwide tropical distribution, and humans are the only known reservoir for the disease. The disease is transmitted by three different mosquito species although usually one species is dominant in a particular geographic area. In the eastern coastal areas of South America, the vectors, in decreasing prominence, include *Culex, Aedes* and *Anopheles* mosquitoes; in Africa, *Anopheles* and *Culex*; in Asia and Micronesia, the primary vector is *Culex* while the *Anopheles* and *Aedes* vectors are dominant in the Polynesian area. Another important agent of lymphatic filariasis is *B. malayi*. The distribution of *B. malayi* is restricted to south and southeast Asia due to the limited range of the *Mansoniodes* mosquito although the *Anopheles* and *Aedes* mosquitoes can also vector the disease. Humans are the primary hosts for *B. malayi,* but zoonotic strains, which infect leaf monkeys and cats, have also been described.

*Wuchereria bancrofti* transmission by the day-feeding *Aedes* mosquito is described as diurnal subperiodicity while transmission by the night-feeding *Culex* and *Anopheles* mosquito is described as nocturnal (between 2200 and 0200 hours) periodicity. *Mansoniodes* mosquitoes are night feeders; therefore, the periodicity of the majority of *B. malayi* infections is nocturnal.

**ETIOLOGY/PATHOLOGY.** Lymphatic filariasis is caused by infection with *W. bancrofti* or *B. malayi* larvae. When an infected mosquito feeds, the larvae, which are about 1 to 2 mm in length, are deposited in or near the bite wound. The larvae enter the lymphatic vessels and mature to adults in a process, which takes 6 to 9 months (Figure 47-1). The adult worms can live for 5 to 10 years in the lymph channels without causing obstruction of the vessels. However, certain individuals, particularly those who have been previously infected or nonnatives mount an inflammatory immune response to the adult worms and their metabolic products, which can temporarily block the infected lymph channels. Symptoms occur during the first 6 months after exposure to *Wuchereria* (first month for *Brugia*) and are generally restricted to the extremities, breasts, and scrotum with tenderness, fever, and swelling of the lymph vessels/nodes (lymphangitis and lymphadenitis) in previously infected persons. The inflammatory response in nonsensitized individuals usually abates after several days. After 6 months the adult female worm begins to periodically produce microfilariae, which are deposited in the peripheral blood. *W. bancrofti* microfilariae can live for up to 2 years in the peripheral blood. The microfilariae and their by-products do not appear to induce a host response. A phenomenon that many speculate is an allergic response to microfilariae sequestered in the lungs known as tropical pulmonary eosinophilia, which is associated with immunologic damage to the host in the absence of microfilariae in the peripheral blood.

The principal pathology in filariasis is caused by the death of the adult worms in the lymph vessels. The death of the adult worm leads to an acute lymphocyte infiltration in and around the vessel, causing blockage.

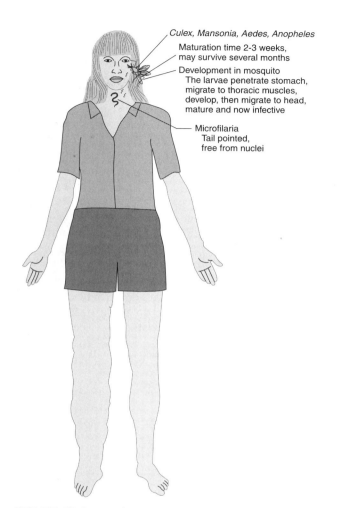

*Culex, Mansonia, Aedes, Anopheles*

Maturation time 2-3 weeks, may survive several months

Development in mosquito
The larvae penetrate stomach, migrate to thoracic muscles, develop, then migrate to head, mature and now infective

Microfilaria
Tail pointed, free from nuclei

**FIGURE 47-1** *Wuchereria bancrofti* and *Brugia malayi.*

Abscesses may develop and are more common with infections by *B. malayi*. If enough collateral vessels are blocked, lymphedema occurs and, in the chronically infected patient, permanent **elephantitis** of the infected area. Elephantitis is usually less pronounced in *Brugia*-infected patients but occurs more rapidly (1 year versus 3 years) and is restricted to the lower extremities. Secondary bacterial abscess formation is a common complication. Visitors to endemic areas may develop a temporary elephantitis without microfilaria. The cause of this temporary elephantitis is believed to be lymph stasis due to a rapid, vigorous inflammatory response to larva in the lymph vessels.

**IDENTIFICATION.**

**Traditional.** The traditional diagnostic test for filariasis is the demonstration of microfilariae in the peripheral blood. Collection of peripheral blood is dictated by the periodicity of the region in which the infection occurred. The gold standard for identification of the microfilariae is still the Giemsa-stained thick smear. The Giemsa stain identification is more effective when the microfilariae are concentrated. Techniques to concentrate microfilariae include membrane filtration of blood, **Knott's technique** (concentration by centrifugation), counting chambers, and quantitative buffy coat fluorescent assay (Wamae, 1994). These concentration techniques increase the chance of parasite detection when using nonperiodic blood samples. The best way to differentiate microfilariae is the examination of the anterior and posterior portions. Both *W. bancrofti* and *B. malayi* microfilariae are sheathed but *Wuchereria* are free of terminal nuclei that are present in *Brugia* (see Table 47-1 and refer to Color Plates 115 through 119). Lymph node biopsy may recover adult worms. The adult *W. bancrofti* female is 80 to 100 mm long and 0.2 to 0.3 mm wide; the adult male is 25 to 50 mm long and 0.1 mm wide. The *B. malayi* adults are approximately one-half the size of those of *Wuchereria.*

*Immunologic.* Lymphatic filariasis induces dramatic increases in total IgM and antigen specific IgG4 antibodies (Eberhard, 1991). The presence of filarial antibody is persistent, and therefore, of little use in determining the disease state unless compared to native serum.

### Loa loa.

**EPIDEMIOLOGY.** Loiasis occurs in focal areas of rain and swamp forest in western equatorial Africa. The disease is transmitted by the female day-biting mango fly (*Chrysops*) and therefore the periodicity of the microfilariae is diurnal. Humans can also be infected with a simian strain of *Loa,* which is transmitted by night-biting *Chrysops langi* and *Chrysops centurionis* flies. The simian *Loa* is thought to be the cause of **Kampala eye worm** seen in Uganda. There are an estimated 13 million cases of loiasis worldwide with the highest prevalence in the Congo river basins.

**ETIOLOGY/PATHOLOGY.** Loiasis is a chronic filarial disease caused by the nematode *L. loa.* The third stage infectious larvae enters the bite wound made by the *Chrysops* fly. These larvae mature while migrating through the subcutaneous tissue. The maturation may take from 6 months to several years. During this time, the immature adults migrate rapidly (1 cm/min) through the subcutaneous tissues. Most infections are asymptomatic but the migrations of immature and mature adult worms in the subcutaneous tissue can produce painful swollen lesions known as **Calabar swelling**. Calabar lesions are caused by allergic reactions to the migration of the worms and are associated with the hypereosinophilia observed in most patients. In addition, the migration of worms in the conjunctiva can produce severe pain and swelling but not blindness. The term "eye worm" is associated with infection by *L. loa* but should not be confused with infection of the eye caused by *Onchocerca volvulus* (see Figure 47-2 and refer to Color Plate 120).

Adult male and female worms eventually mate and, about 18 months after the infection, the females begin to produce sheathed microfilariae. The microfilariae are, like *W. bancrofti* and *B. malayi,* found in the blood. The microfilariae can live up to 2 years in the host and appear to cause no pathology. A rare excep-

## Table 47–1 ▶ Comparison of Human Filarial Infections

| | Geographic Distribution | Vector* | Periodicity[†] | Location of Adults | Location of Microfilaria (Mf) | Length (Mf) | Width (Mf) | Sheath (Mf) | Tail Morphology | Tail Nuclei | |
|---|---|---|---|---|---|---|---|---|---|---|---|
| *W. bancrofti* | World-Wide Tropical/Sub-Tropical areas | *Anopheles* (Mosquito) | N/D | Lymphatics | Blood | 245–295 μm | 7.5–10 μm | + | Tapered to a point | None | A |
| *B. malayi* | South/Southwest Asia and India | *Mansonia* (Mosquito) | N | Lymphatics | Blood | 175–230 μm | 5–6 μm | + | Tapered with a constriction | Nuclei stop anterior of constriction | B |
| *L. loa* | Focal Areas of West/Central Africa | *Chrysops* (Fly) | D/N | Subcutaneous Tissue | Blood | 230–250 μm | 5–7 μm | + | Rounded | Present | C |
| *O. volvulus* | Africa, Mexico, Central/South America | *Simulium* (Black Fly) | None | Subcutaneous Tissue | Skin | 300–315 μm | 5–9 μm | − | Tapered to a sharp point | None | D |
| *M. ozzardi* | Caribbean, Central/South America | *Culicoides* (midge) *Simulium* (Black Fly) | None | Subcutaneous Tissue | Skin/Blood | 160–205 μm | 3–5 μm | − | Tapered to a point | None | E |

*The most prominent vector is listed, consult the text for other possible vectors.

[†]Periodicity: N, nocturnal; D, diurnal. The most prominent periodicity is listed first.

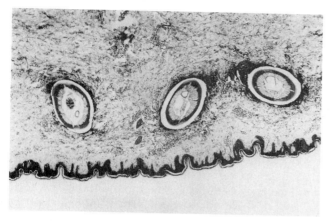

**FIGURE 47-2** Transverse sections of a dying adult male *Loa loa* worm in the dermis, ×110. The dying worm provokes an intense inflammatory reaction. (Courtesy of the Armed Forces Institute of Pathology)

tion is encephalitis caused by the host reaction to dead microfilariae in the brain or spinal cord. The parasite completes its life cycle when it is taken up from the peripheral blood by another biting *Chrysops* fly.

When the adult worms begin to die, major complications may occur. If the adult worm dies in a vital organ such as the heart or other major organ, the subsequent granulomatous response and fibrosis may impair the function of the organ. In addition, the response to the dead adult may increase the hypersensitive response to the remaining adults. The deposition of the resulting immune complexes may cause renal disease; secondary bacterial infections may cause endocarditis or other complications. The primary clinical symptoms include eosinophilia, low-grade pain, and pruritis with or without Calabar swelling. The Calabar lesion is a nonpitting, nonerythematous swelling of the body, which persists for 2 to 3 days. These lesions recur at irregular intervals over the entire body. The tracks of migrating adult worms can be used to differentiate loiais from infections by other migrating larval worms. *L. loa* migrations do not leave visible tracks or cause pain, whereas those caused by migrating human and zoonotic hookworms do. As with other filarial diseases, preventive measures are important to prevent transmission. Diethylcarbamazine (DEC) is the drug of choice for treating loiasis.

**IDENTIFICATION.**

*Traditional.* During the early course of the disease, diagnosis must be based primarily on clinical symptoms. Calabar swelling or the isolation of adult worms from tissue is presumptive for loiasis. Adult worms must be differentiated from other migrating larval/adult helminths such as *Strongyloides*, *Dirofilaria*, *Dracunculus*, *Toxocara*, *Ancyclostoma* species, and *O. volvulus*. Differentiation of some species can be made by size, but generally this task should be left to a refer-

ence laboratory. Microfilariae are 230 to 250 μm long by 5 to 7 μm wide and may not appear in the peripheral blood until 1 to 2 years after infection and must be differentiated from *W. bancrofti* and *B. malayi*. All three genera of microfilariae may be isolated from the peripheral blood and possess sheaths, but *Loa* species are primarily of diurnal periodicity and differ morphologically from the other two because of its rounded tail with terminal nuclei and a sheath that does not stain with Giemsa (see Table 47-1 and refer to Color Plates 121 and 122). The methods for isolation of microfilariae from peripheral blood are similar to those described above for *W. bancrofti* and *B. malayi*.

### *Onchocerca volvulus.*

**EPIDEMIOLOGY.** Onchocerciasis is a significant disease in tropical Africa, the southwest Arabian peninsula, and Central and South America. The disease is focally distributed along fast-moving water, the breeding site of the *Simulium* (black fly) vector. There are approximately 18 million infected people of whom 300,000 are blind. The parasite is only known to infect humans, but the gorilla and other primates have been described as transient reservoirs. The vast majority of the infections occur in Africa. A global strategy for the control of onchocerciasis was reported in a 1995 WHO report and targets the disease for elimination in 10 to 15 years. The strategy for control of the disease is based on epidemiologic maps of endemic areas. The central tenet of the strategy is to first identify and then control morbidity by treatment with the drug ivermectin. Vector control is also important and is practiced when feasible.

**ETIOLOGY/PATHOLOGY.** Onchocerciasis is a disease whose major pathology is immune mediated. The disease is caused by infection with the nematode *O. volvulus*. It usually involves multisystem tissue damage, the most serious of which is blindness. The disease is often referred to by other names such as **"river blindness"** in Africa, **"Robles disease"** in Guatemala, and **"Sowda"** in Yemen. As with other filarial disease, the infection begins with the third stage larva leaving the proboscis of the fly and entering the bite wound after the fly feeds. The larvae migrate in the cutaneous and subcutaneous tissues and mature to adults during the first 3 months following infection. The adults are usually found together in subcutaneous nodules where they mate. About 1 year after infection, the female produces nonperiodic microfilariae. The microfilariae are usually found in the intercellular spaces of the dermis or the eye. The adults usually live about 15 years; the microfilariae last about 2 years. The microfilariae are ingested by a black fly during a blood meal and complete their life cycle.

The major clinical manifestations of onchocerciasis are due to the host reaction to the metabolites of the adult worm and to the antigens released during the death of adult worms or microfilariae. The inflammatory response to these antigens is directly related to the worm burden and productivity (fecundity); more worms lead to increased inflammation. A person's ability to control the inflammation is inversely related to the manifestation of disease pathology (Ottesen, 1995). The initial reactions are usually not observed until several months or years after infection and, if left untreated, may progress to more severe forms. The clinical manifestations of the disease can be diverse and may be progressive. The majority of patients from nonendemic areas experience a limited exposure to the parasite and exhibit a "moderate" reaction that includes severe itching (pruritus), which may include a raised red (erythematous papular) rash. These patients usually have a low level of or no detectable microfilariae. The native population of endemic disease areas usually develop the generalized form of onchocerciasis. People with generalized onchocerciasis display a wide range of clinical symptoms that may include any or all of the following: changes to the skin to include altered pigmentation and loss of elasticity (e.g., hanging groin), formation of nodules, the enlargement of lymph nodes, and infection of the eye and optic nerve. The symptoms of generalized onchocerciasis tend to be progressive if left untreated, but the disease is more easily diagnosed due to the usual abundance of microfilariae.

Onchocerciasis can be prevented by the use of heavy clothing and insect repellent to prevent *Simulium* bites. Spraying or removing vegetation in or near fast-moving water will interrupt the life cycle of the vector by destroying the fly larva habitat. Treatment consists of a combination of ivermectin, to prevent production and kill microfilariae, and suramin to kill adult worms. DEC is no longer recommended for the treatment of onchocerciasis.

**IDENTIFICATION.**

*Traditional.* The adults can be isolated from surgically removed nodules. The female can be up to 500 mm in length by 0.5 mm in width and the male is only about one-tenth the size of the female. The adults are usually identified by immunohistochemical methods at a reference laboratory. A more definitive diagnosis can be made on recovery of microfilariae from aspirates of the nodule. The microfilariae are nonperiodic and can also be recovered from skin snips and sometimes from urine but only rarely from blood. Recovered microfilariae stained with Giemsa are unsheathed, 300 to 315 μm long and 5 to 9 μm wide (see Table 47-1 and refer to Color Plates 123 through 126). They can be differentiated from *Mansonella* microfilariae because of their larger size and more sharply pointed tail. When cultured, living microfilariae demonstrate vigorous motility. But microfilariae do not have to be isolated to make a diagnosis. For example, in patients with eye infections the living microfilariae can be observed in a curled posture in the cornea; dead microfilariae are usually straight.

# CESTODES

Cestodes are tapeworms also known as flatworms. Cestodes are flattened dorsoventrally, are bilaterally symmetrical and lack a body cavity. The adult tapeworm, unlike the adult nematode, has distinct body segments that include a segmented body (**stroblia**), a neck, and a head or scolex. The scolex has specialized hooklets for attachment to the gut mucosa. The neck produces the hermaphroditic (monecious) proglottids that make up the stroblia. The proglottids mature and produce eggs as they become more distal to the neck. Tapeworms may mate with another individual of the same species through their genital pores. The life cycle of most cestodes requires one or more intermediate or definitive hosts. The adult flatworms normally parasitize the intestinal track of definitive hosts. In the intestine, the adults produce eggs, which are passed in the feces. Infectious larvae hatch from the eggs and, depending on the species, infect a nonvertebrate/vertebrate intermediate host. Humans are generally incidental hosts and become infected either by direct ingestion of the egg or consumption of the larvae-containing intermediate host. An interesting cestode pathogen that infects humans worldwide is discussed below.

## *Echinococcus granulosus*

**Epidemiology.** This flatworm is a member of the family *Taeniidae*. *E. granulosus* causes a zoonotic **cystic hydatid disease** in carnivores with humans as an accidental intermediate host. The infection of humans usually occurs by ingestion of fecal material from an infected dog. Because the eggs of *Echinococcus* are very resistant to environmental conditions, they can be spread by handling fomites contaminated by an infected animal. Humans can also become a definitive host for the parasite by directly consuming meat that contains hydatid cysts. The disease has a wide distribution and is endemic in most temperate/semiarid regions of the world. These regions include the Mediterranean, most of the central Asian continent, Australia, Northern Europe, parts of northern Africa, North America, specifically Alaska, Canada, and the south and southeastern United States. The disease occurs in both wild and domesticated carnivore populations but geography dictates which strain the carnivore carries. The northern regions of the world have more wild carnivores that tend to be infected with the sylvatic strain of *E. granulosus*. The pastoral strain infects humans when there is an association between humans-carnivores-herbivores and tends to occur in the southern regions of the temperate zone. Maintenance of the pastoral strain may be due to human behavior. In many parts of the world humans feed their domestic dogs the visceral organs of slaughtered herbivores. If these organs contain hydatid cysts, the dog will become infected and the risk of human exposure will increase. There are believed to be about a million infected humans.

**Etiology/Pathology.** Echinococcosis is a chronic disease caused by incidental ingestion of *E. granulosus* eggs by humans. Adult worms live in the small intestines of definitive hosts, which are primarily canine carnivores. Infected canines are difficult to identify because worms rarely produce symptoms in the definitive host. In the definitive host, adult worms produce gravid proglottids and the resulting eggs are passed in the feces. The eggs are ingested by herbivores, the intermediate host, but omnivores such as humans can also ingest the eggs. The eggs hatch in the small intestine and the **oncosphere** penetrates the intestinal wall and enters the circulation. The circulation then carries the oncospheres to various organs throughout the body. Certain organs are targeted for cyst formation with strain-specific preferences. Pastoral strains favor the liver while the sylvatic strains target the lungs. When the oncosphere reaches the target organ it begins to form a cyst. Infection of humans most commonly leads to production of a single cyst but multiple disseminated cysts also occur. The spherical (unilocular) cyst is an interesting collaboration between the host and parasite. The parasite produces two inner layers that are responsible for the asexual reproduction of scoleces while the host produces an outer granulomatous layer. The parasite's germinal layer produces brood pouches that contain individual scoleces. The brood pouches detach and form internal daughter cysts. The cyst slowly fills with scoleces which, because of their appearance, are called hydatid sand. The original cyst can continue to grow almost indefinitely but will eventually cause obstruction of organ function and may burst.

The major pathology and clinical symptoms are the result of the formation of cysts in the target organs. These symptoms result from the mechanical compression of the organ and disruption of the blood supply. In the liver the biliary flow may be blocked leading to secondary bacterial infection and cirrhosis. The liver cyst (refer to Color Plate 127) can usually be detected by palpation and the patient may have pain, vomiting, and jaundice. Intact cysts in the lung usually do not present any symptoms and are generally detected with an x-ray. Cyst rupture or leakage in the lung may cause breathing difficulties with secondary bacterial pneumonia. An acute allergic reaction to the released scoleces (refer to Color Plate 128) may occur following rupture of the cyst independent of its original location.

Preventive control measures include handwashing to prevent fecal (egg) contamination, disposal of visceral organs to prevent cyst consumption and elimination of wild dog populations coupled with treatment of at-risk domestic dogs with praziquantel. Infected persons should be treated by surgical removal of cysts or administration of the drugs mebendazole or albenda-zole. Patients who have ruptured cysts can be treated with praziquantel to prevent secondary cyst formation.

**Identification.** Radiologic identification of cysts is common, but they must be differentiated from other masses such as tumors or abscesses. Identification of scoleces by acid-fast staining of needle biopsy material from a suspected cyst is useful for differential diagnosis. This infrequently performed procedure is dangerous because there is a possibility of rupturing the cyst. If a cyst has ruptured, scoleces can usually be recovered from the feces (liver cyst) or bronchial washings (lung cyst). Identification of the parasite on the basis of egg morphology (recovered from fomites) is not feasible because *E. granulosus* eggs cannot be differentiated from ova of *Taenia* species.

## TREMATODES

The trematodes can be divided into groups based on the location of the adults during infection. Those that infect the lung and the blood are considered here. Trematodes that infect the liver and intestinal tract are discussed in Chapter 46. Trematodes, like the cestodes, are flatworms. Trematodes have unsegmented, leaf-shaped bodies and are also known as the flukes. Trematodes can be hermaphroditic or, like *Schistosoma,* have separate sexes. Unlike the cestodes, *Schistosoma* have a digestive tract that begins with an oral sucker; an additional ventral sucker is used for attachment. The adults reside as a mating pair in the portal veins of the mesentery or bladder. The female then produces eggs that penetrate the venous walls and enter either the bladder or intestine. The eggs, passed in the feces or urine, contain live ciliated larvae that hatch in water. The *Schistosoma* species that infect humans all require a mollusk that lives in infected water as an intermediate host. The larvae develop in the intermediate host and then depart as infectious cercaria. The cercaria then complete their life cycle by penetrating the skin and entering the circulation of a new host. The three major *Schistosoma* human pathogens are compared below.

### *Schistosoma mansoni, Schistosoma japonicum,* and *Schistosoma haematobium*

**Epidemiology.** An estimated 200 to 300 million persons have schistosomiasis. The three major species that infect humans are *S. mansoni, S. japonicum,* and *S. haematobium.* These species are geographically restricted by the range of the intermediate host snail. *S. mansoni* has the largest range including the tropical areas of continental Africa, Madagascar, the east-central portion of South America and portions of the Caribbean. The range of *S. haematobium* is more restrictive than *S. mansoni* but occurs throughout a greater portion of the African continent to include the Middle East and is the most common etiologic agent of schistosomiasis. *S. japonicum* has the smallest area of endemicity, which includes the Philippines, China, and southeast Asia, but because of the worm's fecundity, it is the parasite that causes the most serious form of schistosomiasis (see Table 47-2). The disease is difficult to eliminate because numerous animals can serve as reservoirs.

**Etiology/Pathology.** The causative agents of schistosomiasis, also known as bilharziasis, are *Schistosoma* worms. The adult worms themselves do not cause notable pathology. Significant pathology can be observed during infection of the skin by invading cercariae, migration of the immature worms, and again in response to the release of eggs. These pathologic responses vary from person to person, but all are host-mediated immune responses. A history of exposure to slow-moving or stagnant water, which contains the free-swimming cercariae, is shared by all three species. Prior sensitization to cross-reactive antigens of avian cercariae seems to be required for cercariae-induced dermatitis. The cercariae penetrate the skin and may cause dermatitis, which, when present, resembles "swimmer's itch" but can be quite extensive with severe itching (pruritus). After penetration, the cercariae lose their forked tail, (now called schistosomules), enter the venous circulation, go though the heart, and then enter the pulmonary circulation. The immature schistosomules begin to develop in the pulmonary circulation and then are taken to the liver, enter the portal circulation, and attach to the portal veins of the mesentery (*S. mansoni, S. japonicum*) or the venous plexuses of the pelvis (*S. haematobium*). The formation of large numbers of immune complexes in response to the immature worms, especially in nonendemic patients, can lead to serum sickness or Katayama fever. This acute serum sickness is associated with eosinophilia, general allergic symptoms, and tissue damage.

The immature worms finish their maturation and pair to sexually reproduce. These adult pairs may live up to 20 years in an appropriate host without inducing any pathology. About 2 months after infection, the female begins to deposit her eggs in the smallest venule that will accommodate her. The eggs can then penetrate the venous wall and mucosa and enter the intestinal lumen (*S. mansoni, S. japonicum*) or the bladder (*S. haematobium*); alternatively, they can become trapped in the tissue or swept to the liver. Eggs in the liver can induce fibrosis, which can lead to internal bleeding (ruptured varices), which is a serious consequence of chronic schistosomiasis. The response to the eggs depends on the burden of infection (number of parasites) and the amount of eggs produced (fecundity). The resulting immune response to the parasite eggs is twofold. First, a vigorous granulomatous response occurs to the eggs, which become trapped in tissue while trying to enter the intestinal lumen or bladder. This is followed by tissue hyperplasia that may ultimately alter the physiology of the affected tissue/organ. The eggs that are passed in the feces or urine must be deposited in water for completion of the parasite's life cycle. The embryonated egg will hatch within minutes of entering the water. The emerging embryo (miracidium) has less than a day to find and enter an appropriate snail. Development within the snail host takes 1 to 2 months. The miracidium gives rise to several daughter sporocysts, which then mature to cercariae. After leaving the snail, the free-swimming cercariae can survive only a few days and must find an appropriate host to complete their life cycle (see Figure 47-3).

Clinical manifestations of the disease vary and may not be sufficiently distinct to make a diagnosis. Acute schistosomiasis or Katayama fever includes several nonspecific symptoms such as fever, chills, weight loss, nausea, vomiting, diarrhea (sometimes bloody), hepatomegaly, eosinophilia, and general aches and pains. The disease must therefore be differentiated from amebic and bacillary dysentery, hepatitis, and colitis. It is important to note that the deposition of immune com-

## Table 47–2 ▶ Comparison of Important Human *Schistosoma* Species

| | Geographic Distribution | Snail Host | Location of Adults | Egg Location* | Length (μm) | Width (μm) Spine | Shape | Fecundity (Ova in Uterus) |
|---|---|---|---|---|---|---|---|---|
| *S. haematobium* | Africa | *Bulinus* | Pelvic venous plexus | Urine | 112–170 | 40–70 Terminal | Ovoid | 20–30 |
| *S. mansoni* | Africa, S. America | *Biomphalaria* | Mesenteric venous plexus | Feces | 140–180 | 45–70 Lateral | Ovoid | 1–4 |
| *S. japonicum* | S.E. Asia | *Oncomelania* | Mesenteric venous plexus | Feces | 70–105 | 50–80 Lateral | Round | 50–100 |

*The most likely location to detect eggs in clinical samples is listed.

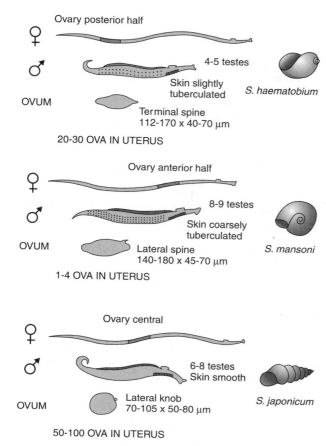

Ovary posterior half

♀

♂                                    4-5 testes

OVUM                                 Skin slightly          *S. haematobium*
                                     tuberculated

                                     Terminal spine
                                     112-170 x 40-70 μm

20-30 OVA IN UTERUS

Ovary anterior half

♀

♂                                    8-9 testes

OVUM                                 Skin coarsely          *S. mansoni*
                                     tuberculated

                                     Lateral spine
                                     140-180 x 45-70 μm

1-4 OVA IN UTERUS

Ovary central

♀

♂                                    6-8 testes
                                     Skin smooth

OVUM                                 Lateral knob           *S. japonicum*
                                     70-105 x 50-80 μm

50-100 OVA IN UTERUS

**FIGURE 47-3** *Schistosoma* species.

plexes can make the acute disease life-threatening. The chronic form of the disease is also nonspecific but includes complications that are also life-threatening. These complications include egg embolization in the lungs leading to heart failure, deposition of eggs in the brain or spinal cord leading to lesions that may cause loss of neural functions, epilepsy and, most commonly, portal hypertension. The chronic complications of schistosomiasis in the liver must be differentiated from other causes of hepatomegaly, which can be eliminated by demonstrating ova in the biopsy sample.

Specific clinical symptoms/pathology are generally associated with each schistosome, although the symptoms are not exclusive to a single causative agent. Infections by *S. haematobium* produce symptoms involving the bladder and ureter including bladder enlargement, blood in the urine (hematuria), and cyst formation. Symptoms of *S. mansoni* infection are generally concentrated in the large intestine, rectum, and liver but can also involve the bladder. The pathologic changes and symptoms include polyp, ulcer, and fistula formation, liver fibrosis with portal hypertension, and splenomegaly. The pathology of *S. japonicum* infections is similar to that of *S. mansoni* but may also include the small intestine and generate more severe

chronic symptomology due to the increased dissemination of eggs throughout the body.

Schistosomiasis can easily be prevented through controlled disposal of human waste. Containment of human waste interrupts the life cycle of the parasites by preventing infection of the host snail. A less practical control measure is the elimination of the host snails. Schistosomiasis can be treated with praziquantel. In addition, some infections by *S. mansoni* or *S. haematobium* respond to oxamniquine or metrifonate, respectively.

**Identification.** The diagnosis of schistosomiasis is usually made by isolation and identification of the egg (refer to Color Plates 129 through 132). The eggs may be found in the feces, urine, or biopsy material 2 months after infection and are sufficiently distinct to identify the three major species. The eggs of *S. mansoni* and *S. haematobium* are oval and roughly equivalent in size, but the eggs of *S. mansoni* have a distinct lateral spine, whereas *S. haematobium* eggs possess a terminal spine. *S. japonicum* eggs are smaller than either of the other two and are round with a discreet lateral knob. The eggs should be collected by concentration techniques such as the Visser filter (Schutte et al., 1994). Occasionally, diagnosis can be made by the identification of adult male and female worms in copula from biopsy samples. The adult males are all approximately the same length and width (9–12 mm × 1–1.5 mm). The adult females are longer and narrower than the males. *S. japonicum* adult pairs are the largest of the three. Together, the adults create a distinctive morphology because the male enfolds the female in his gynecophoral canal. Ultrasonography is useful for the diagnosis and assessment of schistome-induced hepatosplenic and urogenital symptoms to include the detection of granulomas and polyps.

# UNCOMMON HELMINTHS

## *Dracunculus medinensis*

**Epidemiology.** *Dracunculus medinensis* is the largest nematode to infect humans and is also known as the Guinea worm. The parasite has a long history with humans and is depicted in many ancient medical texts. Even today it is a powerful symbol; it is wound around the healer's staff in the modern medical cadusus. The most commonly practiced treatment is, as it has been, to remove the worm by slowly removing the worm from the tissue by winding it around a stick and hence the symbology. This disease still occurs in West-Central Africa, East and Northeast Africa, the Middle East, and India. There are believed to be fewer than 220,000 active infections of this once prevalent disease. The number of reported cases has decreased dramatically since 1977 when the WHO targeted the disease for eradication (Hopkins et al., 1995). Humans are the only known reservoir for *D. medinensis*. The transmission of the disease is seasonal. In dry areas it occurs during the rainy season when collections of water form; in tropical areas it occurs during the dry season when the water levels become lower and stagnate. Prevention of the disease can be accomplished by a combined use of potable (filtered at a minimum) water and the control of exposure to water of those patients with *D. medinensis*-mediated blisters. The copepod host can also be controlled with nontoxic insecticides. Treatment of blisters with topical antibiotics is recommended to prevent secondary bacterial infection.

**Etiology/Pathology.** **Dracunculiasis** is caused by the nematode *D. medinensis*. Humans are infected by drinking water that contains larvae carrying copepods, the vector for the disease. The infectious third stage larvae escapes from the copepod and penetrates the intestine to enter the peritoneal space (see Figure 47-4). During the next 9 to 14 months the larvae mature and the adults mate in the peritoneum. The adult male apparently dies after mating while the gravid female migrates to the subcutaneous connective tissue of the lower extremities. The female eventually forces her anterior end into the dermal tissue of the lower extremity, which induces the formation of a blister. The female does not lay eggs but instead produces live larvae (larviparous), which are released into the blister fluid. The blister is induced to rupture by subsequent exposure to water. The blister fluid, which may contain tens of thousands of first stage larvae, is released in the water. Copepods ingest the first stage larvae,

which then undergo two molts to become infectious for humans. The female will continue to deposit larvae for 2 weeks and is usually expelled or manually removed from the tissue.

The female's migration causes the major pathology by inducing a range of symptoms from an intense granulomatous response to worm metabolites and dying worms to a systemic allergic response. A prodrome syndrome occurs days before the blister forms. This syndrome is believed to be due to a systemic allergic response and includes fever, nausea, vomiting, diarrhea, and an erythematous itching rash. The formed blisters itch and are painful. A frequent complication after the blister ruptures is secondary bacterial infection and abscess formation.

**Identification.** Because the adults are large (50–120 cm in length) and present themselves in such a unique way, the disease is easily diagnosed after the prodrome syndrome (see Figure 47-5). The first stage larvae can also be diagnostic when recovered from the blister fluid. The larvae, though larger (500–700 μm in length by 15–25 μm wide), resemble microfilariae with a round anterior and a pointed tapered tail. ELISA-based assays can be used to identify prepatent infections. These assays can identify individuals that are actively infected versus previously infected because antibody titers rapidly decline after expulsion of the adult worm. The Falcon assay screening test (FAST)-ELISA is very sensitive but less specific because of cross-reactivity to *O. volvulus* serum (Fagbemi & Hillyer, 1990; Garate, Kliks, Cabbera, & Parkhouse, 1990).

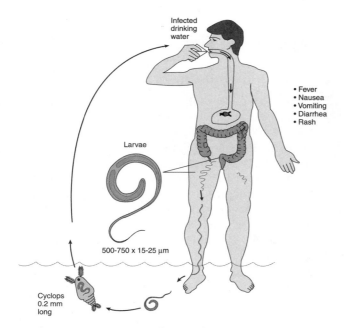

**FIGURE 47-4** *Dracunculus medinensis.*

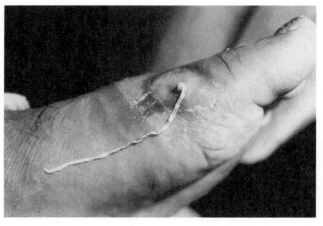

**FIGURE 47-5** *Dracunculus medinensis* clinical presentation. (Courtesy of the Armed Forces Institute of Pathology)

# SUMMARY

▶ The current laboratory tests used to diagnose helminth infections depend heavily on the isolation of the parasite or parasite antigens. To a lesser extent the detection of antibodies to parasite antigens may serve to confirm infection retrospectively.

▶ Insect vectors are important in the transmission of helminth disease. Although the distribution of most helminth disease is restricted to one or a few species of insects, other factors must regulate the areas of disease endemnicity. For instance, certain mosquito vectors are more dominant in transmitting filariasis in different geographic areas even though the same species of mosquitoes are present.

▶ Understanding the phenomenon of periodicity is important for the collection of clinical samples for diagnosis of filarial disease. Blood samples should be collected in conjunction with the periodicity of the suspected disease vector. Alternatively, the appearance of microfilariae in the blood can be induced by the administration of DEC. The risks of DEC treatment must be weighed against the value of its use.

▶ Both wild and domestic dogs are important reservoirs of helminth disease for humans. In particular they serve as reservoirs for echinococcosis, hookworm, toxocariasis, and dirofilariasis.

▶ Geography and weather play an important role in spreading/restricting helminth infections by controlling the multiplication and spread of the vectors and intermediate hosts of helminth disease. It is important to understand the impact of international travel and commerce on the spread of infected humans and helminth vectors in today's world. In addition, human activities and climatic changes can create new niches for the spread of helminth infections.

## CASE STUDY 1

(Adapted from Lucey & Maguire, 1993).

During a trip to Kenya, six American students became ill with diarrhea and fever several weeks after swimming in a slow-moving stream in the Machakos district. All were treated at a hospital in Nairobi where a diagnosis of malaria was considered. One student, a 21-year-old man, developed fever, sweats, and abdominal pain 4 weeks after swimming in the stream. He continued to feel unwell, and 2 weeks later he developed more fever, sweats, chills, and mild nonbloody diarrhea. He received a 4-day course of chloroquine. His symptoms improved, but he developed dull pain in the lumbar region and numbness in his toes. He subsequently became unable to void and he became so weak in his legs that he could not walk. On examination he was unable to lift his legs and had diminished sensation and absent deep tendon reflexes in the legs. The white blood cell (WBC) count was 9,600 with 33% neutrophils and 47% eosinophils. The cerebrospinal fluid WBC count was 44/mm³, the red blood cell count was 36/mm³, and the protein was 84 mg/100 mL. A computed tomography myelogram of the spine showed diffuse enlargement of the lower thoracic spinal cord.

### Questions

1. Name three pathogens or diseases that could cause the above symptoms.

2. Based on the contents of this chapter what is the most likely causative parasite?

3. What clinical samples would you collect and what diagnostic tests would you request?

## CASE STUDY 2

An 18-year-old white boy was admitted to a hospital with fever of unknown origin and nasal catarrh of 1 week duration. During infancy the child had no major illnesses. On numerous occasions, he had been observed eating dirt in the yard. The family had no house pets. On first admission the child was pale, with a temperature of 101°F and a slightly enlarged spleen. His hemoglobin was 7.2% gm, WBC count was 32,000/mm³, with 64% eosinophils. Radiographs of the chest showed streaky, abnormal shadows in the right upper and both lower lobes. A tentative diagnosis was made of iron deficiency anemia and possible visceral larva migrans. He was treated with ferrous sulfate and ampicillin and released. Three weeks later the child was readmitted in a semicomatose state with a 10-day history of shaking spells and ataxia. The WBC count was 9,100/mm³ with 4% eosinophils. Cerebrospinal fluid sugar was 88 mg % and protein 320 mg %. An electroencephalogram was abnormal, but a burr-hole exploration and left carotid angiograph were normal. Convulsions were poorly controlled by antiepileptic agents and the patient died 3 weeks after his second admission and 7 weeks following his first admission.

On autopsy granulomata in various stages of development were found in the liver, heart, and brain. The lungs were edematous and there were numerous granulomata containing infiltrates of eosinophils, neutrophils, lymphocytes, and plasma cells. These were considered to be more chronic lesions. In contrast, the numerous granulomata in the gray and white matter of the cerebral hemispheres, cerebellum, and brain stem appeared to be of more recent origin than those in the visceral organs.

**Questions:**

1. Based on your knowledge of this chapter, what is the most likely causative agent?

2. Explain the reasons for the severity of the clinical symptoms.

## Review Questions

1. You are the microbiologist at a large metropolitan hospital. A patient, who has recently arrived from Africa, is admitted to the hospital and has numerous nonspecific symptoms but also has what the resident-physician describes as Calabar swelling. The astute resident suspects the patient has loiasis but informs you that the patient, due to his religious beliefs, will agree to only one blood sample. It is now 10 PM; you should advise the physician to:
   a. take the blood sample while he can get it.
   b. take the blood sample at 2 PM tomorrow when he comes back on shift.
   c. try to convince the patient that several blood samples must be taken.
   d. take a fecal sample.

2. A man from Brazil is admitted to the hospital with portal hypertension, polyps in the large intestine, and splenomegaly. What is the likely causative agent?
   a. *S. haematobium*
   b. *Schistosoma mansoni*
   c. *S. japonicum*
   d. *Anisakis simplex*

3. You are a cercaria of *S. haematobium*. After secretly entering your favorite human where will you first go to mature?
   a. The venous plexus of the bladder
   b. The pulmonary circulation
   c. The venous plexus of the liver
   d. The venous plexuses of the pelvis

4. Another name for river blindness is:
   a. Elephantiasis
   b. Sowda
   c. Filariasis
   d. All of the above

5. You are an epidemiologist working for the WHO in charge of investigating cystic hydatid disease in Spain. Your most effective advice to the local authorities to help prevent the spread of this disease to humans would include: (1) to increase the chlorine content of the local drinking water; (2) thoroughly educate the public on personal hygiene measures; (3) to stop the feeding of animal organs to other domestic animals; (4) to trap and sample wild carnivores for disease. Then, to recommend extensive hunting of carnivores if they carry the disease. Pick one pair of answers below.
   a. 1, 2
   b. 3, 4
   c. 1, 4
   d. 2, 3

6. The most commonly used diagnostic tests for active trichinosis infections include: (1) biopsy; (2) complement fixation; (3) polymerase chain reaction; (4) antibody detection. Pick one pair of the answers below.
   a. 1, 2
   b. 2, 4
   c. 3, 4
   d. 1, 3

7. (True or False) The definitive diagnosis of filarial infections is complicated by antigenic cross-reactivity between genera/species and the duration of the host's antibody response. This cross-reactivity would be negated by the use of the following assays:
   a. True/False. Detection of circulating antigen.
   b. True/False. Polymerase chain reaction.
   c. True/False. Detection of IgG antibody.
   d. True/False. Detection of IgM antibody.

8. Based on your understanding of epidemiology and the host range of the parasites listed below, which is the parasite most likely to be eradicated by a concerted effort of the WHO?
   a. *Schistosoma japonicum*
   b. *Onchocerca volvulus*
   c. *Dracunculus medinensis*
   d. *Toxocara canis*

9. Which of the following parasites are commonly associated with domestic dogs: (1) *Toxocara canis*; (2) *Dirofilaria* species; (3) *Ancylostoma caninum*. (4) *Echinococcus granulosus*.
   a. 1, 2, 3
   b. 2, 3, 4
   c. 1, 3, 4
   d. 1, 2, 3, 4

10. For the geographic area in which the disease is most prevalent, match the parasite with its most likely vector/intermediate host. Use each answer only once.
   a. *Schistosoma mansoni*     1. *Chrysops* fly.
   b. *Onchocerca volvulus*     2. Copepod.
   c. *Wuchereria bancrofti*     3. *Culex* and *Anopheles* mosquitos.
   d. *Dirofilaria* species     4. Snail.
   e. *Loa loa*     5. *Simulium* (black fly).
   f. *Dracunculus medinensis*     6. *Aedes* mosquito.

## REFERENCES & RECOMMENDED READING

Ash, L. R., & Orihel, T. C. (Eds.). (1990). *Atlas of human parasitology* (3rd ed.). Chicago: ASCP Press.

Babba, H., et al. (1994). Diagnosis of human hydatidosis: Comparison between imagery and six serologic techniques. *American Journal of Tropical Medicine and Hygiene, 50,* 64–68.

Bartlett, J. G. (1996). *Pocket book of infectious disease therapy.* Baltimore: Williams & Wilkins.

Bawden, M., Slaten, D., & Malone, J. (1994). QBC<sup>R</sup>: Rapid filaria diagnosis from blood-*Mansonella ozzardi* and *Wuchereria bancrofti. Transactions of the Royal Society of Tropical Medicine and Hygiene, 88,* 66.

Bradley, J. E., et al. (1993). A sensitive serodiagnostic test for onchocerciasis using a cocktail of recombinant antigens. *American Journal of Tropical Medicine and Hygiene, 48,* 198–204.

Bradley, J. E., & Unnasch, T. R. (1996). Molecular approaches to the diagnosis of onchocerciasis. *Advances in Parasitology, 37,* 57–106.

Brattig, N. W., et al. (1994). Strong IgG isotypic antibody response in Sowdah type onchocerciasis. *Journal of Infectious Disease, 170,* 955–961.

Case definitions for infectious conditions under public health surveillance. (1997). *Morbidity and Mortality Weekly Report, 46,* 40.

Chanekh, M., et al. (1992). Diagnostic value of a synthetic peptide derived from *Echinococcus granulosus* recombinant protein. *Journal of Clinical Investigation, 89,* 458–464.

Charrier-Ferrara, S., Djabali, M., & Goudot-Crozel, V. (1991). *Schistosoma mansoni*: A simple method for the extraction of DNA from single worms for PCR amplification. *Experimental Parasitology, 73,* 384.

De Clercq, D., et al. (1995). Comparison of the circulating anodic antigen detection assay and urine filtration to diagnose *Schistosoma haematobium* infections in Mali. *Transactions of the Royal Society of Tropical Medicine and Hygiene, 89,* 395–397.

Deelder, A. M., et al. (1994). Quantitative diagnosis of *Schistosoma* infections by measurement of circulating antigens in serum and urine. *Trop. Geo. Med., 46,* 233–238.

Dissanayake, S., et al. (1994). Evaluation of a recombinant parasite antigen for the diagnosis of lymphatic filariasis. *American Journal of Tropical Medicine and Hygiene, 50,* 727–734.

Eberhard, M. L. (1991). Laboratory diagnosis of filariasis. *Clinics in Laboratory Medicine, 11,* 977–1010.

Egwang, T. G., Nguiri, C., Kombila, M., Duong, T. H., & Richard-Lenoble, D. (1993). Elevated antifilarial IgG4 antibody levels in microfilaremic and microfilaridermic Gabonese adults and children. *American Journal of Tropical Medicine and Hygiene, 49,* 135–142.

Fagbemi, B. O., & Hillyer, G. V. (1990). Immunodiagnosis of dracunculiasis by falcon assay screening test-enzyme-linked immunosorbent assay (FAST-ELISA) and by enzyme-linked immunoelectrotransfer blot (EITB) technique. *American Journal of Tropical Medicine and Hygiene, 43,* 665–668.

Garate, T., Kliks, M. M., Cabbera, Z., & Parkhouse, M. E. (1990). Specific and cross-reacting antibodies in human responses to *Onchocerca volvulus* and *Dracunculus medinensis* infections. *American Journal of Tropical Medicine and Hygiene, 42,* 140–147.

Gbakima, A. A., Ibrahim, M. S., & Scott, A. L. (1992). Anti-*Onchocerca volvulus* immunoglobulin subclass response in children from Sierra Leone. *Scandinavian Journal of Immunology, 36,* 53–56.

Glickman, L. T., Grieve, R. B., Lauria, S. S., Jones, D. L. (1985). Serodiagnosis of ocular toxocariasis: A comparison of two antigens. *Journal of Clinical Pathology, 38,* 103–107.

Glickman, L. T., & Magnaval, J-F. (1993). Zoonotic roundworm infections. *Infectious Disease Clinics of North America, 7,* 717–732.

Helbig, M., Frosch, P., Kern, P., & Frosch, M. (1993). Serological differentiation between cystic and alveolar echinococcosis by use of recombinant larval antigens. *Journal of Clinical Microbiology, 31,* 3211–3215.

Homan, W. L., Derksen, A. C. G., & van Knapen, F. (1992). Identification of diagnostic antigens from *Trichinella spiralis. Parisitology Research, 78,* 112–119.

Hopkins, D. R., Ruiz-Tiben, E., Ruebush T., II, Agile, A. N., & Withers, P. C., Jr. (1995). Dracunculiasis eradication: March 1994 update. *American Journal of Tropical Medicine and Hygiene, 52,* 14–20.

Hui-Jun, Z., Zheng-Hou, T., Weng-Feng, C., & Piessens, W. F. (1990). Comparison of DOT-ELISA with sandwich-ELISA for the detection of circulating antigens in patients with bancroftian filariasis. *American Journal of Tropical Medicine and Hygiene, 42,* 546–549.

Jeffrey, H. C., & Leach, R. M. (Eds.). (1991). *Atlas of medical helminthology and protozoology* (3rd ed.). New York: Churchill Livingstone.

Khoshoo, V., et al. (1994). Dog hookworm: A cause of eosinophilic enterocolitis in humans. *Journal of Pediatric Gastroenterology Nutrition, 19,* 448–452.

Lewis, J. W., & Maizels, R. M. (Eds.). (1993). *Toxocara and toxocariasis, clinical, epidemiological and molecular perspectives.* London: Institute of Biology.

Loukas, A., Croese, T. J., Opdebeeck, J. P., & Prociv, P. (1992). Detection of antibodies to secretions of *Ancyclostoma caninum* in human eosinophilic enteritis. *Transactions of the Royal Society of Tropical Medicine and Hygiene, 86,* 650–653.

Loukas, A., Opdebeeck, J. P., Croese, T. J., & Prociv, P. (1994). Immunological incrimination of *Ancyclostoma caninum* as a human enteric pathogen. *American Journal of Tropical Medicine and Hygiene, 50,* 69–77.

Lucey, D. R., & Maguire, J. H. (1993). Schistosomiasis. *Infectious Disease Clinics of North America, 7,* 635–653.

Magnaval, J-F., Fabre, R., Maurieres, P. Charlet, J-P., & de Larrard, B. (1991). Application of the Western blotting procedure for the immunodiagnosis of human toxocariasis. *Parasitology Research, 77,* 697–702.

Mahannop, P., Setasauban, P., Morakote, N., Tapchaisri, P., & Chaichmpa, W. (1995). Immunodiagnosis of human trichinellosis and identification of specific antigen for *Trichinella spiralis. International Journal for Parasitology, 25,* 87–94.

Michael, E., Bundy, D. A. P., & Grenfell, B. T. (1996). Reassessing the global prevalence and distribution of lymphatic filariasis. *Parasitology, 112,* 409–428.

Ottesen, E. A. (1995). Immune responsiveness and the pathogenesis of human onchoceriasis. *Journal of Infectious Disease, 171,* 659–671.

Pammenter, M. D., et al. (1991). The value of immunological approaches to the diagnosis of schistosomal myelopathy. *American Journal of Tropical Medicine and Hygiene, 44,* 329–335.

Perera, L., Muro, A., Cordero, M., Villar, E., & Simon, F. (1994). Evaluation of a 22 kDa *Dirofilaria immitis* antigen for the immunodiagnosis of human pulmonary dirofilariosis. *Trop. Med. Parasitol., 45,* 249–252.

Peter, J. B. (Ed.). (1996). *Use and interpretation of tests in infectious disease* (4th ed.). Santa Monica, CA: Specialty Labs.

Pinto, P. L. S., et al. (1995). DOT-ELISA for the detection of IgM and IgG antibodies to *Schistosoma mansoni* worm and egg antigens, associated with egg excretion by patients. *Revista do Instituto de Medicina Tropical de Sao Paolo, 37,* 109–115.

Prociv, P., & Crosse, J. (1990). Human eosinophilic enteritis caused by dog hookworm *Ancyclostoma caninum. Lancet, 335,* 1299–1302.

Rabello, A. L. T., et al. (1995). Humoral immune responses in acute schistosomiasis mansoni: relation to morbidity. *Clinical Infectious Diseases, 21,* 608–615.

Ramachandran, C. P. (1993). Improved immunodiagnostic tests to monitor onchocerciasis control programmes—A multicenter effort. *Parasitology Today, 9,* 76–79.

Ruangkunaporn, Y., et al. (1994). Immunodiagnosis of trichinellosis: Efficacy of somatic antigen in early detection of human trichinellosis. *Asian Pacific Journal of Allergy and Immunology, 12,* 39–42.

Schutte, C. H. J., et al. (1994). Observations on the techniques used in the qualitative and quantitative diagnosis of schistosomiasis. *Annals of Tropical Medicine and Parasitology, 88,* 305–316.

Siridewa, K., Karunanayake, E. H., Chandrasekharan, N. V. (1996). Polymerase chain reaction-based technique for the detection of *Wuchereria bancrofti* in human blood samples, hydrocele fluid and mosquito vectors. *American Journal of Tropical Medicine and Hygiene, 54,* 72–76.

Su, X., Prestwood, A.K., McGraw, R.A. (1991). Cloning and expression of complementary DNA encoding an antigen of *Trichinella spiralis. Molecular Biochemical Parasitology, 45,* 331–336.

Sugane, K., Sun, S., & Matsuura, T. (1992). Molecular cloning of the cDNA encoding a 42 kDa antigenic polypeptide of *Anisakis simplex* larvae. *Journal of Helminthology, 66,* 25–32.

Sun, S., & Sugane, K. (1994). Complete structure of the gene encoding an immunodominant antigen of *Dirofilaria immitis* and larv-specific synthesis of primary transcript. *Journal of Helminthology, 68,* 259–264.

Tsang, V. C. W., & Wilkins, P. P. (1991). Immunodiagnosis of schistosomiasis: screen with FAST-ELISA and confirm with immunoblot. *Clinics in Laboratory Medicine, 11,* 1029–1039.

van Etten, L., Folman, C. C., Eggelte, T. A., Kremsner, P. G., & Deelder, A. M. (1994). Rapid diagnosis of schistosomiasis by antigen detection in urine with a reagent strip. *Journal of Clinical Microbiology, 32,* 2404–2406.

Van Lieshout, L., et al. (1995). Immunodiagnosis of schistosomiasis mansoni in a low endemic area in Surinam by determination of the circulating antigens CAA and CCA. *Acta Tropica, 59,* 19–29.

Villanueva, E. J., & Rodriguez-Perez, J. (1993). Immunodiagnosis of human dirofilariasis in Puerto Rico. *American Journal of Tropical Medicine and Hygiene, 48,* 536–541.

Wamae, C. N. (1994). Advances in the diagnosis of human lymphatic filariases: a review. *East African Medical Journal, 71,* 171–182.

World Health Organization. (1989). Workshop on DNA diagnosis and filariasis and symposium, on filariasis and onchoceriasis. TDR/FIL/DNA/89.1 *Geneva. WHO.1.*

Yagihashi, A., Sato, N., Takahashi, S., Ishikura, H., & Kikuchi, K. (1990). A serodiagnostic assay by microenzyme-linked immunosorbent assay for human anisakiasis using a monoclonal antibody specific for *Anisakis* larvase antigen. *Journal of Infectious Disease, 161,* 995–998.

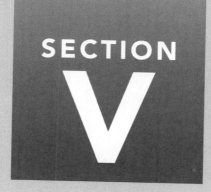

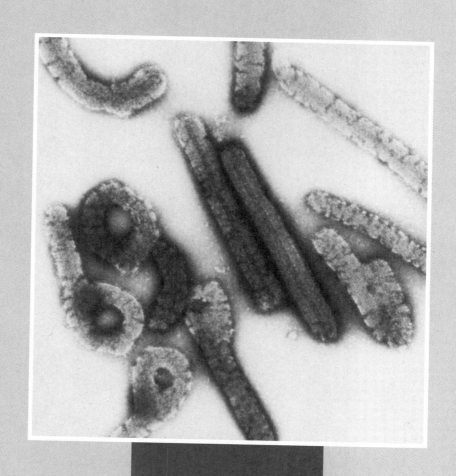

# CHAPTER 48

# Basic Concepts and Techniques in Virology

James D. Kettering, PhD

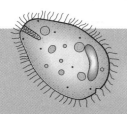

## Microbes in the News

### Hantavirus—Southwest United States

An outbreak of unexplained illness occurred in the southwestern part of the United States in 1993. Hantavirus pulmonary syndrome (HPS) symptoms include fever, muscle aches, headache, and cough, which progress rapidly to severe lung disease, often requiring intensive care treatment. This "new" virus was shown to be a previously undescribed hantavirus that resides in deer mice. Transmission is by inhalation of virus-containing deer mouse feces or urine. As of January 1995, HPS has been recognized in 102 patients in 21 states of the United States, as well as 7 in Canada and 3 in Brazil. The overall mortality rate is 40% (down from 80% in the initial group of patients) due to recognition of the disease and patient management. No specific antiviral chemotherapy is available. *Journal of Virology* (1994); *68*, 592–596.

## KEY TERMS

Antiviral chemotherapy
Capsid
Complement fixation
Cytopathic effect (CPE)
Eclipse phase
Enzyme immunoassay

Hemagglutination
Hemagglutination inhibition
Icosahedral
Interferons
Negative-sense RNA

Neutralization
Nucleic acid probes
Positive-sense RNA
Provirus
Virion

## LEARNING OBJECTIVES

**Upon successful completion of this chapter, the student should be able to:**

1. Explain the significance and usefulness of diagnostic virology to the medical clinician.
2. Describe the general characteristics of animal virus structure, growth, and reaction to environmental reagents.
3. Define the general laboratory approaches used in diagnostic virology.
4. Define how viral cytopathic effect (CPE) in host cells is used in identification of viruses.
5. Describe the various laboratory techniques used in the diagnostic virology laboratory.

## INTRODUCTION

At present most known medically significant human viruses can be isolated in cultured cells, and techniques are continuously being refined to speed up the process of identification. As a result, viral diagnostic facilities are becoming a standard feature of many hospital and most public health laboratories.

There are a number of reasons physicians should use laboratory services to obtain a precise diagnosis of all serious viral diseases, including:

1. The management of the patient and the prognosis often depend on an accurate diagnosis. Some specific examples would include suspected rubella in a pregnant woman (especially in the first trimester), herpes simplex virus infection in a newborn, and cytomegalovirus (CMV) reactivation in a transplant patient.
2. When **antiviral chemotherapy** becomes a practical reality, rapid diagnosis may be required to assist in the selection of the appropriate drug. Acyclovir resistance in herpes simplex viruses has been shown to occur routinely. For example, combinations of antivirals are routinely used in patients with acquired immunodeficiency syndrome (AIDS).
3. Presumably, many viruses remain to be discovered by the alert physician working with cooperative laboratories. The example referred to above in the "Microbes in the News" is an example. A morbillavirus (measles) has recently passed from horses (normal host) to humans (opportunistic) with fatal results.
4. The development of viral vaccines, which has played a key role in controlling a number of serious viral diseases, has also depended on identification of all the serotypes involved. Influenza, measles, and smallpox are good examples.
5. Precise virologic diagnosis is often of considerable importance in the maintenance of the public health, as is the case with dangerous epidemic diseases such as smallpox, yellow fever, rabies, influenza, and viral encephalitis.

## GENERAL CHARACTERISTICS OF VIRUSES

Viruses are among the smallest agents capable of causing infection in higher organisms, with the smallest of these being around 25 nm. A virus has essentially two main parts, a genetic component enclosed in a protein coat. A lipid envelope may surround some viruses. The nucleic acid genome may be either DNA or RNA, but never both. The nucleic acid element contains all the information that the virus needs to infect a host cell, replicate its essential parts, and assemble into mature, infective virus particles (**virions**). The protein coat protects the nucleic acid from nucleases and attaches the virus to host cells. The envelope is also involved in viral attachment. Figures 48-1 and 48-2 depict typical virus structures and terms.

### Growth of Viruses

Viruses are obligate intracellular parasites. In general, DNA viruses mature in the nucleus of the host cell,

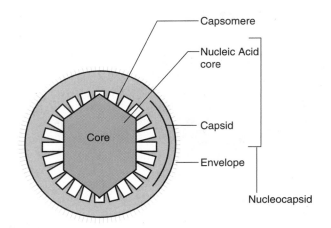

**FIGURE 48-1** Schematic representation of the various components of a typical animal virus. (Adapted from Willet, N. P., White, R. R., & Rosen, S. [1991]. *Essential dental microbiology*. East Norwalk, CT: Appleton & Lange.)

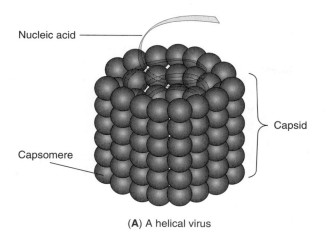

**(A)** A helical virus

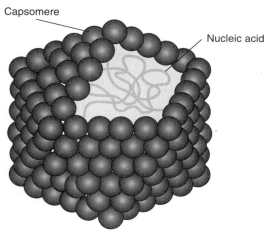

**(B)** A polyhedral virus

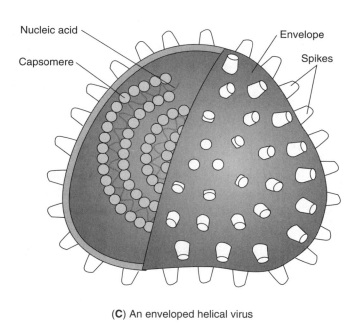

**(C)** An enveloped helical virus

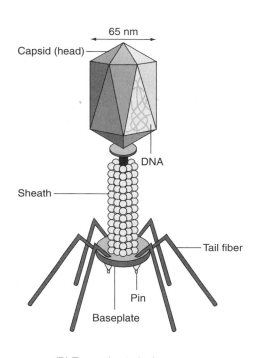

**(D)** T-even bacteriophage

**FIGURE 48-2** Diagrams illustrate the three basic structures found for animal viruses. Cubic, or spherical, viruses appear round due to the icosahedral structure shown here, which illustrates the three axes of symmetry normally found. The nucleic acid is found within the cubic structure. The rod-shaped helical viruses are more simple in construction. The rods are flexible and bend in nature. The complex viruses contain nucleic acid in the center. (Adapted from Willett, N. P., White, R. R., & Rosen, S. [1991]. *Essential dental microbiology*. East Norwalk, CT: Appleton & Lange.)

whereas RNA viruses replicate in the cytoplasm. There are few exceptions. The steps of virus growth include:

1. Attachment—Viral receptors specifically interact with host cell receptors.

2. Entry—Many cells accomplish this by receptor-mediated endocytosis, with the ingested viral particles being contained within endosomes. Others include direct penetration of the cyto-

plasmic membrane. Uncoating of the viral nucleic acid then occurs, allowing viral replication to begin.

3. Synthesis of components (**eclipse phase**)—Production of viral proteins (enzymes and structural) and replication of nucleic acid genomes occur independently.

4. Maturation—**Capsid** proteins autoassemble and nucleic acid genomes are added.

5. Release—Some viruses lyse the host cell and are released. Others are released by a budding process. Envelopes are acquired by the budding process, with the envelope coming from the cytoplasmic membrane of the host cell. Herpesviruses obtain their envelope from the nuclear membrane of the host cell.

**Synthesis of Viral Components.** The productive phase of the viral replicative cycle begins after the uncoating of the viral genome. The essential mechanism that must be accomplished is that specific mRNAs must be transcribed from the viral nucleic acid genome for successful expression and duplication of the genetic information. Once this is accomplished, viruses then use host cell components to translate the mRNA. Groups or classes of viruses use different pathways to synthesize the mRNAs depending on the structure of the viral genome. Some viruses (orthomyxo-, paramyxo-, and rhabdoviruses) carry RNA-dependent RNA polymerases within the virions. These are **negative-sense RNA** viruses because the viral genome is complementary to mRNA. The RNA polymerase is released into the host cell's cytoplasm along with the viral genome to produce viral mRNAs. The viral life cycle could not proceed without this enzyme. **Positive-sense RNA** viruses (polio-, arbo-, and coronaviruses) are so named because their genome functions directly as mRNA, associating with ribosomes for protein production. Purified RNA from positive-sense viruses, if introduced within a host cell's cytoplasm, is able to initiate a viral life cycle sequence. Purified RNA from negative-sense viruses, treated in a similar manner, would not be able to do so. An unusual enzyme exists for the retrovirus grouping. This reverse transcriptase uses single-stranded RNA as a template and produces a double-stranded DNA molecule (termed a **provirus**) that is incorporated into the host cell's chromosome as a necessary step in the replication cycle of these viruses (e.g., human immunodeficiency virus [HIV]). This mechanism is discussed in further detail in Chapter 50.

In the course of viral replication, all the virus-specified macromolecules are synthesized in a highly organized sequence. Viruses containing double-stranded DNA genomes produce early viral proteins soon after infection, which are primarily involved in viral genome replication. Late proteins, consisting primarily of structural components, are made after viral DNA synthesis has occurred. These components migrate to the appropriate compartment of the cell (the nucleus for most DNA viruses), autoassemble into empty viral capsids, and then are packed with viral genomes before maturation. Herpesviruses have three stages of protein production (immediate early, early, and late). Often there are stringent controls on gene expression, with gene products often shutting off earlier gene activity. Figures 48-3 and 48-4 summarize the synthesis steps of an RNA virus and a DNA virus, respectively.

**Antivirals and Vaccines.** Passive immune protection (use of preformed antibodies) has limited use in preventing or modifying viral diseases. Immune serum globulin (ISG) will prevent hepatitis A if given soon after contact with the virus for up to 4 to 5 weeks. ISG and hepatitis B immune globulin (HBIG) have definite benefits in use of postexposure prophylaxis concerning hepatitis B virus (HBV). Rabies immune globulin is used in postexposure management of individuals who may have been exposed.

Antiviral compounds represent natural or synthetic chemicals that prevent viral infections or alter the host-virus interactions in a manner beneficial to the host. Approved antivirals are listed in Table 48-1.

Viral diseases within our population have been mostly controlled through vaccines. Vaccines include live vaccines (host-range mutants, temperature-sensitive mutants, and recombinants incorporating cloned genes from other viruses) and killed or chemically inactivated vaccines. Live, attenuated preparations mimic natural virus infections and provide a more complete immune response than do killed virus vaccines. Some unwanted side effects may be experienced with the use of these materials.

## Table 48–1 ▶ Antivirals and Mechanism of Action

| Virus | Antiviral | Mechanism of Action |
| --- | --- | --- |
| Influenza | Amantidine | Prevents uncoating and inhibits viral RNA polymerase activity |
| Herpes simplex | Foscarnet | Inhibits viral DNA polymerase |
| | Acyclovir | Inhibits viral DNA polymerase |
| Cytomegalovirus | Ganciclovir | Inhibits viral nucleic acid metabolism |
| Respiratory syncytial virus | Ribavirin | Uncertain |
| HIV | Azidothymidine Protease inhibitors | Inhibits viral reverse transcriptase; inhibits protease enzymes |
| Varicella-zoster | Famciclovir | Inhibits viral nucleic acid metabolism |

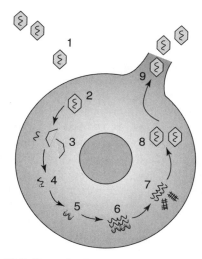

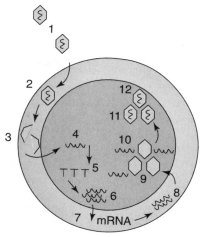

**FIGURE 48-3** Steps in the synthesis of a representative RNA virus (poliovirus). (*1*) Free polioviruses attach to specific receptor sites on the host cell membrane, losing one virus polypeptide (VP4). (*2*) Virions are taken into the cell by viropexis (a cellular function) and (*3*) uncoated, releasing the RNA into the cytoplasm, where it serves as its own mRNA. Early translation occurs (*4*), producing RNA polymerase, nucleases, and other inhibitors, directly causing the formation of double-stranded replicative intermediate RNA molecules (*5*). Inhibitors of cellular RNA and protein synthesis stop these host cell functions. Viral RNA minus and plus strands result in step *6*, with the plus strand either serving as mRNA, a template for continued RNA synthesis, or becoming encapsulated in the protein capsid. Late translation (*7*) generally results in structural proteins being produced at about the same time as RNA synthesis. Step *8* completes the production cycle as RNA molecules are enclosed in the protein capsid, which is released when the cell undergoes lysis (*9*). (Adapted from Willet, N. P., White, R. R., & Rosen, S. [1991]. *Essential dental microbiology*. East Norwalk, CT: Appleton & Lange.)

**FIGURE 48-4** Steps in the synthesis of a representative DNA virus (adenovirus). Attachment (*1*) and penetration (*2*) steps are similar to those described for poliovirus. Uncoating (*3*) is thought to occur through the action of cellular proteolytic enzymes, and the viral DNA is released to migrate into the host cell nucleus (*4*). Specific mRNA is transcribed from viral DNA (*5*), where virus-specific proteins (tumor antigen and enzymes for DNA replication) are produced. Viral DNA is synthesized (*6*), and late mRNA is produced at about the same time. Messenger RNA (*6*) migrates to the cytoplasm (*7*) and is translated into proteins for virus capsids (*8*). These viral proteins now migrate to the nucleus (*9*), where the components are assembled into virus capsids (*10*). Maturation (*11*) occurs when the viral DNA is enclosed by the protein subunits, resulting in complete virions. Releases (*12*) is by cell lysis. (Adapted from Willet, N. P., White, R. R., & Rosen, S. [1991]. *Essential dental microbiology*. East Norwalk, CT: Appleton & Lange.)

**Interferon.** **Interferons** (IFNs) are a group of glycoproteins that interfere with the mutiplication of both DNA and RNA viruses. IFNs are produced by many animal cells and are species specific, meaning they are most effective in the animal species that produces them or in a closely related species. IFNs are not virus specific. An IFN produced in response to one virus will inhibit many other virus species. Humans produce two types and three main groups of IFNs ranging from 20,000 to 40,000 daltons. Type I consists of IFN-α, which is produced by leukocytes, and IFN-ß, produced by fibroblasts. Type II, or IFN-γ, is produced by lymphocytes undergoing an immune response.

Once IFN is released from the virus-infected cell, it binds to the surface of another cell via specific cell receptors and sends a signal to the nucleus of that cell. This signal activates a gene coding from antiviral protein that acts primarily to inhibit the translation of mRNA into proteins. If both viral and cellular mRNAs are blocked, the cell may die. However, the spread of the virus is prevented.

It is now known that IFNs exhibit a wide variety of cell regulatory activities, including cell growth and differentiation. Of greatest significance is the ability of these products to modulate an immune response. For example, natural killer (NK) cells can have enhanced activity when exposed to IFNs. IFNS play significant regulatory roles involving macrophages as well as T and B lymphocytes when the immune system responds to a viral infection. IFNs also have been shown to have potential as anticancer reagents based on their ability to regulate cell functions and to modulate the immune system. Clinical trials testing antiviral and anticancer potentials are being conducted.

**Reaction to Physical and Chemical Agents.** The laboratory, in general, needs to be aware of how viruses will react to a variety of physical and chemical agents. Specimens must be properly treated and stored to ensure that viral viability is retained. Viruses may be transmitted to laboratory personnel by direct contact with a specimen or work space contamination. Procedures for disinfection need to be followed carefully and regularly. This section summarizes how viruses may react to these agents.

**HEAT AND COLD.** There is a great variability in the heat stability of different viruses. **Icosahedral** viruses tend to be stable, losing little viability after several hours at 37°C. Enveloped viruses, on the other hand, rapidly lose infectivity at this temperature. Viral infectivity, in general, may be destroyed by heating at 50° to 60°C for 30 minutes. A clinical specimen submitted for viral isolation may be adversely affected by remaining at room temperature for long periods after collection. Because the number of viruses in such specimens is relatively small, exposure to even room temperature for extended time may make it impossible to isolate any viruses that were originally present.

Viruses can be preserved by storage at low temperatures. The time frame in which a specimen is collected and subsequently delivered to the laboratory will determine the immediate storage temperature need. Most viruses will remain viable for about 24 hours at 4°C. If the laboratory is readily accessible, refrigeration for this time frame should be acceptable. If the specimen must be sent elsewhere, freezing it as cold as possible is the best situation. Storage at −90°C will maintain viability better than −20°C. For shipping, dry ice (−90°C) can be used. Enveloped viruses tend to lose infectivity after prolonged storage at even −90°C and are very sensitive to repeated freezing and thawing. Long-term storage of viruses is best done using liquid nitrogen (−180°C).

**SALTS.** Many viruses can be stabilized by salt concentrations of 1 mol/L. Under these conditions, heating to 50°C for 1 hour will not inactivate the agents. The mechanism is unknown, but may involve protection of the integrity of the protein capsid. This can be especially important in vaccine production and storage. Poliovirus vaccines are normally stored at −20°C or lower to preserve viral potency. Addition of 1 M magnesium salts allows the vaccine to remain viable for weeks at ambient temperatures.

**pH.** Viruses are quite stable over a wide pH range (5.0–9.0). Enteroviruses are resistant to an acidic pH. All viruses appear to be inactivated by alkaline conditions.

**RADIATION.** Ultraviolet, x-rays, and high-energy particles inactivate viruses. The nucleic acid genome is the target of these forces, and infectivity is the most radiosensitive property because replication requires expression of the entire genome.

**ETHER.** Enveloped viruses are inactivated by ether treatment. Ether destroys the lipid envelope, which is necessary for viral attachment to a host cell. Viability of nonenveloped viruses is essentially unaffected by such exposure.

**DETERGENTS.** Nonionic detergents (Triton X-100) solubilize the lipid constituents of viral membranes. Viral proteins would be released in an undenatured state. Anionic detergents (sodium dodecyl sulfate) solubilize viral envelopes and disrupt capsids into polypeptides.

**FORMALDEHYDE.** Formaldehyde destroys viral infectivity by reacting with the viral nucleic acids. Single-stranded genomes are more readily inactivated than double-stranded molecules. Because formaldehyde has minimal effects on proteins, it is often used in killed virus vaccine production.

**PHOTODYNAMIC INACTIVATION.** Viruses may be penetrated to a varying degree by vital dyes (neutral red, proflavine). These dyes bind to the viral nucleic acid, and the virus becomes inactivated when exposed to visible light. Neutral red dye is often used in viral plaque assays to improve visualization of the plaques. If viral progeny will be used from these plates, they need to be protected from bright light to avoid inactivation.

**ANTIBIOTICS.** Antibacterial antibiotics and sulfonamides are ineffective against viruses.

Chemicals that inactivate bacterial enzyme systems (quaternary ammonium compounds) are not effective because viruses contain no enzyme systems to affect.

**HALOGENS.** A 1:10 dilution of household bleach (sodium hypochloride, 5%) is very effective in destroying many viruses. If a great deal of organic material is present, more bleach may be necessary to get complete virus destruction.

# GENERAL APPROACHES TO VIRAL DIAGNOSIS

## Initial Set-up

For years, diagnostic virology was a service that applied primarily to a public health entity or was of epidemiologic interest. The 1980s brought a demand for these services to the local medical care establishment because of the development of high-quality reagents and antivirals, and the time frame from sample submission to final answer was decreased so that such results could be used in patient management decisions.

Viral diseases that commonly require laboratory diagnosis include sexually transmitted diseases, diarrhea, respiratory disease in children and adults, aseptic meningitis, congenital diseases, and infection in individuals who are immunocompromised. Individual viruses that are clinically significant are discussed in Chapter 50. A summary of viral diseases and potential agents that may be isolated in the laboratory is presented in Table 48-2, along with the most useful specimen(s) that would be collected and sent to the laboratory (see Chapter 49).

Those working in a clinical laboratory setting need to be familiar with cell culture, **enzyme immunoassay**, and immunofluorescence procedures, in addition to other common laboratory techniques. Basic equipment should include a laminar flow biologic safety cabinet, fluoresence and regular light microscopes (including an inverted bright-field microscope for cell culture examination), refrigerated centrifuge, refrigerator, freezer (conventional as well as low-temperature models), and carbon dioxide incubators. Although virology can, and probably should be, a component part of the microbiology laboratory section, it would probably be best to dedicate work stations and equipment to this area to avoid contamination of cell cultures by bacteria and mold.

## Isolation of Viruses from Clinical Specimens

Viruses are obligate intracellular parasites that are not capable of replication outside of a living cell. They

### Table 48–2 ► Types of Specimens Needed for Laboratory Diagnosis of Viral Infections

| Disease of Agent | PAIRED BLOODS | STOOL | NASAL SWAB | SPINAL FLUID | VESICLE FLUID | URINE | AUTOPSY/ BIOPSY |
|---|---|---|---|---|---|---|---|
| Adenovirus | x | | x | | | | |
| Aseptic meningitis | x | x | o | x | | | x |
| Chickenpox (varicella) | x | | o | | o | | |
| Colorado tick fever | xh | | | | | | x |
| Congenital rubella | x | | x | | | | |
| Coxsackievirus A | x | x | o | | | | x |
| Coxsackievirus B | x | x | o | o | | | x |
| Cytomegalovirus (CMV) | xh | | x | | | | x |
| Dengue | xh | | | | | x | x |
| Eastern equine | xh | | | | | | |
| Echovirus | x | x | o | o | | | x |
| Encephalitis | x | x | o | o | | | x |
| Enterovirus infections | x | x | o | o | | | |
| Herpes simplex | x | | o | x | | | |
| Influenza A and B | x | | x | | | | x |
| Lymphogranuloma venereum | x | | | | | | x |
| Lymphotic choriomeningitis | xh | | | o | | | |
| Measles (rubeola) | x | | o | x | | | x |
| Mumps | x | | o | x | | | x |
| Parainfluenza I, II, III, IV | x | | x | | | | |
| Pneumonia, viral or atypical | x | | x | | | | x |
| Poliovirus | x | x | o | o | | | x |
| Rabies | | | x | | | | x |
| Respiratory syncytial virus (RSV) | x | | x | | | | x |
| Rotavirus | x | x | x | | | | x |
| Rubella (German measles) | x | | x | | | | |
| Smallpox | xh | | | | | x | x |
| St. Louis encephalitis | xh | | | | x | | x |
| Vaccinia | xh | | | o | | | x |
| Varicella-zoster | x | | o | x | x | | x |
| Western equine encephalitis | xh | | | o | | | |

x, minimal specimen requirements for satisfactory attempt at virologic diagnosis of disease or agent specified; o, specimens not required, but which may be submitted, optionally, for supplemental examinations; h, in addition to paired bloods for antibody determination, heparinized blood for virus isolation.

use living tissue for an energy source and for the building materials necessary for multiplication. A patient's specimen containing a suspect virus is inoculated onto a susceptible tissue culture. Over a period of 1 to 3 weeks, the tissue culture is examined regularly for cytopathic changes that indicate the presence of a virus. This change is commonly referred to as **cytopathic effect (CPE)**. Once CPE is observed, steps are taken to determine the type of virus causing it. Identification procedures include fluorescent antibody procedures and the **neutralization** test.

**Proper Collection of Specimens for Viral Isolation—A Summary.** Specimen collection and processing are discussed in greater detail in Chapter 49. For immediate purposes, the following points are important for samples being inoculated into cell culture systems.

### Specimen Collection Information

| | |
|---|---|
| Urine | Urine is the specimen of choice for the recovery of CMV and should be collected in a sterile container. Collect 10–20 mL of urine. |
| Blood | Collect blood for virus culture in a heparinized tube. |
| Swabs | Samples collected on swabs should be placed in a viral transport medium. Use swabs with plastic shafts. Break off shaft to accommodate the size of the transport tube. Wooden-shafted swabs may contain oils that could be inhibitory to viruses. |
| Timeliness | All samples should be transported to the clinical laboratory as soon as possible. |
| Dr's Order | Read the doctor's orders carefully. |
| Notes | A virus culture for CMV will usually include a fluorescent antibody stain (FA stain). An FA stain for CMV will *NOT* include a culture. |

**Procedures for Handling Positive CPE.** When CPE is observed, the suspected virus should be passed to another tissue tube of the same cell line. Passing is done to ensure that the CPE observed is due to the presence of a virus. Virus will pass, whereas toxic and nonspecific rounding should not. All viruses with the exception of herpes simplex, are passed before proceeding to confirmatory procedures. To pass, the tissue culture is vortexed and 0.2 mL of the tissue culture media in the infected tube is inoculated to a fresh tissue culture tube.

**Confirmation Procedures.** Fluorescent antibody reagents are available in most laboratories for confirmation of the following viruses:

Adenovirus group
Cytomegalovirus
Herpes simplex virus type 1 and type 2
Influenzae A and B
Parainfluenzae I, II, and III
Respiratory syncytial virus
Varicella-zoster

When CPE results suggest one of these viruses, cell spots are made on eight-well microscope slides and stained. Positive and negative controls are made in the same fashion using cells known to be infected with a particular virus and uninfected cells to prepare the slides. Positive/infected cells are placed on the top row of a multiwelled slide and negative/uninfected cells are placed on the bottom row.

## Serologic Techniques

Usually a viral infection elicits immune responses directed against one or more viral antigens. Both cellular and humoral immune responses normally develop, and measurement of either may be used to diagnose a viral infection. Humoral immune responses are of major importance. Antibodies of the IgM class appear initially, followed by IgG antibodies. IgM antibodies disappear within a few weeks, but IgG products may persist for many years. Establishing the diagnosis of a viral infection is accomplished by demonstrating a rise in antibody titer to the virus or by demonstrating IgM antiviral immunoglobulins.

Historically, viral antibodies have been measured by neutralization (Nt), **complement fixation** (CF), **hemagglutination inhibition** (HI), and by immunofluorescence (IF) tests. Currently IF and enzyme immunoassays (EIA) are the most popular mechanisms used and are often available in commercially prepared kit formats. This has the advantage of quality controls being performed by the manufacturer. An important consideration to bear in mind is that measurements of antibodies by different methods do not necessarily give parallel results.

Earlier viral antibody studies used (ideally) two serum samples for comparison. An acute serum sample was drawn as early in the illness as possible, and a convalescent serum sample was drawn from 7 to 14 days later. These sera were diluted in a serial twofold (or 10-fold) pattern and tested at the same time. A fourfold (two dilution tubes) or greater increase in antibody titer between the acute and convalescent sera was and is considered to be diagnostic. Titers, stated as dilutions of the sera that gave positive serologic reactions, were easy to compare for increases or decreases. One problem with EIA procedures is that this familiar dilution pattern is no longer available due to the differences in protocols. EIAs determine whether or not antibody to a viral antigen is present by comparing to a cut-off value and is reported usually as an optical density reading. Comparisons of acute and convalescent antibody concentrations are much more difficult to interpret than those measurements obtained by CF, Nt, or IF tests.

Collection of blood specimens for serologic purposes must be done carefully and processed properly. Specimens should be drawn with aseptic precautions and without anticoagulants. The blood is allowed to clot and the serum separated. Serum is stored at 4°C or

−20°C. For some tests, heat inactivation (56°C for 30 minutes) may be necessary to remove nonspecific interfering or inhibiting substances and complement. Appropriate care should be taken to avoid direct contact with any patient serum due to the possibility of transmission of pathogenic organisms. A summary of serologic methods follows.

**Complement Fixation.** The basic principle in this test is based on the fact that many antibodies to viral antigens require complement for antigen destruction. Strictly standardized procedures must be used. A major problem is preparation of specific viral antigens that are stable and not anticomplementary. Most antigens are derived from viral cell cultures and are available from a variety of reputable companies. Complement, hemolysin, and red blood cells (RBCs) must be treated carefully and precisely titrated for inclusion into the test system.

Diluted patient serum and titered viral antigen are mixed and incubated for 1 hour at 37°C to allow antigen-antibody complexing to occur. Then titrated guinea pig complement is added to the reaction and the test is stored overnight at 4°C. Complement will attach to any antigen-antibody complexes present or remain free in solution if such complexes are absent. The next day, the test system is allowed to come to room temperature. An indicator system (hemolysin-sheep RBCs) is added. If specific viral antibody is present from the patient's serum and complexed with the viral antigen, all the complement will attach to that complex. No complement will be available for the hemolysin-RBC complex and lysis of the RBCs will not occur. No antibody in the patient's serum means that the complement would be available to be complexed by the hemolysin-RBC mixture. Lysis would then occur. CF is a complicated system to run, but many serum samples can be tested against several viral antigens in a single test set-up.

**Neutralization Test.** The principle in this test is that the viral antibody attaches to the virus and neutralizes the CPEs of the virus. It is a time-consuming, expensive test to run, but is very specific in its results. The protocol is used primarily today to specifically identify enteroviruses belonging to the Picornavirus grouping.

**Hemagglutination-Inhibition Test (HI).** Many viruses agglutinate erythrocytes, and this reaction may be specifically inhibited by immune sera. Many respiratory viruses routinely isolated in the diagnostic laboratory will agglutinate specific types of RBCs. To be useful for diagnosis, the RBC suspension must be standardized and the viral antigen standardized and titrated. Positive and negative controls must be included in each test.

Positive **hemagglutination** is indicated by a red, granular layer of RBCs over the entire bottom of the tube or well. Absence of agglutination is indicated by the formation of a compact red button of RBCs at the bottom of the tube or well that must slide or run when the container is tilted. Partial or weak agglutination is a partial layer or ring of RBCs on the tube bottom.

Serial dilutions of the patient sera are made and standard amount of virus (usually 4 hemagglutinating units) is added to each dilution. After mixing, the suspension is incubated at 37°C for 30 minutes. Then appropriate RBCs are added and mixed. This is placed at room temperature for 45 to 60 minutes and periodically examined for hemagglutination. The highest dilution of serum that inhibits hemagglutination is considered the HI titer.

**Fluorescent Antibody Procedures.** Virally infected cells fixed on a glass microscope slide serve as the viral antigen source. Dilutions of the patient serum are made in buffer and applied to a well containing the viral antigen. Incubation is done in a moist atmosphere at 37°C for 30 to 60 minutes. The serum components are removed, and the slide is washed with buffer to remove unreacted serum and antibodies. Antibodies to human IgG or IgM and labeled with fluorescein isothyocianate (FITC) are then added to the cell spot. The steps of incubation at 37°C and washing in buffer are repeated. If human antibody has attached to the viral antigen, antihuman immunoglobulin-FITC will attach to that antibody. This is viewed using a fluorescence microscope. Virally infected cells with human antibody attached will fluoresce a yellow or green color, depending on the microscope's filter system. Uninfected cells can be added to the virally infected ones to serve as an internal negative control. The highest patient serum dilution demonstrating fluorescence is the titer or measure of antibody. This test is specific and sensitive, but requires a special microscope and training in how to read or interpret the staining results.

**Enzyme Immunoassay (ELISA—Enzyme-Linked Immunosorbent Assay).** This method, which has many variations, depends on the conjugation of an enzyme to an antibody. The enzyme is detected by assaying for enzyme activity with its substrate. It is slightly less sensitive than radioimmune assay (RIA) but does not use radioactive materials.

To measure antibody, known viral antigens are fixed to a solid phase (plastic microdilution plate or bead), incubated with test (patient) serum dilutions, washed, and reincubated with antihuman immunoglobulin (IgM or IgG or both) labeled with an enzyme (horseradish peroxidase or alkaline phosphatase). Enzyme activity, measured by adding a specific substrate, results in a color reaction. The color amount can be read in a spectrophotometer and is a direct function of the amount of antibody bound in the test system.

This procedure is highly accurate, sensitive, and easy to perform. It appears to be the current method of choice by companies producing test kits for measuring antibodies to viruses.

## Molecular Diagnostic Techniques

**Direct Antigen Detection.** Several viral diseases provide symptoms that allow for a more rapid diagnosis by use of microscopy and virus staining procedures. Widespread availability of specific monoclonal antibodies has facilitated this method of viral identification. These antibodies may be labeled with such detection systems as FITC or enzymes (horseradish peroxidase or alkaline phosphatase) that greatly enhance the technician's chances of detecting the viral antigen that might be present. Cells containing viral antigen are collected and placed on a microscopic slide (smears or impression imprints or collected exfoliated cells) and can be detected by a direct staining procedure or the more economical indirect staining protocol. Viruses that may be detected by this method include herpes simplex virus, varicella-zoster virus, a variety of respiratory viruses (influenza A and B, adenovirus, parainfluenza viruses 1, 2, and 3, and RSV), and rabies. Mumps and measles viruses and CMV may also be detected by this method if appropriate specimens can be collected and delivered to the laboratory.

Cells or smears are allowed to air dry and fixed in acetone (−20°C overnight or room temperature for 5 minutes). Staining can be accomplished using the protocol similar to the fluorescent antibody detection. Enzyme-labeled antibodies would be detected by addition of an appropriate substrate and development of a specific color. These tests can be performed quickly and allow diagnostic answers to be determined in just a few hours. It is very important that appropriate positive and negative controls be included to determine whether the test procedure has functioned properly and as a comparison for the clinical sample results.

Several companies use EIAs to detect viral antigen in clinical specimens. Kits are available for rotaviruses, adenoviruses, RSV, influenza A virus, and herpes simplex virus. In addition, antibody assay systems for these viruses are also available in the ELISA format. The latest design in ELISA antigen detection kits has been to quantitate viral load for use in evaluating antiviral chemotherapy efficacy.

The final mechanisms use molecular biology procedures. **Nucleic acid probes** are short segments of DNA that are designed to hybridize with complementary viral DNA or RNA segments. The probe is labeled with a fluorescent, chromogenic, or radioactive tag that allows detection if hybridization occurs. The probe reaction can occur in a thin tissue section, in a liquid, or on a reaction vessel surface or membrane. These tests are most useful in situations where the virus load in relatively abundant, viral culture is slow or not possible and other assays (e.g., EIAs) lack sensitivity or specificity. Relatively few commercially available reagents exist for probe assays in diagnostic virology laboratories today. The greatest problem with probe detection of virus appears to be the relative lack of sensitivity compared to conventional detection procedures.

## SUMMARY

- ▶ New viruses continue to appear, causing human infections.
- ▶ Diagnostic virology can be performed in a timely manner so that physicians can make patient management decisions based on appropriate data.
- ▶ Science understands basic information about viruses that enables a laboratory to isolate specific viruses causing diseases and to develop specific antiviral chemicals.
- ▶ There are six DNA viral groups and at least 12 RNA virus families.
- ▶ Many local medical centers have diagnostic virology services directly available to physicians.
- ▶ Proper specimen collection and handling is important for successful laboratory test results.
- ▶ Most human viruses routinely found in the population can be isolated and identified for the physician.
- ▶ Viral serologic information can be a useful diagnostic tool when isolation of viruses cannot be done.
- ▶ Technology is constantly changing, bringing newer methods to diagnostic virology that ensure availability of faster and more accurate information.
- ▶ The technologist must maintain a complete understanding of older and newer diagnostic tests in virology.

## CASE STUDY

An 18-year-old woman, with a sore throat, presented at the college health care facility. She had been well until 3 days ago, when she experienced the gradual onset of malaise, anorexia, and mild sore throat. The symptoms had intensified, and she now felt that her throat was "on fire." She presented as feverish, with a frontal headache, and had lost complete interest in food and cigarettes. She had received the DPT vaccine as a child. Her physical exam showed T 39°C, BP 126/70, P 92, R 18. The patient appeared acutely ill. Her skin showed no rash or jaundice; her throat was intensely red and swollen, with a yellowish exudate on the left tonsil. There was several tender, enlarged lymph nodes, with no signs of meningeal irritation. Chest, heart, abdomen, and neurologic exams were normal. Blood analysis showed a hematocrit of 39%, white cell (WBC) count 14,000, and differential of 52% polymorphonuclear cells (PMNs), 45% lymphocytes, 3% monocytes, and platelets 100,000. Urine and chest x-rays were normal. The following day, the throat culture showed α-hemolytic streptococci and the Monospot was negative. Transaminases were elevated to twice normal levels. WBC, 16,000; differential: 48% PMNs, 50% lymphs (3% are atypical), 2% monos. The patient was treated with aspirin and warm, saltwater gargles. Her throat remained sore for the next 2 days. The following day, her temperature dropped to 38°C and she began to feel somewhat better. The Monospot test was positive by this time.

### Questions:

1. What is your differential diagnosis and what laboratory tests should be ordered to make a microbiologic diagnosis?

2. In view of these laboratory findings, what would be your diagnostic impression?

3. What was this infection and how is this infection transmitted?

## Review Questions

1. The viral structure consisting of the genome and protein coat is called a(n):
   a. envelope.
   b. capsomere.
   c. capsid.
   d. nucleocapsid.

2. Acyclovir inhibits herpes simplex viruses. To do so, it interferes with:
   a. viral protein synthesis.
   b. viral nucleic acid metabolism.
   c. viral envelope development.
   d. viral reverse transcriptase activity.

3. Interferons inhibit viral growth by primarily affecting:
   a. host cytoline production.
   b. host protein synthesis.
   c. viral protein synthesis.
   d. viral nucleic acid production.

4. Which viral disease listed below can be managed, in part, by using passive immunity techniques?
   a. Influenza A infections
   b. Hepatitis A infections
   c. Poliovirus infections
   d. Rotavirus infections

5. Mumps viral infections are best controlled in our population by using:
   a. acyclovir.
   b. amantadine.
   c. ribavirin.
   d. a live vaccine.

6. Multinucleated giant cells are formed as a result of viral infection. They are formed as a result of viral glycoproteins being added to which host cell structure listed below?
   a. Nuclear membrane
   b. Cytoplasmic membrane
   c. Host cell cytoplasm
   d. Endoplasmic reticulum

7. Which viral diseases listed below are currently best controlled by use of vaccines?
   a. Poliovirus and coxsackieviruses
   b. Rubeola and rubella viruses
   c. Mumps and RSV viruses
   d. Hepatitis B and hepatitis C viruses

8. Which respiratory virus listed below can be treated with ribavirin?
   a. Influenza A virus
   b. Influenza B virus
   c. Adenovirus
   d. Respiratory syncytial virus

9. A primary viral isolate from a suspected case of poliomyelitis was inoculated into VERO cells, and a dramatic cytopathic effect (CPE) was noted within 24 hours. The isolate was confirmed as poliovirus by neutralization with polyvalent antibody to poliovirus types I, II, III; however, mono-specific antibody to each type failed to block CPE. This finding suggests that the isolate contained which of the following?
   a. Recombinant of type I and type II viruses
   b. Virus that shares a few antigenic determinants with poliovirus
   c. Mixture of polio and another type of picornavirus
   d. Mixture of two types of poliovirus

10. In a serologic test of acute and convalescent sera during a respiratory disease outbreak, the following results were reported. Influenza A—acute <10 and convalescent 10; influenza B—acute <10 and convalescent 40; RSV—acute 10 and convalescent 80. Which conclusion below is correct?
   a. The data do not allow a diagnosis to be made.
   b. Influenza B caused the disease.
   c. Two viruses were involved in the outbreak.
   d. All three viruses were involved in the outbreak.

## ▶ REFERENCES & RECOMMENDED READING

Arruda, E., Crump, C. E., Rollins, B. S., et al. (1996). Comparative susceptibilities of human embryonic fibroblasts and HeLa cells for isolation of human rhinoviruses. *Journal of Clinical Microbiology, 34*(5), 1277–1279.

Baron, S. (Ed.). (1996). *Medical microbiology* (4th ed.). Galveston, TX: The University of Texas Medical Branch.

Belshe, R. B. (1991). *Textbook of human virology* (2nd ed.). St. Louis: Mosby–Yearbook.

Brooks, G. F., Butel, J. S., & Ornston, L. N. (Eds.). (1995). *Medical microbiology* (20th ed., pp. 303–528. East Norwalk, CT: Appleton & Lange.

Brumback, B. G., & Wade, C. D. (1996). Simultaneous rapid culture for four respiratory viruses in the same cell monolayer using a different multicolored fluorescent confirmatory stain. *Journal of Clinical Microbiology, 34*(4), 798–801.

Burgisser, P., Simon, F., Wernli, M., et al. (1996). Multicenter evaluation of new double-antigen sandwich enzyme immunoassay for measurement of anti-human immunodeficiency virus type 1 and type 2 antibodies. *Journal of Clinical Microbiology, 34*(3), 634–637.

Diaz-Mitona, F., Ruben, M., Sacks, S., et al. (1996). Detection of viral DNA to evaluate outcome of antiviral treatment of patients with recurrent genital herpes. *Journal of Clinical Microbiology, 34*(3), 657–663.

Englund, J. A., Piedra, P. A., Jewell, A., et al. (1996). Rapid diagnosis of respiratory syncytial virus infections in immunocompromised adults. *Journal of Clinical Microbiology, 34*(7), 1649–1653.

Fields, B. N., Knipe, D. M., & Howley, P. M. (Eds.). (1996). *Fields virology* (Vols. 1 and 2, 3rd ed.). Philadelphia: Lippincott-Raven.

Grundy, J. E., Ehrnst, A., Einsele, H., et al. (1996). A three-center European external quality control study of PCR for detection of cytomegalovirus DNA in blood. *Journal of Clinical Microbiology, 34*(5), 1166–1170.

Hsiung, G. D. (1982). *Diagnostic virology, illustrated by light and electron microscopy* (3rd ed.). New Haven, CT: Yale University Press.

Leland, D. S. (1996). *Clinical virology*. Philadelphia: Saunders.

Lennette, E. H. (Ed.). (1985). *Laboratory diagnosis of viral infections*. New York: Marcel Dekker.

Mills, J., Volberding, P. A., & Corey, L. (Eds.). (1996). *Antiviral chemotherapy 4. New directions for clinical application and research*. New York: Plenum Press.

Murray, P. R., Baron, E. J., Pfaller, M. A., et al. (Eds.). (1995). *Manual of medical microbiology* (6th ed.). Washington, DC: ASM Press.

Pagcharoenpol, P., Burgess-Cassler, A., & Schramm, W. (1996). Simplified testing for antibodies to human immunodeficiency virus. *Journal of Clinical Microbiology, 34*(4), 973–974.

Specter, S., & Lancz, G. (Eds.). (1992). *Clinical virology manual* (2nd ed.). New York: Elsevier.

Timbury, M. C. (1991) *Medical virology* (9th ed.). London: Churchill Livingstone.

White, D. O., & Fenner, F. J. (1994). *Medical virology* (4th ed.). San Diego: Academic Press.

Willet, N. P., White, R. R., & Rosen, S. (1991). *Essential dental microbiology*. East Norwalk, CT: Appleton & Lange.

Zuckerman, A. J., Banatvala, J. E., & Pattison, J. R. (Eds.). (1990). *Principles and practice of clinical virology* (2nd ed.). New York: Wiley.

# CHAPTER 49
## Specimen Collection and Processing of Viral Specimens

James D. Kettering, PhD

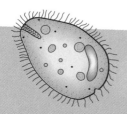

## Microbes in the News
### Mystery Virus Transfer to Humans from Horses

A mysterious virus that killed 14 horses and a horse trainer in Australia recently has the ability to jump from horses (normal host) to humans (opportunistic host). Scientists have no idea where it originated or how big a threat it poses. It is part of a family that includes measles and canine distemper. The virus was isolated from the lungs of the dead horses and the kidney of the late horse trainer. The virus isolates were identical. The virus killed the normal hosts by creating holes in blood vessels that leaked into lungs until the victims drowned in blood. This appears to be the latest in a series of "new" viruses that have been discovered to be maintained naturally in animal hosts and only recently been shown to be able to infect humans also. (*Science,* April 1995)

**INTRODUCTION**

**SPECIMEN COLLECTION AND HANDLING**

Autopsy or Biopsy Specimens—Isolation

Blood (Buffy Coat)

Bone Marrow

Bronchoalveolar Lavage

Genital Swab

Rectal Swab—Isolation

Stool—Isolation

Semen

Cerebrospinal Fluid (CSF)—Isolation

Throat Swab or Washing—Isolation

Urine—Isolation

Vesicular Lesion Material

Vesicular Lesion Smear (Direct Fluorescent Antibody)

**TRANSPORT**

**STORAGE**

**PREPARING SPECIMENS FOR INOCULATION**

Nasopharynx, Throat, Mouth Swab, or Genital Specimens

Tissue Biopsy or Autopsy Specimens

Blood Specimens

Bronchoalveolar Lavage

CSF and Other Body Fluids (Sterile)

Sputum Specimen

Rectal Swabs

Stool Specimens

Urine Specimens

Vesicle Fluid

## KEY TERMS

Acute infection
Anticoagulants

Balanced salt solution
Ficoll-Hypaque

Serology
Viral transport medium

## LEARNING OBJECTIVES

**Upon successful completion of this chapter, the student should be able to:**

1. Describe the various specimens that would/could contain virions responsible for a disease condition.

2. Describe the appropriate procedures to prepare a specimen for inoculation into appropriate cell cultures.

3. List the problems involved in specimen transport and storage that may result in specimen rejection by the laboratorian.

4. List the appropriate specimen(s) that would be collected for a specified disease/clinical manifestation.

5. Discuss the storage of specimens collected for the diagnosis of viral infection.

## INTRODUCTION

Viral diagnosis is a fairly well-established section of many clinical laboratories. Improvements in techniques and timing have allowed information obtained from these results to be used in decisions concerning patient management. Specimens for viral isolation should be obtained from patients in the acute stage of infection and at the same time as those sent to the bacteriology laboratory. This means that the specimens should be collected as soon as possible after the onset of illness.

Blood specimens for serologic testing (**serology**) need to be collected under aseptic conditions and should contain no anticoagulants. Serum should be promptly separated from the clot and frozen, although refrigeration temperature (4°C) will maintain antibody titers for relatively long periods of time. In general, for serologic diagnosis to be clinically useful, at least two specimens of blood should be collected. The first should be taken early during the **acute infection** phase, and the second should be taken 10 to 14 days later. It is often difficult to obtain the second serum sample and only limited diagnostic information can be gained from a single serum sample. Occasionally, a third sample might be desirable and this is usually collected 4 weeks after the first one.

Table 49-1 lists the most common viral diseases encountered routinely in the United States and also notes the most common viral pathogens responsible for those diseases.

Table 49-2 lists the clinical specimens that may be routinely collected from individuals with the specified clinical manifestations and sent to the diagnostic virology laboratory for processing.

## SPECIMEN COLLECTION AND HANDLING

Specimens for viral diagnosis may be collected in a variety of ways, but certain principles need to be kept in mind so that viable virions will be available to be isolated after being inoculated into cell cultures. The following is an overview of the specimens routinely collected, along with appropriate information for proper handling, transport, and storage.

## Autopsy or Biopsy Specimens—Isolation

Collect tissues from probable sites of pathology using a separate, sterile instrument for each sample and place in separate sterile containers to avoid cross-contamination. Collect the autopsy specimen as soon as possible after death. Refrigerate and transport to the laboratory on cold pack within 24 hours. If longer than 48 hours, freeze at –70°C and ship on dry ice to the laboratory. *Specimens placed in a formalin solution are NOT ACCEPTABLE.*

**Central Nervous System Disease.** Submit ½- to 1-inch cube of brain (temporal lobe, cortex, midbrain, medulla) and spinal cord. For the recovery of enteroviruses, submit a 2- to 3-inch segment of descending colon, tied off with contents.

**Influenza or Other Respiratory Disease.** Collect ½- to 1-inch cubes of lung tissue and bronchus or trachea. (Heart muscles, liver, and kidney are less common sources of virus, but may be included if involvement is suspected.) Place small samples (e.g., lung biopsy specimen) into **viral transport medium** (VTM) to prevent drying. Place larger specimens (1–2; e.g., autopsy tissues) into sterile containers. Add 8 to 10 mL VTM to prevent drying.

## Blood (Buffy Coat)

Collect 8 to 10 mL blood in an **anticoagulant** (sodium citrate, ethylenediaminetetra-acetic acid [EDTA], or heparin). Transport to the laboratory as soon as possible. The specimen should be set up within 24 hours of collection. Refrigerate. DO NOT FREEZE.

## Table 49–1 ▶ Viral Diseases and Common Viral Pathogens

| Viral Disease | Common Viral Agent |
|---|---|
| Respiratory—upper—adult | Rhinovirus, coronavirus, adenovirus, influenza, parainfluenza |
| Upper—infants and children | Rhinovirus, coronavirus, parainfluenza, adenovirus, respiratory syncytial virus (RSV), influenza |
| Pneumonia—adult | Influenza, adenovirus |
| Pneumonia—infants and children | SV, adenovirus, influenza, parainfluenza |
| Pharyngitis—infants and children | Adenovirus, coxsackie A, herpes simplex, Epstein-Barr, rhinovirus, influenza, parainfluenza |
| Croup—infants and children | Parainfluenza, RSV |
| Bronchitis—infants and children | Parainfluenza, RSV |
| Bronchiolitis—infants and children | SV, parainfluenza |
| Pleurodynia—adults | Coxsackie B |
| Gastroenteritis | |
| Adults | Calicivirus (Norwalk agents), enteric adenovirus |
| Infants and Children | Rotaviruses, picornaviruses (enterovirus), enteric adenoviruses, caliciviruses |
| All patients | |
| Acute pulmonary syndrome | Hantavirus |
| Cutaneous—rash | Herpes simplex, varicella-zoster, enteroviruses, measles, rubella, parvoviruses, human herpesviruses 6 |
| Encephalitis | Herpes simplex, togaviruses, bunyaviruses, flaviviruses, rabies, enteroviruses, human immunodeficiency virus, JC virus |
| Febrile illness with rash | Echoviruses, coxsackieviruses |
| Hemorrhagic fever | Adenoviruses |
| Hepatitis | Hepatitis A, B, C, D, E viruses (also herpesviruses, rubella, measles, mumps, and others—generalized infections) |
| Infectious mononucleosis | Epstein-Barr, cytomegalovirus |
| Keratitis/conjunctivitis | Herpes simplex, varicella-zoster, adenoviruses, coxsackie A-24, enterovirus 70 |
| Meningitis | Coxsackieviruses, echoviruses, mumps, herpes simplex |
| Myocarditis/pericarditis | Coxsackieviruses, echoviruses |
| Parotitis | Mumps, parainfluenza |
| Pleurodynia | Coxsackie B |

## Bone Marrow

Collect at least 2 mL in anticoagulant (sodium citrate, EDTA, or heparin).

## Bronchoalveolar Lavage

This technique allows the recovery of both cellular and noncellular components from the epithelial surface of the lower respiratory tract and differs from bronchial washings, which refer to the aspiration of either secretions or small amounts of instilled saline from the large airways. In general, sterile buffered saline is infused through the working channel of a bronchoscope in 20- to 50-mL aliquots. After each aliquot is infused, the fluid is withdrawn by hand suction into a syringe. In normal airways, 50% to 60% of the lavage fluid is recovered. Fluids may be kept at room temperature, instead of on ice, with no loss of cell or microorganism viability, if transported to the laboratory for processing within 1 hour. The initial aliquot collected is sometimes discarded on the basis that it does not represent an ideal specimen.

## Genital Swab

Swab cervix or urethra vigorously and place swab in VTM (e.g., Dulbecco's modified Eagle's medium [DMEM]) and refrigerate. Freeze at –70°C only if held longer than 48 hours, en route to the laboratory. Dacron swabs on a plastic shaft are the best to use for collection purposes.

## Rectal Swab—Isolation

Stool samples are more reliable for virus recovery; however, if stool material cannot be obtained, a swab may be used. Moisten a swab with DMEM VTM. Insert swab into the rectum and rub against mucosa and repeat until visible fecal material adheres to the swab.

---

**Table 49–2 ▶ Specimen Collection Based on Symptom-Oriented Guide**

| Clinical Manifestation | Specimen |
|---|---|
| Respiratory tract (pharyngitis, croup, bronchitis, pneumonia) | Nasal wash, throat wash, nasal/throat swab sputum (urine if CMV is suspected) |
| Central nervous system (meningitis, encephalitis) | CFS, throat swab, rectal swab or stool (urine if mumps is expected) (Brain biopsy if herpes simplex is suspected) |
| Genital tract (lesions, vaginitis, cervicitis) | Lesion swab or scraping, cervicovaginal swab |
| Ocular | Conjunctival swab or corneal scraping |
| Gastrointestinal | Stool, rectal swab |
| Hepatitis | Serum (urine if CMV is suspected) |
| Rash—maculopapular | Throat swab, rectal swab |
| Rash—vesicular | Vesicle fluid, lesion swab, throat swab, rectal swab or stool |
| Congenital/neonatal | Nasal/throat swab, urine, stool or rectal swab, CSF |

CMV, cytomegalovirus; CSF, cerebrospinal fluid

---

Place swab into DMEM viral transport medium and refrigerate. Send to the laboratory on cold pack if processing is less than 48 hours; otherwise, freeze at –70°C.

## Stool—Isolation

Collect as soon as possible, no later than 7 to 10 days after onset. Collect 2 to 3 teaspoonsful in a sterile container. Do not use paperboard or unsealed containers for shipment of stool because the specimen may become dessicated. Refrigerate and transport on cold pack if processing is less than 48 hours; otherwise, freeze at –70°C.

## Semen

Collect in sterile container.

## Cerebrospinal Fluid (CSF)—Isolation

As soon as possible after onset, collect 3 to 5 mL of blood-free CSF in a sterile tube. Refrigerate and ship to the laboratory within 48 hours on cold pack. If greater than 48 hours, freeze at –70°C; ship on dry ice to the laboratory. Rarely, CSF may be used for antibody studies.

## Throat Swab or Washing—Isolation

Collect as soon as possible, not later than 5 days after disease onset.

**Swab.** Swab throat and nasopharynx using two separate swabs moistened with sterile saline. Place swab into the DMEM VTM. Refrigerate for up to 48 hours or freeze at –70°C.

**Washing.** Have patient gargle 10.0 mL of sterile saline; expectorate into sterile sputum container and add 10.0 mL DMEM VTM. Refrigerate and process within 48 hours.

## Urine—Isolation

Urine is the specimen of choice for the recovery of CMV or rubella virus in suspected congenitally infected infants, and occasionally for recovery of other viruses. *Urine is not the specimen of choice for general virus isolation.* Collect 10 to 20 mL of urine into a sterile bottle using sterile precautions. CMV in urine is considered to be heat labile and requires special handling. If specimen can be delivered to the laboratory within 24 hours, ship specimen on cold pack to the laboratory, and *DO NOT FREEZE.* If specimen *CANNOT* be delivered to the laboratory within 24 hours, add an equal volume of 70% sorbitol and freeze at –70°C for shipment.

## Vesicular Lesion Material

Collect cellular scrapings from the base of lesions with scalpel or cotton swab, place scrapings or swab-tip in DMEM VTM. Ship refrigerated within 48 hours or freeze at –70°C if transit time is more than 48 hours. Vesicular or pustular fluid should be collected with capillary pipets or swabs and placed in a stoppered tube. Refrigerate or freeze at –70°C.

## Vesicular Lesion Smear (Direct Fluorescent Antibody)

Collect cellular scrapings from fresh lesions (before scab formation) as above. Obtain epithelial cells and avoid pustular exudate. Prepare two slides by making spot smears of cellular scrapings on clean glass slides; concentrate material in three 10 to 15-mm circular areas on each slide. Air dry slides and send to the laboratory in protective metal or plastic container at ambient temperature. Fix slides in acetone. These smears may be infective and should be labeled a biohazard and packaged accordingly.

## TRANSPORT

Swabs are often used for the collection of specimens for viral diagnosis (see Table 50-2). A variety of fibers have been used for the tip of the shaft of commercially available swabs. These have included rayon, cotton, Dacron, polyester, and calcium alginate. Except for the calcium alginate-tipped swabs, all materials have been acceptable for general use for collection of viral specimens. Calcium alginate is toxic to herpes simplex viruses and should not be used. Wooden-shafted swabs should be avoided, if possible. Oils from the wood may diffuse into the transport medium and inhibit viral growth.

Survival times of viruses vary tremendously. Generally, enveloped viruses are more fragile than nonenveloped virions. Viruses, in general, will usually survive for 24 to 48 hours if refrigerated (4°C) after collection. If a specimen has been stored at room temperature for several hours before delivery to the virology laboratory, the chances of isolating viruses diminishes. This aspect must be considered in acceptance-rejection criteria for specimens. Culturettes® (Becton Dickinson Microbiology Systems, Cockeysville, MD) consists of a plastic tube containing a sterile rayon-tipped swab and an ampule of modified Stuart's transport medium. This swab may be used for the specimen collection and transport of organisms involved in bacteriology, mycology, and parasitology, as well as virology.

Hanks' **balanced salt solution** (HBSS) and Leibovitz-Emory medium (LEM) are other examples of transport media that have served well. Some laboratories have found that use of the minimal essential medium (Eagle's or Dulbecco's) used in cell culture maintenance is satisfactory. Comparisons of these materials are reported in the literature and all have been found to be essentially equivalent in regard to virus survival, assuming that factors such as time in transit and temperature are satisfied.

Cost considerations will have to be made as to whether it is more cost effective to purchase commercially available packages compared with laboratory-dispensed tubes.

## STORAGE

Nonenveloped viruses (e.g., adenoviruses and enteroviruses), are capable of surviving freeze-thaw procedures with little loss of viral titer. Herpes simplex virus, on the other hand, may experience a 100-fold decrease in titer after undergoing a single freeze-thaw cycle. Storage at room temperature will generally produce a greater decrease in enveloped virus titers compared to nonenveloped agents. Generally, storage of viruses in transport medium at 4°C will produce no more than a 10-fold loss in infectivity. Therefore, short-term (< 3 days) transport or storage of most virus specimens should be 4°C rather than freezing.

If longer times are involved, freezing at –70°C is recommended. Freezing does reduce the viability of most viruses and should be avoided, if possible. Survival is more likely to occur at the lowest temperatures possible. Minus 70°C is better than conventional freezer temperatures (–20°C), for example, and liquid nitrogen (–168°C) should be considered for long-term storage needs.

## PREPARING SPECIMENS FOR INOCULATION

Specimens collected on swabs and placed in DMEM VTM should have the swab removed as soon as possible because swabs may have a toxic effect on virus. Before removing the swab, the transport tube is vortexed vigorously to remove any viral particles from the swab. Using a pair of forceps that have been flame sterilized, or wiped with alcohol, the swab is pressed firmly against the inside of the transport tube to express all the liquid. The swab is then discarded.

Depending on the source of specimen, treatment with antibiotics, as indicated, may be required before inoculation of tissue cultures.

### Nasopharynx, Throat, Mouth Swab, or Genital Specimens

After removing the swab, 0.9 mL specimen is added to 0.1 mL antibiotic. Vortex and let stand for 30 minutes at room temperature. If a large amount of cellular material is seen in the transport medium (appears cloudy), centrifuge the specimen for 5 minutes at full speed and use the supernatant for tissue culture inoculation.

### Tissue Biopsy or Autopsy Specimens

To prepare tissue specimen for inoculation, place a portion of the tissue in a sterile tissue grinder. Add 1 to 2 mL of tissue culture media as needed, depending on the amount of fluid that may come with the tissue. Remove the homogenized specimen from the tissue grinder and place it in a sterile 12 × 75 mm polystyrene tube. Add 0.1 mL of a penicillin/gentamicin antibiotic solution. Vortex and let stand for 30 to 60 minutes at room temperature. Centrifuge for 5 minutes at 2,500 rpm. Inoculate tissue cultures using the supernatant.

## Blood Specimens

Separation of mononuclear cells (buffy coat) from whole blood is necessary for viral isolation studies. Mononuclear cells are lymphocytes and monocytes and are often the cells that contain the viruses being sought. First, a 50-50% mixture of blood and RMPI medium is made. For each milliliter of blood/RMPI available from above, place 0.6 mL **Ficoll-Hypaque** (F-H) in the bottom of a sterile 15-mL conical polystyrene tube with cap and carefully layer the diluted blood on top of the F-H solution. Centrifuge the tubes for 20 minutes at 1,500 rpm at room temperature. After centrifugation, the tube contains four layers: the top is diluted plasma (may be used for antibody studies), a white layer of mononuclear cells, clear F-H, and at the bottom is a red blood cells layer (which also contains neutrophils). Remove only the mononuclear cell layer with a 1.0-mL pipet. Place cells in a new sterile 15-mL conical polystyrene tube, fill with RMPI medium and mix to wash out F-H residue (wash #1). Then centrifuge at full speed for 5 minutes and repeat the wash two more times. Resuspend the mononuclear button into 0.5 to 0.6 mL tissue culture media for inoculation purposes.

## Bronchoalveolar Lavage

Respiratory viruses are often found associated with epithelial cells of the respiratory tract. The lavage fluids may contain viruses in the liquid component as well. Depending on the volume available, 10 to 50 mL may be submitted for diagnostic virology purposes. Most often only 1 to 5 mL will be submitted. The laboratory may decide to routinely pretreat these specimens with antibiotics to decrease contamination problems in the cell cultures. If the request from the physician is for viral isolation only, appropriate amounts of the specimen can be removed and inoculated into the appropriate cell cultures. If the request is for, or includes, fluorescent antibody tests for direct antigen detection, the specimen is usually mixed with phosphate-buffered saline and centrifuged (1,500–2,000 rpm, 5 minutes) to sediment exfoliated cells. These cells can then be transferred to microscope slides for fixation and appropriate staining.

## CSF and Other Body Fluids (Sterile)

Cerebrospinal fluids are ready for inoculation directly. No antibiotic treatment is necessary. Tissue culture media may be added as needed if less than 0.8 mL of specimen is submitted.

## Sputum Specimen

Add tissue culture media so that at least a 50-50 mixture of specimen and tissue culture media is made.

When there is a large amount of specimen, it may be necessary to place some of it in a 17 × 100 mm polystyrene tube to prepare this mixture. Vortex and use this mixture to inoculate the tissue.

## Rectal Swabs

Remove swab as indicated above in the directions for nasopharyngeal or throat swabs. Treat as a stool specimen and follow the protocol as indicated below.

## Stool Specimens

Place 1 g stool in a sterile 15-mL conical polystyrene tube and add 10 mL tissue culture media. Vortex vigorously until the specimen is broken up into a homogenous mixture. Then centrifuge for 10 minutes at 2,500 rpm. Remove 1 mL of the supernatant and place it into one 12 × 75 mm polystyrene tube. Add 0.1 mL penicillin/gentamicin antibiotic solution to the tube containing 1 mL supernatant. Vortex and allow this to stand at room temperature for 30 to 60 minutes. Inoculate the tissue cultures with the treated supernatants. Supernatants from stool specimens may contain substances toxic to cell cultures. If toxicity occurs, dilute the final supernatant 1:10 with cell culture fluid and inoculate new cells.

## Urine Specimens

Place 10 mL urine in a 17 × 100 mm polystyrene tube with a cap. When less than 10 mL is submitted, use all of the specimen. Centrifuge for 10 minutes at 2,500 rpm. When there is very little sediment, remove all but 1 mL of the supernatant and place it in another 17 × 100 mL tube. Use 1 mL of sediment/supernatant mixture to be treated with an antibiotic mixture.

When a great amount of sediment is present, the sediment may prove toxic to the tissue culture. In this case, it is necessary to remove 1 mL of supernatant from just above the sediment and place it in a 12 × 75 mm polystyrene tube for antibiotic treatment.

For the material from either method described above, add 0.1 mL penicillin/gentamicin antibiotic solution. Vortex and allow this to stand at room temperature for 30 to 60 minutes. Inoculate the tissue cultures with this treated portion of the specimen.

## Vesicle Fluid

This fluid is ready for inoculation. No treatment is necessary. Tissue culture media may be added as needed if less than 0.8 mL of specimen is submitted.

# SUMMARY

- ▶ Viruses causing human diseases continue to be a major cause of morbidity and mortality.
- ▶ Many of these viruses may be isolated from clinical specimens and identified by the laboratory.
- ▶ Specimens need to be properly collected, transported, stored, and processed to maintain viral viability.
- ▶ Some diseases require only one or two specimens for viral isolation; others may require several specimens to ensure successful isolation of the etiologic agent.

- ▶ Many of the viruses causing human diseases can be isolated from a properly collected and handled specimen in a timely manner, allowing patient management decisions to be made with this available information.
- ▶ The variety of specimens for viral diagnosis is similar to those collected for bacteriologic studies and the technologist needs to be aware of unique problems, such as cell culture toxicity, that would not be encountered in bacteriology techniques.

## CASE STUDY

In a medical center performing organ transplants, patients will often have cytomegalovirus (CMV) reactivation due to immune suppression. If such reactivation occurs, this is important for the managing physician to know because antiviral chemotherapy (ganciclovir) can be given. However, early symptoms of CMV reactivation may be similar to early symptoms of graft rejection, prompting an entirely different patient management regimen to be performed. The patient has recently undergone a liver transplantation and appears to be reacting well to the procedure. One morning, however, he develops an elevated temperature and complains of "not feeling very well." The physician, considering the possibility of CMV infection, orders appropriate specimens to be collected from the patient and sent to the medical center's clinical laboratory for viral studies, including CMV detection. The samples were collected and placed on a bedside deck to be transported to the clinical laboratory. Due to a series of events, the specimens were forgotten for more than 2 days when they were discovered by the nursing staff.

### Questions:

1. What specimens are considered appropriate for CMV diagnosis?
2. Are these specimens still useful as diagnostic material?
3. Under what circumstances would the improperly stored specimens be suitable for valid laboratory diagnostic testing?

## Review Questions

1. Cytomegalovirus (CMV) is often isolated from whole blood specimens. The part of the specimen that is inoculated onto the human fibroblast cell cultures is:
   a. plasma or serum.
   b. mononuclear cells.
   c. red blood cells.
   d. polymorphonuclear cells.
   e. unseparated whole blood.

2. Swabs may be used to collect viral isolation samples from all body locations listed below EXCEPT:
   a. throat area.
   b. rectal area.
   c. Vesicular lesion.
   d. Spinal fluid.

3. If viral isolation specimens cannot be delivered to a laboratory in a timely manner for processing, what storage condition listed below will be best to maintain viral viability?
   a. Room temperature
   b. 4°C
   c. −20°C
   d. −70°C

4. Antibiotic pretreatment is usually necessary with some specimens before they can be inoculated into cell cultures. Which specimen listed below MUST be so treated before inoculation?
   a. Cerebrospinal fluid
   b. Vesicular fluid
   c. Biopsy tissue
   d. Stool

5. If specimens must be stored in the laboratory before inoculation into cell cultures, what is the maximum length of time they may be kept at 4°C and still be useful diagnostic materials?
   a. 1 day
   b. 2 days
   c. 4 days
   d. 7 days

6. The best temperature used for long-term storage of viruses is:
   a. room temperature.
   b. 4°C
   c. −20°C.
   d. −168°C.

7. Toxicity to cell cultures will most likely come from which specimen type listed below?
   a. Vesicle fluid
   b. Urine specimens
   c. Stool specimens
   d. Sputum specimens

8. Exfoliated cells may be directly examined for viral antigen. Epithelial cells from the respiratory tract are most efficiently collected by which method listed below?
   a. Throat swab
   b. Saline gargle
   c. Biopsy collection
   d. Bronchial lavage

9. Which of the following specimens is not appropriate for general virus isolation?
   a. Urine
   b. Cellular scraping from a lesion
   c. Genital swab
   d. Bone marrow

10. Why are swabs with calcium alginate tips not appropriate for the collection of spiral specimens?
    a. They contain oils that may inhibit viral growth.
    b. Calcium alginate is toxic to herpes simplex viruses.
    c. Calcium alginate encourages the growth of bacterial normal flora.
    d. Both a and b are true.

## ▶ REFERENCES & RECOMMENDED READING

Brooks, G. F., Butel, J. S., & Ornston, L. N. (Eds.). (1995). *Medical microbiology* (20th ed.). East Norwalk, CT: Appleton & Lange.

Fields, B. N., Knipe, D. M., & Howley, P. M. (Eds.). (1996). *Fields virology* (3rd ed., vols. 1 & 2). Philadelphia: Lippincott-Raven.

Goldstein, R. A., Rohatgi, E. H., Bergosfsky, & Block, E. R. (1990). Clinical role of bronchoalveolar lavage in adults with pulmonary disease. *Annual Review of Respiratory Disease, 142,* 481–486.

Hsuing, G. D. (1982). *Diagnostic virology, illustrated by light and electron microscopy* (3rd ed.). New Haven, CT: Yale University Press.

Leland, D. S. (1996). *Clinical virology.* Philadelphia: Saunders.

Lennette, E. H. (Ed.). (1985). *Laboratory diagnosis of viral infections.* New York: Marcel Dekker.

Murray, P. R., Baron, E. J., Pfaller, M. A., et al. (Eds.). (1995). *Manual of medical microbiology* (6th ed.). Washington, DC: ASM Press.

Specter, S., & Lancz, G. (Eds.). (1992). *Clinical virology manual* (2nd ed.). New York: Elsevier.

# CHAPTER 50
# Clinically Significant Viruses and Their Identification

James D. Kettering, PhD

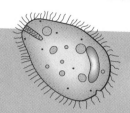

## Microbes in the News
### Kaposi's Sarcoma Virus

Kaposi's sarcoma (KS) is the most common neoplasm that appears in patients with acquired immunodeficiency syndrome (AIDS). Its cause is generally unknown, although a possible viral etiology has been proposed by several research groups. In 1996, workers at the University of California San Francisco School of Medicine identified a suspect virus as the etiologic agent. It is a herpesvirus, showing some similarity to the Epstein-Barr herpesvirus and has been named human herpesvirus 8 (HHV-8). It was found that KS lesions regularly harbor the DNA of this virus. An alternative designation is KS-associated herpesvirus (KSHV). It has been shown that infection precedes tumor development and targets the spindle cells of the tumor, most of which are latently infected. KS tumors also harbor a small subpopulation of productively infected cells. Although little is known concerning the routes of spread of HHV-8, its epidemiology strongly suggests sexual transmission. Mounting evidence supports the view that HHV-8 is the sexually transmitted cofactor predicted by the epidemiology of KS. Latent infection by HHV-8 also occurs in B lymphocytes and is associated with several uncommon lymphoproliferative syndromes in patients with AIDS. HHV-8 infection alone appears to be insufficient for KS tumorigenesis, and an important cofactor role for human immunodeficiency virus (HIV) in this disease still seems likely. (*New England Journal of Medicine* 335, 233–241, 1996; *Lancet* 349, 1133–1138, 1996).

## LEARNING OBJECTIVES

**Upon successful completion of this chapter, the student should be able to:**

1. List the most common viruses causing human illnesses and capable of being isolated in the laboratory.
2. Describe the general characteristics of the seven herpesviruses.
3. Identify the infections caused by herpesviruses and responses available to control these.
4. Describe the properties of and infections caused by enteroviruses.
5. Describe the properties and infections of several viruses that cause respiratory illnesses.
6. Describe the properties and infections of several paramyxoviruses.
7. List the viruses capable of causing hepatitis.
8. Discuss the differences and similarities of the hepatitis viruses and explain the role of the viral diagnostic laboratory in determining which one may be causing disease.
9. Describe the properties of retroviruses, in general, and specific properties of HIV.
10. Define the diagnostic tests available to determine HIV infection.
11. Describe the diagnostic tests available for rabies virus and rotavirus infections.

## INTRODUCTION

Diagnostic virology requires communication between the physician and the laboratory and depends on the quality of specimens and information supplied to the laboratory. Knowledge of the relation of the stage of illness to the presence of virus in the test materials and to the appearance of specific antibody is very important. The laboratory must perform the appropriate tests and return that information to the physician so that it can be used in patient management decisions. It is important to know, for example, that viruses are most likely to be detectable in samples collected during the onset and acute phases of disease and that a specific antibody will be detectable only in the acute, recovery, and convalescence stages of infection. All of this becomes even more significant when one considers that several viral diseases may now be treated with antiviral chemotherapy. The identification of a suspected viral disease needs the combination of physician evaluation and prompt laboratory function and data reporting for the patient to receive the greatest benefit of treatment or management.

### Limitations

Up to the present time, the most effective method of controlling viral infections in the population has been through the use of vaccines. Virus isolation will be required when new epidemics occur (influenza), when serologic tests are not useful (single serum sample collected), and when the same clinical illness may be caused by many different agents (meningitis, respiratory disease). The clinician and technologist need to realize that successful virus isolation may occur from only 10% to 20% of the specimens submitted for examination in many laboratories. A single serum sample will only be able to detect presence or absence of antibody, allowing little or no interpretation of the stage of a disease if some specific antibody is detected. Although timing of test performance and reporting of results from the laboratory have improved dramatically from even a few years ago, 2 or 3 weeks may still be required to determine that a virus is absent from a submitted specimen. Treatment with antivirals before specimen collection may interfere with viral recovery. Although many improvements and advancements have been made in the laboratory in recent years, these limitations must still be acknowledged and serve as a basis for continued improvement and developments in laboratory tests and procedures.

## VIRUSES COMMONLY ISOLATED IN A CLINICAL LABORATORY

### The Herpesviruses—General

The **Herpesviridae** family consists of a large group of DNA-containing viruses that are found worldwide. The name comes from the Greek word, herpin ("to creep"). They are thought to be the most common viruses associated with humans because of their abundance and their tendency to remain latent in the body for life following initial entrance. They often form focal cytopathogenicity, producing vesicles or pocks. The major herpesviruses (see Table 50-1) that infect humans are:

| Common Name | Official Name |
|---|---|
| Herpes simplex virus type 1 (HSV-1) | Human herpesvirus 1 |
| Herpes simplex virus type 2 (HSV-2) | Human herpesvirus 2 |
| Varicella-zoster virus (VZV) | Human herpesvirus 3 |
| Epstein-Barr virus (EBV) | Human herpesvirus 4 |
| Cytomegalovirus (CMV) | Human herpesvirus 5 |
| Human herpesvirus 6 (HHV-6) | Human herpesvirus 6 |
| Human herpesvirus 7 (HHV-7) | Human herpesvirus 7 |
| Human herpesvirus 8 (HHV-8) | Human herpesvirus 8 |

The properties of herpesviruses include large size (120–200 nm), a nucleocapsid with icosahedral symmetry surrounded by a **tegument** (several proteins) and a lipid envelope derived from the host cell's nuclear membrane. The complex, double-stranded DNA is linear and codes for at least 100 proteins, including a **DNA polymerase** and **thymidine kinase**. These enzymes are often the targets in antiherpes chemotherapy.

## Herpes Simplex Viruses— Types 1 and 2

**Properties.** Properties of the HSV are shown in Table 50-2.

### Clinical Findings.

PRIMARY INFECTION. Most primary infections are asymptomatic or mild. Systemic disease is rare and is usually seen in immunosuppressed individuals.

Virus → Mucosal surfaces → Virus replicates at site of
infection causing:
broken skin  "Ballooning" cells
(epithelial cells)  Intranuclear inclusion
bodies
Multinucleated giant
cells
Edema, vesicles filled
with virus
Hemorrhagic necrosis
possible
Usually heals with no
scarring
Latency ← Virus invades local nerve endings an
may be  spreads to ganglia
established

### LATENT INFECTION AND REACTIVATION.
Site of latency:  HSV-1  Trigeminal ganglia
HSV-2  Sacral (dorsal root) ganglia

During latency, little or no virus replication occurs, no symptoms are present, and this persists for lifetime.

Reactivation may occur spontaneously in presence of HSV-specific humoral and cell-mediated immunity,

## Table 50–1 ▶ Herpesvirus Classification—Biologic Properties

| Subfamily | Biologic Properties | | | |
|---|---|---|---|---|
| | GROWTH CYCLE | CYTOPATHOLOGY | LATENT INFECTIONS | EXAMPLE |
| α-Herpesvirinae | Short | Cytolytic | Yes (neurons) | HSV-1 HSV-2 V-ZV |
| ß-Herpesvirinae | Long | Cytomegalic | Yes (glands, kidneys) | CMV |
| γ-Herpesvirinae | Variable | Lymphoproliferative | Yes (lymphatic tissues) | EBV HHV-6 HHV-7 |

## Table 50-2 ► Properties of Herpes Simplex Viruses

| | Types | |
|---|---|---|
| | HSV-1 | HSV-2 |
| Antigenic cross-reactivity | The two types strongly cross-react; glycoprotein G is type-specific (gG-1 and gG-2) | |
| Growth | Both grow in many experimental animals, embryonated eggs, and cell cultures (especially human kidney, rabbit kidney, and human amnion) | |
| Age of primary infection | Young children | Young adults |
| Major site of infection | Oral cavity | Genital area |
| Transmission | Direct contact (saliva) respiratory droplets | Sexual mother-to-offspring |

resulting in asymptomatic viral shedding or mild recurrence of symptoms (usually in the same area as the original infection).

Stimuli that may induce reaction include injury, fever, exposure to ultraviolet radiation, and physical or emotional stress.

**INFECTIONS ASSOCIATED PRIMARILY WITH HSV-1.** Most infections are subclinical. In young children, gingivostomatitis is seen most often, compared with pharyngitis (pharyngotonsillitis) in adults. More complicated manifestations include keratoconjunctivitis, which may result in blindness, and encephalitis, which may have a high (70–80%) mortality rate if untreated.

**SKIN INFECTIONS ASSOCIATED WITH EITHER HSV-1 OR HSV-2.** Herpetic whitlow (lesions on fingers) and eczema herpeticum are most commonly seen.

**INFECTIONS ASSOCIATED PRIMARILY WITH HSV-2.** Genital herpes infections are often very painful and highly contagious. There may be fever, dysuria, and lymphadenopathy. Untreated lesions heal in about 10 days, and complications may include extragenital lesions and meningitis.

Neonatal herpes infections are almost always symptomatic and often severe. Manifestations may be found on the skin, in eye and mouth lesions, as encephalitis, or as a disseminated disease that can include central nervous system (CNS) involvement. There is a high fatality rate of untreated infections, with survivors often having permanent neurologic impairment. The virus is transmitted during the birthing process, not transplacentally. If the mother is actively shedding HSV, with or without evident lesions at this time, cesarean delivery of the infant is recommended.

**Immunity.** Maternal antibody is somewhat protective during the first 6 months of age. The highest susceptibility to transmission of the virus is from 6 months to 2 years of age. Cell-mediated immunity, natural killer cells, and interferon production all appear to be significant in determining whether an initial infection may be subclinical or not.

## Laboratory Diagnosis.

**ISOLATION AND IDENTIFICATION.** Specimens are varied and include material from the skin (lesions), cornea, or brain. Both HSV-1 and HSV-2 infect a wide variety of **cell cultures** and animals. Primary cell cultures (rabbit kidney {RK}), human embryonic kidney (HEK), and guinea pig embryo (GPE) are all very sensitive. Human diploid fibroblasts (HDF) are probably the most widely used cell cultures for HSV isolation, although some continuous cell lines (mink lung, RD, and A549) appear to be more sensitive. HDF cells are readily available from a variety of commercial sources.

The most common sources for virus isolation are vesicular fluids, throat swabs, and genital lesions swabs. HSV produces a rapid destruction of cells with a characteristic CPE (rounding, enlarged cells leading to lysis) within 24 to 72 hours. Multinucleated giant cells may be produced by HSV-2.

Identification and typing is usually done with monoclonal antibodies labeled with fluorescein isothiocyanate or immunoperoxidase labels (see Figure 50-1).

**SEROLOGY.** Antibody levels peak within 2 to 4 weeks and appear to persist for life. Serum antibodies appear to have no effect on recurrent episodes. IgG and IgM

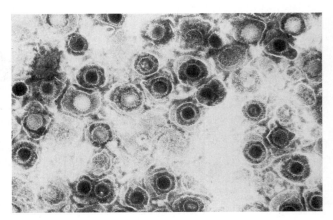

**FIGURE 50-1** Herpes simplex virus. (Courtesy of Centers for Disease Control and Prevention, Atlanta, GA)

antibodies are usually detected by commercial immuno-fluorescence kits. The diagnostic value may be limited because of the widespread infection of HSV in the population.

**Treatment.** **Acyclovir** (acycloguanosine) is the treatment of choice. Vidarabine, idoxuridine, and trifloridine may also be used. Virally coded DNA polymerase and thymidine kinase enzymes are targeted.

## Cytomegalovirus (Salivary Gland Virus)

**Properties.** Cytomegalovirus (CMV) demonstrates typical herpesvirus characteristics in electron micrographs. There appear to be many different strains with a high degree of antigenic cross-reactivity. Monoclonal antibodies are usually targeted to a common antigenic moiety, and no strains of CMV are identified in routine viral diagnosis of this virus.

**Clinical Findings.** In normal hosts, most infections are subclinical. A CMV mononucleosis (infectious mononucleosis-like syndrome) may be experienced. Such individuals will have a mild disease with malaise, myalgia, fever, and liver dysfunction; hematosplenomegaly may occur in young children. Atypical lymphocytes and no heterophile antibody are found. This disease may appear spontaneously or after blood transfusion (postperfusion syndrome).

In immunocompromised hosts, a severe CMV mononucleosis is possible. This may be due to a primary infection or reactivation from a latent state. CMV pneumonia is a frequent complication. Individuals considered to be at an especially high risk include AIDS patients and bone marrow and kidney transplant recipients.

Cytomegalovirus inclusion disease in congenital and perinatal infections is a generalized infection, involving many organs. CMV may be present in severe CNS involvement and is a leading cause of mental retardation in the United States. Other CNS problems include hearing loss, ocular abnormalities and others. In several studies, the mortality rate approached 30%.

**Immunity.** Cytomegalovirus is an excellent antigen and provokes a good antibody response. Maternal antibody does not prevent CMV transmission to an infant, however. Currently, a live attenuated vaccine for immunocompromised children at high risk is being developed.

**Laboratory Diagnosis.**

**ISOLATION AND IDENTIFICATION.** Human diploid fibroblast cells are the primary host for the isolation of CMV. Cell passage must be monitored to ensure continued sensitivity. Virus can be isolated from a variety of body secretions including urine, milk, semen, vaginal or cervical secretions, saliva, tears, stools, and leukocytes. Bronchoalveolar lavage specimens are especially successful for isolating CMV from pulmonary infections or to detect viral antigen directly in exfoliated cells.

Depending on viral load, CPEs may appear in a few days to a few weeks. Usually "no virus isolated" reports are made in 3 to 4 weeks if no viral isolate has appeared.

The shell vial technique for virus isolation was a major improvement in CMV cultures. HDF cells on round cover slips in shell vials are inoculated with viral specimen preparations and centrifuged at low speed (30–60 minutes at 700$g$). The procedure apparently enhances viral attachment to receptors and facilitates viral entry into the host cells. Using monoclonal antibodies to CMV immediate early antigens and labeled with fluorescein isothiocyanate or peroxidase labels allows specific identification of CMV in as few as 24 hours postinoculation. This technique has certainly speeded up the reporting time to physicians and can assist in decisions concerning use of the antiviral, **ganciclovir**. Most laboratories continue to inoculate tubes containing HDF cells (traditional method) because shell vial culture will not detect 100% of all viruses in clinical specimens.

**SEROLOGY.** Serologic determination of CMV antibodies would be similar to that described above for HSV.

**Treatment.** There is a passive immune reagent available for CMV infection. This contains antibodies against CMV. Ganciclovir (a form of acycloguanosine) is the primary anti-CMV chemotherapy currently available. Foscarnet may also be used, either alone or in combination.

## Adenoviruses

**Properties.** Adenoviruses are medium-sized viruses containing linear, double-stranded DNA and no lipid envelope. They have an icosahedral capsid, with fiber-viral receptors that are toxic for host cells. There are currently 41 antigenic types of human adenoviruses recognized. These agents are stable to freezing and thawing (see Figure 50-2).

**Clinical Findings.** The usual mode of transmission is by inhalation, and an average incubation period for

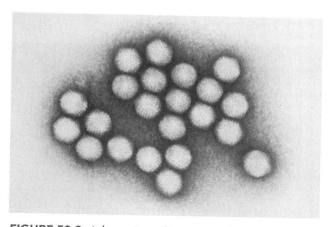

**FIGURE 50-2** Adenovirus. (Courtesy of Centers for Disease Control and Prevention, Atlanta, GA)

adenovirus infection is 5 to 7 days. Human illness is varied. Respiratory infections often present with fever, pharyngitis, cough, and undifferentiated respiratory disease through primary atypical pneumonia. Some strains may cause conjunctivitis along with the upper respiratory infection, and some types may cause an epidemic keratoconjunctivitis. Table 50-3 identifies illnesses associated with certain adenovirus strains or groups.

Adenoviruses causing gastroenteritis often cannot be isolated in the clinical laboratory.

**Immunity.** Adenoviruses are excellent antigens and cause the host to produce high levels of antibodies. Immunity to reinfection is fair, but specific for type. Because no vaccines exist for adenoviruses, any antibodies detected would be from viral infection.

**Laboratory Diagnosis.**

ISOLATION AND IDENTIFICATION. Adenoviruses can be isolated from nasal, throat, conjunctival, and rectal swabs inoculated into human cell cultures. Typical CPE is produced in continuous cells lines (HEp-2 and A549) as well as in HEK and HDF cells. HDF cells are generally less sensitive than the others and have altered CPE, but they are the cells most often available in many viral diagnostic laboratories. Nonhuman cells (rhesus monkey kidney [RhMK]) are of variable sensitivity and virus growth is slower.

Characteristic CPE consists of grapelike clusters of rounded cells with thick edges. CPE may arise in 2 to 7 days or several weeks. Adenoviruses remain cell associated, similar to VZV and CMV.

Identification of isolates is done by immunofluorescence using antibody preparations against the hexon capsomeres (general antigen for adenoviruses). Subgroups based on hemagglutination with rat and rhesus erythrocytes may be done, but usually not in typical viral diagnostic laboratories.

SEROLOGY. Diagnostic serology by complement fixation uses a group-specific antigen shared by all adenoviruses. Paired sera (acute and convalescent samples) are best for diagnostic purposes.

**Treatment.** No antiviral chemotherapy exists for adenovirus infections. Live, attenuated vaccines for respiratory infections are being developed. Chlorination of swimming pools is effective for controlling conjunctivitis strains.

## Enteroviruses—Picornaviruses

**General Properties.** The current classification of human picornaviruses includes the following groups:

▶ Enteroviruses—infect and multiply in the gastrointestinal tract
1. Polioviruses
2. Coxsackieviruses, group A
3. Coxsackieviruses, group B
4. Echoviruses
5. Enteroviruses—68–72
   (enterovirus 72 = hepatitis A virus)
▶ Cardioviruses
▶ Rhinoviruses (respiratory)

Picornaviruses are small (20–30 nm), nonenveloped viruses that contain positive-sense, single-stranded RNA genomes. These agents replicate in the cytoplasm of the host cell and survive fairly well outside the human host. Enteroviruses are stable at pH 3 to 5, whereas rhinoviruses are not. Enteroviruses grow best at 37°C; rhinoviruses grow best at 33°C.

**Polioviruses and Other Enteroviruses.**

PROPERTIES. Polioviruses have a limited host range, infecting humans only. Primates have been infected in the laboratory, and human and monkey kidney cell cultures will support the growth of these agents. Purified RNA genomes (positive sense—can function directly as messenger RNA) can enter and replicate in normally nonpermissive cell lines.

The three antigenic types are designated as 1, 2, and 3. There is little cross-reaction for antibody protection. Although polioviruses are hardy survivors in water sources, they can be destroyed by pasteurization.

### Table 50–3 ▶ Illnesses Associated with Human Adenoviruses

| Group | Disease | Oncogenic Potential |
|-------|---------|---------------------|
| B | Pharyngoconjunctival fever<br>Acute respiratory disease<br>Pneumonia<br>Hemorrhagic cystitis<br>Pneumonia with dissemination | Yes |
| C | Acute febrile pharyngitis in small children, latent infection in lymphatic tissue | Yes |
| D | Epidemic keratoconjunctivitis, cervicitis, urethritis | Yes |
| E | Acute respiratory disease with fever, pneumonia | Yes |
| F, G | Gastroenteritis | Yes |

**Clinical Findings.** Any of the three antigenic types may give rise to any or all of the following:

- ► Inapparent infection
- ► Mild febrile illness
- ► Viral (aseptic) meningitis
- ► CNS paralysis
- ► Progressive postpoliomyelitis muscle atrophy

In all cases, viruses are present and cause antibodies to develop. These will prevent reinfection if contact is made with specific types. Viruses are ingested, grow in the intestinal tract, undergo **viremia**, and may spread to the CNS. Polioviruses are lytic agents, destroying their host cells. This destruction of CNS tissue is responsible for paralysis. Fatalities in the 1950s ranged from 3% to 30%. Two excellent vaccines exist. The multivalent, formalin-killed (Salk) vaccine is recommended for immunodeficient or immunosuppressed individuals. The live, attenuated (Sabin) vaccine is very effective and may eventually be used to eliminate polio from the human population.

Coxsackievirus and echovirus distribution is similar to that of polioviruses. All produce inapparent infections and mild febrile illnesses. Some produce colds and other respiratory illness, viral meningitis, and other systemic infections. Coxsackie B viruses, for example, are important etiologic agents for neonatal disease (acute fatal encephalomyocarditis), pleurodyma, and acute myocardiopathy in adults. It is suggested that coxsackie B4 may even be a cause of diabetes. A rash manifestation is not uncommonly seen in echovirus infections. Even with the CNS involvements, fatalities are generally uncommon.

### Laboratory Diagnosis.

**ISOLATION AND IDENTIFICATION.** In general, enteroviruses will grow on either the HDF or primary monkey kidney (PMK) cells that most laboratories routinely use. Both need to be closely monitored to detect initial CPE because growth may be rapid and the cell monolayer can be destroyed within 24 hours by a rapidly growing isolate.

Poliovirus and coxsackie B viruses grow well in PMK and some established human cell lines (HEp-2). Echoviruses will also do well in PMK, whereas the ideal host for coxsackie A viruses is the newborn mouse. Some coxsackie A strains will grow in HDF, HEK, PMK, RD, or GPE cells.

Enteroviruses can be recovered from feces, throat or rectal swabs, cerebrospinal fluid (CSF), blood, conjunctival swabs, and urine. The typical CPE includes cell rounding that becomes refractile and shrinks in size. The monolayer degenerates and detaches from the vessel surface. Enteroviruses lyse the host cells, and the free viruses in the cell culture supernatant may be easily passed. Initial identification as an enterovirus is done by recognition of the characteristic CPE. A neutralization test in cell culture using antiserum pools is the standard method of specific identification. Unfortunately, it is expensive and time consuming. Frequently, an identification of enterovirus is sufficient for the physician because no specific antiviral chemotherapy exists. Recently, pools of specific monoclonal antibodies labeled with fluorescein isothiocyanate have become available for identification purposes.

**SEROLOGY.** Historically, serology has been done using pools of selected enterovirus antigens by complement fixation for use in diagnosing etiologic agents for meningitis/encephalitis.

**Treatment.** No antiviral chemotherapy agents for enterovirus infections are approved for use at this time. Only the poliovirus has vaccines available for disease prevention.

## Respiratory Viruses

It has been estimated that over 400 million illnesses occur in the United States in 1 year and that approximately 60% of these are respiratory diseases. Most of these respiratory diseases are caused by viruses; some are serious illnesses, others are less so. A syndrome known as the common cold is caused by a number of different viruses in different groups. Although most colds in adults are caused by the 113-plus rhinoviruses and the coronaviruses, other viruses producing similar symptoms are found among the coxsackieviruses, CMV, adenoviruses, respiratory syncytial virus (RSV, especially in children), parainfluenza viruses, and influenza viruses. All of these viruses are endemic with the exception of influenza (epidemic) and parainfluenza, which may be epidemic at times.

**Influenza.** In 1918–1919, one of the worst plagues in the history of man swept the world, killing approximately 20 million people and afflicting a huge portion of the world's population. This was due to the orthomyxovirus, influenza.

There were other influenza pandemics prior to 1918–1919. In the 1889–1890 pandemic, prior to the discovery of viruses, Pfeiffer thought the disease was caused by a bacterium, which was therefore named *Haemophilus influenzae,* a secondary invader. It was not until 1933 that Andrews and his coworkers in England, and Francis and his coworkers at Ann Arbor, Michigan, showed influenza to be caused by a virus. It still occurs in epidemics, which vary in severity. A characteristic of the virus, which creates problems in the development of preventive vaccine, is the fact that the virus changes its antigenic characteristics from one epidemic to the next.

**PROPERTIES.** Influenza is an orthomyxovirus, indicating an affinity for mucous membranes. It contains eight single-stranded, segmented RNA molecules as a genome. The RNA is negative sense. There are three main types (A, B, and C), based on the ribonucleoprotein of the nucleocapsid.

New epidemics of influenza A, and sometimes B, arise because of **genetic reassortment**. Segmented genomes from related viruses may result in mixtures of parental viral genomes in progeny virons resulting from host cells infected with two or more related viruses. The two main molecules responsible for new epidemics include the **hemagglutinin** (HA) and the neuraminidase (NA) enzymes. HAs have an attachment function and NAs assist in the release of virions from a host cell. These enzymes are found in the lipid envelope surrounding the helical viruses. **Antigenic drift** refers to minor antigenic changes (point mutations) in the HA/NA enzymes, and **antigenic shift** is a sudden, major antigenic change brought about by genetic reassortment in the viral growth cycle.

Influenza viruses are fairly stable and do survive for at least a limited time in nature, outside the human host. They are typical RNA viruses, with many steps of the life cycle occurring in the host cell cytoplasm. However, the viral messenger RNA molecules require and obtain cellular capped and methylated termini from the host cell nucleus.

**CLINICAL FINDINGS.** Influenza viruses are spread person to person by airborne droplets or direct contact. Respiratory epithelial cells are infected and eventually killed. The incubation time is very short, averaging only 1 to 2 days. Secretory IgA and the cough reflex are important in the body's mechanism to control spread of the agents. Interferons are produced within a day, and a typical antibody response requires 1 to 2 weeks. Cellular repair may take up to 4 weeks to occur.

Uncomplicated influenza routinely produces chills, headache, dry cough, high fever, muscle aches, malaise, and anorexia. The fever typically lasts 3 to 7 days, but 1 to 3 weeks may be needed for the symptoms to subside. Human infections are most often caused by influenza A strains, with influenza B often involving pediatric patients.

Each influenza epidemic produces an increase in expected deaths in the involved population. The causes are viral, secondary bacterial, or combination infections in the elderly, debilitated, very young, and pregnant individuals. These opportunistic infections occur because the influenza virus infection often results in loss of ciliary function and phagocytic cell dysfunction and because the alveolar exudate supports bacterial growth extremely well. Natural infection is terminated by neutralizing antibodies against the HA and NA. Both IgG and IgA are involved, and these require 1 to 2 weeks to develop. Both natural recovery and vaccination with the killed vaccine provide relatively short (1 year) protection to reinfection.

Reye's syndrome occurs in children during influenza epidemics. It is an acute encephalopathy of children (usually aged 2–15 years old) and fatty degeneration of the liver frequently occurs. The mortality may be high (10–40%) and the cause is unknown. There may be an association of salicylate usage, and, to be safe, compounds containing these compounds should not be used to control fever in children. Such problems may arise during chickenpox (VZV) outbreaks, as well.

**LABORATORY DIAGNOSIS.**

*Isolation and Identification.* The laboratory plays a very essential role at the beginning of a new influenza season or epidemic. The viruses from early cases need to be isolated and the types of HA/NA identified. If new forms are present, the vaccines need to be modified to include them. Once this determination is made and the season or epidemic announced, the clinical presentation is usually sufficient for patient management.

Primary monkey kidney cells are most widely used cell culture for isolation of the influenza virus. Madin-Darby canine kidney (MDCK) cells may be used, but a trypsin treatment may be needed. Both influenza A and B may be isolated in embryonated chicken eggs. Throat swabs, nasal swabs, and nasal washings are good sources for virus and should be collected early in illness. Incubation in a roller drum at 33°C is considered optimal for isolation, but many laboratories are able to isolate these agents using regular tube and shell vial cultures.

Cytopathic effects may appear, but most often virus growth will occur before it is apparent. The virus may be detected by hemadsorption. Many laboratories will routinely stain an inoculated shell vial PMK culture with a pool of antirespiratory monoclonal antibodies labeled with fluorescein isothiocyanate. If a positive test occurs, cell spots may be made from a test tube culture and stained with the specific reagents for identification. One pool currently available contains reagents that will identify influenza A and B, parainfluenza 1, 2, and 3, adenovirus and RSV (see Figure 50-3).

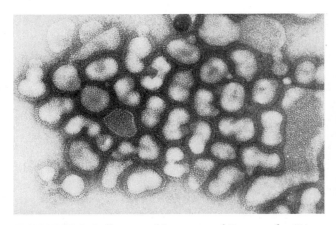

**FIGURE 50-3** Influenza. (Courtesy of Centers for Disease Control and Prevention, Atlanta, GA)

*Serology.* Serologic procedures have been by complement fixation and hemagglutination inhibition. Isolation of the virus is probably most meaningful today.

**TREATMENT. Amantadine** or rimatidine prevents uncoating and replication of influenza A. Optimal use requires that it be given before contact with the virus.

The vaccines in use contain two to three influenza A and one influenza B strains. It is produced by growing viruses in eggs or cell culture and chemically inactivating them for vaccine inclusion. The vaccine should be used in "at-risk" individuals, including health care workers. It must be used yearly for optimal protection. Vaccines prepared in embryonated chicken eggs may be dangerous for individuals with allergies to egg proteins.

### Parainfluenza Viruses.

**PROPERTIES.** Parainfluenza viruses are paramyxoviruses that are helical and surrounded by a lipid envelope. They are larger than influenza viruses and contain a negative-sense RNA genome that is not segmented. All members of the paramyxovirus group are antigenically stable. The envelope contains a glycoprotein spike that possesses both hemagglutinin and neuraminidase (HN) activities. There is also a fusion spike that is absolutely necessary for successful viral entry into a host cell. Parainfluenza viruses usually have minimal effects on host cell metabolism, although multinucleated giant cells (**syncytia**) may form in cell cultures. There are four antigenic types designated by the numbers 1, 2, 3, and 4. Only the first three are important clinically.

**CLINICAL FINDINGS.** Parainfluenza viruses are transmitted in aerosol droplets or by direct contact. Replication of the viruses is limited to the respiratory epithelial cells. Primary infections are most severe and usually occur during the first 5 years of life. Table 50-4 lists the main syndromes seen with parainfluenza infections.

Reinfections are common but usually cause only mild, nonfebrile, upper respiratory infections.

Maternal IgG in infants does not appear to prevent infection or disease. Infection gives rise to secretory IgA antibodies, but these often disappear in a few months. The relative importance of serum antibodies to the HN and fusion proteins are not well understood.

**LABORATORY DIAGNOSIS.**

*Isolation and Identification.* Primary monkey kidney cells are the most sensitive system for the isolation of these viruses. Embryonated chicken eggs are not good host systems. HEK and HDF usually will not support the growth and isolation of the viruses from clinical specimens.

Throat and nasal swabs are good sources for virus. Incubation at 33°C or 36°C in a roller drum is optimal, but many laboratories successfully isolate the virus using tube cultures in racks and shell vials. Viruses may be detected by hemadsorption or use of a pool of antirespiratory virus monoclonal antibodies labeled with fluorescein isothiocyanate. A shell vial cover slip containing PMK cells infected with virus will stain positively with the pooled reagent, and cell spots from an infected tube can be made and stained with specific monoclonal antibodies for identification (see Figure 50-4).

*Serology.* Antibodies may be measured by complement fixation or hemadsorption inhibition.

**TREATMENT. Ribavirin** shows promise of being beneficial when delivered by small-particle aerosol. There are no current live-virus vaccines available.

### Respiratory Syncytial Virus.

**PROPERTIES.** Respiratory syncytial virus is a typical paramyxovirus. It is a medium-sized, helical virus with a lipid envelope. Its genome is a linear RNA molecule of negative polarity. It is surrounded by a lipid envelope.

**CLINICAL FINDINGS.** Respiratory syncytial virus is the most important cause of lower respiratory tract illness in infants and young children. It is the single most important respiratory virus in infants under 1 year of age, causing bronchiolitis and pneumonia. It is responsible for about one-half the cases of bronchiolitis and one-fourth of

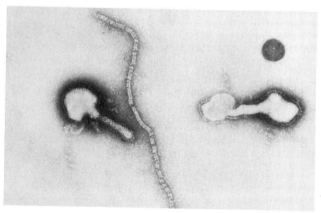

**FIGURE 50-4** Parainfluenza. (Courtesy of Centers for Disease Control and Prevention, Atlanta, GA)

### Table 50-4 ▶ Paramyxovirus Infections in the Respiratory Tract

| Syndrome | Main Symptoms | Infants | Children | Adults |
|---|---|---|---|---|
| Laryngitis/croup | Hoarseness "barking cough" | Yes | Yes | Yes |
| Tracheobronchitis | Cough | Yes | Yes | No |
| Pneumonia | Cough, chest pain | No | Yes | No |

the pneumonia cases in infants in the United States yearly. It causes an estimated 4,000 to 5,000 deaths per year and is present each year in a season or epidemic.

Most RSV infections are symptomatic. Fever, rhinitis, sore throat, and cough are most often seen. It is transmitted by large-droplet aerosol transmission. The virus replicates in the epithelial cells of the nasopharynx and is carried to the lower respiratory tract by secretion. Viremia does not appear to occur. The incubation period is 4 to 5 days, and virus shedding may persist for 1 to 3 weeks. Although the airways of very young infants are narrow and very readily obstructed by inflammation and edema, it is not known why only a small group of young babies develop severe RSV disease.

The immune response may be involved in the pathogenesis of some symptoms seen in RSV infection. Bronchiolitis may especially be caused by an immediate hypersensitivity (type I-IgE involved). Children who received an experimental formalin-killed RSV vaccine developed high titers of serum antibodies, but suffered significantly more severe lower respiratory tract illness when they encountered the wild-type virus that next year. Additional studies are needed to clarify the exact mechanism involved in this episode. RSV does not induce high levels of interferon, and secretory IgA is probably important but does not last long.

Fatal episodes demonstrated an extensive bronchopneumonia, accompanied by the sloughing of the bronchiolar epithelium and monocyte infiltration, accompanied by abundant mucous secretion. The small bronchioles obstruct fairly easily under these conditions. Children who recover may exhibit abnormal pulmonary function for years.

**LABORATORY DIAGNOSIS.** The virus grows well in continuous cell lines of human origin. It will produce a characteristic CPE of multinucleated giant cells (syncytia). Such CPE is variable, however, and viral growth may be missed if cell cultures are several days old when inoculated. Primary MK cells allow growth of the virus and may show CPE. HDF cells support its growth, but seem to be less sensitive than other cells mentioned.

This virus is found in respiratory secretions of the nose and oropharynx. Nasopharyngeal aspirates are more likely to produce viruses than swab samples. Antigen detection tests (enzyme-linked immunosorbent assay [ELISA], immunofluorescence) are rapid and performed directly on clinical specimens. This can allow for rapid diagnosis because it is important to isolate infected infants in the hospital. These can be performed as "stat" tests (especially direct immunofluorescence assays [DFA]). Isolation may require several days for the test to be positive (see Figure 50-5).

*Serology.* Serum antibodies can be measured in a variety of ways. Measurement of serum antibodies are important epidemiologically, but play an insignificant role in immediate patient management.

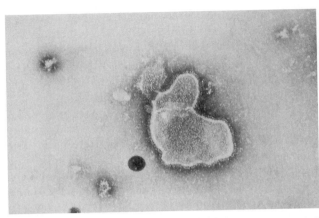

**FIGURE 50-5** Respiratory syncytial virus. (Courtesy of Centers for Disease Control and Prevention, Atlanta, GA)

**TREATMENT.** Treatment of serious RSV disease depends on supportive care (oxygen delivery, removal of secretion) and ribavirin delivered in a continuous small-droplet aerosol for 3 to 6 days. Viral shedding decreases dramatically and little or no systemic toxicity is observed.

Immune globulin with high antibody titers to RSV has been beneficial to individuals at risk, when given as monthly intravenous infusions.

To date, attempts to develop a live, attenuated vaccine have not been successful.

## OCCASIONAL OR DIFFICULT VIRUSES ISOLATED IN THE CLINICAL LABORATORY

In a substantial number of virally caused illnesses each year the etiologic agent may not be easily or routinely isolated and identified. Many times this will not cause a problem in patient management because the clinician will be able to diagnose the illness accurately based on clinical presentation. Often no antiviral chemotherapy exists for many of these agents. Being able to occasionally isolate some of these viruses may be beneficial, however. This section covers viruses that may be fairly common in the population, but do not grow well in the systems routinely used by most viral diagnostic laboratories. The hospital-based laboratory may have a public health laboratory as a reference facility for these more challenging viruses or may need to use large, regionally based commercial reference laboratories to supply the physicians with final answers to their diagnostic problems.

### Measles (Rubeola)

**Properties.** Measles virus is a paramyxovirus. It has a helical nucleocapsid, with a linear single-stranded RNA genome of negative sense. It is surrounded by a lipid envelope with HN and fusion glycoprotein spikes. It may grow, as do other paramyxoviruses, in cells without causing readily apparent CPE. There is only one main antigenic type.

**Clinical Findings.** Measles is an acute, highly infectious disease characterized by a maculopapular rash, fever, and respiratory symptoms. Exposed individuals have about a 99% chance of acquiring the disease. A prominent prodrome precedes the rash phase, and the virus is spread through direct contact with infected droplets from a cough or sneeze or a contaminated fomite. It replicates initially in the respiratory tract and then spreads to the regional lymphoid tissue, where further viral growth occurs. A primary viremia disseminates the virus, which grows in the reticuloendothelial system. A second viremia spreads the virus to the epithelial surfaces of the body, including the skin, respiratory tract, and conjunctiva. Focal lesions are formed and multinucleated giant cells with intranuclear inclusions can be found in the lymphoid tissues throughout the body.

The incubation period may be from 1 to 3 weeks, and the onset of typical measles is usually abrupt. This stage of infection is characterized by coryza, cough, conjunctivitis, fever, and Koplik's spots (small, bluish white lesions on the buccal mucosa) in the mouth. The virus is present in tears, nasal and throat secretions, urine, and blood. The maculopapular rash forms as detectable serum antibody appears and the viremia disappears. The rash appears to be an interaction of immune T cells with virus-infected cells in the small blood vessels and lasts about a week.

A number of very serious complications are known to follow measles infections. Involvement of the CNS is common. Encephalitis occurs in about 1/1,000 cases. The mortality rate is about 15% to 20% and about one-fourth of survivors show sequelae. Subacute sclerosing panencephalitis is a rare late complication, occurring 5 to 15 years following acute measles. It is always fatal.

The most frequent complication of measles involves the lower respiratory tract. Croup, bronchitis, and pneumonias may occur and account for more than 90% of measles-related deaths. Otitis media is a common bacterial complication. Atypical measles (measles without rash) is usually seen in young adults who received an initial killed vaccine that did not have a fusion glycoprotein component as an antigen.

Measles must not be thought of as a common childhood illness with little or no concern. The significant number of possibly life-threatening postinfectious complications make measles one of the most significant agents in the population.

**Laboratory Diagnosis.**

**ISOLATION AND IDENTIFICATION.** Typical measles is reliably diagnosed based on clinical symptoms. Laboratory diagnosis may be necessary in cases of modified or atypical measles. Serologic diagnostic procedures may be preferred because viral isolation methods are slow and inefficient.

Measles virus can be isolated from blood, throat, conjunctivae, and urine. Nasopharyngeal secretion swabs are best for viral collection during the first 4 to 5 days of illness. Urine may have the virus for up to a week. Measles virus grows slowly in PMK, monkey kidney, and human amnion cultures. Typical CPEs include multinucleated giant cells with intranuclear and intracytoplasmic inclusion bodies that form 1 to 2 weeks following inoculation. Specific identity is made using monoclonal antibody labeled with fluorescein isothiocyanate. Measles virus is very sensitive to heat, but stores well at −70°C in a suspension medium containing protein (see Figure 50-6).

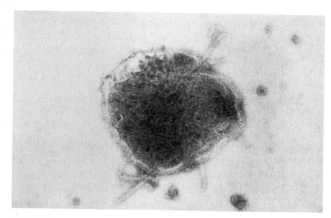

**FIGURE 50-6** Measles. (Courtesy of Centers for Disease Control and Prevention, Atlanta, GA)

**SEROLOGY.** The most practical method of diagnosing measles is to obtain acute and convalescent serum samples and show an increase in measles antibody titer in them. Complement fixation and hemagglutination inhibition tests have been used for this purpose for years. Now, newer methods such as ELISA are available, with greater sensitivity than hemagglutination inhibition. Measles IgM may be difficult to show unless the timing of specimen collection was ideal. IgM antibody peaks 10 days after the rash develops and is undetectable after 30 days.

**Treatment.** No antiviral drugs are available to treat measles or its complications. Bacterial superinfections should be treated with antibiotics. Passive immunity may prevent or modify measles if given early in the incubation period. If given 4 to 6 days postexposure, no benefit is apparent. The best method of disease control is to use the highly effective, safe, live-attenuated vaccine that is available. It is at least 95% effective and provides essentially life-long protection.

# Mumps

**Properties.** Mumps virus is a typical paramyxovirus. It is helical in shape, with a single-stranded negative sense RNA genome. It is surrounded by a lipid envelope with HN and hemolysin spikes. There is a single antigenic type.

**Clinical Findings.** Mumps is an acute contagious disease characterized by nonsupportive enlargement of one or both parotid glands (parotiditis). Man is the only known host and reservoir of the virus. It is endemic worldwide, usually affecting the 6- to 10-year-old age group. More than one-third of cases are asymptomatic.

Transmission is from person to person by large droplets. A primary growth cycle occurs in the upper respiratory tract epithelial cells, and viremia spreads the virus to the salivary glands (parotid glands) and other major organ systems. The incubation period averages 3 weeks, and virus is shed in the saliva for about 2 weeks, centering on the onset of the salivary gland enlargement. Subclinical cases also shed the virus. The parotid gland swelling reaches a maximum in 48 hours and remains so for 7 to 10 days. One or both glands may be involved.

Complications do occur, but these are usually self-limited. The testes and ovaries may be affected, especially after puberty. About 20% of males may develop orochitis, but sterility rarely results. Mumps virus also frequently infects the kidneys. As a result, virus may be detected in urine for up to 14 days following the onset of clinical symptoms. Mumps accounts for 10% to 15% of aseptic meningitis in the United States and occurs in males more often than females. Such involvment in self-limited, although unilateral deafness has been observed and the mortality rate from mumps encephalitis is about 1%.

**Laboratory Diagnosis.**

ISOLATION AND IDENTIFICATION. The diagnosis of mumps infection is fairly simple when typical parotiditis is produced. Laboratory studies are not required in these cases. Enlargement of the parotids due to supporation, drug sensitivity, and tumors and patients with complications of atypical or asymptomatic mumps may require laboratory assistance to make a definitive diagnosis.

A viral isolation from CSF, blood, saliva, or urine confirms the diagnosis of recent infection. Virus can be recovered to within a few days after onset of illness and from the urine for up to 2 weeks. MPK cells are the most sensitive host for isolating the virus. Continuous human cell line (HeLa) and primary human amnion or HEK cells will also support the growth of the virus. The virus produces a characteristic CPE of cell rounding with large syncytia. Some strains do not produce the typical CPE and may be screened for by hemadsorbing with guinea pig erythrocytes. Specific and rapid identification is accomplished by using monoclonal antibodies and immunofluorescent staining.

The virus is stable and retains viability for several days when stored at 4°C. It will remain viable for months at −70°C, especially when buffered with 1% to 2% protein.

SEROLOGY. Serologic diagnosis may be important in cases of meningitis or encephalitis that occur in the absence of parotid swelling. Complement fixation and hemagglutination-inhibition tests have been done of paired sera for best diagnostic results. ELISA is more sensitive and seems to have fewer problems with heterotypical antibodies developed by other paramyxovirus infections. In addition, IgM determinations can be readily done by ELISA.

**Treatment.** No antiviral chemotherapy drugs are currently available for use in mumps infections. Passive immunity appears to have little or no role in preventing mumps disease. An excellent live, attenuated viral vaccine is the best mechanism available for reducing the infection in the population. It is produced in chick embryo cell culture, and individuals allergic to egg protein may not be able to have the vaccine administered. Licensed in 1967, it produces protection in about 95% of recipients.

# Rhinovirus

**Properties.** Rhinoviruses are picornaviruses. They are similar in structure to the enteroviruses (spherical capsid, positive-sense single-stranded RNA genome, no envelope). They are also more acid labile and more heat stable than enteroviruses. A pH of 3 to 5 for 1 hour at 37°C will inactivate rhinoviruses. They grow on human diploid fibroblast cells as well as PMK cells. All strains grow optimally at 33°C. At least 113 or more antigenic types exist that appear to share no common antigen.

**Clinical Findings.** Rhinoviruses are the "common cold" viruses and naturally infect only humans and chimpanzees. The method of transmission is by inhalation of virus-containing secretion droplets. Infections occur year round, with peaks in the early spring and fall months. High titers of virus can be found in nasal secretions, as soon as 1 to 4 days following exposure. Viral titers may fall, with symptoms persisting. The viruses replicate in the cells of the mucous membranes of the nose. Symptoms include rhinorrhea, nasal obstruction, sneezing, sore throat, cough, and headache. Fever does not usually occur. Rhinoviruses do cause otitis media in infants and children and these viruses can be sought in middle ear fluid, if other agents are absent.

Type specific antibodies (IgG and IgA) are produced. These seem to have a short half-life and provide variable protection when challenged by same type viruses.

**Laboratory Diagnosis.**

ISOLATION AND IDENTIFICATION. Rhinoviruses grow in the PMK and HDF cultures that most laboratories use. Such isolation is meaningless in the absence of antiviral chemotherapy agents. Identification of viral etiology might decrease the use of unneeded antibiotics. Virus isolation from nasopharyngeal swabs requires several days, but is very sensitive when samples are collected early in the illness.

**SEROLOGY.** Several test procedures are available on a research basis to measure antibodies to rhinoviruses. None of these are used for routine diagnosis at this time.

**Treatment.** No antiviral chemotherapy drugs or vaccines are available to treat or prevent rhinovirus infections. Interferon has been used, with mixed beneficial results.

## Varicella-Zoster (Chickenpox-Shingles)

**Properties.** Varicella-zoster virus is morphologically identical to HSV. As such, it has an icosahedral capsid, which contains a linear double-stranded DNA genome. A lipid envelope, obtained from the host cell's nuclear membrane, surrounds the nucleocapsid, with tegument proteins located between these two components. VZV has a narrow host range, growing in human fibroblasts or epithelial cell lines. It will grow only moderately in simian cells. It produces intranuclear inclusion bodies. Virions remain cell associated, and passage is facilitated by transferring infected cells and cell culture supernatant to new host cells. VZV does not grow in any laboratory animals. The virus is quite fragile, and care must be taken in the collection, transport, and processing of samples to ensure viral survival.

**Clinical Findings.** Varicella (chickenpox) is a mild, highly contagious disease that usually affects children. It is characterized by a generalized vesicular eruption of the skin and mucous membranes. It is more severe in adults and immunocompromised individuals. Zoster (shingles) is a sporatic, incapacitating disease of adults or immunocompromised individuals. The rash consists of vesicular lesions, limited in distribution to the skin innervated by a single sensory ganglion. In 1965, it was found that zoster represents reactivation of varicella virus that had persisted in a latent form in the sensory ganglia.

The route of infection of VZV is the mucosa of the upper respiratory tract or the conjunctiva. The virus spreads to the local lymphoid tissue and then through the bloodstream to its many target organs (skin, liver, lungs, brain, etc.). Focal cutaneous and mucosal lesions are initiated by viral infection of capillary endothelial cells. The cells enlarge and accumulate tissue fluids that result in vesicle formation. Eosinophilic nuclear inclusions are found in infected cells. Other organs may become involved, with the lung usually most severely damaged. Virus replication and spread is limited by immune responses.

Subclinical varicella is unusual. Malaise and fever are the earliest symptoms, followed by the rash. This starts on the trunk and then appears on the face, the limbs, and the oral mucosa. Vesicles appear in crops. Complications are rare and the mortality rate is very low. Varicella pneumonia is the most common complication in adults and may have a mortality rate of 10% to 40%. Immunocompromised patients are at increased risk of various complications of varicella. Severe, disseminated VZV disease has a mortality rate of about 20%.

Zoster usually starts with severe pain in the area of skin or mucosa supplied by one or more groups of sensory nerves or ganglia. A crop of vesicles appears over the affected area within a few days. The rash is usually unilateral, with the trunk, head, and neck most often involved. Duration and severity of cutaneous eruptions are generally related to the age of the patient. Treatment with antiviral drugs stops virus growth and lesion development. The most common complication of zoster is postherpetic neuralgia. The pain may continue for weeks to months. Zoster tends to disseminate and become more severe in individuals with underlying disease or are immunosuppressed. VZV pneumonia is responsible for a significant number of deaths in these patients.

### Laboratory Diagnosis.

**ISOLATION AND IDENTIFICATION.** The diagnosis of varicella and zoster are predominantly made on clinical grounds. It can be confirmed by one of several laboratory techniques.

If care is taken in sample collection, VSV can be recovered from vesicle fluid relatively easily. It has also been cultured from blood, CSF, or biopsy/autopsy tissues. HDF are the cell lines of choice for this virus. Characteristic CPEs occur between 1 and 2 weeks as an emergence of small and slowly enlarging foci of rounded and swollen refractile cells. The center of the plaque often disintegrates, leaving cellular debris and typical infected cells on the periphery of the focus of infection. Identification is most easily done using monoclonal antibodies in an immunofluorescence assay.

Varicella-zoster virus antigens can be directly detected using the same monoclonal antibody reagents. Stained smears of scrapings or swabs of the base of the vesicle will reveal multinucleated giant cells. Intracellular viral antigens can be demonstrated by directly staining the smears.

**SEROLOGY.** Serology is most often used to assess immunity to VZV rather than to establish a diagnosis. Complement fixing antibodies decline rapidly after convalescence, whereas antibodies are detectable by various immunofluorescence techniques including (fluorescent antibody-to-membrane antigen [FAMA], direct [DFA] and indirect fluorescence [IFA], and anti-complement immunofluorescence [ACIF]). The FAMA test is considered to be the most sensitive serologic tool and the best indicator of prior infection with VZV.

**Treatment.** Varicella in children requires no treatment, if the case is mild. Gamma globulin of high anti-VZV antibody titer can be used to prevent the development of the illness in immunocompromised patients exposed to VZV. Once varicella has started, it has no therapeutic value.

Famciclovir, acyclovir, and vidarabine are all effective anti-VZV drugs that are available for use in various disease situations.

## Rubella

**Properties.** Rubella virus is a member of the Togaviridae family and the only member of the *Rubivirus* genus. As a togavirus, rubella has a positive-sense, single-stranded RNA genome. It has an icosahedral capsid that is surrounded by a lipid envelope. Togaviruses are about 70 nm in diameter. As an RNA virus, rubella viruses replicate in the cytoplasm of the host cell. There is only one antigenic type.

**Clinical Findings.** The disease is quite contagious and is usually transmitted by respiratory secretions. Initial viral replication occurs in the respiratory tract, followed by multiplication in the cervical lymph nodes. Viremia develops in 5 to 7 days and lasts until the appearance of antibody on about day 13 to 15. The rash appears coincidentally with antibody formation, indicating an immunologic basis for its formation. After the rash, the virus is detectable only in the nasopharynx, where it may persist for several weeks. At least one-fourth of the cases are **subclinical infections**.

Initial symptoms include malaise, low-grade fever, and lymphadenopathy. The maculopapular rash emerges first on the face and then on the neck and trunk. Some individuals may have transient arthralgia and arthritis. The signs and symptoms of rubella may be difficult to distinguish from other rash-associated diseases. Therefore, neither the classical presentation nor the absence of classic rubella symptoms can be regarded as definitively diagnostic. The laboratory can assist in this diagnostic uncertainty. Classical rubella in school-age children seldom has any complications. Natural infection and recovery confers a permanent immunity to the disease.

The most signficant complication lies in the clinical rubella syndrome seen in infants born to mothers who have acquired the virus during pregnancy. The mother develops a viremia, and the virus has the ability to cross the placenta. Although a limited number of fetal cells are infected, the growth rate of these cells is reduced. This results in fewer numbers of cells in affected organs at birth, resulting in structural anomalies in the newborn infant. The earlier in pregnancy that the mother acquires the virus, the greater the chance and amount of damage that can develop in the fetus. Inapparent maternal infections can produce these anomalies as well. The most serious consequence is fetal death and spontaneous abortion.

## Laboratory Diagnosis.

**ISOLATION AND IDENTIFICATION.** Viral isolation is seldom attempted for routine diagnosis because the recovery methods are time consuming and relatively insensitive.

Rubella virus can be readily isolated from a variety of specimens obtained from patients with congenital or acquired rubella. Care must be taken in collecting and storing specimens to retain viral viability. Specimen collection should occur as early as possible after the person becomes ill (preferably within 3–4 days). Specimens can be stored at 4°C for up to 48 hours prior to inoculation. Any delay beyond this time would require the sample to be frozen at –70°C immediately after collection. Most body fluids and tissues (placental and aborted material) contain the virus. Nasopharyngeal washings or throat swabs placed in a transport medium should maintain viral viability quite well.

The list of cell cultures that will support rubella virus growth is quite large. These include, in part, RK-13, LLC-RK-1, Vero, GMK-AH-1, BHK-21 and others. The problem arises in the fact that most diagnostic virology laboratories do not routinely carry these cultures and have them readily available for inoculation. Communication between the physician and the laboratory is mandatory to maximize the possiblity to recover the virus. In primary cells, rubella virus seldom produces CPEs, and when they are present the changes are slow to appear and difficult to detect.

Two methods exist for rubella virus detection. The indirect technique is based on the ability of rubella virus to interfere with the growth of enteroviruses, such as ECHO 11. At an established time postinfection, ECHO 11 is inoculated into the cell culture and observed for growth. If no growth of the enterovirus occurs, rubella virus is present. If rubella virus is absent, growth of the enterovirus occurs (see Figure 50-7).

A more specific method would use a monoclonal antibody to rubella virus in an immunofluorescence procedure.

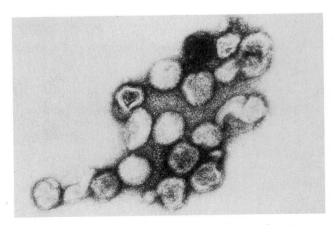

**FIGURE 50-7** Rubella. (Courtesy of Centers for Disease Control and Prevention, Atlanta, GA)

**SEROLOGY.** The hemagglutination inhibition test has been the standard serologic test for rubella. Nonspecific inhibitors must first be removed before it can be performed. Complement fixation tests are of limited usefulness because complement fixation antigens have not been correlated with specific viral proteins. ELISA is very sensitive and can detect rubella antibody where hemagglutination inhibition antibody cannot be found. The presence of any detectable level of antibody or a history of rubella vaccination is accepted presumptive evidence of immunity.

**Treatment.** Rubella is a mild, self-limited illness, and no antiviral chemotherapy is available or needed. Passive immune procedures give limited, if any, protection to the mother or fetus. Proven viral infection in the first trimester may be an indication that pregnancy termination might be considered.

Rubella has an excellent, live attenuated vaccine available. The RA27/3 vaccine, licensed in 1979, provides a permanent protection against the wild-type virus.

## VIRUSES NOT ISOLATED IN THE CLINICAL LABORATORY

### Epstein-Barr Virus

**Properties.** Epstein-Barr virus exhibits typical herpesvirus-like structure and biochemical properties. It has a very narrow host range. In vitro, EBV can be grown in B lymphocytes and, to some extent, in epithelial cells. In B cells, EBV induces a blastogenic transformation and immortalizes (grows indefinitely, but is not an oncogenic transformation necessarily) them. Most of the viral genetic material remains in the form of superhelical circular episomes, but integration into a host chromosome can also occur. Only 10 of the 80-plus genes of the virus can cause host cell transformation. Immortalized B cells express EBV antigens on their membranes and often secrete antibody due to polyclonal activation. EBV remains in a latent state in B cells.

In the 1960s, infectious mononucleosis was shown to be associated with EBV, and an association with Burkitt's lymphoma was demonstrated. Although isolation of the virus is possible using lymphocytes from fetal cord blood, this is not a routine test performed in a viral diagnostic laboratory.

**Clinical Findings.** In developing nations, EBV infection is nearly universal during early childhood. In industrialized countries, half of all EBV infections develop during late adolescence and adulthood. One of the most widespread viruses, adults have an 80% to 90% infection rate. Infection is most likely spread by exchange of infected saliva. The virus does not appear to be easily communicable. Blood transfusion appear to account for a very small percentage of EBV infections.

In children, EBV infection is generally asymptomatic. Pharyngitis and tonsillitis are seen in children (5–15 years of age). No heterophil antibody is usually demonstrable.

With college-age individuals, 33% to 75% of the infections are clinically recognizable and take the form of infectious mononucleosis. The incubation period ranges from 30 to 50 days and symptoms include headache, malaise, fatigue, sore throat, pharyngeal inflammation, enlarged lymph nodes and spleen, with some patients demonstrating a rash. There is an increase in the number and proportion of circulating lymphocytes, with the emergence of large numbers of atypical, antigen-reactive T lymphocytes. Infection of the B lymphocytes by EBV induces polyclonal activation with heterophil antibodies and autoimmune manifestations. Complications are relatively rare, but may include splenic rupture, thrombocytopenia, hemolytic anemia encephalitis, and meningitis. Fatalities are rare.

Chronic EBV infections, producing severe, prolonged disease, are seen in relatively few individuals. Although claimed as a cause of chronic fatigue syndrome, strong evidence for this association is lacking at the present time.

Epstein-Barr virus has been associated with African Burkitt's lymphoma, nasopharyngeal carcinoma, and, possibly, tumors involving intraoral, parotid, and thymic tissues. Organ allograft recipients provide convincing evidence that EBV is involved in the development of lymphoproliferative disorders. Most of the neoplasms are composed of polyclonal B cells and are not true malignancies. Although some evidence of EBV presence (EBV nuclear antigen and EBV DNA) can be demonstrated in neoplastic tissue, the evidence is not clearly at the "cause and effect" stage. EBV DNA, for example, cannot be consistently detected in biopsy specimens of AIDS-associated neoplasia, casting some doubt on the etiologic role of EBV in this setting.

### Laboratory Diagnosis.

**ISOLATION.** Epstein-Barr virus can be detected in saliva, throat wash materials, and peripheral blood mononuclear cells using transformation assays using human umbilical cord lymphocytes. Cord lymphocytes (used within 5 days of collection) are mixed with clinical specimens in cell culture medium and maintained for 6 to 8 weeks. The cultures are examined microscopically, with transformation being indicated by a rapid increase in the number of cells. The cells enlarge and grow in clusters. Infection may be confirmed by anticomplement immunofluorescence staining for Epstein-Barr nuclear antigen. This is not done in most viral diagnostic laboratories.

**SEROLOGY.** Serology is the most common way to confirm a clinical diagnosis of infectious mononucleosis. Nonspecific (heterophil) antibodies and antibodies against specific viral antigens represent a nonspecific response of B cells against a variety of nonviral antibodies to agglutinate or lyse sheep, beef, goat, and horse red blood cells (RBCs) have been used in the preparation of several commercial spot tests that use RBCs in slide agglutination tests. The majority of tests in patients with EBV-caused infectious mononucleosis will be positive in the first week of clinical illness. It may be necessary to test three or four times before a positive rise in heterophil antibody titers can be demonstrated.

Figure 50-8 demonstrates the kinetics of appearance and persistence of antibodies to EBV-specific antigens after a primary infection.

Individuals with recent infection have IgM and IgG antibodies to viral capsid antigen (VCA). Antibodies to early viral antigens [(EA - (diffuse)] develop in 70% to 80% of patients and persist for several months. Several weeks after infection, antibodies to EBNA appear and persist for life. Newer technologies are used to detect EBV nucleic acids in tissues and include DNA amplification by polymerase chain reaction and nucleic acid hybridization with various techniques.

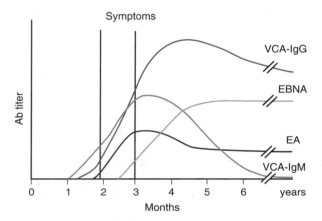

**FIGURE 50-8** Antibody appearances and persistence in Epstein-Barr virus infections. VCA, viral capsid antigen; EA, early antigen; EBNA, Epstein-Barr antigen; Ig, immunoglobulins G and M.

**Treatment.** This is largely supportive. Specific symptoms may be treated with regular analgesics or corticosteroids; EBV does not respond to any antiviral agents that inhibit other herpesviruses.

No effective vaccine has been developed to prevent or modify EBV infection. A vaccine has been used with the gp 340/220 antigen. Although an animal model has shown some protection due to the development of neutralizing antibodies, more work on this system is needed before human trials could be considered.

# Hepatitis Viruses—Hepatitis A, B, C, D, E

Viral hepatitis is a common infection that produces inflammation and necrosis of liver cells. Although most cases are endemic, epidemics are not rare. Hepatitis classically presents with lethargy, loss of appetite, nausea, vomiting, abdominal pain, and, ultimately, jaundice. In children the disease is more benign and jaundice is uncommon. Acute viral hepatitis is caused by one of the following: hepatitis A virus (HAV), hepatitis B virus (HBV), hepatitis C virus (HCV), hepatitis D virus (HDV), hepatitis E virus (HEV), and the hepatitis non-A and non-B (NANB) viruses. These infections may be distinguished by their clinical and epidemiologic features and by serologic tests for definite diagnosis.

Other viruses can cause hepatitis, but the infections often involve other organ systems such as the skin. These viruses include EBV, CMV, rubella, rubeola, mumps, adenovirus, and coxsackievirus. In immunosuppressed hosts and neonates, HSV and VZV can produce a disseminated infection with hepatic involvement.

Chronic hepatitis, an unusual sequela of acute hepatitis, can be traced to HBV, HCV, HDV, and HEV. More than 50,000 cases of viral hepatitis are reported annually in the United States, but the true incidence is probably several times this figure. The mortality rate is about 8/1,000 cases, but it is higher among patients over 30 years of age and recipients of blood transfusions. The distribution of viral hepatitis is worldwide. Over 300 million cases of chronic HBV infection exist. Interferon treatment is the only antiviral treatment, and it appears to be having limited effect.

### Terminology

| | |
|---|---|
| HAV | Hepatitis A virus |
| HBV | Hepatitis B virus |
| $Hb_sAG$ | Hepatitis B antigen, which exists as a separate small 22-nm particle and is also present on the surface of the large HBV particle (a; d/yr; w/r) |
| $HB_cAg$ | Hepatitis B core antigen present within the HBV |
| Anti-$HB_s$ | Antibody to $Hb_sAg$. |
| Anti-$HB_c$ | Antibody to $Hb_cAg$ |
| $Hb_eAg$ | Internal Ag, structural—important for measuring infectivity potential; also called epsilon |
| HCV (NANB) | Non-A, non-B hepatitis agent(s)—transfusion associated |
| δ (HDV) | Delta virus, antigen |
| Anti-D | Antibody to delta antigen |
| HEV | NANB—enterically transmitted |
| NANB | Diagnosis by exclusion—possible two viruses |

### Hepatitis A—Infectious Hepatitis.

**PROPERTIES.** Hepatitis A virus belongs to the enterovirus subgroup of the Picornaviruses. It is a small, nonenveloped virus containing a single-stranded, positive-sense RNA genome. It was once designated as enterovirus 72, but recently a new genus name, *Heprnavirus,* has been proposed.

All enteroviruses are resistant to low pH (pH 3.0) and several proteolytic enzymes. They resist inactivation by several disinfectants (70% alcohol, 5% lysol, 1% quaternary ammonium compounds) and to ether and lipid-destroying detergents. They can be destroyed by formaldehyde (0.3–3.0%), free residual chlorine (0.3–0.5 ppm), drying and heat (50°C for 60 minutes). HAV is more resistant than other enteroviruses (60°C for 10 hours). Storage at –70°C will ensure viability for years; storage at 4°C retains viability for several weeks. Autoclaving and ethylene oxide treatment effectively destroys HAV viability.

The virus replicates in several types of cell cultures of primate origin. It does not induce cytopathic changes and must be detected by immunofluorescence, radioassay, or other methodologies. The virus remains as a persistent infection in cell cultures. Primary isolation is very difficult, with infection lasting several weeks before intracytoplasmic antigen is detectable. This virus is not one that can be routinely isolated by viral diagnostic laboratories. There appears to be a single antigenic type of HAV and a vaccine has recently been approved for human use.

**CLINICAL FINDINGS.** Human enteroviruses have their reservoir in humans and can be isolated from the lower and upper alimentary tracts. Virus is spread primarily by the oral-fecal route, although respiratory transmission has been documented. In areas of poor sanitary conditions, the fecal-oral transmission is predominant. Sexual transmission has not been reported and blood transfusions and insect bites do not appear to be viable routes. Contaminated water transmission is probably most significant and shellfish in such areas are common sources of infection. Nosocomial transmission of HAV in newborn nurseries has been reported.

The virus is found worldwide. The exact incidence is difficult to estimate due to the high proportion of asymptomatic infections. Although serologic surveys suggest that HAV prevalence in industrial countries is decreasing, the infection is almost universal in most countries.

Once transmitted by ingestion, the incubation period of HAV is between 3 and 6 weeks, with a mean of 28 days. Subclinical and anicteric infections predominate. There is a low mortality rate (0.2%), but morbidity may be prolonged. Persistence of infection does not occur and no chronic carriers exist.

All age groups are susceptible to HAV infection. In endemic areas, the incidence is highest among children and adolescents.

Acute HAV infection is frequently found to be initially evidenced by a variety of nonspecific symptoms (fever, chills, headache, malaise, aches, and pains). A few days later anorexia, nausea, vomiting, and right upper quadrant abdominal pains appear. Dark urine

and clay-colored stools are common. The virus grows in liver cells, killing them, and leading to normal liver dysfunction. Jaundice of the skin and sclera of the eyes develop, followed by a rapid, subjective improvement in symptoms. The jaundice may persist for 2 or 3 weeks. Convalescence may be prolonged, taking several months for adults. Symptoms in children are usually less severe. Mortality is low, and fatalities once associated with pregnancy and with HAV are now known to have been caused by HEV. Repair of the liver occurs by regeneration of hepatocytes.

**LABORATORY DIAGNOSIS.** Liver function tests (e.g., increased levels of serum transaminases) were used historically for diagnosis but were nonspecific. Figure 50-9 depicts antibody development during HAV infection and Table 50-5 provides a clinical interpretation for the presence of HAV antibodies. IgM anti-HAV is present early in illness (onset of jaundice) but gone 2 months later. IgG anti-HAV appears 2 weeks later, persists for years, and protects against infection.

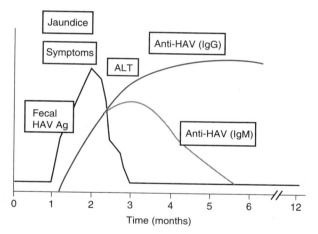

**FIGURE 50-9** Symptoms, antigen, and antibody development during hepatitis A infection. Ag, antigen; ALT, liver transaminase enzyme; IG, immunoglobulins G and M.

| Table 50–5 ▶ Serologic Tests for Hepatitis A Virus Diagnosis | | |
|---|---|---|
| **anti-HAV IgM** | **anti-HAV IgG** | **Interpretation** |
| – | – | Susceptible to HAV |
| + | – | Early acute phase of HAV infection |
| + | + | Acute phase of HAV infection |
| – | + | Convalescent phase of HAV infection or past HAV infection. Immune to HAV reinfection |

**TREATMENT.** Control is difficult because viral load and shedding are highest at the late incubation stage. Spread of HAV is reduced by simple hygienic measures and sanitary disposal of excreta.

Normal human immunoglobulin, containing at least 100 IU/mL of anti-HAV, can be given intramuscularly to prevent or attenuate a clinical illness. Although passive immunity may not prevent infection and excretion of virus, it is effective in often preventing clinical illness. Such treatment appears to be effective up to 4 weeks following exposure to the virus.

No specific antiviral chemotherapy currently is available for HAV infections. A killed vaccine has recently been approved for human use.

### Hepatitis B—Serum Hepatitis.

**PROPERTIES.** Hepatitis B virus belongs to the Hepadnavirus group. The virus particle was once referred to as the "Dane particle." It is a complex, 42-nm double-shelled virion particle. The outer surface (envelope—NOTE: NOT a LIPID envelope) contains the HBV surface antigen ($HB_sAg$) and surrounds a 27-nm inner core that contains core antigen ($HB_cAg$). The genome consists of a double-stranded DNA molecule. One strand is complete, but nicked, and the other strand contains 50% to 90% of the complementary sequences. The virion was thought to contain a DNA-dependent DNA polymerase enzyme, which completed the partial strand and ligated the nicked strand before replication in a host cell could begin. This function is now known to be performed by host cellular enzymes. The virally contained enzyme does possess **reverse transcriptase** activity because an intermediate RNA-DNA hybrid nucleic acid molecule appears to be involved in HBV genome replication. HBV e antigen ($HB_eAg$) is also found in the core of the virion. The e antigen is present when high levels of virions are present and is a marker of a high degree of infectivity.

The virus has not been found to grow in any convenient cell culture system. Studies have relied on infected human volunteers or studies with related Hepadnaviruses in other animal host systems. Isolation of HBV in the viral diagnostic laboratory is not done (see Figure 50-10).

**CLINCIAL FINDINGS.** The incubation period of HBV is usually about 3 months. Although the virus is transmitted primarily by the percutaneous route, $HB_eAg$ has been detected in virtually every body fluid and can be transmitted by oral and genital contact. Transmission in blood transfusions is well documented. HBV preferentially replicates in hepatocytes but has also been reported to replicate in nonhepatocytes and in hemopoietic tissue. Transmission through the placenta can result in in utero infection of the fetus. A carrier state is defined as persistence of the $HB_eAg$ in the blood for more than 6 months. The carrier state may be lifelong and may be associated with liver damage varying from

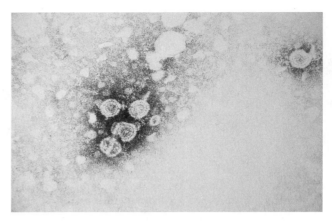

**FIGURE 50-10** Hepatitis B. (Courtesy of Centers for Disease Control and Prevention, Atlanta, GA)

minor changes in the nucleus of hepatocytes to chronic active hepatitis and cirrhosis. A carrier rate in adults ranges from 5% to 10%. In areas with high endemic infection rates, the highest prevalence of $HB_eAg$ is found in children aged 4 to 8 years. The current number of HBV chronic carriers is estimated to be between 300 to 400 million worldwide.

Onset of acute viral hepatitis is often preceeded by nausea, vomiting, severe anorexia, and fever. Jaundice may appear within a few days after these symptoms, but anicteric hepatitis is more common. HBV grows preferentially within hepatocytes. Cell degeneration occurs, with the necrosis of the hepatocytes. There is an accumulation of immunocompetent cells, and the immune system may contribute to cellular destruction to eliminate virus-contaminating cells. Disruption of bile ducts may occur after liver cell enlargement or necrosis. Preservation of the reticulum framework allows for hepatocyte regeneration so that the highly ordered architecture of the liver can be restored. Damaged tissue is usually repaired in 8 to 12 weeks. Figure 50-11 depicts clinical outcomes of HBV infection. Fatalities may range from 0.2% to 10%.

Hepatitis B virus antigens give rise to excellent antibody development. Passive immunity may play a role in disease prevention or modification. Immune serum globulin (ISG) and hepatitis B immune globulin (HBIG—hyperimmunized preparation) contain amounts of anti-$HB_sAg$: 1/100 versus more than 1/100,000 of anti-$HB_sAg$, titer by radioimmunoassay.

Preexposure prophylaxis: Routine passive immunization against hepatitis B is not recommended.

Postexposure prophylaxis: The risk of clinical hepatitis B following exposure to blood known to contain $HB_eAg$ is approximately 1/20.

Table 50-6 provides a summary of recommended uses of these products for passive protection.

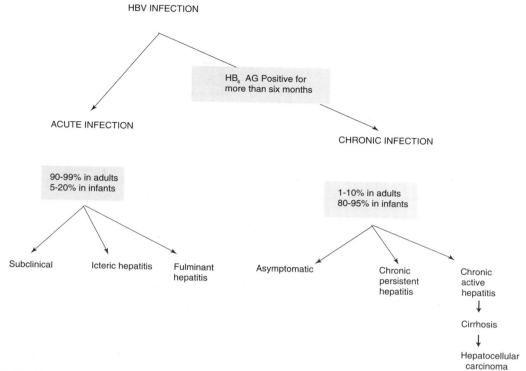

**FIGURE 50-11** Clinical outcomes of hepatitis B virus infection.

| Table 50–6 ► Summary of Postexposure Prophylaxis of Acute Exposures to HBV | |
|---|---|
| **Donor Status** | **Recommended Management** |
| Donor Hb$_s$Ag positive | HBIG (0.06 mL/kg) immediately and 1 month later |
| Donor known Hb$_s$Ag status unknown | Test donor for HB$_s$Ag– |
| | IG (0.06 mL/kg) immediately to recipient |
| High risk (1/20) | If test HB$_s$Ag+ in donor, HBIG as in the first example (above) |
| | If test HB$_s$Ag– in donor, nothing |
| Donor known, HB$_s$Ag negative | No testing of donor necessary |
| Status unknown Low risk (1/2,000) | Nothing or IG (0.06/kg) to Hb$_s$ recipient |
| Donor unknown Status unknown | Nothing or IG (0.06/kg) to HB$_s$Ag recipient |
| Newborn of Hb$_s$Ag positive mother | HBIG (0.5 mL as soon after birth and at 3 and 6 months of age) |
| HBIG, hepatitis B immune globulin; IG, gamma globulin. | |

**LABORATORY DIAGNOSIS.** Attempts to isolate HBV in a cell or organ system have generally not been successful and is not done by diagnostic virology laboratories. Serum transaminase enzyme levels indicate damage to hepatocytes but are nonspecific and may differ according to an acute or a chronic infection. Several generations of laboratory tests have been developed to measure HBV antigens of antibodies to these antigens. Such tests currently available use the enzyme currently available ELISA or radioimmune assay (RIA) formats. Table 50-7 summarizes three tests that can be done to diagnose HBV infections and provides information on virus transmission and probable stage of disease.

**TREATMENT.** Currently, the only licensed antiviral for hepatitis B infection is recombinant α-interferon. It appears to often favorably modify the disease, but once it is discontinued, the infection becomes reestablished.

Hepatitis B virus vaccine is a suspension of inactivated, alum-adsorbed 22-nm surface antigen particles purified from human plasma or prepared from yeast (genetic manipulation). Field trials of the US vaccine have shown 80% to 95% efficacy in preventing infection among susceptible persons. The vaccine should be stored at 2° to 8°C but not frozen. Evidence from serologic studies shows that a booster vaccination every 8 to 10 years may be beneficial.

## Hepatitis C—NANB-Transfusion Associated.

**PROPERTIES.** In recent years since antigens have become available for hepatitis A and hepatitis B and

## Table 50–7 ▶ Serologic Markers for Hepatitis B Virus and Ability to Transmit the Infection

| HB$_s$Ag | anti-HB$_c$ | Anti-HB$_s$ | Contagious | Interpretation |
|:---:|:---:|:---:|:---:|---|
| – | – | – | – | Susceptible to HBV |
| + | – | – | + | Early acute HBV infection |
| + | + | – | + | Acute HBV infection or chronic carrier state |
| – | + | – | + | Convalescent HBV infection or "window phase" |
| – | + | + | – | Late convalescence or past HBV infection. Immune to reinfection. |
| – | – | + | – | Past HBV infection or normal response to HBV vaccine. Immune to reinfection |
| + | + | + | + | Acute HBV infection or chronic carrier state |

– indicates negative test results; + indicates positive test result.

screening of blood serum and plasma for transfusion has become routine, it has been discovered that although the incidence of hepatitis transmitted by transfusion has decreased considerably, there are still significant fractions of transfusions that result in hepatitis. Another hepatitis virus called non-A, non-B (NANB) hepatitis virus has been identified for this and much effort has been put forth to find the virus (see Table 50–8).

Clinical and epidemiologic studies and cross-challenge studies in chimpanzees suggested that there were three **NANB hepatitis** agents, unrelated to HAV or HBV. One of these agents is now called hepatitis C virus (HCV). Studies have shown this to be a positive-stranded RNA virus, now classified as a flavivirus. The expression of **cDNA** clones of the virus yielded proteins that formed the basis of serologic tests for antibodies to HCV. Substantial numbers of individuals with posttransfusion NANB hepatitis have tested positive for HCV. Although the presence of an envelope has been inferred due to sensitivity to organic solvents (lipid envelope destruction), the actual virus particles have only recently been visualized and described. A suggested genus name for HCV is *Hep-c-virus*. A complete analysis and translation of the RNA genome has resulted in a mixture of viral proteins that serve as antigens for the second-generation serologic test.

**CLINICAL FINDINGS.** The virus is estimated to be the cause of approximately 17% to 20% of all viral hepatitis cases in the United States. This includes up to 90% of posttransfusion cases and, possibly, up to 25% of the

sporadic hepatitis cases diagnosed. It is estimated that about 4 million Americans are currently infected with HCV, and this will result in approximately 24,000 deaths annually. Infection spread by shared needles among drug users is also significant.

The incubation period ranges from 5 to 10 weeks. Three features have been associated with the pathogenesis and clinical course of HCV infection. A high serum value of alanine aminotransferase is a meaningful predictor that HCV may be involved (rather than HBV). The histopathologic pattern of liver damage is characterized by a fatty metamorphosis. This suggests a feature of a viral cytopathic form of cell damage, rather than an immunologically induced cellular injury. Finally, 50% to 70% of HCV patients develop chronic liver disease. This chronic involvement is often mild and asymptomatic. Yet 10% to 23% of cases eventually progress to cirrhosis. Chronic cases of HCV may take many years to develop. HCV has been associated with primary hepatocellular carcinoma, as has been HBV.

**LABORATORY DIAGNOSIS.** An ELISA serologic test (second generation) exists for the measurement of antibody to HCV. This version measures antibodies that develop early in disease, overcoming disadvantages of the initial test.

**TREATMENT.** No specific antiviral methods are available for treatment of HCV infections.

### Hepatitis D.

**PROPERTIES.** Hepatitis D virus is a defective virus that will only grow in a cell previously or coinfected with HBV. It contains a single-stranded RNA genome, has an inner protein shell of delta protein, and an outer shell of HBV surface antigen. HDV has been placed in the proposed Deltavirus group for classification.

The morphologic changes seen in NANB hepatitis and HDV appear similar with predominant cytotoxic rather than lymphocytotoxic effects.

**CLINICAL FINDINGS.** The virus can present as an acute or chronic infection. Persons at risk for HBV infection appear to be at similar risk to HDV infection. The primary

## Table 50–8 ▶ Recent Estimated Worldwide NANB Hepatitis

| | |
|---|---:|
| Chronic carriers | 100,000,000 |
| New cases/year, United States | 175,000 |
| New cases/year, Western Europe | 175,000 |
| New cases/year, Japan | 350,000 |

routes of transmission are believed to be similar to those of HBV. Once HDV infection is established, HDV interferes with the expression of HBV gene products and reduces the HBV markers associated with infectivity. The incubation period varies from 2 to 12 weeks.

In Mediterranean countries, HDV infection is endemic among persons with HBV and most transmissions are thought to occur by intimate contact. In nonendemic areas (United States and Northern Europe), HDV infection is usually limited to persons exposed frequently to blood and blood products. HDV is not a new virus because globulin lots prepared from plasma collected in the United States 40 years ago contain antibodies to HDV.

**LABORATORY DIAGNOSIS.** Isolation of HDV is not possible in the diagnostic virology laboratory. The commercial availability of licensed RIA and EIA kits for the detection of antibodies to the delta agent has simplified the diagnosis of this virus.

**TREATMENT.** No antiviral chemotherapy is currently available for HDV infections. Individuals with antibodies to HBV surface antigen will be protected from HDV infection because the outer coat of the virus is $HB_sAg$. Such antibodies would arise from HBV infection or vaccination.

### Hepatitis E—NANB—Enterically Transmitted.

**PROPERTIES.** Hepatitis E virus has a positive-sense, single-stranded RNA genome. It has a diameter of 32 nm and been placed in the Calicivirus classification.

**CLINICAL FINDINGS.** The virus is transmitted enterically and occurs in epidemic form in developing countries, where water supplies may be fecally contaminated. Pregnant women may have a high (20%) mortality rate.

**LABORATORY DIAGNOSIS.** Diagnosis is made by exclusion and epidemiology.

**TREATMENT.** No treatment currently exists for HEV infection.

Table 50-9 summarizes test results and interpretations for acute symptomatic viral hepatitis.

## Human Immunodeficiency Virus

The cause of AIDS, first described in 1981, was declared to be the HIV type-1 (HIV-1) only 3 years later. HIV-1 is the third human retrovirus discovered. Since then, significant advances have been made in understanding the molecular structure of the virus, as well as its interaction with the immune system. The exact origin of HIV-1 is unknown, although one early theory stated that it could have come from Green monkeys in Central Africa. This theory, after numerous studies, is no longer accepted by most experts. There is still no drug for cure of the disease and no vaccine to prevent its spread.

**Properties.** Retrovirus are approximately 130 nm in diameter and have a lipid envelope. They possess an icosahedral or helical symmetry, with HIV having a bar-shaped nucleoid. There are two identical copies of a linear, single-stranded, positive-sense RNA genome. The genome will code for three to nine genes, depending on the virus type. HIV belongs to the Lentivirus subfamily of the Retrovirus classification. This family contains viruses that are nononcogenic generally and cytocidal. This group includes HIV-1, HIV-2, and HIV-3.

The main genes needed for replication include:

▶ Gag gene: —*G*roup *A*ssociated anti*G*ens (core proteins)
▶ Pol gene: —*POL*ymerase (reverse transcriptase, etc.)
▶ Env gene: —*ENV*elope proteins

The ssRNA of the virus is used as a template to synthesize a dsDNA copy. The dsDNA is then circularized

### Table 50–9 ▶ Interpretation of Current Serodiagnostic Test Results for Acute Symptomatic Hepatitis

| | Tests | | | | | |
|---|---|---|---|---|---|---|
| | HB$_s$Ag | TOTAL Anti-HBc | Anti-HCV | IGM Anti-HAV | Anti-HDV* | Most Likely Clinical Diagnosis |
| Single virus | − | − | − | + | | Hepatitis A |
| | + | + | − | − | − | Acute Hepatitis B† |
| | − | − | + | − | | Hepatitis C |
| Combined viruses | + | + | − | + | | Hepatitis A and B† |
| | + | + | − | − | + | Hepatitis B and D coinfection‡ |
| | − | + | − | − | + | |
| | + | − | + | − | − | Hepatitis B and C coinfection† |

*Testing should only be done when serologic evidence of HBV infection exists.

†To distinguish acute from chronic HBV, obtain IgM anti-HBc.

‡Consider coinfection if IgM anti-HBc is positive. A superinfection presumably exists if IgM anti-HBc is negative.

and inserted into cell DNA. This process is highly dependent on reverse transcriptase, which is an unusual multifunctional RNA-dependent DNA polymerase.

► Reverse transcriptase: generates viral RNA:DNA hybrid
degrades RNA in RNA; DNA hybrid
generates viral DNA:DNA copy
helps circularize DNA:DNA copy
► Integrase: integrates DNA:DNA copy into cell DNA
► Protease: cleaves various protein precursors

In the growth cycle, virus attaches via its *gp 120* to *CD4* molecule of cells with high affinity. Entry is by *fusion* of viral envelope and cytoplasmic membrane of cell (fusion is mediated by gp41). Genomic RNA and the reverse transcriptase enzyme is released into the cytoplasm of the host cell. The reverse transcriptase produces a double-stranded DNA copy of the original single-stranded RNA genome. The DNA copy is ligated into a circular molecule and transported to the host nucleus. The reverse transcriptase enzyme integrates the proviral DNA into a host chromosome. By an unknown mechanism and a highly variable latency period, cellular RNA polymerase II produces viral mRNA that is translated into viral components. Viral assembly occurs in the cytoplasm of the host cell, and the lipid envelope is acquired by a budding off process (see Figure 50-12).

T helper cells are infected and destroyed, providing a mechanism for immune dysfunction. Monocytes and macrophages form the major reservoir cells.

The exact number of antigenic types of HIV-1, based on gp120 structure, is unknown. The virus has a high mutation rate, and the virus may change several times within one individual over the course of infection.

**Clinical Findings.** Infection by HIV is followed by a viremia and the virus is disseminated to the lymphoid organs. As HIV growth occurs, the lymphoid organs deteriorate and a second viremia occurs. This correlates with the onset of symptoms and death eventually occurs.

The incubation period appears to range from 2 to 3 weeks to currently more than 15 years. The greatest risk of HIV transmission occurs with semen-to-blood and blood-to-blood interactions. Clinical disease usually is manifested by asymptomatic or mild, transient symptoms (fever, lymphadenopathy, and rash). More serious manifestations include generalized enlargement of the lymph nodes, fever, diarrhea, weight loss, and an increased susceptibility to infections. AIDS occurs with the almost total depletion of CD4+ lymphocytes. There is an increased incidence of opportunistic infections,

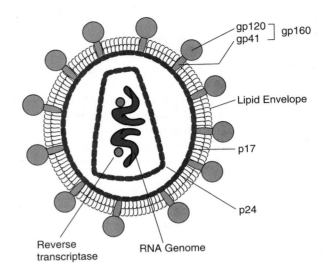

**FIGURE 50-12** HIV viral structure. Gp, glycoprotein; P, protein; ssRNA, single-stranded RNA genome.

malignancies, and degenerative changes in the brain leading to dementia and other neurologic problems.

Currently, more than 90% of AIDS patients die within 3 years of diagnosis, with a mean survival time of 1 year.

Antibodies usually appear 2 to 40 weeks following infection. Anti-gp120, gp41 (gp160)-envelope glycoproteins and anti-p24—a major core protein—are most common. Unfortunately, these possess a low level of neutralizing capacity. The normal, healthy CD4+:CD8+ ratio is 1.8; an AIDS patient has a ratio of less than 1.0 (inverted). Normal CD4+ cell count is 800 to 1,000/μL of blood and an AIDS patient has fewer than 200/μL.

**Laboratory Diagnosis.** Virus can be isolated from blood, T cells, semen, saliva, tears, CSF, and brain tissue. This is a specilized potentially dangerous procedure and is not done routinely.

Diagnosis is usually done by serology. The ELISA is the standard screening test and has a small number of false positives. A positive result is always repeated by ELISA and any sample that has been positive for HIV antibodies both times is subjected to a confirmatory test. The Western blot test consists of purified viral antigens separated on nitrocellulose paper. The strip is mixed with patient serum and positive results are disclosed as solid lines or bands, representing antigen–antibody complexes.

**Treatment.** Approved drugs include AZT (zidovudine), DDI (didanosine), DDC (zalcitabine), and 4dT, all reverse transcriptase inhibitors. Recently protease inhibitors have also been approved. Reverse transcriptase inhibitors are only virostatic, and viral growth recurs once the drugs are withdrawn. Combination treatment using reverse transcriptase inhibitors and protease inhibitors appears to be very effective. The current recommendation is to start AZT treatment when the CD4+ cell count falls below 500/μL.

# Rabies Virus

Rabies is one of the oldest known and most feared of human diseases. Rabies virus has characteristics which place it in the Rhabdoviridae family (> 100 viruses) where the prototype virus is vesicular stomatitis virus (VSV), a virus found in animals. "Rhabdos" (Greek) means rod; "rhabidus" (Latin) means mad.

**Properties.** Rabies viruses have a characteristic bullet (helical) shape, 180 × 75 nm in size. It is surrounded by a lipid envelope containing glycoprotein spikes. The genome is a negative-sense, single-stranded RNA molecule. The virions carry an RNA-dependent RNA polymerase to be capable of initiating a growth cycle, within a host cell. Viral replication occurs in the host cytoplasm, and viruses are released through the cytoplasmic membrane in a budding process.

Rabies virus has a very wide host range. Essentially all warm-blooded animals (dogs, cats, cattle, skunks, racoons, bats in the United States) can be infected. "Street" virus denotes a wild type, freshly isolated strain that will grow in many tissue types and have a highly variable incubation period. "Fixed" virus denotes a strain that has been serially passaged in rabbit brains, grows only in nervous tissue, and has a predictable incubation period of a few days.

Transmission is usually accomplished by the bite of an infected animal. Inhalation of aerosols in bat caves and tissue transplantation are alternative methods that have been described.

Once in the host, rabies virus replicates in muscle and connective tissues and then spreads to peripheral nerves. Eventually it spreads to the CNS for further multiplication. The infection becomes generalized, spreading to other tissues, including salivary glands. No viremia is found. Rabies virus produces a specific eosinophilic cytoplasmic inclusion, called a Negri body in infected nerve cells. It may be absent 20% of the time.

Rabies virus survives well at 4°C. It is rapidly killed by ultraviolet light, heat (50°C for 1 hour), lipid solvents, detergents, and pH extremes. Essentially, a single antigenic type exists.

**Clinical Findings.** Rabies is primarily a disease of animals and is spread to humans by bites of rabid animals. The incubation period varies from 2 to 16 weeks, depending on viral strain, inoculum load, and length of the neural path from the wound to the brain.

Infection results in an acute, fulminating encephalitis. The prodrome is usually manifested by malaise, anorexia, headache, nausea, vomiting, sore throat, and fever. Disease progression includes increasing nervousness, apprehension, hyperventilation, salivation, confusion, hallucinations, and spasms of throat muscles on swallowing (hydrophobia). Final stages include convulsive seizures, coma, and death from respiratory failure. There may be periods of brief hyperactivity (triggered by bright light, sound, or touch) and interspersed with longer periods of quiet. The fatality rate is essentially 100%. Thirty to 50% of individuals with known exposure develop symptoms.

**Laboratory Diagnosis.** Growth of the virus can be achieved only in specialized laboratories. Tissue or saliva can be inoculated intracerebrally into suckling mice. After disease development, virus identification can be made with specific antiserum.

The usual method of diagnosis is by direct immunofluorescence of histologic staining of brain or corneal impressions. The presence of Negri bodies in the cytoplasm of neurons is diagnostic. This requires the sacrifice of the suspected rabid animal for appropriate tissue collection.

Serologic assays (immunofluorescence, complement fixation, or virus neutralization tests) are limited in value because they tend to develop late in disease.

**Treatment.** No effective antiviral chemotherapy exists for rabies virus infection. Based on slow viral growth and timing of protective immunity development, prevention of disease can be attained by using passive immune procedures and vaccination. Postexposure prophylaxis is given to 20,000 to 30,000 individuals each year in the United States.

Suspect bites should be cleaned immediately with soap and water. Human rabies immune globulin (150 IU/mL) is given at 20 IU/kg of body weight. Half is infiltrated into the wound and the other half is injected intramuscularly.

Several types of vaccines are available. The human diploid cell vaccine provides a chemically inactivated preparation free from nerve tissue and is very effective. Only five doses of the material is sufficiently antigenic to obtain a substantial antibody response in most recipients. Some local side effects and mild systemic reactions may be experienced by the recipients.

# Rotaviruses

Human rotaviruses were first observed by electron microscopy, looking at biopsy specimens from the duodenum of children with acute diarrhea. Adult infections are also significant.

**Properties.** Rotaviruses have a segmented (11 pieces) genome of double-stranded RNA. They have a two-layered (double-shelled) capsid configuration and no lipid envelope. They are 60 to 80 nm in diameter, and replication occurs in the cytoplasm of the host cell, where the virions are not completely uncoated. As with other segmented genome viruses, genetic reassortment (see influenza viruses) occurs readily. At least six serotypes have been identified among human rotaviruses.

**Clinical Findings.** Rotaviruses appear to be the single most important worldwide cause of gastroenteritis in young children. Estimates of up to a billion episodes per year occur in children under 5 years of age, resulting in as many as 3 to 4 million deaths. There is no effective antiviral chemotherapy available against rotaviruses, and over half the cases of acute gastroenteritis in hospitalized children are caused by these agents.

Rotaviruses can be found endemically throughout the world, and by school age, up to 90% of children have serum antibodies against one or more types. Secretory IgA antibodies may be important in protection against reinfections. Maternal antibodies are present in mother's milk up to 9 months postpartum. These obviously protect against neonatal infections but do not appear to affect reinfection later.

The incubation period is 1 to 4 days, and typical symptoms include diarrhea, fever, abdominal pain, and vomiting, leading to dehydration. Patients with mild symptoms recover completely; more severely affected individuals should be hospitalized and treated for severe loss of electrolytes and fluids. Infections can occur in adults and nosocomial spread of rotaviruses has been well documented.

**Laboratory Diagnosis.** Diagnosis primarily rests on the demonstration of viruses in the stool collected early in the illness. The most common test format is ELISA, but immune electron microscopy and immunodiffusion have been used. DNA technology with dot hybridization using rotavirus-specific probes may prove to be useful and easy to use. Serology may be determined by ELISA or complement fixation (see Figure 50-13).

**Treatment.** At this time, treatment is supportive, supplying fluid and electrolytes lost by diarrhea and vomiting. Because the viruses are fecally spread, control measures should focus on wastewater treatment and improving community sanitation.

Rotavirus vaccine (bovine and rhesus types) are currently being evaluated as live, attenuated vaccines for human use. The greatest challenge for a successful vaccine will be to induce protective antibodies in very young infants and to include all the important serotypes of the human strains.

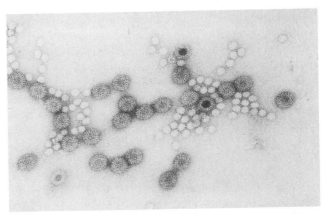

**FIGURE 50-13** Rotavirus. (Courtesy of Centers for Disease Control and Prevention, Atlanta, GA)

## SUMMARY

▶ Viruses that cause human disease and that can be routinely isolated in the diagnostic laboratory include the herpesviruses, adenoviruses, enteroviruses, and several respiratory viruses (influenza, parainfluenza, and respiratory syncytial virus).

▶ Measles, mumps, and rhinoviruses are most often identified on the basis of clinical presentation, with laboratory tests seldom being needed.

▶ Laboratory tests for rubella generally determine presence or absence of specific antibodies in serum and isolation is seldom attempted.

▶ There are five main hepatitis viruses currently recognized, which produce similar clinical manifestations and only appropriate laboratory tests will identify the specific type involved in a disease presentation.

▶ Diagnosis of HIV is done primarily by screening for antibodies by an ELISA technique and confirming with the Western blot test.

▶ Rabies infections are usually detected by identification of viral antigen using a fluorescent antibody technique.

▶ Rotavirus vaccines are currently in development and diagnosis of clinical infection is done by ELISA detection of viral antigen.

## Review Questions

1. Reverse transcriptase is involved in the reproduction cycle of which viruses listed below?
   a. HIV and HAV
   b. HIV and HBV
   c. HIV and HCV
   d. HAV and HCV
   e. HAV and HDV

2. The following serologic tests for hepatitis were reported: HAV IgM positive, HBV$_s$Ag negative, and antibody to HBV$_s$Ag negative. What is your interpretation of the patient's status?
   a. Immune to HBV due to vaccination
   b. Immune to HAV
   c. HBV chronic carrier
   d. Susceptible to HCV infection

## CASE STUDY

A 9-year-old girl was brought to her pediatrician because of fever and rash for 2 days. She also had a headache, sore throat, coryza, and mild cough. On examination she was alert and in mild distress. Her temperature was 38.3°C, her pulse rate was 110 beats/min, and her respiratory rate was 40/min. She had a mild conjunctivitis. Her posterior pharynx was swollen, and petechiae were present on her soft palate. The buccal mucosa also had scattered raised papular lesions. She had a macular rash on her trunk, face, and arms, and her chest x-ray was normal. A throat culture showed absence of group A streptococci. Acute and convalescent blood samples revealed the diagnosis, and the school nurse was notified.

### Questions

1.  Which of the following viral infections can present macular rash? Pick all those that apply.
    a.  Measles virus
    b.  Rubella virus
    c.  Roseola virus
    d.  EBV
    e.  CMV

2.  On the basis of the clinical presentation, what is the most likely etiologic agent in this case?
    a.  Measles virus
    b.  Rubella virus
    c.  Roseola virus
    d.  EBV
    e.  CMV

3.  Which of the following information is most significant for you to pick the answer for Question 2?
    a.  Fever and rash for 2 days
    b.  Headache, sore throat, and mild cough
    c.  Throat culture negative for group A streptococci

    d.  Coryza, conjunctivitis, and fever
    e.  Scattered raised papular lesions on buccal mucosa and palatal petechiae.

4.  Currently available methods for preventing this viral infection are:
    a.  live attenuated vaccine and passive immunity with pooled human IgG.
    b.  killed viral vaccines.
    c.  intravenous antiviral drugs.
    d.  active and passive immunities with specific toxoids.
    e.  nonspecific vaccines to boost cell-mediated immunity.

5.  Which of the following is a *late* complication of this viral infection?
    a.  Severe viral encephalitis following rash
    b.  Spongiform encephalopathy
    c.  Progressive multifocal leukoencephalopathy
    d.  Giant cell pneumonia
    e.  Subacute sclerosing panencephalitis (SSPE)

3.  The most significant respiratory virus for infants less than 6 months old is:
    a.  influenza B virus.
    b.  parainfluenza virus, type 2.
    c.  coxsackieviruses, group A.
    d.  respiratory syncytial virus.
    e.  coronaviruses.

4.  Antigenic shift occurs in which virus–antigen combination below?
    a.  Parainfluenza–envelope antigen
    b.  Hepatitis B virus–surface antigen
    c.  Herpes simplex virus–thymidine kinase
    d.  Mumps virus–fusion protein
    e.  Influenza–hemagglutinin

5. Killed or inactivated viral vaccines exist for all the following human diseases EXCEPT:
    a. hepatitis A virus.
    b. polioviruses.
    c. influenza virus.
    d. rubella virus.
    e. rabies virus.

6. Viruses that can develop a viremia and cross the placenta to infect the fetus include all the following EXCEPT:
    a. rubella virus.
    b. hepatitis B virus.
    c. cytomegalovirus.
    d. respiratory syncytial virus.

7. α-Interferon is approved for use in treating which viral disease listed below?
    a. Hepatitis A
    b. Hepatitis B
    c. Hepatitis D
    d. Hepatitis E

8. Which virus listed below can be accurately described as having a diploid genome?
    a. Hepatitis B virus
    b. Herpes simplex virus
    c. Rotavirus
    d. Human immunodeficiency virus 2

Questions 9 and 10 concern antiviral chemotherapy. Directions: Select the ONE lettered option that is MOST closely associated with the numbered items. Each lettered option may be used once, more than once, or not at all.

    a. Ganciclovir
    b. Acyclovir
    c. Amantadine
    d. Ribavirin
    e. Protease Inhibitors

9. a    b    c    d    e
   Most effective if used prior to viral entry into the patient.

10. a    b    c    d    e
    Effective for varicella-zoster infections

## ▶ REFERENCES & RECOMMENDED READING

Ampel, N. M. (1996). Emerging disease issues and fungal pathogens associated with HIV infection. *Emerging Infectious Diseases, 2*(2), 109–116.

Baron, S. (Ed.). (1996). *Medical microbiology* (4th ed.). Galveston, TX: The University of Texas Medical Branch at Galveston.

Belshe, R. B. (1991). *Textbook of human virology* (2nd ed.). St. Louis: Mosby–Yearbook.

Brooks, G. F., Butel, J. S., & Ornston, L. N. (Eds.). (1995). *Medical microbiology* (20th ed., pp. 303–528). East Norwalk, CT: Appleton & Lange.

Bush, C. E., Donovan, R. M., Markowitz, N., et al. (1996). Gender is not a factor in serum human immunodeficiency virus type 1 RNA levels in patients with viremia. *Journal of Clinical Microbiology, 34*(4), 970–972.

Fields, B. N., Knipe, D. M., & Howley, P. M. (Eds.). (1996). *Fields virology* (3rd ed., vols. 1 and 2). Philadelphia: Lippincott-Raven.

Galana, J. M. D., de Leeuw, N., Wittbol, S., et al. (1996). Prolonged enteroviral infection in a patient who developed pericarditis after bone marrow transplantation. *Clinical Infectious Disease, 22*(6), 1004–1008.

Gruber, W. C., Belshe, R. B., King, J. C., et al. (1996). Evaluation of live attenuated influenza vaccines in children 6–18 months of age: Safety, immunogenicity, and efficacy: *Journal of Infectious Disease, 173*(6), 1313–1319.

Hsiung, G. D. (1982). *Diagnostic virology, illustrated by light and electron microscopy* (3rd ed.). New Haven, CT: Yale University Press.

Khan, A. S., Khabbaz, R. F., Armstrong, L. R., et al. (1996). Hantavirus pulmonary syndrome: The first 100 US cases. *Journal of Infectious Disease 173*(6), 1297–1303.

Leland, D. S. (1996). *Clinical virology.* Philadelphia: Saunders.

Lennette, E. H. (Ed.). (1985). *Laboratory diagnosis of viral infections.* New York: Marcel Dekker.

Leparc-Goffart, I., Julien, J., Fuchs, F., et al. (1996). Evidence of presence of poliovirus genome sequences in cerebrospinal fluid from patients with postpolio syndrome. *Journal of Clinical Microbiology 34*(2), 2023–2026.

Mills, J., Volberding, P. A., & Corey, L. (Eds.). (1996). *Antiviral chemotherapy 4. New directions for clinical application and research.* New York: Plenum Press.

Murray, P. R., Baron, E. J., Pflaller, M. A., et al. (Eds.). (1995). *Manual of medical microbiology* (6th ed.). Washington, DC: ASM Press.

Pujol, F. H., Ponce, J. G., Lema, M. G., et al. (1996). High incidence of hepatitis C virus infection in hemodialysis patients in units with high prevalence. *Journal of Clinical Microbiology, 34*(7), 1633–1636.

Rupprecht, C. E., Smith, J. S., Fekadu, M., and Childs, J. E. (1995). The ascension of wildlife rabies: A cause for public health control or intervention? *Emerging Infectious Diseases, 1*(4), 107–114.

Specter, S., & Lancz, G. (Eds.). (1992). *Clinical virology manual* (2nd ed.). New York: Elsevier.

Spooner, K. M., Lane, H. C., & Masur, H. (1996). Guide to major clinical trials of antiretroviral therapy administered to patients with HIV. *Clinical Infectious Diseases, 23*(1), 15–27.

Timbury, M. C. (1991). Medical virology (9th ed.). London: Churchill Livingstone.

Unicomb, L. E., Faruque, S. M., Malek, M. A., et al. (1996) Demonstration of a lack of synergistic effect of rotavirus with other diarrheal pathogens on severity of diarrhea in children. *Journal of Clinical Microbiology, 34*(5), 1340–1342.

Wang, C.-H., Tschen, S.-Y., Heinricy, U., et al. (1996). Immune response to hepatitis A virus capsid proteins after infection. *Journal of Clinical Microbiology, 34*(3), 707–713.

White, D. O., & Fenner, F. J. (1994). *Medical virology* (4th ed.). San Diego: Academic Press.

Zuckerman, A. J., Banatvala, J. E., & Pattison, J. R. (Eds.). (1990). *Principles and practice of clinical virology* (2nd ed.). New York: Wiley.

# CHAPTER 51
## Emerging Viral Infections

Anne Delaney, MT (ASCP)

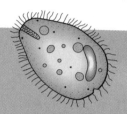

### *Microbes in the News*
#### Ebola Virus

Ebola virus is a member of the Filoviridae classification group. It burst from obscurity with outbreaks of severe hemorrhagic fever. It was first observed in the 1970s as an outbreak of 318 cases (mortality rate of 90%) in Zaire and 250 cases in Sudan (60% mortality). The book *The Hot Zone* describes a 1989 outbreak in the United States. A filovirus closely related to Ebola virus was detected in cynomolgus monkeys imported from the Philippines. Only a few of the 149 persons who came into contact with the infected monkeys, or their tissues, became infected. None became sick. Obviously, variants of virulent forms of filoviruses exist. *Advances in Viral Research* 1994; 43, 2–52.

**INTRODUCTION**

**EMERGING VIRUSES**

Ebola Hemorrhagic Fever
Hantavirus
Dengue Virus

## KEY TERMS

Emerging viral infections
Dengue fever/Dengue hemorrhagic fever/Dengue shock syndrome

Filoviruses
Hantavirus pulmonary syndrome

Hemorrhagic fever
Nosocomial infection
Sin Nombre virus

## LEARNING OBJECTIVES

**Upon successful completion of this chapter, the student should be able to:**

1. Define the term emerging infection.
2. Discuss the factors that contribute to emerging infections.
3. Discuss laboratory methods used to identify these infections.
4. Discuss the differences in the strains of Ebola viruses.
5. List animal reservoirs for each of these emerging infections, and discuss modes of transmission resulting in human infection.

# INTRODUCTION

**Emerging viral infections** include newly described viruses, as well as previously described viral infections that are either occurring at abnormally high incidence, or in unexpected geographic locations. This definition allows many viral infections to be defined as "emerging." A listing of some emerging viruses can be seen in Table 51-1 (Centers for Disease Control and Prevention [CDC], 1994; Institute of Medicine, 1992).

| Table 51-1 ▶ | Examples of Newly Described Viral Pathogens |
|---|---|
| 1977 | Ebola virus |
| 1977 | Hantaanvirus |
| 1977 | Rift Valley fever virus |
| 1979 | Ross River virus |
| 1980 | HTLV-1 |
| 1982 | HTLV-II |
| 1983 | HIV-1 |
| 1986 | HIV-2 |
| 1986 | Human herpesvirus 6 |
| 1989 | Hepatitis C virus |
| 1993 | Sin Nombre virus |
| 1994 | Sabia virus |
| 1995 | Equine morbillivirus |

Several factors in the emergence of these infections include the rapid urbanization of countries that have poor sanitation and water treatment facilities; a relaxation of public health measures that successfully suppressed some of these infections; the effect of "shrinking the world," due to airline travel; changing weather patterns; and the ability of some viruses to mutate rapidly (CDC, 1994; Institute of Medicine, 1992).

# EMERGING VIRUSES

## Ebola Hemorrhagic Fever

The name recognition and dread associated with the **filoviruses** is well deserved, with dramatic **hemorrhagic fevers** and very high mortality rates of 50% to 90%. The filoviruses include Marburg virus and Ebola virus (see Figure 51-1). The first recorded outbreaks of Ebola occurred in 1976 in Nzara, Sudan and Yambuku, Zaire. The name of the virus, Ebola, comes from a river east of Businga, Zaire, near the initial outbreak area (Garrett, 1994a).

Ebola appeared in Nzara during June and July 1976. The people first infected seemed to be associated with a cotton factory. Infected patients affected other areas

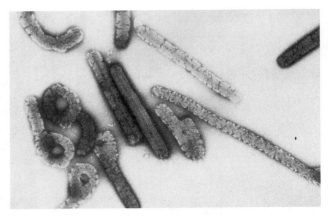

**FIGURE 51-1** Ebola virus. (Courtesy of Centers for Disease Control and Prevention, Atlanta, GA)

by going into the neighboring towns of Maridi, Tembura, and Juba, and transmitting the infections to family members. Patients were treated for fever and bleeding disorders in the hospital in Maridi. Unfortunately, infection control practices were so nonexistent that the hospital was an area of nosocomial transmission of the infections, to include 41 hospital workers. Ultimately, 284 people were infected with Ebola virus, and 151 died. (Bowen, Lloyd, Harris, Platt, Baskerville, & Vella, 1977; Feldmann, Slenczka, & Klenk, 1996; Garrett, 1994b).

About 2 months after the Sudan outbreak had begun, a man was seen in the Yambuku Mission for diarrhea and nosebleeds. He was admitted for 2 days, but his symptoms could not be stopped. He left the hospital. From that point on, several patients who had been at the hospital experienced sudden fever, bleeding from several sites, and diarrhea. The Belgian nuns at Yambuku could do nothing for the patients. In fact, the medical care provided by the nuns, in the form of injections of fluids, vitamins, and antibiotics may have drastically increased the amplitude of the outbreak, due to the lack of proper sterilization of needles and syringes. The circle of infected patients seemed to grow larger each day, until several of the nuns providing care became ill themselves. Most of those patients who became ill died. From October through December, 318 patients contracted hemorrhagic fever, and 280 died, for a mortality rate of 88% (Bowen et al., 1977; Feldmann et al., 1996).

The third outbreak occurred when a man working in Nzara was admitted to the hospital with gastrointestinal symptoms. He died shortly after admission, but not before nosocomial transmission of the Ebola virus had spread the infection throughout the hospital and to the local town. Mortality in this 2-month long outbreak was 65% (Baron, McCormick, & Zubeir, 1983).

Ebola was relatively quiet until 1989 when several cynomolgus monkeys, being held in a quarantine facility in Reston, Virginia, died. A new filovirus, named Ebola Reston, was isolated from the animals. The monkeys had been shipped from the Philippines, and had no association with Africa. This seemed to indicate that Ebola exists outside of Africa, where all other outbreaks had occurred (CDC, 1996; Feldmann et al., 1996).

There have apparently been three independent outbreaks of Ebola-Zaire in Gabon from December 1994 through January 1997. The first outbreak occurred in a camp of gold-panners in northeastern Gabon. The second outbreak, responsible for eight cases, began in February 1996, was localized in Mayibout, Gabon. The third, and most recent outbreak, was the most extensive seen in Gabon. From July 1996 to January 1997, 43 patients died from Ebola hemorrhagic fever. In contrast to the initial outbreak in Zaire in 1976, in which **nosocomial infection** was key, the outbreaks in Gabon seem to involve zoonotic transmission to humans from dead nonhuman primates. Many chimpanzees apparently died from the Ebola-Zaire infection, and humans became accidentally infected after handling the carcasses of the dead animals (Georges-Courbot et al., World Health Organization [WHO], 1997; 1996a, 1996b).

Zaire recently experienced another outbreak of Ebola-Zaire facilitated by nosocomial transmission. A charcoal worker went to a hospital in Kikwit, a city with a population of 400,000. He underwent two laparatomies for suspected typhoid fever. The patient died from complications of intra-abdominal hemorrhage. A few days later, one of his doctors died with typical Ebola symptoms. The infection spread quickly throughout the hospital, infecting many health care providers. During the 7 months of the epidemic (January–August), 315 people developed Ebola infection, and 244 (77%) died (Feldmann et al., 1996; Sanchez et al., 1995).

**Clinical Manifestations.** The incubation period of the infection is 5 to 10 days, after which patients experience sudden onset of high fever, severe headaches, chills, myalgias, nausea, vomiting, and diarrhea. Patients sometimes experience confusion and other central nervous system (CNS) symptoms.

The second week of illness is marked by either recovery or, in the majority of cases, death involving serious hemorrhagic manifestations. The patient may start to bleed from any number of sites, such as the nose, gums, eyes, and gastrointestinal tract. Death usually occurs between days 7 and 16. Postmortem examination shows that death results from hemorrhagic shock and multiorgan failure. The mortality rate for the Sudan subtype is about 50% and approximately 90% with the Zaire subtype (Feldman et al., 1996; Garrett, 1994a, 1994b; Klenck, Slenczka, & Feldman, 1995).

**Taxonomy.** Ebola virus is a member of a family Filoviridae. There are currently four subtypes: Ebola-Zaire, Ebola-Sudan, Ebola-Côte d'Ivoire, and Ebola-Reston. Ebola is an enveloped virus an with enveloped nonsegmented, negative, and single-stranded RNA. The virion is 790 to 900 nm in length and 80 nm in diameter. The surface has protein spikes, approximately 7 nm long, in regular intervals. The filamentous virus is pleomorphic, often appearing curved shapes (Jahrling, 1995; Klenck et al., 1995).

The natural reservoir of the Ebola virus has not yet been discovered. Extensive ecologic studies are currently underway in Cote d'Ivoire, Gabon, and Zaire to identify the reservoir. Since some researchers still have not excluded the possibility that Ebola might be a plant virus, one wide-scale study described results of exposing 24 plant species and 19 different animals to Ebola. None of the plants supported growth; only one bat seroconverted after being inoculated with Ebola. It is yet unclear as to whether bats may be a possible reservoir for the virus (Swanepoel et al., 1996).

**Transmission and Prevention.** The Ebola virus has been transmitted primarily through direct contact with infected fluids and secretions of infected patients. Zoonotic transmission has also occurred, with Ebola-Reston, Ebola-Côte d'Ivoire, and Ebola-Zaire in Gabon (CDC, 1996; WHO, 1996a, 1996b).

Infection control measures, including sterilization of equipment and isolation techniques have been enforced to reduce the possibility of nosocomial transmission of Ebola. Hospital staff are encouraged to wear gowns, masks, gloves, and goggles when caring for patients. Visitors access to hospitalized patients is limited, materials exposed to the patient are incinerated, and all surfaces are disinfected (CDC, 1995).

**Diagnosis and Treatment.** The virus can be cultured from serum during acute febrile phase of the illness. Liver, spleen, heart, and kidney are acceptable specimens for culture. Viral antigens may be detected enzyme-linked immunosorbent assay (ELISA) and polymerase chain reaction (PCR). Viral antibodies can be identified by ELISA and immunofluorescent antibodies (IFA). Virions can also be seen using electron microscopy during peak viremia (Klenck et al., 1995).

## Hantavirus

In May 1993, two Native Americans living in the same house died within 5 days of each other. They had been ill with general respiratory symptoms, including fever, myalgia, headache, and cough. Postmortem examination revealed bilateral pulmonary interstitial infiltrates. Initial cultures and serologies were negative for any known pathogens. Specimens were forwarded to the CDC. Screens for antibodies on the sera of the two patients indicated the pair had been exposed to an Asian hantavirus. This unusual finding led state, federal, and Navajo Nation investigators to conduct serologic testing on local inhabitants and potential vectors, including rodents. A small number of people were also seropositive for hantavirus, as were a significant number of deer mice. Gene amplification confirmed that a new strain of hantavirus was responsible for the two deaths (CDC, 1993a–e).

By the end of July, approximately 2 months since the initial reports, the new agent had been identified, diagnostic tests were available, and 18 cases of this detected. Of those 18 patients, 14 had died (CDC, 1993a). The new virus has had several names, including "Muerto Canyon Virus" and "Four Corners Virus," but is now named "**Sin Nombre**" ("No Name") **virus**. The disease caused by the virus was called **hantavirus pulmonary syndrome** (HPS) (CDC, 1993e). The CDC definition for HPS is defined as:

▶ Either febrile illness (> 38.3°C) in a previously healthy person with:

▶ Adult respiratory distress syndrome, or bilateral pulmonary interstitial infiltrates developing within 1 week of hospitalization with respiratory compromise requiring supplemental oxygen), *OR*

▶ Autopsy findings of noncardiogenic pulmonary edema resulting from an unknown respiratory illness

**Clinical Manifestations.** Hantavirus pulmonary syndrome is a distinctly different infection manifestation than hemorrhagic fever with renal syndrome (HFRS). Patients generally experience a prodrome, lasting 3 to 7 days, which includes sudden onset of fever, headache, malaise, myalgias, and cough. These flulike symptoms are often accompanied by gastrointestinal symptoms, including diarrhea, nausea, and vomiting. Many patients develop respiratory difficulties. Once admitted to a hospital, laboratory tests reveal leukocytosis, thrombocytopenia, hemoconcentration, and a left shift. Chest x-rays show diffuse pulmonary infiltrates consistent with noncardiogenic pulmonary edema. Mortality rates for HPS are 50% to 75%, with patients succumbing to acute respiratory distress syndrome (ARDS) and shock (Khan, Ksiazek, & Peters, 1996; Zaki et al., 1996).

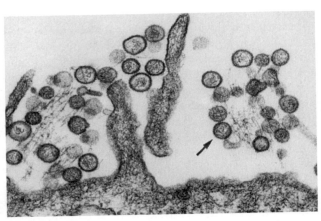

**FIGURE 51-2** Electron micrograph of hantavirus.

**Taxonomy.** The Sin Nombre virus (see Figure 51-2), causative agent for HPS, belongs to the genus *Hantavirus,* family Bunyaviridae (Chu et al., 1994). The recognition of a hantavirus-caused pulmonary syndrome has initiated a large-scale effort to determine how many other patients with pulmonary problems of unknown etiology might have had hantavirus infections. As a result, there have been multiple discoveries of new hantaviruses within the past few years. Some, like Sin Nombre, cause HPS, whereas others seem to be nonpathogenic to humans. Table 51-2 compares the new hantavirus isolates with the older, HFRS-related hantaviruses.

As seen in Table 51-2, the hantaviruses are often endemic to specific areas, generally through the specificity of their rodent reservoirs. In the United States, the reservoirs include different mice, rats, and voles (Rowe et al., 1995; Song et al., 1995). The reservoir for Sin Nombre, the deer mouse (see Figure 51-3), is found in a variety of rural surroundings; it is not typically found in urban population centers (CDC, 1995).

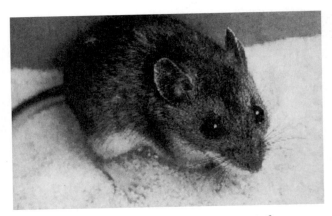

**FIGURE 51-3** The deer mouse is a reservoir for hantavirus.

**Transmission.** Infected deer mice shed Sin Nombre virus in saliva, urine, and feces. Humans usually become infected by inhaling aerosolized virus particles when entering a site containing excreta from infected mice (CDC, 1993e). The virus can also be transmitted via direct inoculation into mucous membranes and broken skin, including bites by infected animals (CDC, 1995). Sin Nombre apparently does not have a human-to-human transmission; however, a Sin Nombre-related hantavirus, the Andes hantavirus, may have been transmitted among 20 patients via person-to-person transmission (Wells et al., 1997).

Outbreaks of HPS in humans may occur indirectly as a result from weather. Navajo tribal elders told investigators that the 1993 outbreak was not the first they had seen of this disease. They recalled outbreaks in 1918 and 1936. The common factor in the years 1918, 1936, and 1993 was uncommonly high rainfalls. The increased

## Table 51–2 ► Clinical Manifestations of Hantaviruses

| Clinical Manifestation | Hantavirus | Geographic Location | Vector |
|---|---|---|---|
| Hemorrhagic fever with renal syndrome | Hantaan | Asia | *Apodemus agrarias* (striped field mouse) |
| | Seoul | Worldwide | *Rattus* spp. (brown rat) |
| | Dobrava/Belgrade | Balkans | *Apodemus flavicollis* (yellow-necked mouse) |
| Hantavirus pulmonary syndrome | Sin Nombre | United States | *Peromyscus. maniculatus* (deer mouse) |
| | Bayou | Louisiana | *Oryzomys palustris* (rice rat) |
| | Black Creek Canal | Florida | *Sigmodon hispidus* (cotton rat) |
| | New York-1 | New York | *Peromyscus leucopus* (white-footed deer mouse) |
| Nephropathia epidemica | Puumala | Europe, western Russia | *Clethrionomys glariolus* (bank vole) |
| Nonpathogenic | El Morro Canyon | United States | *Reithrodontomys megalotis* (harvest mouse) |
| | Isla Vista | California | *Microtus californicus* (California meadow vole) |
| | Thottopalayam | India | *Suncus marinus* (Indian shrew) |
| | Thailand | Thailand | *Bandicota indica* (bandicoot) |
| | Andes | Argentina | ? |
| | Prospect Hill | United States | *Microtus pennsylvanicus* (meadow vole) |

rain in the desert caused an abundance of the pinon nuts, which are a favorite food of deer mice. The high mice populations accounted for more human-mouse interaction, causing outbreaks of HPS during those years (Garrett, 1994c).

**Diagnosis and Treatment.** The prodromal stage of hantavirus infections is nonspecific. Many patients with HPS at first seem to have a flulike syndrome. If the patient admits to contact with rodents or areas where rodent wastes are likely to be found, specific testing can be used to rule out HPS. The CDC offers an enzyme immunoassay that can be used to detect specific IgM and IgG antibodies (Jenison, et al., 1994). Immunohistochemistry can detect hantavirus antigens in a variety of tissue specimens, including lung (Zaki et al., 1996). Reverse-transcriptase PCR can also be used to detect RNA in clinical specimens (CDC, 1993a–e; Hjelle et al., 1994).

The only treatment option for HPS is supportive therapy. Clinical management of symptoms is used, although control of hypotension with fluid administration can worsen pulmonary edema. Although ribavirin shows in vitro activity against Sin Nombre hantavirus, clinical studies are not promising (Khan et al., 1996; Morrison & Rathbun, 1995).

## Dengue Virus

Dengue virus is appropriately named after a Spanish version of the Swahili phrase "ki denga pepo," which implies being suddenly taken over by a spirit (Garret, 1994c). Dengue virus can cause two distinct diseases: **dengue fever** (DF) and **dengue hemorrhagic fever**

(DHF). These infections have become perhaps the most important arthropod-borne viral diseases in the world, with epidemics becoming more severe and geographically widespread (Ramirez-Ronda & Garcia, 1994) (see Figure 51-4). Accurate reporting methods are lacking, but the WHO estimates that there may be as many as 50 to 100 million cases worldwide annually and that 2.5 billion people are living in dengue-endemic areas. In 1995, 41 countries had experienced epidemics of the more severe form of the disease, DHF. Only nine countries had reported epidemics in 1970, which illustrates how dynamically the infection is spreading (Gubler & Clark, 1995; Monath, 1994; WHO, 1996c).

Dengue was first noted about 200 years ago, with epidemics in Cairo, Egypt and in Jakarta, Indonesia in 1779. In 1780 a major epidemic occurred in Philadelphia. It was during that outbreak that Doctor Benjamin Rush first referred to dengue as "breakbone fever," referring to the symptoms of aching joints (Garrett, 1994d; Gubler, 1994).

Dengue infections, often appear following conditions that result in an increase in the population of the mosquitoes, *Aedes aegypti* and *Aedes albopictus*. World War II, with accompanying massive human migrations, aerial bombing campaigns, densely populated refugee camps, and disruptions of mosquito control efforts led to a global pandemic of dengue fever after the war in Southeast Asia (Sabin, 1952). All of these factors resulted in the coexistence of all four dengue serotypes in the region. The number of children being bitten by dengue-carrying *A. aegypti* increased, which ultimately led to the first reported cases of DHF in 1954 (Philip-

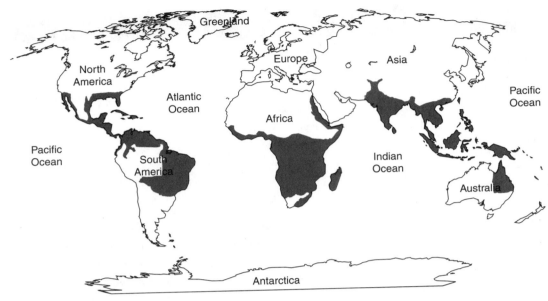

**FIGURE 51-4** Shaded areas indicate areas with endemic dengue.

pines) and 1958 (Thailand) (Hammon, Rudnick, & Sather, 1960). This new form of dengue infection then spread throughout southern Asia and appeared in the Caribbean in 1978. Cuba suffered the first epidemic of DHS in the Americas in 1981, with 24,000 cases and 158 deaths (Monath, 1994; Ramirez-Ronda & Garcia, 1994). Another 13 countries in the Americas have experienced DHF epidemics since then (Gubler & Clark, 1995).

The impact of *A. aegypti*-borne dengue in the United States is minimal because the mosquito cannot tolerate cold winters. However, the mosquito *A. albopictus* invaded the United States in the 1980s. During that time, used car and truck tires from Asia were being shipped to the United States for recapping. Many of the tires collected water while in Asia, and many of the shipments were infested with *A. albopictus*. The potential for future problems is tremendous, in that *A. albopictus* is able to transmit many of the same infections as *A. aegypti*, including dengue, and the mosquito survives winter conditions (Monath, 1994).

**Clinical Manifestations.** Clinical manifestations of dengue vary with age and other host factors (Halstead, 1992). The two distinct syndromes produced by dengue viruses are DF and DHF. Although there are exceptions, DF is usually seen in older children and adults, and DHF is seen primarily in children (Halstead, 1994).

Classic dengue fever is a self-limiting infection with an incubation period of 3 to 15 days. The infection begins as a nonspecific viral syndrome, and may initially be confused with influenza, rubella, measles, mumps, roseola infantum, or other arbovirus infections. Patients experience sudden onset of fever, chills,

myalgia, headache, and malaise. These symptoms usually last a few days, and the patient may begin to feel better before experiencing a second phase of DF, which includes reappearance of the fever, retro-orbital pain that occurs with eye movement, back pain, macular generalized rash, nausea, vomiting, diarrhea, generalized adenopathy, anorexia, and taste aberrations. (Halstead, 1992; Gubler & Trent, 1994; Monath, 1994; Ramirez-Ronda & Garcia, 1994; WHO, 1996c). Younger children, if infected with dengue, will experience either an asymptomatic infection, or a vague, viral syndrome that lacks the characteristic myalgia and arthralgia of dengue fever (Halstead, 1994).

Dengue hemorrhagic fever is the more serious manifestation associated with dengue virus infection, and usually occurs in children under 15 years of age. Symptoms of DHF include fever (possibly reaching 40°–41°C), febrile convulsions, hypovolemia, thrombocytopenia, hemorrhage, and shock. Severity of infection can vary, and the stages of DHF have been defined as: grade I, in which the patient has the symptoms of classical dengue fever along with thrombocytopenia and hemoconcentration due to capillary leakage; grade II, in which the patient may show signs of hemorrhaging; grade III, in which the patient experiences circulatory collapse; and grade IV, in which pulse and blood pressure may be undetectable. Grades III and IV are often referred to as **dengue shock syndrome** (DSS) and may occur in as many as 30% of the patients with DHF (Monath, 1994; Ramirez-Ronda & Garcia, 1994).

Patients with DHF are those who have previously been infected with one serotype of dengue virus earlier in their lifetimes and were reinfected with a different serotype. However, not all secondary exposures lead to

DHF. Some patients who are secondarily exposed to Dengue-1 usually experience signs and symptoms of classical dengue fever, rather than DHF (Halstead, 1994).

**Taxonomy.** There are four different serotypes of dengue (DEN-1, DEN-2, DEN-3, DEN-4), belonging to the genus *Flavivirus*. They are single-stranded positive-polarity RNA viruses (Monath, 1994). There is no cross-protection between serotypes, so a patient could potentially be infected with each serotype in his or her lifetime (Ramirez-Ronda & Garcia, 1994).

**Transmission and Prevention.** Transmission of dengue viruses to humans is by the bite of infected mosquitoes belonging to the genus *Aedes*. The principal mosquito vector, *A. aegypti* (Figure 51-5), is a domesticated urban mosquito that has adapted to living in close association with humans and has a worldwide distribution in the tropics as well as the southeastern United States (Gubler & Trent, 1994; Ramirez-Ronda & Garcia, 1994). *A. aegypti* is a day biting mosquito that breeds in artificial containers such as old tires, water storage vessels, and anything that collects rainwater (Ramirez-Ronda & Garcia, 1994). *A. albopictus,* which has been recently introduced into the United States from Asia, and *A. scutellaris,* complex mosquitoes found in the South and Central Pacific, are also vectors for dengue (Gubler & Trent, 1992).

Female mosquitoes acquire the infection by ingesting blood from a viremic host. The virus multiplies in the salivary glands of the mosquito and then transmits it to the next host while feeding. The mosquito vector suffers no adverse effects from the virus (Ramirez-Ronda & Garcia, 1994).

**Diagnosis and Treatment.** Viral culture is considered the gold standard for detection of dengue virus infections. The virus can be cultured in vitro using mosquito cell lines and in vivo with mosquito inoculation. Antigen capture ELISA and immunofluorescent antibody testing methods are also available. Other tests include IgG ELISA and a dot enzyme immunoassay (Ramirez-Ronda & Garcia, 1994).

Acute and convalescent sera specimens can be collected and used for the diagnosis of dengue. A fourfold increase in antibody titer between acute and convalescent sera is indicative of a dengue infection. Serology can also be used to determine the predominate serotype in a given geographic location (Ramirez-Ronda & Garcia, 1994).

Patients with DF and DHF receive supportive therapy, with bed rest and fluids. Patients are closely monitored for signs of DHF. Aggressive treatment for patients with DHF include blood volume replacement with Ringer's lactate, saline, or plasma. Transfusions may be necessary if hemorrhaging occurs (Ramirez-Ronda & Garcia, 1994).

There are currently no approved vaccines for dengue. The problems that impede vaccine development include the different serotypes, the deficiency of in vitro assays of virulence for humans, and the deficiency of an animal model for assessing viral attenuation (Ramirez-Ronda & Garcia, 1994).

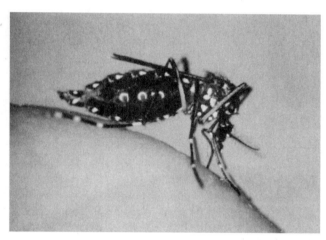

**FIGURE 51-5** *Aedes aegypti.* (Courtesy of Katz et al., *Parasitic diseases,* copyright 1982 by Springer-Verlag, New York)

## SUMMARY

▶ New diseases are emerging as a result of environmental, economic, and geographic factors.

▶ New laboratory technology has been used to resolve issues of origin, reservoirs, and transmission for some of these emerging pathogens, such as Sin Nombre, but has been little help with other emerging viral infections, such as Ebola.

▶ Modes of transmission often limit the scope of outbreaks. For instance, the fact that most serotypes of Ebola are not spread by droplets helps contain these outbreaks. Likewise, the fact that dengue is not spread by person-to-person contact limits the effects of that disease when cases do occur in areas in which the *Aedes* mosquitoes are not endemic.

▶ Outbreaks with these new infections can often be contained by infection control practices and education.

▶ Emerging infections have become a global problem that shows no sign of abating.

## CASE STUDY SEVERE RESPIRATORY ILLNESS

Two weeks after coming home from a camping trip in Arizona, a 21-year-old college student came down with a fever of 102°F and severe muscle aches. She also had a dry cough, headaches, nausea, and vomiting. Four days later the symptoms became progressively worse. Fluid began to accumulate in the lungs. Breathing became more difficult and her blood pressure began to drop. She was then intubated and put on mechanical ventilation.

Serologic and microbiologic tests on various viral and bacterial pathogens were all negative. There was mild thrombocytopenia, leukocytosis, and atypical lymphocytosis. The patient's symptoms were so severe that she had cardiopulmonary arrest and died. Testing of the autopsy specimens were insignificant.

An epidemiologic investigation is conducted. What circumstances should be investigated in regard to her companions, the campsite, and possible related cases?

### Questions:

1. What type of investigation of the deceased patient's companions would be appropriate?

2. What other investigation should be conducted?

3. What would the epidemiologist be looking for at and near the campsite?

## Review Questions

1. Emerging viral infections occur because of:
   a. changes in weather patterns.
   b. the "shrinking" of the world due to airline travel.
   c. a relaxation of public health measures.
   d. All of the above

2. Which of the following is true?
   a. The reservoir in nature for Ebola virus seems to be at least one type of primate.
   b. All of the Ebola viruses seem to be transmitted to humans several ways, including respiratory transmission while patients are hospitalized (nosocomial transmission).
   c. The mortality rates of Ebola vary with the subtypes.
   d. Ebola-Reston cannot infect humans.

3. Hantavirus pulmonary syndrome:
   a. is likely a new disease, resulting from a mutation of hantaviruses, which cause HFRS.
   b. is likely a disease that has appeared sporadically throughout the desert southwest, sometimes occurring during years of high rainfall.
   c. can result in death of the patient as a result of kidney failure, much as in HFRS.
   d. reservoir is the flying foxes.

4. Dengue viruses are:
   a. enveloped filoviruses with single, negative-stranded RNA.
   b. single-stranded RNA viruses that are members of the Bunyaviridae.
   c. members of the Paramyxoviridae; enveloped, pleomorphic virions ranging in size from 38 to 600 nm, with two layers of protein projections on the capsid surface.
   d. single-stranded positive-polarity RNA viruses, belonging to the genus *Flavivirus*.

5. Ebola viruses are:
   a. enveloped filoviruses with single, negative-stranded RNA.
   b. single-stranded RNA viruses that are members of the Bunyaviridae.
   c. members of the Paramyxoviridae; enveloped, pleomorphic virions ranging in size from 38 to 600 nm, with two layers of protein projections on the capsid surface.
   d. single-stranded positive-polarity RNA viruses, belonging to the genus *Flavivirus*.

6. Hantaviruses are:
   a. enveloped filoviruses with single, negative-stranded RNA.
   b. single-stranded RNA viruses that are members of the Bunyaviridae.

c. members of the Paramyxoviridae; enveloped, pleomorphic virions ranging in size from 38 to 600 nm, with two layers of protein projections on the capsid surface.

d. single-stranded positive-polarity RNA viruses, belonging to the genus *Flavivirus*.

7. The natural reservoir of the Ebola virus is:
   a. the Green monkey.
   b. humans only.
   c. one of several avian species.
   d. unknown.

8. Which following statement about dengue is false?
   a. The principal mosquito vector is *A. aegypti*.
   b. There are four different serotypes of Dengue.
   c. There is cross-protection between serotypes.
   d. Female mosquitoes acquire the infection.

9. All of the following statements about Hantavirus are true EXCEPT:
   a. humans become infected by inhaling aerolized virus particles.
   b. transmission may occur via direct inoculation into mucous membranes and broken skin.
   c. infected deer mice shed the virus in saliva, urine, and feces.
   d. vaccine for Hantavirus is now available.

10. Infection control measures for Ebola include:
   a. sterilization of equipment.
   b. isolation.
   c. wearing of protective equipment, i.e. gloves, gowns, and mask.
   d. All of the above.

## ▶ REFERENCES & RECOMMENDED READING

Baron, R. C., McCormick, J. B., & Zubeir, O. A. (1983). Ebola hemorrhagic fever in southern Sudan: Hospital dissemination and intrafamilial spread. *Bulletin of the World Health Organization, 61,* 997–1003.

Bowen, E. T. W., Lloyd, G., Harris, W. J., Platt, G. S. Baskerville, A., Vella, E. E. (1977). Viral hemorrhagic fever in southern Sudan and northern Zaire. *Lancet 1,* 571–573.

Centers for Disease Control and Prevention. (1993a). Outbreak of acute illness—Southwestern United States, 1993. *Morbidity and Mortality Weekly Report, 42,* 421–424.

Centers for Disease Control and Prevention. (1993b). Update: Outbreak of acute illness—Southwestern United States, 1993. *Morbidity and Mortality Weekly Report, 42,* 441–443.

Centers for Disease Control and Prevention. (1993c). Update: Outbreak of acute illness—Southwestern United States, 1993. *Morbidity and Mortality Weekly Report, 42,* 477–479.

Centers for Disease Control and Prevention. (1993d). Update: Outbreak of acute illness—Southwestern United States, 1993. *Morbidity and Mortality Weekly Report, 42,* 570–571.

Centers for Disease Control and Prevention. (1993e). Update: Outbreak of acute illness—Southwestern United States, 1993. *Morbidity and Mortality Weekly Report, 42,* 816–820.

Centers for Disease Control and Prevention. (1994). *Addressing emerging infectious disease threats: A prevention strategy for the United States.* Atlanta, GA: Author.

Centers for Disease Control and Prevention (1995, March). Hanta illness in the United States. http://main.street.net/hantavirus.html

Centers for Disease Control and Prevention. (1996a). Ebola virus hemorrhagic fever: General information. http://www.cdc.gov/ncidod/diseases/virlfvr/ebolainf.htm

Centers for Disease Control and Prevention. (1996b). Filoviruses in nonhuman primates: Overview of the investigation in Texas. URL:http://www.cdc.gov/ncidod/virlfvr/ebola528.htm

Centers for Disease Control and Prevention. (1996c). Hantavirus pulmonary syndrome and Sin Nombre virus. Online: http://www.cdc.gov/ncidod/diseases/hanta/slideset/hanta08f:htm

http://www.cdc.gov/ncidod/disease/hanta/slideset/hanta09f.htm

Chu, Y. K., Rossi, C., LeDuc, J. W., Lee, H. W., Schmaljohn, C. S., & Dalrymple, J. M. (1994). Serological relationships among viruses in the Hantavirus genus, family Bunyaviridae. *Virology, 198,* 196–204.

Feldmann, H., Slenczka, W., Klenk, H.-D. (1996). Emerging and reemerging of filoviruses. *Archives of Virology* (Suppl) *11,* 77–100.

Garrett, L. (1994a). Yambuku. *In the coming plague* (pp 254–259). Penguin Books.

Garrett L. (1994b). N'zara. In *The coming plague* (pp 192–221). Penguin Books.

Garrett, L. (1994c). All in good haste. In *The coming plague* (pp 528–549). Penguin Books.

Garrett, L. (1994d). Microbe magnets. In *The coming plague* (pp. 254–259). Penguin Books.

Georges-Courbot, M.-C., Sanchez, A., Lu, C.-Y., Baize, S., Leroy, E., Lansout-Soukate, J., Bénissan, C., Georges, A. J., Trappier, S. G., Zaki, S. R., Swanepoel, R., Leman, P. A., Rollin, P. E., Peters, C. J., Nichol, S. T., Ksiazek, T. G. (1997). Isolation and phylogenetic characterization of Ebola viruses causing different outbreaks in Gabon. *Emerging Infectious Diseases, 3,* 59–62.

Gubler, D. J. (1994). Perspectives on the prevention and control of dengue hemorrhagic fever. *Kaohsiung Journal of Medical Science, 10,* S15–S18.

Gubler, D. J., & Clark, G. (1995). Dengue/dengue hemorrhagic fever: The emergence of a global health problem. *Emerging Infectious Diseases, 1,* 55–57.

Gubler, D. J., Trent, D. W. (1994). Emergence of epidemic dengue/dengue hemorrhagic fever as a public health problem in the Americas. *Infectious Agents and Disease, 2,* 383–396.

Halstead, S. B. (1994). Dengue in the health transition. *Kaohsiung Journal of Medical Science, 10,* S2–S14.

Halstead, S. B. (1992). Dengue viruses. In S. L. Gorbach, J. G. Bartlett, N. R. Blacklow (Eds.). *Infectious diseases* (pp 1830–1834). Philadelphia: Saunders.

Hammon W., Rudnick, A., & Sather, G. E. (1960). Viruses associated with hemorrhagic fevers of the Philippines and Thailand. *Science, 131,* 1102.

Hjelle, B., Spiropoulou, C. F., Torrez-Martinez, N., Morzunov, S., Peters, C. J., & Nichol, S. T. (1994). Detection of Muerto Canyon virus RNA in peripheral blood mononuclear cells from patients with hantavirus pulmonary syndrome. *Journal of Infectious Disease, 170,* 1013–1017.

Institute of Medicine. (1992). *Emerging infections: Microbial threats in the United States.* Washington, DC: National Academy Press.

Jahrling, P. B. (1995). Filoviruses and arenaviruses. In *Manual of clinical microbiology* (6th ed.) pp 1071–1081. ASM Press, Washington, DC: ASM Press.

Jenison, S., Yamada, T., Morris, C., Anderson, B., Torrez-Martinez, N., Keller, N., & Hjelle, B. (1994). Characterization of human antibody responses to Four Corners hantavirus among patients with hantavirus pulmonary syndrome. *Journal of Virology, 68,* 3000–3006.

Khan, A. S., Ksiazek, T. G., & Peters, C. J. (1996). Hantavirus pulmonary syndrome. *Lancet, 347,* 739–741.

Klenk H-D., Slenczka, W., & Feldmann, H. (1995). In R. G. Webster & A. Granoff (Eds.). *Marburg and Ebola viruses.* Academic Press.

LeDuc J. W., Childs, J. E., & Glass, G. E. (1992). *Annual Review of Public Health 13,* 79–98.

LeGuenno, B., Formentry, P., Wyers, M., Gounon, P., Walker, F., & Boesch, C. (1995). Isolation and partial characterization of a new strain of Ebola virus. *Lancet, 345,* 1271–1274.

Monath, T. P. (1994). Dengue: The risk to developed and developing countries. *Proceedings of the National Academy of Sciences USA, 91,* 2395–2400.

Morrison, Y. Y., & Rathbun, R. C. (1995). Hantavirus pulmonary syndrome: The Four Corners disease. *Annals of Pharmacotherapy, 29,* 57–65.

Murray, K., O'Sullivan, J., Selvey, L., Selleck, P., Hyatt, A., & Gould, A. (1995a). A novel morbillivirus pneumonia of horses and its transmission to humans. *Emerging Infectious Diseases, 1,* 31–33.

Murray, K., Selleck, P., Hooper, P., Hyatt, A., Gould, A., Gleeson, L., Westbury, H., Hiley, L., Selvey, L., Rodwell, B., & Ketterer, P. (1995b). A morbillivirus that caused fatal disease in horses and humans. *Science, 268,* 94–97.

Ramirez-Ronda, C. H., Garcia, C. D. (1994). Dengue in the Western Hemisphere. *Infectious Disease Clinics of North America, 8,* 107–127.

Rowe, J. E., St. Jeor, S. C., Riolo, J., Otteson, E. W., Monroe, M. C., Henderson, W. W., et al. (1995). Coexistence of several novel hantaviruses in rodents indigenous to North America. *Virology, 213,* 122–130.

Sabin, A. B. (1952). Research on dengue during World War II. *American Journal of Tropical Medicine, 1,* 30.

Sanchez, A., Ksiazek, T. G., Rollin, P. E., Peters, C. J., Nichol, S. T., Khan, A. S., & Mahy, B. W. J. (1995). Reemergence of Ebola virus in Africa. *Emerging Infectious Diseases, 1,* 96–97.

Schwartz, D. A., & Bryan, R. T. (1996). Infectious disease pathology and emerging infections. Are we ready? *Archives of Pathology and Laboratory Medicine, 120,* 117–123.

Song, W., Torrez-Martinez, N., Irwin, W., Harrison, F. J., Davis, R., Ascher, M., et al. (1995). Isla Vista virus: A genetically novel hantavirus of the California vole *Microtus californicus. Journal of General Virology, 76,* 3195–3199.

Swanepoel, R., Leman, P. A., Burt, F. J., Zachariades, N. A., Braack, L. E., Ksiazek, T. G., Rollin, P. E., Zaki, S. R., & Peters, C. J. (1996). Experimental inoculation of plants and animals with Ebola virus. *Emerging Infectious Diseases, 2,* 321–325.

Wells, R. M., Estani, S. S., Yadon, Z. E., Enria, D., et al. (1997). An unusual hantavirus outbreak in Southern Argentina: Person-to-person transmission? *Emerging Infectious Diseases, 3*(2) ftp://ftp.cdc.gov/pub/Eid/vol3no2/ascii/wells.txt

World Health Organization. (1996a). Outbreak of Ebola haemorrhagic fever in Gabon officially declared over. *Weekly Epidemiological Record, 71,* 125–126.

World Health Organization. (1996b). Ebola haemorrhagic fever—Gabon. *Weekly Epidemiological Record, 71,* 320.

World Health Organization (1996, May). Dengue and dengue haemorrhagic fever (On-line) available: http://www.who.ch/programmes/inf/facts/fact117.htm

Young, P. L., Halpin, K., Selleck, P. W., Field, H., Gravel, J. L., Kelly, M. A., & Mackenzie, J. S. (1996). Serologic evidence for the presence in Pteropus bats of a paramyxovirus related to equine morbillivirus. *Emerging Infectious Diseases, 2,* 239–240.

Zaki, S. R., Khan, A. S., Goodman, R. A., Armstrong, L. R., Greer, P. W., Coffield, L. M., Ksiazek, T. G., Rollin, P. E., Peters, C. J., & Khabbaz, R. F. (1996). Retrospective diagnosis of hantavirus pulmonary syndrome, 1978–1993. *Archives of Pathology and Laboratory Medicine, 120,* 134–139.

# ►GLOSSARY

**abscess** local purulent reaction in response to infection; localized collection of pus in tissue; localized infection associated with pus.

**acid-alcohol** a combination of acid and alcohol used as a decolorizer in some staining techniques, such as the Ziehl-Neelsen and Kinyoun methods.

**acid-fast bacillus** bacteria having the lipid mycolic acid in their cell walls, for example, *Mycobacterium* and *Nocardia*. These organisms stain "acid-fast" with the Ziehl-Neelsen and other related staining techniques.

**acid-fast stain** differential stain used to distinguish bacteria that are not decolorized by acid alcohol.

**acidic dye** dye consisting of negative charged ions.

**acquired immunity** immunity acquired during the lifetime of the individual to produce antibodies specific to a particular antigen.

**actinomycetoma** mycetomas associated with aerobic actinomycetes.

**acute infection** initial stages of an infection in which symptoms are apparent; not chronic.

**acute meningitis** acute inflammation of the meninges, specifically the leptomeninges and the subarachnoid space in the brain, with clinical signs and symptoms occurring within a matter of a few hours.

**acute urethral syndrome** urinary tract infection characterized by pyuria and a low-level bacteriuria.

**acyclovir** nucleoside analogue (acycloguanasine) used for treating herpes simplex virus infections by interfering with virally coded thymidine kinase and DNA polymerase activities. Acyclovir is virocidal.

**adhesins** structures on the bacterial cell surface by which they adhere to specific receptors (usually glycoproteins or glycolipids) on mammalian cells. Adhesins facilitate bacterial colonization of various parts of the body.

**aerobe, obligate** an organism requiring oxygen for growth.

**aerotolerance** ability of an organism to tolerate oxygen, usually resulting in poor growth.

**aerotolerant anaerobe** those anaerobic bacteria that show limited growth in room air or in a 5% to 10% $CO_2$ incubator but show good growth under anaerobic conditions.

**agar** derivative of algae used to produce a solidifying agent for media.

**alginate polysaccharide** mucoid outer layer of polysaccharide that contains acetylated disaccharide units resembling components that are found in algae. It is often produced by strains of *Pseudomonas aeruginosa* that are isolated from patients with cystic fibrosis.

**α-hemolysis** incomplete lysis of red blood cells seen as greenish discoloration of media.

**amantadine** antiviral approved for use in influenza A infections. It is best when used prophylactically and interferes with viral entry into cells.

**amastigote** nonflagellate, intracellular, morphologic stage in the development of hemoflagellates, resembling the typical adult form of *Leshmania*.

**ambient** referring to the surrounding environment, usually refers to room air.

**amebiasis** infection with *Entamoeba histolytica* that is characterized by abdominal pain and gas, dysentery, fever, and hepatomegaly.

**amebic dysentery** dysentery caused by *Entamoeba histolytica*.

**ameboma** flask-shaped lesion produced by *Entamoeba histolytica* when the intestinal mucosa is penetrated by proteolytic enzymes secreted by the protozoan.

**amnionitis** inflammation of the amnion.

**amniotic fluid** fluid that bathes the fetus inside the amniotic sac of pregnant women.

**anaerobiasis** establishment of an anaerobic environment.

**anaerobic** without oxygen.

**anaerobic culture** inoculation of specimen onto specialized media and incubation in an oxygen-free environment in an effort to isolate bacteria that grow only in the absence of oxygen.

**annellide** a supporting structure giving rise to conidia. As the conidia are produced the annellide elongates, producing a tapered tip.

**anthrax** an infectious disease of cattle, sheep, and other mammals caused by the bacterium *Bacillus anthracis*, transmitted to humans by the handling of wool and other animal products; characterized by dark boils that erupt on the skin of the infected human.

**antibiotic** chemical substance biosynthesized by one organism that can kill or inhibit another organism.

**antibodies** protein substances produced by a host in response to, and designed to inactivate or destroy, an organism or other foreign substance introduced into the host.

**antibody** a glycoprotein produced by B cells in response to a specific antigen.

**anticoagulants** chemical (EDTA, heparin, etc.) that will prevent the clotting reaction in whole blood.

**antigen** a substance that elicits antibody production.

**antigenic drift** minor antigenic changes that occur in the influenza virus hemagglutinin and neuramindase enzymes.

**antigenic shift** major antigenic changes that occur in the influenza virus hemagglutinin and neuraminidase enzymes. Such changes may cause new epidemics to occur.

**antimicrobial** chemotherapeutic agent that is either naturally produced or partially or totally manufactured in a pharmaceutical environment designed for the purpose of killing or inhibiting microorganisms.

**antiviral chemotherapy** clinical use of chemical that inhibits viral growth in such a way as to be beneficial to and tolerated by the patient.

**Apicomplexa** phylum of protozoans having complex life cycles often with alternation of generations.

**apophysis** collar-like structure just below the columella of a sporangiophore.

**arthroconidia** boxcar-like conidia formed by modification of a hyphal cell.

**arthropod vector** insect or arachnid that can transmit disease; insect that can transmit a viral or bacterial organism from one host to another.

**ascariasis** human infection with the nematode, *Ascaris lumbricoides*.

**Aschelminthes** the roundworms.

**Ascomycota** phylum of fungi that produce sexual ascospores.

**ascospore** sexual spore arising from and contained within a sac called an ascus.

**aseptate hyphae** fungal hyphae lacking crosswalls, or septa, between nuclei. This results in a multinucleate structure characteristic of zygomycetes.

**aseptic technique** series of steps used to prevent contamination of microbiologic cultures and personnel.

**aseptically** performed using sterile technique, i.e., in such a manner as to prevent the introduction of contaminants.

**aspiration** withdrawal, by suction, of fluid from a body cavity.

**asymptomatic bacteriuria** urinary tract infection characterized by the lack of pyuria and dysuria.

**ATP-energy parasites** chlamydia are parasitic in eukaryotic host cells because they are unable to produce or store energy in the form of ATP necessary for growth.

**atypical pneumonia** relatively mild pneumonia seen primarily in children and young adults that is caused by *Mycoplasma pneumoniae*. Patients often remain ambulatory, and hence it is sometimes referred to as "walking" pneumonia.

**automated reagin test (ART)** nontreponemal test that detects reagin antibodies in the serum of persons infected with *Treponema*.

**axial filament** flagella-like structure that provides motility to spirochetes.

**babesosis** malaria-like infection caused by *Babesia* species.

**Bacille-Calmette-Guerin** a vaccine made from live *Mycobacterium bovis* used in developing countries primarily to help prevent childhood cases of tuberculosis.

**bacillus** (pl. bacilli) rod-shaped bacterial cells.

**bacteremia** presence of bacteria in the bloodstream.

**bacterial vaginosis (BV)** polymicrobial infection in females characterized by a foul-smelling vaginal discharge; nonspecific vaginitis.

**bacteriocidal** a process that damages the cell in an irreversible manner so that cell death occurs.

**bacteriocins** small substances produced by certain bacteria that kill other strains of the same or similar species.

**bacteriuria** presence of bacteria in the urine; may or may not cause symptoms.

**balanced salt solution** saline-based solution, used in cell culture, that contains additional chemicals to provide a physiologic-like medium that provides optimal protection against cell culture lysis.

**balantidiasis** also called balantidium dysentery. Intestinal infection with *Balantidium coli* that is characterized by dysentery.

**Bancroftian filariasis** human infection with *Wucheria bancrofti* and other filariids.

**Barbour-Stoenner-Kelley (BSK) broth** complex, enriched media used for the cultivation of *Borrelia*.

**basic dye** dye consisting of positive charged ions.

**Basidiomycota** phylum of fungi that produce sexual basidiospores; the "club fungi."

**basidiospore** sexual spore formed on a club-shaped structure called a basidium.

**Bell's palsy** paralysis of the facial nerve due to a variety of causes.

**ß-hemolysis** total lysis or destruction of the red blood cells in a blood agar plate, resulting in a clear area around a colony.

**ß-lactamase** enzyme produced by some species of bacteria that cleaves the ß-lactam ring of penicillin rendering the drug ineffective.

**binomial** "two," as in the binomial system of nomenclature that assigns two names (genus and species) to each organism.

**biofilm** refers to *Pseudomonas aeruginosa* growth in slimy microcolonies along the bronchi of patients with compromised respiratory function.

**biphasic** blood culture media devices that contain both broth and agar.

**black water fever** symptom of some malaria cases in which the urine is darkened due to the presence of the malarial pigment, hemozoin.

**blepharitis** inflammation of the eyelid.

**blind subculture** subculture of blood culture broth onto agar plates performed after about 24 hours of incubation even without visible evidence of growth in the broth.

**blood–brain barrier** barrier in the brain that help to protect the central nervous system from infections by controlling the passage of various blood components into the cerebrospinal fluid.

**blood culture** laboratory cultivation of blood for the recovery of bacteria or fungi, usually in two bottles of broth.

**blue-green pus** pus that has a distinctive blue-green color due to the production of pyocyanin and pyoverdin by *Pseudomonas aeruginosa* infections in wounds and burns.

**bright-field microscope** conventional microscope in which the light source is below the objects being viewed.

**Brownian movement** vibrational movement exhibited by bacteria.

**buboes** swollen lymph glands that occur in the inguinal region, frequently present in genital tract infections.

**budding** type of asexual reproduction exhibited by yeast. After nuclear division a small bulge, or bud, develops on the parent cell. The bud, or daughter cell, enlarges to approximately the same size as the parent cell.

**calabar swelling** a temporary nodule caused by the filarial nematode, *Loa loa*.

**CAMP test** a test that uses the diffusable, heat-stable extracellular streptococcal protein that acts synergistically with staphylococcal ß-hemolysin on sheep or ox erythrocytes; a positive test is an arrowhead pattern of hemolysis adjacent to the staphylococcal streak.

**campy BAP medium** a selective medium that contains 10% sheep blood and cephalothin in addition to the three antimicrobial agents present in Skirrow's agar (see below). It is used for isolation of *Campylobacter* species.

**capnophile** requires high carbon dioxide for optimal growth.

**capnophilic** organisms preferring increased concentrations of carbon dioxide.

**capsid** protein coat surrounding the viral nucleic acid (genome).

**caratae** (aka pinta) skin infection caused by *Treponema carateum*. This disease is commonly seen in Central and South America and without treatment eventually causes a permanent disfiguring mottling of the skin.

**Cary-Blair transport medium** a medium used for prolonging survival of *V. cholerae* and *Campylobacter* species when there is delay between specimen collection and culturing. It is a modification of Stuart's transport medium.

**catalase** an enzyme present in many bacterial species that prevents the toxic buildup of the metabolic end product, hydrogen peroxide.

**catalase test** laboratory test to detect the bacterial production of the enzyme catalase; catalase liberates oxygen from hydrogen peroxide.

**CDC** Centers for Disease Control and Prevention

**cDNA** synthetic strand of DNA that is complementary to the RNA sequence found in a messenger RNA molecule.

**cell cultures** laboratory preparations of mammalian cells growing in vitro, in either a monolayer or suspension condition, and used as a host to propagate viruses for diagnosis, vaccine development or for life cycle studies.

**cell wall active agents** chemotherapeutic agents used to treat microbial diseases that work by disrupting the synthesis or function of microbial cell walls.

**central nervous system (CNS)** system consisting of the brain, spinal cord, and corresponding nerves.

**cercariae** free-swimming larval form of some helminths.

**cerebrospinal fluid (CSF)** fluid in the subarachnoid space that surrounds the brain and the spinal cord.

**cerebrospinal fluid shunt** surgical diversion of abnormal cerebrospinal fluid accumulation in the brain to another area of the body.

**Cestoda** the tapeworms.

**cfu (colony-forming units)** viable organisms that grow and produce visible colonies; used in reporting results of quantitative cultures.

**chagoma** red, raised, painful lesion that is the initial symptom seen in Chagas' disease.

**chancre** primary lesion seen in syphilis that develops at the sight of initial infection.

**chemiluminescent** emission of light as the result of a chemical reaction.

**chemiluminometry** measuring the light energy emitted from the degradation of a labeled chemical compound.

**chitin** a complex carbohydrate that is a component of the cell wall of molds and the exoskeleton of insects; hard polysaccharide substance found within cell walls of some fungi.

**chlamydoconidia** enlarged, round conidia within or at the end of hyphae.

**chlamydospore** an enlarged, thick-walled structure found within or at the end of pseudohyphae of some yeasts. A misnomer as the structure is not actually a spore, but a type of conidium. The term is presently in conventional use when describing the microscopic morphology of yeasts on cornmeal agar.

**cholera toxin** an enterotoxin secreted primarily by the *V. cholerae* O1 serogroup. It is a complex polypeptide that induces the hypersecretion of fluid by increasing the intracellular level of cAMP. The toxin is also known as choleragen.

**cholera** disease caused by the organism *Vibrio cholerae;* symptoms include a severe "rice-water" diarrhea and life-threatening loss of fluids and electrolytes.

**cholesterol** fatty substance found in animal fats and oils. It is incorporated into the triple-layered membrane of mycoplasmas.

**chorioamnionitis** inflammation of the fetal membrane.

**chromatodial body** inclusions found in some cysts of *Entamoeba histolytica* that are made primarily of crystalline RNA. They are elongated and may be short or almost as long as the diameter of the cyst. Chromatodial bodies may have round or squared ends.

**chromatography** a method used to separate components of a mixture and to quantify them.

**chromoblastomycosis** specific verrucose or wartlike skin infection caused by certain dematiaceous (pigmented) fungi.

**chromomycosis** general term referring to any infection caused by dematiaceous (pigmented) fungi.

**chronic ambulatory peritoneal dialysis (CAPD)** fluid that is injected into the peritoneal cavity and removed to eliminate the body's waste products for those with renal disease.

**chronic meningitis** meningitis with clinical symptoms lasting for at least 4 weeks and often occurring in persons who are immunocompromised.

**Ciliophora** phylum of protozoans that are motile by cilia and reproduce by asexual fission or sexual conjugation.

**class** taxonomic group below phylum and above order.

**classic biotype** the original biotype of *V. cholerae* O1. It causes more severe cholera than the more recently identified eltor biotype.

**classification** the placement of organisms into categories with other related organisms.

**CLED medium** a *c*ystine-*l*actose-*e*lectrolyte-*d*eficient medium that inhibits the swarming of highly motile *Proteus* species.

**cleistothecium** a saclike reproductive structure that contains asci and ascospores.

**clinical specimen** substance (blood, urine, stool, swab of infected area, etc.) removed from a patient and submitted to the laboratory for examination.

**clinically significant** microorganism recovered from a blood culture that is interpreted to be the cause of the infections rather than a contaminant.

**clue cells** epithelial cells covered with tiny, gram-variable bacilli, found in vaginal secretions of patients with bacterial vaginosis; vaginal cells covered with the bacterium, *Gardnerella vaginalis* in vaginal fluid.

**coagulase** an enzyme that causes the clotting, or coagulation, of plasma treated with sodium citrate (which prevents the plasma from spontaneously coagulating).

**coagulase-negative staphylococci (CNS)** species of *Staphylococcus* that lack the enzyme to coagulate citrated rabbit plasma.

**coagulase test** laboratory test to detect the bacterial production of the enzyme coagulase; coagulase causes clotting of fibrinogen.

**coccus** (pl. cocci) round bacterial cells.

**coenocytic** fungal hyphae lacking crosswalls (septae) between nuclei.

**cold-agglutinin syndrome** collection of symptoms and signs seen in individuals with high serum titers of agglutinating IgM antibodies that react best in the cold (<37°C). *Mycoplasma pneumoniae* is among the infectious agents that can induce the syndrome.

**cold enrichment** a procedure that is particularly useful for epidimiologic studies when specimens are contaminated with other flora; the specimen is placed at 4°C for several weeks to months, with subculturing at frequent intervals. Useful in isolating *Listeria* from placenta and other tissue.

**colonize (colonization)** the process by which an organism takes up residence in part of the body, but does no immediate harm or damage to the host.

**colony** visible growth on solid media.

**colorimetry** detecting color changes of pH indicators after microbial substrate utilization.

**comma-shaped rods** a term that applies to the curved cellular morphology of gram-negative bacteria that are most commonly classified in the *Vibrionaceae* family.

**commensal** microorganism considered to be nonpathogenic, not causing human disease.

**commensals** organisms that colonize a host.

**complement fixation** serologic test that measures antibodies against viruses and must combine with serum complement proteins to cause destruction of the antigen.

**complicated urinary tract infections** infection usually caused by a structural or medical problem. These infections tend to be difficult to resolve with antimicrobial treatment.

**compound O/129** 2,4-diamino-6,7-diisopropylpteridine phosphate, a compound that inhibits the growth of *V. cholerae,* but not certain other related organisms. However, resistant strains of *V. cholerae* are reported in certain parts of the world.

**congenital syphilis** form of syphilis acquired by transplacental infection of *Treponema pallidum* subspecies *pallidium* from an infected mother to the fetus. If untreated the disease may result in blindness, deafness, or death.

**conidiophore** a stalklike structure arising from the hyphae from which conidia are produced.

**conidium** (pl. conidia) asexual sporelike structures of fungi not formed by cleavage or conjugation.

**conjugation** the transfer of genetic information involving cell-to-cell contact seen in some bacterial and protozoan species.

**conjunctivitis** inflammation of the conjunctiva.

**containment** the process of preventing the spread of harmful agents.

**conventional** standard method of performing a test, on which newer, rapid modifications are based.

**copulatory bursa** specialized reproductive structures found on male pinworms.

**coracidia** larval form of some helminths.

**coryneform** term denoting a club-shaped bacillus or an irregular shaped gram-positive rod.

**cost effective** procedure that, for the cost of labor, supplies, and equipment used, provides a relatively large amount of information that is relevant to the treatment of a patient.

**counterstain** dye used to color items not stained by the primary stain.

**cryptococcal antigen** capsular antigen on *cryptococcus neoformans* that can be detected by the direct antigen detection test.

**cryptosporidiosis** a (usually) self-limiting intestinal disease (in immunocompetent individuals) caused by *Cryptosporidium parvum*. It has become one of the more important opportunistic infections in patients with AIDS.

**culture** growth of microorganisms on media.

**culture media** media used for growth of microorganisms.

**cutaneous** pertaining to the skin.

**cyst** the dormant, often resistant, stage in the life cycle of some protozoans.

**cysticerci** encysted form of some tapeworms.

**cystic fibrosis** inherited disease that is characterized by excessive buildup of mucus in the lungs.

**cystitis** infection of the urinary bladder.

**cytopathic effect (CPE)** damage to host cells as a result of viral growth within those cells.

**dark-field microscope** microscope in which objects are viewed against a dark background using reflected or refracted light.

**decolorized** stain removed.

**decontamination** a method for reducing the number of organisms below that which can produce disease.

**definitive host** (final host) the host in which the adult form (sexually reproducing form) of a parasite resides.

**definitive identification** complete identification of an organism, using confirmatory tests, biochemicals, and other means.

**dematiaceous** fungus that has dark hyphae; fungi that contain melanin pigment in the hyphal walls.

**Dengue fever/dengue hemorrhagic fever/dengue shock syndrome** range of infections, from mildest to most severe, caused by dengue virus.

**dermatophyte** a member of the genus *Trichophyton, Epidermophyton,* or *Microsporum,* which has adapted to keratin and infects skin, hair, and nails.

**dermis** layer of skin underlying the epidermis, consisting of a dense bed of vascular connective tissue.

**descriptive identification** very general categorization of an organism based primarily on microscopic and colony morphology.

**Deuteromycota** phylum of fungi sometimes called the "fungi imperfecta" due to the lack of an observable sexual stage.

**differential media** (indicator media) growth media used to distinguish between types of bacteria; bacteriologic medium that contains sugars or other biochemical substrates and an indicator system showing utilization of the substrates by microorganisms.

**differential stain** stain that distinguishes bacteria with varying cell wall contents.

**dilution streaking** to streak a plate so that the inoculum is dispersed over the surface of the plate to provide isolated colonies.

**dimorphic** two forms of growth seen in some species of fungi that is influenced by environmental factors such as temperature. The saprophytic phase is a mold that is found in the natural habitat. The parasitic phase is found in infected tissues and represents an adaptation to an unfavorable environment, including elevated temperature. The parasitic phase is usually a yeast except for *Coccidioides immitis,* which becomes a spherule with endospores.

**dioecious** species in which the reproduction organs of the different sexes are located in different organisms.

**diphtheria** a toxin-mediated infectious disease caused by *Corynebacterium diphtheriae;* an acute, contagious, febrile illness characterized by inflammation of the oropharynx, formation of a pseudomembrane; can lead to cardiac and nerve damage.

**diphtheroid** microscopic morphology resembling the diphtheria bacillus; resembling diphtheria, or any bacteria that resembles the diphtheria bacillus but does not produce the diphtheria toxin. Chinese letters, due to snapping after cell division.

**direct antigen detection test (DADT)** test used for the rapid detection of bacterial antigens in cerebrospinal fluid, urine, and serum, based on latex agglutination and coagglutination of antigen-antibody reactions.

**direct fluorescent-antibody test for *T. pallidum* (DFA-TP)** procedure used to diagnose syphilis in which the specimen is fixed on a slide and fluorescein-labeled antibodies are added. After a brief incubation the slide is rinsed to remove any unbound antibody and examined under a fluorescence microscope for yellow-green fluorescence.

**disinfection** removal or destruction of harmful or pathogenic organisms.

**disseminated** refers to an infection that has spread from its initial focus to other parts of the body, usually through the bloodstream or lymphatic system.

**diurnal periodicity** microfilariae are present in the bloodstream during the day.

**division** taxonomic category that falls below kingdom and above class; also called phylum.

**DNA polymerase** enzyme used to produce new strands of DNA. These may be coded for by mammalian cells, bacteria, or viruses.

**dracunculisis** infection with a species of worm in the family Dracunculidae.

**droplet nuclei** infectious droplets 1.0 to 5.0 μm in diameter produced when a person with tuberculosis of the lungs sneezes, coughs, or speaks. The droplets may be inhaled by others sharing the airspace with the diseased individual.

**dysentery** diarrheal disease characterized by abdominal pain, inflammation, and presence of blood and mucus in the stool. *Shigella dysenteriae,* as well as a number of other infectious agents, can induce it. In this case, diarrhea is caused by the invasive nature of the microorganism.

**dysuria** occurrence of pain during urination. Indicative of infection.

**early Lyme disease (acute Lyme disease)** occurs 3 days to 1 month after the bite of a *Borrelia*-infected *Ixodes* tick and is characterized by headache, fatigue, chills and fever, myalgia and joint pain, swollen lymph nodes, and a skin rash called erythema migrans.

**eclipse phase** component of the viral life cycle, in which all events are occurring at the molecular level. No evidence of viral particles would be seen if examined by electron microscopy.

**ecthyma gangrenosum** cutaneous syndrome seen in some individuals infected with *Pseudomonas aeruginosa*. It is characterized by the appearance of maculopapular skin lesions that eventually become necrotic in the center because of invasion and destruction of blood vessels by the organisms.

**ectothrix** infection of hair in which the fungus is located on the outer surface of the hair.

**elastase** enzyme produced by *Pseudomonas aeruginosa* that digests elastin in the lung and arterial walls.

**elementary body** infectious unit of *Chlamydia* organisms.

**elephantiasis** body parts grossly swollen, associated with *Wucheria bancrofti* infection.

**Ellinghausen, McCullough, Johnson, and Harris Media (EMJH)** selective, semisolid media used for the cultivation of *Leptospira*.

**Eltor biotype** *V. cholerae* O1 that differs from the original classic biotype in certain biochemical and other reactions. It is the cause of recent pandemics of cholera.

**emerging diseases** new or changing diseases.

**emerging viral infections** infections caused by newly described viruses, or occur in different populations, or in new geographic areas.

**emetic** type of a food-poisoning caused by *Bacillus cereus* characterized by severe nausea and vomiting, as opposed to the diarrheal type; both due to the spores that survive normal cooking temperatures.

**empyema** accumulation of pus in a body cavity; accumulation of pus in the chest cavity, between the chest wall and lung.

**endemic** chronic, low-level presence of disease, or disease-causing agents in a defined area; native, or habitually present in a certain area because of environmental conditions.

**endemic relapsing fever** tick-borne relapsing fever caused by three species of *Borrelia* in the United States.

**endogenous** developing from within the body.

**endospore** spore found within another structure such as a spherule; the thick-walled dormant stage of certain species of gram-positive bacteria including the genera *Bacillus* and *Clostridium*. Endospores are extremely resistant to high temperatures and some toxic substances.

**endothrix** infection of hair in which the fungus has penetrated inside the hair shaft.

**enteric fever** *see typhoid fever.*

**enteroaggregative *E. coli*** (EAEC) strains of *E. coli* that cause acute and chronic diarrheal disease with watery stools. Seen primarily in developing countries. Specific virulence factors have not been well characterized.

**enterobiasis** human infection with the pinworm, *Enterobius vermicularis.*

**enterocolitis** diarrheal disease due to infection with certain *Salmonella* and a few other enteric organisms. Nausea, vomiting, headache, and low-grade fever are characteristic manifestation.

**enterohemorrhagic *E. coli*** (EHEC) these strains of E. coli, especially the O157:H7 serotype, produce a bloody diarrhea (hemorrhagic colitis) and hemolytic uremic syndrome. Verotoxin is a major virulence factor that is produced by the organisms.

**enteroinvasive *E. coli*** (EIEC) strains of *E. coli* that invade the epithelial cells of the intestinal mucosa. They often express the O112 antigen. Infection produces a shigellosis-like disease, especially in children in developing countries.

**enteropathogenic *E. coli*** (EPEC) strains of *E. coli* that are often implicated in diarrheal disease of infants. These organisms frequently express O111 and O125 antigens, as well as adherence factors by which they bind to mucosal cells of the small intestine.

**enterotoxigenic *E. coli*** (ETEC) toxin-producing strains of *E. coli* that are often isolated from cases of diarrheal disease in travelers (i.e., "traveler's diarrhea"). The toxins are enterotoxins in that they enhance the secretion of fluid in the intestinal tract.

**enzootic** endemic disease that occurs in nonhuman hosts that can occasionally infect humans.

**enzyme immunoassay** diagnostic test in which antibodies are labeled with an enzyme (horseradish peroxidase or alkaline phosphatase), which will result in a colored end product that is directly related to the amount of antigen or antibody being sought in the test.

**eosinophilia** elevated numbers of eosinophils, the hallmark of most parasitic infections, that may be present in human patients.

**EPA** Environmental Protection Agency

**epidemic** a disease that affects many people within a given region at the same time and is rapidly spreading.

**epidemic relapsing fever** louse-borne relapsing fever caused by *Borrelia recurrentis.*

**epidemiology** study of the distribution and characteristics of diseases and other conditions in a human population.

**epidermis** outermost layer of skin.

**epididymitis** inflammation of the epididymis, which is the coiled tube that receives sperm from the testes and conveys it to the vas deferens.

**epizootic** epidemic disease outbreak in animals that can also include humans.

**ergosterol** unique sterol found in the plasma membrane of fungus cells. It is the site of action for some antifungal drugs.

**erysipeloid** most common form is a localized cellulitis often on the hand, arm, or fingers characterized by red, painful lesions; acquired by humans subsequent to exposure to animals and animal products; similar to streptococcal erysipelas; some reported cases of septicemic form with cardiac involvement.

**erythema migrans** circular, red rash that appears 3 days to 1 month after the bite of an infected tick. The rash is often spreading and may develop a clearing center and a "bull's-eye" appearance.

**eubacteria** the "true bacteria."

**eucaryotic cells** cells having a true, membrane-bound nucleus and organelles.

**eukaryotic host cells** nucleated cells that serve as hosts for viral chlamydial growth.

**eumycetoma** mycetomas associated with fungi.

**exoantigen immunodiffusion** method for identifying a dimorphic fungus without demonstrating thermal dimorphism. Soluble antigens from the mold form are diffused in agar against known antibodies of control organisms.

**exoenzyme S** enzyme that is secreted by some strains of *Pseudomonas aeruginosa*. It is a virulence factor that functions in adenosine diphosphate-ribosylation of several proteins found in mammalian cells.

**exogenous infection** infection from outside the body.

**exogenously** introduced from outside the body.

**exotoxin A** toxin that is secreted by the majority of *Pseudomonas aeruginosa* isolates from clinical specimens. It inhibits protein synthesis in mammalian cells by catalyzing adenosine diphosphate-ribosylation, thus inactivating elongation factor-2. It is a major virulence factor for the organisms.

**extraintestinal amebiasis** infection with *Entamoeba histolytica* in sites other than the intestine. The liver is the most common site of extraintestinal amoebiasis.

**exudate** discharge.

**exudative** lung lesions in an individual having tuberculosis containing liquid containing neutrophils and monocytes.

**facultative anaerobe** an organism that can grow in the presence or absence of oxygen.

**facultative** organism that can grow either with or without the presence of atmospheric oxygen.

**false-negative** specimens that truly have bacteria in them, but which the instrument fails to detect.

**fascia** fibrous tissue that envelops the body underneath the skin.

**fasciitis** infectious inflammation of the fascia.

**favic chandelier** unusual antler-like hyphae associated with some species of the dermatophytes.

**fecundity** relating to the productivity of ova.

**Ficoll-Hypaque** density gradient material that will allow the separation of mononuclear cells (lymphocytes, primarily) from whole blood. Plasma and red blood cells are also separated in the process and may be collected as separate components.

**filamentous** long, cylindrical, and threadlike; hyphae forming.

**filarial** tissue-dwelling parasites having arthropod intermediate hosts. Slender worms, several of which are important human parasites.

**filariasis** infection with one of several species of filarial worms.

**filoviruses** grouping of extremely virulent viral pathogens that includes Marburg virus and Ebola virus.

**fixing** treating a smear to attach material to a slide.

**Fletcher's media** selective, semisolid media used for the cultivation of *Leptospira*.

**fluorescent microscope** microscope in which objects to be viewed are stained with special dyes that give off light when exposed to ultraviolet radiation.

**fluorescent treponemal antibody absorption (FTA-ABS)** sensitive treponemal test used to confirm infection of patient with *Treponema pallidum,* the causative agent of syphilis.

**fluorometry** measuring the fluorescence given off when a fluorescent-labeled substrate is degraded.

**folliculitis** infection of hair follicles.

**food-borne** disease spread by ingestion of or contact with contaminated food.

**food poisoning** the result of the colonization of the GI tract or production of toxins by any of several bacteria. One example of food poisoning is staphylococcal food poisoning, which is the result of ingestion of a toxin produced by *Staphylococcus aureus.*

**formalin-ethyl acetate sedimentation** concentration method used to detect the presence of cysts in some intestinal protozoan infections.

**"fried egg" colony** refers to the appearance of colonies produced by many mycoplasmas when growing on solid media. The colonies have a dense center (with organisms embedded in agar and piled up) surrounded by a thin layer of growth.

**fulminant infection** severe rapidly progressive infection, often fatal.

**fungemia** presence of viable fungi circulating in the bloodstream.

**fungus ball** mass of fungal hyphae forming a large colony within a cavity, especially in the lung or nasal sinuses.

**fusiform** spindle-shaped.

**γ-bacteriophage** a more specific molecular technique using genetic codes for the toxin, used to identify *Bacillus anthracis,* causative organism of anthrax.

**ganciclovir** nucleoside analogue used to treat cytomegalovirus infections. Like acyclovir, ganciclovir is an acycloguanosine.

**ganglioside GM1** a sialic acid linked to a ceramide lipid that is found on the surface of many cell types, including some that are present in the intestinal lumen. It is the molecule to which the enterotoxin of *V. cholerae* binds.

**gastric carcinoma** a type of stomach cancer that originates from epithelial cells.

**gastritis** inflammation of the stomach.

**gastroenteritis** inflammation of the gastrointestinal tract, usually accompanied by diarrhea.

**genetic reassortment** random inclusion of viral segmented genome (RNA) pieces into a new virus particle. *See influenza.*

**germ theory of disease** the theory that states that microorganisms are the cause of infectious disease.

**ghon complex** tubercle having a fibrous outside and calcified inside containing bacilli that may survive for years or die.

**giardial malabsorption syndrome** impaired ability of host infected with *Giardia lamblia* to absorb some nutrients, especially lipids. This is due to damage to the intestinal mucosa by *Giardia*'s sucking disk and the uptake of bile salts by *Giardia.*

**giardiasis** symptomatic infection with *Giardia lamblia* that is characterized by chronic, abundant, foul-smelling diarrhea and possible malabsorption syndrome.

**Gimenez stain** modification of the Macchiavello stain. Elementary bodies (*Chlamydia*) stain red and the background is greenish.

**gingival pockets** small crevices in the gums where many microorganisms reside.

**glabrous** smooth, with or almost without aerial hyphae.

**glanders** localized pulmonary disease that is caused by *Pseudomonas mallei (Burkholderia mallei).* It is seen primarily in horses and donkeys.

**glomerulonephritis** an immune complex condition that causes inflammatory damage to the kidney glomeruli.

**Gomori-methenamine-silver stain** special stain for screening clinical specimens; stains fungal elements black against a pale green background.

**gram-negative** bacteria with no affinity for the crystal violet stain; stain with the safranin counterstain and appear pink.

**gram-positive** bacteria with an affinity for the crystal violet stain; not decolorized and appear purple.

**Gram stain** differential stain that distinguishes between bacteria with an affinity for crystal violet stain.

**granules** (white, yellow, or red) composed of narrow (0.5–1 μm in diameter) intertwined filaments with coccoid and bacillary forms.

**granuloma** a chronic inflammatory lesion characterized by an accumulation of macrophages, with or without lymphocytes.

**granulomatus amebic encephalitis (GAE)** rare form of encephalitis caused by *Acanthamoeba* species.

**group-reactive antigen** antigenic moiety possessed by all members of a group (e.g., *Chlamydia*).

**"gull-wing" morphology** curved rods that tend to align in such a way as to resemble gulls in flight; often used to describe the appearance of *Campylobacter* species.

**gumma** lesions characteristic of tertiary syphilis.

**halophilic bacteria** bacteria that require at least 2% NaCl for growth (i.e., "salt-loving").

**hantavirus pulmonary syndrome** clinical manifestation caused by Sin Nombre virus, characterized by flulike symptoms, nausea, vomiting, and respiratory difficulties resembling noncardiogenic pulmonary edema.

**heat-labile toxin (LT)** enterotoxin secreted by some strains of ETEC. It activates the adenylyl cyclase enzyme, which, in turn, increases the intracellular level of cyclic adenosine monophosphate. This results in the hypersecretion of fluid into the intestinal lumen and hypermotility of the gut. The toxin is readily inactivated by heat.

**heat-stable toxin (ST)** enterotoxin secreted by some strains of ETEC. Its mechanism of action is similar to that of heat-labile toxin, except that it increases the intracellular level of cycle guanosine monophosphate. It is not readily inactivated by heat.

**hemagglutination** clumping of red blood cells due to viral attachment to receptors on the red cells.

**hemagglutination inhibition** diagnostic test that measures antibodies that attach to viruses capable of causing hemagglutination of red blood cells.

**hemagglutinin** glycoprotein found in the lipid envelope of influenza viruses, which functions as the viral receptor for attachment to host cells.

**hemaphroditic** *see* monecius.

**hematogenously** via the bloodstream.

**hematuria** presence of blood in the urine.

**hemoflagellates** another name for members of phylum Mastigophera that infect the blood and tissues.

**hemorrhagic fever** syndrome seen with some viral infections, characterized by bleeding from any number of surface and interior sites.

**hemozoin** pigment that stains black with Giemsa or Wright's stain. It is produced by *Plasmodium* in infected human erythrocytes.

**HEPA** High Efficiency Particulate Airflow filters

**hepatosplenomegaly** abnormal enlargement and tenderness of the liver and spleen.

**Herpesviridae** suggested family name that would include all known human herpesviruses.

**histone proteins** proteins associated with eucaryotic DNA.

**histopathologic stains** stains used on tissue sections and smears to demonstrate fungal organisms.

**hyaline** clear; hyphae that are not pigmented.

**hyaline hyphomycetes** fungi whose hyphae are clear and not pigmented.

**hyperkeratoses** overgrowth of the cornified epithelial layer of the skin.

**hypha (ae)** long filament of fungal cells.

**hyphae** long filaments of fungal cells.

**icosahedral** virus shape consisting of a polyhedron made up of 20 equilateral triangles.

**id reaction** short for dermatophytid, an allergic reaction on the skin in a patient who has a dermatophyte fungal infection elsewhere on the skin.

**immunity** a reaction to harmful agents such as microbes.

**immunocompromised** the state of having lowered immunity through treatment or disease; an altered state of immunocompetency.

**immunosuppressed** state in which the immune response is inadequate. This may be a primary state or secondary to certain drugs or infections.

**immunosuppressed/immunodeficiencies/immuno-competent/immunocompromised** terms used to describe a person whose immune system has a reduced ability to protect the body from infection.

**impetigo** a local skin infection caused by *Streptococcus pyogenes* that is most often seen in young children. The disease is characterized by localized pustules that crust and rupture.

**inclusion bodies** phagosome body in the cytoplasm of McCoy cells where *Chlamydia* have grown by binary fission. Detected by monoclonal antibodies to *Chlamydia* antigens.

**inclusion conjunctivitis** eye disease, less serious than trachoma, caused by *Chlamydia trachomatis*.

**India ink prep** used to identify the capsule of *Cryptococcus neoformans* in fluids. India ink is repelled by the capsule, producing a clear space against a black background.

**India ink stain** stain used to show the capsule of *Cryptococcus neoformans*.

**infective endocarditis (IE)** infection of the interior lining of the heart or its valves; bacterial growth on rough endothelial tissue or valves of the heart leading to inflammation and damage to those tissues along with continuous shedding of bacteria into the bloodstream.

**inflammatory cells** host cells, such as PMNs, which are drawn to a site of injury or infection in an attempt to repair the damage.

**inhibitory media** culture media with substances added to inhibit growth of contaminating organisms.

**inoculate** to transfer organisms to a growth media.

**inoculum** organisms that are transferred to a growth medium.

**interferons** cytokines (cell products) that directly inhibit virus growth within a host cell.

**intermediate host** the host in which the immature form (larval form, asexually reproducing form) of a parasite resides.

**internal autoinfection** phenomenon that occurs in infection with *Strongyloides* in which asexual reproduction occurs in the host without the usual soil phase of the life cycle.

**International Code of Bacterial Nomenclature** a set of rules that apply to the naming of bacterial species.

**International Journal of Systematic Bacteriology** journal in which new additions and changes in bacterial taxonomy and nomenclature are published.

**interstitial keratitis** inflammation within the layers of the cornea that is sometimes caused by syphilis.

**intertriginous** dermatophyte infection on skin surfaces that have been chafed by rubbing, as between the toes.

**intracellularly** inside of a cell.

**intraerythrocytic** within the red blood cell.

**in vitro** within a glass, observable in a test tube.

**in vivo** within the living body.

**isolated colonies** separate and distinguished colonies on a culture.

**isoniazid** an antituberculosis drug often used in combination with ethambutol and/or rifampin.

**isosporiasis** intestinal infection caused by *Isospora belli* that ranges from asymptomatic and self-limiting to severe.

**Kanawaga-positive strains** refers to strains of *V. parahemolyticus* that produce a heat-stable hemolysin that lysis erythrocytes in Wagatsuma agar. Isolates that produce a positive reaction are usually pathogenic.

**Katayma fever** another name for acute schistomiasis that is characterized by several nonspecific symptoms including fever, chills, and weight loss.

**keratin** protective coating of the skin formed as skin cells mature and die. Hair and nails are modified keratin.

**keratitis** inflammation of the cornea.

**ketoacidosis** state in a patient with uncontrolled diabetes with inadequate insulin for glucose metabolism. Cells switch to utilize fats and proteins for energy resulting in the production of excessive amounts of ketones and organic acids that become toxic. This state may predispose to infection by zygomycetes.

**Kinyoun method** a cold staining method used for the identification of bacteria having the lipid, mycolic acid in their cell wall.

**kissing bug** common name for the blood-sucking arthropod, *Panstrongylus* that vectors *Trypanosoma cruzi* to humans. *See reduviid bug.*

**kissing lesions** pair of lesions where material from the first lesion autoinoculates an adjacent area.

**KOH preparation** technique for direct microscopic examination of specimen for fungal hyphae where cells and debris are first digested or cleared by 10% potassium hydroxide.

**Lancefield antigen** group-specific carbohydrates found on the surfaces of hemolytic streptococci used in serologic classification.

**larviparous** gives birth to live larvae, as opposed to laying eggs.

**late Lyme disease (chronic Lyme disease)** appears weeks, months, or years after the bite of a *Borrelia*-infected *Ixodes* tick and is characterized by arthritis of one or more of the large bone joints, nervous system abnormalities, and sometimes thinning of the skin on the hands and feet.

**latent syphilis** stage of syphilis that usually occurs after the secondary stage. During latent syphilis the patient does not exhibit any symptoms but serological tests are positive.

**leishmaniasis** disease caused by *Leishmania* species that may either be cutaneous, mucocutaneous, or visceral.

**lepromin** a reliable serologic test for leprosy that distinguishes the three forms of the disease.

**leptospiremic** acute phase of leptospirosis that develops after a 1- to 2-week incubation period.

**leptospiruric** immune stage of leptospirosis that occurs at approximately the second week of the disease.

**linin** fibrils in the nucleus of *Entamoeba histolytica* that run from the karyosome to the peripheral chromatin. Linin stains faintly with trichrome or hematoxylin.

**lipophilic** having an affinity for lipids or fat containing compounds.

**lipopolysaccharide** molecule that extends outward from the wall of gram-negative bacteria. It consists of lipid A (the toxic portion), core polysaccharide, and O-specific polysaccharide (antigenic portion).

**Loiasis** infection with the parasitic worm, *Loa loa*.

**lophotrichous flagella** multiple polar flagella that appear tufted; found on *Plesiomonas shigelloides*.

**lumbar puncture** most common method of collecting cerebrospinal fluid, whereby a needle is inserted into the subarachnoid space in the lumbar spine.

**luminometer** instrument that measures the light emitted from degradation of a chemiluminescent compound.

**Lyme disease (Lyme borrelosis)** tick-borne disease caused by the spirochete, *Borrelia burgdorferi*.

**Lyme meningitis** meningitis that occurs when *Borrelia burgdorferi* invades the nervous system and usually occurs within the first few months of infection.

**lymphadenitis** inflammation, usually due to infection, of the lymph node(s).

**macroconidia** large conidia, usually the larger of two types of conidia produced by the same fungus.

**macrogametes** mature female gamete produced by some protozoans such as the coccidians and *Plasmodium*. Macrogametes are fertilized by microgametes producing zygotes.

**macroscopic** visible to the unaided eye.

**macroscopic slide agglutination test** a rapid screening method used to diagnose leptospirosis.

**macule** discolored spot on the skin that is not raised above the surface.

**maculopapular rash** rash seen in secondary syphilis that is characterized by distinctive macules (blemish or discoloration that is flush with the surface of the skin) or papules (small, raised skin lesion) or both.

**mad cow disease** prion disease affecting the central nervous system of cows called bovine spongiform encephalopathy, which resembles Creutzfeldt-Jakob disease in humans.

**Madura foot** destructive fungal abscess (mycetoma) of the foot. The term was originally used to refer to this infection found in India caused by *Madurella mycetomis,* but now is sometimes applied generally to any mycotic mycetoma of the foot; chronic, deep subcutaneous tissue and bone infection of the foot.

**malarial paroxysm** recurring series of shaking chills, followed by fever that is characteristic of malaria.

**malignant jaundice** disease of dogs caused by *Babesia* species.

**Mansonelliasis** infection with *Mansonella ozzardi* or *M. perstans.*

**Mantoux test** a hypersensitivity test to the tuberculin antigen. PPD (purified protein derivative) is intradermally injected into the skin of the arm. The area of application is read and interpreted in 48 to 72 hours after application of the antigen.

**mastitis** infectious inflammation of the breast.

**mastoiditis** inflammation of the mastoid process of the temporal bone.

**mean inhibitory concentration (MIC)** lowest concentration of an antibiotic that will inhibit the growth of a microorganism.

**mebendazole** antihelminthic drug used to treat a number of parasitic infections.

*mecA* **gene** bacterial resistance to the antimicrobial substance, methicillin, is carried on this gene.

**mediastinitis** infectious inflammation of the mediastinum, located behind the sternum and between the lungs.

**melanin** a brown pigment found in the cells of some fungi. Hyphae that have melanin present appear brown and are called dematiaceous.

**melioidosis** acute pneumonia caused by infection with *Pseudomonas pseudomallei (Burkholderia pseudomallei).*

**meningitis** inflammation of the meninges in the brain.

**merosporangium** tubelike sporangium.

**mesenteric adenitis** inflammation of lymph nodes in the abdominal region (mesentery). This is associated with progressive infection due to *Yersinia enterocolitica* and *Yersinia pseudotuberculosis.*

**metacercariae** larval form of some trematodes.

**metallic sheen** refers to the shiny, metal-like appearance of *Pseudomonas aeruginosa* growth on certain types of media.

**methicillin-resistant *Staphylococcus aureus* (MRSA)** strains of *Staphylococcus aureus* having the *mecA* gene.

**metula** supporting structure below a phialide of some species of molds, especially *Aspergillus* and *Penicillium.*

**microaerophile** requires small quantities of oxygen for growth; however, does not grow under strict aerobic or anaerobic conditions.

**microaerophilic** grow best in reduced oxygen concentrations; 85% nitrogen, 10% carbon dioxide, and 5% oxygen; organism that requires reduced oxygen, but not anaerobic conditions, for cultivation.

**microbicide** chemotherapeutic agent that kills microorganisms.

**microbistat** chemotherapeutic agent that inhibits the growth of microorganism.

**microconidia** smaller conidia of fungi that produce two types of conidia.

**microfilariae** the first stage of any ovoviviparous filariid nematode. Usually found in the blood or tissue fluids of the definitive host.

**microgametes** mature male gamete produced by some protozoans such as the coccidians and *Plasmodium*. Microgametes fertilize macrogametes to produce zygotes.

**microhemagglutination test for antibody to *T. pallidum* (MHA-Tp)** easy to perform treponemal test used to confirm syphilis in patients with positive nontreponemal test results.

**Microspora** a phylum of protozoans that possess an organelle called the polar filament that plays a role in infection of the host.

**miliary tuberculosis** a generalized infection with *Mycobacterium tuberculosis* in which tubercle formation occurs in several body organs. The tubercles resemble millet seeds.

**minced** preparation of fresh tissue; chopped up into very small pieces.

**minimum bacteriocidal concentration (MBC)** lowest concentration of an antibiotic that will kill a microorganism.

**miracidium** free-swimming form of some trematodes.

**mold** fungi that display multicellular, filamentous growth, for example, the common bread mold.

**monecious** species in which the reproductive organs of both sexes are located in one organism. These organisms are also referred to as being hemaphroditic.

**mordant** substance used to enhance a stain; acts as a fixative.

**MOTT** mycobacteria other than tuberculosis.

**MRSA** methicillin resistant *Staphylococcus aureus*.

**mucocutaneous relapse** recurrence of symptoms involving the skin and mucous membranes that occurs in approximately 25% of the patients with secondary syphilis.

**mucoid** colony that is viscous and stringy, similar to mucus.

**mucopolysaccharide capsule** mucoid structure surrounding the yeast *Cryptococcus neoformans*.

**mucous membrane** a membrane rich in mucous glands that lines the body passages and cavities.

**MUG test** assay for ß-glucuronidase production using 4-*methylu*mbelliferyl-ß-*g*lucuronide (MUG) as a substrate. The great majority of *E. coli* isolates produce the enzyme, whereas the 0157:H7 serotype does not.

**mushroom** large, multicellular fungus in which a fruiting body grows above the ground.

**mycelium** a tangled mass of fungal hyphae, usually observed in molds.

**mycetoma** a localized chronic cutaneous or subcutaneous infection classically characterized by draining sinuses, granules, and swelling; destructive abscess caused by a mold fungus in which the organisms form visible colonies (granules) in the pus.

**mycology** the study of fungi.

**mycosis (es)** disease caused by a fungus.

**mycotic aneurysm** dilation of the wall of a blood vessel caused by infection.

**myositis** infectious inflammation of muscle.

**NANB hepatitis** non-A, non-B hepatitis viruses. These currently would include viruses now identified as hepatitis C virus (HCV), hepatitis D virus (HDV), and hepatitis E virus (HEV).

**necrosis** cell death caused by the production of degradative enzymes; tissue death.

**necrotizing fasciitis** gas-forming tissue-destroying infection of the fascia, which is a subcutaneous layer of tissue; soft-tissue infection involving superficial fascia that results in extensive damage to surrounding tissue.

**negative-sense RNA** configuration of RNA genome found in some viruses. This term indicates that the genome from these viruses may not function directly as messenger RNA.

**negative stains** staining of the background so that contrast makes bacterial structures visible.

**Nematoda** "roundworms."

**nephropathogenic *E. coli*** (NPEC) strains of *E. coli* that are often isolated from urinary tract infections. They often express certain O antigens, a capsule, and a P pilus.

**neurosyphilis** infection of the central nervous system by *Treponema pallidum* that results in a variety of symptoms.

**neurotropic** fungus organism that is attracted to the nervous system, especially the brain and spinal cord.

**neutralization** diagnostic test in which specific antibody combines with a virus, which results in the inability of the virus to attach to cellular receptors and enter into the host cell in order to grow.

**nocturnal periodicity** microfilariae are concentrated in the small blood vessels of the lungs during the day and are liberated into the periphereal circulation at night.

**nomenclature** the naming of organisms.

**nonfermenter** organisms that do not ferment carbohydrates (e.g., glucose and lactose) that are frequently used to help differentiate gram-negative bacteria.

**nongonococcal urethritis (NGU)** infection of the urethra due to agents other than *Neiserria gonnorrhoeae*. Certain mycoplasmas are implicated in causing this condition.

**nonhistone proteins** a class of proteins associated with DNA.

**nonlactose fermenter** colonies that do not appear to ferment lactose, as indicated by differential media such as MacConkey or EMB agar.

**nonperiodic periodicity** microfilariae are present in the bloodstream both day and night.

**nonphotochromagen** lack of pigment production by a bacterium when grown in the presence of light.

**nontreponemal tests** tests for syphilis that detect reagin antibodies present in the serum of persons infected with *Treponema pallidum*.

**nonvenereal endemic syphilis** disease caused by *Treponema pallidum* subspecies *endemicum* that is seen in the Middle East, Africa, Southeast Asia, and Yugoslavia, and that is usually restricted to cutaneous lesions.

**normal flora** microorganisms that reside on, or in, the body in what is usually a health state of being for the host. Under certain circumstances normal flora may cause opportunistic disease in the host; organisms that are found in particular sites in a healthy host and cause no harm under ordinary circumstances. *See colonization; commensals.*

**normal/resident flora** microorganisms that naturally inhabit areas of the body. In most cases they cause no harm and are beneficial in some way.

**nosocomial infection** infection originating and acquired in a medical facility. *Excludes* infections present or incubating in a hospitalized patient at the time of admission.

**novobiocin test** a test using a filter paper disk impregnated with the antimicrobial substance, novobiocin. This test indicates bacterial resistance or susceptibility to novobiocin.

**nucleic acid probe** small piece of nucleic acid (RNA or DNA) that has been created to specifically hybridize to a target organism's nucleic acid sequence; small segments of nucleic acid sequences that can be labeled with a detection chemical that provides a signal for use in viral identification. The small nucleic acid segment provides the mechanism for viral specificity in the detection process.

**nucleoid** that area in the procaryotic cell where the main chromosome is located.

**O-F media** low-peptone medium to which different carbohydrates are added. It is used to detect acid production by bacteria that metabolize weakly or slowly. It is often used to differentiate nonfermenters from the *Enterobacteriaceae*.

**O, K, H, and Vi antigens** immunogenic components of gram-negative rods that can be identified using antiserum. The O are somatic antigens consisting of polysaccharides, K are capsular antigens that usually consist of polysaccharides, H antigens are flagellar proteins, and the Vi is a special case of a capsular antigen that is produced almost exclusively by *Salmonella typhi*. Some of these antigens, such as the K1 and Vi, are associated with virulence.

**O1 serogroup** *V. cholerae* that possess the O1 antigen. Organisms in this serogroup are responsible for the majority of epidemics and all pandemics of cholera.

**O139 serogroup** a newly identified *V. cholerae* that expresses the O139 antigen. Organisms in this serogroup, like the O1 serogroup, can produce severe diarrheal disease in large numbers of people.

**obligate anaerobe** those anaerobic bacteria that grow in the absence of molecular $O_2$ but fail to multiply in the presence of $O_2$ incubated in room air or in a $CO_2$ incubator (containing 5–10% $CO_2$ in air).

**Onchocerciasis** another name for River blindness. A nonfatal disease caused by the large filarial worm, *Onchocerca volvulus*.

**oncosphere** larval form of the tapeworm, *Taenia solium*.

**oocyst** encysted form of some protozoans such as the coccidia that results from fertilization of the macrogamete by the microgamete; infectious stage of *Cryptosporidium*, *Isospora*, and *Cyclospora*; has a protective shell-like wall and the size varies for each genus.

**opportunistic** an organism that does not cause infection under normal circumstances in a normal host but can cause an infection when the host is abnormal.

**opportunistic fungi** fungi that usually do not cause infections in normal humans, but that can cause infections when the host's resistance is altered.

**opportunistic pathogens** an organism that does not usually cause disease but may become a pathogen under some circumstances.

**osteochondritis** symptom seen in congenital syphilis that effects the epiphyses (bone-forming centers) of the skeleton that results in destruction of the bone.

**osteomyelitis** infection in the bone.

**otitis externa** inflammation of the external ear.

**otitis media** acute, localized inflammation of the middle ear.

**palisades** arrangement of bacilli when viewed on a stained smear in which they are in groups, aligned parallel to each other.

**pandemic** a widespread epidemic disease.

**papule** small, superficial elevated area of the skin.

**parabasal bodies** dark-staining cytoplasmic body found in some flagellates such as *Giardia*.

**paranasal sinuses** any of the mucous-lined air-filled cavities (frontal, ethmoid, sphenoid, maxillary) in the bones of the face, which open into the nasal cavity.

**parapneumonic effusion** accumulation of pleural fluid associated with bacterial pneumonia or lung abscesses.

**parasite** an organism that is metabolically dependent on a host during part or all of its life cycle.

**parasitic phase** morphologic form a dimorphic fungus assumes when it infects a host.

**pasteurization** the process by which a liquid such as beer, wine, or milk, is heated mildly to kill organisms of spoilage or potential pathogens.

**pathogen** a specific causative agent of disease.

**pathogenic** able to cause disease.

**patient population** specific segment of the community that generally seeks treatment at a particular health care facility.

**pectinate body** hyphal form resembling a broken comb associated with some species of dermatophytes.

**pellicle** flexible outer covering that surrounds some protozoans.

**pelvic inflammatory disease (PID)** a collective term for any extensive bacterial infection of the pelvic organs, especially the uterus, uterine tubes, and ovaries.

**penicillin binding protein** mRSA strains have altered penicillin binding proteins that have a decreased affinity for the antimicrobial substance. This makes it impossible for penicillin to bind to the bacterial cell wall.

**peptic ulcers** areas of inflammation of the mucous membranes that line the lumen of the stomach. *Helicobacter pylori* is strongly associated with their development.

**peptidoglycan** a complex molecule consisting primarily of polysaccharide and polypeptide that is a component of the cell wall of most eubacterial species. Also referred to as murein.

**perianal** located around the anus.

**pericardial fluid** fluid that occupies the pericardial cavity located between the membranes surrounding the heart.

**pericarditis** inflammation of the pericardium.

**periodicity** relating to the time of day of the appearance of microfilariae (i.e., nocturnal from 2200–0200 or diurnal). The appearance of microfilariae coincides with the feeding habits of insect vectors.

**peripheral chromatin** chromatin that lines the inside of the nuclear envelope in some protozoans such as *Entamoeba*.

**periplasmic filaments** *see* axial filaments.

**peritoneal fluid** fluid in the peritoneal cavity located between the two layers of the peritoneum.

**peritonitis** infectious inflammation of the abdominal peritoneum.

**phaeohyphomycosis** subcutaneous infection caused by dematiaceous (pigmented) fungi. The prefix *phaeo* refers to dark pigmentation.

**phagosome** cytoplasmic inclusion body, wherein *Chlamydia* organisms divide by binary fission.

**pharyngitis** inflammation of the mucous membrane and underlying tissues of the pharynx.

**phialide** supporting structure giving rise to conidia. It remains fixed in length as the conidia are produced.

**phospholipase C** enzyme produced by many strains of *Pseudomonas aeruginosa* that hyrolyzes phospholipids.

**photochromogen** production of pigment by a bacterium when it is grown in the presence of light.

**phylogeny** the evolutionary relatedness of a species or a group of species.

**phylum** (pl. phyla) taxonomic category that falls below kingdom and above class; same as division.

**PID** collective term for any extensive bacterial infection of the pelvic organs, especially the uterus, uterine tubes, and ovaries.

**pinta** see caratae.

**piperazine** antihelminthic drug used to treat several helminth infections.

**plague** disease due to infection with Yersinia pestis. Bubonic plague is characterized by an intense inflammatory response in the lymph nodes, causing them to become very large ("buboes"), painful, and hemorrhagic, and a variety of systemic symptoms. Pneumonic plague may occur as the result of dissemination or after inhalation of the organisms.

**plasmids** small, circular molecules of DNA found in some bacterial cells in addition to the main chromosome.

**Platyhelminthes** the "flatworms" including phyla Aschelminthes and Platyhelminthes.

**pleimorphic** having many shapes.

**pleomorphic** bacteria whose microscopic appearance is irregular in shape and/or size.

**plerocercoid** larval stage of the tapeworm, Diphyllobothrium, that encysts in the muscle of fish.

**pleural fluid** fluid in the pleural cavity located between the two membranes of the pleura, which encloses the lungs.

**pneumonia** inflammation of lung parenchyma due to microbial infection or chemical inhalation; inflammation of the lungs with exudation. There are numerous causes of pneumonia including several species of bacteria, fungi, and viruses.

**polar flagellum** (pl. flagella) flagellum that is attached to one end of a rod-shaped bacterium. One cell may have one or more polar flagellum.

**polar tube** tube found in microsporidian spores. This structure transfers the infectious content of the spore into host cells.

**polymorphonuclear leukocytes (PMNs)** type of white blood cell which are drawn to the site of infection within the host.

**positive culture** recovery or growth of bacteria or fungi in a blood culture set; the microorganism in the culture is not always clinically significant (the pathogen).

**positive-sense RNA** configuration of RNA genome found in some viruses. Purified viral RNA is capable of directly interacting with ribosomes and functioning as messenger RNA.

**potassium tellurite** a substance reduced by some species of Mycobacterium, a characteristic used to distinguish various species of that genus.

**presumptive identification** identification of an organism, which is not confirmed, but is most likely correct based on all available data.

**primary ameba meningoencephalitis (PAM)** rare form of meningoencephalitis caused by Acanthamoeba species.

**primary infection** initial infection caused by an organism. To be distinguished from disseminated infection.

**primary media** culture media on which the original specimen is cultured.

**primary stain** stain used in the first step of a staining procedure.

**primary syphilis** initial stage of syphilis that develops 10 to 90 days after initial infection. It is characterized by the formation of one or more chancres occurring at the site of infection.

**prion** slow infectious agent confined to the central nervous system, which causes neurologic damage in humans and certain animals.

**procaryotic cells** cells that lack a nuclear membrane and organelles.

**procercoid** second larval stage of Diphyllobothrium that occurs in a suitable crustacean.

**proctitis** inflammation of the rectum.

**productive lesion** lung lesion in individuals infected with tuberculosis consisting of cells but with no liquid, that are organized around the bacilli.

**promastigote** leptomonad stage or form characterized by a free anterior flagellum, resembling the typical form of Leptomonads.

**prophylaxis** measures to preserve health and prevent the spread of disease; chemoprophylaxis: using drugs and related chemicals to improve health; immunoprophylaxis: using immune substances to treat a health condition.

**proteolytic enzymes** enzymes produced by Entamoeba histolytica in invasive infections that destroys host tissue.

**provirus** nucleic acid component of various viruses that may be inserted into host chromosomal material, thereby setting up a latent virus infection. Some proviruses may be present as an uninserted episome.

**pseudohyphae** elongated buds produced by certain yeasts that resemble the hyphae of molds. The false hyphae can be distinguished from true hyphae by constrictions that occur between cells; short chains of yeast cells that fail to separate after budding.

**psittacosis** disease caused by infection with Chlamydia psittaci.

**puerperal sepsis** also called childbed fever. Begins as an infection of the uterus as a result of childbirth or abortion. Often progresses to septicemia. Most often caused by Streptococcus pyogenes.

**pulmonary** pertaining to the lung.

**pure culture** agar plate or broth medium that has growth of only one type of organism.

**purified protein derivative** a dried form of tuberculin used in testing for past or present infection with tubercle bacilli.

**purulent** forming or containing pus.

**pus** accumulated dead bacteria, fluid and dead phagocytes.

**pyelonephritis** infection of the kidney.

**pyocyanin** blue pigment produced by most strains of Pseudomonas aeruginosa. It induces the production of highly unstable oxygen radicals that damage tissues.

**pyogenic** producing pus.

**pyomelanin** brown pigment produced by some strains of Pseudomonas aeruginosa.

**pyorubrin** rust-colored pigment produced by some strains of Pseudomonas aeruginosa.

**pyoverdin** yellow pigment produced by most strains of Pseudomonas aeruginosa. It fluoresces under short-wave ultraviolet light.

**pyrazinamidase** enzyme that hydrolyzes pyrazinamide and is present in most corynebacteria except for three species, used to identify C. diphtheriae, C. ulcerans, and C. pseudotuberculosis.

**pyuria** presence of white blood cells in the urine.

**quality assurance** system that identifies sources of intralaboratory excellence and includes personnel training, performance standards, maintenance of equipment and consumables, calibration, quality control, proficiency testing, and documentation.

**quartan** periodicity of malarial paroxysm that recurs 4 days after the first episode.

**racquet hyphae** hyphal forms resembling a club or racquet.

**rapid plasma reagin (RPR)** screening test for syphilis that detects reagin antibodies present in infected persons.

**rapid screening methods** test procedures designed to identify those specimens requiring further testing by conventional culture; results are generally available in just a few minutes or hours.

**rectal prolapse** an outward displacement of the rectum.

**redia** larval stage of some trematodes.

**reducing media** culture media containing substances that will combine with any dissolved oxygen in the media.

**reduviid bug** common name for the blood-sucking arthropod, *Panstrongylus* that vectors *Trypanosoma cruzi* to humans. *See kissing bug.*

**reference laboratory** large, often private, commercial laboratory providing extensive services and more complex test methods not usually available in small or medium sized laboratories.

**relapsing fever** louse- or tick-borne disease caused by several species of *Borrelia*.

**reticulate body** also called "initial body" reorganized elementary body, whereby *Chlamydia* organisms undergo division by binary fission.

**reverse transcriptase** RNA-dependent DNA polymerase. This enzyme is found in all retroviruses, from which the viral name was derived. HIV is a retrovirus.

**rheumatic fever** an infection caused by *Streptococcus pyogenes* that is usually considered to be an immune complication.

**rhizoid** rootlike structure along the hyphae of some zygomycetes.

**ribavirin** chemotherapeutic compound used to treat respiratory syncytial virus (RSV) infections.

**"rice-water" stools** refers to the appearance of the excreted bowel contents of patients with cholera. The small flecks of mucus in the large volume of excreted fluid look like rice.

**rickettsemia** rickettsial organisms in the bloodstream.

**ringworm** common term for skin infection due to a dermatophyte fungus. The term refers to the ringlike shape of the infection as it spreads.

**river blindness** *See onchocerciasis.*

**Robert Whittaker** developed the five kingdom system of classification.

**Robles disease** another name for river blindness.

**R plasmids** circular pieces of extrachromosomal DNA that carry genes conferring resistance to one or more antibiotics. They are the most common cause of acquired antibiotic resistance in bacteria.

**rugose** wrinkled or folded.

**Runyon classification** a method used to group mycobacteria based on pigment production, the effect of light on pigment production, and growth time.

**rust** a mold that exhibits a powdery form of growth. Several species are plant pathogens.

**salpingitis** inflammation or infection of a tube, usually the fallopian tubes between the ovaries and the uterus.

**sandfly** common name for blood-sucking arthropods of the genera *Lutzomyia* and *Plebotomus* that vector *Leishmania* species to humans.

**saprophyte** heterotrophic organisms that use dead organic material for their nutritional needs. They are generally not pathogenic under normal circumstances.

**saprophytic phase** morphologic form a dimorphic fungus assumes in its natural habitat.

**Sarcomastigophora** phylum of protozoans that are motile by pseudopods, flagella, or both. Reproduction is by asexual binary fission.

**scalded skin syndrome** also known as Ritter's disease. This disease most often affects children less than 5 years old and is the result of exfoliative toxin A and B produced at a localized infected site. Large areas of blistered skin develop. The toxins are produced by *S. aureus*.

**sclerotic bodies** round, thick-walled, brown bodies that reproduce by splitting. It is the form of fungi causing chromoblastomycosis assumed in the infected tissue.

**scotochromogen** production of a particular pigment when a bacterium is grown in the dark.

**secondary syphilis** second stage of syphilis that occurs approximately 2 to 10 weeks after primary syphilis. It is marked by the development of a maculopapular rash on the palms, soles, oral mucosa, and genitals.

**selective media** bacteriologic media that contains substances such as dyes, bile salts, or antibiotics. These substances inhibit one or more groups of bacteria, while allowing other groups to grow.

**sepsis and septicemia** clinical evidence of a systemic response to microorganisms that are present in and causing the bloodstream infection.

**septate hyphae** elongated fungal filaments that possess crosswalls or septa that divide the cells.

**septic arthritis** arthritis associated with infections that are usually bacterial in origin, but may be caused by viral, fungal, or mycobacterial pathogens.

**septicemia** infection of the bloodstream. Microorganisms are actively growing in the normally sterile blood.

**serology** science of serum reactions, diagnosis, and treatment; the location of antibodies (immunoglobulins) that arise as a result of the humoral immune system being exposed to an antigen.

**serous exudate** serum-like fluid that is slowly discharged from the chancre seen in primary syphilis. This fluid is rich in spirochetes and is highly infectious.

**sharps** needles, scalpel blades, glass slides, broken glass and plastic that could puncture the surface of the skin.

**Sheather's sugar concentration flocculation** method used to increase the chances of recovering cysts from fecal specimens.

**Shiga toxin** heat-labile exotoxin that is produced by *Shigella dysenteriae*. It inhibits protein synthesis in mammalian cells by inactivating the 60S ribosomal subunit. Its action in the intestinal tract results in bloody diarrhea; it also has neurotoxic effects.

**significant bacteriuria** concentration of bacteria in the urine at which the organisms are considered to be causative of the symptoms or require antimicrobial therapy.

**simple stain** single dye to color structures of an organism.

**Sin Nombre virus** correct name for the causative agent for the epidemic of hantavirus pulmonary syndrome in the desert southwest United States in 1993. The virus has also been called Muerto Canyon virus and Four Corners virus.

**Skirrow's medium** a selective medium with a 5% horse blood agar base that contains vancomycin, polymyxin B, and trimethoprim. It is used for isolation of *Campylobacter* and *Helicobacter*.

**slime layer** outer capsule-like layer that is produced by certain bacteria. *Pseudomonas aeruginosa* produces a slime layer that is of mixed composition, but is primarily polysaccharide in nature.

**slow growing** rate of growth of the organism on solid media (> 4 days).

**smears** film of substance on a slide.

**smut** a mold that exhibits a powdery form of growth. Several species are plant pathogens.

**sowda** another name for river blindness.

**special stain** stain to emphasize specific structures.

**species** in reference to the bacteria a species is a type strain and all other strains that warrant inclusion of it in the species.

**spectrophotometer** instrument that measures the transmittance of light at a specific wavelength through a suspension and compares it to a control suspension.

**spherule** large, round, saclike, thick-walled structure produced by *Coccidioides immitis*. It becomes filled with endospores.

**spiral hyphae** curled hyphae form associated with some species of dermatophytes.

**spirillum** (pl. spirilla) helical bacterial cells.

**spirochete** helical bacterial cells with axial filaments.

**spontaneous recovery** refers to the recovery of a patient with an infectious disease without any treatment.

**sporangiophore** stalklike structure arising from the hyphae of zygomycetes supporting the sporangium.

**sporangiospore** asexual spore of zygomycetes formed by cleavage in a sporangium.

**sporangium** (pl. sporangia) saclike structure containing asexual sporangiospores. Characteristic of zygomycetes; case or sac in which the spores are produced, the appearance of which is used in the differentiation of *Bacillus* species.

**spores** usually possess a thick wall enabling the cell to withstand unfavorable environmental conditions. Difficult to destroy because of resistance to heat.

**sputum** secretions from the lower respiratory tract, usually coughed up and expectorated through the mouth.

**staining** color structures and organisms.

**Standard Precautions** guidelines recommended by the CDC to protect health care workers from blood- and body fluid-borne disease such as HIV and hepatitis; include the use of gloves and other protective clothing to avoid infection and the spread of infection.

**staphylococci** clusters of round bacterial cells.

**stasis** standing still, stoppage, unchanged.

**STD** sexually transmitted disease.

**sterilization** any process that will kill all forms of life (may not remove bacteria or their products).

**strain** the descendants of a single cell, isolated from a pure culture.

**streaking** spread inoculum over the surface of a culture plate using an inoculating loop or swab.

**strep throat** pharyngitis due to *Streptococcus pyogenes*.

**streptococci** chains of round bacterial cells.

**string of pearls test** simple test that reflects the susceptibility of a strain to penicillin, modified for use in presumptive identification of *Bacillus anthracis;* a positive test is the presence of strings of spherical cellular forms of the organism resembling a string of pearls under microscopic examination of growth on Mueller-Hinton agar.

**strobilation** a type of continuous replication of reproductive organs occurring in most tapeworms. Segments differentiate at a zone near the scolex.

**subclinical infection** infection wherein the microorganism (bacterial or viral) grows in the host, but no clinical manifestation of disease is present. The host's immune system will respond to the presence of the microorganism.

**subculture** to transfer an organism from one growth medium to another, to obtain fresh growth of a pure culture.

**subcutaneous** situated or occurring directly under the skin.

**superantigen** protein present on *Mycoplasma arthritidis* that activates an unusually large number of T lymphocytes by a unique pathway, i.e., by binding simultaneously to the T-cell antigen receptor and the class II molecule on an antigen-presenting cell. Superantigens may contribute to acute and chronic inflammatory effects observed after infection with mycoplasmas and certain other infectious agents.

**suppurate** to form and then discharge pus.

**suprapubic aspirate** method of collecting urine with a needle and syringe, in which the bladder is punctured through the skin above the bladder.

**swarming motility** refers to the ability of highly motile *Proteus* species to "swarm" over the surface of solid media, thereby forming a thin, transparent film of growth, rather than discrete colonies.

**swimmer's ear** the popular (nonmedical) name used for *Pseudomonas aeruginosa* infections of the external auditory canal. It is equivalent to otitis externa.

**syncytia** aggregations of cells, usually as a result of viral infection. Syncytia may develop into multinucleated giant cells.

**synovial fluid** fluid found in the joints.

**synovitis** inflammation of the synovium.

**systemic** affecting the body as a whole, not localized.

**systemic infection** an infection affecting the body as a whole.

**tachyzoite** another name for the trophozoite of *Toxoplasma gondii.*

**taxa** a group of similar organisms; a taxonomic category.

**taxonomy** the classification, nomenclature, and identification of organisms.

**TCBS agar** *t*hiosulfate-*c*itrate-*b*ile-*s*ucrose agar; a medium used for selective growth of vibrios. *V. cholerae* ferments sucrose and forms yellow colonies; most other vibrios do not ferment sucrose and form olive-green colonies on this medium.

**Tcp pili** *t*oxin-*c*o-regulated *p*ili that are produced V. cholerae; they adhere to microvilli of cells within the intestinal tract and assist in colonization.

**tegument** component of the herpesvirus virion, comprising protein material between the lipid envelope and the protein coat of the whole virus.

**teichoic acid** a polysaccharide found in gram-positive cell walls.

**teleomorphic** referring to a sexual state of an organism.

**tendinitis** infectious inflammation of a tendon.

**tenesmus** spasmodic contraction of anal or vesicle sphincter with pain and persistent desire to empty the bowel or bladder, with involuntary ineffectual straining efforts.

**tenosynovitis** inflammation of the tendon sheath.

**terminal subculture** subculture of blood culture broth onto agar plates performed at the end of the incubation period for the broth, even without visible evidence of growth in the broth.

**tertian** periodicity of malarial paroxysm that recurs 3 days after the first episode.

**tertiary syphilis** final stage of syphilis that may occur after months to over 40 years of latency. Gummas are one symptom that is characteristic of tertiary syphilis.

**Texas cattle fever** a bovine disease caused by *Babesia.*

**texture** the quality of a surface related to touch.

**thiabendazole** antihelminthic drug used to treat several helminth infections.

**thick smear** concentrated blood film prep in which the red blood cells are lysed during the staining process for the detection of all parasites in the blood.

**thin smear** blood film prep that allows for species identification of the blood or tissue parasite and red blood cell morphology.

**thymidine kinase** enzyme involved in DNA synthesis. It adds a phosphate group to a nucleoside, creating a nucleotide that will eventually have three phosphate groups and can be incorporated into a growing DNA chain. The enzyme may be coded for by mammalian cells or viruses.

**tine test** a tuberculin skin test in which dried antigen on metal tines are imbedded in a round plastic head. The tines are pressed against the skin for intracutaneous application of the tuberculin antigen. Each tine unit is used once and discarded.

**tinea** wormlike. Medical term referring to ringworm infections caused by a dermatophyte fungus.

**tissue culture** involves the use of cells grown in dishes to cultivate microorganisms such as *Chlamydia* and viruses, which are more difficult to isolate than bacteria.

**topography** detailed description of a surface.

**toxic shock syndrome** caused by a toxin produced by *S. aureus*. The disease was first identified in the 1980s and is associated with menstruating women using hyperabsorbent tampons.

**toxins** for the gram-positive bacilli, proteins secreted as *exotoxins* into the surrounding environment exhibiting a cytopathic effect on host cells.

**toxoid** toxin that has been treated to destroy its toxicity. A *toxoid vaccine* is still capable, however, of eliciting a protective antibody response to the toxin.

**trachoma** eye disease that may develop into blindness, caused by *Chlamydia trachomatis* (serotypes A-C).

**transduction** the transfer to genetic material between cells by a bacteriophage.

**transformation** the transfer of genes between bacterial cells as "naked DNA" in solution.

**Trematoda** leaf-shaped platyhelminthes having complex life cycles.

**trends** set of sequential values to a single test that are compared.

**treponemal tests** tests used to confirm syphilis in patients with positive nontreponemal test results.

**trichomoniasis** infection with *Trichomonas vaginalis*. This organism is often transmitted by sexual contact. Infected women are often asymptomatic as are most infected men. Symptoms in women include an abnormal vaginal discharge, pain, itching, and redness of the vaginal mucosa.

**trophozoite** the vegetative, or active stage of a protozoan.

**tropism** the growth of a nonmotile organism, away from, or toward an external stimulus.

**true pathogen** organism that has the capacity to cause infection in a normal host.

**tsetse fly** blood-sucking arthropod of the genus *Glossina* that vectors the two subspecies of *Trypanosoma brucei* to humans.

**T strains** designation sometimes used for *Ureaplasma urealyticum* because it forms very small or *t*iny colonies on solid media.

**tubercle** a small round nodule produced by infection with tuberculosis.

**tuberculate macroconidia** large conidia that have a rough or bumpy surface. Characteristic of *Histoplasma capsulatum*.

**tuberculate** having a rough or bumpy surface.

**tuberculin** an extract prepared from killed tuberculosis bacilli used in the tuberculin skin test.

**tumefaction** swelling.

**turbidometry** measuring the decrease in transmitted light that occurs when light is blocked by particles.

**TWAR strain** alternate, older name for *Chlamydia pneumoniae*.

**tween 80** a detergent hydrolyzed by some species of *Mycobacterium*. Tween 80 hydrolysis assists in separating the Runyon classification organisms into species.

**tympanocentesis** aspiration of fluid from the middle ear with a needle inserted through the tympanic membrane.

**type strain** the strain of a species that serves as the example of the species.

**typhoid fever** disease due to infection with *Salmonella typhi* and, to a much lesser extent, *Salmonella paratyphi*. It is characterized by fever, headache, and constipation followed by bloody diarrhea. Dissemination of the organisms via the blood circulation may result in focal hemorrhagic lesions in various organs. The disease is also known as enteric fever.

**ubiquitous** found everywhere, prevalent in the environment.

**ulcer** depression in the skin (or elsewhere) caused by the sloughing of necrotic tissue.

**ulcerative acanthameba keratitis** uncommon disease of the eye caused by *Acanthamoeba* species and that is contracted by swimming in contaminated water, swimming with contact lenses, or improperly disinfecting contact lenses.

**umbonate** having a rounded projection or knob.

**undulant fever** brucellosis.

**unit membrane** triple-layered cytoplasmic membrane of the mycoplasmas that contains large amounts of cholesterol and other lipids.

**Universal Standards** series of steps to protect health care workers from biohazard exposure.

**urethritis** infection of the urethra.

**urinary tract infection** broad term encompassing infection of the kidneys, ureters, bladder or urethra.

**urine screen** any of a number of rapid laboratory tests used to detect pyuria and bacteriuria.

**vaccination** the process by which a vaccine is administered to stimulate the development of immunity.

**valley fever** common name given to the primary flu-like clinical infection of coccidioidomycosis. Valley refers to the San Joaquin Valley in California.

**Venereal Disease Research Laboratory (VDRL)** nontreponemal test that detects reagin antibodies in patients infected with syphilis.

**venereal syphilis** syphilis that is contracted by direct, sexual contact with a person having active primary or secondary lesions.

**verotoxin** toxin produced primarily by *E. coli* that are associated with bloody diarrhea and hemorrhagic uremic syndrome (i.e., the EHEC). Its mechanism of action is similar to that of the Shiga toxin.

**verrucose** covered with wartlike protrusions.

**vesicle** small bladder or sac containing liquid; blister.

**viral transport medium** sterile solution (e.g., sterile, minimal essential cell culture medium) in which specimens may be placed for transport and storage and will allow viral survival to occur.

**viremia** viruses present in the bloodstream.

**virions** term used to refer to an individual virus particle.

**virulence** degree of pathogenicity or disease-producing ability of a microorganism.

**vulva** collective term for the external female genital structures, including the pubic symphysis, the labia majora, the labia minora, and the clitoris.

**Wasserman test** nontreponemal test used to detect reagin antibodies in patients infected with syphilis.

**water-borne** infectious disease spread by ingestion of or contact with contaminated water.

**Weil-Felix reaction** diagnostic test for rickettsial infections. It is an agglutination test, based on shared antigens on rickettsia and OX-19, OX-2, and OX-K strains of *Proteus*.

**Widal test**  tube agglutination assay used to detect antibodies against certain O and H antigens of the salmonellae.

**yaws**  a nonvenereal infection caused by *Treponema pertenue* contracted by direct contact with lesions on the skin of an infected person. This disease is associated with poor hygiene and is most often seen in tropical climates.

**yeast**  ovoid, unicellular fungi that reproduce by budding or fission.

**Ziehl-Neelsen method**  staining method using heat and the primary stain, carbolfuchsin. It is one staining method used to identify bacteria having mycolic acid in their cell walls.

**zoonosis/zoonotic**  human disease acquired from a nonhuman source; an infection related to a nonhuman animal.

**Zygomycota**  phylum of fungi that produce sexual zygospores.

**zygospore**  sexual spore formed by fusion of two compatible hyphae of the zygomycetes.

# ► INDEX

Page numbers followed by *f* and *t* represent figures and tables respectively.